ENVIRONMENTAL HEALTH

From Global to Local

Howard Frumkin, Editor

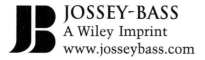

JOSSEY-BASS
A Wiley Imprint
www.josseybass.com

Published by Jossey-Bass
A Wiley Imprint
989 Market Street, San Francisco, CA 94103-1741 www.josseybass.com

Jossey-Bass books and products are available through most bookstores. To contact Jossey-Bass directly call our Customer Care Department within the U.S. at 800-956-7739, outside the U.S. at 317-572-3986, or fax 317-572-4002.

Jossey-Bass also publishes its books in a variety of electronic formats. Some content that appears in print may not be available in electronic books.

Library of Congress Cataloging-in-Publication Data

Environmental health : from global to local / Howard Frumkin, editor.
p. ; cm.
Includes bibliographical references and index.
ISBN 0-7879-7383-1 (alk. paper)
1. Environmental health. 2. Health risk assessment. I. Frumkin, Howard.
[DNLM: 1. Environmental Health. 2. Environmental Exposure. WA 30 E915 2005]
RA565.E482 2006
616.9'8—dc22
2005010360

Printed in the United States of America
FIRST EDITION
HB Printing 10 9 8 7 6 5 4 3 2

CONTENTS

Tables and Figures ix

The Editor xvii

The Contributors xix

Introduction xxix

Howard Frumkin

PART ONE: METHODS AND PARADIGMS 1

1 Ecology and Human Health 3

John Wegner

2 Toxicology 24

Jason R. Richardson, Gary W. Miller

3 Epidemiology 46

Kyle Steenland, Christine Moe

4 Exposure Assessment, Industrial Hygiene, and Environmental Management 72

P. Barry Ryan

5 Environmental Psychology 96
Daniel Stokols, Chip Clitheroe

6 Genetics and Environmental Health 128
Samuel H. Wilson

7 Environmental Health Ethics 143
Andrew Jameton

8 Environmental Justice 170
Charles Lee

9 Religious Approaches to Environmental Health 197
Daniel J. Swartz

PART TWO: ENVIRONMENTAL HEALTH ON THE GLOBAL SCALE 219

10 Population Pressure 221
Don Hinrichsen

11 Climate Change 238
Jonathan A. Patz

12 War 269
Barry S. Levy, Victor W. Sidel

13 Developing Nations 288
Jerome Nriagu, Jaymie Meliker, Mary Johnson

PART THREE: ENVIRONMENTAL HEALTH ON THE REGIONAL SCALE 329

14 Air Pollution 331
Michelle L. Bell, Jonathan M. Samet

15 Energy Production 362
Richard Rheingans

16 Urbanization 387
Sandro Galea, David Vlahov

17 Transportation and Health 414
John Balbus, Dushana Yoganathan Triola

18 Water and Health 454
Timothy Ford

PART FOUR: ENVIRONMENTAL HEALTH ON THE LOCAL SCALE 517

19 Solid and Hazardous Waste 519
Sven Rodenbeck, Kenneth Orloff, Harvey Rogers, Henry Falk

20 Pest Control and Pesticides 544
Mark G. Robson, George C. Hamilton

21 Food Safety 581
David McSwane

22 Indoor Air 625
Michael J. Hodgson

23 Workplace Health and Safety 648
Melissa Perry, Howard Hu

24 Radiation 683
Arthur C. Upton

25 Injuries 715
Junaid A. Razzak, Jeremy J. Hess, Arthur L. Kellermann

26 Disaster Preparedness 745
Eric K. Noji, Catherine Y. Lee

27 Nature Contact: A Health Benefit? 781
Howard Frumkin

28 Children 805
Maida Galvez, Joel Forman, Philip J. Landrigan

PART FIVE: THE PRACTICE OF ENVIRONMENTAL HEALTH 847

29 Prevention 849
Joel A. Tickner

30 The Practice of Environmental Health 895
Sarah Kotchian

31 Geographic Information Systems 926
Lance A. Waller

32 Risk Assessment 940
Scott Bartell

33 Environmental Health Policy 961
Barry L. Johnson

34 Risk Communication 988
Vincent T. Covello

35 Health Care Services 1010
Robert Laumbach, Howard M. Kipen

36 Legal Remedies 1032
Douglas A. Henderson

Name Index 1067

Subject Index 1081

TABLES AND FIGURES

Tables

1.1 Estimates of the Value of Various Ecosystem Services 20
2.1 Examples of Toxic Compounds in Three Classifications 28
3.1 Rate Ratios for Lung Cancer Mortality, Silicosis Mortality, and End-Stage Kidney Disease Incidence in a Cohort of 4,626 Silica-Exposed Workers 62
5.1 Levels of Environmental Analysis 101
5.2 Functions of Both Real and Virtual Neighborhoods 106
5.3 The Presence of Nature 116
8.1 Examples of Community-Based Environmental Justice Issues 175
11.1 The Main Greenhouse Gases 240
11.2 Mortality from the 2003 Heat Wave in Europe 245
13.1 Attributable Mortality by Risk Factor, Level of Development, and Gender, 2000 292
13.2 Attributable DALYs by Risk Factor, Level of Development, and Sex, 2000 293
13.3 Effects of Globalization on the Health of People in Developing Countries 297
13.4 Changes in Environmental Health Risk Factors Associated with Agricultural Development 302

13.5 Population with and Without Access to Safe Drinking Water (Free of Disease-Causing Microbes), 2000 316
13.6 Estimated Population Exposed to Arsenic in Drinking Water at Concentrations >50 μg/L, the MCL in Many Countries 319
13.7 Global DALYs Due to Injuries, 2002 322
14.1 Major Ambient Air Pollutants: Sources, Health Effects, and Regulations 336
15.1 Per Capita Energy Use by Sector and Region, 1999 364
15.2 Overall Energy Use and Source by Region, Current and Projected, Million Oil-Ton Equivalents 366
15.3 Electricity Generation Sources by Region (in Terawatt Hours, TWH), 2000 366
15.4 Fossil Fuel Types and Uses 368
15.5 Air Emissions from Traditional Fuels Used in Cookstoves in India 379
15.6 U.S. Emissions and Costs of Electricity Production by Fuel Type, 2000 380
17.1 Mode Share of Trips in Urban Areas by Country (Proportion of Total), 1990 418
17.2 Fatality Rates per Million Passengers by Travel Mode, Great Britain, 1992 425
17.3 Representative Federal Emissions Standards for Automobiles and Trucks, 1970–2010 431
17.4 Energy Expenditure (in METS) During Various Modes of Travel 432
17.5 Safety Benefits of Various Transportation Demand Management (TDM) Strategies 443
18.1 Hot Spots: Past and Potential Future Water Resource Conflicts 461
18.2 Examples of Health Consequences of Engineering Schemes 462
18.3 Classes of Chemical Contaminants in Water 464
18.4 Examples of Studies Linking Exposure to Chemicals in Drinking Water with Increased Health Risk 471
18.5 Pathogens in Drinking Water: Infectious Doses, Diseases, and Additional Comments 473
18.6 The Indicator Approach 478
18.7 Examples of Vector-Borne Diseases with Risk Factors Associated with Water 484
18.8 Approaches to Disinfection 496
22.1 Specific Building-Related Illnesses and Their Causes 629
22.2 Typical Symptoms in Sick Building Syndrome 630
22.3 Determinants of Indoor Air Quality and People's Symptoms 631
24.1 Radiation Injuries Following Roentgen's 1895 Discovery of the X-Ray, 1896–1912 685

24.2 Quantities and Dose Units of Ionizing Radiation 687
24.3 Average Amounts of Ionizing Radiation Received Annually by a Resident of the United States 688
24.4 Major Forms and Features of Acute Radiation Syndrome 694
24.5 Estimated Lifetime Risks of Fatal Cancers from Acute Exposure to Ionizing Radiation 697
25.1 Ranking of Injury-Related Mortality and Burden of Disease (DALYs Lost), 1990 and 2020 718
25.2 The Haddon Matrix Applied to Motor Vehicle Crashes 721
25.3 Options Analysis in Injury Control 721
25.4 Countermeasures for Intentional Injuries 730
25.5 Countermeasures for Burns 730
25.6 Countermeasures for Poisoning 731
25.7 Countermeasures for Falls 732
25.8 Countermeasures for Drowning 733
25.9 Countermeasures for Workplace Injuries 734
25.10 Countermeasures for Playground Injuries 735
25.11 Countermeasures for Road Injuries 737
25.12 Countermeasures for Home Injuries 739
26.1 Selected Natural Disasters, 1970–2004 746
26.2 Short-Term Effects of Major Natural Disasters 749
30.1 The Ten Essential Services of Public Health 902
30.2 The PACE-EH Process 905
30.3 Core Competencies for Local Environmental Health 921
32.1 Carcinogenic Effects of Chloroform on Male Rats 944
34.1 Template for Risk Communication Message Map 998
34.2 Sample Risk Communication Message Map 1005
35.1 Categories of Environmental and Occupational Diseases 1012

Figures

I.1 The DPSEEA Model xlviii
1.1 Population Growth Patterns: A Comparison of Exponential and Logistic Growth 7
1.2 Possible Population Age Structures for Human Populations 10
1.3 Basic Components of an Ecosystem 11
1.4 Energy Flow Through a Heterotrophic Population 14
1.5 Generalized Nutrient Cycle 16
1.6 Simplified Carbon Cycle 17
1.7 Generalized Nitrogen Cycle 19

2.1 Interdisciplinary Nature of Toxicology 25
2.2 Biotransformation Pathways of Chlorpyrifos 41
2.3 Tiered Approach to Toxicity Testing 43
3.1 Job-Exposure Matrix for a Retrospective Cohort Study of 4,626 Silica-Exposed Workers 59
4.1 Air Pollution Sampling Apparatus for Ozone and Particulate Matter 81
4.2 Personal Protective Equipment for Solvent Exposure 83
4.3 Assessing Exposure in an Occupational Setting 87
5.1 Airplane Coming in for Landing over an Elementary School in Los Angeles 107
5.2 The Space Needle in Seattle, Washington 112
5.3 Cars Waiting in Line for "Fast Food" Service 113
5.4 Ghirardelli Square in San Francisco 114
5.5 The Plaza Mayor in Madrid, Spain 115
5.6 Neighborhood Green Space in Irvine, California 117
5.7 A Neighborhood Park in Whistler, British Columbia, Canada 118
6.1 Determinants of Individual Response to an Environmental Exposure 130
6.2 Research Approaches to Link Environmental Exposures with Disease 137
8.1 Relationship Between Environmental Hazards, Vulnerability, and Health Disparities 183
9.1 What Would Jesus Drive? 198
11.1 The Greenhouse Effect 239
11.2 Variations of the Earth's Surface Temperature Across Two Time Frames 241
11.3 Projected Changes in Global Temperature: Global Average 1856–1999 and Projection Estimates to 2100 243
11.4 Urban Heat Island Profile 247
11.5 Landslides in California Reported from 1998 Storms 248
11.6 Potential Impact of Sea-Level Rise on Bangladesh 249
11.7 The Projected Increase in Ozone Exceedance Days Associated with Global Warming 252
12.1 Nagasaki After Detonation of a Nuclear Bomb, August, 1945 274
12.2 This Girl, at the Indira Gandhi Children's Hospital in Kabul, Afghanistan, Lost Both Her Legs After Stepping on a Landmine Near Her Village Outside Kabul in 1989 280
13.1 Age-Standardized Rates of Years Lived with Disability (YLDs), Developed and Developing Countries, 2002. 294
14.1 Mortality and Air Pollution Levels During 1952 London Fog 332

14.2 Cardiac Emergency Bed Service Applications and SO_2 Levels During the 1952 London Fog 333
14.3 Particulate Matter Mass Distribution 342
14.4 U.S. Air Lead Concentrations, 1977–1996 349
14.5 Change in U.S. Blood Lead Levels, 1976–2000 350
15.1 The Energy Ladder 367
16.1 Global Urban Population Growth in Wealthy Versus Less Wealthy Countries 388
16.2 Urban Versus Rural Populations in Less Wealthy Countries 389
16.3 Urban Sprawl in the New York Metropolitan Area 392
16.4 Urban Sprawl: In the Top Photo Denver Spreads to the Foot of the Rocky Mountains; in the Bottom Photo a Suburban Residential Subdivision Adopts a Typical Loop and Lollipop Pattern 394
16.5 Caracas: A Glittering Modern Business District in the Background and Substandard Housing in the Foreground Reflect Rapid Rural-Urban Migration That Strains Urban Services 401
16.6 Manila: Substandard Housing Near Contaminated Water Is Evident But So Are Signs of Electricity and Televisions in Homes 402
17.1 Mode Share of Commuting to Work in the United States, 1960–2000 418
17.2 Percentage of Trips in Urban Areas Made by Bicycling and Walking, Selected Countries of North America and Europe, 1995 419
17.3 Trends in Emissions of Criteria Air Pollutants from Transportation-Related Sources, 1970–1997 427
17.4 Relative Contribution of On-Road, Nonroad, and Stationary Sources to Six Priority Mobile Source Air Toxics, in California's South Coast Air Basin, 1999 427
18.1 The Hydrologic Cycle 455
18.2 Schematic of the Interconnections Between Water and Health 456
18.3 The Ogallala Aquifer 458
18.4 Pesticide Movement in the Hydrologic Cycle, Including Pesticide Movement to and from Sediment and Aquatic Biota Within the Stream 469
18.5 Sanitation Options 474
18.6 An Idealized Wastewater Treatment System, Based on Boston's Deer Island System 475
18.7 Emergence of New Epidemic Serogroups of *Vibrio Cholerae* 489
18.8 New York City's Water Supply System 492
18.9 A Multibarrier Approach to Maximize the Microbiological Quality of Water 495

18.10 Idealized Scheme for Safe Drinking Water 506
19.1 Composition of the 229 Million Tons of Municipal Solid Waste Produced in the United States (Before Recycling), 2001 521
19.2 Total and Per Capita Amounts of Municipal Solid Waste Produced in the United States (Before Recycling), 1960–2001 522
19.3 Labeling on Medical Waste Container 524
19.4 Total Amounts and Percentages of Municipal Solid Waste Recycled in the United States, 1960–2001 528
19.5 Waste Tires 529
19.6 Generalized Depiction of a State-of-the-Art Landfill 532
19.7 Generalized Diagram of Incineration Material and Process Flow 535
19.8 Leachate Collection Ponds at the Kin-Buc Landfill in Edison, New Jersey 538
19.9 This Mine Tailings Pile Is the Legacy of Sixty Years of Lead and Zinc Mining in Ottawa County, Oklahoma 539
20.1 Application of Lead Arsenate in the Early 1900s 546
20.2 Modern Pesticide Application Equipment 547
20.3 A Corn Borer, an Example of an Insect Pest, Causing Damage in the Stalk of a Corn Plant 547
20.4 Workers in Ghana Mixing and Loading an Organophosphate Insecticide Without Adequate Personal Protective Equipment 565
21.1 Common Sources of Food Contamination 584
21.2 Food Temperature Danger Zone 603
21.3 The Proper Hand Washing Procedure 605
21.4 The 2001 FDA Food Code 613
21.5 Fight BAC! Campaign Logo 615
22.1 Schematic of a Generic HVAC System 634
23.1 Alice Hamilton, Pioneer in Occupational Health in the United States 651
23.2 Incidence Rate of Nonfatal Occupation Injury Cases by Private Sector, 2001 657
23.3 The Karasek Job Strain Model 661
23.4 Occupational Health in India: A Child Worker in a Marketplace 667
23.5 Foundry Worker Pours Molten Metal 669
23.6 Workers in an Automobile Battery Plant, a Source of Occupational Lead Exposure 676
24.1 The Electromagnetic Spectrum 684
24.2 A Pioneer Radiologist Testing His Fluoroscope by Examining His Own Hand, Fully Exposing Himself and His Patient in the Process 685

24.3 A Basal Cell Carcinoma of the Skin of Twenty Years Duration in a Fifty-Eight-Year-Old Man 700
24.4 Cell Phones, Now Virtually Ubiquitous, Increase the Level of Radiofrequency Radiation Throughout the Environment 704
25.1 The Injury Pyramid 719
25.2 Typology of Violence 729
26.1 Kosovo War Refugee Camp Outside the Village of Cegrane, Macedonia, 1999: An Example of the Social Displacement and Poor Environmental Conditions That Can Follow Disasters of Natural or Human Origin 748
26.2 Debris and Damaged Buildings in Pensacola, Florida, Resulting from Hurricane Ivan, September 2004 754
26.3 Destruction of North Carolina Hwy 12 Along Hatteras Island, Resulting from Hurricane Isabel, September 2003 755
26.4 Malibu, California, Wildfire, 1996: State Office of Emergency Services Firefighters Monitor the Fire's Spread Across the Dry Brush on a Hillside 763
27.1 Three Views of Robert Taylor Homes: Aerial View (Top), Barren Surroundings (Middle), and Surroundings with Trees (Bottom) 790
28.1 A Children's Playground Located Near a Source of Toxic Emissions 814
28.2 Children Bathing in a Drum That Once Held a Toxic Chemical 815
29.1 An Environmental Health Intervention Model 851
29.2 The Product Life Cycle 879
29.3 Clean Production Is Based on a Circular Vision of the Economy 880
31.1 Hypothetical Example of the GIS Layering Operation 929
31.2 Examples of Buffers Around Point (Top), Line (Middle), and Area (Bottom) Features 931
31.3 Map of Genesee County, Michigan, Showing 1990 Census Block Groups and Minimill Location 936
32.1 Risk Assessment Framework 942
32.2 Normal Tolerance Distribution (Probit Model) 951
32.3 Three Dose-Response Models (Logit, Probit, and Three-Parameter Multistage) Fit to the Chloroform Dose-Response Data in Rats 952
32.4 Cubic Smoothing Spline, Logit Model, and Categorical Model Fit to Nested Case-Control Data on Silica Exposure and Lung Cancer 953
35.1 Determining Causation 1018

THE EDITOR

Howard Frumkin is professor and chair of the Department of Environmental and Occupational Health at the Rollins School of Public Health of Emory University (where he teaches the survey course in Environmental Health), professor of medicine at Emory Medical School, and director of the Southeast Pediatric Environmental Health Specialty Unit. He has been president of the Association of Occupational and Environmental Clinics, chair of the science board of the American Public Health Association, and a member of the board of directors of Physicians for Social Responsibility, where he cochaired the environment committee. He has served on the Institute of Medicine Roundtable on Environmental Health Sciences, Research, and Medicine; the Environmental Protection Agency's Children's Health Protection Advisory Committee, where he chaired the Smart Growth and Climate Change workgroups; and the National Toxicology Program Board of Scientific Counselors, and he is a member of Collegium Ramazzini. He was named the 2004 Georgia Environmental Professional of the Year by the Georgia Environmental Council. He is the author of *Urban Sprawl and Public Health* (with Lawrence Frank and Richard Jackson, Island Press, 2004) and the editor of *Emerging Illness and Society* (with Randall Packard, Peter Brown, and Ruth Berkelman, Johns Hopkins

Press, 2004) and *Safe and Healthy School Environments* (with Leslie Rubin and Robert Geller, Oxford University Press, 2006). He received his AB degree from Brown University, his MD degree from the University of Pennsylvania, his MPH and DrPH degrees from Harvard, his internal medicine training at the Hospital of the University of Pennsylvania and Cambridge Hospital, and his occupational medicine training at Harvard.

THE CONTRIBUTORS

John Balbus, MD, MPH
Senior Scientist and Program Director
Environmental Health
Environmental Defense
Washington, D.C.

Scott Bartell, PhD
Assistant Professor of Environmental and Occupational Health
Rollins School of Public Health of Emory University
Atlanta, Georgia

Michelle L. Bell, MS, MSE, PhD
Assistant Professor of Environmental Health
Yale School of Forestry & Environmental Studies
New Haven, Connecticut

Chip Clitheroe, PhD
Lecturer
School of Social Ecology
University of California, Irvine
Irvine, California

Vincent T. Covello, PhD
Director
Center for Risk Communication
New York, New York

Henry Falk, MD, MPH
Director
Coordinating Center for Environmental Health and Injury Prevention
Centers for Disease Control and Prevention
Atlanta, Georgia

Timothy Ford, PhD
Professor and Chair
Department of Microbiology
Montana State University
Bozeman, Montana

Joel Forman, MD
Assistant Professor of Pediatrics and Community and Preventive Medicine
Mount Sinai School of Medicine
New York, New York

Sandro Galea, MD, MPH, PhD
Associate Director
Center for Urban Epidemiologic Studies
New York Academy of Medicine
New York, New York

Maida Galvez, MD
Instructor of Pediatrics and Community and Preventive Medicine
Mount Sinai School of Medicine
New York, New York

George C. Hamilton, PhD
Extension Specialist in Pest Management
Rutgers University
New Brunswick, New Jersey

Douglas A. Henderson, PhD, JD
Partner
Troutman Sanders LLP
Atlanta, Georgia

Jeremy J. Hess, MD, MPH
Emergency Medicine Resident
Department of Emergency Medicine
Emory University School of Medicine
Atlanta, Georgia

Don Hinrichsen, docent
Multi-Media Consultant on Environment and Population
New York and London

Michael J. Hodgson, MD, MPH
Director
Occupational Health Program
Veterans Health Administration
Washington, D.C.

Howard Hu, MD, MPH, ScD
Professor of Occupational and Environmental Medicine
Harvard School of Public Health
Boston, Massachusetts

Andrew Jameton, PhD
Professor and Section Head, Humanities and Law
Department of Preventive and Societal Medicine
University of Nebraska Medical Center
Omaha, Nebraska

Barry L. Johnson, PhD
Adjunct Professor
Rollins School of Public Health of Emory University
Atlanta, Georgia

Mary Johnson, BA
Graduate Student
Department of Environmental Health Sciences
University of Michigan School of Public Health
Ann Arbor, Michigan

Arthur L. Kellermann, MD, MPH
Professor and Chair
Department of Emergency Medicine
Emory University School of Medicine
Director
Center for Injury Control
Rollins School of Public Health of Emory University
Atlanta, Georgia

Howard M. Kipen, MD, MPH
Professor and Director
Clinical Research and Occupational Medicine Division
Environmental & Occupational Health Sciences Institute
UMDNJ-Robert Wood Johnson Medical School
Piscataway, New Jersey

Sarah Kotchian, EdM, MPH, PhD
Associate Director for Planning
Institute for Public Health
University of New Mexico School of Medicine
Albuquerque, New Mexico

Philip J. Landrigan, MD, MSc
Ethel H. Wise Professor and Chairman
Department of Community and Preventive Medicine
Mount Sinai School of Medicine
New York, New York

Robert Laumbach, MD, MPH, CIH
Assistant Professor
Clinical Research and Occupational Medicine Division
Environmental & Occupational Health Sciences Institute
UMDNJ-Robert Wood Johnson Medical School
Piscataway, New Jersey

Catherine Y. Lee, MPH
Research Consultant
Unconventional Concepts Inc.
Arlington, Virginia

Charles Lee
Associate Director for Policy and Interagency Liaison
Office of Environmental Justice
U.S. Environmental Protection Agency
Washington, D.C.

Barry S. Levy, MD, MPH
Adjunct Professor of Community Health
Tufts University School of Medicine
Boston, Massachusetts

David McSwane, HSD, REHS, CFSP
Professor of Public and Environmental Affairs
School of Public and Environmental Affairs
Indiana University-Purdue University
Indianapolis, Indiana

Jaymie Meliker, MS
Graduate Student
Department of Environmental Health Sciences
University of Michigan School of Public Health
Ann Arbor, Michigan

Gary W. Miller, PhD
Associate Professor of Environmental and Occupational Health
Rollins School of Public Health of Emory University
Atlanta, Georgia

Christine Moe, PhD
Associate Professor of Global Health
Rollins School of Public Health of Emory University
Atlanta, Georgia

Eric K. Noji, MD, MPH
Medical Officer
Centers for Disease Control and Prevention
Atlanta, Georgia

Jerome Nriagu, PhD, DSc
Professor
Department of Environmental Health Sciences
University of Michigan School of Public Health
Ann Arbor, Michigan

Kenneth Orloff, PhD, DABT
Assistant Director for Science
Division of Health Assessment and Consultation
Agency for Toxic Substances and Disease Registry
Atlanta, Georgia

Jonathan A. Patz, MD, MPH
Associate Professor of Environmental Studies and Population Health Sciences
Gaylord Nelson Institute for Environmental Studies
University of Wisconsin
Madison, Wisconsin

Melissa Perry, ScD, MHS
Assistant Professor of Occupational Epidemiology
Harvard School of Public Health
Boston, Massachusetts

Junaid A. Razzak, MD
Assistant Professor of Emergency Medicine
Emory University School of Medicine
Atlanta, Georgia
Assistant Professor of Emergency Medicine
Department of Medicine
Aga Khan University
Karachi, Pakistan

Richard Rheingans, PhD
Research Assistant Professor of Global Health
Rollins School of Public Health of Emory University
Atlanta, Georgia

Jason R. Richardson, PhD
Postdoctoral Fellow in Toxicology
Department of Environmental and Occupational Health
Rollins School of Public Health of Emory University
Atlanta, Georgia

Karl-Henrik Robèrt
Professor
Blekinge Technical Institute
Karlskrona, Sweden
Founder and Chair
The Natural Step International
Stockholm, Sweden

Mark G. Robson, PhD, MPH
Chair
Department of Environmental and Occupational Health
University of Medicine and Dentistry of New Jersey
School of Public Health
Piscataway, New Jersey

Sven Rodenbeck, ScD, PE, DEE
Environmental Engineer
National Center for Environmental Health/Agency for Toxic Substances and Disease Registry
Centers for Disease Control and Prevention
Atlanta, Georgia

Harvey Rogers, MS
Engineer
National Center for Environmental Health/Agency for Toxic Substances and Disease Prevention
Centers for Disease Control and Prevention
Atlanta, Georgia

P. Barry Ryan, PhD
Professor of Environmental and Occupational Health
Rollins School of Public Health of Emory University
Atlanta, Georgia

Jonathan M. Samet, MD
Professor and Chair, Epidemiology
Bloomberg School of Hygiene and Public Health
Johns Hopkins University
Baltimore, Maryland

Victor W. Sidel, MD
Distinguished University Professor of Social Medicine
Department of Epidemiology and Social Medicine
Montefiore Medical Center and Albert Einstein College of Medicine
Bronx, New York

Kyle Steenland, PhD
Professor of Environmental and Occupational Health
Rollins School of Public Health of Emory University
Atlanta, Georgia

Daniel Stokols, PhD
Professor of Planning, Policy and Design
School of Social Ecology
University of California, Irvine
Irvine, California

Rabbi Daniel J. Swartz, MHL
Coordinator
Greater Washington Interfaith Power and Light
Washington, D.C.

Joel A. Tickner, ScD
Assistant Professor
Department of Department of Community Health and Sustainability
University of Massachusetts Lowell
Lowell, Massachusetts

Dushana Yoganathan Triola, MD
Clinical Instructor of Community and Preventive Medicine
Mount Sinai School of Medicine
New York, New York

Arthur C. Upton, MD
Clinical Professor of Environmental and Community Medicine
University of Medicine and Dentistry of New Jersey
Robert Wood Johnson Medical School
Piscataway, New Jersey

David Vlahov, PhD
Director
Center for Urban Epidemiologic Studies
New York Academy of Medicine
New York, New York

Lance A. Waller, PhD
Associate Professor of Biostatistics
Rollins School of Public Health of Emory University
Atlanta, Georgia

John Wegner, PhD
Campus Environmental Officer and Senior Lecturer
Department of Environmental Studies
Emory University
Atlanta, Georgia

Samuel H. Wilson, MD
Deputy Director
National Institute of Environmental Health Sciences
Research Triangle Park, North Carolina

INTRODUCTION

Howard Frumkin

Please stop reading.

That's right. Close this book, just for a moment. Lift your eyes and look around. Where are you? What do you see?

Perhaps you're in the campus library, surrounded by shelves of books, with carpeting underfoot and the heating or air-conditioning humming quietly in the background. Perhaps you're home—a dormitory room, a bedroom in a house, a suite in a garden apartment, maybe your kitchen. Perhaps you're outside, lying beneath a tree in the middle of campus, or perhaps you're on a subway or a bus or even an airplane. What is it like? How does it feel to be where you are?

Is the light adequate for reading? Is the temperature comfortable? Is there fresh air to breathe? Are there contaminants in the air—say, solvents off-gassing from newly laid carpet or a recently painted wall? Does the chair fit your body comfortably?

If you're inside, look outside. What do you see through the window? Are there trees? Buildings? Is the neighborhood noisy or tranquil? Are there other people? Are there busy streets, with passing trucks and busses snorting occasional clouds of diesel exhaust?

Now imagine that you can see even farther, to a restaurant down the block, to the nearby river, to the highway network around your city or town, to the factories and assembly plants in industrial parks, to the power plant in the distance supplying electricity to the room you're in, to the agricultural lands some miles away. What would you see in the restaurant? Is the kitchen clean? Is the food stored safely? Are there cockroaches or rats in the back room? What about the river? Is your municipal sewage system dumping raw wastes into the river, or is there a sewage plant discharging treated, clean effluent? Are there chemicals in the river water? What about fish? Could you eat the fish? Could you swim in the river? Do you drink the water from the river?

As for the highways, factories, and power plant . . . are they polluting the air? Are the highways clogged with traffic? Are people routinely injured and killed on the roads? Are workers in the factories being exposed to hazardous chemicals or to noise or to machines that may injure them or to stress? Are trains pulling up to the power plant regularly, off-loading vast piles of coal? And what about the farms? Are they applying pesticides, or are they controlling insects in other ways? Are you confident that you're safe eating the vegetables that grow there? Drinking the milk? Are the farmlands shrinking as residential development from the city sprawls outward?

Finally, imagine that you have an even broader view. Floating miles above the earth, you look down. Do you notice the hundreds of millions of people living in wildly differing circumstances? Do you see vast megacities with millions and millions of people, and do you see isolated rural villages three days' walk from the nearest road? Do you see forests being cleared in some places, rivers and lakes drying up in others? Do you notice that the earth's surface temperature is slightly warmer than it was a century ago? Do you see cyclones forming in tropical regions, glaciers and icecaps melting near the poles?

OK, back to the book.

Everything you've just viewed, from the room you're in to the globe you're on, is part of your environment. And many, many aspects of that environment, from the air you breathe to the water you drink, from the roads you travel to the wastes you produce, may affect how you feel. They may determine your risk of being injured before today ends, your risk of coming down with diarrhea or shortness of breath or a sore back, your risk of developing a chronic disease in the next few decades, even the risk that your children or your grandchildren will suffer from developmental disabilities or asthma or cancer.

What Is Environmental Health?

Merriam-Webster's Collegiate Dictionary defines *environment,* first, in a straightforward manner as "the circumstances, objects, or conditions by which one is surrounded." The second definition it offers is more intriguing: "the complex of physical, chemical, and biotic factors (as climate, soil, and living things) that act upon an organism or an ecological community and ultimately determine its form and survival." If our focus is on human health, we can consider the environment to be all the external (or nongenetic) factors—physical, nutritional, social, behavioral, and others—that act on humans.

A widely accepted definition of *health* comes from the constitution, crafted in 1948, of the World Health Organization (2005): "A state of complete physical, mental, and social well-being and not merely the absence of disease or infirmity." This broad definition goes well beyond the rather mechanistic view that prevails in some medical settings to include many dimensions of comfort and well-being.

Environmental health has been defined in many ways (see Box I.1). Some definitions make reference to the relationship between people and the environment, evoking an ecosystem concept, and others focus more narrowly on addressing particular environmental conditions. Some focus on abating hazards, and others focus on promoting health-enhancing environments. Some focus on physical and chemical hazards, and others extend more broadly to aspects of the social and built environments. In the aggregate the definitions in Box I.1 make it clear that environmental health is many things: an interdisciplinary academic field, an area of research, and an arena of applied public health practice.

Box I.1: Definitions of Environmental Health

"[Environmental health] [c]omprises those aspects of human health, including quality of life, that are determined by physical, chemical, biological, social and psychosocial factors in the environment. It also refers to the theory and practice of assessing, correcting, controlling, and preventing those factors in the environment that can potentially affect adversely the health of present and future generations" (World Health Organization [WHO], 2004).

"Environmental health is the branch of public health that protects against the effects of environmental hazards that can adversely affect health or the ecological balances essential to human health and environmental quality" (Agency for Toxic Substances and Disease Registry, cited in U.S. Department of Health and Human Services [DHHS], 1998).

"Environmental health comprises those aspects of human health and disease that are determined by factors in the environment. It also refers to the theory and practice of assessing and controlling factors in the environment that can potentially affect health. It includes both the direct pathological effects of chemicals, radiation and some biological agents, and the effects (often indirect) on health and well-being of the broad physical, psychological, social and aesthetic environment, which includes housing, urban developmental land use and transport" (European Charter on Environment and Health; see WHO, Regional Office for Europe, 1990).

"Environmental health is the discipline that focuses on the interrelationships between people and their environment, promotes human health and well-being, and fosters a safe and healthful environment" (National Center for Environmental Health, cited in DHHS, 1998).

The Evolution of Environmental Health

Human concern for environmental health dates from ancient times, and it has evolved and expanded over the centuries.

Ancient Origins

The notion that the environment could have an impact on comfort and well-being—the core idea of environmental health—must have been evident in the early days of human existence. The elements can be harsh, and we know that our ancestors sought shelter in caves or under trees or in crude shelters they built. The elements can still be harsh, both on a daily basis and during extraordinary events, as the tsunami of 2004 reminded us.

Our ancestors confronted other challenges that we would now identify with environmental health. One was food safety; there must have been procedures for preserving food, and people must have fallen ill and died from eating spoiled food. Dietary restrictions in ancient Jewish and Islamic law, such as bans on eating pork, presumably evolved from the recognition that certain foods could cause disease. Another challenge was clean water; we can assume that early peoples learned not to defecate near or otherwise soil their water sources. In the ruins of ancient civilizations from India to Rome, from Greece to Egypt to South America, archeologists have found the remains of water pipes, toilets, and sewage lines, some dating back more than 4,000 years (Rosen, [1958] 1993). Still another environmental hazard was polluted air; there is evidence in the sinus cavities of ancient cave dwellers of high levels of smoke in their caves (Brimblecombe, 1988), foreshadowing modern indoor air concerns in homes that burn biomass fuels or coal.

An intriguing passage in the biblical book of Leviticus (14:33–45) may refer to an environmental health problem well recognized today: mold in buildings. When a house has a "leprous disease" (as it is translated in the Revised Standard Version),

> . . . then he who owns the house shall come and tell the priest, "There seems to me to be some sort of disease in my house." Then the priest shall command that they empty the house before the priest goes to examine the disease, lest all

> that is in the house be declared unclean; and afterward the priest shall go in to see the house. And he shall examine the disease; and if the disease is in the walls of the house with greenish or reddish spots, and if it appears to be deeper than the surface, then the priest shall go out of the house to the door of the house, and shut up the house seven days. And the priest shall come again on the seventh day, and look; and if the disease has spread in the walls of the house, then the priest shall command that they take out the stones in which is the disease and throw them into an unclean place outside the city; and he shall cause the inside of the house to be scraped round about, and the plaster that they scrape off they shall pour into an unclean place outside the city; then they shall take other stones and put them in the place of those stones, and he shall take other plaster and plaster the house. If the disease breaks out again in the house, after he has taken out the stones and scraped the house and plastered it, then the priest shall go and look; and if the disease has spread in the house, it is a malignant leprosy in the house; it is unclean. And he shall break down the house, its stones and timber and all the plaster of the house; and he shall carry them forth out of the city to an unclean place."

As interesting as it is to speculate about whether ancient dwellings suffered mold overgrowth, it is also interesting to consider the "unclean place outside the city"—an early hazardous waste site. Who hauled the wastes there, and what did that work do to their health?

Still another ancient environmental health challenge, especially in cities, was rodents. European history was changed forever when infestations of rats in fourteenth century cities led to the Black Death (Zinsser, 1935; Herlihy and Cohn, 1997; Cantor, 2001; Kelly, 2005). Modern cities continue to struggle periodically with infestations of rats and other pests (Sullivan, 2004), whose control depends in large part on environmental modifications.

Industrial Awakenings

Modern environmental health further took form during the age of industrialization. With the rapid growth of cities in the seventeenth and eighteenth centuries, "sanitarian" issues rose in importance. "The urban environment," wrote one historian, "fostered the spread of diseases with crowded, dark, unventilated housing; unpaved streets mired in horse manure and littered with refuse; inadequate or nonexisting water supplies; privy vaults unemptied from one year to the next; stagnant pools of water; ill-functioning open sewers; stench beyond the twentieth-century imagination; and noises from clacking horse hooves, wooden wagon wheels, street railways, and unmuffled industrial machinery" (Leavitt, 1982, p. 22).

The provision of clean water became an ever more pressing need, as greater concentrations of people increased both the probability of water contamination and the impact of disease outbreaks. Regular outbreaks of cholera and yellow fever in the eighteenth and nineteenth centuries (Rosenberg, 1962) highlighted the need for water systems, including clean source water, treatment including filtration, and distribution through pipes. Similarly, sewage management became a pressing need, especially after the provision of piped water and the use of toilets created large volumes of contaminated liquid waste (Duffy, 1990; Melosi, 2000).

The industrial workplace—a place of danger and even horror—gave additional impetus to early environmental health. Technology advanced rapidly during the late eighteenth and nineteenth centuries, new and often dangerous machines were deployed in industry after industry, and mass production became common. Although the air, water, and soil near industrial sites could become badly contaminated, in ways that would be familiar to modern environmental professionals (Hurley, 1994; Tarr, 1996; Tarr, 2002), the most abominable conditions were usually found within the mines, mills, and factories.

Charles Turner Thackrah (1795–1833), a Yorkshire physician, developed an interest in the diseases he observed among the poor in the city of Leeds. In 1831, he described many work-related hazards in a short book with a long title: *The Effects of the Principal Arts, Trades and Professions, and of Civic States and Habits of Living, on Health and Longevity, with Suggestions for the Removal of many of the Agents which produce Disease and Shorten the Duration of Life.* In it he proposed guidelines for the prevention of certain diseases, such as the elimination of lead as a glaze in the pottery industry and the use of ventilation and respiratory protection to protect knife grinders. Public outcry, and the efforts of early Victorian reformers such as Thackrah, led to passage of the Factory Act in 1833 and the Mines Act in 1842. Occupational health did not blossom in the United States until the early twentieth century, pioneered by the remarkable Alice Hamilton (1869–1970). A keen firsthand observer of industrial conditions, she documented links between toxic exposures and illness among miners, tradesmen, and factory workers, first in Illinois (where she directed that state's Occupational Disease Commission from 1910 to 1919) and later from an academic position at Harvard. Her books, including *Industrial Poisons in the United States* (1925) and *Industrial Toxicology* (1934), helped establish that workplaces could be microenvironments that threatened worker health.

A key development in the seventeenth through nineteenth centuries was the quantitative observation of population health—the beginnings of epidemiology. With the tools of epidemiology, observers could systematically attribute certain diseases to certain environmental exposures. John Graunt (1620–1674), an English merchant and haberdasher, analyzed London's weekly death records—the *bills of mortality*—and published his findings in 1662 as *Natural and Political Observations Upon the Bills of Mortality.* Graunt's work was one of the first formal analyses of this data source and a pioneering example of demography. Almost two centuries later, when the British Parliament created the Registrar-General's Office (now the Office of Population Censuses and Surveys) and William Farr (1807–1883) became its compiler of abstracts, the link between vital statistics and environmental health was forged. Farr made observations about fertility and mortality patterns, identifying rural-urban differences, variations between acute and chronic illnesses, and seasonal trends, and implicating certain environmental conditions in illness and death. Farr's 1843 analysis of mortality in Liverpool led Parliament to pass the Liverpool Sanitary Act of 1846, which created a sanitary code for Liverpool and a public health infrastructure to enforce it.

If Farr was a pioneer in applying demography to public health, his contemporary Edwin Chadwick (1800–1890) was a pioneer in combining social epidemiology with environmental health. At the age of thirty-two, Chadwick was appointed to the newly formed Royal Commission of Enquiry on the Poor Laws, and helped reform Britain's Poor Laws. Five years later, following epidemics of typhoid fever and influenza, he was asked by the British government to investigate sanitation. His classic report, *Sanitary Conditions of the Labouring Population* (1842), drew a clear link between living conditions—in particular overcrowded, filthy homes, open cesspools and privies, impure water, and miasmas—and health, and made a strong case for public health reform. The resulting Public Health Act of 1848 created the Central Board of Health, with power to empanel local boards that would oversee street cleaning, trash collection, and water and sewer systems. As sanitation commissioner, Chadwick advocated such innovations as urban water systems, toilets in every house, and transfer of sewage to outlying farms where it could be used as fertilizer (Hamlin, 1998). Chadwick's work helped establish the role of public works—essentially applications of sanitary engineering—to protecting public health. As eloquently pointed out by Thomas McKeown (1979) more than a century later, these interventions were to do far more than medical care to improve public health and well-being during the industrial era.

The physician John Snow (1813–1858) was, like William Farr, a founding member of the London Epidemiological Society. Snow gained immortality in the history of public health for what was essentially an environmental epidemiology study. During an 1854 outbreak of cholera in London, he observed a far higher incidence of disease among people who lived near or drank from the Broad Street pump than among people with other sources of water. He persuaded local authorities to remove the pump handle, and the epidemic in that part of the city soon abated. (There is some evidence that it may have been ending anyway, but this does not diminish the soundness of Snow's approach.) Environmental epidemiology was to blossom during the twentieth century (see Chapter Three) and provide some of the most important evidence needed to support effective preventive measures.

Finally, the industrial era led to a powerful reaction in the worlds of literature, art, and design. In the first half of the nineteenth century, Romantic painters, poets, and philosophers celebrated the divine and inspiring forms of nature. In Germany painters such as Caspar David Friedrich (1774–1840) created meticulous images of the trees, hills, misty valleys, and mercurial light of northern Germany, based on a close observation of nature, and in England Samuel Palmer (1805–1881) painted landscapes that combined straightforward representation of nature with religious vision. His countryman John Constable (1776–1837) worked in the open air, painting deeply evocative English landscapes. In the United States, Hudson River School painters such as Thomas Cole (1801–1848) took their inspiration from the soaring peaks and crags, stately waterfalls, and primeval forests of the northeast. At the same time, the New England transcendentalists celebrated the wonders of nature. "Nature never wears a mean appearance," wrote Ralph Waldo Emerson (1803–1882) in his 1836 paean, *Nature.* "Neither does the wisest man extort her secret, and lose his curiosity by finding out all her perfection. Nature never became a toy to a wise spirit. The flowers, the animals, the mountains, reflected the wisdom of his best hour, as much as they had delighted the simplicity of his childhood." Henry David Thoreau (1817–1862), like Emerson a native of Concord, Massachusetts, rambled from Maine to Cape Cod and famously lived in a small cabin at Walden Pond for two years, experiences that cemented his belief in the "tonic of wildness." And America's greatest landscape architect, Frederick Law Olmsted (1822–1903), championed bringing nature into cities. He designed parks that offered pastoral vistas and graceful tree-lined streets and paths, intending to offer tranquility to harried people and to promote feelings of community. These and other strands of cultural life reflected yet another sense of "environmental health," forged in response to industrialization: the idea that pristine environments were wholesome, healthful, and restorative to the human spirit.

The Modern Era

The modern field of environmental health dates from the mid-twentieth century, and perhaps no landmark better marks its launch than the 1962 publication of Rachel Carson's *Silent Spring. Silent Spring* focused on DDT, an organochlorine pesticide that had seen increasingly wide use since the Second World War. Carson had become alarmed at the ecosystem effects of DDT; she described how it entered the food chain and accumulated in the fatty tissues of animals, how it indiscriminately killed both target species and other creatures, and how its effects persisted for long periods after it was applied. She also made the link to human health, describing how DDT might increase the risk of cancer and birth defects. One of Carson's lasting contributions was to place human health in the context of larger environmental processes. "Man's attitude toward nature," she declared in 1964, "is today critically important simply because we have now acquired a fateful power to alter and destroy nature. But man is a part of nature, and his war against nature is inevitably a war against himself. . . . [We are] challenged as mankind has never been challenged before to prove our maturity and our mastery, not of nature, but of ourselves" (Carson, 1963 [2005]).

The *recognition of chemical hazards* was perhaps the most direct legacy of *Silent Spring.* Beginning in the 1960s, Irving Selikoff (1915–1992) and his colleagues at the Mount Sinai School of Medicine intensively studied insulators and other occupational groups and showed that asbestos could cause a fibrosing lung disease, lung cancer, mesothelioma, and other neoplasms. Outbreaks of cancer in industrial workplaces—lung cancer in a chemical plant near Philadelphia due to bis-chloromethyl ether (Figueroa, Raszkowski, and Weiss, 1973; Randall, 1977), hepatic hemangiosarcoma in a vinyl chloride polymerization plant in Louisville (Creech and Johnson, 1974), and others—underlined the risk of carcinogenic chemicals. With the enormous expansion of cancer research, and with effective advocacy by such groups as the American Cancer Society (Patterson, 1987), environmental and occupational carcinogens became a focus of public, scientific, and regulatory attention (Epstein, 1982).

But cancer was not the only health effect linked to chemical exposures. Herbert Needleman (1927–), studying children in Boston, Philadelphia, and Pittsburgh, showed that lead was toxic to the developing nervous system, causing cognitive and behavioral deficits at levels far lower than had been appreciated. When this recognition finally helped achieve the removal of lead from gasoline, population blood lead levels plummeted, an enduring public health victory. Research also suggested that chemical exposures could threaten reproductive function. Wildlife observations such as abnormal genitalia in alligators in Lake Apopka, Florida, following a pesticide spill (Guillette and others, 1994), and human observations such as an apparent decrease in sperm counts (Carlsen, Giwercman, Keiding, and Skakkebaek, 1992; Swan, Elkin, and Fenster, 1997) suggested that certain persistent, bioaccumulative chemicals (persistent organic pollutants, or POPs) could affect reproduction, perhaps by interfering with hormonal function. Emerging evidence showed that chemicals could damage the kidneys, liver, and cardiovascular system and immune function and organ development.

Some knowledge of chemical toxicity arose from toxicological research (see Chapter Two) and other insights resulted from long-term epidemiological research (see Chapter Three). But catastrophes—reported first in newspaper headlines and only later in scientific journals—also galvanized public and scientific attention. The discovery of accumulations of hazardous wastes in communities across the nation—Love Canal in Niagara Falls, New York (Gibbs, 1998; Mazur, 1998); Times Beach, Missouri, famous for its unprecedented dioxin levels; Toms River, New Jersey, and Woburn, Massachusetts, where municipal drinking water was contaminated with organic chemicals; "Mount Dioxin," a defunct wood treatment plant in Pensacola, Florida; and others—raised concerns about many health problems, from nonspecific symptoms to immune dysfunction to cancer to birth defects. And acute disasters, such as the isocyanate release that killed hundreds and sickened thousands in Bhopal, India, in 1984, made it clear that industrialization posed real threats of chemical toxicity (Kurzman, 1987; Dhara and Dhara, 2002; Moro and Lapierre, 2002).

Even as the awareness of chemical hazards grew, supported by advances in toxicology and epidemiology, environmental health during the second half of the twentieth century was developing in a different direction altogether: *environmental psychology.* As described in Chapter Five, this field arose as a subspecialty of psychology, building on advances in perceptual and cognitive psychology. Scholars such as Stephen Kaplan and Rachel Kaplan at the University of Michigan carried out careful studies of human perceptions and of reactions to various environments. An important contribution to environmental psychology was the theory of *biophilia,* first advanced by Harvard biologist E. O. Wilson in 1984. He defined biophilia as "the innately emotional affiliation of human beings to other living organisms." He pointed out that for most of human existence, people have lived in natural settings, interacting daily with plants, trees, and other animals. As a result, Wilson maintained, affiliation with these organisms has become an innate part of human nature (Wilson, 1984). Other scholars extended Wilson's concept beyond living organisms, postulating a connection with other features of the natural environment—rivers, lakes, and ocean shores; waterfalls; panoramic landscapes and mountain vistas (Kellert and Wilson, 1993; Kellert, 1997). Environmental psychologists studied not only natural features of human environments but also such factors as light, noise, and way-finding cues to assess the impact of these factors. They increasingly recognized that people responded to various environments, both natural and built, in predictable ways. Some environments were alienating, disorientating, or even sickening, whereas others were attractive, restorative, and even salubrious.

A third development in modern environmental health was the continued *integration of ecology with human health.* Ancient wisdom in many cultures had recognized the interrelationships between the natural world and human health and well-being. But with the emergence of formal complex systems analysis and modern ecological science, the understanding of ecosystem function advanced greatly (see Chapter One). As part of this advance the role of humans in the context of ecosystems was better and better delineated. On a global scale, for example, the concept of *carrying capacity* (Wackernagel and Rees, 1995) helped clarify the impact of human activity on ecosystems and permitted evaluation of the ways ecosystem changes, in turn, affected human health and well-being (Rappaport and others, 1999; McMichael, 2001; Aron and Patz, 2001; Martens and McMichael, 2002; Alcamo and others, 2003; Waltner-Toews, 2004; Brown, Grootjans, Ritchie, and Townsend, 2005). Ecological analysis was also applied to specific areas relevant to human health. For example, there were advances in medical botany (Lewis and Elvin-Lewis, 2003; van Wyk and Wink, 2004), in the understanding of biodiversity and its value to human health (Grifo and Rosenthal, 1997), and in the application of ecology to clinical medicine (Aguirre and others, 2002; Ausubel with Harpignies, 2004). These developments, together, reflected a progressive synthesis of ecological and human health science, yielding a better understanding of the foundations of environmental health.

A fourth feature of modern environmental health was the expansion of *clinical services* related to environmental exposures. Occupational medicine and nursing had been specialties in their respective professions since the early twentieth century, with a traditional focus on returning injured and ill workers to work and, to some extent, on preventing hazardous workplace exposures. In the last few decades of the twentieth century, these professional specialties incorporated a public health paradigm, drawing on toxicological and epidemiological data, using industrial hygiene and other primary prevention approaches, and engaging in worker education (see Chapter Thirty-Five). In addition, the occupational health clinical paradigm was broadened to include general environmental exposures. Clinicians began focusing on such community exposures as air pollutants, radon, asbestos, and hazardous wastes, emphasizing the importance of taking an environmental history, identifying at-risk groups, and providing both treatment and preventive advice to patients. Professional ethics expanded to recognize the interests of patients (both workers and community members) as well as those of employers, and in some cases even the interests of unborn generations and of other species (see Chapter Seven). Finally, a wide range of alternative and complementary approaches arose in occupational and environmental health care. For example, an approach known as *clinical ecology* postulated that overloads of environmental exposures could impair immune function, and offered treatments including "detoxification," antifungal medications, and dietary changes purported to prevent or ameliorate the effects of environmental exposures (Randolph, 1976, 1987; Rea, 1992–1998).

Environmental health policy also emerged rapidly. With the promulgation of environmental laws beginning in the 1960s, legislators at the federal and state levels created agencies and assigned them new regulatory responsibilities (see Chapter Thirty-Three). These agencies issued rules that aimed to reduce emissions from smokestacks, drainpipes, and tailpipes; control hazardous wastes; and achieve clean air and water. Although many of these laws were oriented to environmental preservation, the protection of human health was often an explicit rationale as well. Ironically, the new environmental regulations created a schism in the environmental health field. Responsibility for environmental health regulation had traditionally belonged to health departments, but this was now transferred to the new environmental departments. At the federal level, the U.S. Environmental Protection Agency (EPA) assumed some of the traditional responsibilities of the Department of Health, Education, and Welfare (now Health and Human Services), and corresponding changes occurred at the state level. Environmental regulation and health protection became somewhat estranged from each other.

Environmental regulatory agencies increasingly attempted to ground their rules in evidence, using quantitative risk assessment techniques (see Chapter Thirty-Two). This signaled a sea change in regulatory policy. The traditional approach had been simpler; dangerous exposures were simply banned. For example, the 1958 Delaney clause, an amendment to the 1938 federal Food, Drug, and Cosmetic Act, banned carcinogens in food. In contrast, emerging regulations tended to set permissible exposure levels that took into account anticipated health burdens, compliance costs, and technological feasibility.

At the dawn of the twenty-first century, then, the environmental health field had moved well beyond its traditional sanitarian functions. Awareness of chemical toxicity had advanced rapidly, fueled by discoveries in toxicology and epidemiology. At the same time, the complex relationships inherent in environmental health—the effects of environmental conditions on human psychology, and the links between human health and ecosystem function—were better and better recognized. In practical terms, clinical services in environmental health had developed, and regulation had advanced through a combination of political action and scientific evidence.

Emerging Issues

Environmental health is a dynamic, evolving field. As the twenty-first century unfolds, traditional sanitarian functions remain critically important, and chemical hazards will continue to be a focus of scientific and regulatory attention. Looking ahead, we can identify at least five trends that will further shape environmental health: environmental justice, a focus on susceptible groups, scientific advances, global change, and moves toward sustainability.

Beginning around 1980, African American communities identified exposures to hazardous waste and industrial emissions as matters of racial and economic justice. Researchers documented that these exposures disproportionately affected poor and minority communities, a problem that was aggravated by disparities in the enforcement of environmental regulations. The modern *environmental justice* movement was born, a fusion of environmentalism, public health, and the civil rights movement (Bullard, 1994; Cole and Foster, 2000; see also Chapter Eight). Historians have observed that environmental justice represents a profound shift in the history of environmentalism (Shabecoff, 1993; Gottlieb, 1993; Dowie, 1995). This history is commonly divided into waves. The first wave was the conservation movement of the early twentieth century, the second wave was the militant activism that blossomed on Earth Day, 1970, and the third wave was the emergence of large, "inside-the-beltway" environmental organizations such as the Sierra Club, the League of Conservation Voters, and the Natural Resources Defense Council, which had gained considerable policy influence by the 1980s. Environmental justice, then, represents a fourth wave, one that is distinguished by its decentralized, grassroots leadership, its demographic diversity, and its emphasis on human rights and justice. The vision of environmental justice—eliminating disparities in economic opportunity, healthy environments, and health—is one that resonates with public health priorities. It emphasizes that environmental health extends well beyond technical solutions to hazardous exposures to include human rights and equity as well. It is likely that this vision will be an increasingly central part of environmental health in coming decades.

Environmental justice is one example of a broader trend in environmental health—a *focus on susceptible groups.* For many reasons, specific groups may be especially vulnerable to the adverse health effects of environmental exposures. In the case of poor and minority populations, these reasons include disproportionate exposures, limited access to legal protection, limited access to health care, and in some cases compromised baseline health status (see Chapter Eight). Children make up another susceptible population, for several reasons (see Chapter Twenty-Eight). They eat more food, drink more water, and breathe more air per unit of body weight than adults do and are therefore heavily exposed to any contaminants in these media. Children's behavior—crawling on floors, placing their hands in their mouths, and so on—further increases their risk of exposure. With developing organ systems and immature biological defenses, children are less able than adults to withstand some exposures. And with more years of life ahead of them, children have more time to manifest delayed toxic reactions. These facts have formed the basis for research and public health action on children's environmental health. Women bear some specific environmental exposures risks, both in the workplace and in the general environment, due both to disproportionate exposures (for example, in health care jobs) and to unique susceptibilities (for example, to reproductive hazards). Elderly people also bear some specific risks, and as the population ages, this group will attract further environmental health attention. For example, urban environments will need to take into account the limited mobility of some elderly people and provide ample sidewalks, safe street crossings, and accessible gathering places to serve this population. People with disabilities, too, require specific environmental health attention to minimize the risks they face. In the coming decades environmental health will increasingly take account of susceptible groups as the risks they face and their needs for safe, healthy environments become better recognized.

A third set of emerging issues in environmental health is being introduced by *scientific advances.* In toxicology better detection techniques have already enabled us to recognize and quantify low levels of chemical exposure and have supported major advances in the understanding of chemical effects (see Chapter Two). Advances in data analysis techniques have supported innovative epidemiological analyses and the use of large databases. In particular the use of geographic information systems (GISs) has yielded new insights on the spatial distribution of environmental exposures and diseases (see Chapter Thirty-One). Perhaps the most promising scientific advances are occurring at the molecular level, in the linked fields of genomics, toxicogenomics, and proteomics (Schmidt, 2003; Mattes and others, 2004; Pesch and others, 2004; Pognan, 2004; Waters and Fostel, 2004; see also Chapter Six). New genomic tools such as microarrays (or *gene chips*) have enabled scientists to characterize the effects of chemical exposures on the expression of thousands of genes. Databases of genetic responses, and the resulting protein and metabolic pathways, will yield much information on the effects of chemicals and on the variability in responses among different people. Scientific advances related to environmental health will have profound effects on the field in coming decades.

Moving from the molecular scale to the global scale, a fourth set of emerging issues in environmental health relates to *global change.* This broad term encompasses many issues, including population growth, climate change, urbanization, and the increasing integration of the world economy. These trends will shape environmental health in many ways.

The world population is currently just over six billion and is expected to plateau at something like nine billion during the twenty-first century (see Chapter Ten). Most of this population growth will occur in developing nations, and much of it will be in cities. Not only this population growth but also the increasing per capita demand for resources such as food, energy, and materials will strain the global environment, in turn affecting health in many ways. For example, environmental stress and resource scarcity may increasingly trigger armed conflict, an ominous example of the links between environment and health (Homer-Dixon, 1999; Klare, 2001; see also

Chapter Twelve). Global climate change, which results in large part from increasing energy use (see Chapter Fifteen), will threaten health in many ways, from infectious disease risks to heat waves to severe weather events (see Chapter Eleven). As more of the world's population is concentrated in dense urban areas, features of the urban environment—noise, crowding, vehicular and industrial pollution—will come to be important determinants of health (United Nations Centre on Human Settlements, 2001; see also Chapter Sixteen). And with integration of the global economy—the complex changes known as *globalization*—hazards will cross national boundaries (Ives, 1985; see also Chapter Thirteen), trade agreements and market forces will challenge and possibly undermine national environmental health policies (Low, 1992; Sand, 1992; Runge, 1994; Brack, 1998; Victor, Raustiala, and Skolnikoff, 1998), and global solutions to environmental health challenges will increasingly be needed.

Sustainability has been a part of the environmental health vernacular since the 1980s. In 1983, the United Nations formed the World Commission on Environment and Development to propose strategies for sustainable development. The commission, chaired by then Norwegian prime minister Gro Harlem Brundtland, issued its report, *Our Common Future,* in 1987. The report included what has become a standard definition of sustainable development: "development that meets the needs of the present without compromising the ability of future generations to meet their own needs." In 1992, several years after the publication of *Our Common Future,* the United Nations Conference on Environment and Development (UNCED), commonly known as the Earth Summit, convened in Rio de Janeiro. This landmark conference produced, among other documents, the Rio Declaration on Environment and Development, a blueprint for sustainable development. The first principle of the Rio declaration placed environmental health at the core of sustainable development: "Human beings are at the centre of concerns for sustainable development. They are entitled to a healthy and productive life in harmony with nature" (United Nations, 1992).

Like environmental justice the concept of sustainable development blends environmental protection with notions of fairness and equity. As explained on the Web site of the Johannesburg Summit, held ten years after the Earth Summit:

> The Earth Summit thus made history by bringing global attention to the understanding, new at the time, that the planet's environmental problems were intimately linked to economic conditions and problems of social justice. It showed that social, environmental and economic needs must be met in balance with each other for sustainable outcomes in the long term. It showed that if people are poor, and national economies are weak, the environment suffers; if the environment is abused and resources are over consumed, people suffer and

economies decline. The conference also pointed out that the smallest local actions or decisions, good or bad, have potential worldwide repercussions [United Nations Department of Economic and Social Affairs, 2003].

The concept of sustainability has emerged as a central theme, and challenge, not only for environmentalism but for environmental health as well. In the short term sustainable development will permit improvement in the living conditions and therefore the health of people across the world, especially in the poor nations. In the long term sustainable development will protect the health and well-being of future generations. Some of the most compelling thinking in environmental health in recent years offers social and technical paths to sustainable development (Hawken, Lovins, and Lovins, 1999; Brown, 2001, 2003; McDonough and Braungart, 2002; Ehrlich and Ehrlich, 2004; Brown, Grootjans, Ritchie, and Townsend, 2005). These approaches build on the fundamental links among health, environment, technological change, and social justice. Ultimately, they will provide the foundation for lasting environmental health.

Spatial Scales, from Global to Local

The concept of spatial scale is central to many disciplines, from geography to ecology to urban planning. Some phenomena unfold on a highly local scale—ants making a nest, people digging a septic tank. Some phenomena spread across regions—the pollution of a watershed from an upstream factory, the sprawl of a city over a 100-mile diameter. And some phenomena, such as climate change, are truly global in scale. Al Gore, in describing environmental destruction in his 1992 book, *Earth in the Balance,* borrowed from military categories to make this point, distinguishing among "local skirmishes," "regional battles," and "strategic conflicts."

Spatial scale is important not only in military and environmental analysis but also in environmental health. Some environmental factors that affect health operate locally, and the environmental health professionals who address them work on a local level; think of the restaurant and septic tank inspectors who work for the local health department or the health and safety officer at a manufacturing facility. Other environmental factors affect health at a regional level, and the professionals who address these problems work on a larger spatial scale; think of the state officials responsible for air pollution or water pollution enforcement. At the global level such problems as climate change require responses on a national and international scale. These are crafted by professionals in organizations such as the Intergovernmental Panel on Climate Change. So useful is the concept of spatial scales in environmental health that it provides the framework for this book. After introducing the methods and paradigms of environmental health in the first nine chapters, we address specific issues, beginning with global scale problems in Chapters Ten to Thirteen, moving to regional scale problems in Chapters Fourteen to Eighteen, and ending with local problems in Chapters Nineteen to Twenty-Eight. The final eight chapters describe the practice of environmental health, ranging from tools such as geographic information systems to activities such as risk communication and health care services.

It is clear that environmental health professionals work on different spatial scales, but it is not always so clear who is an environmental health professional. Certainly, the environmental health director at a local health department; the director of environment, health, and safety at a manufacturing firm; an environmental epidemiology researcher at a university; or a physician working at an environmental advocacy group would recognize himself or herself and be recognized by others as an environmental health professional. But many other people work in fields that have an impact on the environment and human health. The engineer who designs power plants helps protect the respiratory health of asthmatic children living downwind if she includes sophisticated emissions controls. The transportation planner who enables people to walk instead of drive also protects public health by helping clean up the air. The park superintendent who maintains urban green spaces may contribute greatly to the well-being of people in his city. In fact much of environmental health is determined by "upstream" forces that seem at first glance to have little to do with environment *or* health.

The Forces That Drive Environmental Health

Public health professionals tell the emblematic story of a small village perched alongside a fast-flowing river. The people of the village had always lived near the river, they knew and respected its currents, and they were skilled at swimming, boating, and water rescue. One day they heard desperate cries from the river and noticed a stranger being swept downstream past their village. They sprang into action, grabbed their ropes and gear, and pulled the victim from the water. A few minutes later, as they rested, a second victim appeared, thrashing in the strong current and gasping for breath. The villages once again performed a rescue. Just as they were commenting on the coincidence of two near drownings in one day, a third victim appeared, and they also rescued him. This went on for hours. Every available villager joined in the effort, and by midafternoon all were exhausted. Finally, the flow of victims stopped, and the villagers collapsed, huffing and puffing, in the town square.

At that moment one of the villagers strode whistling into the town square, relaxed and dry. He had not been seen since the first victims were rescued and had not helped with any of the rescues. "Where were you?" his neighbors challenged him. "We've been pulling people out of the river all day! Why didn't you help us?"

"Ah," he replied. "When I noticed all the people in the river, I thought there must be a problem with that old footbridge upstream. I walked up to it, and sure enough, some boards had broken and there was a big hole in the walkway. So I patched the hole, and people stopped falling through."

Box I.2: A Prevention Poem

Like the story of the villagers who saved drowning victims, this poem emphasizes that prevention may lie with root causes. These root causes are often environmental—like the hole in the village's bridge or, in this case, an unguarded cliff edge.

'Twas a dangerous cliff, as they freely confessed, though to walk near its crest was so pleasant;

But over its terrible edge there had slipped a duke, and full many a peasant;

So the people said something would have to be done, but their projects did not at all tally.

Some said: "Put up a fence round the edge of the cliff;" Some, "An ambulance down in the valley."

But the cry for the ambulance carried the day, for it spread through the neighboring city.

A fence may be useful or not, it is true, but each heart became brimful of pity,

For those who slipped over that dangerous cliff; and dwellers in highway and alley,

Gave pounds or gave pence, not to put up a fence, but an ambulance down in the valley.

"For the cliff is all right if you're careful," they said, "And if folks even slip and are dropping,

It isn't the slipping that hurts them so much as the shock down below when they're stopping."

So day after day as those mishaps occurred, quick forth would those rescuers sally,

To pick up the victims who fell off the cliff with the ambulance down in the valley.

Then an old sage remarked, "It's a marvel to me that people gave far more attention

To repairing results than to stopping the cause, when they'd much better aim at prevention.

Let us stop at its source all this mischief," cried he; "Come, neighbors and friends, let us rally;

If the cliff we will fence, we might also dispense with the ambulance down in the valley."

"Oh he's a fanatic," the others rejoined; "Dispense with the ambulance? Never!

He'd dispense with all charities too if he could. No, no! We'll support them forever!

Aren't we picking up folks just as fast as they fall? And shall this man dictate to us? Shall he?

Why should people of sense stop to put up a fence while their ambulance works in the valley?"

But a sensible few who are practical too, will not bear with such nonsense much longer.

They believe that prevention is better than cure; and their party will soon be the stronger.

Encourage them, then, with your purse, voice, and pen, and (while other philanthropists dally)

They will scorn all pretense and put a stout fence on the cliff that hangs over the valley.

Better guide well the young than reclaim them when old, for the voice of true wisdom is calling;

To rescue the fallen is good, but 'tis best to prevent other people from falling;

Better close up the source of temptation and crime than deliver from the dungeon or galley;

Better put a strong fence 'round the top of the cliff, than an ambulance down in the valley.

Upstream thinking has helped identify the root causes of many public health problems (also see Box I.2), and this is nowhere more true than in environmental health. Environmental hazards sometimes originate far from the point of exposure. Imagine that you inhale a hazardous air pollutant. It may come from motor vehicle tailpipes, from power plants, from factories, or from any combination of these. As for the motor vehicle emissions, the amount of driving people do in your city or town reflects urban growth patterns and available transportation alternatives, and the pollutants generated by people's cars and trucks vary with available technology and prevailing regulations. As for the power plants, the amount of energy they produce reflects the demand for energy by households and businesses in the area they serve, and the pollution they emit is a function of how they produce energy (are they coal, nuclear, or wind powered?), the technology they use, and the regulations that govern their operations. Hence a full understanding of the air pollutants you breathe must take into account urban growth, transportation, energy, and regulatory policy, among other upstream determinants. This book contains chapters on many of the upstream forces that affect environmental health, including population growth, transportation, and energy.

These ideas are at the core of a useful model created by the World Health Organization (Figure I.1) (WHO, Regional Office for Europe, 2004). The DPSEEA (driving forces—pressures—state—exposure—effects—actions) model was developed as a tool both for analyzing environmental health hazards and for designing indicators useful in decision making. The *driving forces* are the factors that motivate environmental health processes. In our air pollution example, these factors might include population growth; consumer preferences for energy-consuming homes, appliances, and vehicles; and sprawl that requires driving long distances. The driving forces result in *pressures* on the environment, such as the emission of oxides of nitrogen, hydrocarbons, particulate matter, and other air pollutants. These emissions, in turn, modify the *state* of the environment,

FIGURE I.1. THE DPSEEA MODEL.

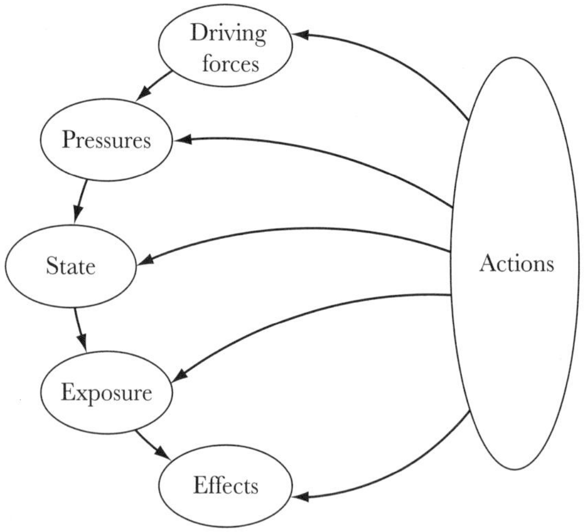

Source: WHO, Regional Office for Europe, 2004.

accumulating in the air and combining to form additional pollutants such as ozone. However, this deterioration in the state of the environment does not invariably threaten health; human *exposure* must occur. In the case of air pollutants, exposure occurs when people are breathing when and where the air quality is low. (Some people, of course, sustain higher exposures than others; an outdoor worker, an exercising athlete, or a child at play receives relatively higher doses of air pollutants than a person in an air-conditioned office.) The hazardous exposure may lead to a variety of health *effects,* acute or chronic. In the case of air pollutants, these effects may include coughing and wheezing, asthma attacks, heart attacks, and even early death.

Finally, to eliminate or control environmental hazards and protect human health, society may undertake a wide range of *actions,* targeted at any of the upstream steps. For example, protecting the public from the effects of air pollution might include encouraging energy conservation to reduce energy demand and designing *live-work-play* communities to reduce travel demand (addressing driving forces); providing mass transit or bicycle lanes to reduce driving, requiring emissions controls on power plants, or investing in wind turbines to reduce emissions from coal-fired power plants (addressing pressures); requiring low-sulfur fuel (addressing the state of the environment); warning people to stay inside when ozone levels are high (addressing exposures); and providing maintenance asthma medications (addressing health effects). The most effective long-term actions, however, are those that are preventive, aimed at eliminating or reducing the forces that drive the system (see Chapter Twenty-Nine). This theme is universal in public health, applying both to environmental hazards and to other health hazards.

Acknowledgments

In many religions and cultures teachers are revered. I honor that tradition, as well I should: I have been blessed with more superb teachers than I had any right to expect when I first marched off to school. They didn't know it, but they were all preparing me to envision this book and pull it together. One of the sweetest privileges of an editor—and there have been many—is the chance to thank them.

I express my deep and lasting gratitude to my high school teacher Barbara Leventer, who taught me that writing a research paper means specifying a hypothesis, organizing an outline, finding good sources, and writing clearly (and all of that before the Internet!); my college teachers Ed Beiser, who taught me that there is no excuse for muddled thinking and unclear expression, and Steve Lyons and Hunter Dupree, who taught me the majesty and endless relevance of history; my medical school teachers Paul Stolley, who taught me the power of epidemiological data and who set a standard for principled advocacy, and the late John Eisenberg, who modeled a formidable combination of clinical excellence, astute policy analysis, and great kindness; my residency teacher Bob Lawrence, who taught me that primary care extends from the bedside to the global commons; and my graduate school teachers Richard Monson, John Peters, and David Wegman, who taught me the interface of public health and the environment.

I thank my colleagues and students at Emory University's Rollins School of Public Health, who for fifteen years have provided a challenging, convivial, and exciting intellectual environment, and my colleagues across campus, at other universities, and in organizations from the Centers for Disease Control to the Environmental Protection Agency, from environmental community groups to law firms to manufacturing companies, who have taught me more than I can say about the many facets of environmental health. In particular, I thank my friends and colleagues at Physicians for Social Responsibility; the Institute of Medicine Roundtable on Environmental Health, Research, and Medicine; the Clean Air Campaign; the EPA Children's Health Protection Advisory Committee; the Association of Occupational and Environmental Clinics; and the American Public Health Association.

I thank the chapter authors of this book, all of them highly expert and exceedingly busy people. They willingly shared their expertise and time (and gracefully tolerated my prodding and editing) to help compile the kind of book that we would all want to use in our own teaching.

I thank my editors at Jossey-Bass, Andy Pasternack and Seth Schwartz, who believed in this project, generously tolerated delays, and kept me on track. If there is a special place for editors in heaven, Andy and Seth will certainly end up there (although they would probably prefer to stay in San Francisco). And I thank production editor Susan Geraghty and copyeditor Elspeth MacHattie, who are consummate professionals, a pleasure to work with, and an enormous asset to the book.

I thank Hope Jackson, who served as editorial assistant on this book during her transition between Emory College and medical school. She managed hundreds of files and thousands of tasks big and small with skill and professionalism. Hope's patients will be as lucky as I have been. I also thank the dedicated and hard-working staff, past and present, in Emory's Department of Environmental and Occupational Health—especially Robin Thompson, Adrienne Tison, Erica Weaver, Rachel Wilson, and Suzanne Mason—who have made it possible for all of our students and faculty to thrive.

And I thank my family. During the year I edited this book, our house burned down, we moved away, rebuilt the house, and came back. Meanwhile life went on—classes, dissertation research, seeing clients, a Bat Mitzvah, scouting meetings, soccer games, recycling trips, homework, dog care, you name it. I thank Beryl for shouldering more than her share and for supporting this project. Every chapter edited, every source consulted, every reference checked, was borrowed from our family time. That's a loan I can never repay adequately, but if a book like this is an investment in the future, I know that Gabe and Amara will compound it, making giant contributions to a safer, healthier, and more sustainable world.

References

Aguirre, A. A., and others (eds.). *Conservation Medicine: Ecological Health in Practice.* New York: Oxford University Press, 2002.

Alcamo, J., and others. *Ecosystems and Human Well-Being: A Framework for Assessment.* Millennium Ecosystem Assessment. Washington, D.C.: Island Press, 2003.

Aron, J. L., and Patz, J. A. *Ecosystem Change and Global Health: A Global Perspective.* Baltimore, Md.: Johns Hopkins University Press, 2001.

Ausubel, K., with Harpignies, J. P. (eds.). *Ecological Medicine: Healing the Earth, Healing Ourselves.* San Francisco: Sierra Club Books, 2004.

Brack, D. (ed.). *Trade and Environment: Conflict or Compatibility?* London: Earthscan, 1998.

Brimblecombe, P. *The Big Smoke.* London: Routledge, 1988.

Brown, L. R. *Eco-Economy: Building an Economy for the Earth.* New York: Norton, 2001.

Brown, L. R. *Plan B: Rescuing a Planet Under Stress and a Civilization in Trouble.* New York: Norton, 2003.

Brown, V. A., Grootjans, J., Ritchie, J., and Townsend, M. *Sustainability and Health: Supporting Global Ecological Integrity in Public Health.* London: Earthscan, 2005.

Bullard, R. D. *Dumping in Dixie: Race, Class, and Environmental Quality.* (2nd ed.) Boulder, Colo.: Westview Press, 1994.

Cantor, N. *In the Wake of the Plague: The Black Death and the World It Made.* New York: Free Press, 2001.

Carlsen, E., Giwercman, A., Keiding, N., and Skakkebaek, N. "Evidence for Decreasing Quality of Semen During Past 50 Years." *British Medical Journal,* 1992, *305,* 609–613.

Carson, R. Oral statement on "The Silent Spring of Rachel Carson," *CBS Reports,* April 3, 1963. [http://www.rachelcarson.org/index.cfm?fuseaction=obituary]. 2005.

Cole, L. W., and Foster, S. R. *From the Ground Up: Environmental Racism and the Rise of the Environmental Justice Movement.* New York: New York University Press, 2000.

Creech, J. L., and Johnson, M. N. "Angiosarcoma of the Liver in the Manufacture of PVC." *Journal of Occupational Medicine,* 1974, *16,* 150–151.

Dhara, V. R., and Dhara, R. "The Union Carbide Disaster in Bhopal: A Review of Health Effects." *Archives of Environmental Health,* 2002, *57,* 391–404.

Dowie, M. *Losing Ground: American Environmentalism at the Close of the Twentieth Century.* Cambridge, Mass.: MIT Press, 1995.

Duffy, J. *The Sanitarians: A History of American Public Health.* Urbana: University of Illinois Press, 1990.

Ehrlich, P., and Ehrlich, A. *One with Nineveh: Politics, Consumption, and the Human Future.* Washington, D.C.: Island Press, 2004.

Epstein, S. *The Politics of Cancer.* New York: Random House, 1982.

Figueroa, W. G., Raszkowski, R., and Weiss, W. "Lung Cancer in Chloromethyl Methyl Ether Workers." *New England Journal of Medicine,* 1973, *288,* 1096–1097.

Gibbs, L. M. *Love Canal: The Story Continues.* Gabriola Island, B.C.: New Society, 1998.

Gore, A. *Earth in the Balance.* Boston: Houghton Mifflin, 1992.

Gottlieb, R. *Forcing the Spring: The Transformation of the American Environmental Movement.* Washington, D.C.: Island Press, 1993.

Grifo, F., and Rosenthal, J. (eds.). *Biodiversity and Human Health.* Washington, D.C.: Island Press, 1997.

Guillette, L. J., and others. "Developmental Abnormalities of the Gonad and Abnormal Sex Hormone Concentrations in Juvenile Alligators from Contaminated and Control Lakes in Florida." *Environmental Health Perspectives,* 1994, *102,* 680–688.

Hamlin, C. *Public Health and Social Justice in the Age of Chadwick: Britain, 1800–1854.* New York: Cambridge University Press, 1998.

Hawken, P., Lovins, A., and Lovins, L. H. *Natural Capitalism: Creating the Next Industrial Revolution.* Boston: Little, Brown, 1999.

Herlihy, D., and Cohn, S. K. *The Black Death and the Transformation of the West.* Cambridge, Mass.: Harvard University Press, 1997.

Homer-Dixon, T. F. *Environment, Scarcity and Violence.* Princeton, N.J.: Princeton University Press, 1999.

Hurley, A. "Creating Ecological Wastelands: Oil Pollution in New York City, 1870–1900." *Journal of Urban History,* 1994, *20,* 340–364.

Ives, J. H. (ed.). *The Export of Hazard: Transnational Corporations and Environmental Control Issues.* New York: Routledge, 1985.

Kellert, S. R. *Kinship to Mastery: Biophilia in Human Evolution and Development.* Washington, D.C.: Island Press, 1997.

Kellert, S. R., and Wilson, E. O. (eds.). *The Biophilia Hypothesis.* Washington, D.C.: Island Press, 1993.

Kelly, J. *The Great Mortality: An Intimate History of the Black Death, the Most Devastating Plague of All Time.* New York: HarperCollins, 2005.

Klare, M. T. *Resource Wars: The New Landscape of Global Conflict.* New York: Henry Holt, 2001.

Kurzman, D. *A Killing Wind: Inside Union Carbide and the Bhopal Catastrophe.* New York: McGraw-Hill, 1987.

Leavitt, J. W. *The Healthiest City: Milwaukee and the Politics of Health Reform.* Princeton, N.J.: Princeton University Press, 1982.

Lewis, W. H., and Elvin-Lewis, M.P.F. *Medical Botany: Plants Affecting Human Health.* (2nd ed.) New York: Wiley, 2003.

Low, P. (ed.). *International Trade and the Environment.* World Bank Discussion Papers 159. Washington, D.C.: World Bank, 1992.

Martens, P., and McMichael, A. J. (eds.). *Environmental Change, Climate and Health: Issues and Research Methods.* London: Cambridge University Press, 2002.

Mattes, W. B., and others. "Database Development in Toxicogenomics: Issues and Efforts." *Environmental Health Perspectives,* 2004, *112,* 495–505.

Mazur, A. *A Hazardous Inquiry: The Rashomon Effect at Love Canal.* Cambridge, Mass.: Harvard University Press, 1998.

McDonough, W., and Braungart, M. *Cradle to Cradle: Remaking the Way We Make Things.* New York: North Point Press, 2002.

McKeown, T. *The Role of Medicine: Dream, Mirage, or Nemesis?* Princeton, N.J.: Princeton University Press, 1979.

McMichael, T. *Human Frontiers, Environments and Disease.* New York: Cambridge University Press, 2001.

Melosi, M. *The Sanitary City: Urban Infrastructure in America from Colonial Times to the Present.* Baltimore, Md.: Johns Hopkins University Press, 2000.

Moro, J., and Lapierre, D. *Five Past Midnight in Bhopal: The Epic Story of the World's Deadliest Industrial Disaster.* New York: Warner, 2002.

Patterson, J. T. *The Dread Disease: Cancer and Modern American Culture.* Cambridge, Mass.: Harvard University Press, 1987.

Pesch, B., and others. "Challenges to Environmental Toxicology and Epidemiology: Where Do We Stand and Which Way Do We Go?" *Toxicology Letters,* 2004, *151*(1), 255–266.

Pognan, F. "Genomics, Proteomics and Metabonomics in Toxicology: Hopefully Not 'Fashionomics.'" *Pharmacogenomics,* 2004, *5,* 879–893.

Randall, W. *Building 6: The Tragedy at Bridesburg.* Boston: Little, Brown, 1977.

Randolph, T. G. *Human Ecology and Susceptibility to the Chemical Environment.* Springfield, Ill.: Thomas, 1976.

Randolph, T. G. *Environmental Medicine: Beginnings and Bibliographies of Clinical Ecology.* Fort Collins, Colo.: Clinical Ecology, 1987.

Rappaport, D. J., and others. "Ecosystem Health: The Concept, the ISEH, and the Important Tasks Ahead." *Ecosystem Health,* 1999, *5,* 82–90.

Rea, W. J. *Chemical Sensitivity.* 4 vols. Boca Raton, Fla.: Lewis, 1992–1998.

Rosen, G. *A History of Public Health.* (Expanded ed.) Baltimore, Md.: Johns Hopkins University Press, 1993. (Originally published 1958.)

Rosenberg, C. *The Cholera Years: The United States in 1832, 1849, and 1866.* Chicago: University of Chicago Press, 1962.

Runge, C. F. *Freer Trade, Protected Environment: Balancing Trade Liberalization and Environmental Interests.* New York: Council on Foreign Relations Press, 1994.

Sand, P. H. (ed.). *The Effectiveness of International Environmental Agreements: A Survey of Existing Legal Instruments.* Cambridge, UK: Grotius, 1992.

Schmidt, C. W. "Toxicogenomics: An Emerging Discipline." *Environmental Health Perspectives,* 2003, *110,* A750–A755.

Shabecoff, P. *A Fierce Green Fire: The American Environmental Movement.* New York: Hill & Wang, 1993.

Sullivan, R. *Rats: Observations on the History and Habitat of the City's Most Unwanted Inhabitants.* New York: Bloomsbury, 2004.

Swan, S. H., Elkin, E. P., and Fenster, L. "Have Sperm Densities Declined? A Reanalysis of Global Trend Data." *Environmental Health Perspectives,* 1997, *105,* 1228–1232.

Tarr, J. A. *The Search for the Ultimate Sink: Urban Pollution in Historical Perspective.* Akron, Ohio: University of Akron Press, 1996.

Tarr, J. A. "Industrial Waste Disposal in the United States as a Historical Problem." *Ambix,* 2002, *49,* 4–20.

United Nations. *Report of the United Nations Conference on Environment and Development: Annex I: Rio Declaration on Environment and Development.* [http://www.un.org/documents/ga/conf151/aconf15126-1annex1.htm]. 1992.

United Nations Centre for Human Settlements (Habitat). *Cities in a Globalizing World: Global Report on Human Settlements 2001.* London: Earthscan, 2001.

United Nations Department of Economic and Social Affairs. "Johannesburg Summit 2002." [http://www.johannesburgsummit.org/html/basic_info/unced.html]. 2003.

U.S. Department of Health and Human Services. "An Ensemble of Definitions of Environmental Health." [http://web.health.gov/environment/DefinitionsofEnvHealth/ehdef2.htm]. Nov. 1998.

van Wyk, B.-E., and Wink, M. *Medicinal Plants of the World: An Illustrated Scientific Guide to Important Medicinal Plants and Their Uses.* Portland, Ore.: Timber Press, 2004.

Victor, D. G., Raustiala, K., and Skolnikoff, E. B. (eds.). *The Implementation and Effectiveness of International Environmental Commitments: Theory and Practice.* Cambridge, Mass.: MIT Press, 1998.

Wackernagel, M., and Rees, W. *Our Ecological Footprint: Reducing Human Impact on the Earth.* Gabriola Island, B.C.: New Society, 1995.

Waltner-Toews, D. *Ecosystem Sustainability and Health: A Practical Approach.* New York: Cambridge University Press, 2004.

Waters, M. D., and Fostel, J. M. "Toxicogenomics and Systems Toxicology: Aims and Prospects." *Nature Reviews: Genetics,* 2004, *5,* 936–948.

Wilson, E. O. *Biophilia.* Cambridge, Mass.: Harvard University Press, 1984.

World Commission on Environment and Development. *Our Common Future.* New York: Oxford University Press, 1987.

World Health Organization. "Protection of the Human Environment." [http://www.who.int/phe/en]. 2004.

World Health Organization. "Governance: Constitution of the World Health Organization." [http://www.who.int/governance/en]. 2005.

World Health Organization, Regional Office for Europe. *Environment and Health: The European Charter and Commentary.* WHO Regional Publications European Series no. 35. Copenhagen: World Health Organization, Regional Office for Europe, 1990.

World Health Organization, Regional Office for Europe. "Environment and Health Information System: The DPSEEA Model of Health-Environment Interlinks." [http://www.euro. who.int/EHindicators/Indicators/20030527_2]. 2004.

Zinsser, H. *Rats, Lice and History: Being a Study in Biography, Which, After Twelve Preliminary Chapters Indispensable for the Preparation of the Lay Reader, Deals with the Life History of Typhus Fever.* Boston: Little, Brown, 1935.

ENVIRONMENTAL HEALTH

PART ONE

METHODS AND PARADIGMS

CHAPTER ONE

ECOLOGY AND HUMAN HEALTH

John Wegner

The term *ecology* was coined in the mid-1860s by the German scientist Ernst Haeckel and is derived from the Greek word *oikos,* which means "house" or "home." Therefore ecology is the study of an organism's home (Odum, 1971). *Oikos* also forms the root of *economics,* which literally means home finance. Over the last 150 years, ecology as a scientific discipline has evolved from natural history. Natural history is the simple study of nature and relies heavily on the use of observation to interpret the behavior of organisms. It also explores their life history strategies, or *lifestyles.*

Today there are about as many definitions of *ecology* as there are ecology textbooks (for example, Odum, 1971; Krohne, 1998; Bush, 2000). However, all the definitions have a common theme: that ecology is the study of organisms and their environment. *Environment* includes both animate and inanimate factors. At the core of ecology, therefore, is the study of the abundance and distribution of an organism. Ecologists ask questions like these: Why are some species rare and others common? and, Why do some species occur over large geographic areas whereas others have very limited distributions?

Ecologists today look to both the physical environment and the presence of other species to answer these questions. For example, ecologists can use average annual precipitation and average temperature in a geographic area to predict the types of plants that can be found there. In the eastern United States where the average precipitation is >50 inches per year and the average temperature is 50°F

(Chapin, Matson, and Mooney, 2002), ecologists conclude that historically the area was forested, and that indeed is the case. This is the deciduous forest zone. There is sufficient moisture to support trees. Plants use water for conveying nutrients from the roots to the leaves and also need water for photosynthesis. A large tree requires thousands of gallons of water per year to survive and the precipitation in the eastern United States is sufficient to support the growth of very large trees. Descriptions of the forests by early travelers indicate that some trees, like the tulip poplar, commonly attained a diameter of nine feet! The ecologist would predict that the trees that grow in this zone are deciduous—they shed their leaves every year—because of the average yearly temperature. The temperature is too low to support tropical evergreen forests but not cold enough to favor the evergreen conifers that grow in the northern boreal forest.

Another example is the arctic, the region at the northern extreme of the northern hemisphere continents. Here the total precipitation is less than six inches per year and the average yearly temperature is around freezing. Ecologists characterize the arctic as *wet desert.* Although it doesn't seem to make sense for a desert to be wet, this is indeed the case in the arctic. The land is relatively flat, and more important, much of the soil is permanently frozen, or permafrost. Thus the small amount of precipitation that falls on the land has nowhere to go, so it puddles on the surface. If you are going to go to this desert, you need to remember to bring along your rubber boots! There are few trees in the arctic because it is so cold, and exposed plant twigs and leaves would not survive the cold winters. The only place where trees can be found in the arctic is in snow beds that may be several feet deep. In fact, one can predict the yearly depth of the snow in these areas by looking at the height of the trees in the summer. The height of the trees equals the depth of the snow.

The Ecosystem Concept

One of the most important advances in ecology in the twentieth century was the development of the ecosystem concept (Golley, 1993; Aber and Melillo, 2001; Chapin, Matson, and Mooney, 2002). Alfred Tansley defined the term *ecosystem* in 1935 to alleviate a problem that was developing in ecology. Until that time, ecologists who studied plant communities (a *plant community* is all the species of plants found in a particular location) had focused only on how the presence of one plant species affected the distribution and abundance of other plant species. An extreme form of this approach was the discipline called *phytosociology,* which literally studied social relations among plants. Phytosociologists would discuss which species of plants "got along with" other species and which ones didn't, and they considered plant communities analogous to *surpraorganisms* (organisms made up of other organisms). They viewed individual species in a community as, for example, the "heart" or the "lungs" of the community and thus saw all the species as essential to the existence of the whole community. Ecology had become a holistic discipline (Odum, 1971) in which the whole—in this case the plant community—was considered greater than the sum of its parts and communities were considered to have *emergent properties,* attributes that emerged from the interactions of all the species. Tansley was uncomfortable with this approach and put the ecosystem concept forward as a substitute for the community concept.

An *ecosystem* is defined as all the species found in an area plus the physical environment in which they reside. One of the important aspects of this concept is that it views the ecology of an organism as determined not only by the presence of other species but also by the characteristics of the physical environment. Another aspect of this concept is that an ecosystem is a heuristic tool. It is not an entity in the sense that an organism is an entity; it is an entity by definition. Tansley recognized that what defines a particular ecosystem is the ecological question one is asking at the moment. Tansley was one of the first ecologists to recognize that ecology is hierarchical, and that ecosystems occur on a variety of spatial and temporal scales, ranging from very small to very large.

Let's examine the ecosystem concept further by posing two questions and exploring the ecosystem scale that is appropriate for each of the questions. The first question is, Is the amount of carbon dioxide in the atmosphere changing, and what are the factors that might explain such changes? For this question, our ecosystem would be the whole biosphere—all the layers of the earth and its atmosphere where life occurs. In answering this question we would find that forests can be an important source of carbon dioxide and that the destruction by burning of tropical rainforests has released large amounts of carbon dioxide to the atmosphere. We would also discover that other human activities also affect the amount of carbon dioxide in the atmosphere. The burning of fossil fuels is the largest anthropogenic contribution of carbon dioxide to the atmosphere. Another important source of carbon dioxide is the manufacturing of cement. However, if we added up all the carbon dioxide that is released to the atmosphere every year from both human and natural sources, and added that amount to the current amount of carbon dioxide in the atmosphere (which also derived from both sources), we would find that there is less carbon dioxide in the atmosphere than our math predicts. The question then becomes, Where has the extra carbon dioxide gone? The answer appears to be the oceans. About half of the carbon dioxide entering the atmosphere every year ends up being dissolved in the ocean and eventually comes to reside in the deep ocean.

The second question comes from the observation that some frog species in the genus *Rana* freeze during the winter (Storey and Storey, 1990). Why do some species of *Rana* freeze and survive while others don't? To answer this question, we need to look at the characteristics of the ecosystem where each species spends the winter. For example, the leopard frog (*Rana pipiens*) overwinters in the bottom of ponds. Ponds typically do not freeze to the bottom, and therefore leopard frogs are not exposed to freezing temperatures and have not evolved the ability to freeze. Wood frogs (*Rana silvatica*) overwinter terrestrially. Typically, they burrow into the soil along tree roots, tunneling to depths where the soil temperature does not go below −10°C. As a result they have evolved the ability to freeze, thaw, and hop another day.

Population Ecology

Ecologists not only study where species occur; they also ask questions about changes in the number of individuals in a species over time. To predict how populations change through time, ecologists use population growth models (Meyer, Yung, and Ausubel, 1999). A population is considered to be all the individuals of a species for which it is reasonable to assume a common birthrate and death rate. The simplest growth model that ecologists use is the exponential growth model. This model assumes that a population can grow continuously without any limit (that is, nothing impedes the growth of the population). It can be described this way: the change in the population over time is equal to the current population size times the rate of increase for the population:

$$dN/dt = r(N)$$

or

$$N_t = N_o(e^{rt}).$$

Where dN/dt is the change in the population (N) over time (t), r is the rate of increase (births minus deaths), N_t equals the population at time t, N_o equals the population at some previous time, and e is a constant equal to 2.72.

In 1798, Thomas Malthus used this equation to argue that the human population was outstripping the rate at which food was being produced and that the population in Europe would soon decrease dramatically (Smith and Smith, 2003). The curve labeled "exponential" in Figure 1.1 graphs a population that is growing exponentially. Exponential growth predicts a J-shaped curve that shows the population constantly expanding. Although this equation is very simple to use, it is not ecologically realistic. Eventually, all species will face some limit on population

FIGURE 1.1. POPULATION GROWTH PATTERNS: A COMPARISON OF EXPONENTIAL AND LOGISTIC GROWTH.

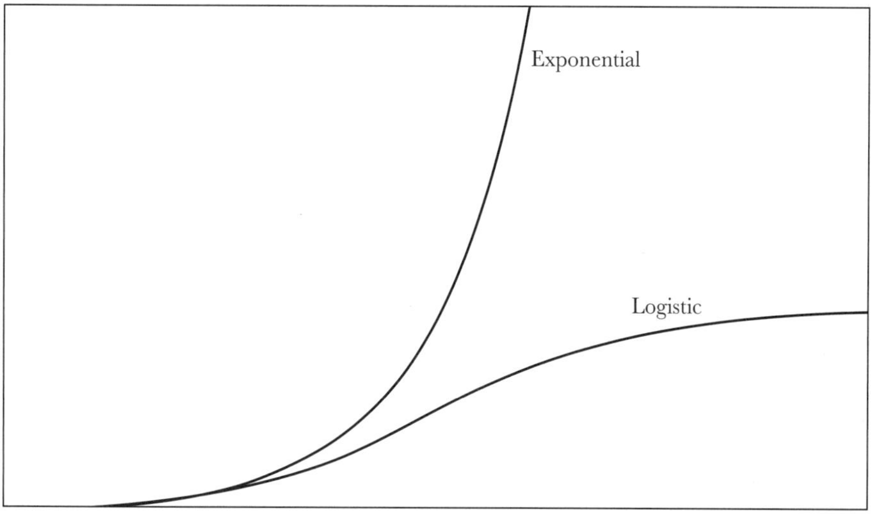

Source: Adapted from Meyer, Yung, and Ausubel, 1999.

size, be it food, space, or some other resource. The best use for this equation is to predict growth over those short periods of time when the population is not significantly limited by any resource. The exponential growth model has been widely used to make predictions about *doubling time:* that is, the amount of time that it takes a population to double in size. Doubling time is equal to 0.69 divided by *r.* Doubling time is commonly used to predict how fast the human population will grow. Currently, the doubling time for the U.S. population is sixty-five years (Carrying Capacity Network, 2004). Historically, the exponential growth model has been a good predictor of human population size; however, that may soon be changing as we use more and more of the earth's resources.

Doubling time is also used to characterize the use (and depletion) of resources. For example, between 1989 and 1999, U.S. use of energy increased by about 1.6 percent per year (World Resources Institute, 2004). At that rate the total amount of energy consumed in the United States would be projected to double in just twenty-seven years.

A more realistic population growth model is the logistic model. This model assumes that some resource or resources will limit the size of the population, implying a maximum population size, or a *carrying capacity* (K), for the population. The change in the population over time is thus predicted to be

$$dN/dt = r(N)((K - N)/K).$$

Where $(K - N)/K$ varies from near 1 when the population is small to 0 when the population is at its carrying capacity.

The curve labeled "logistic" in Figure 1.1 illustrates that the predictions of the logistic equation take the form of an S-shaped growth curve, where the population eventually levels off at the carrying capacity. Note that even with the same starting population and the same growth rate, the exponential and logistic growth models always predict different population sizes and that the difference in the predictions increases with time. Although the logistic growth model is more realistic than the exponential one, it still is an oversimplification of how population size changes. For example, the equation does not account for gender or age distribution and assumes that the population is closed, that is, there is no inmigration or outmigration.

K- Versus r-Species

Ecologists use the terms used in the growth equations to distinguish between two types of life history strategy for organisms (Pianka, 2000). *K-species* are species that live at or near their environmental carrying capacity in the ecosystem. Individuals in these species reach sexual maturity late and have a long life span, are large organisms at maturity, produce few offspring over a lifetime, have a large parental investment in each offspring, and reproduce multiple times over a lifetime. These species have a relatively low population growth rate and tend to live in stable environments. Elephants and oak trees are good examples of K-species.

Conversely, *r-species* live in unstable environments and where the species is far below its carrying capacity. Individuals in these species tend to reach sexual maturity very rapidly and be short lived, are relatively small organisms, tend to reproduce only once, and have a small parental investment in each offspring. These species have the capability for explosive population growth. Mice and ragweed are good examples of r-species.

Ecologists have noticed that successful invasive species tend to be r-species. *Invasive* species are species that arrive in a new environment and are successful in establishing populations there. Goats in the Galapagos and starlings in North American are good examples of r-species that have been highly successful in the environments into which they have been introduced. Unfortunately, these species can have profound negative impacts on their new ecosystems. For example, goats have denuded the Galapagos of vegetation. Starlings compete with native birds for nest cavities and have virtually wiped out bluebirds in eastern North America.

Carrying Capacity and Humans

Does the concept of carrying capacity apply to the human population? Logically, one might say yes, but determining the carrying capacity for humans is a daunting task. For example, when most human populations were hunter-gatherer societies, the carrying capacity of the earth was much lower than it became after agricultural societies developed. With the development of each new agricultural technology (such as mechanized agriculture, inorganic fertilizers, pesticides, and most recently, genetically modified organisms), the carrying capacity of the earth has increased. The same has been true for other technological advances. In addition, changing human behavior can also affect carrying capacity. If all humans became vegetarians, we could support more people from the land once used to produce animal feed. Therefore, although we might agree that carrying capacity applies to us as a species, it is a very difficult number to predict accurately. In the last section of this chapter we will look at one way that ecologists have attempted to apply carrying capacity to humans.

Importance of Population Age Structure for Predicting Population Growth

As mentioned earlier the exponential and logistic growth models do not account for *population age structure,* the relative proportions of a population that are in the prereproductive, reproductive, and postreproductive age categories (Smith and Smith, 2003). Interestingly, few species besides humans have a postreproductive age category, and this may be a recent addition, with the advent of public health and medicine extending the human life span.

Replacement rate (R_0) measures population growth rate. It compares the number of female offspring produced for the next generation relative to the females in the population in the current generation. Therefore a replacement rate greater than 1 means that the population is growing, and a replacement rate less than 1 means that the population is declining. Figure 1.2 shows the three possible types of population age structure. Common sense suggests that if we want the human population to stabilize, on average each female should have one female offspring (out of two children altogether). However, this will not be the case if the population age structure is like that on the far left in Figure 1.2. With one female child per female it would take a few generations for this population to stabilize, owing to what is called *population momentum.* Population momentum is an important consideration when predicting future population size.

FIGURE 1.2. POSSIBLE POPULATION AGE STRUCTURES FOR HUMAN POPULATIONS.

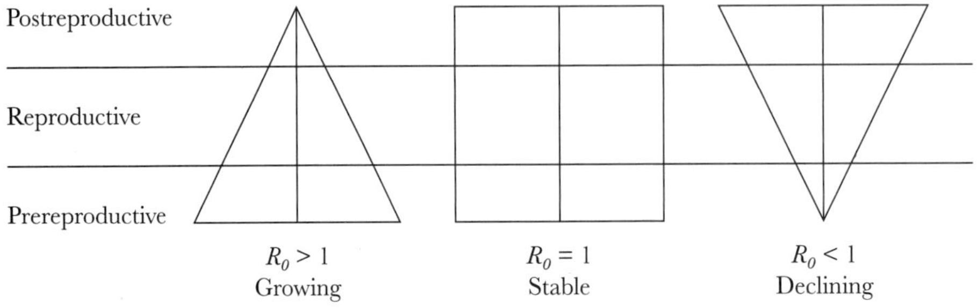

Reproductive category is on the *y*-axis and each figure is divided vertically in two for males and females in the population. *Ro* equals the net replacement rate of a female from one generation to the next.

Perhaps the most important advance in the last twenty years in our understanding of population growth is our recognition of the role of immigration and emigration, particularly for small populations (Smith and Smith, 2003). This recognition has led to the development of the concept of a *metapopulation,* or a population of populations. This population growth model recognizes that few local populations last forever; whole populations frequently go extinct. If a species is to survive in a geographic area, as local populations go extinct the area needs to be recolonized from other local populations. This concept has been important in conservation biology, the area of ecology that investigates the conservation of species. Frequently, one of the impacts of humans on a species' environment is to fragment it, dividing larger local populations into smaller ones. These smaller local populations are more likely than larger ones to go extinct, and recolonization from other local populations may be difficult due to the insertion of other habitat types between the local populations. A species extinction is most commonly the result of local extinctions that accumulate until they lead to the loss of the whole species from the planet.

Ecosystem Ecology

The ecosystem concept has been such a potent tool that it has given rise to a subdiscipline of ecology called *ecosystem ecology* (Golley, 1993). Ecosystem ecology takes the basic components of the ecosystem and applies systems thinking. Simply

FIGURE 1.3. BASIC COMPONENTS OF AN ECOSYSTEM.

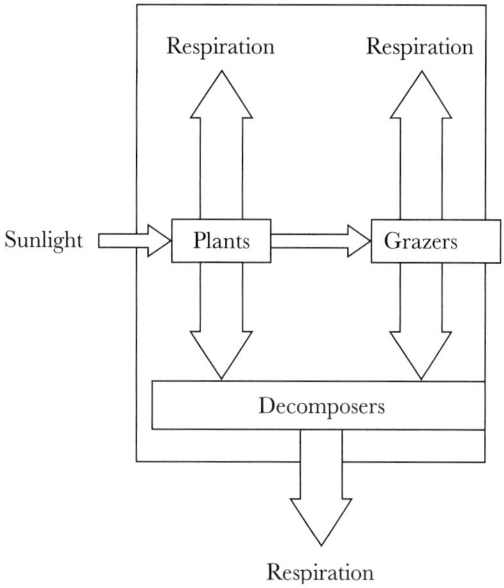

put, ecosystem ecology views an ecosystem in the same way that one might think about a stereo system. A system has a common function or functions, a boundary, inputs and outputs across the boundary, system components, and interactions between those components. The two most common functions in an ecosystem in this systems view are energy flow and nutrient cycling. Figure 1.3 illustrates the basic components of an ecosystem. The components are categories of organisms and the flows represent movement of energy or nutrients from one component to another. This paradigm is also a powerful tool for thinking about human health in an environmental context, as discussed later in this book (Box 29.7).

Energy Flow Through Ecosystems

Virtually all ecosystems (excluding those in the deep ocean vents) get their primary energy from the sun (Smith and Smith, 2003). In the presence of sunlight, plants convert carbon dioxide and water through photosynthesis into sugars that provide the energy necessary for the plant's respiration. Ecologists refer to this as *fixing* energy (taking sunlight and storing it in chemical bonds) and to plants as *autotrophs* ("self-feeders"). Of course plants don't really feed themselves; they are dependent on sunlight and nutrients to produce the sugars and other products they need to survive. Most plants respire (metabolize) about 50 percent of the energy they produce via photosynthesis. Of the remaining energy, some may be used for plant growth (for example, trees get taller and larger in diameter), and some may be used in reproduction (producing seeds).

Animals that feed on plants are called *heterotrophs* ("other feeders"). Therefore they are organisms that are dependent on plants for food. If the animals eat living plants, they are herbivores and form part of the grazing *food chain* comprising plants, herbivores, carnivores (animals that eat animals), and omnivores (animals that eat both plants and animals). Each of these types of organism may be considered a different component in the ecosystem. As feeding relationships within the food chain become more complex, we may refer to the *food web* instead of the food chain. In most ecosystems, less than 10 percent of the energy available to animals flows into the grazing food chain.

Interestingly, there are no organisms visible to the naked eye that can digest the cellulose that forms the cell walls of plants. Most of the herbivorous animals that come to mind, such as cows and rabbits, depend on microorganisms in their digestive tracts to digest plant cell walls. For example, cows are ruminants; they have a four-part stomach, each part having specific environmental conditions favoring different species of bacteria. In addition, cows chew their cud, that is, they regurgitate food and chew the partly digested plant material with their massive molars, thus breaking open additional plant cells. This material is swallowed and is digested, and eventually undigested food passes out of the colon as feces. Rabbits use coprophagy to digest food. Microorganisms capable of digesting cellulose occur in a portion of the rabbit intestine that follows the portion where nutrients are absorbed. Rabbits recover this digested cellulose by eating their fecal pellets. Even with these elaborate digestive systems, herbivores rarely can digest more than 20 percent of the food they consume.

Animals that eat plants that have died are called *decomposers.* The most common decomposers are bacteria and fungi, but invertebrates such as earthworms, roundworms, and many insects also feed on dead plant material. Of course other animals may feed on these decomposer animals, thus forming the decomposer food chain. In most terrestrial ecosystems, more than 90 percent of all the available plant material passes through the decomposer food chain, or food web. Currently, ecologists know very little about species composition and decomposition pathways in the decomposer component of the ecosystem, as most research has focused on the grazing food web. From an ecosystem perspective, one of the most important results of decomposition is the production of humus, which is nothing more than partly digested plant material. Humus performs a very important role in terrestrial ecosystems. One of its characteristics is that its colloidal particles are negatively charged. In contrast many plant nutrients are positively charged and therefore can be adsorbed to the humus in the soil, a process that keeps nutrients from being leached (removed) from the soil as rainwater percolates through it.

One of the ways that ecologists characterize the energy flow in an ecosystem is to calculate the system's *P*/*R* ratio:

$$P/R = \frac{\text{Total amount of photosynthesis in the ecosystem}}{\text{Total amount of respiration of all organisms in the ecosystem}}.$$

The value of the *P*/*R* ratio can fit into one of three categories that tell ecologists something important about the overall flow of energy in that ecosystem. If *P*/*R* is greater than 1, then the plants are photosynthesizing more energy than is being metabolized in the ecosystem. In this case energy, in the form of organic matter, is accumulating in the ecosystem. A young, actively growing forest is an example of an ecosystem with a *P*/*R* greater than 1. Agricultural plant crops (for example, wheat, corn, sugar cane) all have *P*/*R* ratios greater than 1. These ecosystems are called *autotrophic* systems because plants dominate them.

In the second category *P*/*R* is equal to 1. This ratio indicates an ecosystem that is neither accumulating organic material nor losing it. For example, the *P*/*R* ratio of a mature deciduous forest might be 1.007 (Odum, 1971).

In the final category *P*/*R* is less than 1. In an ecosystem with this ratio the plants are not providing sufficient energy to meet the needs of all of the organisms in the ecosystem. A couple of things may occur as a result. First, the amount of organic matter in the ecosystem may be declining. This could occur in an ecosystem that is suffering from an infectious disease or an outbreak of defoliating insects that is killing the plants in the ecosystem. The other, more common reason for an ecosystem to have a *P*/*R* ratio of less than 1 is that this ratio is a natural or normal feature of that ecosystem. A woodland stream is an example of such a system. Because the stream is underneath the canopy of the forest, little photosynthesis occurs in the stream itself. The heterotrophs living in the stream are therefore dependent not on plants growing in the stream but on the input of organic matter in the form of tree leaves as their energy source. Sewage treatment plants and cities are other examples of this type of ecosystem. These ecosystems are called heterotrophic systems because plants play a less important role and heterotrophs dominate the systems.

Linking a heterotrophic ecosystem to an autotrophic one is called *ecosystem coupling*. For example, white-tailed deer spend the day in forests, ruminating and hiding from predators. However, the forest may have a very low production to respiration ratio, especially near the ground, where deer have to feed. Therefore at night the deer forage in meadows, which have a higher production to respiration ratio. Similarly, cities are dependent on agricultural land for their survival.

Energy Flow Through Populations and Individuals

We can also look at the energy flow in a population within an ecosystem. The general form for looking at energy flow through a heterotrophic population is outlined in Figure 1.4.

If the diagram represents energy flow through an herbivore population, then the available food would be all the living plant material in the ecosystem. Let's imagine that Figure 1.4 is the energy flow diagram for a population of white-tailed deer. Not all of the available plant material can or will be eaten by these herbivores. Some of it, such as tree trunks, is inedible, and other material, such as the canopy, is out of the deer's reach. Of the material that is ingested, a portion is not digested and is excreted as feces and urine. What remains is the energy that is actually assimilated by the organism. In a deer population 98 to 99 percent of all the assimilated energy goes toward metabolism, leaving only 1 to 2 percent for the growth of individuals or reproduction.

Ecologists use the respiration to assimilation ratio (R/A) to categorize organisms. For *endotherms* (species that thermoregulate, like deer and humans), this ratio is typically between 0.98 and 0.99. Although thermoregulation has many advantages, it has a high energy cost. For these species, reproductive rates are relatively low because only 1 to 2 percent of the energy is available for that purpose.

Ectotherms (species that are dependent on their environment for the control of body temperature) on the other hand have a significantly lower R/A, typically in the 0.65 to 0.70 range. These species may have one-third of the energy they assimilate available for reproduction and as a result are capable of explosive population growth. All invertebrates, fishes, and reptiles and amphibians fit into this category.

FIGURE 1.4. ENERGY FLOW THROUGH A HETEROTROPHIC POPULATION.

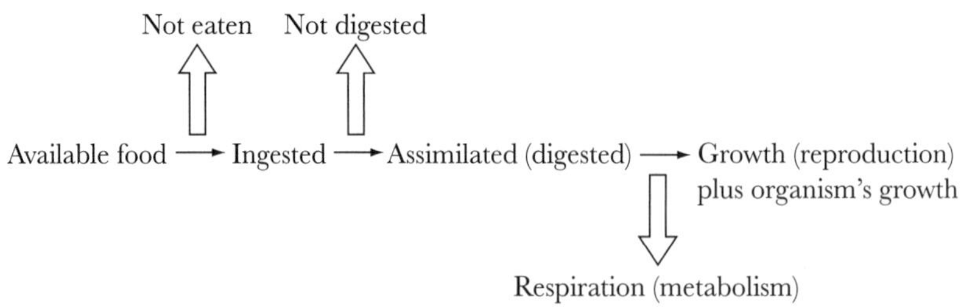

Source: Adapted from Odum, 1983.

Ecologists can use R/A to explore the life history strategy of a species. For example, the immature spittlebug (an insect) has an R/A of 0.98, although a typical insect would have a ratio much lower. What distinguishes spittlebugs from other insects? It turns out that spittlebugs, as their name suggests, produce a mucus-like material that coats the surface of the insect. This coating provides two advantages. First, it decreases the rate of evaporation from the surface and enables the insect to live in drier habitats than it otherwise could. Second, as you might imagine, it provides protection from predators.

There are two particularly important properties of energy flow in ecosystems. First, energy *flows* through the ecosystem; it does not *cycle*. Energy enters the ecosystem as sunlight and eventually it all leaves the system as metabolic energy, which is not a useful form of energy for organisms. This principle is related to the second property of energy flow through an ecosystem: the transfer from one level in the food chain to the next is not 100 percent efficient. Energy is lost, in terms of availability, at each transfer. Both of these principles flow from the laws of thermodynamics and are immutable properties of energy flow through all ecosystems, food chains, and populations.

Humans, Fossil Fuels, and Energy Flow

Humans are the only species on earth that can rely on an energy source other than the sun to power their ecosystems. In the last several decades, fossil fuels have been used to subsidize human ecosystems (see Chapter Fifteen). However, we must not forget that this energy is energy from photosynthesis in autotrophic ecosystems that was stored millions of years ago. In a sense, using fossil fuels is like spending down the capital in your bank account instead of using only the interest (that is, sunlight) from the account. Some common obvious uses of fossil fuels are burning gasoline to power cars and burning coal to produce electricity. However, other common uses of fossil fuels are less obvious. For example, fossil fuels are used in producing the food that we eat. They are needed not only to power the machinery that the farmer drives but also for making fertilizer, processing food, transporting the food to the store, and preparing the food in the home. It may take as much as thirty to forty kilocalories to produce one kilocalorie of food energy. Therefore, although the P/R ratio of an agricultural system may be substantially greater than 1, this value is inflated due to the fossil fuel subsidy used to supplement the sunlight used for photosynthesis in the ecosystem (Odum, 1971).

The Concept of Nutrient Cycles

All nutrients in ecosystems flow from nonliving components of the system (for example, the soil or atmosphere) into living components of the system and then back

FIGURE 1.5. GENERALIZED NUTRIENT CYCLE.

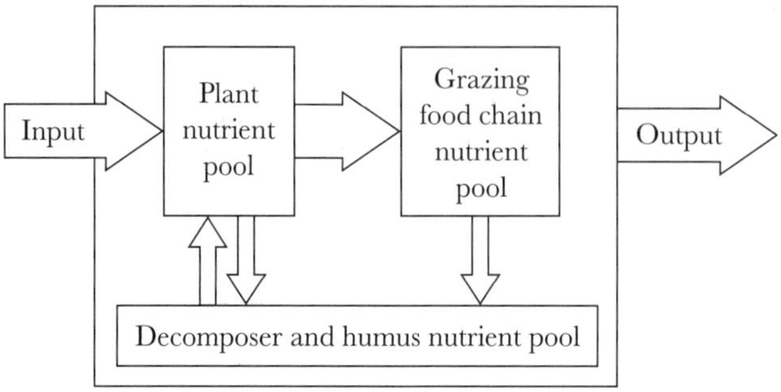

into nonliving components, in what are referred to as *biogeochemical cycles,* or *nutrient cycles.* A generalized nutrient cycle is shown in Figure 1.5. All nutrient cycles can be characterized by their pools (amount of nutrients in a ecosystem component), nutrient flows (the amount of nutrients moving between ecosystem components), and the input to and output from nutrients to the ecosystem. Nutrient cycles tend to be either *open,* with many inputs and outputs, or *closed,* with most of the nutrients used by the system coming from recycling within the system. One of the significant impacts that humans have had on most nutrient cycles is to make them more open.

The Carbon Cycle

Figure 1.6 represents a simplified *carbon cycle.* An important characteristic of the carbon cycle is that it has an atmospheric pool, unlike the phosphorus and sulfur cycles, whose nutrients only truly cycle on a geological time scale. Carbon is a fundamental molecular building block of life and as a result is intimately connected to energy flow. Carbon dioxide is removed from the atmosphere by plants and, with water and with sunlight as an energy source, produces sugars via photosynthesis. This fixed energy then supplies the energy and carbon needs of the rest of the ecosystem. Through other organisms' metabolism, carbon dioxide is released back into the atmosphere. In the past the uptake of carbon dioxide from the atmosphere by plants was balanced with the release of carbon dioxide back into the atmosphere via plant and animal metabolism. However, with our species' increased dependency on fossil fuels for energy, that balance has been upset. When carbon dioxide concentrations in the atmosphere were first measured, in the late 1800s, they were found to be 280 parts per million (ppm) (Houghton and

FIGURE 1.6. SIMPLIFIED CARBON CYCLE.

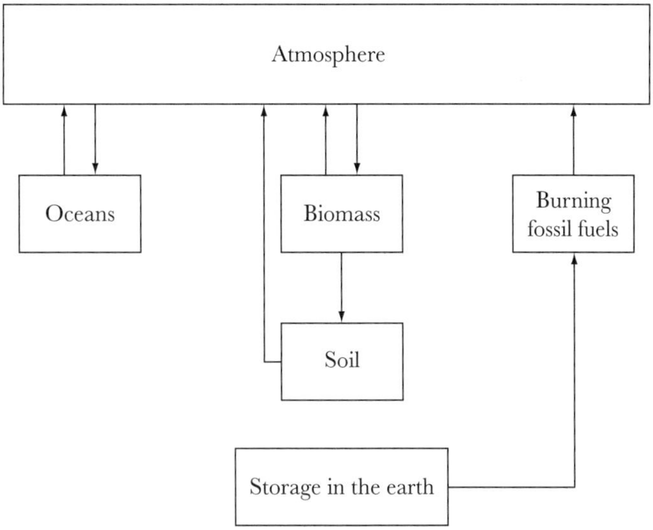

others, 1996). Now the carbon dioxide levels in the atmosphere are close to 380 ppm. Another factor affecting the amount of carbon dioxide in the atmosphere is the clearing of tropical rain forests for agriculture and other human activities. Some estimates suggest that the amount of carbon dioxide released into the atmosphere by the burning of tropical rain forests is equal to the amount released via burning of fossil fuels. In any case humans are having an impact on the carbon dioxide concentration in the atmosphere. Interestingly, the increase in carbon dioxide in the atmosphere is less than predicted when anthropogenic release of carbon dioxide is estimated. Where does the excess carbon dioxide go? Scientists now think that the oceans are an important sinks (that is, storage areas) for carbon dioxide. Without these sinks, concentrations of carbon dioxide in the atmosphere would be much higher.

Why should we worry about the amount of carbon dioxide in the atmosphere? Carbon dioxide accounts for only about 0.03 percent of the atmosphere, whereas oxygen accounts for 20 percent and nitrogen accounts for 79 percent. Why should we worry about a change from 0.028 percent to 0.038 percent? The answer lies in one of the properties of carbon dioxide; it absorbs heat energy that is reradiated from the earth's surface and thus it acts to retain heat in the lower atmosphere. This phenomenon is called the *greenhouse effect.* Since the 1970s, the greenhouse effect has been in the news as scientists have debated the relationship between carbon dioxide increases in the atmosphere and warming at the earth's surface (that is, *global warming,* or global climate change). The consensus among atmospheric scientists now is that we are experiencing global change as a result of the increase in carbon dioxide concentration in the atmosphere. Because we have been collecting temperature data for only a little over 100 years, it has been difficult to show exactly how much temperatures have increased, but reasonable estimates are from one to a few degrees Fahrenheit. Apart from the current increase, however, the greenhouse effect is not a bad thing. Without it the surface of the earth would be at least 70°F cooler, and all of us would be complaining of the cold. But excessive warming may have immense public health consequences, as discussed in Chapter Eleven.

Thus, by changing the way in which carbon cycles, we have affected the earth's energy balance. This illustrates an important principle of ecology: *you can't do just one thing,* or, *everything is connected to everything else.*

The Nitrogen Cycle

Although nitrogen is available in large quantities in the atmosphere (79 percent), large amounts of energy are needed to convert this nitrogen gas into a form that plants can use (Odum, 1971). This conversion process is called *nitrogen fixation,* and it is accomplished primarily by microorganisms in the soil. Many of the species of nitrogen fixers are associated with the roots of plants in a symbiotic relationship. The plant provides sugars to the nitrogen fixers, and the nitrogen fixers in turn provide a useful form of nitrogen to the plant. It takes about ten grams of sugar to convert one gram of nitrogen into a form usable to a plant. Nitrogen fixation also occurs via lightning, but this is a relatively small amount. Figure 1.7 shows the nitrogen cycle.

Since the introduction of inorganic fertilizers, human fixation of nitrogen, using processes requiring fossil fuels, has equaled all other types of nitrogen fixation. The Haber-Bosch process, invented in 1914, has led to a dramatic increase in the use of fertilizer. This reaction is carried out at pressures ranging from 200 to 400 atmospheres and at temperatures ranging from 400°C to 650°C (750°F to 1200°F). Estimates are that 1 percent of all energy use worldwide goes to producing fertilizer in this fashion.

Due to the energy costs of producing usable nitrogen, once nitrogen enters an ecosystem, keeping it from being lost back to the atmosphere or to the groundwater has important ecological consequences. Most terrestrial ecosystem nitrogen cycles are closed cycles. This is due primarily to the form in which nitrogen occurs in the soil. The primary decomposition pathway produces positively charged

FIGURE 1.7. GENERALIZED NITROGEN CYCLE.

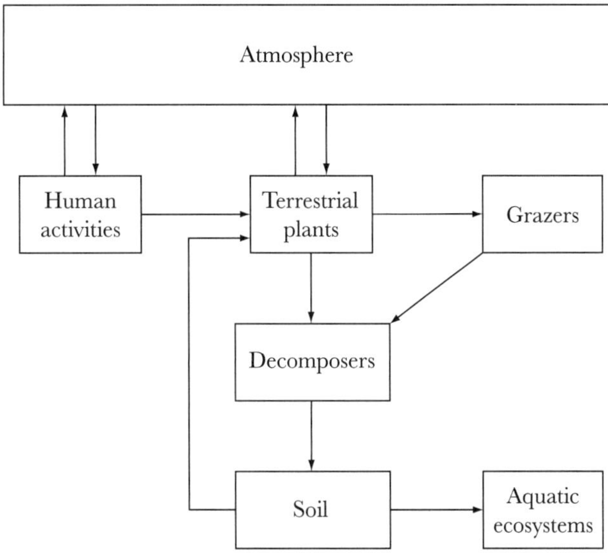

ammoniacal nitrogen. This form of nitrogen can be adsorbed to the negatively charged soil organic matter. If this nitrogen is converted to nitrate nitrogen, which is negatively charged, it will be leached from the soil when water percolates through the soil. In an experimental clear cut of a forest at Hubbard Brook, New Hampshire, researchers showed that loss of the plants from this ecosystem had a dramatic impact on the nitrogen cycle. Prior to clear cutting, nitrogen was accumulating in the system (that is, a closed cycle existed) and the form found in the soil was primarily ammoniacal nitrogen. After clear cutting, the system lost large quantities of nitrogen (that is, it became an open cycle), and the main form of nitrogen being lost was nitrate nitrogen. These researchers hypothesized that the plants may have been inhibiting the microorganisms that convert ammoniacal nitrogen to nitrate nitrogen to obtain energy (Aber and others, 2002).

Humans have also disrupted the nitrogen cycle by using inorganic nitrogen fertilizer on agricultural crops. Not only have we tremendously increased the amount of nitrogen that is fixed, but we also have affected the amount of nitrogen present in water running off the agricultural fields. Nitrate concentrations in the runoff may be higher than the standard for drinking water (10 ppm). Excess nitrate in drinking water may cause methemoglobinemia, or blue baby syndrome, which may be fatal (Criss and Davisson, 2004).

Ecosystem Services

Ecological systems perform essential functions for humans. They may produce ecosystem goods (for example, food) or ecosystem services (for example, nutrient recycling). Recently, economists and ecologists (Costanza and others, 1997) have attempted to place a dollar value on these goods and services (sometimes collectively referred to as services) that represent the benefits received by humans from ecosystem functions. Many of these services are outside the traditional capital economy. Examples of services provided by aquatic ecosystems include wetlands that transform nutrients and energy into valuable outputs like fish and shellfish; floodplains along rivers that provide flood protection, pollution abatement, and recreation; and mountain watersheds that provide hiking opportunities and recreation. The Catskill/Delaware watershed provides 90 percent of the drinking water for New York City. In the mid-1960s, the city had a choice between building a new water filtration plant at a cost of up to $6 billion dollars and protecting the watershed at a cost of $1 to 1.5 billion dollars. Water managers decided to protect the watershed instead of constructing a new water plant (Heal and others, 2004). Another essential ecosystem service is the supplying of medicinal products (Daily and others, 1997). Eighty percent of the world's population relies on natural products for medicine. In fact, of the top 150 prescription drugs used in the United States, 118 originate from natural sources.

Estimating the values of such ecosystem services is difficult and fraught with potential errors; however, Costanza and others (1997) used a conservative approach that assigns a minimum estimate to service value. Table 1.1 lists the major

TABLE 1.1. ESTIMATES OF THE VALUE OF VARIOUS ECOSYSTEM SERVICES.

Ecosystem Service	Value (in trillions of dollars)
Soil formation	$17.1
Recreation	3.0
Nutrient cycling	2.3
Water regulation and supply	2.3
Climate regulation	2.3
Habitat	1.4
Flood and storm protection	1.1
Genetic resources	0.8
Atmosphere gas balance	0.7
Pollination	0.4
All other services	1.6
Total value of ecosystem services	33.3

Source: Adapted from Costanza and others, 1997.

ecosystem service categories for which Costanza and colleagues estimated the value. Their estimate of the total annual value of the services provided is over $33 trillion dollars, which is 1.8 times the annual global gross national product (GNP). Topping the list is the formation of soil necessary for agricultural production, at $17.1 trillion. Without the continual recycling of nutrients, producing food for the world's population would be impossible. More difficult to estimate, but equally important for agriculture, is the value of pollination of plants. Over 100,000 animal species, including bats, bees, flies, and birds pollinate plants and one third of all human food derives from plants pollinated by wild pollinators (Daily and others, 1997). It is difficult to imagine substituting human pollination of these plants.

Another way of valuing ecological systems is to look at the proportion of the earth's energy flow that goes directly to humans (Vitousek, Mooney, Lubchenco, and Melillo, 1997). From 10 to 15 percent of the earth's land surface area is dominated by agriculture and urban development. Another 6 to 8 percent is used as pastureland. It is estimated that over 40 percent of the earth's land surface has been transformed by humans and that over 50 percent of all available freshwater is used by humans. Between 40 and 50 percent of all terrestrial biological production is used by humans. On a more subtle level, 100 percent of the earth has been influenced by humans via the burning of fossil fuels and the related increase in the carbon dioxide concentration in the atmosphere. As Bill McKibben (1989) eloquently discussed in *The End of Nature*, there are no longer any ecosystems on earth that are not influenced by humans.

Ecological Footprints

If McKibben's assertion is correct, then how do we estimate the total impact of humans on the earth? Wackernagel and Rees (1996) developed the *ecological footprint* concept to do just that. It provides a way of translating the energy and matter used by humans into the land or water area necessary to support those flows. It estimates the amount of productive land necessary for the resource consumption and waste assimilation of a human population. The ecological footprint reinforces the notion that humans are dependent on nature. Because the total land surface area of the earth is fixed, this may be a way to calculate the carrying capacity of the earth for humans. Currently, there are approximately four acres of productive land available for every person. However, this figure does not include land for other species.

For each category of resource use, Wackernagel and Rees maintain that we need to determine the amount of land area necessary to sustainably produce that resource or energy. In considering the gasoline (the fossil fuel energy) we use in our cars, for example, we would either estimate the amount of land necessary to store the carbon dioxide released by burning that gas or the amount of land necessary to produce the ethanol equivalent of that gas. The categories that Wackernagel and Rees use in their analysis are food production, housing (both operation and construction), transportation (for ourselves and for goods), consumer goods, and services such as health care and social services. They estimate that the average North American requires ten to twelve acres a year to produce the resources and energy he or she consumes. If all the world's population were to have a North American lifestyle, we would need at least three earths to produce the necessary resources. In light of this analysis the North American lifestyle is not sustainable. In large part this overshooting of our planet's carrying capacity is a result of our dependence on fossil fuels, a resource we are using faster than it is being produced.

Ecological footprint analysis can be used to explore ways that we could reduce our impact on the earth and bring into balance our resource use and the land available to produce those resources.

Thought Questions

1. Calculate your ecological footprint, taking into account what you eat, how you travel, and how you use energy.
2. Explain at least three ways in which degradation of the ecosystem could threaten human health.
3. What is the Gaia hypothesis? Is it consistent with ecological principles? Is it informative with regard to human health?
4. Explain the concept of ecosystem services and what these services have to do with human health.

References

Aber, J. D., and Melillo, J. M. *Terrestrial Ecosystems.* (2nd ed.) San Diego: Harcourt Academic Press, 2001.

Aber, J. D., and others. "Inorganic Nitrogen Losses from a Forested Ecosystem in Response to Physical, Chemical, Biotic and Climatic Perturbations." *Ecosystems,* 2002, *5*(7), 648–658.

Bush, M. B. *Ecology of a Changing Planet.* Upper Saddle River, N.J.: Prentice Hall, 2000.

Carrying Capacity Network. "Doubling Time." [http://www.carryingcapacity.org/doubling.html]. 2004.

Chapin, F. S., III, Matson, P. A., and Mooney, H. A. *Principles of Terrestrial Ecology.* New York: Springer, 2002.

Costanza, R., and others. "The Value of the World's Ecosystem Services and Natural Capital." *Nature,* 1997, *387,* 253–260.

Criss, R. E., and Davisson, M. L. "Fertilizers, Water Quality, and Human Health." *Environmental Health Perspectives,* 2004, *112,* A536.

Daily, G. C., and others. *Ecosystem Services: Benefits Supplied to Human Societies by Natural Ecosystems.* Issues in Ecology, no. 2. Washington, D.C.: Ecological Society of America, 1997.

Golley, F. B. *A History of the Ecosystem Concept in Ecology.* New Haven, Conn.: Yale University Press, 1993.

Heal, G. M., and others. *Valuing Ecosystem Services.* Washington, D.C.: National Academy of Sciences, 2004.

Houghton, J., and others (eds.). *Climate Change 1995: The Science of Climate Change.* Contribution of Working Group I to the Second Assessment Report of the Intergovernmental Panel on Climate Change. New York: Cambridge University Press, 1996.

Knutson, R. M. *Furtive Fauna.* New York: Penguin Books, 1992.

Krohne, D. T. *General Ecology.* Belmont, Calif.: Wadsworth, 1998.

McKibben, B. *The End of Nature.* New York: Anchor Books, 1989.

Meyer, P. S., Yung, J. W., and Ausubel, J. H. "A Primer on Logistic Growth and Substitution: The Mathematics of the Loglet Lab Software." *Technological Forecasting and Social Change,* 1999, *61*(3), 247–271.

Odum, E. P. *Fundamentals of Ecology.* (3rd ed.) Philadelphia: Saunders, 1971.

Odum, E. P. *Basic Ecology.* Philadelphia: Saunders, 1983.

Pianka, E. R. *Evolutionary Ecology.* (6th ed.) San Francisco: Cummings, 2000.

Smith, R. L., and Smith, T. M. *Elements of Ecology.* (5th ed.) San Francisco: Cummings, 2003.

Storey, K. B., and Storey J. M. "Frozen Alive." *Scientific American,* 1990, *263,* 92–97.

Tansley, A. G. "The Use and the Abuse of Vegetational Concepts and Terms." *Ecology,* 1935, *16,* 284–307.

Vitousek, P. M., Mooney, H. A., Lubchenco, J., and Melillo, J. M. "Human Domination of Earth's Ecosystems." *Science,* 1997, *227,* 494–499.

Wackernagel, M., and Rees, W. *Our Ecological Footprint: Reducing Human Impact on the Earth.* Gabriola Island, B.C.: New Society, 1996.

World Resources Institute. "EarthTrends Data Tables: Energy and Resources." *Energy,* 2004. [http://earthtrends.wri.org/pdf_library/data_tables/eng1_2003.pdf].

For Further Information

Aber, J. D., and Melillo, J. M. *Terrestrial Ecosystems.* (2nd ed.) New York: Harcourt Press, 2001.

Chambers, N., Simmons, C., and Wackernagel, M. *Sharing Nature's Interest: Ecological Footprints as an Indicator of Sustainability.* London: Earthscan, 2000.

Golley, F. B. *A Primer for Environmental Literacy.* New Haven, Conn.: Yale University Press, 1998.

Odum, E. P . *Ecological Vignettes: Ecological Approaches to Dealing with Human Predicaments.* Amsterdam: Harcourt Academic Publishers, 1998.

Pimentel, D. *Food, Energy. and Society.* Boulder: University of Colorado Press, 1966.

Smith, R. L., and Smith, T. M. *Elements of Ecology.* (5th ed.) San Fancisco: Cummings, 2003.

CHAPTER TWO

TOXICOLOGY

Jason R. Richardson
Gary W. Miller

Toxicology is the study of the adverse effects of chemicals on biological systems. These adverse effects can range from mild skin irritation to liver damage, congenital anomalies, or even death. The chemicals that are studied come from natural as well as industrial sources. The breadth of topics in toxicology requires the field to take an interdisciplinary approach, borrowing techniques and methods from numerous scientific fields (Figure 2.1). The term *biological system* can be broadly defined, and so a toxicologist might study the effects of pesticides on insect physiology, herbicides on plant development, or antibiotics on bacterial growth; however, most work in the field of toxicology is focused on human health. This chapter focuses on the toxicological effects of environmental agents on human health, such as the deleterious effects of chlorine gas on pulmonary function, environmental estrogens on reproductive function, and chemical weapons or pesticides on neuronal function.

Typically, a toxicologist has earned a PhD degree in toxicology or a related field (such as biochemistry, pharmacology, or environmental health) and has received additional training in laboratory science during postdoctoral fellowships. Toxicologists are employed in academia, industry, and government positions. Academic toxicologists perform basic research on the adverse effects of chemicals, train the next generation of toxicologists, and teach toxicology to public health, medical, pharmacy, and veterinary students. Toxicologists in pharmaceutical companies seek to identify adverse effects of new drugs before these drugs move into clinical trials, and they may suggest ways these drugs can be modified to minimize toxicity. A toxicologist at an

FIGURE 2.1. INTERDISCIPLINARY NATURE OF TOXICOLOGY.

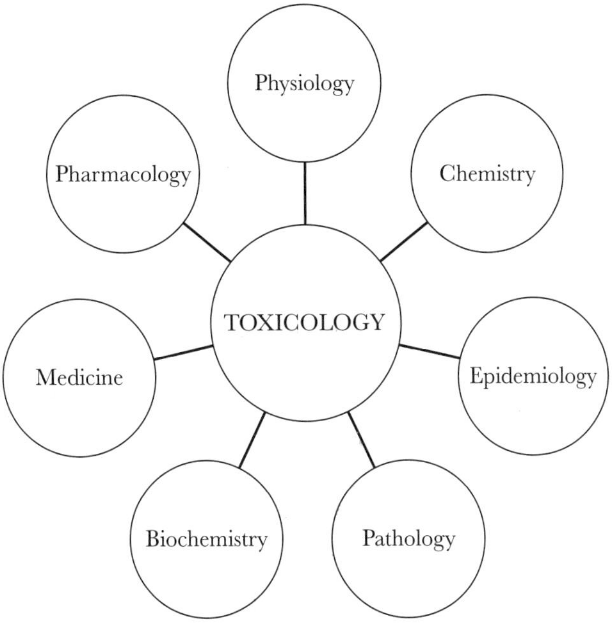

Toxicology borrows from several disciplines to characterize the adverse effects of chemicals.

agricultural company may work to develop safer and more effective pesticides. On the government side, toxicologists at the Food and Drug Administration, the Environmental Protection Agency, and the Centers for Disease Control and Prevention ensure that companies are following federal regulations, determine the relative safety of drugs or chemicals, provide resources to the general public regarding toxic exposures, and advise the government on policy decisions regarding industrial products.

A conceptual starting point for toxicology is that all substances have the potential to be toxic. Paracelsus, the father of toxicology, was the first to articulate this concept (Box 2.1).

Box 2.1. "The Dose Makes the Poison"—Paracelsus

Philippus Aureolus Theophrastus Bombastus von Hohenheim (1493–1541; his friends called him Paracelsus) was a respected physician of his day. He stated, "Alle Ding sind Gift und nichts ohn Gift; alein die Dosis macht das ein Ding kein Gift ist" (All things are poison and not without poison; only the dose makes a thing not a poison). This may be paraphrased as, All substances are toxic; the dose differentiates a remedy from a poison, or even more simply, The dose makes the poison.

Although poisons such as strychnine, cyanide, or nerve gas come readily to mind, every compound can cause toxicity. Of course all compounds are not equally toxic; some have effects at minuscule doses and others require very high doses. On the one hand, table salt (sodium chloride) used in moderation is fine in the human diet, but consuming half a cup of salt a day would eventually cause significant electrolyte and kidney problems and possibly death (Box 2.2). On the other hand, ingestion of a small amount of potassium cyanide (one gram) can kill a human. It is the job of the toxicologist to determine the relative toxicity of various compounds. This toxicity information, when combined with information about the potential benefits of a compound, permits us to decide whether a compound is acceptable for a particular use and what doses (for a medication) or exposures (for other chemicals) would be permissible. For example, the general public (and regulatory agencies) would not tolerate a cold remedy that caused mild liver or kidney damage in 10 percent of users or a food additive that caused cancer in 1 in 1,000 consumers. However, if a new chemotherapeutic agent cured cancer in 80 percent of the cases, some mild liver or kidney damage might be tolerated. Toxicology helps characterize the adverse effects that form part of the risk-benefit balance for a given chemical.

Box 2.2. LD_{50} for Various Compounds

The LD_{50}, or lethal dose for 50 percent, is the dose of a chemical that kills 50 percent of those exposed to it. A low LD_{50} for a chemical indicates that compared to other compounds less of this chemical is needed to cause toxicity—that it is more potent, or in common terms, that it is more poisonous. Here, for example, are the LD_{50}s for several chemicals, expressed in terms of dose per kilogram of body weight.

Glyphosate (Roundup)	5,600 mg/kg
Table salt (sodium chloride)	2,400 mg/kg
Pseudoephedrine	660 mg/kg
Acetaminophen (Tylenol)	500 mg/kg
Chlorpyrifos (Dursban)	18 mg/kg
Sodium cyanide	10 mg/kg
VX nerve gas	1 mg/kg
Sea anemone toxin	0.001 mg/kg

How Does Toxicology Fit into Environmental Public Health?

Toxicology is an essential part of environmental health and of public health more generally. Public health professionals manage resources necessary to maintain health, prevent disease, and treat illnesses. A chemical or other environmental contaminant that harms humans at levels found in the environment raises obvious public health concern.

The field of toxicology helps determine the conditions under which a given compound may cause adverse effects. It is important for public health professionals to understand key concepts that toxicologists use to make these determinations. Once exposure has occurred, through what routes does the compound enter the body? How much of the compound enters? Where in the body does it go? What does it do once it reaches a particular organ? What physiological effects follow, and if appropriate, what forms of treatment exist? How does the body handle the compound? Is it stored in particular organs, and is it metabolized and cleared? Armed with the scientific principles of toxicology, the public health professional can make prudent decisions on how to manage a particular exposure.

Decades ago many compounds could be detected only at relatively high concentrations—say, in parts per million. Today's detection systems, such as gas and liquid chromatography, mass spectrometry, and atomic absorption spectrometry, are up to a million times more sensitive. As a result, dangerous chemicals are now often detected in environmental samples; however, they usually occur at very low levels. It is essential to remember that the dose, and not the mere presence of a toxicant in a sample, makes the poison. If it takes a concentration of 10 parts per billion of a particular compound to cause any toxicity and if that compound is detected at 1 part per trillion, it is very unlikely to cause an adverse effect. Thus one of the most important questions to be asked is, How much of the compound is in the environment? As described in Chapter Four, this is the domain of an exposure assessment professional, often working in conjunction with a toxicologist or chemist.

Toxicology is integrated into public health practice in several ways. For example, in providing safe drinking water to a community, it is important to understand both the adverse effects of organisms found in the water and the adverse effects of chemicals used to kill the organisms. As discussed in Chapter Eighteen, chlorination is an effective means of reducing microbiological contamination in water, but it can result in the presence of chlorinated organic compounds known as disinfection byproducts. Toxicology can help in identifying these compounds, assessing the risk they pose, and balancing that risk against the risk of microbiological contaminants.

Another reason that a student in any discipline, especially environmental health, should develop an appreciation for toxicology is that it is highly relevant to one's own health. We are exposed to a myriad of chemicals every day. We ingest chemical residues in the food we eat, and we inhale particles in the air we breathe. Many people voluntarily ingest pharmaceutical and recreational drugs with little or no knowledge of the potential adverse effects. An understanding of toxicology can clarify some of these issues and help us make healthy choices. For example, a student who has a basic understanding of toxicology will realize that a claim that a product—whether a vitamin, an herbal supplement, an agricultural chemical, a medication, or an illegal drug—has no side effects is erroneous and misleading. Virtually no agent is completely free of adverse effects, given sufficient doses and circumstances. Similarly, a student who thinks in terms of toxicological action will realize that *natural* is not the same as *safe*. Nature produces some highly toxic compounds, such as arsenic, some snake venoms, and the carcinogenic toxins produced by some molds. Natural is not necessarily better.

How Are Toxicants Classified?

There are three major ways to categorize toxic compounds: by chemical class, by source of exposure, and by the effects on human health (Table 2.1). Each helps in understanding toxicology.

TABLE 2.1. EXAMPLES OF TOXIC COMPOUNDS IN THREE CLASSIFICATIONS.

Chemistry	Alcohols Solvents Heavy metals Oxidants Acids
Source	Industrial wastes Agricultural chemicals Waterborne toxicants Air pollutants Food additives
Organ system	Kidney (nephrotoxins) Liver (hepatotoxins) Heart (cardiotoxins) Nervous system (neurotoxins) DNA (mutagens, carcinogens)

Chemical Class

Examples of chemical classes are heavy metals, alcohols, and solvents. In essence the rules of chemistry create the classes, based on such features as functional groups, the presence of metallic elements, and physical properties such as vapor pressure. Classification may also address physical state, that is, whether a toxicant exists as a liquid, solid, gas, vapor, dust, or fume.

Source of Exposure

The second system of categorization is functional and is based on the source of exposure. Examples are industrial pollutants, waterborne toxicants, air pollutants, and pesticides (Box 2.3). These categories are useful in identifying the source of a problem and are commonly used by environmental health professionals. However, chemicals used in similar ways may vary greatly in their mechanism of toxicity. Because this categorization system groups chemicals with little in common, together, it makes it difficult for users to see connections based on molecular structure. To the toxicologist this system ignores the biological mechanisms that underlie toxicity.

Box 2.3. A Rail Crash That Released Chlorine Gas

On January 6, 2004, a train hauling forty-two cars, three of which were tankers filled with chlorine gas, collided with a locomotive with two cars parked on a side track near a mill in Graniteville, South Carolina. The crash derailed sixteen cars, including the three chlorine tankers. Fortunately, only one of the chlorine tankers was damaged, but it sustained a four-inch hole in its side. A cloud of chlorine gas spread throughout the area, exposing hundreds of people in the following hours.

Chlorine is a yellow-greenish gas with intermediate water solubility. Chlorine gas can combine with water to form hydrochloric acid and hypochlorous acid:

$$Cl_2 + H_2O \rightarrow HCl + HOCl$$

Thus, when chlorine gas is inhaled, it can react with the moisture in a person's eyes, mouth, and airways to form corrosive acids. The initial symptoms include irritation and pain of the conjunctivae of the eye and the mucosal lining of the nose, pharynx, larynx, trachea, and bronchi. The irritation of the airway mucosa leads to local edema. When the reaction is severe, pulmonary edema can occur, with the lungs filling with fluid, impairing breathing. This is precisely what was seen in the people exposed in Graniteville. Those exposed to low levels of the gas complained of eye and throat irritation, and those closer to the accident scene had significant breathing difficulties.

Fortunately, local and federal response teams had information on how to deal with the chlorine release. Much of our knowledge of the toxicological consequences of chlorine gas has, sadly, come from dramatic human suffering. During World War I, at Ypres, the German army used chlorine gas (and a related chemical, phosgene) as a chemical weapon to kill over 40,000 soldiers. Chlorine gas is heavier than air, so it settled into the trenches. The soldiers trapped there died of massive pulmonary edema. Since then, there have been several industrial incidents in which storage tanks or railcars have released significant quantities of chlorine gas.

The response included several components. A hazardous materials (HAZMAT) team, wearing suitable protective equipment, was able to patch the leak before all the chlorine escaped. The exposed area was cleared, and chlorine levels were monitored until the gas had dissipated. Affected individuals were taken to medical facilities where they were clinically evaluated with physical examinations, chest X-rays, and pulmonary function testing, and treated when necessary with such interventions as supplemental oxygen and bronchodilators. Clinical follow-up monitored them for the presence of persistent respiratory problems, including a condition called reactive airways dysfunction syndrome, which can follow acute irritant inhalation exposures.

From a historical perspective the incident at Graniteville stands out as one of the worst chlorine gas releases in the United States. Over 5,000 people were evacuated, 250 people were injured, and 9 people died. Those who were injured may continue to have breathing difficulties for years. This incident illustrates the acute toxicity of irritating inhaled materials and how they may occur both in the workplace and the general environment. It also illustrates the trade-offs inherent in environmental health; although chlorine gas is highly toxic, chlorine has an important public health role in water purification (see Chapter Eighteen).

Target Organ

The last system of categorization is based on the organ system where the toxic effects are most pronounced. For example, toxins that damage the liver are referred to as *hepatotoxins* and those that target the kidney are called *nephrotoxins.* Compounds that damage the nervous system, whether peripheral or central, are *neurotoxins.* Chemicals that disrupt DNA structure or function are classed as genetic *toxicants, mutagens,* or *carcinogens,* depending on their specific effects. Other organ systems that can be the targets of toxicity include the respiratory system, cardiovascular system, skin, reproductive system, endocrine system (Box 2.4), immune system, and blood. Fetal development is more a process than an organ system, but it too is often viewed as a target of toxic exposures.

Box 2.4. Endocrine Disruptors

Recently, toxicologists' attention has focused on the observation that chemicals in the environment may act in a manner analogous to that of endogenous hormones in wildlife and humans. One group of potential *endocrine disrupters* is a group of chemicals thought to mimic endogenous estrogen and termed *environmental estrogens* or *xenoestrogens.* Estrogen is the predominant female reproductive hormone. It exerts its physiological actions by binding to nuclear receptors and activating gene transcription in target tissues such as the breast, uterus, and brain. Environmental estrogens may disrupt normal estrogen function by binding to these same receptors and eliciting a similar, although usually smaller, response than the endogenous hormone or by blocking normal estrogen binding to these receptors. Chemicals that may act this way include the pesticide DDT, polychlorinated biphenyls (PCBs), and bis-phenol A. Evidence of this phenomenon in the environment includes observations of feminized male fish downstream from pulp mills, associated with high concentrations of chlorophenolic compounds produced during the pulp bleaching process, and male feminization and reproductive failure among alligators in Lake Apopka, Florida, associated with elevated levels of DDT and its metabolite DDE following a pesticide spill. There is some evidence linking human trends, such as menarche at younger ages and declining sperm counts, with environmental estrogens, although this finding remains controversial.

In addition to man-made chemicals that may act as estrogen mimics, there are also naturally occurring estrogen mimics, such as the isoflavones that are synthesized by plants as a defense against pathogens and herbivores. Indeed, high levels of isoflavones in clover have been linked to the infertility in sheep termed *clover disease.* High levels of isoflavones have also been found in soy milk. Excretion of natural hormones, the use of estrogen-containing pharmaceuticals, and the use of veterinary medication may also contribute to the levels of estrogens in the environment.

Estrogens are not the only hormones whose action may be disrupted by environmental chemicals. Potential antiandrogens include phthalates, vinclozolin, and DDE; these may interfere with androgen-mediated events such as formation of the male genitalia during embryogenesis. In addition, various chemicals are known to interfere with thyroid function; these may be especially important to intrauterine development of the nervous system.

(For further information, see Baccarelli, Pesatori, and Bertazzi, 2000; Cheek and others, 1998; Choi, Yoo, and Lee, 2004; Fox, 2004; Golden and others, 1998; Safe and others, 2001; Sonnenschein and Soto, 1998; Zoeller and others, 2002.)

Organ system classification is favored by most toxicologists. When considering human health, one needs to consider how a chemical will affect a particular physiological function, whether it be blood pressure, respiration, memory, or urine production. Because each of these functions is controlled by a particular organ system (or systems), organ system classification provides a logical framework for toxicologists, who often specialize in the actions of compounds on a specific organ system. Also, although compounds that affect a specific system may differ in their chemical composition, they often share features that lead them to target that system. For example, hepatotoxic compounds often share features that lead them to target the liver. A public health professional should not be satisfied with knowing that a particular substance is toxic, but should ask, What does it do to the body? What system is it disrupting? What are the expected effects? Because symptoms (discomfort felt by a patient) and physiological dysfunction derive from disruption of an organ system, this is where the organ system approach is especially helpful.

To evaluate the toxic effects on a particular organ system, one needs a general understanding of how that system works. For example, the main function of the kidneys is to maintain fluid and electrolyte homeostasis in the body. This is accomplished by the reabsorption of filtered material from the blood, including water, ions, and nutrients, and by the excretion of waste material. The kidneys receive a disproportionate amount of the body's blood flow, approximately 20 percent of cardiac output, considering that they represent less than 1 percent of the total body weight. This high blood flow, in combination with the numerous transport mechanisms within the kidney, renders the kidneys exquisitely sensitive to damage by blood-borne toxicants. Of all the cell types in the kidney, one of the most common targets of toxicant-induced injury is the proximal tubule. The renal proximal tubule is divided into three morphologically distinct segments, designated S1, S2, and S3. S1 is characterized by a thick brush border and high rates of metabolism and transport. S2 contains fewer mitochondria than S1 and has a less developed brush border. S3 contains sparse amounts of mitochondria and the brush border is shorter than that of S2 in most species. The proximal tubule reabsorbs 99 percent of the glomerular filtrate. The numerous transport mechanisms in the proximal tubule allow reabsorption of amino acids, sugars, proteins, bicarbonate, sodium, potassium, chloride, phosphate, and other solutes. Damage to the proximal tubules by toxicant exposure can lead to deterioration of renal function and ultimately renal failure. Exposure to mercury, for example, is known to damage S3 segments of the proximal tubule. Enzymes involved in S3 brush border functions may slough off into the urine, providing a biomarker of the type of injury. A toxicologist interested in identifying how mercury alters renal function would isolate proximal tubules in the laboratory and perform toxicity tests on these isolated cellular sections. Another approach would be to study animals, evaluating renal function from urine clearance studies and postmortem examination.

How is it that a compound can selectively target a particular cell type in a particular organ and in a particular species? Specificity of action is a central theme in toxicology.

What Is Toxicological Specificity?

The most dramatic differences in specificity are found between species. Glyphosate (Roundup) is used to kill unwanted or nuisance vegetation (for example, grass in sidewalk cracks). This compound was specifically designed to inhibit 5-enolpyruvylshikimate-3-phosphate synthase, an enzyme involved in a biochemical pathway (the *shikimate* pathway) for the production of the aromatic amino acids. This pathway is essential for plant function, and when it is blocked, the plant dies. Animals, in contrast, rely on their diet for aromatic amino acids; they therefore do not have the molecular target of glyphosate and do not exhibit toxicity until extremely high exposures occur.

A different example is the piscicide rotenone, which is used to kill unwanted fish. Rotenone targets mitochondrial function, perhaps by disabling complex I of the mitochondrial electron transfer chain (ETC). It exerts this action in humans just as it does in fish. Thus, unlike glyphosate, rotenone is not species specific. Species specificity therefore relates closely to the mechanism of toxic action.

Another kind of specificity is target organ specificity, as mentioned earlier and discussed further later in this chapter.

What Happens After Exposure to a Toxicant?

After exposure to a *xenobiotic* (a chemical foreign to the body), a sequence of steps ensues that determines the response to the chemical: absorption into the body, distribution throughout the body, metabolism, and excretion. Along the way, toxic effects may occur. Understanding the risks of a chemical exposure and how to reduce these risks requires understanding *toxicokinetics,* that is, the processes in this toxicological sequence.

Absorption

Once a person has come in contact with a toxic compound, that compound may gain access to the body. It is not enough for this compound to contact the skin, be inhaled into the lungs, or enter the intestinal track; it must actually traverse the biological barrier. Each of these pathways exhibits characteristics that affect absorption.

The *gastrointestinal system* is designed for nutrient absorption, and it has a large surface area with numerous transport mechanisms. Unfortunately, many toxicants can take advantage of this system to enter the body. Toxicants can also be absorbed through the *pulmonary alveoli.* The alveoli are the functional units of the lung and the sites of gas exchange between the air and the blood supply. Alveoli allow diffusion of most water-soluble compounds. In addition, water-soluble compounds dissolve in the mucous lining in the airways, and may be absorbed from there. Lipid-soluble (fat-soluble) gases can also cross into the bloodstream in the alveoli. Large particles and aerosol droplets may be deposited in the upper part of the lungs, where cilia attempt to excrete them. Smaller particles and aerosols penetrate more deeply, reaching the alveoli where absorption is very efficient. The *skin* represents a third key route of toxicant exposure. Many occupational exposures occur via this route. Although intact skin provides an effective barrier against water-soluble toxicants, fat-soluble toxicants can readily penetrate the skin and enter the bloodstream.

Distribution

Once in the bloodstream a toxicant can be distributed throughout the body. If the toxicant is lipid soluble, it is often carried through the aqueous environment of the bloodstream in association with blood proteins such as albumin. Toxicants generally follow the laws of diffusion, moving from areas of high concentration to areas of low concentration. Chemicals absorbed in the intestine are shunted to the liver through the portal vein, in a process termed *first-pass,* and may undergo metabolism promptly. A limited number of chemicals may be excreted unchanged by the kidneys or into bile.

Metabolism

Most toxicants undergo a metabolic conversion or *biotransformation,* a process mediated by enzymes. The majority of biotransformations occur in the liver, which is rich in metabolic enzymes. However, nearly all cells in the body have some capacity for metabolizing xenobiotics. In general, metabolic transformations lead to products that are more polar and less fat soluble. The metabolic product is therefore more soluble in urine, which facilitates its excretion. For example, benzene is oxidized to phenol, and glutathione combines with halogenated aromatics to form nontoxic and more polar mercapturic acid metabolites. However, metabolic transformations sometimes yield increasingly toxic products. One example is the oxidation of methanol (a relatively nontoxic compound in its native form) to formaldehyde (a compound that is quite toxic, especially to the optic nerve).

The idea that metabolism may increase the toxicity of a compound is well established in the field of carcinogenesis (Box 2.5). Vinyl chloride, known to cause liver and other tumors, is oxidized to a reactive epoxide intermediate, which is actually the proximate carcinogen. Similar transformations probably occur with trichloroethylene, vinylidene chloride, vinyl benzene, and chlorobutadiene. In fact a major mechanism of carcinogenicity in aromatic compounds is conversion to reactive epoxides, which in turn combine with cellular nucleophiles, like DNA and RNA.

Box 2.5. Chemical Carcinogenesis

Cancer resulting from chemical exposure has been known for hundreds of years. Cancer is pathologically defined as uncontrolled cell growth, reflecting alterations in the cell's genome or gene expression (or in both). Chemically induced carcinogenesis is thought to proceed in stages. The first stage is termed *initiation* and is associated with an irreversible change in cell genotype or phenotype. At this time the cell either moves to the next stage in the process or is destroyed, typically through programmed cell death. In the initiation stage the chemical carcinogen may act through a genotoxic mechanism and directly damage DNA. However, chemical carcinogens may not directly damage DNA but rather may alter signal transduction pathways, resulting in altered phenotype. Chemicals that act in this manner are termed epigenetic. The second stage is *promotion* and involves factors that facilitate cell growth and replication, such as dietary and hormonal factors. Promotion is not required for all chemical carcinogens and, unlike initiation, it is reversible. An example of a promoting agent is the hormone estrogen, which activates gene expression pathways in target organs such as the breast and thereby promotes tumor growth. Another example of a promoter is any chemical that inhibits the programmed cell death that would normally terminate an initiated cell. The third stage is *progression.* Progression is irreversible and involves morphological alterations in the genomic structure and growth of altered cells. The final stage is *metastasis,* in which the affected cell population spreads from its immediate microenvironment to invade other tissues.

Many of the known environmental chemical carcinogens must be bioactivated in order to exert their damaging effects. An example is benzo(a)pyrene, which must be converted to its epoxide metabolite in order to damage DNA. Other chemical carcinogens include metals (such as arsenic, chromium, and nickel), minerals (such as asbestos), aliphatic compounds (such as formaldehyde and vinyl chloride), and aromatic compounds (such as coke oven emissions and naphthylamines).

Although many chemicals have the potential to induce cancer, a number of defense mechanisms can mitigate cell damage. Many enzyme systems can detoxify reactive toxicants before they can interact with their target molecules. DNA repair mechanisms can often repair damage caused by toxicants. If DNA is not repaired, the cell may undergo programmed cell death before the altered DNA can be replicated. Finally, the immune system can seek out and destroy transformed cells that have escaped the other mechanisms of defense.

Classically, metabolic transformations are divided into four categories: oxidation, reduction, hydrolysis, and conjugation. Transformations in the first three reaction categories, known as *phase I reactions,* increase the polarity of substrates and can either increase or decrease toxicity. In conjugation, the only *phase II reaction,* polar groups are added to the products of phase I reactions. Most chemicals are handled sequentially by the two phases, although some are directly conjugated. The spectrum of reactions of each type can be found in any toxicology text, and only a few examples, of environmental health interest, are presented here.

Oxidation is the most common biotransformation reaction. There are two general kinds of oxidation reactions: direct addition of oxygen to the carbon, nitrogen, sulfur, or other bond, and dehydrogenation. Most of these reactions are mediated by microsomal enzymes, although there are mitochondrial and cytoplasmic oxidases as well. *Reduction* is a much less common biotransformation than oxidation, but it does occur with substances whose redox potentials exceed that of the body. *Conjugation* involves combining a toxin with a normal body constituent. The result is generally a less toxic and more polar molecule, which can be more readily excreted. However, conjugation can be harmful if it occurs in excess and depletes the body of an essential constituent. *Hydrolysis* is a common reaction in a variety of biochemical pathways. Esters are hydrolyzed to acids and alcohols, and amides are hydrolyzed to acids and amines.

As mentioned earlier, various combinations of these reactions may be assembled in response to the same toxicant. Metabolic strategies for a particular toxin may vary widely among species, so an animal study, to be applicable to humans, should use a species with pathways similar to those of humans. The most prominent enzyme system for performing phase I reactions is the cytochrome 450 system, also known as the mixed-function oxygenase system. These enzymes are found in the endoplasmic reticulum of hepatocytes and other cells. In recent years advances in molecular biology have greatly expanded our understanding of cytochrome P450. Dozens of distinct P450 genes have been identified and sequenced. They have been grouped into eight distinct families, and for many, specific functions have been identified. For example, the enzyme CYP1A1 metabolically activates PAHs (polycyclic aromatic hydrocarbons); the enzyme CYP2D6 is responsible for metabolizing such medications as beta-blockers, tricyclic antidepressants, and debrisoquin; and the enzyme CYP2E1 bioactivates vinyl chloride, methylene chloride, and urethane.

These insights in turn have helped explain why people may vary widely in their metabolic activity following similar exposures. Polymorphism in the genes that code for various P450 proteins has been shown to result in different metabolic phenotypes (see Chapter Six). For example, people whose CYP2D6 phenotype makes them poor metabolizers of debrisoquin are at risk of various adverse drug reactions, whereas extensive metabolizers are at increased risk of lung cancer, probably because of carcinogenic metabolites they produce.

Any enzyme system has a finite capacity. When a preferred pathway is saturated, the remaining substrate may be handled by alternative pathways. (Most substrates can be metabolized by more than one enzyme system.) However, in some instances when a preferred metabolic pathway is saturated, the substrate may persist in the body and exert toxic effects. One form of enzyme saturation is *competitive inhibition.* This may be a mechanism of toxicity, as when organophosphate pesticides compete with acetylcholine for the binding sites on cholinesterase molecules, or when metals such as beryllium compete with magnesium and manganese for enzyme ligand binding. However, competitive inhibition is important as well in metabolizing toxins. For example, methyl alcohol is oxidized by the enzyme alcohol dehydrogenase to the optic nerve toxin formaldehyde. This process can be blocked by large doses of ethanol, which competes for the binding sites of the enzyme and slows the formation of the toxic metabolite. The drug fomepizole acts in the same way, by selectively inhibiting alcohol dehydrogenase. This drug has been used to treat ethylene glycol poisoning, preventing the formation of the toxic metabolites glycolic acid and oxalic acid.

The enzyme systems that metabolize xenobiotics are not static. When the demand is high, their synthesis can be enhanced in a process called *enzyme induction.* The resulting increase in enzyme activity helps the organism respond to subsequent exposures not only to the original xenobiotic but to similar substances as well. DDT and methyl cholanthrene are examples of substances known to induce metabolic enzymes. People vary in their capacity for biotransformation in several ways. Two types of difference have already been mentioned: genetic and enzyme induction. Other factors also account for interindividual differences in metabolism; among them are general health, nutritional status, and concurrent medications.

Excretion

Because biotransformation tends to make compounds more polar and less fat soluble, the beneficial outcome of this process is that toxins can be more readily excreted from the body. The major route of excretion of toxins and their metabolites is through the kidneys. The kidneys handle toxins in the same way that they handle any serum solutes: passive glomerular filtration, passive tubular diffusion, and active tubular secretion. Smaller molecules can reach the tubules through passive glomerular filtration, because the glomerular capillary pores will allow molecules of up to about 70,000 daltons to pass through. However, this excludes substances bound to large serum proteins; these substances must undergo active tubular secretion to be excreted. The tubular secretory apparatus apparently has separate processes for organic anions and organic cations, and, like any active transport system, these processes can be saturated and competitively blocked. Finally, passive tubular diffusion out of the serum probably occurs to some extent, especially for certain organic bases. Passive diffusion also occurs in the opposite direction, from the tubules to the serum. As in any of the membrane crossings discussed previously, lipid-soluble molecules are reabsorbed from the tubular lumen much more readily than polar molecules and ions are, which explains the practice of alkalinizing the urine to hasten the excretion of acids. The daily volume of filtrate produced is about 200 liters—five times the total body water—in a remarkably efficient and thorough filtration process.

A second major organ of excretion is the liver. The liver occupies a strategic position because the portal circulation promptly delivers compounds to it following gastrointestinal absorption. Furthermore, the generous perfusion of the liver and the discontinuous capillary structure within it facilitate its filtration of the blood. Thus excretion into the bile is potentially a rapid and efficient process. Biliary excretion is somewhat analogous to renal tubular secretion. There are specific transport systems for organic acids, organic bases, neutral compounds, and possibly metals. These are active transport systems with the ability to handle protein-bound molecules. Finally, reuptake of lipid-soluble substances can occur after secretion, in this case through the intestinal walls. Toxicants that are secreted with the bile enter the gastrointestinal tract and, unless reabsorbed, are secreted with the feces. Materials ingested orally and not absorbed and materials carried up the respiratory tree and swallowed are also passed with the feces. All of this may be supplemented by some passive diffusion through the walls of the gastrointestinal tract, although it is not a major mechanism of excretion.

Volatile gases and vapors are excreted primarily by the lungs. The process is one of passive diffusion, governed by the difference between plasma and alveolar vapor pressure. Volatiles that are highly fat soluble tend to persist in body reservoirs and take some time to migrate from adipose tissue to plasma to alveolar air. Less fat-soluble volatiles are exhaled fairly promptly, until the plasma level has decreased to that of ambient air. Interestingly, the alveoli and bronchi can sustain damage when a vapor such as gasoline is exhaled, even if the initial exposure occurred percutaneously or through ingestion.

Other routes of excretion, although of minor significance quantitatively, are important for a variety of reasons. Excretion into mother's milk obviously introduces a risk to the infant, and because milk is more acidic (pH 6.5) than serum, basic compounds are concentrated in milk. Moreover, owing to the high fat content of breast milk (3 to 5 percent), fat-soluble substances such as DDT can also be passed to the infant. Some toxins, especially metals, are excreted in sweat or laid down in growing hair, which may be of use in diagnosis. Finally, some materials are secreted in the saliva and may then pose a subsequent gastrointestinal exposure hazard.

Toxicokinetics

It is a useful exercise to track a potential toxic compound from the environment (water, air, soil, food), into the body and throughout the body, all the way to its molecular site of action. This process is often termed *toxicokinetics.* For example, suppose that compound X is generated as a by-product of a particular industrial process. Whereas an exposure assessor measures the concentrations of compound X in the air and an epidemiologist studies the incidence of certain diseases in the surrounding community, the toxicologist is concerned with how the compound gets into the body and what it does once it is there. For example, compound X may be inhaled into the lungs. Once there, it rapidly crosses the alveolar membrane and enters the pulmonary circulation. It travels through the pulmonary vein to the left side of the heart and is then sent throughout the entire body. A large percentage of the compound goes to the liver where it is activated into a reactive epoxide. This compound then finds its way to the kidney, where it is reabsorbed along with salts and other polar compounds and transported across the cellular membrane of the proximal tubule. There it accumulates and damages cellular macromolecules.

If the toxicologist can show that compound X damages the kidney and the epidemiologist identifies an exposure-related increase in the incidence of renal failure in a population, regulatory steps may be taken to eliminate or limit the use of this compound. Toxicology can also be very useful in monitoring the development of new compounds. If a toxicologist shows that a new compound (compound Z) has an action in rats or mice similar to the action of compound X, it is very likely to show the same toxicity in humans, so a manufacturer would be very wise to discontinue development of that compound. The understanding of mechanisms can lead to the development of safer chemicals and drugs.

What Makes Toxic Compounds Toxic?

The mere presence of a toxic compound in a particular location in the body does not guarantee that there will be an adverse effect. The toxicant must interact with a biological target to cause harm.

Toxicants, whether endogenous or exogenous, are distributed to many cells and tissues but often cause toxicity in only a specific type of cell or organ. This may be due in part to greater accumulation of the toxicant in a particular cell type or organ. Some cells may be specifically affected owing to their genetic or biological makeup or the level of activity at which they function. For example, the heart and lung may be particularly vulnerable because they receive the largest blood volumes of all the organ systems. Conversely, the brain and testes may be protected from a number of toxicants because of the presence of the blood-brain and blood-testes barriers. However, the brain is extremely sensitive to toxicants that affect energy metabolism, due to its high requirement for ATP (adenosine triphosphate), the primary cellular energy source.

Some toxicants interact with targets that are shared by a number of different cells, tissues, or organs. Good examples of this type of toxicant are compounds such as carbon monoxide and cyanide, which affect the cellular utilization of oxygen or the supply of high energy compounds such as ATP. Because every cell and tissue requires oxygen and energy, these compounds have the ability to damage many cell and tissue types. However, the organ systems that require the most oxygen and energy are the most vulnerable to these toxicants. Thus the heart and brain are considered uniquely sensitive to the toxic effects of cyanide and carbon monoxide.

In contrast, some toxicants are more selective, and are especially toxic for particular cell types or organ systems. For example, the herbicide paraquat specifically targets the lung via selective uptake by the diamine/polyamine transporter. Once in the lung, paraquat readily undergoes oxidation-reduction reactions generating free radicals. This can result in lung fibrosis and ultimately in death because of reduced respiratory capacity. Exposure of humans to less than three grams of paraquat has been demonstrated to be lethal. In an analogous manner the dopaminergic neurotoxin MPTP (1-methyl-4-phenyl-1,2,3,6-tetrahydropyridine) is converted in the brain to its toxic metabolite MPP+ (1-methyl-4-phenylpyridinium), which is then taken up into dopamine neurons by the dopamine transporter. Once inside dopamine neurons, MPP+ can be concentrated in the mitochondria and can reduce cellular ATP, resulting in the death of dopamine neurons.

Other toxicants are specifically designed to target a particular organ system, as is the case with insecticides. Most insecticides are designed to kill insects through hyperexcitation of the nervous system. For example, the oxon metabolites of organophosphate insecticides inhibit the enzyme acetylcholinesterase, with predictable physiological effects (Box 2.6). Unfortunately, humans have the same acetylcholinesterase enzyme as the insects targeted for eradication, giving rise to the possibility of harm to humans.

Box 2.6. Organophosphate Insecticides

Organophosphorus insecticides, commonly referred to as organophosphates, were first synthesized by Gerhardt Schrader, in Germany, prior to World War II. Although Schrader's interests were in the development of effective pesticides, the high toxicity and volatility of some of the early compounds led to their development by the German army as chemical warfare agents. After the war the interest in organophosphates as insecticides was renewed. Following the banning of organochlorine pesticides in the 1970s, the organophosphates became the primary class of pesticides, with numerous uses in agricultural and household settings (see Chapter Twenty). Recently, for example, the organophosphorus insecticide malathion was used in New York City to combat mosquitoes thought to carry the West Nile virus.

Organophosphorus insecticides exert their toxicity by inhibiting the enzyme acetylcholinesterase, which elevates levels of the neurotransmitter acetylcholine. This results in hyperstimulation of cholinergic receptors in the central and peripheral nervous system, leading to the characteristic signs of cholinergic poisoning: hypersecretion (including diarrhea and excess production of saliva, tears, and urine), constricted pupils, and spasm of the airways. With severe acute intoxication, organophosphates cause death through depression of the respiratory center of the brain and paralysis of the diaphragm.

Most organophosphorus insecticides are converted to their oxon metabolites, the active compound. This conversion occurs primarily in the liver and is catalyzed by the cytochrome P450 family of enzymes. An example of this conversion, starting with the pesticide chlorpyrifos, is shown in Figure 2.2. Chlorpyrifos may be converted to the active oxon (chlorpyrifos-oxon), in a reaction termed *desulfuration*. Alternatively, a detoxication reaction called *dearylation* may occur giving rise to 3,5,6-trichloropyridinol and either diethyl phosphate or diethyl phosphorothioate.

The organophosphates provide a good example of trade-offs in environmental health. Many of them are highly toxic and have had their uses restricted. However,

FIGURE 2.2. BIOTRANSFORMATION PATHWAYS OF CHLORPYRIFOS.

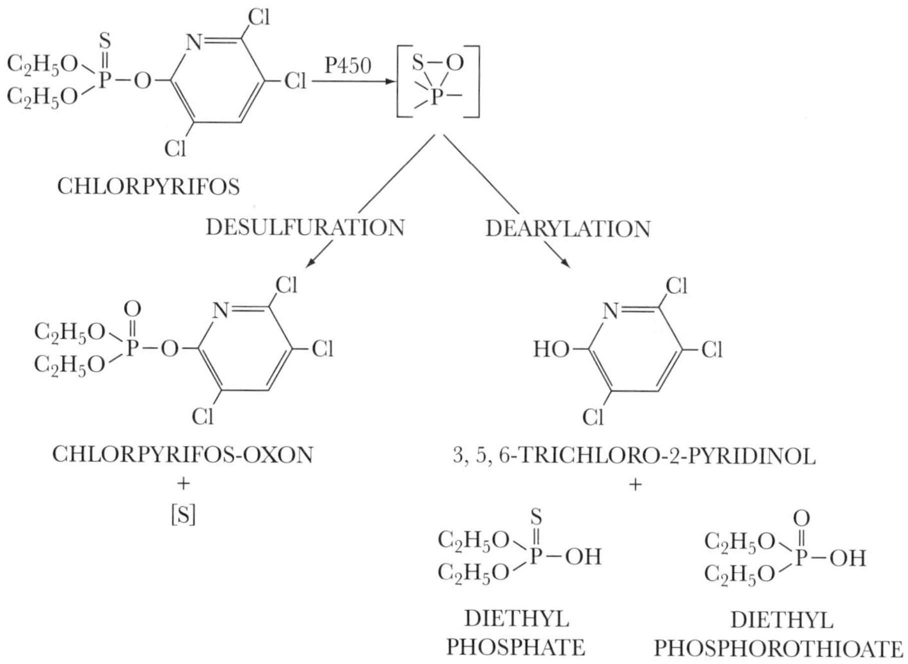

this class of pesticides has helped reduce insect-borne disease and insect-related crop losses over the past fifty years. Maximizing crop yield and safety and minimizing disease require a combination of toxicological knowledge and systems thinking, as described in Chapter Twenty-Nine.

All of the previous examples have involved the idea of acute toxicity, often at high doses. However, humans are more commonly exposed to low levels of toxicants for long periods of time, raising the possibility of chronic toxicity as opposed to acute toxicity. An example of chronic toxicity is the development of emphysema or lung cancer following years of cigarette smoking. In this situation the compounds contained in cigarette smoke do not cause an immediate acute toxic outcome. However, years of exposure to the compounds in cigarette smoke may overwhelm the protective defenses of the body and result in damage to the lung. Another example is the possible outcome of long-term exposure to the chemical acrylamide, which is often used as a waterproofing agent and to remove solids from water, as in sewage treatment plants. Acrylamide is a neurotoxicant that attacks the sensory and motor nerves, primarily in the extremities. It may cause damage following a single high exposure; however, it has been demonstrated in laboratory animals and in some occupationally exposed individuals that longer-term, lower-level exposures can result in similar damage. (In 2002, considerable concern followed media reports of acrylamide in french fries; see, for example, Gorman, 2002. Subsequent research by Becalski, Lau, Lewis, and Seaman, 2003, found that amino acids and glucose in potatoes, under the conditions found in commercial frying, could combine to form acrylamide. Some public health advocates have called for more stringent regulation of acrylamide levels in food.)

How Are Compounds Tested for Toxicity?

How does a toxicologist determine that one compound is more toxic than another?* Several decades ago, toxicologists used a rather crude method for determining the relative toxicity of compounds. By exposing laboratory animals to compounds and determining the dose that killed half the animals, they calculated the "lethal dose for 50 percent," or LD_{50}, an index that allowed comparisons among several unrelated compounds. Although crude, the LD_{50} has some important scientific strengths. The exposure is well defined (unlike the exposure in most human situations), the outcome is unambiguous, the LD_{50} is a measure that can be applied across different compounds, and it can lead to a useful practical conclusion: if a compound is lethal at very low doses then human exposures should be prevented or strictly controlled.

Animal testing is also used to study chronic toxicities, such as cancers. In a typical study, animals are exposed to a suspected carcinogen at several dose levels. There is also a placebo group. The animals are observed for a defined period of time and then sacrificed to check for evidence of neoplasm. If, for example, a compound causes excess liver cancer in rats at a relatively low dose, it is prudent to restrict human exposures. Conversely, if rodent studies show no adverse effects at doses orders of magnitude higher than humans experience, then a chemical may be approved to proceed through development.

Animal studies have several disadvantages. They use higher doses than people typically experience in the environment, a necessity for maximizing the sensitivity of the testing. Species-to-species differences make extrapolation from animals to humans difficult. Human life spans are longer than those of rodents, so long-term outcomes in humans may not be evident in animals. And critics have pointed to animal welfare considerations, urging that alternatives to animal testing be developed and used (Meyer, 2003).

A tiered approach to toxicological testing has now emerged, with at least two approaches used alongside (and often before) animal testing (Figure 2.3).

FIGURE 2.3. TIERED APPROACH TO TOXICITY TESTING.

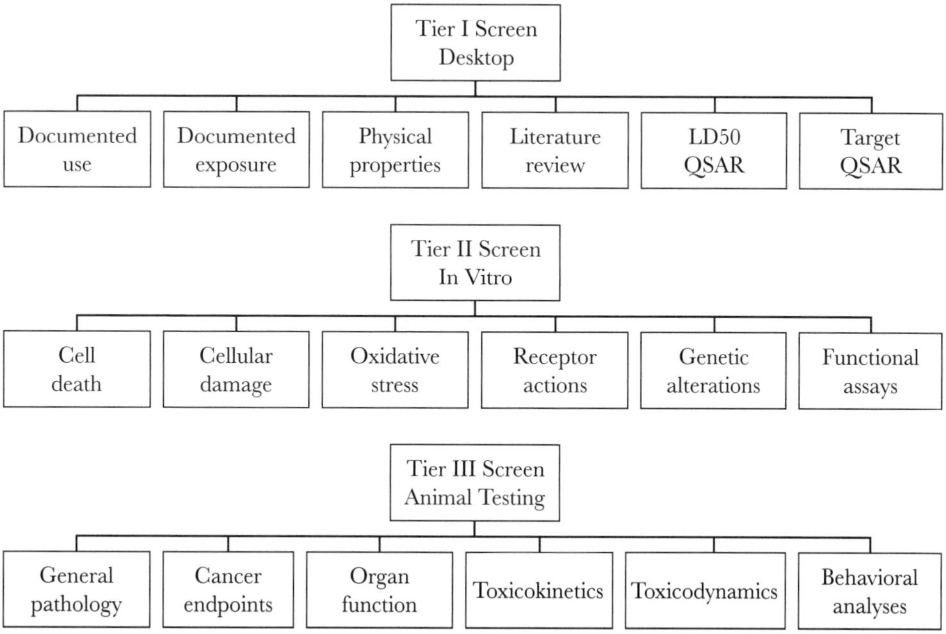

Desktop analysis relies on *quantitative structure-activity relationships* (QSARs); if the toxicologist notes that a particular chemical structure has a particular toxicity, then other chemicals with related structures are assessed for the potential to cause similar effects. *In vitro* testing involves exposure of cell systems, such as bacteria or cultured human cells, to a potential toxin. Cellular responses such as mutation are observed and help predict human responses. Desktop and in vitro studies are less expensive and more rapid than animal testing, but the need to extrapolate to human responses, with all the assumptions required in that exercise, make them less definitive methods than animal testing and epidemiological studies.

Conclusion

Toxicology is the study of the adverse effects of chemicals on biological systems. Environmental and occupational toxicology is the study of how chemical exposures in the workplace, air, water, food, and other environmental media may threaten human health. Toxicologists think in terms of an exposure sequence, from exposure to absorption to distribution to metabolism to excretion, and analyze the end-organ effects that may occur during this process. They are interested in identifying mechanisms of toxicity and levels of exposure that are safe or unsafe. This information is directly informative to regulators and others who work to identify the safest chemicals for our use and to set acceptable levels of exposure for chemicals that may be dangerous.

Thought Questions

1. Toxicologists use several methods to test the toxicity of a compound. Name each method, and describe its advantages and disadvantages.
2. Toxicologists study both *acute* and *chronic* toxic effects. Acute effects are easier to study, and regulations have traditionally been based on acute toxicity, although in recent years more emphasis has been given to chronic outcomes. Why do you think the initial emphasis was on acute effects?
3. Explain why you and your classmates may have different responses to the same exposure to a chemical.
4. Pick a toxic effect that interests you—such as reproductive toxicity, endocrine disruption, or another effect—look up the methods toxicologists use to test for this outcome, and describe these methods.

References

Baccarelli, A., Pesatori, A. C., and Bertazzi, P. A. "Occupational and Environmental Agents as Endocrine Disruptors: Experimental and Human Evidence." *Journal of Endocrinological Investigation,* 2000, *23,* 771–781.

Becalski, A., Lau, B. P., Lewis, D., and Seaman, S. W. "Acrylamide in Foods: Occurrence, Sources, and Modeling." *Journal of Agricultural and Food Chemistry,* 2003, *51*(3), 802–808.

Cheek, A. O., and others. "Environmental Signaling: A Biological Context for Endocrine Disruption." *Environmental Health Perspectives,* 1998, *106* (suppl. 1), 5–10.

Choi, S. M., Yoo, S. D., and Lee, B. M. "Toxicological Characteristics of Endocrine-Disrupting Chemicals: Developmental Toxicity, Carcinogenicity, and Mutagenicity." *Journal of Toxicology and Environmental Health Part B: Critical Reviews,* 2004, *7*(1), 1–24.

Fox, J. E. "Chemical Communication Threatened by Endocrine-Disrupting Chemicals." *Environmental Health Perspectives,* 2004, *112,* 648–653.

Golden, R. J., and others. "Environmental Endocrine Modulators and Human Health: An Assessment of the Biological Evidence." *Critical Reviews in Toxicology,* 1998, *28,* 109–227.

Gorman, C. "Do French Fries Cause Cancer?" *Time,* 2002, *159*(18), 73.

Meyer, O. "Testing and Assessment Strategies, Including Alternative and New Approaches." *Toxicology Letters,* 2003, *140–141,* 21–30.

Safe, S. H., and others. "Toxicology of Environmental Estrogens." *Reproduction, Fertility, and Development,* 2001, *13,* 307–315.

Sonnenschein, C., and Soto, A. M. "An Updated Review of Environmental Estrogen and Androgen Mimics and Antagonists." *Journal of Steroid Biochemistry and Molecular Biology,* 1998, *65*(1–6), 143–150.

Zoeller, T. R., and others. "Thyroid Hormone, Brain Development, and the Environment." *Environmental Health Perspectives,* 2002, *110* (suppl. 3), 355–361.

For Further Information

Aldridge, W. N. *Mechanisms and Concepts in Toxicology.* New York: Taylor & Francis, 1996.

Klaasen, C. D. (ed.). *Casserrett and Doull's Toxicology: The Basic Science of Poisons.* New York: McGraw-Hill, 2001.

Timbrell, J. *Introduction to Toxicology.* (3rd ed.) New York: Taylor & Francis, 2002.

CHAPTER THREE

EPIDEMIOLOGY

Kyle Steenland
Christine Moe

Epidemiology is the study of exposures in relation to disease. The key question is whether a given exposure, or set of exposures, causes a certain disease. Obviously, if we can show that an exposure causes disease, we have a chance to intervene and prevent disease occurrence, which is our ultimate goal.

Epidemiology can give us the tools, the techniques of study design and analysis, to determine whether a given exposure is *associated* with a given disease. How do we judge that an association is *causal* (sometimes called *causal inference*)?

A general philosophical framework exists for judging causality. It is accepted by most epidemiologists, and it stems from the writings of philosopher Karl Popper (for a good discussion, see Rothman and Greenland, 1998, pp. 16–28). In this framework, observations (especially repeated observations) that one event is followed by another enable the epidemiologist to form a hypothesis, to posit that A causes B. The key to Popperian philosophy is that all hypotheses (or theories of causation) are tentative and may be disproved by further testing. Hypotheses that are tested many times and hold up tend to become accepted as scientific facts (for example, we now accept that cigarettes cause lung cancer), but over the course of time many accepted hypotheses are also overthrown by new scientific insights (we now accept that miasma, or foul air, does not cause cholera).

On the practical level, epidemiologists commonly use a famous set of criteria, set out by Hill (1965), to judge whether a particular causal hypothesis is plausible, whether the observed association between A and B makes it seem likely that in fact A causes B. Hill set out nine criteria. Only one is absolutely required, and it is that the exposure precedes the disease. Although it seems that this should always be easy to know, sometimes this is not clear. Other commonly used Hill criteria that argue in favor of causality include consistency (the association is repeated in many studies), a large effect size (the exposed have much more disease than the nonexposed), a positive dose-response (more exposure causes more disease), and biological plausibility (a biological explanation makes it reasonable that A causes B).

Regulators and risk assessors must conclude from the weight of the epidemiological evidence, using criteria such as these, whether an association is likely to be causal. A number of agencies, such as the International Agency for Research on Cancer (IARC), the National Toxicology Program (NTP), the Institute of Medicine (IOM), and the Environmental Protection Agency (EPA), regularly review epidemiological evidence and publish summaries in which they evaluate whether associations are likely to be causal. Epidemiology has provided evidence judged to show that a large number of environmental and occupational exposures are associated with diseases: lead is now associated with cognitive impairment in children, trihalomethanes (in water) with bladder cancer, air pollution (particulates) with cardiorespiratory disease, radon gas with cancer, and ergonomic stress with low back pain, to name just a few.

Epidemiological Studies: Types and Issues

In this section we describe the major kinds of studies that epidemiologists design and conduct, and we examine issues relating to bias and analysis.

Descriptive Studies

Epidemiological studies may be divided into categories according to their design. At the simplest level are the *descriptive* studies, which characterize a disease by factors such as age, sex, time, and geographic region. These studies do not formally test a hypothesis about the association between a specific exposure (or *risk factor*) and a disease but rather describe patterns in disease occurrence in terms of broad demographic and other variables. These studies are often first steps and may provide clues about factors that cause disease. For example, the fact that malaria occurs mainly in tropical areas provides a clue that warm climate may play a role in its transmission. The fact that heart disease occurs at a later age in women than in men may provide a clue about endogenous estrogen playing a protective role.

Correlational, or Ecological, Studies

Descriptive studies are a close cousin to *correlational,* or *ecological,* studies, which study the correlation between disease rates and some specific exposure, but at the level of the group rather than of the individual. For example, one can correlate breast cancer rates in countries around the world with degree of socioeconomic development; rates are higher in richer, more urban countries. Such studies will often provide clues about possible risk factors for disease, which can then be examined further in studies of individuals. Generally, ecological studies are viewed as weaker than studies of individuals, and they are often called *hypothesis-generating* studies. However, in some instances an ecological design is the design of choice. One example is the use of time series studies of air pollution, in which pollution levels are correlated with disease rates on a day-to-day basis. Such studies have the advantage of looking at a presumably stable population over time and thus comparing it to itself (eliminating most confounding). The only variables that are changing on a daily basis are the exposure variables of interest (air pollution levels) and the outcomes of interest (daily disease rates), although seasonal variation in temperature also needs to be taken into account.

Etiologic, or Analytical, Studies

Etiologic, or *analytical,* studies are generally studies of individuals in which the investigators seek to test a specific hypothesis about exposure and disease: for example, whether pesticide exposure is associated with Parkinson's disease. Such studies are often undertaken after descriptive and correlational studies have indicated that they are worth doing, that is, after a plausible hypothesis has emerged that needs to be tested.

Analytical studies can in turn be divided into two types, observational studies and clinical trials. *Clinical trials,* usually called *randomized clinical trials,* are in a sense the model for rigorous epidemiological studies. They are often done to compare one medication or treatment to another. They are controlled experiments, because they assign treatment (or exposure) randomly to one group and not another. The treated and untreated groups are therefore usually assumed to be comparable with regard to other variables (such as age, weight, sex, education, and the like) that might affect the disease outcome; therefore any difference in subsequent disease rates can be assumed to be due to exposure. Then both treated and untreated groups are followed over time.

However, randomized clinical trials are generally impractical for studying the effects of toxic exposures, simply because one cannot ethically administer a suspected toxin to a human population. Clinical trials are therefore restricted to studying treatments or other responses after toxic exposures have occurred. Lead has been well studied in this regard; clinical trials have suggested that dimercaptosuccinic acid (DMSA) is not useful as a treatment for lead-exposed children (Dietrich and others, 2004), that education of mothers is only slightly helpful in maintaining low blood lead levels in their children (Jordan and others, 2003), that dietary calcium supplementation is not useful in lowering blood lead levels in children with adequate calcium stores (Markowitz, Sinnett, and Rosen, 2004), and that lead dust control in urban homes is not effective in reducing children's blood lead levels (Lanphear, Eberly, and Howard, 2000). This is useful information. However, the epidemiologist interested in studying suspected occupational and environmental toxins to determine if they cause disease needs to conduct observational studies.

Observational studies are uncontrolled, or natural, experiments, of which the epidemiologist takes advantage. For example, the epidemiologist wants to study the effect of lead on cancer, so he or she follows a cohort of lead-exposed workers over time and compares them to the general population for cancer rates. However, the workers and the general population are likely to differ with respect to other characteristics, such as smoking habits or diet that may in turn affect cancer rates (such variables are called *confounders*). The epidemiologist may be able to adjust or control for the effects of such confounders, but if not, they may distort the findings about the effect of exposure on disease. For this reason observational studies are viewed as less definitive than clinical trials. A famous recent example of different findings resulting from clinical trials and from observational studies is the case of postmenopausal estrogen replacement therapy and its relationship to the risk of heart disease (Whittemore and McGuire, 2003).

Observational Study Designs

The three principal designs for observational studies are cohort, case-control, and cross-sectional. *Cohort* studies start with an exposed group and a nonexposed group, both disease free, and follow them forward in time to observe disease incidence or mortality rates. Disease rates or risks in the exposed and nonexposed can then be compared to produce a rate (or risk) ratio or a rate (or risk) difference. The observation period in cohort studies may start in the past and move forward to the present (*retrospective*) or start in the present and move into the future (*prospective*). The former is obviously quicker and usually cheaper; for example, to study lung cancer among welders and nonwelders one can identify a cohort as of 1950 and trace cohort members' lung cancer mortality until the present. The disadvantage of the retrospective approach is that one is dependent on historical information about exposure levels and about other variables that might be potential confounders (smoking habits, for example). Although prospective studies take a long time and are often expensive, they are more appropriate when one wants to measure exposure levels and confounding variables at the study baseline or when biological samples (such as blood) are required. They may also be needed to study diseases that are difficult to ascertain in retrospect, such as spontaneous abortions (whose occurrence, and date of occurrence, may be difficult for individuals to remember accurately). Cohort studies can consider disease events per person (cumulative incidence, or risk) or disease events per person-time (rates). The former are appropriate for short follow-up periods and *fixed* cohorts, where everyone is followed for the whole follow-up period. The latter are appropriate for long follow-up periods and *dynamic* cohorts, where people may enter the follow-up period at different times, and may be lost to follow-up at any time and therefore are followed for different periods of time. Cohort studies are good for rare exposures and common diseases, because one begins with assembling an exposed group and hence can assemble a large number of exposed subjects (for example, welders); however, when the disease that might result from exposure is rare, a *very* large number of subjects may need to be assembled.

Case-control studies are the opposite of cohort studies in that one begins with diseased and nondiseased groups and looks backward in time. For example, bladder cancer cases and controls can be asked about their past consumption of water treated with chlorine (this treatment results in trihalomethane formation and trihalomethanes are suspected bladder carcinogens). The investigator determines the odds of exposure in each group, and these odds are then compared (if a is the number exposed, and b is the number nonexposed, then $a/(a + b)$ is the proportion exposed, and a/b is the odds of exposure). If the odds of exposure are higher among the diseased group (the cases) than among the nondiseased group (the controls), then one judges that the exposure is associated with the disease. The usual measure of effect is the odds ratio. Case-control studies are more subject to bias than are cohort studies because it is sometimes difficult to choose the cases and controls so that they are representative of the overall diseased and nondiseased populations (this is particularly true for the controls) and because it is often difficult to measure exposure in the past accurately. *Recall bias,* for example, can occur if cases tend to remember more about past exposures than controls. However, if cases and controls are chosen properly, a case-control study should give the same answer about the exposure-disease relationship as a cohort study.

Case-control studies are useful for rare diseases and common exposures, the opposite of cohort studies. Case-control studies can be done within the general population or within hospitals, or they can be nested within cohorts.

Cross-sectional studies, or *prevalence* studies, tend to measure exposure and disease at the same time. For example, lead exposure in relation to children's performance on intelligence tests may be studied by measuring lead in the blood at the time of neurological testing, or cadmium levels in the urine of smelter workers may be measured at the same time as small protein in the urine (a measure of kidney damage). Cross-sectional studies are often done when the outcome of interest is subclinical or asymptomatic disease. In the workplace, cross-sectional studies miss symptomatic cases if workers with the disease leave employment.

A typical problem of cross-sectional studies is determining whether exposure in fact preceded the health outcome. For example, in the case of the smelter workers, if those with higher levels of cadmium in their urine were also excreting more small protein, it would not be known whether the protein excretion preceded or followed the presence of cadmium in the urine. The same would be true for neurological tests and lead in children. The interpretation of positive findings in the latter study would be made even more difficult by the fact that socioeconomic status (SES) is an important confounder that is difficult to control; children of low SES have higher lead exposure and perform worse on neuropsychological tests. Cross-sectional studies tend to be seen as a somewhat weaker design than cohort and case-control studies, although they are often the only possible design and they can provide valid results, which may then be confirmed or disconfirmed in cohort or case-control studies.

Bias Issues

Bias refers to the distortion of the true relationship between exposure and disease. The most important types of bias are selection bias, confounding, and information bias.

Selection bias occurs when the relationship between exposure and disease in the study population is not representative of the true relationship between exposure and disease in the general population because the study population has been selected in a nonrepresentative way. For example, in a study of ethylene oxide (a sterilant gas) and breast cancer, suppose only 20 percent of the target population answers a questionnaire about breast cancer occurrence. These self-selected study participants may differ from the rest of the target population—perhaps, for example, they have had higher exposure and higher breast cancer rates—so the association that they demonstrate between exposure and disease would not have been found if the entire target population had participated. This kind of bias cannot be fixed in the analysis. In fact one cannot even be sure of the direction of selection bias, because the occurrence of the disease (breast cancer in this case) among the rest of the target population cannot be known. The study will thus be suspect. The *healthy worker effect* is another kind of selection bias. Here, workers are compared to the general population. However, workers as a group are healthier than the general population, so study results will be biased against finding adverse health effects among the workers. This is another example of a selection bias that cannot be readily fixed at the analysis stage.

Confounding refers to the distortion of the exposure-disease relationship by a third variable, one that is associated both with exposure and with disease. For example, in a study of welders in relation to lung cancer, if the welders smoke more than nonwelders, then smoking (strongly associated with lung cancer) could act as a confounder. Adjustment for the effect of smoking can be made by stratifying the analysis into smokers and nonsmokers, determining the exposure-disease relationship in each group, and then forming a weighted average of the exposure-disease relationship across both groups. However, this can be done only when adequate data on smoking have been collected in both exposed and nonexposed groups.

Another possibility is that a third variable modifies the effect of the exposure variable of interest. This is not confounding but instead is called *effect modification*. For example, one could imagine that the welding–lung cancer relationship might differ between smokers and nonsmokers in that only smokers might show a welding effect, perhaps because smoking injures the lung epithelium, permitting a carcinogenic effect from the metal fumes. In this circumstance the investigator cannot calculate the weighted average of exposure-disease associations across both strata of the third variable and instead must report results for each stratum separately. No adjustment for confounding occurs, as no weighted average of exposure effect across levels of the confounder should be conducted.

Finally, once the study population has been selected, *information bias* can occur when information obtained about either exposure or disease is incorrect. One of the main sources of information bias in epidemiological studies is mismeasurement or misclassification of exposure. When exposure is measured incorrectly (for a continuous exposure variable) or misclassified (for a categorical exposure variable), one might expect that the exposure-disease association will be distorted. Usually, when exposure is equally poorly measured or classified for both diseased and nondiseased groups (*nondifferential error* or *misclassification*), then the effect is to bias the exposure-disease association toward the null (toward finding no association). If, however, the mismeasurement or misclassification is greater for the diseased or the nondiseased, biases away from the null can occur. This problem is typical of retrospective exposure assessment in case-control studies, when cases may recall past exposures more often than controls (recall bias), which will bias the study toward finding an association (away from the null).

Analysis Issues

The choice of methods of analysis in epidemiology typically depends on whether the exposure variable and the disease variable are continuous or categorical. Most of the examples cited so far in this chapter consider disease as a categorical (yes/no) variable (a yes/no variable is called a *dichotomous* variable). This is typically true of symptomatic disease: you either get the disease or you don't. However, many studies consider a continuous disease variable, such as blood pressure or the concentration of a small protein in the urine. In some instances continuous variables might be transformed into categorical variables (for example, a study might define high blood pressure as a systolic pressure greater than 140), especially when medical guidelines suggest such cutpoints. Exposure variables may also be continuous (for example, cadmium in the urine) or categorical (for example, welder or nonwelder).

When both exposure and disease variables are dichotomous, then one usually calculates the measures referred to earlier, such as a rate ratio or an odds ratio. These categorical analyses may be stratified to control for confounding, as also indicated earlier. However, when the disease and exposure are continuous variables, typically a regression analysis (for example, linear regression) is conducted, in which the outcome is disease and the predictors include the exposure variable as well as any other confounder variable about which the investigator has data. One seeks to know if the exposure is a significant predictor of disease: that is, is the regression coefficient for the exposure variable significantly different from the null value of zero?

Mixtures of these situations may be employed. A linear regression analysis for a continuous outcome may also be calculated with the exposure variable categorized in the regression. Furthermore, even when the disease variable is dichotomous, there is a type of regression called logistic regression in which the measure of interest remains the odds ratio and either categorical or continuous variables may be included as predictors.

One important feature of the analysis is the precision of the estimate of effect (that is, of the rate ratio, the odds ratio, or the regression coefficient for the exposure variable). Large sample sizes lead to high precision, and vice versa. Precision is often presented as a confidence interval (CI), which represents a range of plausible values for the measure of effect. For example, an odds ratio in a case-control study of bladder cancer in relation to water supply (public water versus private wells) might be 2.00, indicating that those who use public water (more trihalomethanes) versus private wells (fewer trihalomethanes) have a doubling of bladder cancer risk. If the study is based on twenty cases and twenty controls, it will have low precision, and the 95 percent confidence interval for the odds ratio of 2.00 might be 0.50–8.00, indicating a wide range for plausible values. If the study is based on 2,000 cases and 2,000 controls, the 95 percent confidence interval might be 1.90–2.30, indicating a narrow range of plausible values. The precision of the estimate is a reflection of what is called *random error*, the error likely to result when choosing a sample of the total population of interest (all users of water in this case).

Precision is related to statistical significance. *Statistically significant* usually means that the estimate of effect is different from the null value and that the difference is unlikely to have occurred by chance. Typically, a finding is judged to be statistically significant when the probability that the difference from the null value is likely to have occurred by chance is .05 or less (usually stated as a *p* value of less than .05). A 95 percent confidence interval that excludes the null value (for example, the null value of 1.00 for an odds ratio, indicating no difference in risk of disease between exposed and nonexposed) will correspond to a *p* value of less than .05. Epidemiologists now prefer to express the precision of study results with confidence intervals rather than *p* values (or statistical significance), partly because a range of plausible values is more informative than a single test of statistical significance.

Environmental and Occupational Epidemiology

Environmental epidemiology and occupational epidemiology do not use any special epidemiological techniques but simply refer to areas of epidemiology defined by the exposures involved.

Environmental epidemiology studies environmental agents to which large numbers of people are exposed involuntarily. This usually excludes voluntary exposures to things such as alcohol, cigarettes, medications, and infectious agents transmitted person-to-person. However, environmental tobacco smoke (secondhand smoke) and infectious agents in water supplies would be included. Although this definition is a bit arbitrary, and although environmental epidemiology thus defined may sometimes overlap with other areas of epidemiology, nonetheless it is useful. Other examples of environmental agents (and their associated outcomes) are radon in homes in relation to lung cancer, environmental tobacco smoke in relation to lung cancer, arsenic in water in relation to low birthweight, chlorination by-products in water supplies in relation to bladder cancer, pesticide residues in food in relation to cancer, particulate matter in the air in relation to cardiovascular disease, and lead in soil in relation to neurological deficits. These exposures are often low-level and relatively homogenous across large numbers of people, making them particularly difficult to study. Furthermore, relative risks between those with more exposure and those with less exposure are usually low and therefore hard to detect reliably, often requiring large sample sizes.

Environmental exposures can be thought of as contributing to either epidemics or endemics. *Epidemics* are unusual outbreaks of disease, clearly above a normal level. The causative agents are sometimes familiar, as in the cholera outbreaks in Peru in the early 1990s. However, other recent outbreaks have not initially had a known cause, including the 1981 outbreak of neuropathy in Madrid (due to an oil contaminant), the 1993 gastrointestinal illness outbreak in Wisconsin (due to cryptosporidium in the water), and the 1976 pneumonia outbreak in Philadelphia (Legionnaires' disease). In contrast, *endemics* are constant, low (*background*) levels of disease that may or may not have an environmental cause. Examples are the possible contribution of radon in homes to lung cancer, the contribution of dioxin in the diet to cancer rates, the contribution of low-level air pollution to cardiovascular disease, and the contribution of lead in the environment to neurological deficits in children. Possible associations between environmental agents and background levels of disease are more and more often the subject of environmental epidemiology, especially in developed countries, and these associations are difficult to detect.

Occupational epidemiology is the epidemiological study of illness or injury associated with workplace exposures. It includes, for example, a focus on the associations between stressful repetitive motion and carpal tunnel syndrome, welding and lung cancer, silica exposure and kidney disease, and poor office ventilation and respiratory illness among office workers. Occupational epidemiology often involves relatively high exposures in relatively small numbers of people, often geographically isolated at a worksite. This context makes for easier studies from a scientific standpoint (the workplace exposure is a *natural* experiment). However, workplace studies also involve vested economic interests and are sometimes politically controversial. It may be difficult to gain access to the workers or the worksite, for example.

Historically, occupational studies were carried out in the context of very high exposures. Early studies revealed silicosis and asbestosis resulting from silica and asbestos exposures. These earlier occupational studies were responsible for the discovery of many carcinogens. For example, occupational studies have implicated asbestos, aniline dyes, silica, nickel, cadmium, arsenic, dioxin, beryllium, acid mists, radon gas, and diesel fumes in the causation of cancer (Steenland, Loomis, Shy, and Simonsen, 1996; Rom, 1998). Most of these agents occur in the general environment as well, where people are exposed at much lower levels. Whether associations seen in the workplace also occur in the general environment is controversial. For example, on the one hand it is unclear whether dioxin or diesel fumes in the general environment cause cancer. On the other hand radon in homes and arsenic in water are believed to be environmental carcinogens.

Today, workplace exposures to suspected toxins are much lower than in the past, at least in industrialized countries, and they are less often the focus of occupational epidemiology. For example, occupational cancer is less commonly studied today, as many of the most obvious suspected carcinogens in the workplace have already been studied and controlled. Current occupational studies more commonly involve issues more difficult to study, such as job stress and heart disease or lifting and back strain.

Clusters

One aspect of both environmental and occupational epidemiology that deserves special mention is the occurrence of clusters. A *cluster* is an apparently elevated number of cases of disease in a limited area over a limited period of time, suggesting some common cause (Rothman, 1990); typically, the number of cases in the cluster is small, on the order ten or twenty rather than hundreds. Clusters typically come to the attention of public health authorities, who must first determine whether they in fact represent an unusually high occurrence of disease. This is more difficult than it might seem, particularly for environmental clusters where the geographic and temporal boundaries are not clear. For example, three cases of childhood leukemia on the same street might be unusual if the denominator at risk is taken to be all the children on that street, but three cases might not appear excessive if the boundary is the neighborhood of a dozen different streets. Assuming investigators can determine that a cluster does represent a high rate of disease, the next step is to determine whether there is a common cause. Finding a common cause is more likely when the cases of disease are restricted to a specific diagnosis, such as childhood leukemia, rather than falling into a general category, such as childhood cancer; cancer includes many diseases with many different causes. But even when the cases represent a narrow and specific diagnosis, they still will often have many possible causes, and an epidemiological study will often not be able to pinpoint a specific cause. One reason for this is that such a study is typically restricted to a small number of cases (often using a case-control design), and the power to detect an association is therefore low, even if that association is quite strong.

Most investigations of environmental clusters do not find a common cause for the cluster. Caldwell (1990) summarized 108 cancer clusters investigated by the Centers for Disease Control and Prevention and concluded that no clear single cause was found for any of them. Similarly, Schulte, Ehrenberg, and Singal (1987) summarized 61 occupational clusters and found that only 16 were confirmed, and in none was a specific cause discovered.

Nonetheless, despite the long odds, cluster investigations have historically provided important clues that have later been confirmed in larger studies. Among the famous clusters that have led to discovery of new associations are the 1976 cluster of Legionnaires' disease cases in a hotel in Philadelphia (environmental), the clusters of asthma cases in Barcelona in the early 1980s that were eventually tied to soybean dust (environmental), the 1973 cluster of angiosarcoma cases among workers in a single vinyl chloride plant (occupational), and the 1977 cluster of infertility in a plant making a pesticide called dibromochloropropane (DBCP) (occupational). The discovery of a specific cause for a cluster is more likely when the disease in question is extremely rare. Compared to environmental clusters, occupational clusters have a somewhat higher chance of representing a common cause because they have a natural boundary (the worksite) and therefore avoid the boundary problem inherent in environmental clusters.

Measuring Exposure

Measuring exposure with as much accuracy as possible is key to valid epidemiological studies (for a fuller discussion see Chapter Four). Misclassification of dichotomous exposure status (exposed versus nonexposed) can severely bias results toward the null, and mismeasurement of a continuous exposure variable also often biases dose-response trends toward the null. In cross-sectional or prospective studies current exposure can be measured more or less easily, depending on the agent of interest. However, it is often difficult to measure exposure accurately when it occurred in the past and must be estimated, as in case-control studies, retrospective cohort studies, and cross-sectional studies in which one wishes to assess the impact of past exposures on current outcomes. Therefore we focus here on the problem of retrospective exposure assessment. In case-control studies of bladder cancer and drinking water, for example, subjects may be asked to remember their pattern of drinking-water consumption over the past fifty years. In cross-sectional studies of lead and neurological deficits in children, one may wish not only to measure current lead levels via the blood but to also assess prior exposure to lead via its measurement in bone. In retrospective cohort studies, investigators may be estimating past silica exposure for workers in a specific plant. As can be seen in these examples, in some instances investigators attempt to measure external exposure (water-drinking patterns, silica in the breathing zone of workers), and in others they seek a biomarker of internal exposures (blood and bone lead). In the following paragraphs we discuss both these scenarios.

First, let us consider more thoroughly the example of assessment of past exposure to silica among workers in a retrospective cohort study. Suppose there are some existing silica exposure measurements taken at various times during the past twenty years for some workers in some jobs. This is a typical situation, as exposure measurements were not routinely made in earlier periods. However, the cohort may have been employed over the past forty or fifty years, and the investigators may be seeking to conduct an exposure-response analysis and therefore require an estimate of past exposure for all workers across all jobs at all points in time. This may not be possible at all in many retrospective cohort studies. However, in some instances it may be possible to construct a *job-exposure matrix* (JEM), which is simply a cross classification of jobs and exposure levels across time. This requires an industrial hygienist to extrapolate beyond the more recent exposure data and to make a good guess about exposure further back in time, taking process changes at the plant into consideration because, typically, plants were dirtier further back in time. The industrial hygienist will also need to group similar jobs into a small number of categories, looking for groupings for which there are similar exposure levels and at least some past measurements. Then all workers in all jobs in each category, at any given point in time, can be assigned the same exposure level. If all this is possible, a JEM can be constructed, and all workers in a given job at a given point in time can be assigned a level of exposure by the JEM. This will in turn enable an estimate of cumulative exposure to silica for each worker. Cumulative exposure is often the measure of interest for chronic disease outcomes like silicosis, lung cancer, or kidney disease. An example of the construction of a job exposure matrix is given in Figure 3.1.

An alternative to estimating external exposure is the use of biomarkers of exposure (for example, dioxin or cotinine, a metabolite of nicotine, in the blood and lead in bone). Such biomarkers can be useful because they measure internal dose rather than external exposure. They may therefore take into account variation in metabolism and absorption of the external dose, possibly providing a more accurate estimate of the biologically relevant dose that can cause disease. However, many factors may make internal dose less desirable than external exposure, including wide individual variation, difficulty in obtaining accurate laboratory measurements of the biomarker, and choice of the wrong biomarker in a metabolic pathway in which several candidates exist for the toxin that causes disease. Perhaps more important, in retrospective exposure assessment, few biomarkers of exposure persist long enough to be useful.

For example, in a case-control study of Parkinson's disease in which serum is available, it would be ideal to be able to measure past exposure to pesticides (organophosphates and organochlorines) and also to organochlorines such as polychlorinated biphenyls (PCBs). Organophosphate pesticides, thought to play a role in chronic neurological disease partly because of their acute effects on the nervous system, are rapidly metabolized. Therefore blood levels of these compounds cannot be used to measure exposure beyond a few days in the past. Organochlorine pesticides and PCBs are also of interest because they have been shown to decrease dopamine levels in the brain in animal studies, and dopamine loss is the hallmark of Parkinson's disease. Organochlorines have half-lives that are measured in years. Some may be measured routinely in the serum long after exposure has ceased,

FIGURE 3.1. JOB-EXPOSURE MATRIX FOR A RETROSPECTIVE COHORT STUDY OF 4,626 SILICA-EXPOSED WORKERS.

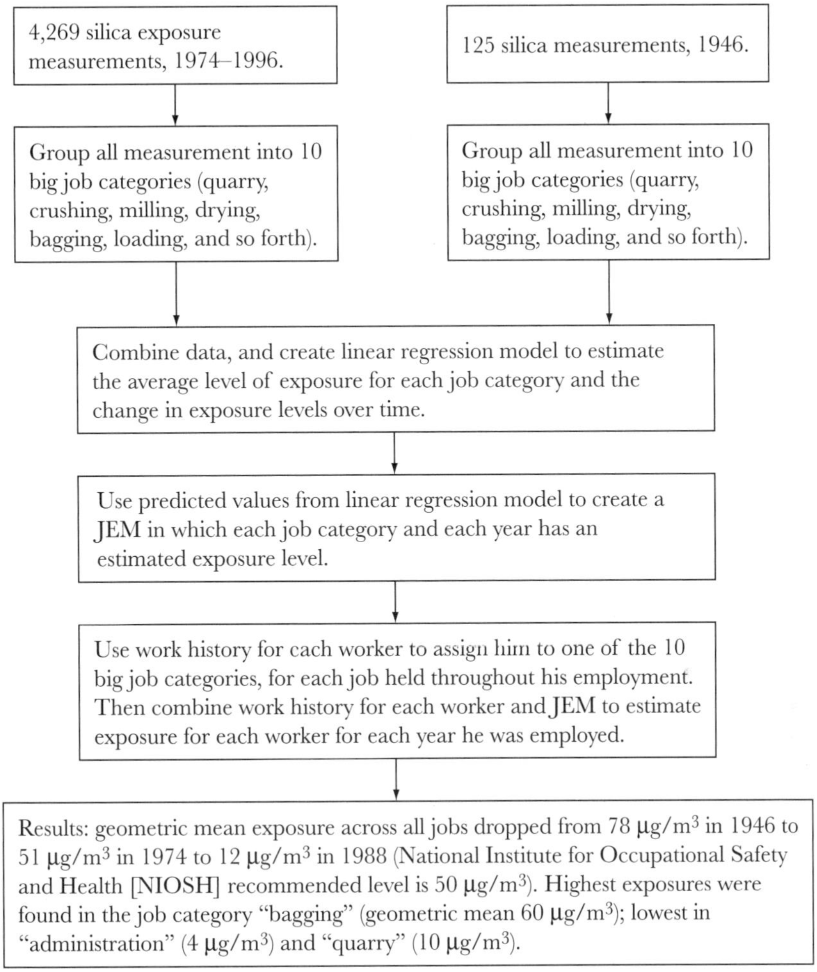

Source: Adapted from Steenland, Sanderson, and Calvert, 2001; Sanderson, Steenland, and Deddens, 2000.

and therefore this measurement may be more useful in detecting exposures above background level. DDE, for example, the principal metabolite of the pesticide DDT, can be measured today in the serum of most of the U.S. population even though DDT use was phased out in the 1970s. In contrast many other organochlorine pesticides phased out at the same time, such as dieldrin and aldrin, have shorter half-lives and are nondetectable in most of the U.S. population. PCBs were also phased out in the 1970s. The heavier PCBs (more highly chlorinated) can be measured in older Americans, but the lighter ones are usually nondetectable.

Another important example is lead, often measured in the blood, where its presence reflects exposure over the previous two or three months. However, lead also accumulates in the bone, where it provides a good measure of cumulative exposure over time, even long after exposure ceases. This has been important in measuring the association between lead and neurological deficits in children. This subject has been controversial for several reasons. Most studies are cross-sectional, and current blood lead levels may not reflect past exposure. Lead and SES are closely related, and SES in turn is closely related to performance on cognitive tests. Lead in teeth shed by children has been useful in establishing prior lead exposure and can act as a measure of the levels of exposure in groups that are identical in SES. Similarly, bone lead, measured by radiographic techniques, has been important in studies of past lead exposure in adults in relation to blood pressure and other long-term effects of lead.

Boxes 3.1 and 3.2 present detailed examples of occupational and environmental epidemiology studies.

Box 3.1. Occupational Epidemiology: An Example

We will use the example of the retrospective cohort study of silica-exposed workers, introduced earlier, to review and expand on the concepts we have been discussing. It has long been known that silica causes silicosis, a nonmalignant respiratory disease. This cohort presented two additional outcomes of interest, lung cancer and kidney disease (Steenland, Sanderson, and Calvert, 2001; Steenland and Sanderson, 2001). There was considerable debate about whether silica could cause these diseases.

There were 4,626 workers in the cohort, exposed to silica while producing industrial sand from the 1940s to the 1980s. The average length of exposure was nine years. Complete work history on these workers was obtained from company personnel records, which also provided information on social security numbers, birth dates, race, and sex. The cohort was 99 percent male. Follow-up began at the time of first exposure and continued through 1996. Cause of death, needed to determine who died of lung cancer, was obtained from death certificate information, using the National Death Index, a national registry of deaths. In addition to lung cancer mortality, incidence of nonmalignant kidney disease was studied by matching the cohort with a national registry of patients with end-stage kidney disease. (These are patients whose kidneys have failed; in the United States the government pays for the expensive treatment, either dialysis or transplant, for these patients. As a result there is a national registry of end-stage kidney patients, virtually the only national disease registry in the United States. Other countries have many such national registries, facilitating epidemiology.)

The silica-exposed workers cohort was dynamic; workers could enter the cohort at any time and exit at any time. Exit occurred at death or at the end of the study in 1996. Note that these workers were followed and were at risk of lung cancer and kidney disease after they left work. For acute outcomes, such as work-related injuries, the follow-up period may end when employment ends. Because these workers were followed for different amounts of time, the investigators studied lung cancer *rates* (rather than *risks*) in the exposed cohort, so that the denominator was person-time rather than people.

The comparison population was the U.S. population, with stratification used to control possible confounding by age, race, sex, and calendar time. Lung cancer death rates for the United States were available from national vital statistics. U.S. kidney disease incidence rates are available from the same U.S. registry of end-stage kidney disease used to determine who in the cohort had had kidney disease.

There were 109 deaths from lung cancer, with 68 deaths expected, resulting in a rate ratio of 1.60 (95 percent CI: 1.23–1.93). The workers had a 60 percent higher lung cancer death rate than the U.S. population of similar age, race, and sex. Given that workers smoke more than the general population and that smoking is by far the most important known risk factor for lung cancer, one might question whether the excess lung cancer rate was due to smoking or to silica. Limited smoking data on 346 men were available from the cohort for the years 1978 to 1989. (Such limited data are typical for retrospective studies based on company personnel records.) These data indicated that among cohort members aged twenty-four to sixty-four, 24 percent were never smokers, 41 percent were current smokers, and 35 percent were former smokers. The corresponding percentages for the U.S. male population aged twenty-five to sixty-four in the 1980s were 37 percent, 35 percent, and 28 percent. These smoking differences would be expected to account for an approximately 10 percent higher lung cancer rate among silica-exposed workers as compared to the U.S. population, suggesting that silica exposure rather than cigarette smoking was responsible for most of the observed 60 percent higher lung cancer rate among the workers.

Twenty-three cases of end-stage kidney disease occurred in the cohort versus 11.7 expected for the U.S. population of similar age, race, and sex (rate ratio: 1.97; 95 percent CI: 1.25–2.06).

The availability of exposure estimates enabled the study investigators to conduct detailed exposure-response analyses, which were important in assessing causality as well as quantitative risk. Exposure-response data for lung cancer, silicosis, and kidney disease are shown in Table 3.1, in relation to estimated cumulative exposure to silica. Cumulative exposure was divided into quartiles for analysis, and male workers in the lowest quartile served as the comparison population (rate ratio: 1.0). For lung cancer, cumulative exposure was estimated using a fifteen-year lag, under the assumption that the last fifteen years of exposure before the end of follow-up would not be the cause of the lung cancer seen at the end of follow-up (that is, allowing for a fifteen-year latency period). All three outcomes show a positive trend in rate ratios with increased cumulative exposure, strengthening the case for causality. Silicosis deaths are included as a kind of validity check on the exposure estimates, because they would

TABLE 3.1. RATE RATIOS FOR LUNG CANCER MORTALITY, SILICOSIS MORTALITY, AND END-STAGE KIDNEY DISEASE INCIDENCE IN A COHORT OF 4,626 SILICA-EXPOSED WORKERS.

	Exposure Levels			
Outcomes	**Lowest Quartile**	**Quartile 2**	**Quartile 3**	**Highest Quartile**
Lung cancer (15-year lag)	1.00 (17 deaths)	0.78 (21 deaths)	1.51 (20 deaths)	1.57 (16 deaths)
End-stage kidney disease	1.00 (2 cases)	3.09 (5 cases)	5.22 (6 cases)	7.79 (5 cases)
Silicosis	1.00 (1 death)	1.22 (2 deaths)	2.91 (4 deaths)	7.39 (7 deaths)

Source: Data from Steenland, Sanderson, and Calvert, 2001; Steenland and Sanderson, 2001.

be expected to show a positive trend (note that although the numbers of silicosis deaths are small, many more workers had silicosis than died from it). The probabilities that the observed positive linear trends in lung cancer, end-stage kidney disease, and silicosis occurred by chance (trend tests) were .07, .0004, and .00001.

Box 3.2. Environmental Epidemiology: An Example

Studies of recreational water quality provide an interesting example of many of the principles and challenges of environmental epidemiology. The number of gastroenteritis outbreaks associated with recreational water exposure has been steadily increasing since 1989 (Lee and others, 2002) and has prompted closer examination of the risk factors leading to both endemic and epidemic waterborne disease associated with exposure to recreational waters (also see Chapter Eighteen). Many epidemiological studies of recreational water quality and gastrointestinal illness have been conducted (reviewed in Pruss, 1998; Wade, Pai, Eisenberg, and Colford, 2003). The basic research approach is typically a cohort study. Swimmers and nonswimmers are recruited into the study at a recreational water site and are interviewed about their swimming exposure on that day. Water samples may be collected. Participants are later interviewed regarding disease incidence following the swimming, and swimmers are compared to nonswimmers.

Gastroenteritis is the most common adverse health outcome due to water contamination and has been the most frequently studied. Most studies have collected data on self-reported symptoms by means of a standardized questionnaire or interview. The exposure of interest is water with fecal contamination, because of the fecal-oral transmission route of enteric pathogens.

Misclassification or mismeasurement of exposure is likely to be the most common problem in these studies and can be due to error in assessing water quality (owing to the use of poor microbial indicators or poor water sample storage and analyses) or to error in classifying the degree of individual water contact. These biases are likely to be random and nondifferential, biasing results toward the null.

Selection bias may occur in several ways. Recruitment of the study population at a beach may result in a study population that is not representative of the general population. For example, regarding external validity, tourist populations at a beach may have higher attack rates than local populations have, affecting the generalizability of results. Regarding internal validity, selection of a nonexposed group that systematically differs from the exposed group may cause bias that cannot be corrected by controlling for measured confounders in the analysis. There is a debate whether the nonexposed group should be nonswimmers or swimmers in cleaner water.

Confounding may occur, for example, due to exposures to enteric pathogens through alternative routes (food and drink) or due to socioeconomic factors that may be related both to exposure and to disease. Seasonality and water temperature may also act as confounders if the study takes place over different seasons or over different days with different water temperatures.

A recent study by Haile and others (1999) illustrates these concepts. The purpose of this study was to examine the risks of gastrointestinal illness associated with swimming in marine waters that received untreated runoff from storm drains in Santa Monica Bay, near Los Angeles. The specific study questions were

> "Are there different risks of adverse health outcomes among subjects swimming at different distances from the storm drains?"
>
> "Are risks of specific health outcomes associated with the concentration of specific bacterial indicators of water quality or with the presence of enteric viruses?"

The study team interviewed subjects at three Santa Monica Bay beaches. These beaches had a wide range of microbial indicator counts and high swimmer density. A total of 22,085 subjects were interviewed between June 25 and September 14, 1995, and 17,253 of them were eligible and able to participate. Subjects were eligible if they had a telephone, spoke English or Spanish, and had not been swimming at the study beaches or in heavily polluted areas within the seven days before the beach interview. A total of 15,492 subjects (90 percent of the eligible subjects) agreed to participate in the study and were asked to provide information about their age, residence, and swimming experience on that day (whether they swam and if so where, and whether they immersed their heads into the water). The locations of the storm drains were identified, and the interviewer categorized the swimmer's location by distance from the storm drains (the categories were 0, 1–50, 51–100, and 400 yards from a drain) and noted gender and race of each subject. Follow-up interviews were conducted by telephone nine to fourteen days after the beach interview and asked about the occurrence of fever, chills, eye discharge, earache, ear discharge, skin rash, infected cuts, nausea, vomiting, diarrhea, diarrhea with blood, stomach pain, coughing, nasal congestion, and sore throat. *Highly credible gastrointestinal illness* (HCGI) was defined as having one or more of the following: (1) vomiting, (2) diarrhea and fever, or (3) stomach pain and fever. The investigators were able to contact 13,278 subjects (86 percent) for follow-up interviews. During these interviews, 1,485 subjects were excluded because they swam at a study beach or in heavily polluted waters between the day of the beach interview and the telephone follow-up and it would not be possible to determine whether any symptoms they reported at the interview were due to their exposure on the day of the beach interview (when the water quality was measured) or due to subsequent exposures. An additional 107 subjects were excluded because they did not immerse their faces in the ocean water during swimming.

Water samples were collected on the same days that subjects were recruited at the beaches. Samples were collected from each exposure category location (distance from drains) and were analyzed for commonly used microbial indicators of water quality: total coliforms, fecal coliforms, enterococci, and *E. coli,* using standard membrane filtration techniques. Additional water samples were collected on weekends from three storm drain sites and analyzed for culturable enteric viruses.

Because the study population was restricted to swimmers, the analyses compared symptom rates and HCGI rates among groups of swimmers: comparing swimmers >400 yards away from the storm drains to swimmers closer to the storm drains and comparing swimmers in waters with different prespecified levels of microbial indicators. For example, enterococci exposure categories were set to ≤35 colony forming units (cfu) per 100 ml (the EPA guideline for marine recreational water; U.S. EPA, 1986), 35–104 cfu/100 ml, and >104 cfu/100 ml. The investigators reported that distance was a "reasonably good" surrogate for bacterial indicator levels and that higher concentrations of indicators were observed near the storm drains (although these data were not shown). All analyses adjusted for the following potential confounders: age (categorical), sex, beach, race, place of residence (California versus out of state), and concern about potential health hazards at the beach (categorical).

The rates of several symptoms and HCGI (331 cases) were higher among people who swam near the drains compared to the rates for those who swam at least 400 yards away from the drains. The adjusted relative risks ranged from about 1.2 for eye discharge, sore throat, and HCGI to 2.3 for earache. Positive associations were also observed between various symptoms and higher levels of specific microbial indicators. Swimmers within 50 yards of the storm drains on days when enteric viruses were detected in the water samples (386 swimmers) reported elevated rates of HCGI and several other symptoms compared to the rates for those who swam near the storm drains on days when enteric viruses were not detected (3,168 swimmers). Adjusted relative risks ranged from about 1.2 for cough, diarrhea, and chills to 1.9 to 2.3 for eye discharge, vomiting, and HCGI. However, there were no clear dose-response patterns across increasing levels of microbial indicators, and none of the elevated relative risks was statistically significant. The investigators concluded that the strength and consistency of the associations they observed across several measures of exposure suggest that there is an increased risk of adverse health effects associated with swimming in marine waters that receive untreated urban runoff, despite the lack of dose-response patterns (possibly due to misclassification of exposure) and the lack of statistical significance.

Although this study had the advantage of a large sample size, it seems likely that there were problems with misclassification of exposure. No data were provided on the results of the microbiological analyses of the beach water. What was the range of water quality to which study subjects were exposed? How much variation was there between water samples taken at different locations from a single beach on a single day, and how well do these samples reflect the water quality to which a swimmer is actually exposed at the location and time he or she is swimming? There can be substantial temporal and spatial variations in water quality, especially open bodies of water with currents. How frequently were high levels of microbial contamination measured, and how closely did that reflect the presence of fecal contamination and microbial pathogens?

There may have been individuals in the low-exposure reference group (those who reported swimming at the greatest distance from the drains) who may have been exposed to high levels of pathogens either because they swam near the drains without observing that they did so or because water currents had moved slugs of contaminants to the area where they were swimming. It is also possible that classification of exposure on the basis of bacterial indicator organisms, especially total and fecal coliforms, is a poor surrogate for exposure to viral and protozoan pathogens that move differently and persist longer in the aquatic environment. Several previous studies have reported no significant relationships between symptom rates and fecal indicator bacteria, and Pruss (1998) asserts that the use of microbial indicators is one of the major sources of bias in epidemiological studies of recreational water quality and health. In the study discussed here, Haile and others (1999) attempted to measure enteric viruses but did not show any data on how frequently they detected viruses in the water samples or on the efficacy of their virus detection methods. Detecting enteric viruses in environmental water samples is difficult.

A recent meta-analysis of twenty-seven studies of recreational water quality and gastrointestinal illness concluded that despite significant heterogeneity among the studies, the results generally supported the EPA guideline levels for *E. coli* in freshwater and enterococci in marine waters (Wade, Pai, Eisenberg, and Colford, 2003). The authors noted that the studies that reported elevated relative risks tended to be those that used a nonswimming control group, focused on children, or used study populations from athletic or other recreational events instead of populations recruited at a beach. This observation shows how study design features can affect the observed association between water quality and gastrointestinal illness, presumably by introducing selection biases affecting either external or internal validity. Wade, Pai, Eisenberg, and Colford (2003) argue that if measuring the risks associated with swimming is the goal of the study, then nonswimmers are the appropriate control group and that using a control group of swimmers may underestimate the risk of recreational water contact and result in regulatory guidelines that are too high (lenient). Nonswimming controls used by other studies have been family members or others at the beach who did not swim (parents and so forth), bystanders at or organizers of athletic or recreational water events, or participants in a related recreational event that did not include swimming (Wade, Pai, Eisenberg, and Colford, 2003). However, Haile and others (1999) defended their use of a swimming control group (those who swam >400 yards away from the storm drains or those in the lowest bacterial indicator exposure category) on the grounds that restricting the study to swimmers reduced the potential for confounding (that is, subjects who swim are different from subjects who choose not to swim). Future studies could attempt to collect more information on swimmers and nonswimmers in order to ensure that these groups have similar age distributions and risk factors.

Epidemiology and Risk Assessment: Determining Permissible Levels of Exposure

The results of occupational and environmental epidemiological studies can affect public health by alerting policymakers to new hazards and possibly by triggering regulations about permissible levels of exposure. Sometimes a single large and definitive study is deemed sufficient to change public policy, but in other instances regulators want to see the study's results replicated (recall Hill's criterion of consistency). When a number of studies point in the same direction, public authorities are more likely to act.

In the past, qualitative literature reviews were used to summarize the evidence across many studies. Today one is more likely to see a quantitative meta-analysis that provides a weighted average of quantitative results across studies. Meta-analyses were originally used to examine results of clinical trials, but they have been used extensively for observational studies in the last decade. Meta-analyses can combine results from different study designs: for instance, rate ratios from cohort studies and odds ratios from case-control studies. For example, a meta-analysis may give a weighted average of lung cancer rate ratios or odds ratios across many studies of silica and lung cancer (actually, the logarithms of the ratio measures are used and then converted back to the original scale at the end). The weights are typically the inverse of the variance of each study's result; this means that the largest studies with the narrowest confidence intervals, those that are estimated more precisely, will have the lowest variance and the most weight.

Meta-analyses do not require access to the original study data; results from the published literature can be used. A variant method of summarizing data across studies is a pooled analysis, in which the raw data for each study are obtained and the combined data are then reanalyzed. Pooled analyses are much more time consuming but have the advantage of providing more flexibility in the analysis.

Meta-analyses are most often done to determine a common ratio measure (such as a rate ratio) of disease rates in the exposed versus the nonexposed. However, they may also be done to determine a common exposure-response coefficient across a number of exposure-response analyses.

Exposure-response analyses are of particular interest to public health authorities who seek to determine a permissible exposure level for the public or for workers. The determination of a permissible exposure level relies on risk assessment (discussed in detail in Chapter Thirty-Two). Risk assessment may be based on animal data or human data. The former requires extrapolation from animals to humans, and hence involves a considerable amount of uncertainty. For this reason human (epidemiological) data are preferred, but they may not exist for the agent in question. When epidemiological data do exist, results giving the increased rate of disease per unit of exposure (exposure-response data) for an exposed population must typically be converted to the excess risk of disease over a lifetime for an individual exposed to a specific agent. The level of exposure that limits excess lifetime risk to a specific level, typically somewhere in the range of 1 in 100,000 to 1 in 1,000, is then determined to be permissible. For workers the Occupational Safety and Health Administration (OSHA) typically seeks to limit risk to 1 in 1,000, a higher risk than is usually accepted by the EPA, under the assumption that workers voluntarily accept a somewhat higher risk. The conversion of rates to risk can be done with simple formulas.

There are often two issues of particular concern to risk assessors working with epidemiological exposure-response models. The first is the shape of the exposure-response curve. When data are sparse, or sometimes even when they are not, it may be difficult to choose between competing models that have very different consequences for permissible limits. Typical questions involving model selection might be whether the exposure-response shows a linear increase in disease rates per unit of exposure, whether or not there is a threshold below which there is no risk followed by an increase, or conversely, whether there is a cutpoint above which disease risk begins to flatten out or even decrease. The threshold question usually involves the nature of the exposure-response relationship in the low-dose region, where there may be few data. This question often occurs when occupational epidemiological studies (involving high exposure) are used in risk assessment for general environmental exposures (to diesel fumes, dioxin, asbestos, and so forth).

For example, a risk assessment in which these issues occurred examined cancer subsequent to dioxin exposure, based on a study of 3,538 workers (Steenland, Deddens, and Piacitelli, 2001). Most workers were exposed to dioxin several orders of magnitude above typical environmental levels, raising questions about the extrapolation of results to low-dose levels. However, there were some data in the low-dose range, allowing some confidence in such an extrapolation. A model using the log of cumulative exposure produced estimated risks in the low-dose region that were ten times higher than the risks that the linear model predicted in that region. A doubling of background levels in the serum (10 parts per trillion [ppt] versus 5 ppt), such as might occur due to high fish consumption (dioxin intake in the general public is due primarily to the diet), resulted in an increase in lifetime risk of cancer mortality of about 0.9 percent using a model with the log of cumulative exposure and of about 0.05 percent using a linear model. The background risk of death from cancer by age seventy-five is 12 percent for males and 11 percent for females.

Conclusion: Future Directions in Environmental and Occupational Epidemiology

Occupational epidemiology is becoming less concerned with exposures to toxins, which are less and less prevalent in the workplace. Instead, interest has focused more on exposures that affect a large number of workers. One such exposure is job stress, which is difficult to measure but may have large consequences via increasing blood pressure or cardiovascular disease. Results to date for a link between job stress and blood pressure are tantalizing but far from conclusive; potential confounding by socioeconomic status is a major issue in studies of job stress. Shift work and noise exposure are related exposures that may result in stress and increased blood pressure. Another related exposure is the loss of employment, which may in turn increase stress.

Another area of large concern is ergonomics. Musculoskeletal injuries such as low back pain and carpal tunnel syndrome are extremely common in the workplace and result in a large economic burden of disability. Epidemiological studies relating specific work practices to these musculoskeletal outcomes are difficult to design and conduct. Nonetheless, the evidence to date clearly implicates forceful repetitive motion in carpal tunnel syndrome. The epidemiological evidence for low back pain is somewhat less conclusive but also points to awkward lifting postures as a contributor.

When toxins do continue to be of concern in the workplace, epidemiologists are increasingly concerned with risks of subclinical outcomes among the exposed workers, outcomes that may or may not have long-term consequences. Examples of these outcomes are cytogenetic changes such as sister-chromatid exchange and chromosomal aberrations (future cancer risk?), excess small protein in the kidney (future kidney disease?), and the presence of autoantibodies in the serum (future autoimmune disease?).

Another trend is the assessment of gene-environment interactions. For example, subjects with high levels of PCBs in their serum may be at risk for Parkinson's disease only if they have a certain genetic polymorphism.

These trends are occurring primarily in developed, industrialized countries (where epidemiology is more commonly practiced). In less developed countries large numbers of people are still experiencing very high levels of exposure to classic occupational toxins. In many of these situations what is needed is hazard surveillance and control rather than new epidemiological studies.

One problem that affects occupational epidemiology in the United States, and to some extent all countries, is the increasing difficulty of conducting workplace studies at all. In many instances permission from the employer is required, and the spread of market economies, coupled with the relative weakness of organized labor, has meant decreased emphasis on workplace health and safety and increased difficulty in conducting occupational studies.

As for environmental epidemiology, low-level exposure to common toxins continues to be of interest in determining whether such exposure contributes to background endemic disease rates. Arsenic in the water, PCBs in the diet, mercury in the air, and small particulates in the air are just a few of the agents of interest. The difficulty of conducting conclusive epidemiological studies of such agents and the potentially large public health consequences continue to lead to increasingly sophisticated studies. In addition to these by now classic problems, newer issues are arising. Global warming is now largely accepted as a real trend by the scientific community (see Chapter Eleven). However, the health effects of such warming have yet to be documented. Indeed, it is not clear what the endpoints are for such studies (the presence of malaria in previously unaffected regions?), and often the appropriate study designs may not be apparent. Lack of a protective ozone layer in certain parts of the world is another recent issue. Other issues are even newer, such as how to measure the health effects of an urban environment with more parks and less pavement (see Chapter Twenty-Seven).

Thought Questions

1. Suppose you want to determine whether dioxin causes cancer in humans. (It is a strong animal carcinogen.) Dioxin was a contaminant of some herbicides commonly used in the past in the United States and also in Vietnam during the Vietnam War. These herbicides have not been made since the 1970s. However, dioxin persists in human tissues for a long time (half-life is seven years). It

can be found in the blood in very low levels in the general population (largely from dietary consumption of low levels), and in high levels in Air Force personnel who sprayed herbicides in Vietnam, and in high levels in workers who made the herbicides. What population might you study? Who would be the exposed and who the nonexposed, and how would you define or measure "exposure"? How would you measure cancer occurrence? What study design would you use?

2. Suppose you want to study whether environmental tobacco smoke (ETS) causes heart disease. ETS exposure occurs among both smokers and nonsmokers who are around tobacco smoke. However, smokers have much higher levels of chemicals from cigarettes than do nonsmokers who are exposed to ETS. In what population would you choose to study ETS? Who would be the exposed and who would be the nonexposed? How would you measure exposure? What would be your heart disease outcome and how would you measure it? What would be your study design?
3. We rely on both human evidence (from epidemiology) and animal evidence (from toxicology) to clarify the health effects of toxic exposures. Although each provides valuable information, each has advantages and disadvantages. Please compare and contrast the two kinds of evidence and explain their relative merits.

References

Caldwell, G. "Twenty-Two Years of Cancer Cluster Investigations at the Centers for Disease Control." *American Journal of Epidemiology,* 1990, *132* (suppl. 1), S43–S47.

Dietrich, K. N., and others (Treatment of Lead-Exposed Children Clinical Trial Group). "Effect of Chelation Therapy on the Neuropsychological and Behavioral Development of Lead-Exposed Children After School Entry." *Pediatrics,* 2004, *114*(1), 19–26.

Haile, R. W., and others. "The Health Effects of Swimming in Ocean Water Contaminated by Storm Drain Runoff." *Epidemiology,* 1999, *10,* 355–363.

Hill, A. B. "The Environment and Disease: Association or Causation?" *Proceedings of the Royal Society of Medicine,* 1965, *58,* 295–300.

Jordan, C. M., and others. "A Randomized Trial of Education to Prevent Lead Burden in Children at High Risk for Lead Exposure: Efficacy as Measured by Blood Lead Monitoring." *Environmental Health Perspectives,* 2003, *111,* 1947–1951.

Lanphear, B. P., Eberly, S., and Howard, C. R. "Long-Term Effect of Dust Control on Blood Lead Concentrations." *Pediatrics,* 2000, *106*(4), e48.

Lee, S. H., and others. "Surveillance for Waterborne-Disease Outbreaks—United States, 1999–2000." *Morbidity and Mortality Weekly Report: CDC Surveillance Summaries,* 2002, *51*(SS08), 1–28.

Markowitz, M. E., Sinnett, M., and Rosen, J. F. "A Randomized Trial of Calcium Supplementation for Childhood Lead Poisoning." *Pediatrics,* 2004, *113*(1, pt. 1), e34–e39.

Pruss, A. "Review of Epidemiological Studies on Health Effects from Exposure to Recreational Water." *International Journal of Epidemiology,* 1998, *27,* 1–9.

Rom, W. (ed.). *Environmental and Occupational Medicine.* (3rd ed.) Philadelphia: Lippincott-Raven, 1998.

Rothman, K. "A Sobering Start for the Cluster Busters' Conference." *American Journal of Epidemiology,* 1990, *132* (suppl. 1), S6–S13.

Rothman, K., and Greenland, S. *Modern Epidemiology.* (2nd ed.) Philadelphia: Lippincott-Raven, 1998.

Sanderson, W., Steenland, K., and Deddens, J. "Historical Respirable Quartz Exposures of Industrial Sand Workers: 1946–1996." *American Journal of Industrial Medicine,* 2000, *38,* 389–398.

Schulte, P., Ehrenberg, R., and Singal, M. "Investigation of Occupational Cancer Clusters: Theory and Practice." *American Journal of Public Health,* 1987, *77,* 52–56.

Steenland, K., Deddens, J., and Piacitelli, L. "Risk Assessment for 2,3,7,8-*p*-Dioxin (TCDD): Based on an Epidemiologic Study." *American Journal of Epidemiology,* 2001, *154,* 451–458.

Steenland, K., Loomis, D., Shy, C., and Simonsen, N. "Review of Occupational Lung Carcinogens." *American Journal of Industrial Medicine,* 1996, *29,* 474–490.

Steenland, K., and Sanderson, W. "Lung Cancer Among Industrial Sand Workers Exposed to Crystalline Silica." *American Journal of Epidemiology,* 2001, *153,* 695–703.

Steenland, K., Sanderson, W., and Calvert, G. "Kidney Disease and Arthritis Among Workers Exposed to Silica." *Epidemiology,* 2001, *12,* 405–412.

U.S. Environmental Protection Agency. *Bacteriological Water Quality Criteria for Marine and Fresh Recreational Waters.* EPA-440/5-84-002. Cincinnati, Ohio: Office of Water Regulations and Standards, U.S. Environmental Protection Agency, 1986.

Wade, T. J., Pai, N., Eisenberg, J.N.S., and Colford, J. M., Jr. "Do US Environmental Protection Agency Water Quality Guidelines for Recreational Waters Prevent Gastrointestinal Illness? A Systematic Review and Meta-Analysis." *Environmental Health Perspectives,* 2003, *111,* 1102–1109.

Whittemore, A., and McGuire, V. "Observational Studies and Randomized Trials of Hormone Replacement Therapy: What Can We Learn from Them?" *Epidemiology,* 2003, *14,* 8–10.

For Further Information

Checkoway, H., Pearce, N., and Kriebel, D. *Research Methods in Occupational Epidemiology.* (2nd ed.) New York: Oxford University Press, 2004.

Rothman, K., and Greenland, S. (eds.). *Modern Epidemiology.* (2nd ed.) Philadelphia: Lippincott-Raven, 1998.

Steenland, K., and Savitz, D. (eds.). *Topics in Environmental Epidemiology.* New York: Oxford University Press, 2000.

CHAPTER FOUR

EXPOSURE ASSESSMENT, INDUSTRIAL HYGIENE, AND ENVIRONMENTAL MANAGEMENT

P. Barry Ryan

This chapter introduces a set of concepts and activities that are at the core of environmental health: recognizing, measuring, and ultimately controlling hazardous exposures. Our account begins with industrial hygiene, a technical field that evolved in industrial workplaces. Then it moves beyond industrial hygiene to describe a modern field active both in the workplace and the general environment: exposure assessment.

Industrial hygiene and exposure assessment share a common task: quantifying hazardous exposures. This task is relevant both to public health practice and to research. In public health practice, quantifying exposures helps people to assess potential problems, direct preventive efforts and check their success, and monitor compliance with regulations. Quantifying exposures is also essential in research, because it allows investigators to quantify the association between the exposures and health outcomes. Knowing, for example, that carbon monoxide is an asphyxiant is only so useful. Knowing *how much* carbon monoxide exposure can be tolerated and how much is dangerous, and knowing how to measure the exposures where and when they occur, enables us to understand the biological effects more completely, identify acceptable levels and set standards accordingly, and monitor environments to be sure they are safe.

But even though they share a common task, industrial hygiene and exposure assessment differ in an important way. Industrial hygiene has traditionally moved beyond measuring exposures to controlling them. An industrial hygienist in a factory would typically monitor air levels of, say, hazardous solvents, and if they were excessive in a particular part of the factory, she or he would implement controls, such as substituting a safer solvent, upgrading the ventilation system, or providing personal protective equipment for affected workers. An exposure assessor, in contrast, would specialize only in measuring and quantifying exposures (often in a research setting), and responsibility for controlling excessive exposures would rest with other professionals.

Anticipation, Recognition, Evaluation, and Control

Industrial hygiene has been defined as the . . . "science and art devoted to the anticipation, recognition, evaluation, and control of those environmental factors or stresses arising in or from the workplace that may cause sickness, impaired health and well-being, or significant discomfort among workers or among citizens of the community . . . " (American Industrial Hygiene Association, quoted in Plog, Niland, and Quinlan, 1996, p. 3). Industrial hygienists are the professionals who manage workplace risks, together with allied professionals such as occupational physicians and nurses. Industrial hygiene has been practiced in the United States for almost 100 years. Historically, the profession's paradigm was summarized as "recognition, evaluation, and control," but in recent years this has been expanded to "anticipation, recognition, evaluation, and control." Under this paradigm the industrial hygienist aims to predict and then recognize hazards in the workplace, measure the magnitude of exposure, and implement appropriate control strategies. Koren and Bisesi (1996) have developed concise definitions of each part of this paradigm. They define *anticipation* of occupational hazards as "proactive estimation of health and safety concerns that are commonly, or at least potentially, associated with a given occupational or environmental setting" (p. 471). *Recognition* of occupational hazards is the "identification of potential and actual hazards in a workplace through direct inspection" (p. 471), which emphasizes that empirical observation is at the heart of industrial hygiene. *Evaluation* includes measuring exposures through "visual or instrumental monitoring of a site" (p. 472). Finally, *control* is the "reduction of risk to health and safety through administrative or engineering measures" (p. 473). Industrial hygiene is by its nature a field discipline, and industrial hygienists spend much of their time in workplaces, observing, measuring, and problem solving. As they do so, each element of the paradigm is part of their approach.

Anticipation

Anticipation may be viewed as the *pre-preliminary* assessment before going into the field. Prior to visiting a workplace the industrial hygienist typically receives some information about it, such as the history of the site, the manufacturing processes in place, the job titles employed, and the chemicals in use. Given this information and a general knowledge of the industry, the hygienist can develop a preliminary list of potential health and safety hazards, including those confined to the workplace (occupational hazards) and those that may migrate over the fence line to nearby rivers, woodlands, or communities, becoming environmental hazards.

Industrial hygienists divide occupational hazards into two focus areas: safety and health. Examples of *safety hazards* are insufficient emergency egress, slippery surfaces and other risks of trips and falls, and chemical storage that poses a fire or explosion risk. Moving machinery, unguarded catwalks, and moving vehicles such as forklifts come under this safety hazard heading. Although these concerns are also the domain of a related profession, *safety engineering*, many industrial hygienists handle safety concerns as part of their job, especially at smaller facilities where they need to be jacks of all trades.

Health hazards in the workplace are highly varied. They may include *physical hazards*, such as high noise levels, elevated temperatures and humidity, and radiation. Physical hazards may also include repetitive motion such as typing or hand tool use, which can increase the risk of work-related musculoskeletal injuries such as shoulder pain or carpal tunnel syndrome. *Chemical hazards* can result from many workplace processes and may be acute or chronic. Acute high-level exposures to certain highly toxic chemicals, such as chlorine gas, may result in acute and chronic health effects, disability, and even death. Such events must be clearly anticipated and controlled. More common are long-term exposures leading to chronic effects. Some effects, such as neurological damage from solvent exposure, have been well established through occupational epidemiological investigations. For example, long-term exposure to benzene increases the risk of bone marrow dysfunction and aplastic anemia, a blood disease characterized by reduced amounts of several lines of blood cells. Other examples are the increased risk of asbestosis in asbestos workers, silicosis in foundry workers, and lung cancer in uranium miners.

In modern industrial hygiene the industrial hygienist is often called on to anticipate *environmental hazards* as well as those in the workplace. Environmental hazards may endanger safety (as when a chlorine tank ruptures and neighbors are exposed to toxic gas), health (as when a plume of organic wastes from improper disposal at a factory contaminates groundwater and enters people's wells), and welfare (as when smokestack emissions damage nearby trees or homes). Environmental effects may also include ecological damage (as when the oxygen-carrying ability of a local water supply is harmed) and economic damage (as when industrial discharges contaminate nearby land with heavy metals, industrial solvents, or pesticides, to the point that the land can no longer be used for residential or recreational purposes). The industrial hygienist should anticipate such possibilities and design a preliminary investigation to address such concerns. This may include reviewing many aspects of a factory's operations. For example, if records or employee interviews suggest that hazardous materials were stored inappropriately in years past, then these materials may have seeped into the ground and migrated off site, contaminating groundwater. The hygienist who suspects widespread contamination may consult an environmental specialist with expertise in environmental exposure assessment.

Boxes 4.1 and 4.2 present examples of evaluations performed by an industrial hygienist, emphasizing the opportunities to anticipate hazards. These examples show that even with minimal information, the industrial hygienist can anticipate hazards and devise a reasonable plan of attack prior to visiting a facility. This strategy requires examining all available information before visiting the site: the industrial process description, the job titles of workers in the facility, the chemicals in use at the facilities (often available on *material safety data sheets*), and the history of the site. With this information in hand, the industrial hygienist can develop a list of potential health and safety hazards, perhaps in checklist form to permit the recording of observations during her or his *walk-through* visit. During this plant visit, unanticipated hazards may of course become apparent as well.

Box 4.1. An Electronics Manufacturing Facility

An industrial hygienist is asked to evaluate an electronic manufacturing facility and to focus on occupational hazards. She is told of several operations performed at this workplace that may have health impacts. Solvent degreasing (to clean metal pieces) and acid etching may expose workers to chemicals, various machines and cutting tools are in use, and some workers perform repetitive operations with their hands and arms.

Solvents such as trichloroethylene, acetone, and stoddard solvent are used extensively for degreasing in industry. Most facilities have a single room in which these materials are used. The industrial hygienist, taking a prudent approach, anticipates the potential in this room for spillage, respiratory exposure (perhaps due to inadequate ventilation), and skin contact (perhaps due to improper handling or inadequate personal protective equipment). Further, on-site storage areas for solvents may result in occupational exposure and, over time, contamination of the surrounding environment. The industrial hygienist plans for close inspection of solvent use and storage areas in this facility. Her anticipated concerns with acid-etching activities are similar, even though the occupational and environmental outcomes are likely to be different. The industrial hygienist is also concerned with the specific activities associated with acid etching, the storage of used materials and acids on site, and the potential for environmental contamination and effects.

At least some workers perform repetitive operations as part of their jobs. The industrial hygienist anticipates problems associated with such activities. She arranges to observe the repetitive activities to assess the potential for associated musculoskeletal damage. This will be an essential part of the walk-through she does at the facility. Similarly, she plans to inspect machine operations for electrical safety, the presence of unguarded cutting edges, risks of crush injury, and so on.

The industrial hygienist will also review administrative procedures that may bear on risk. Are workers trained in safety procedures? Do records of injuries on the job suggest that injuries are excessive in this facility? Are chemical inventories carefully tracked and accounted for?

Finally, the industrial hygienist anticipates that there may be hazards not mentioned in the initial request, hazards of which the company may be unaware or that personnel may take for granted. Examples are safety hazards involving fire exits, fire potential, and potential for trips and falls. Her walk-through visit will include attention to all such hazards.

This facility may be looked on as a prototype of an industrial manufacturing setting. In such a case the industrial hygienist may visit the facility with a checklist of potential or expected hazards. Some of the potential hazards may be present in a specific situation, others may be absent, and still others may be controlled. Only direct inspection (or evaluation, as discussed later in this chapter) can lead to a direct conclusion about control strategies.

Box 4.2. Leaking Underground Storage Tanks at an Old Gas Station

An industrial hygienist is asked to evaluate an abandoned gas station in a residential setting where, he is told, gasoline and oil leakage has been noted. Further, he is told that there is housing nearby and associated with this housing is a drinking-water well field that supplies drinking water for some part of the local area. How does he anticipate potential hazards in such a situation?

This is not a classical industrial hygiene problem, but more and more industrial hygienists are seeing such problems in their daily work. The facility is no longer in operation and therefore does not have any occupational hazards associated with it; its hazards are now in the realm of *environmental hygiene.* Because of this, the industrial hygienist may wish to contact an environmental consultant for added insight. However, the industrial hygienist can identify numerous anticipated hazards.

Judging by the information given to the hygienist, the most important consideration is the leakage of gasoline and oil from the facility. It is critical then for him to evaluate the magnitude of the leakage and determine how long this leaking has been going on. Underground storage tanks may leak undetected for months or even years. Because housing and a superficial well field are close to the location, such leakage has the potential for serious environmental consequences, such as property damage, well contamination, and even closure of the wells. The industrial hygienist therefore prepares to evaluate the extent of the contamination upon reaching the site. Has the contaminant plume migrated off site? If so, how far? Are homes in danger? Is there sufficient hazard to merit evacuation and immediate cleanup? Has the well field been affected? If so, are all the wells contaminated? Time is of the essence in addressing these concerns.

Recognition

Once an industrial hygienist has anticipated the potential hazards associated with a facility, the next step is recognition of the hazards. The initial recognition phase is usually accomplished during a site visit or walk-through, a visual inspection of the facility. The purpose of the walk-through is to gather both qualitative and quantitative information about occupational and environmental hazards. The industrial hygienist reviews the various processes and procedures at the facility, the job categories, the number of workers in each job category and their job descriptions, and any health and safety programs in place at the plant. She or he identifies hazardous physical, chemical, and biological exposures and the ergonomic, mechanical, and psychological factors affecting the workplace. Visual inspection might reveal such hazards as exposed machinery, pinch points, sharp edges or blades, unsecured tip-over hazards, high noise levels, and the presence of chemicals. A similar review of environmental hazards might be undertaken with an emphasis on off-site emissions.

Another important aspect of the walk-through is recognition of the subpopulations in the facility. For example, certain workers may be exposed to ergonomic hazards because they perform lifting activities or repetitive movements as part of their jobs. A second group may experience few of these hazards but may work in a high-temperature area and may be subject to heat stress. A third group may confront neither of these exposures but may work with industrial machinery and be exposed to safety hazards. During a walk-through the industrial hygienist notes these subpopulations and might choose to evaluate hazards differently for each group.

At the end of the recognition phase, the industrial hygienist should have a detailed picture of the manufacturing processes and of the associated hazards and a plan for evaluating these hazards. This plan is written down, and a detailed protocol is developed for the next phase, the *evaluation* of the hazards.

Evaluation

At this point the industrial hygienist has a list of potential hazards in the facility but no quantitative information about the degree of worker exposure. Even when a metalworking facility uses toxic degreasing solvents, the risk of exposure may be minimal with proper storage and handling and appropriate ventilation. The evaluation phase actually begins during the walk-through, and there is a smooth transition from the recognition of hazards to their evaluation.

The evaluation component focuses on quantifying the degree of exposure. As described later in the section on exposure assessment, the hygienist may choose to measure exposures in a particular part of the workplace (*area sampling*), in the immediate vicinity of individual workers (*personal sampling*), or even in the bodies of individual workers (*biological sampling*).

Population Sampling for Exposure Evaluation. Initially, the hygienist needs to determine which workers' exposures to study. The focus may be on certain workers with specific job titles. For example, degreasers may be monitored for solvent exposure, and forklift drivers or package handlers may be monitored for ergonomic exposures. In some industries, especially those with widespread or serious hazards, evaluation may involve all employees at a facility or even all workers in a specific industry, such as workers in asbestos-related industries or in industries where radiation is present, such as nuclear power generation. In industrial settings monitoring is sometimes performed at the request of a local union. In this case the union may have specific concerns and may ask for monitoring of all its members. Although the industrial hygienist may offer guidance and suggest monitoring only specific subpopulations, she or he may have to defer to the requirements of the union.

Once the population has been selected, the next choice is the type of population sample to be taken. For small facilities, or in facilities where regulation requires it, a *census* sample should be taken. In such a sample, all potentially exposed individuals are monitored. However, in larger facilities this can be very expensive, and a statistically representative subsample can characterize the exposure of all the individuals in the group. Each individual monitored represents a known number of individuals in the same class. For example, if a given airline has 10,000 flight attendants, it may be impractical to monitor each of them for exposure to ozone during flights. So the industrial hygienist may instead choose to monitor a subset of, say, 500 individuals, selected to be statistically representative of the full 10,000. This type of measurement is subject to sampling error because not all the exposed people are monitored. However, techniques are available for determining the magnitude of this error. The industrial hygienist, working with statistician colleagues, can determine the adequacy of any sample size for predicting exposures for the entire population.

A third type of population often used is the *anecdotal,* or *convenience,* sample. Often such a sample consists of volunteers or individuals with a particular complaint. This type of sampling is subject to bias; there is no reason to believe that volunteers or those with complaints typify the other members of the group. This sampling strategy should be avoided. However, a related sampling strategy may have a role. The hygienist may select *worst case* sampling. This involves sampling those workers at highest risk of exposure or sampling at times when exposure is most likely (or doing both), on the theory that if these worst case exposures are shown to be well controlled, then the remaining workers or workers present at other times are also unlikely to be overexposed.

Instruments for Exposure Evaluation. Two general types of instruments are available for measuring environmental exposures: direct reading instruments and sample collection instruments. *Direct reading instruments* provide real-time measurements of the parameter of interest, and *sample collection instruments,* as the name implies, collect samples for later analysis.

Direct reading instruments are useful for measuring many physical hazards, such as temperature, noise, and radiation. These instruments typically have a dial or digital readout, and some have the ability to store data collected over a period of time for later downloading. Common examples are digital thermometers, to measure temperature; hygrometers, to measure relative humidity; noise monitors; and radiation monitors based on the Geiger counter principal. Such instruments are portable, often weighing less than a kilogram, and are usually enclosed in a rugged carrying case, allowing easy transport to field sites.

Direct reading instruments are also available for measuring levels of many airborne pollutants, including gases, vapors, and particles. For example, organic vapors are measured with photoionization detectors, and particulate matter with light-scattering devices. Other types of monitors are also available for specific compounds. A limitation in using these instruments is that the character of the airborne pollutant must be known before monitoring can be carried out. In industrial hygiene applications this often offers no difficulty as one specific compound is of concern or a particle of a specific size is produced by the process under investigation.

Sample collection instruments are used instead of direct reading instruments when multiple airborne pollutants are present or further analysis of samples is desirable. In this case the instrument collects a sample of air—with whatever contaminants are in it—on an absorbing medium. The absorbing medium is then taken to the laboratory, and the amounts of the compounds of interest are determined.

The air delivery-absorber system is generally one of two types, active or passive. In an *active* system, air is drawn through the absorbing medium by an electric pump. The amount of air drawn through is controlled by the pump and can be varied. The total volume of air sampled can be calculated by multiplying the air flow rate by the duration of sampling, and when the mass of contaminant on the sampling medium is later quantified, its concentration in the air, in units of mass per volume, can be readily calculated. The sampling time period can be shortened by increasing the pump flow rate, thereby delivering the same amount of air in less time—a useful maneuver when exposure durations are short or are highly variable.

There are distinct disadvantages to active sampling. Chief among them is the presence of the pump, which requires electricity to run and is often bulky. Both of these drawbacks make such devices unsuited to many kinds of personal sampling. Often, active sampling is limited to area sampling, which means that the samples are not identical to what the individual worker experiences as contaminant exposure. Two active sampling devices are shown in Figure 4.1. The sampling devices themselves (for ozone and particulate matter) and the pump are located inside the box at the bottom of the apparatus. The vertical pipe with the metal cone on top is a device designed to collect particles that are inhalable deeply into the lung. The device includes as size-selection sampling head designed to allow particles smaller than a certain diameter to pass through to the particulate sampler. Ozone is sampled off the same air stream.

Passive sampling devices require an absorbing medium that removes the compound of interest from the air by reaction or absorption. This process takes advantage of the concentration gradient between the air to be sampled and the surface of the absorbing medium. Because of this concentration gradient, the compound of interest diffuses from the air to the surface of the absorbing medium, from which it is then removed. Analysis of the concentration is accomplished in a manner similar to that used in active sampling; the amount of the compound gathered in the absorbing medium is determined in the laboratory, and the amount of air delivered to the surface is computed using Fick's law of diffusion. The concentration in the air during the sampling period is then calculated by dividing the amount of material on the absorbing medium, as determined in the laboratory, by the volume of air passed through the system to the absorber. Most industrial hygiene applications use this type of system.

Passive devices have the advantage of not requiring a pump but the disadvantage of slow sampling rates, often 1,000-fold slower than active samplers. Thus the amount of material sampled in a given time is substantially lower. However, in occupational settings, concentrations are often sufficiently high to allow the industrial hygienist to use passive devices and still achieve excellent results. When

FIGURE 4.1. AIR POLLUTION SAMPLING APPARATUS FOR OZONE AND PARTICULATE MATTER.

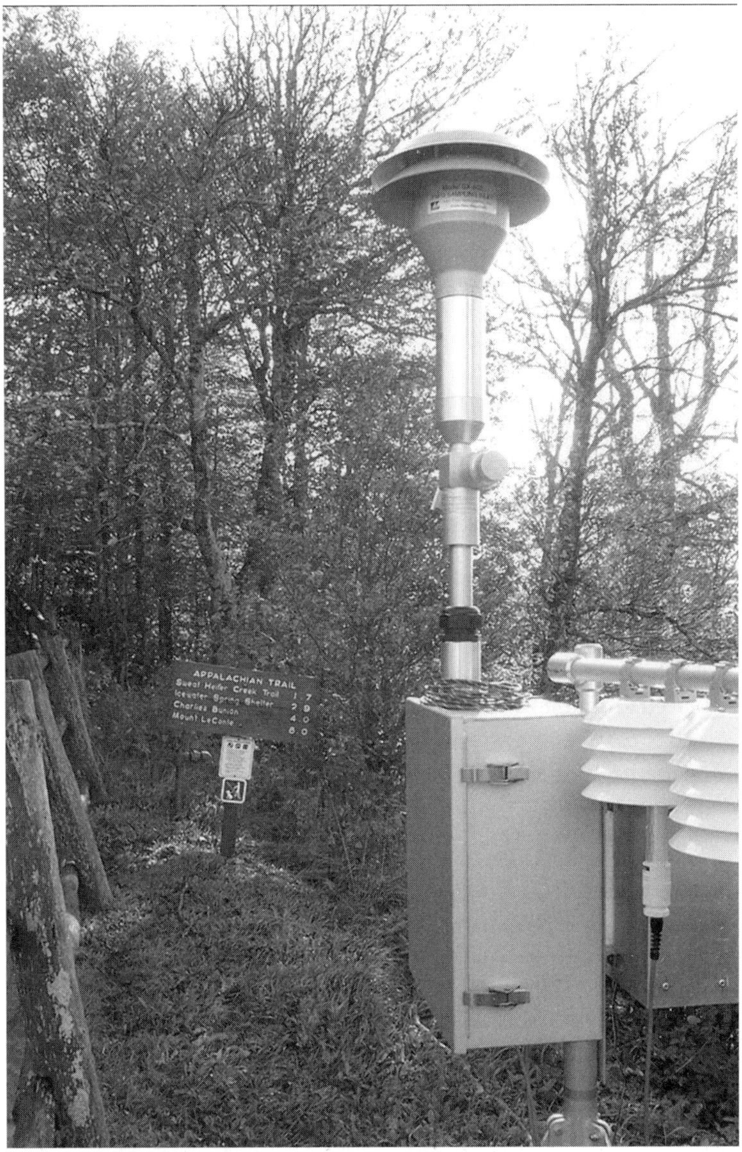

available, and of sufficient precision and accuracy, passive sampling devices can be the method of choice. The industrial hygienist developing a monitoring system should be cautious, however. Passive devices do not exist for every contaminant of interest. In particular, passive devices for particulate matter are not yet of sufficient precision and accuracy to merit their use in typical occupational settings, although this too is changing.

Biological monitoring, discussed later, is of interest to the industrial hygienist as well. In such monitoring programs, biological samples, such as hair, saliva, blood, or urine, are collected from potentially exposed individuals and analyzed for either the compound of interest or a metabolite of that compound. Such techniques are well established for only a few compounds, but in the circumstances where such techniques exist, they often offer the best solution for a monitoring program.

Control

The final component of the industrial hygiene paradigm is the control of the hazards. In public health terms this corresponds to *primary prevention,* a central goal. Industrial hygienists take several approaches to modifying the workplace environment: substitution, isolation, and ventilation. *Substitution* involves replacing a hazardous material or process with a less hazardous one. For example, benzene (a bone marrow toxin) might be replaced by toluene. *Isolation* involves containing or limiting access to the hazardous process. For example, a metal cage might be placed around moving parts to reduce the likelihood of clothes catching on a part and causing injury to the worker. For certain hazards, most notably chemical and heat-related hazards, *ventilation* offers a viable control strategy. Introduction of fresh air, local exhaust ventilation, or introduction of cool air to a hot location may significantly alter the risk associated with exposure.

Protective devices are often used to control safety hazards. For example, a worker operating a cutting machine may need to push two buttons, one with each hand, to initiate a cut; this guarantees that neither hand will be in the cutting zone when the machine functions. Similarly, a power cutoff may be installed that automatically shuts off the supply of electricity to a machine when it is entered for maintenance. This prevents unintentional start-up of the machine, which would be hazardous to maintenance workers. *Personal protective equipment,* such as respirators, gloves, safety glasses, hard hats, safety harnesses, and steel-toed boots, may also be recommended, although this approach is less preferable than the environmental changes just described. Figure 4.2 shows an example of personal protective equipment in use. Working at a solvent degreasing tank, the worker is subjected to elevated levels of vapor exposures if not protected. The worker wears personal

FIGURE 4.2. PERSONAL PROTECTIVE EQUIPMENT FOR SOLVENT EXPOSURE.

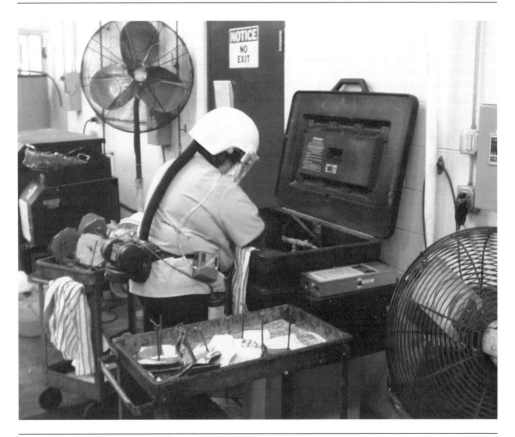

Source: Courtesy of Dr. Philip Williams, University of Georgia.

protection equipment consisting of a face shield to protect the face from splashed solvent and a fresh air supply supplied by a pump (on the worker's back), which is delivered through a plastic hose to dilute the solvent vapors being breathed. The exposure is monitored using the pump and collection device mounted on the worker's hip.

Administrative strategies, such as rotating workers through dangerous jobs to limit any individual's aggregate exposures (used, for example, with radiation workers), sometimes have a role as well. These strategies, and the philosophy that guides choosing among them, are discussed in further detail in Chapter Twenty-Nine.

Exposure Assessment

Industrial hygiene focuses on workplace exposures. Although such exposures are often quite high and therefore of great scientific and public health interest, they affect only a subset of the population. Environmental health scientists are also concerned about exposures among the community as a whole. The study of exposures in nonoccupational settings grew out of the industrial hygiene experience. As early as the 1950s, environmental health scientists turned their attention from high-level workplace exposures to lower-level community exposures to the same chemicals. These efforts gave rise to the science of *exposure assessment.*

Exposure assessment focuses on quantifying the contaminant exposures experienced by individuals as they go about their daily activities. In performing this quantification, key concepts include concentration, exposure, and dose. These concepts are defined in Box 4.3.

Box 4.3. Concentration, Exposure, and Dose

A starting point for exposure assessment is to ask how much of a contaminant is found in environmental media—what, for example, is the level of lead in workplace air or the level of pesticides in food? These parameters are usually measured as *concentration,* expressed in units of mass per mass or mass per volume. Air contaminants, for example, may be quantified in units of micrograms (μg) of contaminant per cubic meter (m^3) of air ($\mu g/m^3$). In measures of air concentrations of gases, the units often express a mixing ratio—the fraction of total air that is made up of the contaminant gas, usually expressed as parts per million (ppm) or parts per billion (ppb). For example, suppose a carbon monoxide (CO) level is measured at 1 ppm. This means that in a given volume of air divided into one million portions of equal volume, one part would be CO and the remaining 999,999 parts something else. In one cubic meter of air, for example, one cubic centimeter (cm^3 or cc) would be CO (and nitrogen and oxygen would be about 780,000 cc and 210,000 cc, respectively). Of course all these parts are mixed together—there is not 1 cc of pure CO; rather, the CO molecules are dispersed throughout the entire cubic meter. Although 1 ppm sounds like a very low concentration, for many air contaminants it is sufficient to threaten health.

Concentrations are measured similarly in other environmental media, including water, soil, and food. Contaminant concentrations in water are expressed in terms of either micrograms of contaminant per cubic meter of water or micrograms of contaminant per gram of water. The first is similar to expressing air concentrations, and the second is analogous to the mixing ratio in air (because 1 μg of contaminant per gram of water is a ratio of masses, corresponding to 1 ppm). Similarly, soil or food, both being solids, can be described using either unit.

But concentration is different from exposure; the mere presence of a contaminant at some concentration does not necessarily imply that people will be exposed. *Exposure* is defined as contact between the environmental contaminant and a boundary of the subject of interest. Although ecological exposure assessment is an important area, this discussion focuses on human exposures. Thus the boundaries of interest are tissues such as skin, alveolar surfaces, and the gastrointestinal tract lining, which separate the "inside" of a human receptor from the "outside," the rest of the environment. Exposure requires the simultaneous presence of a contaminant and a human receptor in the same environment.

If a person is indeed exposed, the exposure is a function of the concentration and of time. Therefore exposures are expressed in units of concentration multiplied by time, such as (μg/m^3)(hours). When a contaminant is ingested, the temporal component appears in the computation as the number of meals or the total mass taken into the body.

Just as concentration is different from exposure, exposure is different from dose. The *dose* is the amount of contaminant that crosses the epithelial barrier and gets inside the body. Suppose a person is exposed to an air contaminant concentration of 100 μg/m^3 for a period of 10 hours (and suppose that inhalation is the only significant exposure route; ingestion and dermal contact do not contribute to exposure). The concentration then is 100 μg/m^3, and the exposure is (100 μg/m^3)(10 hours)= (1000 μg/m^3)(hours of exposure). What is the dose? Here additional information is needed. The dose is delivered to the lungs through breathing. A typical breathing rate (depending on the person's size, level of activity, and other factors) might be 1100 cc/breath and 15 breaths per minute, or approximately 1 m^3 of air per hour. During a 10-hour period, this person would breathe in 10 m^3 of air. The dose is the product of the concentration, the duration of exposure, and the rate at which the material reached the appropriate boundary:

$$Dose = \frac{\mu\text{g(contaminant)}}{\text{m}^3\text{(air)}} \times 10\text{(hours of exposure)} \times \frac{1\ \text{m}^3\ \text{(air breathed)}}{\text{hour of exposure}}.$$

$$Dose = 1000\ \mu\text{g (contaminant breathed)}.$$

In this case, 1000 μg of contaminant has reached the body boundary. This is the potential dose. Assuming all the material crosses the boundary, this is the dose. Note that the units correspond to the amount of mass delivered across the boundary. There is no explicit time dimension.

From an exposure assessment point of view, investigators often stop at the potential dose, that is, the amount of material that reaches the body boundary over a fixed period of time. However, absorption is typically incomplete, and the *biologically relevant dose* or *dose to the target organ* may be lower than the entire potential dose. Toxicologists, physicians, and other health scientists may focus on the actual dose absorbed as they study the relationship between exposure and health effects (see Chapter Two).

Suppose a worker is required to enter a tank that was formerly filled with a volatile solvent. The enclosed space is saturated with the solvent vapor. What is the concentration in the tank, the worker's exposure, and her dose?

The concentration in the tank is relatively simple to understand; it is the saturation vapor pressure of the organic solvent. This can be readily measured using appropriate instrumentation.

What is her exposure? This is a more difficult question. In this occupational setting the worker would doubtless be fitted with a respirator that supplied air from outside the tank, as it would be much too dangerous to send an individual into such an enclosed space without such a device. Under these conditions (assuming a functioning respirator), her inhalation exposure would be zero because no solvent vapor would reach her lung epithelium. However, she might receive an exposure to her skin, and dermal exposure may be an important route. It is important to consider all routes and attempt to identify all pathways to exposure.

And what is her dose? Understanding the dose requires understanding how much material actually crosses the boundary and gets inside the body. If the worker did not wear a respirator, one could infer the inhaled dose by knowing the concentration and breathing rate. One would also need information regarding the efficiency of transfer across the alveolar membranes in the lungs. Similarly, calculating the dermal dose would combine information about the concentration in the air, the amount of exposed skin area, and the efficiency of skin absorption. A biomarker of exposure—say, blood levels of the solvent or urinary levels of its metabolite—would provide an estimate of the dose that integrated all this information.

Figure 4.3 shows an example of exposure measurement. Here a worker is using a sandblaster to remove silica-containing material from a pipe. Because inhalation of silica can cause severe respiratory problems, the worker is using an airline respirator that supplies fresh air through the pipe going off to the right; the worker receives no exposure to silica dust. However, the worker is still exposed to potentially hazardous noise from the sandblaster. To test for this hazard, the worker wears a noise monitor (the small rectangular box attached near the small of the worker's back).

Exposure Magnitude, Frequency, and Duration

An important aspect of exposure is its time course, sometimes referred to as the exposure profile. Intuitively, one might infer that a brief but very high-level exposure to a contaminant would have a different impact on health than would exposure to a modest concentration over an entire work shift, even assuming equivalent total exposures. For example, a worker welding for 15 minutes in an enclosed space might be subjected to a concentration of metal fumes of 40 mg/m^3. He thus receives an exposure of $40 \text{ mg/m}^3 \times 0.25 \text{ h} = 10 \text{ mg/m}^3 \times \text{h}$. After welding,

FIGURE 4.3. ASSESSING EXPOSURE IN AN OCCUPATIONAL SETTING.

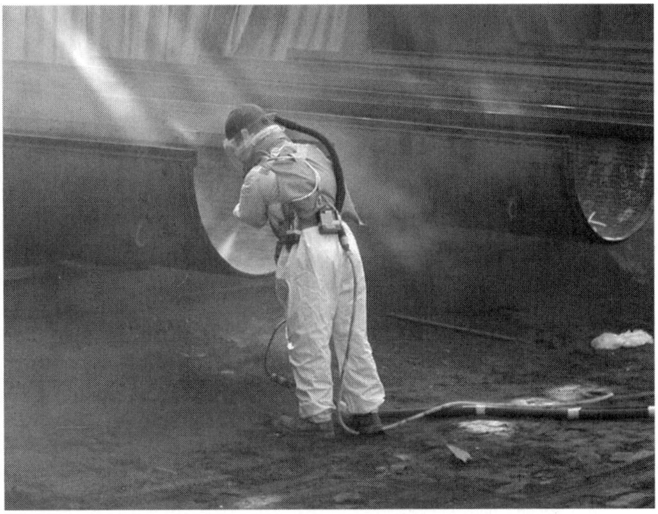

Source: Courtesy of Dr. Philip Williams, University of Georgia.

he goes on to different activities in a different part of the facility in which he experiences no concentration of welding fumes and thus receives no further exposure during the shift. His coworker, working in the welding area but not exposed directly to the fumes, remains there for the entire 8-hour shift. Measurement of metal fume concentrations over the course of the day in the location of the second worker gives 1.25 mg/m^3. The worker in this location receives an identical exposure: 1.25 mg/m^3 $\times$ 8 h = 10 mg/m^3 $\times$ h, but the pattern is different.

This issue is important because some contaminants are relatively readily metabolized, or cleared, at low levels of exposure but toxic at higher levels of exposure. In other words, the *dose rate* may affect the health outcome. To account for such differences, exposure assessors focus on the magnitude, frequency, and duration of exposure, asking such questions as: What is the *peak concentration* experienced during the monitoring period? Does it differ significantly from the mean concentration? How frequently are high concentration peaks found? Are the concentrations relatively stable, or is there variability from minute to minute or hour to hour? Do the peaks recur regularly, or episodically? What is the duration of the exposure? Is it short followed by no exposure, or does it occur at moderate levels for a long period? Such information can prove invaluable in addressing potential effects and control strategies.

Exposure assessors distinguish acute exposures from chronic exposures. *Acute* exposures are brief, and when they occur at high levels, poisoning or other acute responses may follow. *Chronic* exposures occur over months, years, or even decades. Chronic exposures at low levels may manifest nonacute health outcomes: carcinogenesis or long-term lung damage, for example. Intermediate between these two exposure categories are *subchronic* exposures, which may occur over intermediate time scales, often weeks or months, and also may be episodic and recurring.

Exposure Routes and Pathways

As explained in Chapter Two, environmental contaminants enter the body through one of three principal *routes of exposure*: inhalation, ingestion, and dermal contact. (Other routes, such as injection or ocular absorption, may be important in some circumstances, and transplacental transfer is important for the fetus.) It is important to distinguish between these routes of exposure and a related term, the *exposure pathway*, or the path by which the contaminant moves from a source to a human receptor. For example, sulfur dioxide exposure may result from distinct pathways. It may be generated through the combustion of sulfur-containing coal, followed by the concomitant release of this gas from the combustion facility and advection and dispersion in the air. Alternatively, an industrial process might use sulfurous acid with the concomitant release of sulfur dioxide at an individual workstation, exposing the worker directly. These two pathways differ substantially and require entirely different control strategies to reduce exposure.

Exposure Assessment Methods

Just as there is a continuum from concentration to exposure to dose (see Box 4.3), there is a corresponding continuum of exposure assessment methods. The ideal method quantifies the amount of contaminant reaching the target organ of interest in each individual of interest, but this is of course not feasible in most cases. Four broad categories of exposure assessment methods can be identified, forming a continuum from least to most accurate: imputing or modeling exposures, measuring environmental exposures, measuring personal exposures, and measuring biomarkers. In general as the methods become increasingly accurate they also become increasingly expensive.

Imputing or Modeling Exposures. To impute exposures, researchers use *indirect exposure assessment methods* that either forgo direct measurements of the exposures of interest or that use partial data. For example, in a study of air pollution exposure, researchers might identify various microenvironments thought to have relatively homogeneous concentrations and measure those concentrations. Research subjects could record the amount of time they spent in each of the microenvironments (or the researchers could estimate this time). The researchers would then multiply the concentrations by the amount of time spent in each microenvironment, and sum the results for an estimate of each subject's overall exposure. For other routes of exposure, a similar approach can be used. For example, for ingestion, concentrations of selected contaminants can be measured in each of many foods. A research subject can then record types and amounts of foods eaten, using a food diary. Summing the concentrations over all the foods eaten gives the dietary exposure.

An alternative strategy, called *exposure scenarios,* does without direct measurement. In this strategy an activity pattern for an individual is assumed, perhaps based on observational data about population activity patterns. Available monitoring data for each activity and location can then be combined with activity data to model estimates of individual exposures. This approach is less expensive to implement because no individuals actually have their exposures measured and no specific activities are recorded. Exposure scenarios are used extensively in risk analysis.

A special case of indirect exposure assessment is the *job-exposure matrix.* Suppose an occupational epidemiologist wants to study the health effects of silica exposure in a working population, using a retrospective cohort approach. Consulting old employment records the epidemiologist might identify ten different job categories, each with characteristic tasks, and fifteen different workplace zones, each with its own silica concentrations. (Historical industrial hygiene monitoring results may help the epidemiologist to reconstruct this information and to estimate concentrations in each part of the workplace.) The epidemiologist could then construct a job-exposure matrix that retrospectively assigns an exposure level for each worker, based on his or her job assignment and location in the workplace (see Chapter Three). If the workplace changed over time, as is typical, then the epidemiologist would create a *job-time-exposure matrix,* classifying each worker's exposure according to job title, location in the plant, and calendar year. In this fashion the epidemiologist could impute an exposure profile to each member of the cohort. This method is often the only available way to assess exposures in retrospective epidemiological studies. However, it is painstaking and time consuming, and records are not always accurate or complete enough to support accurate exposure assessment.

Although less satisfying than direct exposure assessment, these indirect approaches are often substantially easier to implement, and large populations can be studied more effectively in this manner.

Measuring Environmental Exposures. Direct exposure assessment methods may occur at the area level or at the individual level, as described earlier. An example of environmental measurements is air pollution monitoring, which is carried out in most major cities. Not only does ongoing measurement of air pollutants (such as ozone, nitrogen oxides [NO_x], sulfur oxides [SO_x], and particulate matter) monitor compliance with regulations, it also provides exposure information that can be used to warn the public of dangerous exceedances, to monitor the success of interventions, and to support health research.

Measuring Personal Exposures. Personal exposure assessment involves outfitting an individual with a monitor that measures exposures during daily activities, exactly as is done in the workplace. This procedure is most easily visualized for airborne contaminants. In this case an air monitor collects a sample of the air breathed by the individual over a period of time, and that air sample is analyzed for the contaminant of interest, either on a real-time or time-integrated basis. Similar monitors may be envisioned for exposures occurring via the ingestion or dermal pathways as well. With such direct methods, actual exposures experienced by an individual can be observed. This is a major strength in accessing exposure and is generally desirable. However, portable monitors may not exist for the particular contaminant under investigation, or the presence of the monitor may influence the individual to alter activity patterns, with the result that the activities monitored are not her or his typical ones.

Measuring Biomarkers. Exposure to environmental contaminants requires the simultaneous presence of a contaminant concentration and a human subject to *receive* the exposure. The methods described previously assume that exposure occurs if these two conditions exist. However, the only way to verify this assumption is to measure contaminant levels in humans themselves. This is what exposure assessors do when they use biological markers (sometimes referred to as biomarkers) of exposure. Biological markers of exposure to a given contaminant sample biological material, such as exhaled breath, urine, blood, feces, or hair. These samples are analyzed for the contaminant in question (called the *parent compound*), a metabolite of the contaminant, or a biological response known to reflect exposure. For example, blood lead levels are measured to quantify lead exposure, levels of urinary cotinine (a metabolite of nicotine) are measured to quantify exposure to environmental tobacco smoke, and blood carboxyhemoglobin levels are measured to quantify exposure to carbon monoxide (see Box 4.4). Pesticide exposure offers another example. Blood samples can be taken from individuals and analyzed for organochlorine pesticide parent compounds to ascertain exposure to this class of compound. For organophosphate pesticides, the direct parent compound can be determined in serum, or alternatively, metabolites produced through hydrolysis (for example, dialkyl phosphates) can be used to infer the magnitude and timing of exposures.

Box 4.4. Exposure Assessment of Carbon Monoxide

Carbon monoxide (CO) is a colorless, odorless gas that competes with oxygen for binding sites on hemoglobin. CO binds avidly with hemoglobin, effectively disabling the hemoglobin's oxygen-carrying capacity. If enough CO is inhaled, death can ensue due to asphyxiation.

CO exposure occurs through a single route, inhalation. The pathways are numerous, but all involve incomplete combustion; CO is produced when too little oxygen is present to permit complete conversion of hydrocarbons and oxygen to carbon dioxide and water. Specific pathways often associated with CO poisoning are improperly vented combustion appliances such as gas heaters, improperly vented gasoline engines (automobiles running in closed spaces, for example), or inhalation of cigarette smoke.

Exposure to CO is easily measured in two different ways. Relatively simple air samplers are available that sample for CO in either active mode or passive mode. In active mode, real-time analyzers can give second-by-second readings of CO concentration. Exposure is determined by noting the amount of time spent in the location being measured.

An alternative strategy is to use a biological marker of exposure, namely the blood concentration of carboxyhemoglobin, the CO adduct to hemoglobin. Unexposed individuals typically have about 1 percent carboxyhemoglobin in their blood, due to endogenous production of CO. Smokers carry a higher percentage, as high as 4 percent, due to inhalation of CO in cigarette smoke. Symptoms such as headaches are observed in most individuals with levels above about 10 percent, and levels above 40 percent are not compatible with survival.

Exposure thus defined does not tell the full story of CO's effects, however. Individuals in industrial societies are exposed to modest levels of CO. Regulations are in place to ensure that these levels are kept low enough to hold carboxyhemoglobin levels below the threshold at which effects would be felt. However, multiple scenarios could give rise to the same exposure level. Exposure to 1 ppm of CO for 10,000 hours would give the same exposure as 10,000 ppm of CO for 1 hour. However, the effects would be completely different. Exposure to the former scenario would case no problems at all, whereas exposure to the latter scenario would surely result in death.

This illustration emphasizes the importance of considering the magnitude and duration of the exposure when estimating effects. Further, it emphasizes the importance of understanding the toxicology of the effect under investigation. CO binds reversibly to hemoglobin, albeit with a very long half-life. If only a little CO is around, there is still plenty of hemoglobin left to bind oxygen and carry it to the cells. However, if there is a lot of CO around and it displaces a lot of oxygen from hemoglobin, then there may not be enough oxygen delivered to the cells, and asphyxiation will ensue.

The use of biological markers of exposure has received great attention in the scientific community in the last ten to fifteen years. Biomarkers have the advantage of integrating over all routes of exposure. Further, exposures determined through the use of this method explicitly incorporate the concept of *bioavailability*. Many compounds may enter the body through, for example, ingestion, but the transfer across the gut epithelium may be inefficient, so the relationship between exposure and health outcome is masked. Biological markers overcome this difficulty in that in order for the compound to be measured in the biological medium it must have crossed the boundary, the exposure must have been "effective" in delivering a dose to the body.

Exposure Assessment for Ingestion and Skin Absorption

Much of exposure assessment methodology developed around inhalation exposures. However, the two remaining principal routes of entry, ingestion and skin absorption, are important in many circumstances and pose special challenges for exposure assessment.

One approach to assessing ingestion exposure is to collect duplicate portions of food that is eaten, through what is called a *duplicate diet study*, and analyze the food for contaminant levels. Typically, a researcher would homogenize all of the food eaten, creating a single sample, which is then weighed to determine total mass. An aliquot (fraction) of this food is then analyzed for contaminant content, and the concentration determined. Multiplication of the concentration in the food by the amount eaten yields the total amount of contaminant eaten during the time period—the exposure. (This is not yet a dose, because it measures only what was ingested, not what was absorbed across the epithelial layer, the gut lining.) This straightforward method is an example of the direct method of exposure assessment.

In a second approach to ingestion exposure assessment, people are asked to keep dietary diaries. Simultaneously, various foods are purchased at local grocery stores and brought back to the laboratory for analysis. A data set is then compiled, listing each type of food and its contaminant concentration. The food diary data set can then be combined with the concentration data set to determine the amount of contaminant ingested by the individual. Because the food actually eaten by the individual is never measured, this method is an example of the indirect method of exposure assessment. This technique is quite useful in that food diaries are much easier to administer than duplicate diet studies and thus this technique can be implemented on a large scale. Further, fewer food samples have to be analyzed, as once all the various food items purchased have been assessed, no further analysis is needed. The principal disadvantage of this method is that the individual food items consumed by the participant are not analyzed. If the concentrations in those items differ from the concentrations in the items purchased at the grocery store, then the researcher makes an error in the exposure estimate proportional to the variability in the pollutant concentrations.

Dermal exposures are quite difficult to study. In one method, individuals are asked to wear a patch placed on the skin that absorbs the material of interest, such as a pesticide. The individual then carries out activities while exposed to air containing the pesticide. This may occur for research purposes in a laboratory setting, with known concentrations of pesticide in the air, or it may occur in the individual's normal exposure situations. Either way, the patches are removed from the individual's skin following exposure and analyzed for pesticide concentration. Knowing the size of the patch relative to the total exposed skin surface of an individual, one can estimate overall skin exposure. A second method uses cadaver skin. Pesticide is placed on one side of the cadaver skin, and the penetration of the material through the skin surface is measured.

Each of these techniques has limitations. Experimental use of the patch method is contrived and offers few insights about real-world exposures. Use of the patch in the real world, however, suffers in that many exposures will be below the detection limit of the analytical process yet will still incur the large costs associated with that process. Although of interest, the cadaver skin method measures dose and provides little information on exposure. Further, cadaver skin may not act the same way living skin does with a given exposure level, calling into question the dose determination also.

Conclusion

Industrial hygiene, the anticipation, recognition, evaluation, and control of workplace hazards, presents a paradigm for the study of the more general discipline of environmental exposure assessment. Many of the tools of industrial hygiene are easily transferable to environmental exposure assessment, but the latter requires some new tools as well. The four-step paradigm must be integrated into the community setting. Sampling strategies, compliance with monitoring protocols, and field implementation are often more difficult in community exposure assessment studies, and call for statistical sampling techniques more commonly found in epidemiological studies. Exposure assessment is a rapidly growing area, ripe for contributions from professionals in many areas of environmental health. Research and professional practice in this area will continue to grow for the foreseeable future.

Thought Questions

1. Exposure assessment faces challenges in the community setting that differ from the challenges encountered in the workplace setting. Describe the differences.
2. Exposure assessment is essential to environmental epidemiology. Agree or disagree, and explain your answer.
3. Biomarkers of exposure offer many advantages over environmental sampling. Explain these advantages.
4. Biomarkers of exposure may function very differently in the age of genomics. Do a literature search on the role of genetic polymorphisms in interpreting biomarker data, and summarize your findings.

References

Koren, H., and Bisesi, M. (eds.). *Handbook of Environmental Health and Safety: Principles and Practices.* 2 vols. (3rd ed.) Boca Raton, Fla.: CRC Press, 1996.

Plog, B. A., Niland, J., and Quinlan, P. J. *Fundamentals of Industrial Hygiene.* (4th ed.) Itasca, Ill.: National Safety Council, 1996.

For Further Information

A standard reference in industrial hygiene, in addition to the two works cited above, is

Harris, R. L. (ed.). *Patty's Industrial Hygiene.* 4 vols. (5th ed.) Hoboken, N.J.: Wiley, 2000.

Overview of Exposure Assessment

Zartarian, V. G., Ott, W. R., and Duan, N. "A Quantitative Definition of Exposure and Related Concepts." *Journal of Exposure Analysis and Environmental Epidemiology,* 1997, *7*(4), 411–437.

Biomarkers of Exposure

Gil, F., and Pla, A. "Biomarkers as Biological Indicators of Xenobiotic Exposure." *Journal of Applied Toxicology,* 2001, *21*(4), 245–255.

Godschalk, R. W., Van Schooten F. J., and Bartsch, H. "A Critical Evaluation of DNA Adducts as Biological Markers for Human Exposure to Polycyclic Aromatic Compounds." *Journal of Biochemistry and Molecular Biology,* 2003, *36*(1), 1–11.

Metcalf, S. W., and Orloff K. G. "Biomarkers of Exposure in Community Settings." *Journal of Toxicology and Environmental Health Part A,* 2004, *67*(8–10), 715–726.

Wessels, D., Barr, D. B., and Mendola, P. "Use of Biomarkers to Indicate Exposure of Children to Organophosphate Pesticides: Implications for a Longitudinal Study of Children's Environmental Health." *Environmental Health Perspectives,* 2003, *111,* 1939–1946.

Job-Exposure Matrices

Coughlin, S. S., and Chiazze, L., Jr. "Job-Exposure Matrices in Epidemiologic Research and Medical Surveillance." *Occupational Medicine,* 1990, *5*(3), 633–646.

Plato, N., and Steineck, G. "Methodology and Utility of a Job-Exposure Matrix. *American Journal of Industrial Medicine,* 1993, *23*(3), 491–502.

CHAPTER FIVE

ENVIRONMENTAL PSYCHOLOGY

Daniel Stokols
Chip Clitheroe

Environmental psychology focuses on behavior in its sociophysical environment. The field of environmental psychology assumes that a dynamic and reciprocal relationship exists between individuals and groups and the environments in which they live, work, play, learn, recreate, and travel (see Box 5.1). To an environmental psychologist, environmental health and well-being are the result of an appropriate and supportive *fit* between an individual or group and the places and people with whom they interact as they go about their lives.

Box 5.1. A Trio of Tripping Pedestrians

Pat tripped first. She had stepped off this curb hundreds of times, and if you'd asked her, she would have told you that it was a little higher than the normal curb. But today she'd been seriously distracted—she was deeply involved in a conversation with her boyfriend who had asked her to marry him the night before.

Joe stumbled next. He was new to the big city. He had been gawking at the fast-moving traffic, tall buildings, and rushing throngs on their way to work. In the quiet suburbs where he lived, there weren't many pedestrians, and the curbs were all exactly the same height.

Mark was the last to stumble. He considered himself an excellent athlete but had twisted his ankle last night sliding into second base, trying to stretch a single into a double in the recreational softball league, and was using one of his father's canes this morning. He didn't misgauge the height of the curb—he planted the cane awkwardly in the street and almost lost his balance.

The street maintenance workers watching these behaviors concluded that the curb was unsafe and needed modification because it was a public health hazard.

Environmental psychologists study the myriad ways in which sociophysical milieus, or *contexts,* affect individuals and groups, including affecting their health. The factors involved may include the kind of dwelling in which an individual resides, social and physical aspects of his or her neighborhood, and features of his or her commute between home and work. But environmental psychology is about more than objective descriptions of these factors. An individual's perceptions or feelings about each of these factors are likely to have an important bearing on his or her emotional and physical well-being. An understanding of environmental perceptions and feelings is also within the province of environmental psychology.

Environmental psychologists approach *contexts* as holistic, complex, naturally occurring, time-dependent entities. Moreover, they view the social and physical dimensions of *settings* as highly interdependent (hence the term *sociophysical* environment) and as jointly influencing an individual's psychological and physical well-being. As opposed to traditional approaches to public health, environmental psychology focuses on *all* those factors that might influence an individual's health, including aspects of the physical and ambient environments, social relationships, and anything else that might result in environmental stress. A more encompassing term, *environment and behavior studies (EBS),* is sometimes used to refer to this field (Stokols, 1995).

This chapter explores key concepts, methods, and findings in the field of environmental psychology and their relevance to environmental health. The following approaches are typical of the field of environmental psychology:

- Research in the field of environmental psychology is centrally concerned with the behavioral, emotional, and health outcomes of people's transactions with their everyday environments (called *settings*). These environments may include residential, occupational, educational, recreational, public, and virtual places (Barker, 1968; Bechtel, 1997; Gifford, 1997; Proshansky, Ittelson, and Rivlin, 1976; Stokols and Montero, 2002).
- Research in this field favors naturalistic field studies over controlled laboratory experiments.
- Environmental psychology emphasizes a multidisciplinary perspective, including all the branches of psychology, environmental design (architecture, landscape architecture, interior design, and urban planning), geography,

sociology, human ecology, natural resources management, government, and public health.

- Environmental psychologists study behavioral and health outcomes in relation to both the objective features and subjective meanings of built and natural environments.
- Environmental psychology focuses on *users*—anyone who comes in contact with or interacts with a context.
- Environmental psychologists examine behavior within relevant time intervals. These *events* have naturally occurring beginnings and endings, and the relationship between contextual factors and health conditions and outcomes can change during the event (Clitheroe, Stokols, and Zmuidzinas, 1998).
- Environmental psychologists emphasize a holistic approach to understanding the environment's impact on individuals; that is, they consider the effects of multiple settings and contextual factors over time and these factors' cumulative or joint influences on health.
- The field of environmental psychology has always been committed to understanding and responding to important societal issues, including public health.

The field of environmental psychology thus offers a valuable reservoir of conceptual insights, methodological tools, and empirical findings for broadening the scope of environmental health practice and assisting it in becoming even more relevant to the present and future concerns of the field of public health.

Box 5.2. The Trio of Tripping Pedestrians Revisited

Pat's, Joe's, and Mark's well-beings were apparently threatened by a curb. But was this an accurate conclusion? Pat had stepped off that curb successfully hundreds of times—her well-being was in fact threatened this morning by a lack of attention that had nothing to do with the physical setting. Joe's well-being was threatened by his being a first-time visitor to the big city—in environmental psychological terms, by his lack of an adequate cognitive schema describing a dense urban setting and his status as a first-time wayfinder. Mark's health had already been affected by his recreational escapades of the night before. His stumbling had nothing to do with the curb but rather with his temporary disabled status and inability to plant the cane tip firmly in the street. The environmental psychologists who had also been observing this behavior had chosen to observe the interaction between the setting and its users from a distance, so that they wouldn't affect the natural interaction occurring in the context. They concluded that the curb at this location was not really the problem but that modifying it and adding wheelchair-accessible, curb-cut ramps would facilitate safer interactions between the curb and all its users.

Environmental Psychology: Expanding the Perspective of Environmental Health

The field of environmental health has focused largely on the deleterious effects of people's exposure to toxins, pathogens, radiation, and other hazardous conditions of the physical environment (Detels, McEwen, Beaglehole, and Tanaka, 2002; Koren and Bisesi, 2002; Yassi, Kjellström, de Kok, and Guidotti, 2001). Environmental psychology is more broadly concerned with conceptualizing, measuring and evaluating complex environmental settings such as buildings, neighborhoods, and public places and the ways these influence behavior, health, and well-being. Environmental psychologists consider health to be more than the absence of illness or injury and, to include both physical and psychological well-being, or wellness.

The field of environmental health began to expand beyond its longstanding concern with the negative health effects of physical hazards, toxins, and pathogens at the same time as the field of environmental psychology began to emerge as a viable discipline—in the turbulent social change and ecological awareness of the 1960s. During this period, for example, Cassel (1964, 1976) urged public health researchers to give greater attention to the crucial role of social relationships in moderating individuals' resistance to hazardous environments. Cassel's research signaled a shift from *germ theory* accounts of health and illness (focusing on the adverse effects of specific pathogens once they invaded a human *host*) toward a social epidemiological model of public health and disease prevention.

During the 1980s, Lindheim and Syme (1983) reiterated Cassel's call for greater emphasis on social factors in health and highlighted the joint influence of multiple environmental dimensions (that is, the natural, social, symbolic, and built environment) on emotional and physical well-being. More recently, Frumkin (2001, Chapter Twenty-Nine) described the "greening of environmental health" and underscored the importance of documenting the positive health outcomes associated with people's exposure to natural landscapes and wilderness settings. He has also identified several facets of healthy places and cited evidence suggesting that individuals' *sense of place* substantially affects their mental and physical well-being (Frumkin, 2003).

These and other efforts among researchers to broaden the scope of the field of environmental health reflect a convergence with some of the basic principles and themes of environmental psychology—especially an emphasis on *salutogenic* as well as *pathogenic* processes (Antonovsky, 1987) as they occur in relation to natural as well as built, social as well as physical, and subjective as well as objective dimensions of human environments (Bechtel and Churchman, 2002; Stokols and Altman, 1987).

Mapping the Sociophysical Context of Health

Environmental psychology assumes that the health effects of our surroundings are the result of the confluence of a variety of contextual factors. The negative health effects of routine exposure to residential density and noise, for example, are more severe in poor households than in affluent ones due to the cumulative effects of multiple environmental stressors faced by low-income families (Evans, 2004). Field experiments, similarly, have shown that persons exposed to cold viruses are much more likely to develop cold symptoms when they are experiencing high levels of stress in one or more areas of their lives (for example, in their relationships with family members, friends, or coworkers) than when they are reporting low levels of chronic stress (see, for example, Cohen and others, 1997a, 1998).

Clearly, a large number of life circumstances can affect the ways in which people respond to particular environmental demands. Yet identifying the many contextual factors that influence a person's health is a dauntingly complex task due to the large number of settings in which individuals participate on a day-to-day basis and the diverse physical and social factors they encounter in each one. Moreover, each of these environmental factors can be considered in relation to diverse health criteria, ranging from the absence of physical injury and illness to states of complete wellness reflected in exceptionally high levels of emotional, physical, spiritual, and social well-being (O'Donnell, 1989; World Health Organization, 1986, 1997).

In establishing a basis for mapping the environmental contexts of health, it is useful to begin by identifying a relatively small number of analytical categories, each of which subsumes a much larger set of environmental variables (Clitheroe, Stokols, and Zmuidzinas, 1998; Magnusson, 1981). The basic units of environmental analysis are arrayed on different levels, or scales, ranging from specific stimuli that are part of the situations immediately experienced by persons in a particular setting or place (for example, being stuck in rush hour traffic, with horns honking and tempers flaring)—to the more complex life domains (for example, residential, employment, and educational environments) that are themselves clusters of multiple situations and settings (Table 5.1).

Stimuli are defined as observable features of objects or discrete conditions in an environment, such as the color of a table, the temperature level in a room, a sudden flash of light, or the occurrence of a loud noise (Pervin, 1978). *Situations* are sequences of individual or group activities and events that occur at a particular time and place (Forgas, 1979). *Settings* are socially structured and geographically bounded locations where certain kinds of activities and events recur on a regular basis—for example, the college classroom where one attends a particular course at the same time each week or the favorite coffee shop where one visits several

TABLE 5.1. LEVELS OF ENVIRONMENTAL ANALYSIS.

Elemental	Water, air, earth, food, germs, physical substances
Individual	An individual's (1) body and physical, perceptual, and cognitive abilities and (2) intellectual abilities, personal beliefs, values, attitudes, emotions, and experiences
Stimuli	Observable (by any sense) features of an environment that cause a personal perception or physical or psychological reaction, or both
Situation	Sequences of individual or group activities and events that occur at a particular time and place
Setting	Socially structured and geographically bounded locations where certain kinds of activities and events recur on a regular basis
Life domain	Spheres of a person's life that encompasses multiple situations and settings, for example, home, work, or school
Societal	Overarching system of beliefs and values, social and cultural norms, and social, political, and economic institutions

times each month for a mocha malt Frappuccino (Barker, 1968; Schoggen, 1989; Stokols and Shumaker, 1981). *Life domains* are more encompassing spheres of a person's life, such as family, education, religion, recreation, and employment (Campbell, 1981). An even broader unit of contextual analysis can be defined, usually referred to as a person's *overall life situation,* that encompasses all the major life domains in which the individual is involved during a particular period of his or her life (Chapin, 1974; Magnusson, 1981; Michelson, 1985).

Three Principles of Contextual Analysis

The environmental units outlined previously reflect three basic principles of contextual analysis common to environmental psychology.

1. *The relationship between environment and health is influenced by interdependencies among immediate situations, settings and more remote environmental conditions.*

Stimuli and situations are nested within larger units such as organized settings and places that are themselves subsumed by individuals' life domains, activity systems, and conditions (for example, economic, political, or cultural trends) that are widespread throughout whole communities and geographic regions. As environmental analyses shift their focus from smaller and more detailed to larger and more holistic levels, the potential range of contextual influences on mental and physical health expands dramatically due to the hierarchically nested structure of human environments.

For instance, when unemployment rates in a community are high, the psychological and organizational stress associated with job insecurity is more prevalent and disruptive among coworkers based at one or more companies in that region (Dooley, 2003; Dooley, Fielding, and Levi, 1996). At the same time, the occupational health and safety of workplaces at the local level is directly influenced by state and national regulations aimed at protecting environmental quality and employee health (Stokols, McMahan, Clitheroe, and Wells, 2001). A more dramatic and tragic example of the interdependencies between local and remote environments is the syndrome of chronic emotional stress and health impairment triggered by the terrorist attacks of September 11, 2001, not only among Americans residing in or near New York City, Washington, D.C., and Shanksville, Pennsylvania, but also among those living hundreds or thousands of miles away from the attack sites (Silver and others, 2002).

These examples suggest a second principle of contextual analysis.

2. *The different environments in which an individual participates exert a cumulative, synergistic effect on his or her health.*

Bronfenbrenner (1979) emphasized the ways in which functional linkages between two or more settings (such as family and occupational environments) and connections with other more distant settings in which an individual does not directly participate (for example, the workplaces of a child's parents) can affect development and well-being. Such multilevel, integrative analyses can result in recognition of subtle health relationships (for example, stressful experiences at work that impair the quality of parents' interactions with their children at home). Particularly important in a world of expanding communication and entertainment media, Bronfenbrenner also identified an overarching societal system of beliefs, social and cultural norms, political and economic institutions and events that also influence the health and well-being of individuals and groups.

The combined influence of multiple settings and life domains on individuals' health has been observed in several studies, and this reality is recognized in the third general principle of contextual analysis.

3. *Health is the result of an interaction among the objective features of the environments in which individuals participate, individuals' perceptions of those features, and individuals' personal attributes.*

That is, the impact of particular stimuli, situations, settings, and life domains on a person's health depends not only on the objective features of an environment but also on individual attributes (for example, genetic heritage, psychological dispositions, coping resources) and on the person's subjective interpretation of the environments in which he or she participates.

For instance, children's exposure to environmental stressors (such as high levels of spatial density and noise) in both their residential and elementary school environments revealed additive effects of those conditions on their physiological health (for example, systolic and diastolic blood pressure) and academic performance (Cohen, Evans, Stokols, and Krantz, 1986). In other studies, employees' perception that they lacked the flexibility to schedule children's doctor visits during working hours led to their underutilization of employer-provided family health benefits (Fielding, Cumberland, and Pettitt, 1994), with long-term negative health consequences for the family. Studies have also documented both the negative health consequences of *work-family conflict* and the positive effects of spousal support in buffering work-related stressors (O'Neil and Greenberger, 1994).

To derive more precise hypotheses about the links between environmental factors and their effects on health, it is useful to consider more specific theories of the relationship between persons and their environment that identify (a) those situations and settings in a person's life that have the greatest impact on their health and (b) the ways in which personal attributes or *individual differences* (for example, related to personality, cognition, gender, age, education, and income) mediate the effects of environmental conditions on emotional and physical well-being.

These multiple settings and environments and their interaction and interdependencies constitute a daunting research challenge that "require[s] data sets including individuals nested within areas or neighborhoods" (Diez Roux, 2001, p. 1784). Analytical methods able to assess these complex relationships are emerging from the fields of environmental health (*multilevel analysis*), urban planning (*geographic information systems,* or GIS), and the behavioral sciences (*hierarchical linear analysis*).

The Changing Neighborhood and Its Influence on Health

Many settings and situations have been extensively studied by researchers in the field of environmental psychology, including home and work environments and natural and technological disasters. In this chapter we have chosen to use the concept of *neighborhood* as a focus for exploring the links between environmental psychology and public health. The neighborhood is an especially appropriate context in which to consider the links between environment, behavior, and health for at least three reasons. First, the neighborhood is a sufficiently broad contextual unit to encompass a variety of stimuli, situations, settings, and life domains relevant to health. Second, the concept of neighborhood is not peripheral to people's day-to-day activities and concerns but plays a central and meaningful role in determining the substance, quality, and health of their life. And third, although the neighborhood has been long regarded as a psychologically and socially meaningful unit of analysis in the fields of sociology, public health, and community and environmental psychology, the concept of neighborhood is currently undergoing fundamental rethinking and change among scholars in several fields due to the advent of digital and mobile communications.

The neighborhood is no longer simply viewed as a contiguous, geographically delimited, relatively stable arena of daily activities. Rather, people now participate in multiple, geographically defined places and socially defined networks concurrently, some of which are *real* (involving a physical space or place) and others of which are less real (involving a *virtual* space) and more mobile. Thus consideration of contemporary changes in the structure and functions of the neighborhood offers us an opportunity to explore some exciting new lines of research concerning the impact of digital communications and virtual communities on people's psychological attachment to places and their overall well-being (see, for example, Blanchard and Horan, 1998; Meyrowitz, 1985; Stokols, 1999; Wellman and Haythornthwaite, 2002).

Traditional definitions of *neighborhood* emphasize geographic location, unique physical features (such as architectural styles and public parks), the social attributes of residents, and residents' objective participation in and subjective identification with the area (Altman and Wandersman, 1987). For instance, Rivlin (1987) states:

> When we speak of contemporary neighborhoods, we are talking about a very heterogeneous unit based on the nature of the geography, the numbers and kinds of people there, the socioeconomic status of these people, their ages, cultural background, and housing form. . . . The criterion of a neighborhood is the acknowledgment by residents, merchants, and regular users of an area that a locality exists. It presumes some agreement on boundaries and a name and the recognition of distinguishing characteristics of the setting. . . . The recognition by people of a bounded territory as having an integrity and personal meaning is, in my view, the necessary requirement of a neighborhood [pp. 2–3].

More recently, scholars in urban sociology, information science, and other fields have challenged the traditional view that a neighborhood is both geographically bounded and psychologically central to an individual's life. Researchers are beginning to recognize that "neighborhood contexts may be related to public health, independently of individual-level attributes" (Diez Roux, 2001, p. 1783). According to this emerging view, people's communications and relationships with others are no longer constrained by geography but occur instead within highly personalized digital communication networks unbounded by space and time (Negroponte, 1995; Rheingold, 1993). For instance, Wellman (2001) observes:

> The importance of a communication site as a meaningful place will diminish even more. The person—not the place, household, or workgroup—will become

> even more of an autonomous communication node. Contextual sense and lateral awareness will diminish. . . . People usually obtain support, companionship, information, and a sense of belonging from those who do not live within the same neighborhood or even within the same metropolitan area. People maintain these community ties through phoning, writing, driving, railroading, and flying. . . . Neighborhoods are not important sources of community. They have become variably safe and salubrious milieus from which people sally forth in their cars, telephone from their kitchens, or email from their dens [p. 233].

Rather than adopt the traditional view that local neighborhoods are the most important context of people's day-to-day transactions with their surroundings or the revisionist view that place-based neighborhoods are no longer important sources of community and well-being, the present discussion offers a more integrative conceptualization of neighborhood that recognizes the complementarity of geographically bounded and virtually dispersed neighborhood functions.

Specifically, we define the *new neighborhood* as those people, places, and technologies that enable the sociophysical interactions that define everyday life. This definition assumes that people's psychological ties with local, place-based environments are an important source of their identity and well-being (Proshansky, Fabian, and Kaminoff, 1983; Unger and Wandersman, 1985), but it also recognizes that the number and the scope of individuals' psychologically meaningful neighborhoods (such as those based at home, at school, at work, in public community settings . . .) have expanded and that in addition to physical proximity individuals can now be closely linked with each other through the Internet and mobile digital communications (Brill and Weidemann, 2001; Wellman and Haythornthwaite, 2002). Both real and virtual neighborhoods respond to the same basic human needs (Table 5.2).

Features of Neighborhoods

Place-based neighborhoods have defined geographic boundaries and identifiable physical features. The extent of a neighborhood can be mapped from a personally defined central reference point (for example, a student's desk in a dormitory room on a college campus) out toward more distant areas that are located within the neighborhood's boundaries (for example, the community park located three blocks from the campus). The student's room, the dormitory building, the college campus, and the community settings surrounding the campus are situated along continuums ranging from immediate to more remote areas and from completely known to less known parts of the neighborhood.

TABLE 5.2. FUNCTIONS OF BOTH REAL AND VIRTUAL NEIGHBORHOODS.

Affiliation	Facilitate communication and interaction between individuals and groups
Identity	Provide a definable group character (name, style, real or virtual landmarks) for assimilation by individuals and an opportunity to contribute to the development of that character and to the individual's own self-concept
Social support	Offer psychologically reinforcing interactions between individuals or within groups
Community	Offer a connection to the opportunities provided and demands made by larger social units
Information	Provide awareness of and access to information the individual finds essential to successful daily life and personal goals
Daily life	Assist with the basics: acquisition and maintenance of food, shelter, safety, convenience, and comfort
Recreation	Supply opportunities to physically or mentally refresh, to play, to explore, to challenge oneself, to learn and grow

In contrast, virtual neighborhoods arise when people routinely communicate and congregate electronically, with no need for a physical, geographically defined place in which to come together. Thus a person's neighborhood would include all those physical and virtual settings he or she uses regularly. Some of these settings are located inside buildings, some are located outdoors, and some are in cyberspace. The following discussion of neighborhood settings presents several examples of environmental psychological concepts and research that describe contextual factors related to public health. We start with physical settings and conclude with virtual ones.

Indoor Neighborhood Settings

Indoor neighborhood settings include dwellings, classrooms, workspaces, indoor recreation facilities, places for socialization, places for worship, and neighborhood resources such as markets, shops, and restaurants. Physical conditions include building design and furnishing, entrance, egress, and windows. Ambient conditions include lighting, air quality, temperature, humidity, sound, and color.

Environmental stress is any demand made on an individual by an environment (physical or social). Thus environmental stressors may be considered stimuli, requiring a physical or psychological response. Pioneering work by Selye (1956) defined the physiological reactions of an individual to injury, illness, or environmental stressors:

elevated blood pressure, enlarged adrenal glands, gastrointestinal ulcers, and impaired immune function. *Psychological stress* can occur when perceived environmental demands exceed the individual's perceived ability to cope with them. Such stress may be caused by experiences of isolation, irritability, or interpersonal conflict, for example. The individual's subjective interpretation of an environment (for example, whether or not its demands seem overwhelming or manageable) plays a major role in determining the severity and persistence of psychological stress reactions.

Research on environmental stress has shown, for example, that chronic exposure to high levels of *noise* leads to a variety of health impairments. For instance, when children living in noisy dwellings near congested roadways or attending schools under the flight path of a busy airport (Figure 5.1) were compared to children occupying quieter environments, chronic noise exposure was found to be associated with impaired hearing and reading skills, lower levels of academic achievement, and elevated blood pressure (Bronzaft, 2002; Cohen, Evans, Stokols,

FIGURE 5.1. AIRPLANE COMING IN FOR LANDING OVER AN ELEMENTARY SCHOOL IN LOS ANGELES.

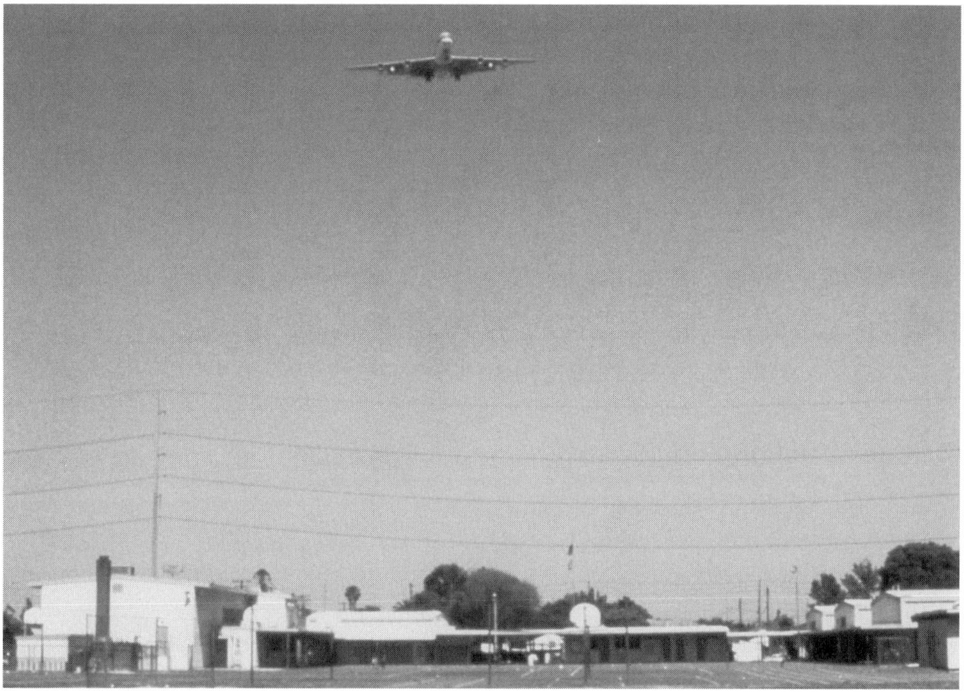

and Krantz, 1986; Cohen, Glass, and Singer, 1973; Evans and others, 2001; Hygge, Evans, and Bullinger, 2002). In addition, prolonged experiences of *crowding* in dormitories, apartments, and homes have been linked to dysfunctional social behavior, feelings of isolation, and emotional distress (Baum and Epstein, 1978; Baum and Valins, 1977; Evans and Lepore, 1993).

One of the reasons that noisy or crowded interior spaces provoke psychological stress among their occupants is that they typically lead to prolonged feelings of stimulation overload, distraction, frustration, and fatigue (Baum and Epstein, 1978; Evans and Johnson, 2000; Milgram, 1970). In settings with large numbers of people (*spatially dense* settings), an additional source of psychological stress is the difficulty occupants encounter in their efforts to regulate interpersonal *privacy* and *personal space* (Altman, 1975; Sommer, 1969). Coresidents and coworkers who are able to establish and maintain effective guidelines for the use of shared spaces (for example, through personalization and decoration of spaces in a shared residence or workspace) are better able to remain individually and collectively productive and to avoid interpersonal conflict and distress (Brill and Weidemann, 2001; Sundstrom and Sundstrom, 1986; Taylor, 1988).

To the extent that individuals can gain some measure of real or perceived control over environmental stressors such as noise, crowding, and infringements on privacy, they are able to avoid both the immediate and delayed effects of these stressors on their performance and well-being (Cohen, 1980; Evans, 2001; Glass and Singer, 1972). Perceptions of environmental controllability and predictability enable individuals to maintain high levels of emotional and physical well-being, even in the context of highly demanding settings. For instance, elderly persons living in institutionalized residential care facilities who were encouraged by staff members to take personal responsibility for the maintenance and beautification of their own living spaces (for example, by caring for plants placed in their bedrooms) exhibited higher levels of emotional and physical well-being than those who were not encouraged to assume those responsibilities (Langer and Rodin, 1976; Rodin and Langer, 1977; also see Schulz and Hanusa, 1978).

Outdoor Neighborhood Settings

Immediately outside a home, apartment building, dormitory, classroom, or workplace lies the realm of transitional areas that link personalized indoor environments with more public areas of the neighborhood, such as sidewalks, streets, and commercial and recreational settings (Alexander and others, 1977; Altman, 1975). Just as physical conditions such as noise and high spatial density influence the quality of social interactions indoors, an interdependence between physical and social conditions is evident in outdoor spaces. For instance, loud noise (at or above

85 decibels) from a lawnmower operating near the sidewalk in a suburban neighborhood significantly reduced pedestrians' attentiveness to the needs of others (specifically, to the needs of a person wearing an arm cast who had dropped a stack of books near his car) and their willingness to stop and render assistance (Mathews and Canon, 1975).

In another study the linear distance between the front doors of apartments in a Massachusetts Institute of Technology student housing complex (a physical dimension) reliably predicted which residents happened to meet each other and eventually became friends (Festinger, Schachter, and Back, 1950). Moreover, neighbors whose apartments were further apart but who met regularly at group mailboxes, a basketball court, or in the parking lot (social dimensions) were more likely to form friendships than those who lived far apart and did not "run into" each other regularly. Interestingly, the residents who formed friendships also developed similar political attitudes and consumer behaviors (for example, deciding to purchase the same brands of appliances for their apartments).

The influence of sociophysical environmental factors on friendship formation has important health implications. Most immediately, the presence of friends who live close by and can render assistance when called upon improves the sociability, or *social climate,* of the neighborhood (Moos, 1979). A positive social climate is in turn seen as a form of *social capital* and can contribute to residents' perceptions of security and neighborhood safety (Putnam, 2000). Other research suggests that socially isolated individuals are more susceptible to illnesses of various kinds—even premature death—than those who are actively involved in mutually supportive friendship, family, religious, and professional networks (Berkman and Syme, 1979; Cohen and others, 1997b, 2003).

Certain conditions of outdoor environments have been found to curtail social contacts among neighbors dramatically. One of these constraining factors is a high daily volume of vehicular traffic. Appleyard (1981), in his now classic study of livable streets, found that compared to streets with low or moderate traffic levels, residential streets in San Francisco with high traffic volumes were characterized by substantially lower self-reported rates of neighborliness among residents living in the same building or on the same block. Residents living on high-volume streets also complained more strongly about the inconveniences of roadway noise, dust and fumes, and traffic-related threats to pedestrian safety (especially among children and the elderly). When asked to sketch and describe their "home territory," residents of high-volume streets usually described only their bedroom or immediate apartment, whereas those living on lightly and moderately traveled streets described areas outside their apartment buildings and along both sides of their block in addition to their personal living space and building. Thus two very different perceptions of neighborhood emerged in response to a dominant sociophysical condition—vehicular traffic.

The sociability of neighborhoods is also undermined by the presence of physical and social *incivilities. Physical incivilities* include the presence of litter, graffiti, protective bars on windows, evidence of street disrepair (for example, broken curbs and potholes), poor building and exterior maintenance (for example, peeling paint, unkempt yards, and overgrown landscaping), and damage to buildings (for example, broken windows) (Nasar and Fisher, 1993; Perkins, Wandersman, Rich, and Taylor, 1993). *Social incivilities* include displays of public drunkenness, the presence of gangs or prostitutes, excessive numbers of liquor outlets, stores offering pornography, and a generally unfriendly or threatening atmosphere in the neighborhood (Holman and Stokols, 1994).

One consequence of these environmental incivilities is the stigmatization of a neighborhood, accompanied by reduced social and economic investment in the area, greater fear of crime, and higher rates of victimization and injury among residents and visitors. Neighborhoods such as South Central Los Angeles that have experienced widely publicized civil violence are particularly prone to this downward spiral of stigmatization, disinvestment, and crime. Concerted efforts to remove physical cues such as disrepair and to encourage the development of prosocial events, including street and cultural fairs, drama or music festivals, and community gardening programs, can reverse this negative trend (Garland and Stokols, 2002; Lewis, 1979).

Other architectural and site-planning strategies can be applied to create outdoor spaces that enhance the social climate and security of residential and commercial areas. *Defensible space* (Newman, 1973) refers to those features of an environment that "combine to bring it under the control of its residents" (p. 3). For instance, apartment buildings can be sited on blocks so as to create natural buffer zones easily surveyed by residents, and apartment windows can be positioned to facilitate surveillance of semipublic areas adjacent to the building. Changes in elevation, landscaping, and signage also can be used to mark transitions between public and private areas (Alexander and others, 1977). In a study of Salt Lake City neighborhoods, Brown (1985) found that homes characterized by defensible space design (for example, the presence of actual or symbolic barriers such as fences or hedges surrounding the property and physical traces of residents' presence (such as lights on in the home) were less likely to have been burglarized than were residences lacking those features. This body of environmental psychology research has become institutionalized in the form of guidelines promoted by police departments and adopted by cities and counties throughout the United States (Newman, 1966) (see Chapter Twenty-Five).

Neighborhoods as Wholes

We next consider larger-scale qualities of neighborhoods such as the coherence of their spatial organization; the diversity of their recreational, cultural, and commercial settings; and their overall *sense of place.* A neighborhood can be described not only in terms of buildings, sidewalks, open areas, parks, shops, and streets but also in terms of larger factors that contribute to its distinctive identity or overall atmosphere (Ittelson, 1973). For instance, Lynch (1960) defines *imageability* as an environment's memorability, its capacity to evoke strong visual memories of its physical features among residents and visitors. According to Lynch, the likelihood that an environment will evoke a vivid image in an observer depends on its visual clarity, or "*legibility*—the ease with which its parts can be recognized and organized into a coherent pattern" (p. 3). Lynch also defines the environmental features that strongly contribute to this legibility. The legible environment has (1) a *path* system (for example, roadways and walking paths) that is arrayed in a logical and easy-to-remember fashion; (2) unique *districts* (for example, cultural, residential, recreational, and commercial areas) that are bounded by (3) clearly defined *edges* such as major streets, seashores, riverfronts, or cliffs; (4) strategic *nodes* of social interaction (for example, a train station, a bus depot, or a street corner at a busy intersection) in various parts of the neighborhood; and (5) distinctive physical *landmarks* (for example, a tall building, a monument, a colorful sign) that serve as visual reference points (as do the Space Needle in Seattle (Figure 5.2), the Eiffel Tower in Paris, the Washington Monument in the District of Columbia, and the Gateway Arch in St. Louis). The imageability and legibility of a place derive not only from its physical features but also from social meanings. In a study of Parisians' *cognitive maps,* Milgram and Jodelet (1976) found that certain areas of the city were remembered more for their social and historical meanings than their distinctive physical or visual attributes.

Both the social and the physical imageability of a neighborhood can affect residents' and visitors' well-being in at least two ways. First, visually legible environments are less confusing and easier to navigate than others, enabling pedestrians and drivers to feel more secure, to arrive at their destinations more efficiently, to enjoy their experience of the neighborhood, and to avoid potentially unsafe areas; these are all experiences that decrease environmental stress. Second, the presence of widely recognized and shared cultural or symbolic meanings can contribute positively to the sociability and supportive climate of a place, thereby increasing social capital and promoting norms of cooperativeness, trust, and engagement with others (see, for example, Putnam, 2000) while also reducing crime rates and fear of crime in the area. All of these factors contribute to the health of the neighborhood and of the people who live, work, and play there.

FIGURE 5.2. THE SPACE NEEDLE IN SEATTLE, WASHINGTON.

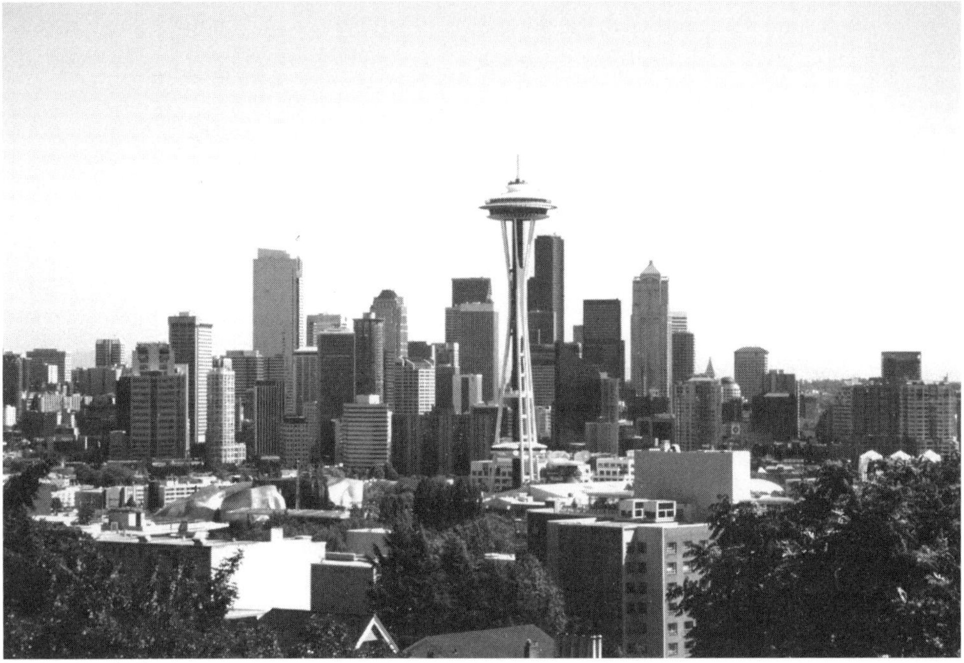

An important neighborhood quality that contributes to its social climate is the number and diversity of its *behavior settings,* including recreational, commercial, cultural, educational, and civic places (Barker and Schoggen, 1973; Jacobs, 1961). The presence of multiple settings geared to the interests and activities of diverse groups of residents and visitors (children, adolescents, young adults, elderly persons, and different cultural and ethnic groups) promotes active interchange among these groups and contributes to the overall vitality of the neighborhood. At the same time, an overabundance of certain settings, such as fast-food restaurants, may have a negative influence on residents' well-being. In a recent study of the "economics of obesity," Rashad and Grossman (2004) found that a major factor in the rise of obesity in the United States between 1980 and the present is the dramatic growth in the per capita number of fast-food and full-service restaurants during those years. According to this research, as much as two-thirds of the increase in adult obesity since 1980 can be explained by the rapid expansion of the restaurant industry and the increasing tendency of U.S. adults and children to eat their meals at fast-food and full-service restaurants (Figure 5.3). Thus a prevalence

FIGURE 5.3. CARS WAITING IN LINE FOR "FAST FOOD" SERVICE.

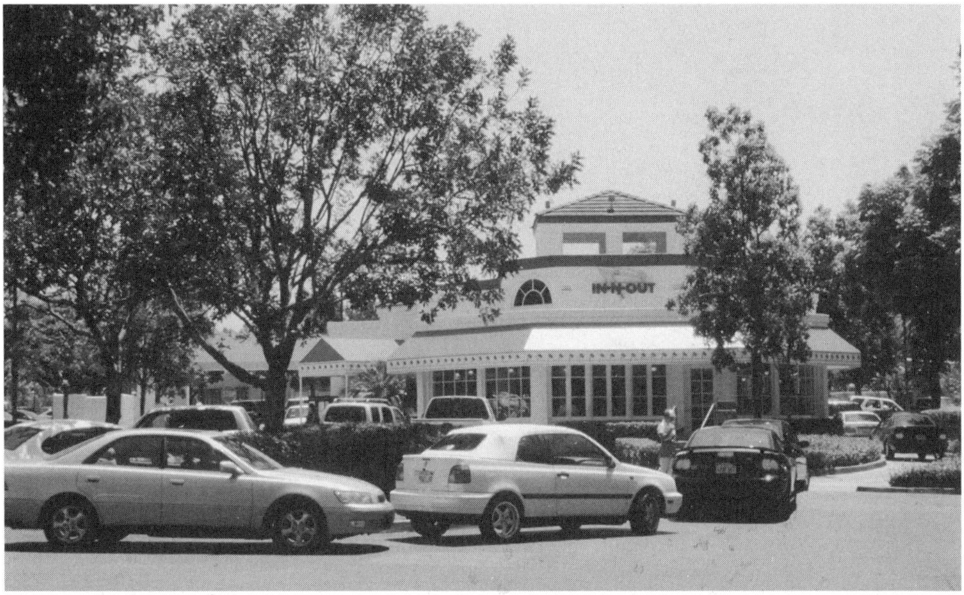

of fast-food settings (which generally serve high-fat, high-calorie meals) and abundant opportunities for families to dine out in a neighborhood may have a deleterious effect on residents' health.

Among the most important neighborhood settings are what Oldenburg (1999) refers to as *third places*—"the variety of public places that host the regular, voluntary, informal, and happily anticipated gatherings of individuals beyond the realms of home and work" (p. 16). (Home settings and work settings are, respectively, individuals' *first places* and *second places*.) Third places such as local bookstores, coffee shops, parks, and other popular hang-outs (such as Ghirardelli Square in San Francisco) (Figures 5.4 and 5.5) serve as "core settings of informal life." Oldenburg contends that third places offer people escape and relief from the psychological stress of work and family responsibilities and strengthens their sense of belonging to the community and thus their overall well-being. Interestingly, Florida's (2002) research on the *creative class* suggests that regional economic growth and job opportunities in the United States are fueled by where the creative people, who represent 30 percent of the workforce, choose to live. One of the things creative people look for when deciding whether to move to a particular area is a diverse mix of third places—neighborhood settings that

FIGURE 5.4. GHIRARDELLI SQUARE IN SAN FRANCISCO.

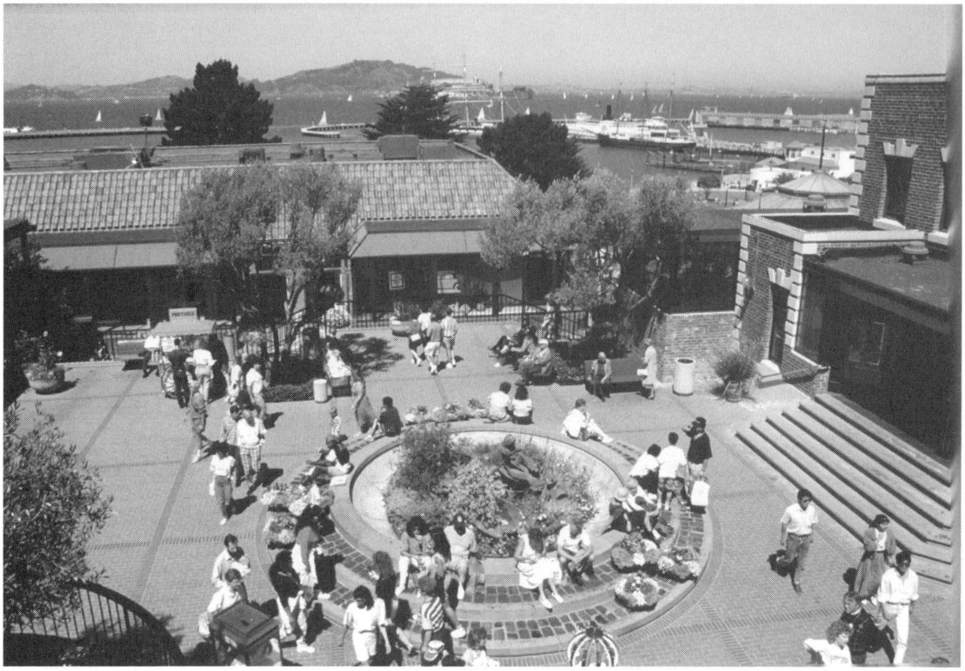

offer recreational resources such as vibrant nightlife and opportunities for social and cultural exchange.

In some localities schools may become third places. A recent positive example of neighborhood change involves the conceptualization of neighborhood public schools as places that can "improve overall health in densely populated communities" when they are designed as "mixed-use, neighborhood-centered" facilities that provide "much needed, neighborhood-based health and human services . . . [and] safe, convenient spaces for children and their families to walk, run, participate in sports and otherwise enjoy being outdoors" (Abel and Fielding, 2004, p. M2).

In addition to third places, the aesthetic quality of neighborhood environments, the presence of nature (for example, lakes or forested parks) at all environmental levels (Table 5.3; Figure 5.6), and the provision of resources for physical activity (for example, bike trails and public parks) (Figure 5.7) all contribute positively to residents' mental and physical health and to the neighborhood's sense of place. Natural areas in a neighborhood offer residents a respite from their daily

FIGURE 5.5. THE PLAZA MAYOR IN MADRID, SPAIN.

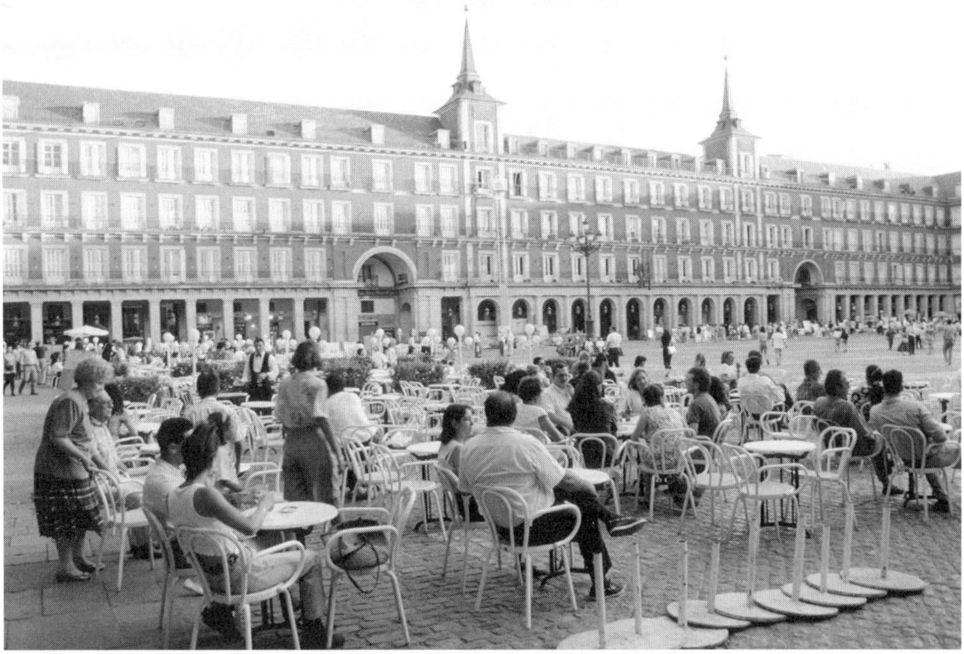

work routines as well as opportunities for emotional restoration and recovery from mental fatigue (Kaplan and Kaplan, 1989). Similarly, urban design features can either encourage or discourage residents' engagement in physical activity as an antidote to the obesity pandemic currently rampant in the U.S. population (Frank, Engelke, and Schmid, 2003). (The links between access to nature and well-being and between urban design and physical activity patterns are discussed more fully in Chapters Sixteen and Twenty-Seven.)

Virtual Neighborhoods

Having discussed some of the physical features and subjective qualities of place-based neighborhoods that influence health, we now consider the ways in which the Internet and digital communications have given rise to fundamentally new categories of neighborhoods—*virtual communities,* located in cyberspace, that complement (and sometimes complicate) people's transactions with their place-based environments.

TABLE 5.3. THE PRESENCE OF NATURE.

Elemental	• Natural scents (incense) • Natural objects (driftwood, shells, stones, plants)
Individual	• Clothing choices • Eating choices
Stimuli	• Natural sounds (birdsong, rain, wind in trees) • Natural surfaces (wood, rock, grass, sand, water) • Natural colors and textures (earth tones, burlap) • Views of nature through windows • Natural images (pictures of natural places)
Situation	• Outdoor meetings, meals, entertainment • Gardening
Setting	• Outdoor recreation • Outdoor relaxation or meditation
Life domain	• Outdoor occupations • Location of residence and workplace • Mode of transportation and routes
Societal	• Nature preserves and wilderness areas • Protected seashores, rivers and lakes • Regional, national and international ecological conventions and agreements

The computing revolution and the rapid expansion of the Internet during the 1980s and 1990s (Kiesler, 1997; Kling and Iacono, 1991) have dramatically altered people's transactions with their environments in at least three ways. First, the emergence of the Internet and digital communications has made it much easier for individuals to be in contact even when they are geographically or temporally remote from each other. Second, the Internet has facilitated the development of virtual behavior settings and virtual neighborhoods such as chat rooms, Listservs, bulletin boards, and electronic commerce sites like eBay and Amazon.com, each located at a particular "address" in cyberspace. Like real places, these virtual settings are frequented by members on a regular basis, and the members develop widely shared norms concerning appropriate social behavior and etiquette (Blanchard, 1997; Blanchard and Horan, 1998). Moreover, the members of virtual communities (such as the Palace and the Well) tend to identify strongly with these sites and fellow members (Rheingold, 1993). Third, because individuals are in or at a specific physical place at the same time that they are participating in a virtual setting via computer contact or cell phone conversations, they must simultaneously pay attention to information from both their immediate sociophysical environment and their virtual environment.

This concurrent processing of information generated by place-based and virtual settings raises the possibility that certain conflicts between these two realms

FIGURE 5.6. NEIGHBORHOOD GREEN SPACE IN IRVINE, CALIFORNIA.

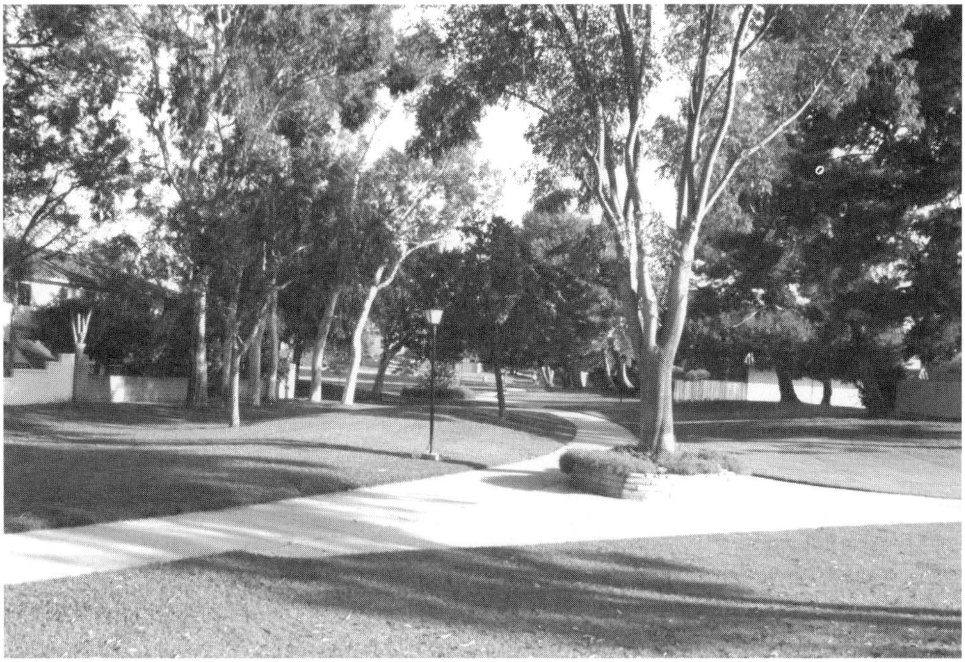

of experience will occur and that negative health impacts (such as traffic crashes caused by the use of cell phones while driving) may be a consequence of those conflicts. The proliferation of *r-v* situations, incorporating at least one *r*eal (place-based) and one *v*irtual setting (accessed from a desktop computer, laptop, hand-held device, or cell phone), raises novel questions about the relationships between environment, behavior, and health (see, for example, Stokols, 1999). For example, r-v conflicts arise when parents engage in chat room activities on a home computer and become less responsive to the needs of their children and when employees inappropriately "surf the Internet" from their workplaces, arousing the resentment of coworkers and supervisors who are more focused on job-related tasks. These examples illustrate the kinds of interpersonal and organizational strains that may result from a conflict between real and virtual settings.

Social strains and interpersonal conflicts are not the only health problems prompted by the overlap of real and virtual settings. Another major threat to an individual's well-being is the *stimulation overload* (see, for example, Milgram, 1970) that results from chronic *multitasking,* such as simultaneously communicating with a person situated in a real setting and a person in a virtual setting in an attempt

FIGURE 5.7. A NEIGHBORHOOD PARK IN WHISTLER, BRITISH COLUMBIA, CANADA.

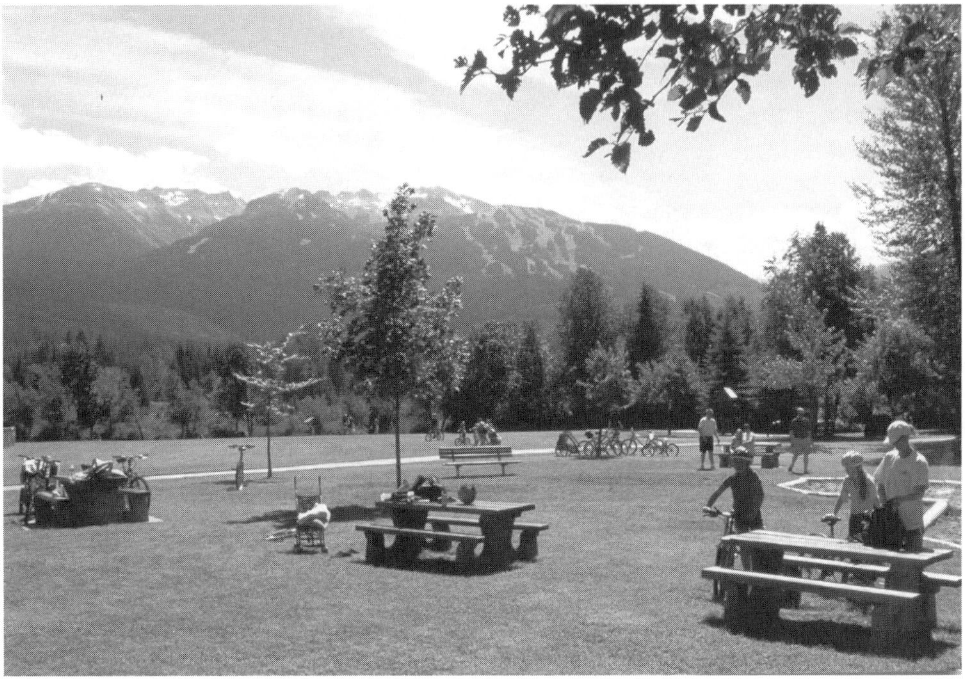

to accomplish diverse tasks in a short period of time. The digital electronic revolution has subjected large segments of the population to an onslaught of communications transmitted via desktop and laptop computers, hand-held devices, cell phones, and fax machines. The rapid rise in Internet use and digital communications, including both more users and more e-mail messaging per user, has been recorded in a number of recent studies (for example, International Technology and Trade Associates, 2000; Lyman and Varian, 2000; Nie and Erbring, 2000; Wellman and Haythornthwaite, 2002; Messagingonline, 2000). This communications explosion has resulted in individuals' becoming more susceptible to distraction, information overload, and mental fatigue. When these conditions persist, individuals can experience attentional fatigue, which has been closely linked to greater irritability, reduced sensitivity to the needs of others, and health-threatening errors in occupational settings—for example, among physicians, nurses, air traffic controllers, and automobile drivers (Cohen, 1980; Kaplan and Kaplan, 1989; Kohn, Corrigan, and Donaldson, 2000).

Although conflicts between real and virtual settings are common, place-based neighborhoods can benefit from residents' participation in virtual communities. Blanchard and Horan (1998), for instance, distinguish two types of these locally beneficial virtual *communities of interest:* place-based and geographically dispersed. Place-based communities of interest are exemplified by the Blacksburg Electronic Community (www.bev.net), an Internet site developed by the residents of Blacksburg, Virginia, for the purposes of facilitating social and commercial exchange among individuals and groups in the city and enhancing the sense of community and sense of place in Blacksburg. Other cities have followed Blacksburg's lead by developing Internet sites that reinforce their place-based neighborhoods (Cohill and Kavanaugh, 2000). Geographically dispersed communities of interest are those in which most participants do not communicate face-to-face or even by telephone. Examples include health support groups on the Internet as well as Web sites featuring hobbies or shared intellectual, political, artistic, literary, or recreational interests. Even though these virtual communities do not directly reinforce a sense of place, they do enrich the quality of life in place-based neighborhoods by delivering valuable information, services, and support to neighborhood residents.

Connections between virtual and place-based neighborhoods can have both positive and negative consequences for participants' well-being. Not all members of place-based neighborhoods, however, have access to virtual settings, due to limited financial resources or educational backgrounds. The growing rift between information-rich and information-poor segments of the population is referred to as the *digital divide* (Castells, 1998; Garces, 2000; National Telecommunications and Information Administration, 2000). Individuals who find themselves on the wrong side of this divide are frequently caught in a downward spiral of increasing poverty because they have little access to job opportunities that require training in information technology. If this problem is not redressed, the resulting social divisions and inequity may provoke the same sort of social conflict, community destabilization, and health impairments (including lack of access to care) that led to widespread social upheaval in the 1960s. Thus, narrowing the digital divide remains an important priority for future environmental and health research.

Conclusion

This chapter has presented the contours of environmental psychology as an interdisciplinary field that offers a useful vantage point for understanding the relationships between environment and health. Several important topics that expand the conceptualization of environmental health have been introduced:

- Theory and research in environmental psychology are providing a broader conceptualization of the sociophysical context of health relative to the traditional focus of the field of environmental health on the adverse effects of exposure to specific toxins, pathogens, and hazardous conditions of the physical environment.
- Similarly, environmental psychology is adopting a broader stance toward health itself, incorporating both the absence of injury or illness and the presence of well-being in the idea of health.
- Environmental psychology is also adopting a concept of the environment that includes both objective and subjective perspectives and physiological and psychological health outcomes.
- A revised understanding of *neighborhood* has been developed in this chapter and used to introduce a wide range of concepts, research, and findings related to environmental and public health.
- The discussion of real and virtual settings and communities in this chapter has revealed several potential conflicts and benefits with consequences for the health of neighborhood residents.

Environmental psychology concepts and research results can enrich future research on environment and health and provide a basis for enlarging the scope and effectiveness of public health programs and policies. Studies of environment and health should give greater attention to health-enhancing as well as pathogenic processes as they occur in relation to the natural and built environments, and to the cumulative influence of conditions experienced by individuals across multiple settings and life domains. This more fully contextual perspective, incorporating the joint influence of multiple environmental settings and factors on health, is exemplified by recent studies of the adaptive burdens faced by individuals—especially members of low-income and ethnic minority groups—resulting from their chronic exposure to multiple environmental stressors (Bullard, 1990; Evans, 2004; McEwen and Stellar, 1993; Taylor, Repetti, and Seeman, 1997). Chapter Eight in this volume provides more extensive coverage of these environmental justice concerns. Finally, the rapidly expanding prevalence of virtual communities (incorporated here into the definition of neighborhood) and the multifaceted role of the Internet as both a resource for health promotion and a source of health problems have emerged as important topics for future environmental health research.

Thought Questions

1. Make a list of the ways that you communicate with your friends and acquire information about the world. Then make lists of the ways your parents and grandparents communicated and acquired information when they were your

age. Then add to your lists the places that facilitate or enable (in your case) and facilitated or enabled (in your grandparents' case) these communication and information activities. What are the potential health consequences of the changes you note in these lists?

2. What are the physical and social factors that differ between low-income and high-income neighborhoods that have implications for the health of residents? (Hint: Think about the quantity, variety, and quality of the first, second, and third places available to residents of each type of neighborhood.)
3. Draw a large circle on a piece of paper. Around the edge of the circle, write words or phrases that describe important aspects of your current home environment (for example, "comfortable," "quiet," "no privacy," "safe"). Then, draw lines going through the circle (note: all lines will go through the circle) that connect items that are strongly related to each other (for example, "garden" and "relaxing"). How complex are the relationships between these sociophysical factors in your residential setting? Which seem most important; that is, which exhibit the most connections to other factors? Which factors might be related to the health of the residents of your home environment?
4. Consider the route you take to get to and from school. Do you consider it stressful or relaxing? Why? What do you listen to, that is, what kind of information do you absorb along the way? What options are available to you: fast-food restaurants, natural views, dense urban scenes, light traffic, and so forth? How does each of these contextual factors affect your mood, your expectations about the day ahead, your readiness to learn, and your overall health?

References

Abel, D., and Fielding, J. "If You Want to Build a Better Community, It Takes a School." *Los Angeles Times,* Jan. 25, 2004, p. M2.

Alexander, C., and others. *A Pattern Language.* New York: Oxford University Press, 1977.

Altman, I. *The Environment and Social Behavior.* Pacific Grove, Calif.: Brooks/Cole, 1975.

Altman, I., and Wandersman, A. (eds.). *Neighborhood and Community Environments.* New York: Plenum, 1987.

Antonovsky, A. *Unraveling the Mystery of Health: How People Manage Stress and Stay Well.* San Francisco: Jossey-Bass, 1987.

Appleyard, D. *Livable Streets.* Berkeley: University of California Press, 1981.

Barker, R. G. *Ecological Psychology: Concepts and Methods for Studying the Environment of Human Behavior.* Stanford, Calif.: Stanford University Press, 1968.

Barker, R. G., and Schoggen, P. *Qualities of Community Life.* San Francisco: Jossey-Bass, 1973.

Baum, A., and Epstein, Y. M. *Human Response to Crowding.* Mahwah, N.J.: Erlbaum, 1978.

Baum, A., and Valins, S. *Architecture and Social Behavior: Psychological Studies of Social Density.* Mahwah, N.J.: Erlbaum, 1977.

Bechtel, R. B. *Environment & Behavior: An Introduction.* Thousand Oaks, Calif.: Sage Publications, 1997.

Bechtel, R. B., and Churchman, A. (eds.). *Handbook of Environmental Psychology.* Hoboken, N.J.: Wiley, 2002.

Berkman, L. F., and Syme, S. L. "Social Networks, Host Resistance, and Mortality: A Nine-Year Follow-Up Study of Alameda County Residents." *American Journal of Epidemiology,* 1979, *109,* 186–204.

Blanchard, A. "Virtual Behavior Settings: An Application of Behavior Setting Theories to Virtual Communities." Unpublished manuscript, Center for Organizational and Behavioral Sciences, Claremont Graduate University, 1997.

Blanchard, A., and Horan, T. "Virtual Communities and Social Capital." *Social Science Computer Review,* 1998, *16,* 293–307.

Brill, M., and Weidemann, S. *Disproving Widespread Myths About Workspace Design.* Buffalo, N.Y.: BOSTI Associates, 2001.

Bronfenbrenner, U. *The Ecology of Human Development: Experiments by Nature and Design.* Cambridge, Mass.: Harvard University Press, 1979.

Bronzaft, A. L. "Noise Pollution: A Hazard to Physical and Mental Well-Being." In R. B. Bechtel and A. Churchman (eds.), *Handbook of Environmental Psychology.* Hoboken, N.J.: Wiley, 2002.

Brown, B. "Residential Burglaries: Cues to Burglary Vulnerability." *Journal of Architectural Planning and Research,* 1985, *2,* 231–243.

Bullard, R. D. *Dumping in Dixie: Race, Class, and Environmental Quality.* Boulder, Colo.: Westview Press, 1990.

Campbell, A. *The Sense of Well-Being in America.* New York: McGraw-Hill, 1981.

Cassel, J. "Social Science Theory as a Source of Hypotheses in Epidemiological Research." *American Journal of Public Health,* 1964, *54,* 1482–1488.

Cassel, J. "The Contribution of the Social Environment to Host Resistance." *American Journal of Public Health,* 1976, *104,* 107–123.

Castells, M. *End of Millennium.* Malden, Mass.: Blackwell, 1998.

Chapin, F. S. *Human Activity Patterns in the City: Things People Do in Time and in Space.* Hoboken, N.J.: Wiley, 1974.

Clitheroe, C., Stokols, D., and Zmuidzinas, M. "Conceptualizing the Context of Environment and Behavior." *Journal of Environmental Psychology,* 1998, *18,* 103–112.

Cohen, C., Evans, G. W., Stokols, D., and Krantz, D. S. *Behavior, Health, and Environmental Stress.* New York: Plenum, 1986.

Cohen, S. "Aftereffects of Stress on Human Performance and Social Behavior: A Review of Research and Theory." *Psychological Bulletin,* 1980, *88,* 82–108.

Cohen, S., Glass, D. C., and Singer, J. E. "Apartment Noise, Auditory Discrimination, and Reading Ability in Children." *Journal of Experimental Social Psychology,* 1973, *9,* 407–422.

Cohen, S., and others. "Chronic Social Stress, Social Status, and Susceptibility to Upper Respiratory Infections in Nonhuman Primates." *Psychosomatic Medicine,* 1997a, *59*(3), 213–221.

Cohen, S., and others. "Social Ties and Susceptibility to the Common Cold." *Journal of the American Medical Association,* 1997b, *277,* 1940–1944.

Cohen, S., and others. "Types of Stressors That Increase Susceptibility to the Common Cold in Healthy Adults." *Health Psychology,* 1998, *17*(3), 214–223.

Cohen, S., and others. "Sociability and Susceptibility to the Common Cold." *Psychological Science,* 2003, *14*(5), 389–395.

Cohill, A., and Kavanaugh, A. *Community Networks: Lessons from Blacksburg, VA.* (2nd ed.). Norwood, Mass.: Artech House, 2000.

Cooper, C. "The House as Symbol of the Self." In J. Lang, C. Burnette, W. Moleski, and D Vachon (eds.), *Designing for Human Behavior.* Stroudsburg, Penn.: Dowden, Hutchinson, and Ross, 1974.

Detels, R., McEwen, J., Beaglehole, R., and Tanaka, H. (eds.). *Oxford Textbook of Public Health.* (4th ed.) New York: Oxford University Press, 2002.

Diez Roux, A. V. "Investigating Neighborhood and Area Effects on Health." *American Journal of Public Health,* 2001, *91,* 1783–1789.

Dooley, D. "Unemployment, Underemployment, and Mental Health: Conceptualizing Employment Status as a Continuum." *American Journal of Community Psychology,* 2003, *32*(1–2), 9–20.

Dooley, D., Fielding, J., and Levi, L. "Health and Unemployment." *Annual Review of Public Health,* 1996, *17,* 449–465.

Evans, G. W. "Environmental Stress and Health." In A. Baum, T. Revenson, and J. E. Singer (eds.), *Handbook of Health Psychology.* Mahwah, N.J.: Erlbaum, 2001.

Evans, G. W. "The Environment of Childhood Poverty." *American Psychologist,* 2004, *59*(2), 77–92.

Evans, G. W., and Johnson, D. "Stress and Open-Office Noise." *Journal of Applied Psychology,* 2000, *85*(5), 779–783.

Evans, G. W., and Lepore, S. J. "Household Crowding and Social Support: A Quasi-Experimental Analysis." *Journal of Personality and Social Psychology,* 1993, *65,* 308–316.

Evans, G. W., and others. "Community Noise Exposure and Stress in Children." *Journal of the Acoustical Society of America,* 2001, *109*(3), 1023–1027.

Festinger, L., Schachter, S., and Back, K. *Social Pressures in Informal Groups.* New York: HarperCollins, 1950.

Fielding, J. E., Cumberland, W. G., and Pettitt, L. "Immunization Status of Children of Employees in a Large Corporation." *Journal of the American Medical Association,* 1994, *271,* 525–530.

Florida, R. *The Rise of the Creative Class.* New York: Basic Books, 2002.

Forgas, J. P. *Social Episodes: The Study of Interaction Routines.* New York: Academic Press, 1979.

Frank, L. D., Engelke, P. O., and Schmid, T. L. *Health and Community Design: The Impact of the Built Environment on Physical Activity.* Washington, D.C.: Island Press, 2003.

Fried, M. "Grieving for a Lost Home." In L. Duhl (ed.), *The Urban Condition.* New York: Basic Books, 1963.

Frumkin, H. "Beyond Toxicity: Human Health and the Natural Environment." *American Journal of Preventive Medicine,* 2001, *20*(3), 234–240.

Frumkin, H. "Healthy Places: Exploring the Evidence." *American Journal of Public Health,* 2003, *93,* 1451–1456.

Garces, R. F. *Experts Propose Policies to Bridge California's Digital Divide, Improve Health.* California Center for Health Improvement. [http://www.cchi.org/pdf/WrkHlth2.pdf]. 2000.

Garland, C. A., and Stokols, D. "The Effect of Neighborhood Reputation on Fear of Crime and Inner City Investment." In J. I. Arragones, G. Francescato, and T. Garling (eds.), *Residential Environments: Choice, Satisfaction, and Behavior.* Westport, Conn.: Greenwood, 2002.

Gifford, R. *Environmental Psychology: Principles and Practice.* (2nd ed.) Boston: Allyn and Bacon, 1997.

Glass, D. C., and Singer, J. E. *Urban Stress.* New York: Academic Press, 1972.

Holman, E. A., and Stokols, D. "The Environmental Psychology of Child Sexual Abuse." *Journal of Environmental Psychology,* 1994, *14,* 237–252.

Hygge, S., Evans, G. W., and Bullinger, M. "A Prospective Study of Some Effects of Aircraft Noise on Cognitive Performance in Schoolchildren." *Psychological Science,* 2002, *13*(5), 469–474.

International Technology and Trade Associates. "State of the Internet 2000." [http://www.itta.com/internet2000.htm]. 2000.

Ittelson, W. H. *Environment and Cognition.* New York: Seminar Press, 1973.

Jacobs, J. *The Death and Life of Great American Cities.* New York: Random House, 1961.

Kaplan, R., and Kaplan, S. *The Experience of Nature: A Psychological Perspective.* New York: Cambridge University Press, 1989.

Kiesler, S. (ed.). *Culture of the Internet.* Mahwah, N.J.: Erlbaum, 1997.

Kling, R., and Iacono, S. "Making a 'Computer Revolution.'" In C. Dunlop and R. Kling (eds.), *Computerization and Controversy: Value Conflicts and Social Choices.* New York: Academic Press, 1991.

Kohn, L. T., Corrigan, J., and Donaldson, M. S. *To Err Is Human: Building a Safer Health System.* Washington, D.C.: National Academies Press, 2000.

Koren, H., and Bisesi, M. (eds.). *Handbook of Environmental Health.* 2 vols. (4th ed.) Boca Raton, Fla.: CRC Press, 2002.

Langer, E. J., and Rodin, J. "The Effects of Choice and Enhanced Personal Responsibility for the Aged: A Field Experiment in an Institutional Setting." *Journal of Personality and Social Psychology,* 1976, *34,* 191–198.

Lewis, C. A. "Comment: Healing in the Urban Environment: A Person/Plant Viewpoint." *Journal of the American Planning Association,* 1979, *45,* 330–338.

Lindheim, R., and Syme, S. L. "Environments, People, and Health." *Annual Review of Public Health,* 1983, *4,* 335–359.

Lyman, P., and Varian, H. R. "How Much Information?" Berkeley School of Information Management and Systems, University of California. [http://www.sims.berkeley.edu/how-much-info]. Oct. 20, 2000.

Lynch, K. *The Image of the City.* Cambridge, Mass.: MIT Press, 1960.

Magnusson, D. "Wanted: A Psychology of Situations." In D. Magnusson (ed.), *Toward a Psychology of Situations: An Interactional Perspective.* Mahwah, N.J.: Erlbaum, 1981.

Mathews, K.E.J., and Canon, L. K. "Environmental Noise Level as a Determinant of Helping Behavior." *Journal of Personality and Social Psychology,* 1975, *32,* 571–577.

McEwen, B. S., and Stellar, E. "Stress and the Individual: Mechanisms Leading to Disease." *Archives of Internal Medicine,* 1993, *153,* 2093–2101.

Messagingonline. "AOL Per-User Email Figures Climb 60 Percent in 1999." [http://www.messagingonline.net/mt/html/feature020400.html]. Oct. 29, 2000.

Meyrowitz, J. *No Sense of Place: The Impact of Electronic Media on Social Behavior.* New York: Oxford University Press, 1985.

Michelson, W. H. *From Sun to Sun: Daily Obligations and Community Structure in the Lives of Employed Women and Their Families.* Lanham, Md.: Rowman & Littlefield, 1985.

Milgram, S. "The Experience of Living in Cities." *Science,* 1970, *167,* 1461–1468.

Milgram, S., and Jodelet, D. "Psychological Maps of Paris." In H. M. Proshansky, W. H. Ittelson, and L. G. Rivlin (eds.), *Environmental Psychology.* (2nd ed.) Austin, Tex.: Holt, Rinehart and Winston, 1976.

Moos, R. H. "Social Ecological Perspectives on Health." In G. C. Stone, F. Cohen, and N. E. Adler (eds.), *Health Psychology: A Handbook.* San Francisco: Jossey Bass, 1979.

Nasar, J. L., and Fisher, B. "'Hot Spots' of Fear and Crime: A Multimethod Investigation." *Journal of Environmental Psychology,* 1993, *13,* 187–206.

National Telecommunications and Information Administration. "Americans in the Information Age Falling Through the Net." [http://www.ntia.doc.gov/ntiahome/digitaldivide]. 2000.
Negroponte, N. P. *Being Digital.* New York: Vintage Books, 1995.
Newman, O. *Creating Defensible Space.* Rockville, Md.: U.S. Department of Housing and Urban Development, 1966.
Newman, O. *Defensible Space.* New York: Macmillan, 1973.
Nie, N. H., and Erbring, L. *Internet and Society: A Preliminary Report.* Stanford Institute for the Quantitative Study of Society. [http://www.stanford.edu/group/siqss/Press_Release/Preliminary_Report.pdf]. 2000.
O'Donnell, M. P. "Definition of Health Promotion, Part III: Expanding the Definition." *American Journal of Health Promotion,* 1989, *3,* 5.
Oldenburg, R. *The Great Good Place: Cafes, Coffee Shops, Bookstores, Bars, Hair Salons, and Other Hangouts at the Heart of a Community.* (2nd ed.) New York: Marlowe, 1999.
O'Neil, R., and Greenberger, E. "Patterns of Commitment to Work and Parenting: Implications for Role Strain." *Journal of Marriage and the Family,* 1994, *56,* 101–112.
Pastalan, L. A. "Environmental Displacement: A Literature Reflecting Old Person-Environment Transactions." In G. D. Rowles and R. J. Ohta (eds.), *Aging and Milieu: Environmental Perspectives on Growing Old.* New York: Academic Press, 1983.
Perkins, D., Wandersman, A., Rich, R., and Taylor, R. "The Physical Environment of Street Crime: Defensible Space, Territoriality, and Incivilities." *Journal of Environmental Psychology,* 1993, *13,* 29–49.
Pervin, L. A. "Definitions, Measurements, and Classifications of Stimuli, Situations, and Environments." *Human Ecology,* 1978, *6,* 71–105.
Proshansky, H. M., Fabian, A. K., and Kaminoff, R. "Place Identity: Physical World Socialization of the Self." *Journal of Environmental Psychology,* 1983, *3,* 57–83.
Proshansky, H. M., Ittelson, W. H., and Rivlin, L. G. (eds.). *Environmental Psychology.* (2nd ed.) Austin, Tex.: Holt, Rinehart and Winston, 1976.
Putnam, R. D. *Bowling Alone: The Collapse and Revival of American Community.* New York: Simon & Schuster, 2000.
Rashad, I., and Grossman, M. *The Economics of Obesity.* [http://www.thepublicinterest.com/archives/2004summer/article3.html]. 2004.
Rheingold, H. *The Virtual Community: Homesteading on the Electronic Frontier.* Reading, Mass.: Addison-Wesley, 1993.
Rivlin, L. G. "The Neighborhood, Personal Identity, and Group Affiliations." In I. Altman and A. Wandersman (eds.), *Neighborhood and Community Environments.* Vol. 9. New York: Plenum, 1987.
Rodin, J., and Langer, E. J. "Long-Term Effects of a Control-Relevant Intervention with the Institutionalized Aged." *Journal of Personality and Social Psychology,* 1977, *35,* 897–902.
Schoggen, P. *Behavior Settings: A Revision and Extension of Roger G. Barker's Ecological Psychology.* Stanford, Calif.: Stanford University Press, 1989.
Schulz, R., and Hanusa, B. H. "Long-Term Effects of Control and Predictability-Enhancing Interventions: Findings and Ethical Issues." *Journal of Personality and Social Psychology,* 1978, *36,* 1194–1201.
Selye, H. *The Stress of Life.* New York: McGraw-Hill, 1956.
Silver, R. C., and others. "Nationwide Longitudinal Study of Psychological Responses to September 11." *Journal of the American Medical Association,* 2002, *288,* 1235–1244.
Sommer, R. *Personal Space: The Behavioral Basis of Design.* Upper Saddle River, N.J.: Prentice Hall, 1969.

Stokols, D. "The Paradox of Environmental Psychology." *American Psychologist*, 1995, *50*, 821–837.

Stokols, D. "Human Development in the Age of the Internet: Conceptual and Methodological Horizons." In S. L. Friedman and T. D. Wachs (eds.), *Measuring Environment Across the Lifespan: Emerging Methods and Concepts*. Washington, D.C.: American Psychological Association, 1999.

Stokols, D., and Altman, I. (eds.). *Handbook of Environmental Psychology*. 2 vols. Hoboken, N.J.: Wiley, 1987.

Stokols, D., McMahan, S., Clitheroe, H.C.J., and Wells, M. "Enhancing Corporate Compliance with Worksite Safety and Health Legislation." *Journal of Safety Research*, 2001, *32*, 441–463.

Stokols, D., & Montero, M. "Toward an Environmental Psychology of the Internet." In R. Bechtel & A. Churchman (eds.), *Handbook of Environmental Psychology* (pp. 661–675). New York: Wiley, 2002.

Stokols, D., and Shumaker, S. "People in Places: A Transactional View of Settings." In J. Harvey (ed.), *Cognition, Social Behavior, and the Environment*. Mahwah, N.J.: Erlbaum, 1981.

Sundstrom, E., and Sundstrom, M. G. *Work Places: The Psychology of the Physical Environment in Offices and Factories*. New York: Cambridge University Press, 1986.

Taylor, R. B. *Human Territorial Functioning*. New York: Cambridge University Press, 1988.

Taylor, S. E., Repetti, R. L., and Seeman, T. "Health Psychology: What Is an Unhealthy Environment and How Does It Get Under the Skin?" *Annual Review of Psychology*, 1997, *48*, 411–447.

Unger, D. G., and Wandersman, A. "The Importance of Neighbors: The Social, Cognitive, and Affective Components of Neighboring." *American Journal of Community Psychology*, 1985, *13*(2), 139–160.

Wellman, B. "Physical Place and Cyberplace: The Rise of Personalized Networking." *International Journal of Urban and Regional Research*, 2001, *25*(2), 227–252.

Wellman, B., and Haythornthwaite, C. A. (eds.). *The Internet in Everyday Life*. Malden, Mass.: Blackwell, 2002.

World Health Organization. *The Ottawa Charter for Health Promotion (Declaration from the 1st International Conference on Health Promotion)*. [http://www.who.int/hpr/archive/docs/ottawa.html]. 1986.

World Health Organization. *The Jakarta Declaration on Leading Health Promotion into the 21st Century (Declaration from the 4th International Conference on Health Promotion)*. [http://www.who.int/hpr/archive/docs/jakarta/english.html]. 1997.

Yassi, A., Kjellström, T., de Kok, T., and Guidotti, T. *Basic Environmental Health*. New York: Oxford University Press. 2001.

For Further Information

Academic Journals

Environment and Behavior. Sage Publications. [http://www.sagepub.co.uk/journals/details/j0163.html].

Journal of Environmental Psychology. Academic Press. [http://www.hbuk.co.uk/ap/journals/ps]. Ltd.

Journal of Architectural and Planning Research. Locke Science Publishing. [http://archone.tamu.edu/pressroom/japr/japr_index.html].

Professional Organizations

American Psychological Association, Division 34, Population and Environmental Psychology. E-mail: DIV34@LISTS.APA.ORG

American Sociological Association, Environment and Technology Section. [http://www.asanet.org/sections/environ.html]; Community and Urban Sociology Section. [http://www.asanet.org/sections/commun.html].

Canadian Psychological Association, Environmental Section. [http://www.cpa.ca/environmental/].

City University of New York, Graduate Training Programs in Environmental Psychology, Environmental Psychology Doctoral Training Program, Graduate Center. [http://web.gc.cuny.edu/dept/psych/environmental/index.htm].

Environment-Behaviour Research Association of China. [http://www.ebra2004.com/home.htm].

Environment, Behaviour, and Society Research. Department of Architecture, University of Sydney. [http://www.arch.usyd.edu.au/web/research/ebr.html].

Environmental Design Research Association (EDRA). [http://www.edra.org/].

Environmental Psychology Division of the International Association for Applied Psychology [http://www.psy.gu.se/iaap/envpsych.htm].

Environmental Psychology in the UK. [http://www.envpsy.org.uk/index.php].

International Association for People-Environment Studies (IAPS). [http://www.iaps-association.org].

University of California-Irvine, School of Social Ecology, Ph.D. Program in Social Ecology. [http://www.seweb.uci.edu].

University of Wisconsin-Milwaukee, School of Architecture and Urban Planning, Ph.D. Program in Architecture, Environment-Behavior Studies. [http://www.uwm.edu:80/dept/phd-arch-ebs/toc.htm].

CHAPTER SIX

GENETICS AND ENVIRONMENTAL HEALTH

Samuel H. Wilson

The solution of a medical mystery in England in 1775 provided the first scientific documentation that exposure to environmental chemicals can cause human disease. Percival Potts, who is today considered the father of epidemiology, noticed that chimney sweeps (young boys small enough to shimmy down chimneys) were contracting scrotal cancer at an unusually high rate. Potts correctly deduced that exposure to the coal tar in the soot they were removing was causing the malignant lesions. When the youngsters were given the opportunity to bathe regularly, the incidence of the lesions decreased (Doll, [1955] 1993).

Knowledge of environmental health science is far more sophisticated today than it was in Percival Potts's time. We understand that the interaction between our environment and our genes is often at the root of disease, an insight that makes scientific questions, issues, and investigations infinitely more complex. For example, some people are more susceptible than others to organophosphate pesticide poisoning, as well as to vascular disease, because of variations in a gene involved in toxicant metabolism (Davies and others, 1996; Jarvik and others, 2003; Li and others, 2000). In other words, a dose that is harmless to one person can

The author wishes to thank science writer Ernie Hood for his instrumental role in the preparation of this chapter.

make another person sick. This is one of the many examples of *gene-environment interaction*—a concept that has gained wide acceptance in the scientific community and is central to the future of both genetics and environmental health (Collins, 2004; Potter, 2004). These two fields, once separate and distinct, are now inextricably entwined. *Genetics,* the study of individual genes, has expanded to include *genomics,* which is the study of all the genes that make up an organism; a complete genome is present in every cell and governs an individual's unique characteristics and responses. Similarly, the definition of what constitutes the environment has evolved. Currently, and particularly as it relates to gene-environment interactions, the *environment* is considered to be anything outside the body that can affect an individual's health. This includes of course our air, water, soil, and climate, but also takes into account elements such as the food, drink, and medicine we ingest, behavioral choices such as tobacco and alcohol consumption, infectious agents, socioeconomic status, age or developmental status, stress, and even the structures and infrastructure around us (the so-called built environment) (Hanna and Coussens, 2001; also see Chapter Sixteen).

Gene-Environment Interactions: Susceptibility, Risk, and Exposure

The questions of what causes disease and what can we do to prevent it, cure it, or minimize its impact on quality of life have been medicine's central questions from time immemorial. Today they are the central questions that propel the mission of biomedical science to understand and characterize gene-environment interactions. The vast majority of human disease arises when something is wrong in the relationship between our body and the environment. Such miscues can occur in the blink of an eye, as in the case of acute exposures to toxic agents, or can take decades to develop, in illnesses such as cancer or Alzheimer's disease.

Although certain inherited disorders, such as Huntington's disease, cystic fibrosis, and Tay-Sachs disease, arise from mutation in a single gene, these are relatively rare, accounting for no more than 5 percent of human disease. Thus the risk of such a disease for a person with a specific disease gene variant (referred to as an *allele*) is relatively high, but the incidence of such *monogenic* diseases in the general population is low. However, many common human diseases appear to be *polygenic,* resulting from complex interactions of several genes. A variant of one gene might not be detrimental, but it might become detrimental in combination with specific alleles of other genes. Such susceptibility conferring genes increase disease risk only a fewfold, but they can have a large effect on the incidence of a disease in the human population because of their frequency. Susceptibility genes alone are not sufficient to cause disease; they modify risk in combination with other genes and with exposure to environmental agents.

Every organism is continually exposed to hazardous agents in its environment. As a result organisms have evolved sophisticated pathways that can minimize the biological consequences of such exposures. These pathways constitute what we term the *environmental response machinery.* All human genes, including those that encode components of the environmental response machinery, are subject to genetic variability, which can be associated with altered efficiency of the gene product (usually an enzyme or protein) and ultimately with a biological pathway. So a person's risk for developing an illness as a result of an environmental exposure might depend on the efficiency of his or her own unique set of environmental response genes. These genes might, for example, determine how an individual responds to and metabolizes drugs or carcinogenic compounds after exposure (Figure 6.1).

Determining how genetic susceptibility contributes to disease risk from environmental exposures is a main focus of today's environmental health research. In the quest to characterize gene-environment interactions, however, the picture is immensely complicated. Not only are combinations of genes typically involved but there are also issues of combinations of exposures, the time periods over which exposures have occurred (relative to physiological development and age), and the detection and identification of chronic low-level exposures. The panoply of variables affecting gene-environment interactions is dauntingly large. But advances in research technologies and methods and in computational abilities have given environmental health scientists new tools that should spawn major improvements in public health. (Box 6.1 reviews some of the issues beyond health issues that this genetic research is raising.)

FIGURE 6.1. DETERMINANTS OF INDIVIDUAL RESPONSE TO AN ENVIRONMENTAL EXPOSURE.

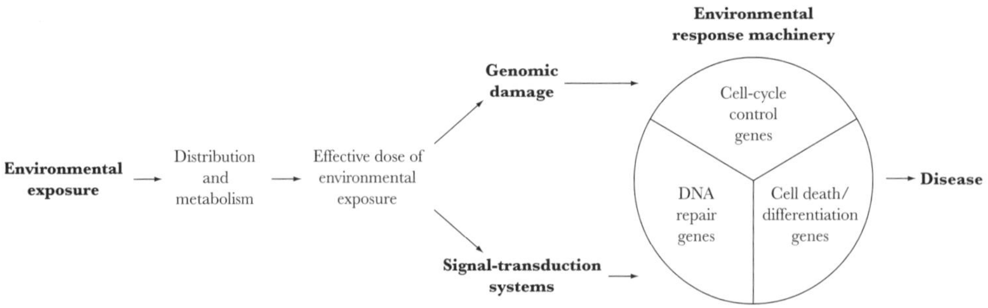

Box 6.1. What About ELSIs?

Most people today are at least nominally familiar with the ethical, legal, and social implications (ELSIs) of genetics, such as the potential for genetic discrimination by employers or insurers, the confidentiality issues, and so on. As science and technology rapidly progress and the fields of genomics and environmental health converge, many thorny issues will need to be dealt with forthrightly in the public debate.

Advancing knowledge of risk and susceptibility, which will eventually enable routine determination of an individual's susceptibility to a wide variety of environmentally induced diseases, will require real-world answers to ELSI questions that today are still largely anticipatory and theoretical. For example, if you are found through genotyping to have an increased susceptibility to a specific disease, a risk that is increased by exposure to a specific material, do you have the right to be employed in a workplace in which you might be likely to suffer that exposure? Does the employer have the right to deny you employment based on your genotype, or is the employer obligated to provide a workplace, potentially at great expense, in which you will be protected from occupational exposure to the agent? This is just one among many lines that will soon need to be drawn to ensure that all stakeholders are adequately, responsibly, and ethically informed and protected.

The Human Genome Project recognized the need to address these issues from its inception in 1990 and allocated a significant percentage of its overall budget to the research and outreach activities undertaken by its ELSI program. The ELSI program was a successful instance of the scientific community taking its responsibility to the public seriously. It stands today as a model for future initiatives (including a proposed independent, nonprofit genomic policy organization) designed to ensure that as we learn more and more about gene-environment interactions and as that learning influences public and private policies, the rights of every person to privacy, personal freedom, and fair treatment will not be compromised (for review, see Sharp, Yudell, and Wilson, 2004).

The Human Genome Project and Beyond

The last half of the twentieth century and the early years of the twenty-first century were a period of extraordinarily rapid progress in biomedical research. In 1953, the structure of the DNA double helix was reported (Watson and Crick, 1953). Just fifty years later, scientists in the Human Genome Project (HGP) completed sequencing the genome, providing a complete roadmap to the locations of the approximately 30,000 human genes (an event hailed by special issues of the journals *Nature* [Feb. 15, 2001], and *Science* [Feb. 16, 2001]). The sequencing of the human genome will probably stand as one of the most significant achievements in the history of science; nonetheless it is clear that the genomic information has not, in and of itself, resulted in answers to the many questions about the genetic basis of disease. The genome sequence can be viewed as a dictionary that gives researchers the framework needed to flesh out "the grammar and syntax of the language of disease." As National Human Genome Research Institute director Francis Collins (2001) put it when the project was nearing completion, "[This is] the end of the beginning . . . the true payoff from the HGP will be the ability to diagnose, treat, and prevent disease, and most of those benefits to humanity still lie ahead." The genome sequence information will be used as a reference to learn about individual human genetic variations. The extent of genetic variation, or *polymorphism,* between human beings is still unknown, as is the question of how much variation is acquired as we age.

Genetic Variation

Although the completed human genome sequence is vital to achieving an understanding of disease, it is the characterization of genetic variations among individuals or groups that will provide the most useful information. Variations in genes or groups of related genes result in *phenotypes.* Phenotypes can describe physical traits such as hair color, behavioral features such as anxiety, and specific physiological susceptibilities or responses to gene-environment interactions. Our collective individual phenotypes make us who we are—determining whether we are at greater risk than the general population of contracting a disease or whether a particular drug will work, prove ineffective, or even be toxic for us.

The genetic variation among individuals is typically due to single nucleotide polymorphisms (SNPs) and insertions and deletions of DNA known as *indels.* Identifying these DNA sequence variations, and characterizing how they determine or influence phenotypes, is the focus of an enormous amount of current research and is the starting point for arriving at a useful understanding of gene-environment interactions and their myriad effects on human health (Box 6.2).

Box 6.2. Genetic Variability and Susceptibility to Lead Toxicity

Lead has long been recognized to be highly toxic to humans. Although environmental levels of the metal have been greatly reduced over the past few decades, due in large measure to its elimination from gasoline and paint, lead toxicity is still a major public health problem, especially in children who live in housing retaining lead-based paint residues or who reside in lead-contaminated localities, such as areas close to smelters or battery factories. The problem is exacerbated by the fact that lead accumulates in the body and that lead acquired early in life can be released into the bloodstream to wreak physiological havoc much later in life—during menopause, for example.

Environmental health scientists have determined that polymorphisms in certain genes can make some individuals far more susceptible to the damaging effects of lead poisoning by affecting the absorption, accumulation, and transport of the toxin. Variants of the gene coding for δ-aminolevulinic acid dehydratase (ALAD), an enzyme involved in heme biosynthesis, for example, appear to adversely affect bone and blood levels of lead. Polymorphisms of the vitamin D receptor (VDR) gene have been implicated in increased accumulation of lead in bone. Also variants of the hemochromatosis gene coding for the HFE protein, which is involved in iron transport in the body, may also influence lead absorption and transport (Onalaja and Claudio, 2000). Discovery and characterization of these and other genetic markers of increased susceptibility to lead toxicity are key scientific milestones in the effort to reduce, treat, or prevent gene-environment interactions that cause disease and dysfunction associated with lead poisoning.

It has been estimated that there are roughly 11 million SNPs in the human population (Kruglyak and Nickerson, 2001), of which several million have been identified and catalogued by various research efforts. To be recognized as a SNP, a single-letter variation in DNA sequence must occur in at least 1 percent of the population. SNPs with a frequency of 10 percent or more are thought of as *common.* SNPs tend to occur in patterns, or blocks, of associated, inherited alleles called *haplotypes.* The identification of haplotypes can in some cases obviate the need to document individual SNPs, as the haplotype is considered to be the inherited functional unit that ultimately influences physiology. A public-private research consortium called the International HapMap Project (2005) aims to map all the haplotypes in the human genome. The HapMap, to be completed by 2006, will be a powerful new tool for researchers to identify genetic variations in disease susceptibility, drug response, infectious disease resistance, and longevity. Although initiatives designed to establish comprehensive databases of SNPs, indels, and haplotypes take the genome sequence data compiled by the HGP a step farther, they still do not yield directly applicable information, that is, knowledge that will translate directly into beneficial new treatments, prevention, or therapeutic paradigms. That step will require more information about how human genetic variation is associated with phenotypes.

The New Generation in Environmental Health Research

Polymorphisms in an individual's environmental response genes can modify the risk of environmentally induced disease. To achieve an understanding of that relationship and its implications in gene-environment interactions, the National

Institutes of Health launched an initiative in 1997 called the Environmental Genome Project (EGP, 2005). The EGP uses the *candidate gene* approach to identify and characterize human genetic variability in selected genes thought to be involved in susceptibility to toxicant-induced disease (Olden and Wilson, 2000; Wilson and Olden, 2004). By resequencing the selected candidate genes in a set of DNA samples representative of the U.S. population, the project aims to discover SNPs and other variants that are relevant to environmental responses, and eventually to yield knowledge that will have implications for medical and environmental policymaking and regulation (Box 6.3).

Box 6.3. EGP Cases in Point

Using the candidate gene approach the EGP has already engendered significant information about genes implicated in gene-environment interactions at the root of human disease. As briefly alluded to earlier, EGP investigators Clement Furlong and colleagues have conducted detailed studies of polymorphisms in the paraoxanase gene PON1 (Davies and others, 1996; Jarvik and others, 2003; Li and others, 2000). The gene regulates production of the enzyme paraoxanase (PON1), which metabolizes toxic organophosphates and some pharmaceutical agents, such as the cholesterol-lowering statin drugs. Furlong's group discovered that certain SNPs influence PON1 activity, altering production of the enzyme. Their study clearly demonstrated that an individual's PON1 status has implications for susceptibility to environmentally associated diseases, including organophosphate toxicity and cardiovascular disease. PON1 status also is suspected to be involved in susceptibility to Gulf War syndrome (as well as Parkinson's disease), although studies of that association have shown conflicting results (Kelada and others, 2003; Kondo and Yamamoto, 1998; Taylor, Le Couteur, Mellick, and Board, 2000; Akhmedova, Anisimov, Yakimovsky, and Schwartz, 1999; Akhmedova, Yakimovsky, and Schwartz, 2001; Wang and Liu, 2000).

EGP researcher Martyn Smith, of the University of California at Berkeley, examined gene-environment interactions in blood-related cancers, including leukemia, lymphoma, and myeloma. Many leukemia cases are thought to be induced by environmental factors, including exposure to benzene, radiation, and chemotherapeutic agents. Genetic factors are also thought to play a significant role, especially in pathways controlling DNA repair and oxidative DNA damage. Smith and his collaborators identified one candidate gene that appears to be involved in the etiology of leukemia, namely, the gene encoding NAD(P)H:quinone acceptor oxireductase 1 (NOQ1). This enzyme plays a role in preventing oxidative damage caused by exogenous and endogenous quinines, which are biologically active compounds found in natural substances such as vitamins, aloe, and henna and in chemicals such as photographic fixatives and dyes. The C609T polymorphism of that gene, which occurs in 5 to 20 percent of the population, results in complete loss of enzyme activity in homozygotes (people with two copies of the variant gene). Case-control studies indicate a 1.5- to 2.5-fold increased odds ratio for several types of leukemia in association with the 609T variant (Smith and others, 2001, 2002; Krajinovic and others, 2002). Although this effect is relatively small, adverse environmental exposure may interact with this genetic variant and lead to significantly increased risk of disease.

The concept of environmentally responsive genes is illustrated in Figure 6.1, and those genes selected for study by the EGP tend to fall into eight categories: cell cycle, DNA repair, cell division, cell signaling, cell structure, gene expression, apoptosis, and metabolism. Cell cycle and cell division genes regulate the ability of a cell to proliferate, grow, and differentiate. Changes in the progression of a cell through the cell cycle can increase the cell's ability to survive stress, for example, by allowing cellular damage to be repaired prior to cell division. Cell signaling and gene expression pathways have effects on all cellular functions, including cell proliferation and differentiation. Metabolic pathways are crucial determinants of the outcome of exposure. An innocuous compound may be metabolically converted into a reactive species that causes cellular damage; alternatively, some metabolic pathways destroy toxic compounds by changing the compound's chemical structure. DNA repair genes can influence the outcome of exposure to environmental agents that cause DNA damage. Individuals with higher or lower capacity for DNA repair have decreased or increased risk, respectively, of certain types of environmentally induced disease. Heavily damaged cells often die by the process known as apoptosis, or programmed cell death. This process protects the organism by removing damaged or aberrant cells, and failure to execute the process is associated with adverse health effects, such as cancer.

To date about 400 candidate genes, mostly metabolism, DNA repair, and cell cycle genes, have been resequenced by the EGP. Another accomplishment was compilation of the publicly accessible GeneSNPs database, which lists the thousands of new SNPs made available for research use (GeneSNPs, 2005; EGP, 2005). The EGP has also turned researchers' attention to the functional significance of polymorphisms in an effort to establish whether or not each polymorphism is an active component in exposure-associated disease. One method of tying SNPs and indels to function is to develop and examine mouse models of human gene variants, and the EGP is currently doing this in a project known as the Comparative Mouse Genomics Centers Consortium. The mouse models produced in this project will be subject to phenotypic analysis in tests of susceptibility to environmental exposures.

Beyond the laboratory, the significance of individual polymorphisms can be elucidated by population-based research, in which large numbers of people are screened for variants and the data are analyzed to determine associations between polymorphisms, disease susceptibility, and exposures (Altshuler, Kruglyak, and Lander, 1998). The effects of solitary gene polymorphisms are believed to be relatively weak, and the environmentally induced diseases under study are believed to be polygenic, involving interactions of multiple genetic variants and exposures. Due to these factors the population studies will need to be very large to identify subgroups at increased risk of disease because of their particular genotypes. This will undoubtedly be a challenging aspect of the EGP, but it is this type of knowledge that will yield the largest public health benefits.

Linking Genes and Environmental Exposures

As already noted in this chapter, most human disease is understood to involve complex interactions among genetic predispositions (due to genetic variants), environmental exposures (both acute and chronic—that is, both short- and long-term), and aging or physiological development. Although characterizing the relationships among these elements in a useful way is an extraordinarily complicated undertaking, this is the pathway that will eventually lead to a new age of medicine and disease prevention. An era of personalized medicine is possible, but the road toward achieving it is still very long, most realistically measured in decades. The assurance of progress requires that multiple research approaches be used for linking exposures with clinical disease (Figure 6.2).

The traditional approach to environmental exposure assessment, working from the release of a toxicant into the general environment to human exposure to internal dose to biological effect and eventually to disease, has proven to be an extremely effective framework for environmental health research (Suk and Wilson, 2002). Its component methodologies have matured, and innovative measurement and assessment techniques continue to be developed. In the hazard assessment approach to exposure, advanced techniques are employed to characterize the relationship between the dose of an agent and the adverse response of a model organism. Obviously, the starting point for this type of investigation is the agent itself, along with a variety of questions: Is the agent toxic? At what levels of exposure is it toxic? What are the biological effects of such exposures? How do genotypes modulate the impacts of those effects? And the ultimate question of course is, How can this information be interpreted to accurately predict human health outcomes following exposure to environmentally relevant doses? These can be extremely complicated questions, but methodologies are emerging to characterize dose-response curves at the molecular level (such as gene expression, protein expression, metabolism, and so forth). High-throughput analytical tools along with the computational tools necessary to interpret massive amounts of data have

FIGURE 6.2. RESEARCH APPROACHES TO LINK ENVIRONMENTAL EXPOSURES WITH DISEASE.

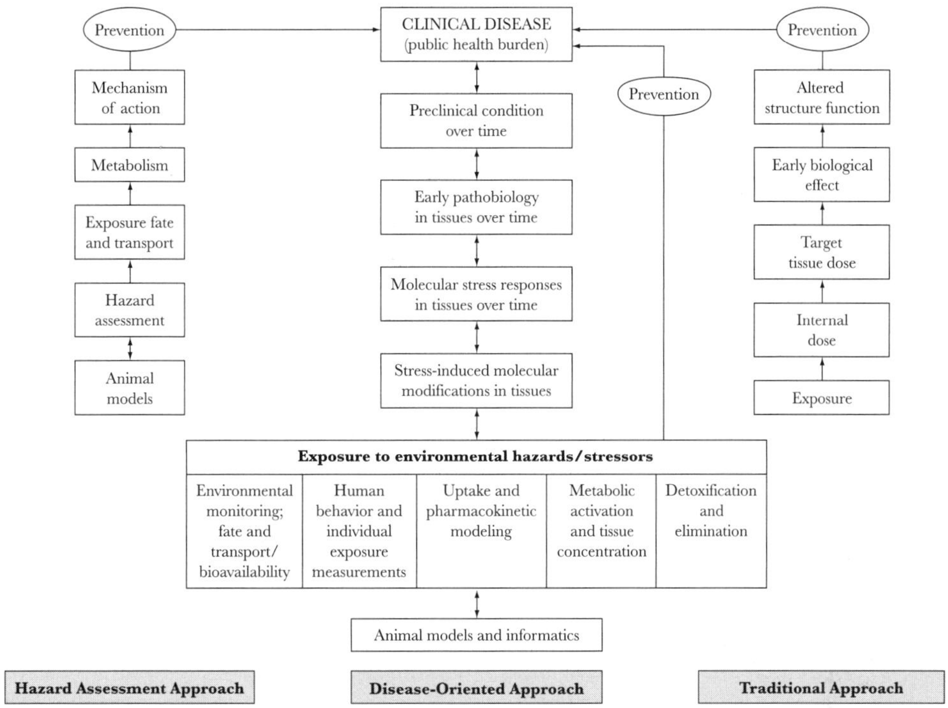

allowed the development of the scientific paradigm known as *systems biology.* In systems biology the goal is to understand the functioning and responses of the entire organism by integrating information about its elements (such as genes and proteins) with knowledge about the elements' interrelationships. Many laboratories are using high-throughput tools to gain an understanding of how the system operates, while refining information about dose-response relationships.

To understand linkages between disease and environmental exposures, several distinct categories of information must be pursued simultaneously, such as the measurement of general atmospheric pollutants and toxicants, the fate and transport of hazardous agents in the ecosystem, the human body burden and metabolism of such agents, and the biomarkers of exposure. Yet all this information needs to be clearly related to the disease burden. This creates the need for another exposure-disease approach that can provide accurate, consistent health status endpoints that can be measured precisely over many years. The disease-oriented approach, which is currently emerging as a new construct in the field, takes a clinical disease and the public health burden it represents as its starting point, or surrogate of exposure, and then facilitates inquiry toward the molecular characterization of disease and the underlying exposure responses (Figure 6.2). This approach is presently being used to investigate gene-environment interactions in major diseases influenced by environmental exposures, such as breast cancer, Parkinson's disease, and autism. The disease-oriented approach relies on both exposure research and large-scale studies of the health status of the general population over long periods of time, to identify subpopulations at risk and groups of unaffected individuals for comparison. Research initiatives using this approach will of necessity be large scale and lengthy.

The -Omics Technologies

Many significant advances seen in environmental health sciences over the past several years have been facilitated by the availability of an improved scientific toolbox: improved cellular and animal models; new, more precise experimental methods, materials, and computational tools; and perhaps most of all, new scientific specialties known collectively as the *-omics* technologies. Just as genetics has embraced genomics, many of the traditional fields in biology have now embraced an -omics component, each with the capability of studying biological phenomena on the genome scale. For example, *pharmacogenetics,* which examines the response of individual genes to medicines, now includes *pharmacogenomics,* which looks at drug response over the entire genome and is in widespread use to identify drug targets, screen compounds for medicinal activity, and characterize response phenotypes. Pharmacogenomics is part of the push toward personalized medicine. Although such an application of pharmacogenomics is still over the horizon, even today the field is having some impact on individuals' medical care. The breast cancer drug trastuzumab (trade name Herceptin) is marketed in tandem with a diagnostic test that determines whether it will work in individual patients; if a patient's tumor is found to be of a type that will respond to the drug, therapy is commenced; if not, other treatments are employed. Individualized response (or lack of response or hyperresponse) to medication is certainly one very important manifestation of gene-environment interaction. But given the broad definition of environment there are many more. The investigation of relationships between environmental exposures and genotypes has engendered the relatively new field called *toxicogenomics.* Toxicogenomics has its roots in traditional toxicology, but again, the ability to examine (or *interrogate*) all of the genes in a genome simultaneously, allows researchers to take a systems biology approach to an organism's response to an environmental insult. Genomewide screenings, which document which genes are expressed in response to a particular exposure, can shed light on the pathways and signaling networks that are relevant to outcomes. Due to the increasing number of animal genomes that have been sequenced, such as mouse, rat, yeast, zebra fish, nematode, and other genomes, researchers are also pursuing inquiries in the field known as *comparative toxicogenomics.* Comparing genomic responses to identical exposures among animal species and humans is a fruitful method of discovering and describing cellular mechanisms in the environmental response machinery (Mattingly and others, 2004).

Each step along the pathway of cellular response has its own specialized field of study within the -omics universe (for a complete glossary of the -omics, see Cambridge Healthtech Institute, 2005). For the purposes of this chapter's broad overview of genomics and environmental health, two additional -omics areas should be described: proteomics and metabolomics (also referred to as metabonomics and metabolic profiling). *Proteomics* is the study of the proteome, the global expression of proteins in a cell. Unlike the genome, which is more or less static, finite, and can be completely mapped, the proteome is constantly changing in response to the cellular environment, and proteins are constantly interacting with one another in a highly complex fashion. So a cellular proteome is unlikely ever to be fully mapped; it is too dynamic and almost infinitely variable. But a point of proteomics is to gain information about which proteins are expressed by which genes, when and where in the cell and at what level, and in response to what stimuli. Vast amounts of useful information are expected to emerge from the field as these questions are addressed, protein-protein interactions are characterized, and signature patterns of response are derived. Proteomics also aims to classify differences in protein expression between known samples, such as diseased and nondiseased or exposed and unexposed. Unique proteomic patterns of disease can be identified, without necessarily identifying the specific proteins involved. This approach appears promising in the area of clinical diagnostics, as encouraging results have already been seen in the early detection of some forms of cancer (Petricoin and others, 2002) and the ability to predict the metastatic fate of lung tumors (Yanagisawa and others, 2004).

Functional proteomics seeks to uncover the functions of proteins and subsets of proteins by describing their interactions and functional importance in signaling networks, disease mechanisms, and various other biological processes. *Structural proteomics* involves mapping of the three-dimensional structures of proteins as they exist within the architecture of the cell. Such information can elucidate disease states and cellular functions and also can point to strategies for the design of therapeutic agents. And finally, *toxicoproteomics* is a field in its own right, with researchers using the methodologies of proteomics to uncover cellular and subcellular mechanisms behind responses to environmental toxicants and other stressors at the protein level. Each proteomics specialty uses extremely sophisticated bioinformatics to accomplish its tasks.

Metabolomics is another step in the pathway from disease to exposure, or vice versa. Enzymes govern the production of metabolites, which are often the biochemical endpoints in the response process. Metabolomics involves the identification of metabolites, or suites of metabolites, in body fluids as they relate to particular responses. This information can provide fingerprints that serve as biomarkers of response, in which the identity of the compounds themselves is a secondary consideration.

All of these -omics pursuits play an important role in the grand design to achieve a grasp of systems biology and systems toxicology. As the experimental technologies continue to advance, along with the bioinformatics tools required to glean useful knowledge from the enormous data sets generated, the field of environmental health sciences should move closer to an understanding of the entire range of gene-environment interactions, on both sides of the gene × environment equation.

Thought Questions

Information on a gene (allele) linked to human disease susceptibility is likely to be developed and quantified in terms of a "risk factor" established through epidemiology studies. Consider the following questions:

1. How does one communicate the concept of increased or decreased risk factor to the lay public?
2. How does one translate information obtained from a large epidemiology cohort to the task of providing advice to an individual patient or client?
3. With what degree of certainty can one translate risk factor data obtained from a large epidemiology cohort to the issue of causation in the courtroom?

References

Akhmedova, S., Anisimov, S., Yakimovsky, A., and Schwartz, E. "Gln—>Arg 191 Polymorphism of Paraoxonase and Parkinson's Disease." *Human Heredity,* 1999, *49,* 178–180.

Akhmedova, S. N., Yakimovsky, A. K., and Schwartz, E. I. "Paraoxonase 1 Met-Leu 54 Polymorphism Is Associated with Parkinson's Disease." *Journal of the Neurological Sciences,* 2001, *184,* 179–182.

Altshuler, D., Kruglyak, L., and Lander, E. "Genetic Polymorphisms and Disease." *New England Journal of Medicine,* 1998, *338,* 1626.

Cambridge Healthtech Institute. "-Omes and -Omics Glossary." [http://www.genomicglossaries.com/content/omes.asp]. 2005.

Collins, F. S. "Contemplating the End of the Beginning." *Genome Research,* 2001, *11*(5), 641–643.

Collins, F. S. "The Case for a US Prospective Cohort Study of Genes and Environment." *Nature,* 2004, *429,* 475–477.

Davies, H. G., and others. "The Effect of the Human Serum Paraoxonase Polymorphism Is Reversed with Diazoxon, Soman, and Sarin." *Nature Genetics,* 1996, *14,* 334–336.

Doll, R. "Mortality from Lung Cancer in Asbestos Workers." *British Journal of Industrial Medicine,* 1993, *50*(6), 485–490. (Originally published 1955)

Environmental Genome Project. Home page. [http://www.niehs.nih.gov/envgenom/home.htm]. 2005.

GeneSNPs. Home page. [http://www.genome.utah.edu/genesnps]. 2005.

Hanna, K., and Coussens, C. *Rebuilding the Unity of Health and the Environment, A New Vision of Environmental Health for the 21st Century: A Workshop Summary for the Institute of Medicine's Roundtable on Environmental Health Sciences, Research, and Medicine.* Washington, D.C.: National Academies Press, 2001.

International HapMap Project. Home page. [http://www.hapmap.org]. 2005.

Jarvik, G. P., and others. "Novel Paraoxonase (PON1) Nonsense and Missense Mutations Predicted by Functional Genome Assay of PON Status." *Pharmacogenetics,* 2003, *13,* 291–295.

Kelada, S. N., and others. "Paraoxonase 1 Promoter and Coding Region Polymorphisms in Parkinson's Disease." *Journal of Neurology, Neurosurgery, and Psychiatry,* 2003, *74*(4), 546–547.

Kondo, I., and Yamamoto, M. "Genetic Polymorphism of Paraoxonase 1 (PON1) and Susceptibility to Parkinson's Disease." *Brain Research,* 1998, *806,* 271–273.

Krajinovic, M., and others. "Role of NOQ1, MPO and CYP2E1 Genetic Polymorphisms in the Susceptibility to Childhood Acute Lymphoblastic Leukemia." *International Journal of Cancer,* 2002, *97,* 230–236.

Kruglyak, L., and Nickerson, D. A. "Variation Is the Spice of Life." *Nature Genetics,* 2001, *27,* 234–236.

Li, W. F., and others. "Catalytic Efficiency Determines the in-Vivo Efficacy of PON1 for Detoxifying Organophosphorus Compounds." *Pharmacogenetics,* 2000, *10,* 767–779.

Mattingly, C. J., and others. "Promoting Comparative Molecular Studies in Environmental Health Research: An Overview of the Comparative Toxicogenomics Database (CTD)." *Pharmacogenomics Journal,* 2004, *4*(1), 5–8.

Olden, K., and Wilson, S. "Environmental Health and Genomics: Visions and Implications." *Nature Reviews: Genetics,* 2000, *1,* 149–153.

Onalaja, A., and Claudio, L. "Genetic Susceptibility to Lead Poisoning." *Environmental Health Perspectives,* 2000, *108* (suppl. 1), 23–28.

Petricoin, E. F., and others. "Use of Proteomic Patterns in Serum to Identify Ovarian Cancer." *Lancet,* 2002, *359,* 572–577.

Potter, J. D. "Toward the Last Cohort." *Cancer Epidemiology, Biomarkers, and Prevention,* 2004, *13,* 895–897.

Sharp, R. R., Yudell, M. A., and Wilson, S. H. "Shaping Science Policy in the Age of Genomics." *Nature Reviews: Genetics,* 2004, *5,* 311–316.

Smith, M. T., and others. "Low NAD(P)H:Quinone Oxidoreductase 1 Activity Is Associated with Increased Risk of Acute Leukemia in Adults." *Blood,* 2001, *97,* 1422–1426.

Smith, M. T., and others. "Low NAD(P)H:Quinone Oxidoreductase Activity Is Associated with Increased Risk of Leukemia with MLL Translocations in Infants and Children." *Blood,* 2002, *100,* 4590–4593.

Suk, W. A., and Wilson, S. H. "Overview and Future of Molecular Biomarkers of Exposure and Early Disease in Environmental Health." In S. H. Wilson and W. A. Suk (eds.), *Biomarkers of Environmentally Associated Disease, Technologies, Concepts, and Perspectives.* Boca Raton, Fla.: Lewis, 2002.

Taylor, M. C., Le Couteur, D. G., Mellick, G. D., and Board, P. G. "Paraoxonase Polymorphisms, Pesticide Exposure and Parkinson's Disease in a Caucasian Population." *Journal of Neural Transmission,* 2000, *107,* 979–983.

Wang, J., and Liu, Z. "No Association Between Paraoxonase 1 (PON1) Gene Polymorphisms and Susceptibility to Parkinson's Disease in a Chinese Population." *Movement Disorders,* 2000, *15,* 1265–1267.

Watson, J. D., and Crick, F.H.C. "The Structure for Deoxyribose Nucleic Acid." *Nature,* 1953, *171,* 737–738.

Wilson, S. H., and Olden, K. "The Environmental Genome Project: Phase 1 and Beyond." *Molecular Interventions,* 2004, *4*(3), 147–156.

Yanagisawa, K., and others. "Proteomic Patterns of Tumour Subsets in Non-Small-Cell Lung Cancer." *Lancet,* 2004, *362,* 433–439.

For Further Information

These articles provide further background on genomics in general, and on gene-environment interactions.

Hunter, D. J. "Gene-Environment Interactions in Human Disease." *Nature Reviews Genetics,* 2005, *6*(4), 287–298.

Thayer, A. M. "The Genomics Evolution." *Chemical and Engineering News,* December 8, 2003.

The Environmental Genome Project (EGP) was initiated by the National Institute of Environmental Health Sciences (NIEHS) in 1998 to improve understanding of human genetic susceptibility to environmental exposures. Its Web site provides a good overview of current research in this field [http://www.niehs.nih.gov/envgenom/home.htm].

CHAPTER SEVEN

ENVIRONMENTAL HEALTH ETHICS

Andrew Jameton

We most often discuss ethics when a controversy or dilemma arises. However, ethical concerns are unobtrusively and globally present in the everyday fabric of life: Everyday actions by environmental health professionals typically depend on a commitment to such ethical values as service, human health, and concern for the environment.

Ethics and Morals

Ethics can be defined most readily by contrasting it with *morals. Morals,* or *morality,* is the set of core beliefs or commitments of a person or society that identifies what is most important, valuable, or right with regard to conduct and character. *Ethics* refers to a more formal version of morality. *Ethics* can mean

- A reasoned or systematic approach to figuring out what is the right or wrong thing to do or to stand for

The author thanks Susanna von Essen, M.D., professor, Internal Medicine, Section of Pulmonary and Critical Care, University of Nebraska Medical Center, and Kenneth W. Goodman, Ph.D., director, Bioethics Program, co-director, Ethics Programs, University of Miami, for their help.

- Professional morality as expressed in codes and statements, in contrast to personal morality
- The scholarly study of morality by philosophers

When faced with an ethical problem in professional life, one may visit some or all of these concepts of formal morality. Ethics is not simply about *describing* the morality of a person, association, or culture. Instead, it is a *normative* process of deciding what we should do or ought to do: "Philosophers have only *interpreted* the world in various ways;" wrote Marx and Engels ([1845] 1983, p. 158); "the point is to change it."

Ethics is essentially a connecting or interpretive vocabulary that helps us understand our daily actions in the light of a larger picture of society and the world around us. So, when we use an ethical concept such as *justice,* we may refer to a single fair action by an individual, a nationwide project to reduce health disparities, an initiative to reduce international debt, or even a belief that the universe keeps all events in harmony. Using a concept such as justice highlights the analogies between individual actions (such as one person keeping a promise) and larger entities (such as a government establishing a fair system of taxes). By using basic ethical concepts such as justice to refer to actions in relationship to a broad scale of groups and institutions, we maintain a feeling of coherence with regard to a broad range of actions.

Beginning students of ethics often think of moral beliefs as essentially private and consider it inappropriate to make moral judgments about the conduct of others, but they soon learn that friends and professional colleagues often have genuinely useful and justifiable ideas as to what is right for themselves and others. Similarly, most environmental health decisions involve and affect many people, and so what is "right" in environmental health can never be simply the opinion of a single individual. So most statements of ethics in environmental health practice represent the consensus of professional groups and committees authorized to compose principles that will guide practice.

Because discussions of ethics are normative, when we make decisions with others we always go beyond the bare facts and use language and ideas that cannot be resolved entirely by scientific or objective methods. Nevertheless, we can think objectively to some degree in ethics. Thinking objectively in ethics is usually characterized by

- Being reasonable and not doctrinaire
- Listening actively to others
- Letting the best reasons determine judgments
- Remaining calm and optimistic in the face of controversy

- Being realistic about the situations and choices that we face
- Considering the approaches of other cultures involved in the situation

Ethics has a downside in that it tends to be discussed in language that is less precise than the language of scientific discussion and that is open to a wide variety of interpretations. The upside is that we all need to have a sense of integrity and meaning in our daily lives, and there is no way to achieve this without considering our actions in a broad moral context.

Ethics in Environmental Health

The environmental health professions are diverse and in the process of acquiring a common sense of identity, and so environmental health ethics, as a unified concept, is in formation and draws on a wide variety of sources. This section sketches a little of the history of environmental health ethics and identifies some of its sources.

Reflection on environmental health and ethics has an ancient history. In classical times, scholars reflected on the relationship of humans to the earth and debated the extent to which the earth was created to provide its bounty for human welfare and the extent to which humans have a responsibility to perfect nature for human use. Medieval reflection considered whether environmental damage to the earth resulted from human sins; and early modern reflection considered the prospects for human dominance over nature as science and industry entered their infancy (Glacken, 1973).

In modern times the work of environmental health occupations diversified with the growth of statistics and health surveillance in the seventeenth century; the study of population growth and macroeconomics in the early nineteenth century; the growth of the occupational health, sanitarian, and public health movements throughout the nineteenth century; and the modern medical revolution of the early twentieth century (Porter, 1999; Rosen, [1958] 1993). The twentieth century was also marked by rapid growth in the number and specializations of all health professions. Many currently existing environmental health professional organizations experienced their birth during the early to middle twentieth century. Most were associated with industrial and occupational health. One of the first medical subspecialty associations to be founded was the American College of Occupational and Environmental Medicine (ACOEM) in 1916. The American Association of Occupational Health Nurses (AAOHN) was established in 1942 (as the American Association of Industrial Nurses, AAIN). As the environmental revolution took off in the 1970s, many new environmental agencies were founded (such as the Environmental Protection Agency). Environmental regulation widened, along with rapidly increasing recognition of environmental problems. These developments spurred the creation of many new environmental health professions.

The development of ethics in environmental health is thus closely associated with the growth of ethics in the health professions generally. Although each profession has its own approach to codes, oaths, and ethics statements, all tend to share a set of common concerns and principles (see Box 7.1).

Box 7.1. Typical Elements of Professional Codes of Ethics

1. Dedication to service to the client
2. Respect for other professionals
3. Assurance of high levels of competence
4. Protection of confidentiality
5. Performance with honesty and integrity
6. Avoidance of conflicts of interest
7. Informed consent and cooperation with clients
8. Service to the community
9. Promotion of the profession itself

Inevitably, professions adopt ethical codes because professionals

- Provide a socially valued service, such as protecting the health of the community
- Possess a high degree of autonomy at work as result of their special expertise, and are not easily supervised by others
- Have a skill or craft that if not directed to the right goals could be harmful
- Depend on the trust and confidence of others to function effectively
- Need to cooperate with others toward common goals

Each professional ethics code, or statement, represents a consensus among leading members of the profession and so reflects the values and goals of many environmental health professionals. Although such statements are useful in organizing the profession and public support for it, they are subject to interpretation and improvement. Over the years such statements continue to be revised and crafted to clarify their meaning and to help professionals in making decisions.

Several ethics codes exist for professionals in environmental health. The "Code of Ethics for Members" of the National Environmental Health Association (NEHA, 2004) states that the goal of the environmental health profession is, "To prolong life, eliminate and/or control disease, and create and maintain an environment that is conducive to humankind's full development."

The ACOEM's "Code of Ethical Conduct" (1993) sets a high priority on safety, scientific integrity, and honesty. Like many professional codes it emphasizes confidentiality and privacy of the individual while balancing this with appropriate but limited information to employers. It accepts a responsibility to let individuals and groups know of work-related health risks and discusses chemical dependency and abuse.

The "Code of Ethics" of the AAOHN (2004) reads very much like the "Code for Nurses" of the American Nurses Association (ANA). It contains a nondiscrimination statement, urges collaboration with other professions, protects privacy, champions community service and public health, and urges members to maintain competence and to participate in educational and scientific efforts. Like many nursing professional codes, it promises that the professional will safeguard patients from the unethical or illegal actions of others.

Ethical codes are valuable and should be read and consulted often. Their main purpose is to indicate the general direction of professional purpose and commitment and to express professional idealism while at the same time setting criteria that define minimal standards of conduct. So an idealistic environmental health professional could, for instance, use such a code to support championing tighter limits on the release of particulates into the air while a licensing board could refer to the same code when criticizing a professional who accepted bribes in order to suppress health data potentially costly to an industry.

Because all health professions must address similar ethical issues, a reflection by a clinical nurse, for instance, may be useful to environmental health professionals. Similarly, statements made by historical authorities can lend weight to current actions—consider, for example, Florence Nightingale's observation that "[n]o amount of medical knowledge will lessen the accountability for nurses to do what nurses do, that is, manage the environment to promote positive life processes" (Nightingale Institute for Health and the Environment, 2002).

When professionals are making decisions on hard cases, however, ethics codes are sometimes limited in their application. These codes represent a broad consensus, and realms of controversy tend to be omitted. Because the codes have this limitation, additional fields of ethics have been developed to address broad issues of controversy and change.

Two of these fields arose during the 1970s. The first of these, *bioethics,* was given that label around 1969 by Van Rennselaer Potter (Potter, 1971; Reich, 1995). Potter's thesis was that biology and the humanities need to be brought together to respect and to integrate human health and the environment in order for humans to be able to survive the environmental crisis with dignity. Intense theoretical and case study of the ethics of the health professions and clinical care grew under the rubric of bioethics. This field of study has brought about the realization that codes of professional ethics need to be grounded in larger principles of ethics (see Box 7.2 for selected ethical theories). It has also been influential in specifying details, laws, and procedures that refine the concepts of respect for patients, confidentiality, informed consent, care of the dying, and so on. As a result, codes of professional ethics now tend to address these issues with increasing care.

Box 7.2. Selected Ethical Theories

Deontology. The position that individual autonomy is key, but that responsible choice requires obedience to a common moral law (Kant, [1785] 1998).

Utilitarianism. The position that that act is right which maximizes the likely balance of happiness over unhappiness (Mill, [1863] 1998).

Bioethics. A set of principles for health care ethics that emphasizes beneficence (doing good), nonmaleficence (avoiding harm), respect for patient autonomy, and justice (Beauchamp and Childress, 2001).

Feminist ethics. The principle of care, with a priority that process and relationships, not abstract principles, should dominate ethics (Clement, 1996; Tong, 1997).

The second field that addresses broad issues of controversy and change is *environmental ethics.* Stimulated by the increasing rate of environmental change and decline, those concerned with human values have begun to articulate new and revolutionary ideas about the human relationship with nature. Two important concepts in this field are

- *Sustainability,* which places strong demands on human activity to respect long-term consequences to the natural world
- *Global health,* which places local health concerns in a broad global context

Because environmental consciousness is recent and changing rapidly, the environmental health professions are just beginning to integrate these ideas into professional codes and position statements. In 1990, for example, McCally and Cassel published arguments to show that the medical profession must begin to accept environmental responsibilities. The environmental health professions are beginning to take the same position (World Health Organization, 1989).

A number of health-related civic groups have also formed to promote environmental awareness in the health professions and sciences, such as the Canadian Association of Physicians for the Environment (CAPE), Health Care Without Harm (HCWH), the Science and Environmental Health Network (SEHN), Hospitals for a Healthy Environment (H2E), Physicians for Social Responsibility (PSR), and many others.

The environmental responsibilities of health professions are often expressed in position statements separate from codes of ethics, sometimes by the professions themselves and sometimes by activist groups. Statements by major social groups on environment and health are especially useful, inspiring, and clarifying. For example, the "Declaration of the Environment Leaders of the Eight on Children's Environmental Health" (Environment Leaders of the Eight, 1997) states, "We increasingly understand that the health and well-being of our families depends upon a clean and healthy environment." The Earth Charter provides an important statement promoting a unified struggle for both human and environmental health, as does the Rio Declaration on Environment and Development (see Box 7.3). Such statements not only add specificity and idealism to the profession, they also lend authority to its actions and recommendations.

Box 7.3. Consensus Statements

"The resilience of the community of life and the well-being of humanity depend upon preserving a healthy biosphere with all its ecological systems, a rich variety of plants and animals, fertile soils, pure waters, and clean air. The global environment with its finite resources is a common concern of all peoples. The protection of Earth's vitality, diversity, and beauty is a sacred trust" (The Earth Charter; see Earth Charter Initiative, 2000).

"Human beings are at the centre of concerns for sustainable development. We are entitled to a healthy and productive life in harmony with nature" (*Rio Declaration on Environment and Development;* see United Nations Conference on Environment and Development [UNCED], 1992).

Indeed, the world is in a great environmental bottleneck and it will continue to be so for many years to come. With a large human population living at a level beyond the earth's capacity to sustain itself (Wackernagel and others, 2002) and a deteriorating global environment (United Nations Development Programme . . . , 2000), a global public health decline of the first order should be of concern to every environmental health occupation. What, in these circumstances, should the broader ethical principles of environmental health work look like?

General Principles of Ethics

Most environmental health work involves population health and the relationships of populations to the environment. And so, environmental health ethical principles tend to emphasize general ecological and population impacts rather than immediate and individual impacts. Accordingly, environmental health ethics needs to be somewhat different from traditional individual-centered professional ethics, as illustrated by the seven principles outlined in the following sections.

Sustainability

Conduct environmental health work in such a way that it allows future generations to meet their health needs as well (see also Box 7.4).

Box 7.4. Ethics and Sustainability

"An acceptable system of ethics is contingent on its ability to preserve the ecosystems which sustain it" (Elliott, 1997).

This is one way to state the principle of sustainability. A more common definition of sustainability comes from the language of the World Commission on Environment and Development (1987), often referred to as the Brundtland Commission: "development that meets the needs of the present generation without compromising the needs of future generations." Both of these statements indicate that ethical discussion needs to consider the long term, that is, a period of several generations. Why is this principle important to environmental health?

- The significant environmental health technologies and projects—such as those dealing with sewage, agriculture, energy production, and nature restoration—are designed to serve multiple generations.
- Human health needs are lifelong and relatively stable, and so considering health over the normal life span commits us to planning for most of a century.
- We care about the future welfare of humanity, and future people will have similar health needs and concerns.
- Currently, earth's declining ecosystems are profoundly reducing the ability of the environment to support human health. These declines are taking place in time frames of decades to centuries, and so environmental health professionals must think for the future as well as the present.

A concern for sustainability has three immediate implications for environmental health practice.

First, methods of cost accounting that discount future risks must be reconsidered. Discounting tends to diminish the significance of events a few decades ahead to nothing, when in fact they are significant and may become irremediable unless we take present action.

Second, the full life cycle cost of environmental health measures must be considered. Life cycle costs stretch from costs of extracting and processing the materials used in making or building something through the costs of transporting, packaging, and using materials and products to the costs of disposing of supplies, tools, equipment, and buildings when they are retired. So, for example, if a municipality plans to build a sewage plant, it must consider not only local health benefits but also the carbon cost to the atmosphere of fuel expenditures to process the sewage and the environmental costs of mining and harvesting materials, producing energy, and shipping in order to build the plant in the first place. Or a community might determine that the best way to prevent an old munitions plant from polluting a local aquifer is to blow it up (as is being done in Nebraska), but the community must first consider whether explosively spreading those toxic materials into the atmosphere is really a sound alternative. Once the full life cycle environmental costs are considered, it is not always clear that large physical projects are the best approaches to health problems in the long run.

Third, many have observed a strong correspondence between the wealth of a nation and the average health of its citizens (World Bank, 1993). However, if in maintaining the current welfare of its population, a nation overburdens its environment or the environments of other nations and of the globe, that nation will undermine everyone's health in the long run. Thus immediate health gains must be judged within limits set by sustaining environmental health in the long run. Finding the right economic and public policy measures to address sustainability is a challenge. As Garret Hardin (1968) pointed out in a classic article, sharing the global commons without rules limiting consumption inevitably results in a decline of the commons. Some have argued that privatization of parcels of the commons will tend to protect resources better, but ownership of property in a market society does not necessarily protect resources because resources must ultimately be sold to pay for investment in the property.

Healthfulness

The health of humans and the environment needs to be restored, balanced, and harmonized (see also Box 7.5).

Box 7.5. Ecological Medicine

"Ecological medicine is a new field of inquiry and action to reconcile the care and health of ecosystems, populations, communities, and individuals" (SEHN, 2002).

We should think not just of improving human health but of improving human health in the setting of a healthy global environment. Careful thinkers have rightly noted that the meaning of the term *health* cannot be as readily applied to the natural environment as to humans. It is not immediately clear what a healthy polar landscape should be like, nor is a polar landscape locally friendly to humans. Yet, as noted earlier, ethics concepts are meant to link values into a coherent whole, and the bottom line is that healthy ecosystems are necessary to maintain human health in the long run.

Thus the use of such toxic substances as cleaners, pesticides, and herbicides poses a dilemma for environmental health practice. Although these substances may protect human health in the short run, they are likely in the long run to damage the environment. So, in addition to their indirect toxic effects on humans, their impact on the environment can also harm human health in the long run.

Moreover, we should think in terms of the restoration of human and environmental health. In many parts of the world, human and environmental health are declining in tandem. For example, Africa bears the cost of many of the environmental practices of the developed nations and has fallen to radically low levels of environmental health. Some island nations are experiencing hurricanes, floods, and chronic salinization of agricultural and forest land due to climate change.

Environmental health professionals should recognize that healthiness is good in itself. It is a feature of the abundance and thriving of life and not just a means to accomplish other social ends. There are limits to the value of health, however. It is only one value in the panoply of ethical values. Many individuals have willingly sacrificed their own health to serve larger community purposes. Most societies generally give higher status to other values, such as liberty, justice, and community service. Limited though health is in relationship to other values, it is still one of the most basic human values and is especially important as a measure of the welfare of the population as a whole. Thus an environmental health professional should speak to the key value of health and the dependency of achieving other values on health while recognizing that health is not the only value. This means that environmental health work requires collaborating with others to harmonize health values with other cultural and community goals.

Interconnection

Environmental health actions have far-reaching consequences. As Evans and Stoddart (2003, p. 374) wrote, "Health depends on everything, all the time."

A strong sense of interconnection does not so much constitute a rule of ethical rightness and wrongness as it speaks to the basic concept of moral responsibility. Much of modern ethical philosophy has been dominated by the notion that each individual and his or her interests can readily be separated from the needs and concerns of others (Mill, [1869] 2003; Lane, Rubinstein, Cibula, and Webster, 2000). Indeed, much has been achieved and won on the basis of individualism and individual rights. And the protection of the individual, and his or her capacity to meet his or her needs, from the weight of collective social needs continues to be essential.

However, the doctrine of individualism has overemphasized the satisfaction of personal wants as a basis of happiness. In actuality most of us are happiest when we feel connected with others and work with others in the service of our families, communities, and meaningful social goals. So a substantial element of an individual's life is a sense of responsibility and connectedness. Probably, if we had thought more carefully about it, modern ethics would have been based on the idea of the maternal-child bond or of families rather than on the image of the isolated single (male) individual (Ruddick, 1989). At the root of individual choice are our responsibilities and our interest in the care of others, not simply our personal satisfaction.

This importance of a strong sense of responsibility has been greatly amplified by our increasing understanding of the earth as a coherent ecological system (Lovelock, 1979). For many in the environmental movement, this is largely expressed by awareness of the strong biological and physical interconnections of earth's ecosystems:

- Carbon released from smokestacks in the Northern Hemisphere spreads to the Southern Hemisphere.
- Fertilized agricultural areas of the Midwest release nitrogen into rivers; this nitrogen then overloads and kills areas of the Gulf of Mexico.
- Toxic chemical pollutants, such as dioxins, can be found in the ice and snow of polar regions.
- Streams and groundwater in the United States show detectable levels of antibiotics, caffeine, fire retardants, estrogens, and other complex medical, agricultural, and industrial chemicals (Kolpin and others, 2002).
- Much of the lead pollution in Europe is attributable to its use in pipes and other technologies in ancient Roman times. Not only is the world spatially interconnected, it is interconnected over long periods of time as well.

Interconnection is not only biological and physical. It is social and economic as well. No longer can physicians diagnose fevers, rashes, and diarrhea in the Midwestern United States without considering the possibility of distant sources of disease. The combination of travel, immigration, trade, and transportation has led to a high level of exposure in all populations to diseases that may have had their origins anywhere on the globe.

Likewise, global environmental problems require international and global political and economic solutions. One of the important achievements in environmental health in recent decades was the 1987 Montreal Protocol on Substances That Deplete the Ozone Layer (United Nations Environment Programme, 2000), which limited the use of chlorofluorocarbons (CFCs) and other chemicals damaging to stratospheric ozone. Although the earth's protective ozone layer is still vulnerable, it is believed that this international agreement has done much to reverse an extremely dangerous situation. Many other international treaties, agreements, and statements have addressed environmental and health issues. Numerous international nongovernmental organizations (NGOs) are active in environmental health areas and are significantly influencing environmental health globally.

Respect for All Life

Environmental health work should be conducted with respect for both human and nonhuman life.

Respect for human life and proscriptions against taking it are nearly universal in human culture. Similarly, respect for animal life is widespread and ancient. It appears strongly in Hindu and Buddhist doctrines. And respect for all life is experiencing a rebirth in Western ethical traditions, which have tended during the modern period to subordinate the natural world to the needs of humans and to permit its open-ended exploitation (White, 1967; see also Chapter Nine).

A debate has raged among environmental philosophers in recent decades over whether the value of nature is *anthropocentric* and depends on nature's value to humans or whether nature can be valued in a nonanthropocentric way, independent of the welfare of humans. This is a complex and significant debate with consequences for choices that environmental health professionals must make.

On the side of anthropocentrism is a perspective that views us humans as focused on meeting our own needs and limited in our ability to care for nature in itself. This perspective holds that however much we may emphasize the needs of nature, it is not reasonable to expect us to respect ethical rules that consider earth's welfare apart from our own. Anthropocentric arguments in defense of nature ultimately rest on the impact of the natural world on humans.

The nonanthropocentric approach places humans more clearly as one species among others in earth's larger ecosystems. Like theological approaches to the cosmos that subordinate humans to a larger sense of theistic order, nonanthropocentric approaches to nature emphasize its complexity, long history, capacity for adaptation and change, beauty and splendor, and potential for growth and change far into the future. Humans, such a theory might claim, are on earth in part to care for the natural world, much as Plato ([c. 360 BCE], 1992) argued that a guardian class was expected to care for the society it served.

Some nonanthropocentric theories emphasize the sentience of other species (why should the pain of a baby octopus be inconsiderable?) and that many animals seem to act with intention or purpose, such as to protect themselves and their young. However, nonanthropocentric theories do not necessarily rest on the sentience of individual animals. They may also rest on a sense of the coherence of the natural world as a whole and as a changing, reactive network of many beings, sentient or not. Indeed the vast bulk of living things are (apparently) not conscious. Microorganisms alone outweigh humans by tens of thousands of times. Plant biomes, plankton, fungal structures, nematodes in the soil, and the many senseless creatures of nature make up most of the biological world. It would be foolish of humans to underestimate the importance of these organisms, not only to human health but to the health of other sentient earthly beings as well (Darwin, 1966 [1881]; Quammen, 1988, pp. 10–16).

The anthropocentric versus nonanthropocentric debate is heartfelt and often leads to differing positions on environmental health issues. Nonanthropocentrists are likely to favor nature restoration even where human health risks are involved. Good examples are the debates over major carnivores. Some naturalists would like to see wolf and tiger habitats preserved and restored, even though this involves risks to human beings. Another good example is wetlands restoration. For environmental and health reasons, including protection of the hydrologic cycle, one may want to restore wetlands. But wetland restoration also tends to encourage the breeding of mosquitoes, notorious vectors of disease. The anthropocentrist would likely take fewer risks on behalf of mosquitoes than would the nonanthropocentrist.

Both sides, however, also have much in common. Whether for the sake of humans in the long run or for nature in itself, both consider maintenance of a healthy natural world a key element of environmental health. Both sides oppose the notion that human health is best protected by eliminating all predators and oppose using any means, however toxic, to promote human development. So the anthropocentrism debate need not be resolved for environmental health activists to speak strongly on behalf of the natural world.

The middle ground in this debate takes various forms. One course, as discussed in Chapter Twenty-Seven, is to emphasize the positive effects of exposure to the natural world on human health. This view can be seen as arising in part from humans' love of the living world, what E. O. Wilson (1984) has termed *biophilia* (see also Chapter Twenty-Seven). If it is in our nature to love the natural world, then it is simultaneously in our interest and our duty to care for it. Another middle course is to set a simple ordering of priorities (Shrader-Frechette, 1991). We should first seek to meet the needs of humans, which include basic human health. Then we should meet the needs of nature. Then, if it does not damage the needs of nature, we can also seek nonnecessary goods for humans. However, there are two important limitations to this approach:

- Meeting human needs must be undertaken in a way that treads as lightly as possible on the needs of nature.
- Basic human health needs are best met by means of healthy natural services.

Global Equity

Everyone is entitled to just and equal access to the basic resources needed for an adequate and healthy life.

Modern theories of ethics do not privilege the needs of one person or community over another. Because humans are basically interconnected on a limited planet and have roughly equal needs and capacities (all humans have the same number of hours in the day), it is difficult to justify anything but equal access to basic resources, especially those in the global commons, such as the atmosphere, the oceans, our genetic heritage, and the wilderness.

Arguments that justify differential access to resources usually rest on our local power to influence events close to us, our history of ownership and contribution to society, the specific needs and handicaps of individuals, and the role each of us plays in neighborhoods and communities. Most philosophers would justify some level of difference in deservingness of resources in order to reward meritorious contributions to the community and to discourage harming it. How much difference to tolerate and how to reconcile conflicts over activities that allocate environmental benefits and burdens is subject to debate. Environmental justice is discussed in detail in Chapter Eight, so only a few issues are mentioned here.

Inequality is harmful to public health. Stratified societies excite envy, hinder self-expression, and tend to create conditions so limited that some of us are unable to meet basic health needs. Thus among First World nations the average level of public health corresponds less to the average level of wealth than to the average level of economic equality (Wilkinson, 1996). Overprivileging one group in relationship to another is probably unhealthy for both groups. For the group left in poverty the environmental health risks are obvious. But for the wealthy there are the risks of obesity, overconsumption, inactivity, anxiety, and so on. Equality, even apart from its ethical strength, is a public health measure. As a result, environmental health professionals need to consider

- How economic schemes to promote health, such as major factory developments, also affect income inequality.
- What the costs are to others of environmental measures that benefit specific populations.

For example, if a hospital is to be kept clean with strong antibacterial agents, it is important that these agents not be caustic or carcinogenic to the workers who handle and apply them.

Ethically, considerations of equity do not stop at national borders. Everyone has an equal entitlement to earth's resources. Similarly, everyone has a similar obligation not to overburden them. Global health and income inequality are among the greatest problems the world now faces (Farmer, 2003). In the last several decades, health and income disparities have increased substantially. For example, in the American Midwest this might mean that an environmental health activist not only should fight to have filters and scrubbers placed on a new coal-fired electric power plant but also should oppose building the plant at all. A new coal-fired plant would increase the burden that Midwesterners place on the earth's atmosphere, which the developed world already exploits disproportionately. Further, greater local public health gains might be achieved by stressing a reduction in the consumption of electricity and restoration of prairie regions to support wildlife.

Respectful Participation

Respect the considered and responsible choices of stakeholders, whether individuals or organizations (Lambert and others, 2003).

Those with and for whom environmental health professionals work need to participate in the decisions of environmental health professionals. We can generalize about common human health needs, but individuals and organizations have widely varying, and sometimes myopic, interpretations of their own environmental health needs. This presents difficulties for environmental health professionals asked by their clients to support unwise choices.

Perhaps the problem of disagreement with patients, employers, and stakeholders is best resolved through the concept of leadership. When consulted, a professional with environmental health expertise is expected to lead others to what the profession would recommend as the healthiest course of action. However, leadership must be balanced. One must chart a balanced course between paternalism, that is, coercive leadership, and abandonment, that is, failing to give direction. Working with stakeholders with whom one disagrees calls upon a professional's deepest skills and sensitivities.

One key way to reconcile potential conflicts between individual choices and professional recommendations is to press for the *right to know.* Although the principle of the right to know takes many forms, its main thrust is to urge that people who are affected by environmental hazards and toxins should be made aware of the nature of the risks to which they are exposed. This principle has many advantages. Because most of us are reasonable, we can make our own decisions about the risks to which we are exposed. This encourages both cooperation and reasonable disagreement. Such communication builds trust among all parties. It also affords the opportunity for those of us who prefer to do so, to operate more independently. The principle of the right to know strengthens when the hazards to which individuals are exposed are great.

The principle does, however, have some weakness and complexities. Not all who receive knowledge are rational, and realistic risk assessment is often intellectually and emotionally difficult (see Chapters Five and Thirty-Two). Some information is proprietary and confidential, so the right to know must be weighed against the rights of those who "own" information or who feel exposed to legal or economic risk if information is shared. Moreover, some information involves complex and unpredictable risks for a wide community, as in the case of environmental genomics, and so it is difficult to know who should be informed and whether some would prefer not to know or hear about dangers from which we can do little to protect ourselves (Beritic, 1993; Michaels and others, 1992; Sattler, 1992; Jardine and others, 2003; Beierle, 2004).

Moreover, what is known or discovered may affect those with whom the environmental health professional lacks a relationship. Although the needs of those who employ or consult the environmental health professional should presumptively be foremost in the professional's judgment, professionals can educate patients, employers, stakeholders, and corporations about the need to weigh seriously the environmental costs to others and the need to make responsible choices. More difficult, the environmental health professional may face client needs that conflict with community needs. Although some ethicists argue that professional ethics requires the environmental health professional to insulate the client as much as possible from outside concerns, the spirit of environmental health recommends striving to work in an interconnected manner with the larger community.

Realism

Environmental health ethics should be founded on a realistic understanding of the health sciences and the risks and benefits of proposed activities and investments (Weed and McKeown, 2003).

This discussion concludes with this principle because the strong emphasis in the earlier sections on the fate of the earth's environment may make the principles discussed so far seem idealistic and unrealistic. However, they are realistic; the earth and its human population are facing a wrenching crisis of declining capacities of nature, increasing poverty among humans, and declining human health. A realistic ethics takes these concerns into account and expresses them explicitly in the ethical commitments of the environmental health professions. And even if these principles are somewhat idealistic, we must remember that ethical principles are *supposed* to be idealistic, so that we can strive to do better than we would otherwise do. Not being perfect or not achieving the maximal good is not a failure; it is ethically adequate to do the best one can.

Critics of health activists often argue that economic and political realities stand in the way of health improvements. A company may argue that it is "too expensive" to protect workers' health or to make a safer product. Indeed, these arguments are sometimes valid. However, the history of many activist campaigns has shown that economic and political enterprises can adapt to the needs of the public and the environment. The point of economics and politics is not that humans should serve the economy and the state first. The responsibility is the other way: economics and politics need to adapt to serve the health needs and ideals of communities.

Limits to the earth are real; appreciating the earth's limits is thus part of realism and not simply a defeatist provocation against ever-expanding visions of economic profit and development. Meeting the basic health needs of humans is not necessarily elaborate or economically expensive. It is ethically more fundamental that these needs be met than that grander visions be realized (Maslow, 1970).

It is clear that humans now consume more in a year than the earth's natural processes can replace during the year. Some societies clearly consume more than others. A rough measure, the *ecological footprint,* estimates each person's share of global resources. Judging by their footprint, North Americans consume on average three to five times what the earth can provide for the entire human population at the same level of resource consumption (Redefining Progress, 2004). As global population grows, the environment declines, climate change continues apace, and energy resources become more expensive, it will become very difficult to maintain the environmentally costly lifestyle of North Americans.

This will be very challenging for environmental health professionals and activists. Those aware of environmental health and the human dependence on nature will need to educate the population in how to continue to maintain health in a less abundant environment. This will require creative technological innovations, but it will also involve shifting to philosophies of wellness that include not only a philosophy of prevention but also a more global sense of how to live well on limited resources.

Realistic risk assessments are also needed in environmental health ethics. The history of modernity, for all humans have achieved, has not taken into account modernity's full costs nor the difficulty in managing the environmental risks of otherwise beneficial activities. For instance, many people believe more oil and coal are needed to promote public health and welfare, but the resulting climate change from greater oil and coal consumption is likely to diminish global health status as oceans rise and droughts and large storms become more common (Martens and McMichael, 2002; also see Chapter Eleven). Some believe that nuclear power will be needed to replace fossil fuels; yet the proliferation of nuclear waste materials is a dangerous and unsolved health and security risk. Technological optimists should examine whether the risks of new technologies can be managed over the vast time scales demanded by these technologies.

Such revision in modern technological progressivism has already resulted in the increasingly widespread adoption of the *precautionary principle* as a mode of realistic risk assessment (see Chapter Thirty-Two). The precautionary principle states that "when an activity raises threats of harm to human health or the environment, precautionary measures should be taken even if some cause and effect relationships are not fully established scientifically" (SEHN, 1998; Raffensperger and Tickner, 1999). This principle

- Recommends better study of the risks of industrial innovations before each new practice or new chemical becomes widespread. For example, those opposed to the development of genetically modified organisms (GMOs) are concerned that these may make potentially disastrous non-point sources of toxins if not properly managed.
- Shifts the burden of proof so that proponents (such as manufacturers) must demonstrate that a practice is sustainable, whereas before the burden was on critics to prove it was not sustainable.
- Assumes that it is more important to avoid harm than to incur benefits.
- Takes a long-term view.
- Presumes a certain amount of historical and sociological knowledge about the management of toxic materials and risks. Although the risks of a technology may be readily managed in a tightly controlled test environment, they often become greater when the technology becomes widely used.

Controversies in Environmental Health Ethics

Because environmental and health concerns are involved in most human activities, many ethical questions, dilemmas, and controversies arise in environmental health ethics (see Box 7.6 for a brief list).

Box 7.6. Case Problem Areas

Air pollution. How should we balance the health costs and the benefits of air-polluting activities, and deal with the politics of risk estimation, the involvement of multiple jurisdictions, and uncertainties about health risks?

Water pollution. How can the focus on upstream and downstream ownership be turned to a focus on clean water for all? How should we apply what we are learning about the tensions between groundwater and surface water? How do we face the reality that human uses of water are in conflict with natural habitats?

Vegetarianism. This is the healthiest way and easiest on the environment, but how do we cope with the fact that it is culturally unacceptable in many parts of the world?

Cultural conflict. Many cultures value highly activities that are in conflict with both health and the environment. How should health be prioritized in relationship to other cultural values? How do we deal with the dilemma that, for example, driving automobiles and watching television at current levels is not good for us or our world?

Fossil fuels and climate change. How should the short-term gains of using fossil fuels be weighed against major long-term losses (not only from climate change but also from the toxicity of fossil fuels)? As the environmental urgency to limit fossil fuel use increasingly challenges our capacity for rapid social change, how shall we maintain active advocacy for change in balance with increasing pessimism that it is too late?

Genetically modified organisms. Is it acceptable to copyright living material? Are particular modifications appropriate? How will we deal with unexpected health risks and confront the lack of trust among all the parties involved? How can we direct genetic modifications in directions that reduce human conflict with the environment, and how can we prevent their deliberate misuse as new weapons technologies?

Nuclear power. This would be the solution to our energy problems except that we need to ask, What are the risks of nuclear materials being used for war or terrorism, and Can we solve the problem of safely sequestering radioactive wastes for tens of thousands of years?

Pesticides. Sure, we need an ample food supply and we compete with weeds and insects for food, but what are the many costs of releasing billions of pounds of toxic materials into the environment?

Obesity, undernutrition, starvation. The existence of these conditions reveals a problem in environmental justice. Indeed, should we be regarding many of the conflicts of the world as between the fat and the thin?

Human environmental genome. Should we conduct genetic testing of job applicants and allow only those most resistant to toxic materials to work in certain occupational environments?

Confidentiality, informed consent, and the right to know. How shall we collect needed epidemiological information without invading the privacy of individuals? To what extent should individuals be able to consent to surveillance for environmental health purposes?

War. Is there any way to conduct human conflict without wrecking the public health and environmental conditions in a region for decades thereafter?

Research ethics. When we ask individuals to subject themselves to experiments for long-term health gains, are we unfairly using them as a means to an end? What is appropriate consent? What is appropriate oversight? Is it fair to use individuals in particular communities for research when those communities may never see the benefits of the research?

A few general observations can be made, however, about similarities among these controversies. Ethical doubts, dilemmas, and struggles tend to arise when the following elements are present:

- *New technologies with uncertain risks.* It is a notorious principle that new technologies are likely to bring with them unexpected effects (Tenner, 1996). People may reasonably differ over whether the risks are known, whether they can be well managed, and whether those developing the technology can be trusted.
- *Social relationships with expectable conflicts.* Confidentiality, informed consent, and environmental justice problems all arise from controversies over respectful treatment of others. These problems are by no means confined to environmental health issues.
- *The rational balancing of risks and benefits.* Some of these debates involve disagreements over the value of activities (Do we really need another suburban hospital when the proposed design wipes out precious prairie and forest?). Some of the debates are simply over how to weigh risks rationally: How much more important is safety and avoiding harm than finding new ways to benefit people?

And mistrust among groups with different interests makes it difficult to rely on common estimates of risks.

- *Competing goods.* Health is one of many goods. All environmental health discussions must take place in the context of commitments to other values, some of which are difficult to harmonize with health.
- *Cultural differences.* Although there are many human universals, from the maternal-child bond to poetry (Brown, 1991), different cultures tend to use slightly different social concepts and to set out problems and arguments in differing styles. Moreover, different geographic locations tend to expose people to different environmental risks. So, understanding each other's needs across cultures can be challenging.
- *Our place in and relationship to nature.* While we debate our place in nature, the global environment is sliding downhill at an increasing pace. Environmental health professionals need to consider how to balance service to humans with protection of the environment.
- *Complexity.* Many of the chronic ethical debates persist simply because they are complex and involve many of these factors.

There is no magic formula, no final or ultimate ethical theory to resolve moral problems. Although those with expertise in ethics are useful in facilitating debates, ethics involves everyone, whether or not he or she is trained in ethics. Because most environmental health issues involve a community of people and the natural world, there will inevitably be many people involved in ethical disputes in this arena. This means that environmental health professionals need to work respectfully and persistently with others to achieve the environmental health ideals for which they stand. Because the natural world is in decline and maintaining human population health globally is becoming more challenging, environmental health professionals occupy an increasingly important place in the world and need to speak out clearly and actively for their professions' ethical ideals.

Thought Questions

1. Why are some ethical principles stated in the professional codes of ethics while other principles are not? Look over one of the codes of ethics relevant to environmental health. Would you add anything? Would you leave anything out? Why?
2. Should there be sanctions for those professionals who violate the organizational code of ethics? How might such sanctions be administered?
3. What are some analogies between human health and the health of the environment? What are some ways in which they are not analogous?

4. What are some cases in which it would be ethical to encourage a stakeholder to think past his or her immediate needs and to consider broader human and environmental needs? What are some cases in which it would be unethical to do so?
5. A hospital creates some public health risks (from power production, incineration, cleaning agents, disposal of drugs and supplies, and so on). How should these risks be balanced against health gains?
6. Select a debated issue in environmental health ethics, and offer some reasons why the debate persists (suggest reasons on both sides of the issue).
7. In reference to any of the debates in environmental health ethics, are there any scientific facts that, if you knew them for certain, would settle the issue for you?
8. Do you have some personal values that harmonize well with, or that may conflict with, the professional ethics of environmental health?
9. How might you go about reducing the ecological footprint of your personal life? How might you relate your efforts to reduce your personal environmental impact to reducing the impact of your professional work and that of your clients?
10. What are the broader social responsibilities of environmental health professionals to advocate environmental health in the political, social, and economic spheres?

References

American Association of Occupational Health Nurses. "Code of Ethics." [http://www.aaohn.org/practice/ethics.cfm]. 2004.

American College of Occupational and Environmental Medicine. "Code of Ethical Conduct." [http://www.acoem.org/code/default.asp]. Aug. 1993.

Beauchamp, T. L., and Childress, J. F. *Principles of Biomedical Ethics.* (5th ed.) New York: Oxford University Press, 2001.

Beierle, T. C. "The Benefits and Costs of Disclosing Information About Risks: What Do We Know About the Right-to-Know?" *Risk Analysis,* 2004, *24*(2), 335–346.

Beritic, T. "Workers at High Risk: The Right to Know." *Lancet,* 1993, *341,* 933–934.

Brown, D. E. *Human Universals.* Philadelphia: Temple University Press, 1991.

Clement, G. *Care, Autonomy, and Justice: Feminism and the Ethic of Care.* Boulder, Colo.: Westview Press, 1996.

Darwin, C. *Darwin on Humus and the Earthworm; the Formation of Vegetable Mould through the Action of Worms with Observations on their Habits.* London: Faber and Faber, 1966. (Originally published 1881.)

Earth Charter Initiative. *The Earth Charter.* [http://www.earthcharter.org/files/charter/charter.pdf]. Mar. 2000.

Elliott, H. "A General Statement of the Tragedy of the Commons." [http://www.dieoff.com/page121.htm]. Feb. 26, 1997.

Environment Leaders of the Eight. "Declaration of the Environment Leaders of the Eight on Children's Environmental Health." [http://www.g8.utoronto.ca/environment/1997miami/children.html]. 1997.

Evans, R. G., and Stoddart, G. L. "Models for Population Health: Consuming Research, Producing Policy?" *American Journal of Public Health,* 2003, *93,* 371–379.

Farmer, P. *Pathologies of Power: Health, Human Rights, and the New War on the Poor.* Berkeley: University of California Press, 2003.

Glacken, C. J. *Traces on the Rhodian Shore: Nature and Culture in Western Thought from Ancient Times to the End of the Eighteenth Century.* Berkeley: University of California Press, 1973.

Hardin, G. "The Tragedy of the Commons." *Science,* 1968, *162,* 1243–1248.

Jardine, C., and others. "Risk Management Frameworks for Human Health and Environmental Risks." *Journal of Toxicology and Environmental Health Part B: Critical Reviews,* 2003, *6*(6), 569–720.

Kant, I. *Groundwork of the Metaphysics of Morals.* New York: Cambridge University Press, 1998. (Originally published 1785.)

Kolpin, D. W., and others. "Pharmaceuticals, Hormones, and Other Organic Wastewater Contaminants in U.S. Streams, 1999–2000: A National Reconnaissance." *Environmental Science & Technology,* 2002, *36,* 1202–1211.

Lambert, T. W., and others. "Ethical Perspectives for the Public and Environmental Health: Fostering Autonomy and the Right to Know." *Environmental Health Perspectives,* 2003, *111,* 133–137.

Lane, S. D., Rubinstein, R. A., Cibula, D., and Webster, N. "Towards a Public Health Approach to Bioethics." *Annals of the New York Academy of Sciences,* 2000, *925,* 25–36.

Lovelock, J. E. *Gaia: A New Look at Life on Earth.* New York: Oxford University Press, 1979.

Martens, P., and McMichael, A. J., (eds.). *Environmental Change, Climate and Health: Issues and Research Methods.* New York: Cambridge University Press, 2002.

Marx, K., and Engels, F. "Theses on Feuerbach." In E. Kamenka (ed.), *The Portable Karl Marx.* New York: Penguin Books, 1983. (Originally published 1845.)

Maslow, A. H. *Motivation and Personality.* (2nd ed.) New York: HarperCollins, 1970.

McCally, M., and Cassel, C. K. "Medical Responsibility and Global Environmental Change." *Annals of Internal Medicine,* 1990, *113,* 467–473.

Michaels, D., and others. "Workshops Are Not Enough: Making Right-to-Know Training Lead to Workplace Change." *American Journal of Industrial Medicine,* 1992, *22*(5), 637–649.

Mill, J. S. *Utilitarianism.* New York: Oxford University Press, 1998. (Originally published 1863.)

Mill, J. S. *On Liberty.* New Haven, Conn.: Yale University Press, 2003. (Originally published 1869.)

National Environmental Health Association. "Code of Ethics for Members." [http://www.neha.org/member]. 2004.

Nightingale Institute for Health and the Environment. *Environmentally Responsible Health Care: Nurses Can Make a Difference.* Burlington, Vt.: Nightingale Institute for Health and the Environment, 2002.

Plato. *Republic.* Indianapolis: Hackett, 1992. (Written c. 360 BCE.)

Porter, D. *Health, Civilization, and the State: A History of Public Health from Ancient to Modern Times.* New York: Routledge, 1999.

Potter, V. R. *Bioethics: Bridge to the Future.* Upper Saddle River, N.J.: Prentice Hall, 1971.
Quammen, D. *The Flight of the Iguana: A Sidelong View of Science and Nature.* New York: Simon & Schuster, 1988.
Raffensperger, C., and Tickner, J. (eds.). *Protecting Public Health and the Environment: Implementing the Precautionary Principle.* Washington, D.C.: Island Press, 1999.
Redefining Progress. "Ecological Footprint Analysis." [http://www.redefiningprogress.org/footprint]. 2004.
Reich, W. T. "The Word 'Bioethics': The Struggle Over Its Earliest Meanings." *Kennedy Institute of Ethics Journal,* 1995, *5*(1), 19–34.
Rosen, G. *A History of Public Health.* (Expanded ed.) Baltimore, Md.: Johns Hopkins University Press, 1993. (Originally published 1958.)
Ruddick, S. *Maternal Thinking: Toward a Politics of Peace.* Boston: Beacon Press, 1989.
Sattler, B. "Rights and Realities: A Critical Review of the Accessibility of Information on Hazardous Chemicals." *Occupational Medicine,* 1992, *7*(2), 189–196.
Science and Environmental Health Network. "The Wingspread Statement on the Precautionary Principle." [http://www.sehn.org/state.html#w]. Jan. 1998.
Science and Environmental Health Network. "Ecological Medicine: A Call for Inquiry and Action." [http://www.sehn.org]. Feb. 2002.
Shrader-Frechette, K. "Ethics and the Environment." *World Health Forum,* 1991, *12,* 311–321.
Tenner, E. *Why Things Bite Back: Technology and the Revenge of Unintended Consequences.* New York: Knopf, 1996.
Tong, R. *Feminist Approaches to Bioethics: Theoretical Reflections and Practical Applications.* Boulder, Colo.: Westview Press, 1997.
United Nations Conference on Environment and Development. *"Rio Declaration on Environment and Development."* [http://www.un.org/documents/ga/conf151/aconf15126-1annex1.htm]. 1992.
United Nations Development Programme, United Nations Environment Programme, World Bank, and World Resources Institute. *World Resources 2000–2001: People and Ecosystems, the Fraying Web of Life.* Amsterdam: Elsevier Science, 2000.
United Nations Environment Programme, Ozone Secretariat. "Montreal Protocol on Substances That Deplete the Ozone Layer: As Either Adjusted and/or Amended in London 1990, Copenhagen 1992, Vienna 1995, Montreal 1997, Beijing 1999." [http://www.unep.org/ozone/pdfs/Montreal-Protocol2000.pdf]. 2000.
Wackernagel, M., and others. "Tracking the Ecological Overshoot of the Human Economy." *Proceedings of the National Academy of Sciences of the United States of America,* 2002, *99*(14), 9266–9271.
Weed, D. L., and McKeown, R. E. "Science and Social Responsibility in Public Health." *Environmental Health Perspectives,* 2003, *111,* 1804–1808.
White, L., Jr. "The Historical Roots of Our Ecological Crisis." *Science,* 1967, *155,* 1203–1207.
Wilkinson, R. *Unhealthy Societies: The Afflictions of Inequality.* New York: Routledge, 1996.
Wilson, E. O. *Biophilia.* Cambridge, Mass.: Harvard University Press, 1984.
World Bank. *World Development Report 1993: Investing in Health.* New York: Oxford University Press, 1993.
World Commission on Environment and Development. *Our Common Future.* New York: Oxford University Press, 1987.
World Health Organization, Regional Office for Europe. *European Charter on Environment and Health.* [http://www.euro.who.int]. 1989.

For Further Information

Publications

American Public Health Association (APHA). "Code of Ethics." [http://www.apha.org/codeofethics/ethics.htm].

Athanasiou, T. *Divided Planet: The Ecology of Rich and Poor.* Boston: Little, Brown and Company, 1996.

Attfield, R. *Environmental Ethics: An Overview for the Twenty-First Century.* Cambridge, U.K.: Polity Press, 2003.

Barlett, P. F., and Chase, G. W. (eds.). *Sustainability on Campus: Stories and Strategies for Change.* Cambridge, Mass.: MIT Press, 2004.

Beauchamp, D. E., and Steinbock, B. (eds.). *New Ethics for the Public's Health.* New York: Oxford University Press, 1999.

Brown, N. J., and Quiblier, P. (eds.). *Ethics and Agenda 21: Moral Implications of a Global Consensus.* New York: United Nations Environment Program, United Nations Publications, 1994.

Callahan, D. *False Hopes: Why America's Quest for Perfect Health Is a Recipe for Failure.* New York: Simon & Shuster, 1998.

Case Western University, Online Ethics Center for Engineering and Science. "Environmental Ethics and Sustainable Development." [http://onlineethics.org/environment].

Chesworth, J. (ed.). *The Ecology of Health: Identifying Issues and Alternatives.* Thousand Oaks, Calif.: Sage, 1996.

Costanza, R., Norton, G. B., and Haskell, B. D. (eds.). *Ecosystem Health: New Goals for Environmental Management.* Washington, D.C.: Island Press, 1992.

Crocker, D. A., and Linden, T. (eds.). *Ethics of Consumption: The Good Life, Justice, and Global Stewardship.* Lanham, Md.: Rowan & Littlefield, 1998.

Daily, G. (ed.). *Nature's Services: Societal Dependence on Natural Ecosystems.* Washington, D.C.: Island Press, 1997.

Diamond, J. *Collapse: How Societies Choose to Fail or Succeed.* New York: Viking, 2005.

Durning, A. *How Much Is Enough? The Consumer Society and the Future of the Earth.* In L. Starke (series ed.), The Worldwatch Environmental Alert Series. New York: Norton, 1992.

Farmer, P. *Infections and Inequalities.* Berkeley: University of California Press, 1999.

Fox, W. (ed.). *Ethics and the Built Environment.* New York: Routledge, 2000.

Gorz, A. *Ecology as Politics.* Boston: South End Press, 1980.

Harvard Medical School, Center for Health and the Global Environment (CHGE). *Human Health and Global Environmental Change.* [http://www.med.harvard.edu/chge/textbook/index.htm]. 2004.

International Commission on Occupational Health (ICOH). "International Code of Ethics for Occupational Health Professionals." [http://www.icoh.org.sg]. 2004.

Jamieson, D. (ed.). *A Companion to Environmental Philosophy.* Malden, Mass.: Blackwell Publishers, 2001.

Light, A., and Rolston, H. (eds.). *Environmental Ethics: An Anthology.* Malden, Mass.: Blackwell Publishers, 2003.

Lubchenco, J. "Entering the Century of the Environment: A New Social Contract for Science." *Science,* 1998, *279,* 491–497.

McCally, M. (ed.) *Life Support: The Environment and Human Health.* Cambridge, Mass.: The MIT Press, 2002.

McKeown, T. *The Role of Medicine: Dream, Mirage, or Nemesis?* Princeton, N.J.: Princeton University Press, 1979.

McKibben, B. *The End of Nature.* New York: Doubleday, 1989.

Meadows, D., Randers, J., and Meadows, D. *Limits to Growth: The Thirty Year Update.* White River Junction, Vt.: Chelsea Green, 2004.

Newton, L. *Ethics and Sustainability: Sustainable Development and the Moral Life.* Upper Saddle River, N.J.: Prentice Hall, 2003.

Partridge, E. (ed.). *Responsibilities to Future Generations: Environmental Ethics.* Buffalo, N.Y.: Prometheus Books, 1981.

Pedersen, D. "Disease Ecology at a Crossroads: Man-Made Environments, Human Rights and Perpetual Development Utopias." *Social Science and Medicine,* 1996, *43,* 745–758.

Pierce, J., and Jameton, A. *The Ethics of Environmentally Responsible Health Care.* New York: Oxford University Press, 2004.

Pimentel, D., and Lehman, H. (eds.). *The Pesticide Question: Environment, Economics, and Ethics.* New York: Chapman and Hall, 1993.

Ponting, C. *A Green History of the World: The Environment and the Collapse of Great Civilizations.* New York: St. Martin's Press, 1991.

Proctor, R. N. *Cancer Wars: How Politics Shapes What We Know and Don't Know About Cancer.* New York: Basic Books, 1995.

Rachels, J. *The Elements of Moral Philosophy.* (4th ed.) Boston: McGraw-Hill Humanities, 2002.

Shiva, V. *Staying Alive: Women, Ecology and Development.* London: Zed Books, 1989.

Shrader-Frechette, K., and McCoy, E. D. *Method in Ecology: Strategies for Conservation.* New York: Cambridge University Press, 1993.

Singer, P. "Famine, Affluence, and Morality." In W. Aiken and H. LaFollette (eds.), *World Hunger and Morality* (pp. 26–38). (2nd ed.) Upper Saddle River, N.J.: Prentice Hall, 1996.

Wackernagel, M., and Rees, W. E. *Our Ecological Footprint: Reducing Human Impact on the Earth.* Gabriola Island, B.C.: New Society, 1996.

Westra, L. *Living in Integrity: A Global Ethic to Restore a Fragmented Earth.* Lanham: Rowman & Littlefield, 1998.

Zwaan, van der, B., and Petersen, A. (eds.). *Sharing the Planet: Population, Consumption, Species: Science and Ethics for a Sustainable and Equitable World.* Delft, The Netherlands: Eburon, 2003.

Organizations

American Association of Occupational Health Nurses (AAOHN) [http://www.aaohn.org].

American College of Occupational and Environmental Medicine (ACOEM) [http://www.acoem.org].

American Society for Bioethics and Humanities (ASBH) [http://www.asbh.org].

Canadian Association of Physicians for the Environment (CAPE) [http://www.cape.ca].

CleanMed, Conferences for Greening Health Care [http://www.cleanmed.org].

Climate Action Network (CAN) [http://www.climatenetwork.org].

Collaborative on Health and the Environment [http://www.cheforhealth.org].

Doctors for Global Health (DGH) [http://www.dghonline.org].

Environmental Health Perspectives (EHP) [http://ehp.niehs.nih.gov].

Environmental Working Group (EWG) [http://www.ewg.org].

Health Care Without Harm (HCWH) [http://www.noharm.org].

Hospitals for a Healthy Environment (H2E) [http://www.h2e-online.org].

International Association for Environmental Philosophy (IAEP) [http://www.environmentalphilosophy.org].
International Association of Bioethics (IAB) [http://www.bioethics-international.org].
International Society for Ecology and Culture [http://www.isec.org.uk].
International Society of Environmental Ethics (ISEE) [http://www.cep.unt.edu/ISEE.html].
National Environmental Health Association (NEHA) [http://www.neha.org].
National Wildlife Federation (NWF), Campus Ecology [http://www.nwf.org/campusecology].
The Natural Step (TNS) [http://www.naturalstep.org].
Nightingale Institute for Health and the Environment (NIHE) [http://www.nihe.org].
Northwest Environment Watch [http://www.northwestwatch.org].
Partners in Health [http://www.pih.org/index.html].
Physicians for Human Rights (PHR) [http://www.phrusa.org].
Physicians for Social Responsibility (PSR) [http://www.psr.org].
Rachel's Environment and Health News [http://www.rachel.org/home_eng.htm].
Redefining Progress [http://www.rprogress.org].
Science and Environmental Health Network (SEHN) [http://www.sehn.org].
Second Nature, Education for Sustainability [http://www.secondnature.org].
University of Nebraska Medical Center, Green Health Center Project [http://www.unmc.edu/green].
University of Pennsylvania, Center for Bioethics [http://www.bioethics.upenn.edu].
World Resources Institute [http://www.wri.org].

CHAPTER EIGHT

ENVIRONMENTAL JUSTICE

Charles Lee

Environmental justice represents the convergence of two of the greatest social movements of the latter half of the twentieth century: the civil rights movement and the environmental movement. (Other social movements also considered roots of the environmental justice movement include public health, labor, farmworker, and native land rights movements; see Faber and McCarthy, 2001.) It is appropriate therefore that a statement attributed to the venerable civil rights activist Fannie Lou Hamer has come to embody the feelings of communities within the environmental justice movement: "I am sick and tired of being sick and tired." This poignant plea by environmentally overburdened communities of people of color and low-income and tribal communities in the United States reflects profound disappointment with the status of their health, frustration with the public health community's failure to assist in improving health, anger with the many businesses complacent about their regulatory obligations and unresponsive to the health problems their neighbors face, and bewilderment at the government's failure to understand and correct these shortcomings. For many communities facing stresses from factors beyond their control, living with a myriad of

The views expressed in this chapter are solely those of the author. No official support or endorsement by the Environmental Protection Agency or any other agency of the federal government is intended or should be inferred.

polluting facilities, this affront is compounded by the impacts of racial and economic discrimination (National Environmental Justice Advisory Council, 2004).

This chapter begins with a short description of the roots of the environmental justice movement. It then explores three core concepts of environmental justice, concepts at the nexus of civil rights and environmentalism:

- *The meaning of disproportionate impacts*, a concept originally centered on disproportionate exposure and since expanded to encompass cumulative environmental hazards, vulnerability, inequities in regulatory enforcement, and disparities in socioeconomic status, power, and health
- *The legal, public policy, and research challenges* inherent in the concept of environmental justice, particularly those related to integrating civil rights and social justice concepts into an environmental law paradigm
- *The community-based collaborative problem-solving strategies and tools* needed to address the interrelated environmental, health, economic, and social concerns of disadvantaged, underserved, and overburdened communities

These three concepts are key to integrating environmental justice into the mainstream of environmental and public health practice. (In addition, the environmental and public health fields themselves need to unify; see Lee, 2002.) The first concept deals with issues of assessment—assessment of environmental exposures, of community assets and liabilities, and of disparities. It illuminates the underlying complexities that the second and third concepts must address. The second reflects the paradigmatic conflicts between civil rights law and environmental law. If these conflicts are not recognized and addressed, then civil rights and social justice concepts may be marginalized in environmental policy. The third concept is strategic. As communities address complex environmental justice issues with many stakeholders, collaborative problem-solving strategies and tools are needed. These three concepts have presented conundrums during the evolution of environmental justice theory and practice, and they have enormous historical implications for the future viability of environmental justice.

The Roots of Environmental Justice

Although the concept of environmental justice is relatively recent, many would argue that environmental injustice has existed in the Western Hemisphere since the first European settlement more than 500 years ago (Mankiller, 1992). For example, the trans-Atlantic slave trade began as a West-to-East passage, with

Christopher Columbus, on his return from his second journey to the Western Hemisphere, bringing 500 Arawak Indians from the island of Puerto Rico to Spain for sale (Konig, 1976). The workplace environment has long confronted workers with disparate hazardous exposures. For example, the disaster at Gauley Creek, West Virginia, during the Great Depression of the 1930s, was perhaps the worst occupational health disaster in U.S. history. Some 500 African American workers died and more than 1,500 were disabled due to silicosis while they were digging a tunnel for the New Kanawha Power Company, a subsidiary of the Union Carbide Corporation. The deceased were buried in unmarked graves, sometimes two and three to a hole (Cherniak, 1987).

The modern environmental justice movement dates from around 1980. In 1979, the African American community of North Hollywood, in Houston, Texas, filed suit to prevent the siting of a solid waste landfill in *Bean* v. *Southwestern Waste Management.* In 1982, the predominantly African American community in Warren County, North Carolina, protested the siting of a PCB landfill. This incident brought together the environmental and civil rights communities and attracted national attention (Box 8.1). It gave rise to the landmark 1987 United Church of Christ (UCC) study *Toxic Wastes and Race in the United States,* the first national study of the demographic patterns associated with the location of hazardous waste sites (UCC, 1987; Lee, 1993). The reverend Benjamin F. Chavis Jr., director of the UCC Commission for Racial Justice, introduced the term *environmental racism* to describe the tendency to locate toxic waste sites and emitters near communities of color. The UCC study found that race was the most significant variable for differentiating between areas with and without treatment, storage, and disposal facilities (TSDFs).

Box 8.1. Warren County, North Carolina

[E]ven in 1982 we knew that where we lived, where we worked, and where we played was really our environment. When the state of North Carolina decided that it was going to put PCB into a community that was 65 percent African Americans, we said 'No.' We said we will put our lives on the line.

And we did it by laying our bodies in front of the trucks, but as we lay there we knew that we were neither politically or economically empowered enough to stop the trucks. . . . As we lay our bodies in front of the trucks and were hauled off to jail by the bus load, we didn't know that the media was going to publicize [our plight]. . . . We didn't know that hundreds of people were going to come and demonstrate with us.

We only knew in our hearts that we were doing the right thing. We knew in our hearts that God required of us to do justice. We hoped and prayed that our going to jail would not be in vain. And we feel that it was not in vain because many good things happened as a result of our going to jail. For the first time, blacks and whites in Warren County united. African Americans determined that henceforth and forever more we will have some say in the government that was controlling our destiny.

Source: Burwell, 1992, p. 126.

In late October 1991, the First National People of Color Environmental Leadership Summit coalesced a national movement on environmental justice. Leaders and activists gathered for the first time in a dramatic display of community-based environmental and social justice activism. To the planners of the conference the juxtaposition of the words *people of color, environment,* and *leadership* provided a synergy that spoke for itself. When District of Columbia congresswoman Eleanor Holmes Norton spoke at this summit of defining great movements, she said, "We have all the names we need in there" (Norton, 1992). In the eyes of many people, both persons of color and whites, the summit was a historic turning point in the environmental movement in the United States (Lee, 1992). Less than three years later, the U.S. Environmental Protection Agency (EPA) had established the Office of Environmental Equity (now the Office of Environmental Justice) and the president of the United States had signed Executive Order 12898, titled "Federal Actions to Ensure Environmental Justice in Minority Populations and Low-Income Populations." (See also Box 8.2.)

Box 8.2. Would Dr. King Have Become an Environmental Justice Advocate?

I think all of you know the answer to that question. Dr. King dedicated his life to fighting racial discrimination and social inequity in the United States. He fought racial discrimination during the Birmingham bus boycotts. He fought racial discrimination in education, in employment, in housing, in health care, in the courts, and at the ballot box. Dr. King went to jail to secure for African Americans and other people the right to participate in the political process. Given all this, there is absolutely no doubt in my mind that, if he were living today, Dr. King would be a staunch and committed advocate for environmental justice.

In fact, Dr. King gave his life in 1968 around an environmental justice struggle to advance the rights and working conditions of sanitation workers in Memphis, Tennessee. Were he living today, Dr. King not only would have become an outspoken advocate for environmental justice but, as history tells us, he *always was* an environmental justice advocate and his historical legacy *includes* environmental justice. Indeed, Dr. King gave his life *as a champion for environmental justice.*

Source: Lee, 1994.

These events gave impetus to the emerging consciousness about environmental conditions in low-income and tribal communities and communities of people of color. A groundswell of activity began to take place in these communities around a vast array of issues, including but not limited to toxicants, lead poisoning, housing, land use, air quality, workplace heath and safety, transportation, and economic development (Bullard, 1994). Some examples of these struggles are described in Table 8.1.

In a little over a decade a loose alliance of community-based activists, church-based civil rights leaders, and academic researchers grew into a vibrant social movement. Members of this movement sought to examine systematically the environmental degradation in communities of color and poor and tribal communities and to develop proactive strategies to address these problems. Initially, the focus was on the siting of hazardous waste sites and other polluting facilities, with the emphasis on demonstrating that they were located disproportionately in communities of color. However, as public discourse over issues of race, poverty, and the environment expanded, environmental justice concerns ranged more widely. For example, a landmark article in the *National Law Journal* in 1994 documented inequities in the enforcement of environmental laws. "There is a racial divide," the authors declared, "in the way the U.S. government cleans up toxic waste sites and punishes polluters. White communities see faster action, better results and stiffer penalties than communities where blacks, Hispanics, and other minorities live. The unequal protection occurs whether the community is wealthy or poor" (Lavalle, Coyle, and MacLachlan, 1994, p. S1). Communities of the poor and of people of color demanded that the issues they confronted—such as unemployment, poor public services, and poor housing—be linked to environmental policy. As the environmental justice paradigm matured, it became more holistic, increasingly viewing individual and community health as a product of physical, social, cultural, and spiritual factors.

Environmental justice represents a vision born out of a community-driven process whose essential core is a transformative public discourse over what constitutes truly healthy, livable, sustainable, and vital communities for all peoples. It has given birth to a broad definition of the environment as "the place where we live, where we work, and where we play" (Gauna, 1991). It sees the ecosystem that forms the basis for life and well-being as composed of four interrelated environments: natural, built, social, and cultural and spiritual (Lee, 1996). It has made clear the necessity for public participation and accountability in formulating environmental policy. It has expanded environmental health discourse to include issues of multiple, cumulative, and synergistic risks. It has pressed for a new paradigm that features community-driven science and holistic, placed-based, systems-wide environmental protection. It is searching for concepts and tools that

TABLE 8.1. EXAMPLES OF COMMUNITY-BASED ENVIRONMENTAL JUSTICE ISSUES.

Community	Location	Organization(s)	Demographics	Issues
Altgeld Gardens	Chicago, Illinois	People for Community Recovery	African American, poor, urban, industrial	Public housing project, with population of 10,000, built on top of landfill in 1940s and now surrounded by polluting industries, landfills, incinerators, smelters, steel mills, chemical companies, paint manufacturing plant, municipal sewage treatment facility. Also known as Chicago's *toxic donut*. Led to formation of the nation's first environmental organization in a public housing project.
Barrio Logan	San Diego, California	Environmental Health Coalition	Latino, urban, border	City zoning decisions of 1950s made neighborhood a repository for incompatible noxious land uses (metal plating, auto body shops, highways) and air pollution. In 2002, community-led effort resulted in a city council resolution to develop new land use and zoning plan for area.
West Harlem	New York, New York	West Harlem Environmental Action	African American, urban	Northern Manhattan is the site of the North River sewage treatment plant and hosts 5 of the 6 bus depots in Borough of Manhattan; it has high rates of asthma and respiratory illness. The partnership between WE ACT and Columbia University School of Public Health is a leading example of community-based participatory research.
Norco	Norco, Louisiana	Concerned Citizens of NORCO	African American, industrial	Homes within feet of a mammoth Shell oil refinery and chemical plant were concerned about health and safety. Area is subject to major explosions and spills. After community residents traveled to the Netherlands to confront company executives at a conference, Shell agreed to relocate residents in 2002.
Alaska Native villages	Alaska	Alaska Federation of Natives	Alaska Native, rural villages	More than 648 military installations, active and abandoned, pollute land, groundwater, wetlands, streams, and air with fuel spills, pesticides, solvents, munitions, and radioactive materials. Unique and intractable cleanup issues confront the Alaska Native population of approximately 100,000.

(*Continued*)

TABLE 8.1. EXAMPLES OF COMMUNITY-BASED ENVIRONMENTAL JUSTICE ISSUES. (*Continued*)

Community	Location	Organization(s)	Demographics	Issues
Triana	Triana, Alabama	(Not applicable)	African American, rural	DDT and PCB contamination of Alabama River affected nearly 1,200 local residents who use the river for subsistence fishing. Some of the highest levels of DDT in humans ever recorded. In 1982, lawsuit against Olin Corporation resulted in a $24 million settlement.
Townships of North Carolina	North Carolina	Concerned Citizens of Tillary	African American, rural	Proliferation of "hog farms" in concentrated animal feeding operations (CAFOs) throughout the state led to major multiple health and environmental impacts. A study by Concerned Citizens of Tillary and University of North Carolina found CAFOs more likely to be located in poor and nonwhite areas of North Carolina.
Asian immigrant women workers	San Francisco, California	Asian Immigrant Women Advocates	Asian, urban	Non-English-speaking immigrant workers in garment, hotel, and electronics industries suffer assorted health impacts ranging from exposure to toxic substances, poor work conditions, long hours, and accidents. Participatory action research conducted by hotel workers, union, and University of California Labor Occupational Health Program led to demands at contract negotiations for workload reductions.
Barrio Boca	Guayanilla, Puerto Rico	Centro de Accion Ambiental	Puerto Rican, rural	Pesticide drift results from aerial spraying on mango and banana plantation owned and operated by Tropical Fruit Company. Community actions resulted in court order to restrict spraying to only optimal weather conditions.
Tucson International Airport Area Superfund Site	Tucson, Arizona	Tucsonians for a Clean Environment	Latino, urban	Trichlorethylene (TCE), an industrial solvent, seeped into aquifer and created a toxic groundwater plume 5 miles long and 2 miles wide. Designated by the EPA as a Superfund site. Class action lawsuit resulted in a settlement with Hughes Missile Systems Company of $84.5 million. Local residents also secured a health clinic.

are at the same time holistic, bottom-up, community-based, multi-issue, cross-cutting, interdependent, integrative, and unifying.

Historians of the environmental movement have referred to environmental justice as the defining feature of the fourth wave of environmentalism. The first and longest wave grew out of the conservation movement of the late nineteenth and early twentieth centuries. The second wave resulted in the era of protective legislation in the early 1970s. During the third wave well-funded mainstream environmental groups operated primarily in Washington, D.C. ("inside the Beltway"), relying heavily on legal and political strategies. In the fourth wave environmental justice emerged as the first truly grassroots form of environmentalism, one that links environmental issues to social and economic inequality and has the potential to be socially transformative (Shabecoff, 1993; Dowie, 1995).

The Meaning of Disproportionate Impacts

The concept of environmental justice arose out of evidence that hazardous environmental exposures and their health consequences differed among populations differentiated by race, ethnicity, and income. This pattern was first described in racial terms (hence the term *environmental racism*), after early studies suggested that people of color communities were disproportionately exposed to environmental hazards. Later studies focused on poverty as an additional risk factor for disproportionate exposures. The concept of disproportionate impacts, however, is far more complicated than exposures alone. There is a complex interplay of factors at work in communities with a history of social and economic disadvantage, inadequate services, and environmental exposures. Thus *disproportionate impacts* may refer to inequities in levels of harmful environmental exposures, deficiencies in services or benefits, or differentials in communities' ability to withstand or mitigate harms. This section briefly discusses the components of disproportionate impact and their implications for the theory and practice of environmental justice.

Proximity to Pollution Sources

At the simplest level, adverse human health and environmental effects can be understood in terms of differential proximity to environmental hazards. During the 1980s, most environmental justice research focused on the proximity of people of color and low-income populations to environmental hazards. These studies examined a wide spectrum of exposures, including exposures to waste sites, industrial facilities, ambient air pollution, transportation thoroughfares, garbage transfer stations, hog farms, and all types of noxious and incompatible land uses.

Over time the studies established a pattern of disproportionate exposure that convinced even skeptical observers. For example, political scientists Lester, Allen, and Hill (2001) wrote that "[w]e must admit that at the outset in 1994 we were skeptical of many of the *strident* claims regarding environmental injustice. However, our analyses (as well as our findings) over the past five years have caused us to reconsider our original positions" (p. vx).

These proximity studies became highly sophisticated over time, deploying locational data in geographic information systems (GIS) (Maantay, 2002; also see Chapter Thirty-One). Geographic information systems have proved helpful in performing multistressor, multimedia, and multi-issue analyses of communities. For example, recent studies have considered not just the presence of hazards but also the lack of amenities in characterizing disproportionate environmental impacts. A Whittier College GIS environmental justice project, for instance, is evaluating land use change and recreation access in California's San Gabriel Valley (Swift and Henderson, 1997).

However, proximity to an exposure source may be an inexact surrogate of actual contact with a toxicant (Institute of Medicine, 1999; see also Chapter Four). For a full and accurate picture of human health and environmental effects, proximity data must be augmented with exposure studies employing such approaches as modeling and actual monitoring. In its first report on environmental justice, the EPA concluded:

> There are clear and dramatic disparities among ethnic groups for death rates, life expectancy, and disease rates. There is also a surprising lack of data on human exposure to environmental pollutants for Whites as well as for ethnic and racial minorities. One exception is lead exposures in children, and the data are unequivocal. Black children have disproportionately higher blood lead levels than White children even when socioeconomic variables are factored in. For other pollutants, available information suggests that racial minorities may have a greater *potential* for exposure to some pollutants because they tend to live in urban areas, are more likely to live near a waste site, or exhibit a greater tendency to rely on subsistence fishing for dietary protein [EPA, 1992, vol. II, p. 15].

Unique Exposure Pathways

Some communities sustain unique environmental exposures because of practices linked to socioeconomic status or cultural background. A good example is subsistence fishing. For some indigenous peoples and some Asian and Pacific Islander immigrant populations, this is a culturally specific practice based on a worldview that values human connection to the environment for both physical and spiritual well-being (Arquette and others, 2002). In addition, economic deprivation may compel rural or urban poor people to fish in polluted waters to supplement their diets. West, Fly, and Marans (1992) found that African Americans in Detroit engaged in higher levels of subsistence fishing from the contaminated Detroit River than did others in the population. Another example is pica, the habit among malnourished young children of eating dirt or paint chips because they are hungry. Issues of socioeconomic status and racial discrimination are embedded in such unique exposure pathways. In describing a famous 1982 case involving contamination and subsistence fish consumption in Triana, Alabama, a resident called the situation yet another example of how "pollution follows the path of least resistance" (Taylor, 1982).

Susceptible and Sensitive Populations

From the perspective of environmental justice, it is necessary to look not only at *intrinsic* factors related to susceptibility, like age, sex, genetics, and race or ethnicity, but also at *acquired* factors, which may include chronic medical conditions, health care access, nutrition, fitness, other pollutant exposures, and drug and alcohol use (Sexton, 1997). Box 8.3, for example, presents an excerpt from a recent review paper explaining how susceptibility to air pollution may be related to social position.

Box 8.3. Social Position and Susceptibility to Air Pollution Exposure

People in lower socioeconomic circumstances may be more susceptible to air pollution for reasons directly related to their relative disadvantage and psychosocial stress. For example, they may lack access to grocery stores that sell fresh fruits and vegetables or the income to buy them, resulting in reduced intake of anti-oxidant vitamins that can protect against adverse consequences of air pollution exposure. Another possibility is reduced access to medical care, so poor people may not have the appropriate prescription for a respiratory condition such as asthma. Medication can alleviate symptoms aggravated by pollution exposure, and more consistent use of corticosteroids lowers baseline inflammation, potentially lowering responsiveness to proinflammatory pollutants. An additional hypothesis is that psychosocial stress and violence, which can be higher among those of low SEP [socioeconomic position], can increase susceptibility.

Characteristics of neighborhoods can affect susceptibility. In four U.S. communities, residence in a disadvantaged neighborhood was associated with coronary heart disease (CHD) incidence, even after controlling for established CHD risk factors and personal income, education, and occupation. With current emphasis on cardiac effects of air pollution, this finding is particularly relevant to the study of air pollution and socioeconomic interaction. Because lower-income people are more likely to live near roadways, there is also evidence that increased traffic density has been associated with lack of neighborhood communication and collaboration (thereby reducing available social networks).

Another potential mechanism of susceptibility directly related to social position is coexposure to other pollutants, including indoor pollutants. A person with a relatively high dose of other pollutants may be "weakened" and less able to withstand the additional insult of ambient air pollution. People with less wealth are more likely to be employed in dirtier occupations and in developing countries, they may also be more likely to be exposed to pollutants indoors from heating and cooking. Workers in blue-collar occupations may also be more exposed to environmental tobacco smoke than are white-collar workers in cases where regulations limiting indoor smoking in the workplace are not applied consistently. Housing stock in poorer communities with high rates of crowding can have higher levels of certain allergens as well as other risk factors for asthma sensitization and exacerbation.

Source: O'Neill and others, 2003, p. 1865; article references have been omitted.

Multiple and Cumulative Effects

Disadvantaged and underserved communities are likely to suffer a wide range of environmental burdens, from poor air to poor housing. For example, a recent study by the Columbia Center for Children's Environmental Health found that African American women in the South Bronx exposed to auto exhaust, cigarette smoke, and incinerators in the third trimester of pregnancy tended to give birth to smaller babies with smaller head circumferences (Perera and others, 2004). The label *toxic hotspots* is often associated with environmental justice. Traditional risk assessment and risk management have not addressed these pockets of multiple and cumulative exposures because they have been geared toward controlling sources of pollution through technology-based regulation or a chemical-by-chemical approach (see Chapter Thirty-Two). In this context the Environmental Protection Agency's 2003 framework for cumulative risk assessment represents a milestone for both cumulative risk assessment and environmental justice. It is significant for environmental justice because of the following features:

- It takes a broad view of risk, including areas outside the EPA's regulatory authority, and poses questions for which quantitative methods do not yet exist.
- It employs a population-based and place-based analysis, rather than an agent-to-receptor analysis.

- It promotes a comprehensive and integrated assessment of risk.
- It recognizes multiple stressors, including both chemical and nonchemical, as well as social factors that may affect risk.
- It expands the definition of *vulnerability* to include both biological and social factors.
- It places a premium on community involvement and partnerships.
- It emphasizes the importance of planning, scoping, and problem formulation.
- It links risk assessment to risk management in the context of prevention and intervention strategies to meet community health goals.

Fundamental to the framework's contribution to the discourse on risk assessment and environmental justice is its recognition that assessment requires an iterative process that involves the affected community and all relevant stakeholders, including government and business, as articulated in the National Academy of Sciences report *Understanding Risk* and the report of the Presidential/Congressional Commission on Risk Assessment and Risk Management (1997; see also Stern and Fineberg, 1996).

Social Vulnerability

Underserved and disadvantaged communities have numerous liabilities that may contribute to the way environmental exposures affect health. These factors may affect a community's ability to prevent, withstand, or recover from the effects of environmental insult. Research by Pastor, Sadd, and Hipp (2001) has revealed an intriguing example. They found a strong correlation between periods of greatest community demographic change and the introduction of noxious land uses. These transition periods seem to be low points for community social capital in terms of stable leaders, networks, and institutions. Pastor and his colleagues coined a term to describe this phenomenon, *ethnic churning.*

Social factors such as employment status, access to health insurance, language ability, and access to social capital, can play a major role in determining the response to environmental insult. Lack of health care can be a major factor. Poverty, poor nutrition, and psychosocial stress may affect the strength of one's coping systems. Isolation, whether economic, racial, linguistic, or otherwise, leads to fewer connections, less access to information or influence, and thus less ability to prevent, withstand, or recover from environmental stressors. Social problems such as these may significantly limit meaningful involvement in the environmental decision-making process. Indices that measure such isolation, such as disparity and dissimilarity indexes, may be useful in this area. (In the following discussion, I am indebted to a definition of *vulnerability* developed by Roger Kasperson and adopted in the EPA's 2003 framework for cumulative risk assessment. Kasperson posits four categories: susceptibility/sensitivity, differential exposure, differential preparedness, and differential ability to recover.)

Two major issues are highlighted by this discussion. First, disproportionate impacts cannot be characterized solely or primarily according to disparities in exposure to environmental hazards. It is necessary to look at both sides of the risk equation—the magnitude and severity of exposures and the nature of the receptor population. Both biological and social aspects of vulnerability must be taken into account. Second, there is a functional relationship between socioeconomic and cultural factors and environmental risk. Disadvantaged, underserved, and environmentally overburdened communities confront both physical and social vulnerability. Environmental justice is predicated on the fact that certain communities come to the table with preexisting physical and social deficits that make the effects of environmental pollution more, and in some cases unacceptably, burdensome. In other words the concept of vulnerability is central to the meaning of environmental justice.

If cumulative effects are viewed in a temporal context, then the legacy of racial and economic discrimination is one dimension of environmental injustice, and it results in a high prevalence of certain diseases and conditions, which in turn increases the population's susceptibility to environmental harms. These diseases and conditions are commonly known as *health disparities,* and the United States has made a national commitment to eliminate them. Vulnerability and health disparities are thus integrally related concepts, and linking them can produce a very powerful analytical tool for understanding the complex relationships that contribute to disproportionate environmental risk. Figure 8.1 shows this relationship, illustrating that health disparities are both an outcome of and a contributor to vulnerability.

Two important conclusions are embedded in the concept of disproportionate impacts. First, although the concept of disproportionate impacts is a cornerstone for understanding environmental justice, researchers and practitioners are only now appreciating its complexity. A comprehensive, robust, conceptual framework for understanding disproportionate impacts—one that includes disparities in exposure, susceptibility, law enforcement, and health and that accounts for multiple and cumulative impacts—is just beginning to emerge. This conceptual framework will greatly enhance the development of the research and policy agendas needed to redress such impacts. Second, a narrow focus on controlling and preventing pollution may be ineffective; it is necessary to address the myriad social, economic, and cultural realities of disadvantaged, underserved, and overburdened communities concurrently. A community's well-being depends on the health of many different sectors, including economic development, housing, transportation,

FIGURE 8.1. RELATIONSHIP BETWEEN ENVIRONMENTAL HAZARDS, VULNERABILITY, AND HEALTH DISPARITIES.

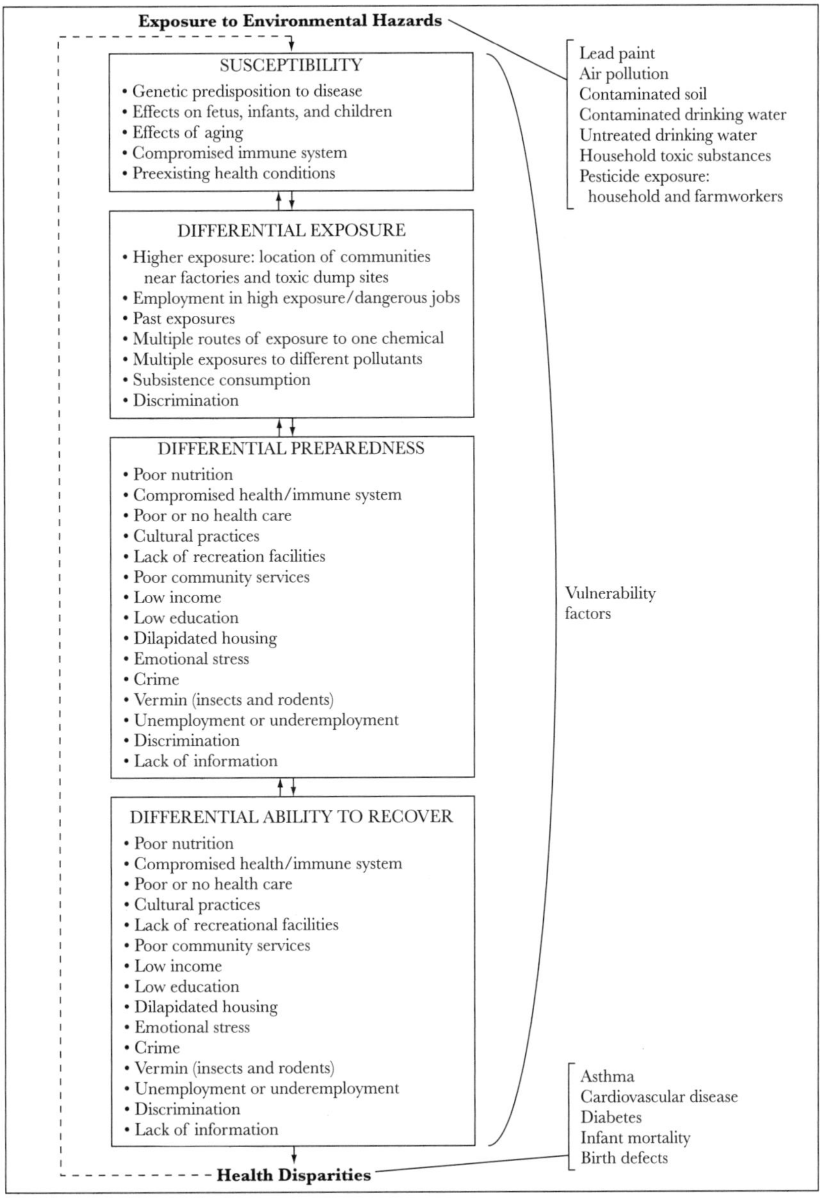

Exposure to Environmental Hazards
SUSCEPTIBILITY
• Genetic predisposition to disease
• Effects on fetus, infants, and children
• Effects of aging
• Compromised immune system
• Preexisting health conditions
DIFFERENTIAL EXPOSURE
• Higher exposure: location of communities near factories and toxic dump sites
• Employment in high exposure/dangerous jobs
• Past exposures
• Multiple routes of exposure to one chemical
• Multiple exposures to different pollutants
• Subsistence consumption
• Discrimination
DIFFERENTIAL PREPAREDNESS
• Poor nutrition
• Compromised health/immune system
• Poor or no health care
• Cultural practices
• Lack of recreation facilities
• Poor community services
• Low income
• Low education
• Dilapidated housing
• Emotional stress
• Crime
• Vermin (insects and rodents)
• Unemployment or underemployment
• Discrimination
• Lack of information
DIFFERENTIAL ABILITY TO RECOVER
• Poor nutrition
• Compromised health/immune system
• Poor or no health care
• Cultural practices
• Lack of recreational facilities
• Poor community services
• Low income
• Low education
• Dilapidated housing
• Emotional stress
• Crime
• Vermin (insects and rodents)
• Unemployment or underemployment
• Discrimination
• Lack of information
Health Disparities
Lead paint
Air pollution
Contaminated soil
Contaminated drinking water
Untreated drinking water
Household toxic substances
Pesticide exposure: household and farmworkers
Vulnerability factors
Asthma
Cardiovascular disease
Diabetes
Infant mortality
Birth defects

Source: National Environmental Justice Advisory Council, 2004.

arts, green space, and recreation. Public health and environmental justice advocates must think holistically, seeking comprehensive, integrative paradigm changes to promote truly healthy and sustainable communities for all peoples.

Legal, Public Policy, and Research Implications

Once disproportionate impacts are more fully understood, environmental justice researchers and advocates face a second challenge: crafting legal and policy responses. An important barrier to meeting this challenge has been a divergence between the civil rights and environmental law paradigms.

Just seven years after the 1987 publication of *Toxic Wastes and Race,* on February 11, 1994, President Clinton signed Executive Order 12898, "Federal Actions to Address Environmental Justice in Minority Populations and Low-Income Populations." Because Executive Order 12898 was one of the first public policy statements in the arena of environmental justice, it is worth analyzing various interpretations of its key clause, which reads as follows: "To the greatest extent practicable and permitted by law . . . each Federal agency shall make environmental justice part of its mission by identifying and addressing, as appropriate, the disproportionately high and adverse human health and environmental effects of its programs, policies, and activities on minority populations and low-income populations."

Under the prevailing interpretation this Executive Order has been viewed as a directive to identify minority and low-income populations. These would be defined as *protected groups,* on whose behalf protective actions could presumably then be taken. This interpretation is understandable given the legal framework of civil rights, which is premised on the notion of *protected classes,* such as people of color, women, and the disabled. However, the intent of Executive Order 12898 extended well beyond identifying target populations; it was action oriented. The order directed agencies to "identify and address disproportionately high and adverse human health and environmental effects." Moreover, it called for actions to be pursued "to the greatest extent practicable and permitted by law." The order created no new rights or obligations, but an often overlooked accompanying Presidential Memorandum referred to the use of existing statutes to achieve the goals of the order. (Also see Box 8.4.)

Box 8.4. Science and Environmental Justice at the EPA

In 1992, a number of environmental justice advocates, including this chapter author, met as members of the "Michigan Coalition" with then EPA administrator William Reilly. He informed us of the EPA's plans to establish an Office of Environmental Equity (renamed the Office of Environmental Justice in 1994). I asked Reilly, "How will EPA ensure that the Office of Environmental Equity not be marginalized like the Office of Civil Rights was?" This encounter presaged the historical significance of the proper interpretation of the language in Executive Order 12898 and the challenges of operationalizing civil rights and social justice concepts within the mission of an environmental agency like the EPA.

It is instructive to recount the testimony of William Rucklehaus, the first EPA administrator, before Congress at the time when the agency was being established. He was asked how the EPA was going to address matters of civil rights and social equity. As I recall, he said that as important as these issues were, the Environmental Protection Agency was primarily a science agency, and its first priority was to build its science foundation. (Two decades later the United Church of Christ Commission for Racial Justice sent a copy of *Toxic Wastes and Race* to the EPA, to which the agency's response was, "EPA addresses issues of technology, not sociology.") I wonder where we would be today if Rucklehaus's answer to Congress had been that the EPA would systematically incorporate concerns of civil rights and social equity into its "sound science base" and make such concerns a part of the analytical and operational paradigm within the context of the laws the agency is authorized to administer.

Thus it is not surprising that during the decade after the Executive Order, most community activists, advocates, researchers, industry groups, and governmental agencies operated from the premise of identifying the *environmental justice community*—that is, identifying disproportionately high-minority and low-income populations. This interpretation fails to recognize that the nation's environmental laws are premised not on the concept of a "protected class" but on "human health and environmental effects." (Interestingly, the U.S. Department of Justice, charged with enforcing the nation's laws, focuses on the concept of "disproportionately high and adverse human health and environmental effects.")

This distinction is important because it bears directly on the use of environmental laws. The designation *environmental justice communities,* although descriptive, does not trigger specific provisions of applicable laws. Hence it is often unclear what actions, other than more study or efforts to ensure public participation, an agency should undertake once a determination that a community is an environmental justice communities is made. *Environmental justice issues* is a far more useful analytical concept, as it incorporates disproportionate and adverse human health and environmental effects. The more clear the nexus between identifying such effects and triggering specific provisions in law, the more readily legal remedies can follow. This emphasizes the importance of fully characterizing disproportionately high and adverse human health and environmental effects of the kind discussed earlier.

The notion of environmental justice as a convergence of the civil rights and environmental movements does not mean simply transplanting civil rights premises to the environmental arena. Rather it requires an understanding that civil rights law and environmental law bring different paradigms to environmental justice issues (Targ, 2002). Making them mesh properly requires a focus not on environmental justice communities but on environmental justice issues, with reliable indicators of disproportionate impacts. This issue has tremendous historical significance and helps to explain why the concepts advanced by the civil rights movement have been largely marginalized by U.S. federal and state environmental protection regimes. Although this issue will surely unfold over time, its significance should not be underestimated, as the cautionary tale in Box 8.4 points out.

Issues of vulnerability bear directly on developing a research agenda that meets the needs of policymakers. It is not surprising that most environmental justice research in the first twenty years focused on proximity studies, demonstrating that communities of color and low-income communities are disproportionately located near environmental hazards. However, the next generation of research should focus on understanding the functional relationships between socioeconomic factors and environmental exposure and on devising innovative measures of disproportionate health and environmental effects. The Health Disparities Research Program of the National Institute of Environmental Health Sciences (NIEHS) offers an example of such research:

> The purpose of the Health Disparities Research Program is to foster multidisciplinary research that will elucidate underlying mechanisms by which the interaction of physical exposures and the social environment leads to health disparities. Physical exposures include physical agents (e.g., radiation), chemical agents (e.g., pesticides) and biological agents (e.g., pathogens, harmful algal blooms). The social environment includes socioeconomic status (SES), residential factors, education, cultural variables, institutional and political forces, familial factors, and media influences. The ultimate goal of this research is to understand the sources of disparities in health among the U.S. population, especially between lower SES groups and higher SES groups. Via this initiative the National Institutes of Health (NIH) seeks to clarify biological, social, and behavioral processes that lead to health disparities stemming from the interaction of social and physical environments as a basis for ultimately developing intervention strategies [NIEHS, 2004].

Collaborative and Integrated Problem Solving

The growing theoretical and practical understanding of disproportionate impacts, as well as the related legal, public policy, and research challenges, is helping to identify the strategies and tools best suited to addressing the complex issues of achieving environmental justice. As noted earlier, communities of color and indigenous and low-income communities often suffer adverse and disproportionate exposure to environmental and occupational hazards. Moreover these populations tend to be more vulnerable by virtue of deficiencies in their social environments involving housing, land use, transportation, health care, and other factors. Finally, the inability to use a range of capacities (that is, human, technical, financial, social, and political capital) within affected communities presents great obstacles to positive change. How can communities and public health professionals work both to improve environmental health and to eliminate disparities related to disproportionate impacts?

The vision of environmental justice is the development of a holistic, community-based, participatory, and integrative paradigm for achieving healthy and sustainable communities for all peoples. This holistic approach aligns with the World Health Organization's view of community health as a positive concept that "encompasses all the environmental, social, and economic resources as well as the emotional and physical capacities that enable people in a geographic area to realize their aspirations and satisfy their needs" (quoted in Lasker and Weiss, 2003, p. 55). Environmental justice also calls for a holistic analysis of the problems that impair the health of people in communities, including social, economic, environmental, political, emotional, and biological determinants, as noted earlier. (Box 8.5 offers one example of a broadly conceived revitalization project.)

Box 8.5. ReGenesis Revitalization Project, Spartanburg, South Carolina

Harold Mitchell grew up in a house near an abandoned hazardous waste site in the impoverished Arkwright section of Spartanburg, South Carolina. Members of his family, like others in the neighborhood, suffered what seemed to be a disproportionately high number of cancers, respiratory diseases, and miscarriages. Mitchell's leadership helped to transform this concern over environmental insults into a broad vision for community revitalization. Since its inception, the ReGenesis Revitalization Project has grown to include more than 100 partners. Its vision encompasses housing, health facilities, recreation facilities and green space, transportation, job creation, and green business development. By the end of 2003, the project had leveraged more than $5 million in public and private funding. In February 2004, a Swiss bio-technology firm announced that it was going to locate a plastics alternatives plant in the area. The project is a prime example of what Mary Nelson calls "turning a corner in the fight for environmental justice." Nelson is executive director of Bethel New Life, Inc., a renowned faith-based community development corporation in the West Garfield section of Chicago. She believes that communities now understand that "it is not enough to stand against something. We are now moving to the stage where we can say what we want and formulate a vision for healthy, sustainable communities."

Roz Lasker and Elisa Weiss (2003), of the New York Academy of Medicine, build on this point when introducing the concept of collaboration in community problem solving. They write that the "growing interest in using collaboration stems from the fact that many of these problems are complex; consequently, they go beyond the capacity, resources, or jurisdiction of any single person, program, organization, or sector to change or control. Without sufficiently broad-based collaboration, it has been difficult for communities to understand the underlying nature of these kinds of problems or to develop effective and locally feasible solutions to address them" (p. 18). Problems that require comprehensive actions have been difficult to solve when essential participants are not involved or when programs, organizations, and policies work at cross-purposes. The tremendous diversity in populations affected by health problems and in the local contexts in which these problems occur limits the effectiveness of top-down, one-size-fits-all solutions.

Both affected communities and public health practitioners must engage in a dialogue that seeks to apply collaborative problem solving to the task of achieving environmental justice and healthy communities (Lee, 2005). Three premises motivate this conclusion:

1. Environmental justice advocates and practitioners must develop a conceptual framework that moves the environmental justice discourse from a focus primarily on problem identification to a focus that is also solution oriented.
2. Environmental justice issues are enormously complex. Environmentally, economically, and socially distressed communities require human, technical, legal, institutional, and financial resources to address them properly. Environmental justice groups must harness these necessary resources. This speaks to the need for social capital, consensus building, dispute resolution, collaborative problem solving, and civic capacity.
3. Environmental justice strategies need to address economic and social factors such as housing, transportation, economic development, job creation, green space and recreation—factors that make up the larger environment and contribute to overall well-being.

Collaborative and integrative problem solving arose because it is a better way of dealing with complex ecological and organizational systems and the information needs associated with complex societal problems. There is an emerging literature on collaborative problem solving in arenas such as environmental health, community development, planning, law, and natural resource management. For example, Kathryn Kohm and Jerry Franklin (1997), of the University of Washington, apply this approach to natural resource management; appreciating the complexity of systems and managing for wholeness rather than for the efficiency of individual components places forestry in the context of a much broader movement toward systems thinking.

This message is highly resonant, because a recurring theme of this chapter is the complex nature of environmentally, economically, and socially distressed communities and tribes. Such complexity requires holistic and integrated problem solving. Julia Wondolleck and Steven Yaffee (2000), writing about collaboration in natural resource management, call for strategies that "focus on the problem in new and different ways." They suggest "rethinking" problems in ways that integrate geographically, integrate functionally, and integrate different elements of the problem.

To apply these lessons to environmental justice will require community-based experience and authentic partnerships. It will also require an appreciation of the power imbalances and tensions that exist when trying to work through complex problems that may require both confrontational and collaborative approaches.

One goal of such collaborations is to build the strategic thinking, planning, and problem-solving capacity of communities and other involved parties. Strategic approaches should build on community visioning and local planning processes. Such collaborative models should employ asset-building and asset-mapping methods, recognizing that no matter how deficit-laden and problem-ridden a given community may be, there are still many untapped resources to harness. For example, in 2003, Bethel New Life—the organization whose director has called for "turning environmental liabilities into community assets and opportunities"—broke ground on a transit-oriented commercial development that will incorporate photovoltaics, a living roof, recycled materials, super insulation, and energy efficiency measures. The location is a formerly contaminated brownfield site.

Environmental justice collaborative models would employ community-based participatory research (CBPR) efforts, as the two approaches share many principles and methods (see Box 8.6). Moreover, these collaborative models would expand the reach of CBPR by providing the venues and stakeholders that could apply research results to real problems. These models would also make use of consensus building and dispute resolution methods, including the *mutual gains approach to negotiations* (Susskind, Levy, and Thomas-Larmer, 2000). Such models would build on the concepts in the EPA's new cumulative risk framework by promoting proactive, comprehensive, and multimedia risk reduction efforts. They would have wide applicability for areas including, but not limited to, community development, transportation, brownfield redevelopment, smart growth, and comprehensive community revitalization initiatives.

Box 8.6. Community-Based Participatory Research

- *Promotes active collaboration and participation at every stage of research:* CBPR fosters equal participation from all partners. It provides all participants with an equal sense of ownership over the research and the outcomes.
- *Fosters co-learning:* CBPR provides an environment in which both community residents and researchers contribute their respective expertise and where partners learn from each other. Community members acquire new skills in conducting research, and researchers learn about community networks and concerns—information that can be used to inform hypothesis generation and data collection.
- *Ensures projects are community-driven:* Research questions in CBPR are guided by the environmental health issues or concerns of community members. NIEHS recognizes that for research and prevention/intervention strategies to be successful, they must address the concerns of community residents.
- *Disseminates results in useful terms:* Upon completion of CBPR projects, results are communicated to all partners in culturally appropriate, respectful, and understandable terms.
- *Ensures research and intervention strategies are culturally appropriate:* With active participation of community residents from the beginning, research and prevention/intervention strategies are likely to be based in the cultural context of the community in which such work is intended to benefit.
- *Defines community as a unit of identity:* NIEHS Translational Research programs promote collaboration among academic scientists and community partners from underserved communities. In the case of these projects, community is typically characterized by a sense of identification and emotional connection to other members through common interests and a commitment to address shared concerns, such as harmful environmental exposures or environmental injustice.

Source: O'Fallon and Dearry, 2002.

Social capital—the social networks, norms, and social trust that facilitate coordination and cooperation for mutual benefit (Putnam, 2000)—is critically important to environmental justice collaborative problem solving. The challenge of linking resources with needs, an apt practical definition of collaboration, is especially salient in disadvantaged and underserved communities, where groups must harness necessary human, technical, legal, institutional, and financial resources to address complex issues. Marshaling the necessary resources requires the efforts of different people from different backgrounds representing the different sectors of the society. It is hard for people not to work toward resolving issues once they have sat at a table together, engaged in dialogue, and come to know each other on a human level. Once social capital is built, it leverages other forms of capital investments—financial, institutional, infrastructural, and environmental. In Robert Putnam's words: "Social connections are also important for the rules of conduct that they sustain. Networks involve (almost by definition) mutual obligations; they are not interesting as mere *contacts*. Networks of community engagement foster sturdy norms of reciprocity. . . . A society characterized by generalized reciprocity is more efficient than a distrustful society. . . . Trustworthiness lubricates social life. Frequent interaction among a diverse set of people tends to produce a norm of generalized reciprocity. Civic engagement and social capital entail mutual obligation and responsibility for action" (Putnam, 2000, pp. 20–21).

Indeed, the emergence of the idea of collaborative models to achieve environmental justice and healthy communities reflects a similar movement in many arenas, including community development and community health. In public health, for example, the *social determinants of health* are such factors as income distribution, discrimination, access to education, and housing policies. Public health professionals increasingly recognize that addressing these social influences on well-being will require innovative research and intervention strategies, collaboration across disciplinary groups, and engagement of community members (Schulz, Galea, and Kreiger, 2002). The following appraisal of public health practice, from which the areas of community-based participatory research and social determinants of health emerged, resonates strongly with the vision of environmental justice:

> Recognition of the inequities in health status associated with, for example, poverty, inadequate housing, lack of employment opportunities, racism, and powerlessness, has led to calls for a focus on an ecological approach that recognizes that individuals are embedded within social, political, and economic systems that shape behaviors and access to resources necessary to maintain health. Researchers and practitioners alike have called for increased attention to the complex issues that compromise the health of people living in marginalized communities; for more integration of research and practice; for greater community involvement and control, for example, through partnerships among academic, health practice, and community organizations; for increased sensitivity to and competence in working with diverse cultures; for expanded use of both qualitative and quantitative research methods; and for more focus on health and quality of life, including the social, economic, and political dimensions of health and well-being [Israel, Schulz, Parker, and Becker, 1998, p. 174].

Indeed, it is enlightening to ponder the vast array of prevention and intervention strategies that a holistic understanding of the natural, built, social, and cultural and spiritual environments—the approach implicit in the concept of environmental justice—would offer public health practitioners.

Conclusion

Nobel laureate Amartya Sen's work has made it clear that vulnerability to environmental change is a major shaper of global risk. Risk is closely tied to vulnerability and can be viewed as a product of environmental stress and human and ecological vulnerability. Authoritative bodies such as the World Commission on Environment and Development have underscored the intertwined nature of poverty and environmental threat. These are the same complex and multidimensional issues, albeit on a global scale, that have given rise to the concept of environmental justice. In a very short period of time the theory and practice of environmental justice have evolved to include an impressive array of concepts, players, and endeavors. These endeavors include new models of community organizing and empowerment, community-based participatory research, environmental impact assessment, use of existing laws, and other strategies for achieving healthy and sustainable communities, domestically and internationally. Issues of environmental justice form a complex web of public health, environmental, economic, and social concerns that require multiple, holistic, integrative, and unifying strategies. The achievement of a vision of healthy and sustainable communities for all peoples not only necessitates the articulation of new concepts, new strategies, new models, and new partnerships but calls as well for a critical appraisal of where progress has been made and what obstacles still stand in the way. It will require committed individuals willing and able to provide foresight, analysis, and leadership.

Thought Questions

1. What evidence exists to show that race and poverty contribute to negative environmental health effects?
2. What factors can exacerbate the effect of environmental exposures on populations with low socioeconomic status?
3. Why is involving the affected community important to achieving solutions to environmental justice issues?
4. What are some global implications of environmental justice?

References

Arquette, M., and others. "Holistic Risk-Based Environmental Decision Making: A Native Perspective." *Environmental Health Perspectives,* 2002, *110*(suppl. 2), 259–264.

Bullard, R. D. *People of Color Environmental Groups: 1994–95 Directory.* Atlanta, Ga.: Environmental Justice Resource Center, Clark-Atlanta University, 1994.

Burwell, D. "Reminiscences from Warren County, North Carolina." In C. Lee (ed.), *Proceedings of the First National People of Color Environmental Leadership Summit.* New York: United Church of Christ, Commission for Racial Justice, 1992.

Cherniak, M. *The Hawk's Nest Incident: America's Worst Industrial Disaster.* New Haven, Conn.: Yale University Press, 1987.

Dowie, M. *Losing Ground: American Environmentalism at the Close of the Twentieth Century.* Cambridge, Mass.: MIT Press, 1995.

Executive Order no. 12898. "Federal Actions to Address Environmental Justice in Minority Populations and Low-Income Populations." *Federal Register* 59 (1994), 7629.

Faber, D. R., and McCarthy, D. *Green of Another Color: Building Effective Partnerships Between Foundations and the Environmental Justice Movement.* Boston: Philanthropy and Environmental Justice Research Project, Northeastern University, Apr. 10, 2001.

Gauna, J. Presentation at the First People of Color Environmental Leadership Summit National Advisory Committee meeting, Washington, D.C., May 20, 1991.

Institute of Medicine. *Toward Environmental Justice: Research, Education, and Health Policy Needs.* Washington, D.C.: National Academies Press, 1999.

Israel, B. A., Schulz, A. J., Parker, E. A., and Becker, A. B. "Review of Community-Based Research: Assessing Partnership Approaches to Improve Public Health." *American Review of Public Health,* 1998, *19,* 173–202.

Kohm, K. A., and Franklin, J. F. *Creating a Forestry for the 21st Century: The Science of Ecosystem Management.* Washington, D.C.: Island Press, 1997.

Konig, H. *Columbus: His Enterprise.* New York: Monthly Review Press, 1976.

Lasker, R. D., and Weiss, E. S. "Broadening Participation in Community Problem Solving: A Multidisciplinary Model to Support Collaborative Practice and Research." *Journal of Urban Health,* 2003, *80,* 14–57.

Lavelle, M., Coyle, M., and MacLachlan, C. "Unequal Protection: The Racial Divide in Environmental Law." *The National Law Journal,* Sept. 21, 1994, p. S1.

Lee, C. "Introduction." In C. Lee (ed.), *Proceedings of the First National People of Color Environmental Leadership Summit.* New York: United Church of Christ, Commission for Racial Justice, 1992.

Lee, C. "Beyond Toxic Wastes and Race." In R. D. Bullard (ed.), *Confronting Environmental Racism: Voices from the Grassroots.* Boston: South End Press, 1993.

Lee, C. "Would Dr. King Have Become an Environmental Justice Advocate?" Speech presented at a U.S. Department of Justice Symposium, "A Dream Deferred: 30 Years After the Passage of the Civil Rights Act of 1964." Washington, D.C.: Nov. 30, 1994.

Lee, C. "Environmental Justice, Urban Revitalization, and Brownfields: The Search for Authentic Signs of Hope." Presentation at the U.S. Environmental Protection Agency National Brownfields Workshop, Washington, D.C., Feb. 13–14, 1996.

Lee, C. "Environmental Justice: Building a Unified Vision of Health and Environment." *Environmental Health Perspectives,* 2002, *110*(suppl. 2), 141–144.

Lee, C. "Collaborative Models to Achieve Environmental Justice and Healthy Communities." In D. Pellow and R. Brulle (eds.), *Power, Justice, and the Environment: A Critical Appraisal of the Environmental Justice Movement.* Cambridge, Mass.: MIT Press, 2005.

Lester, J. P., Allen, D. W., and Hill, K. M. *Environmental Injustice in the United States: Myths and Realities.* Boulder, Colo.: Westview Press, 2001.

Maantay, J. "Mapping Environmental Injustices: Pitfalls and Potential of Geographic Information Systems in Assessing Environmental Health and Equity." *Environmental Health Perspectives,* 2002, *110*(suppl. 2), 161–171.

Mankiller, W. "Native American Historical and Cultural Perspectives on Environmental Justice." In C. Lee (ed.), *Proceedings of the First National People of Color Environmental Leadership Summit.* New York: United Church of Christ, Commission for Racial Justice, 1992.

National Environmental Justice Advisory Council. *Ensuring Risk Reduction for Communities with Multiple Stressors: Environmental Justice and Cumulative Risks/Impacts.* Washington, D.C.: United States Environmental Protection Agency, 2004.

National Institute of Environmental Health Sciences. "Health Disparities Research." [http://www.niehs.nih.gov/translat/hd/healthdis.htm]. 2002.

Norton, E. H. "Perspectives from the District of Columbia." In C. Lee (ed.), *Proceedings of the First National People of Color Environmental Leadership Summit.* New York: United Church of Christ, Commission for Racial Justice, 1992.

O'Fallon, L. R., and Dearry, A. "Community-Based Participatory Research as a Tool to Advance Environmental Health Sciences." *Environmental Health Perspectives,* 2002, *110*(suppl. 2), 155–159.

O'Neill, M. S., and others. "Health, Wealth, and Air Pollution: Advancing Theory and Methods." *Environmental Health Perspectives,* 2003, *111,* 1861–1870.

Pastor, M., Jr., Sadd, J., and Hipp, J. "Which Came First? Toxic Facilities, Minority Move-In, and Environmental Justice. *Journal of Urban Affairs,* 2001, *23*(1), 1–21.

Perera, F. P., and others. "Molecular Evidence of an Interaction Between Prenatal Environmental Exposures on Birth Outcomes in a Multiethnic Population." *Environmental Health Perspectives,* 2004, *112,* 626–630.

Presidential/Congressional Commission on Risk Assessment and Risk Management. *Framework for Environmental Risk Assessment: Final Report.* Vol. 1. Washington, D.C.: Presidential/Congressional Commission on Risk Assessment and Risk Management, 1997.

Putnam, R. D. *Bowling Alone: The Collapse and Revival of American Community.* New York: Simon & Schuster, 2000.

Schulz, A. J., Galea, S., and Kreiger, J. (eds.). "Community-Based Participatory Research—Addressing Social Determinants of Health: Lessons from the Urban Research Centers." *Health Education and Behavior,* 2002, *20*(3, special issue).

Sexton, K. "Sociodemographic Aspects of Human Susceptibility to Toxic Chemicals: Do Class and Race Matter for Realistic Risk Assessment?" *Environmental Toxicology and Pharmacology,* 1997, *4,* 261–269.

Shabecoff, P. *A Fierce Green Fire: The American Environmental Movement.* New York: Hill & Wang, 1993.

Stern, P. C., and Fineberg, H. V. (eds.). *Understanding Risk: Informing Decisions in a Democratic Society.* Washington, D.C.: National Academies Press, 1996.

Susskind, L., Levy, P., and Thomas-Larmer, J. *Negotiating Environmental Agreements: How to Avoid Escalating Confrontations, Needless Costs, and Unnecessary Litigation.* Washington, D.C.: Island Press, 2000.

Swift, C. C., and Henderson, J. A. "Using GIS to Evaluate Land Use Change and Recreation Access in the San Gabriel Valley: A Study in Environmental Justice." Paper presented at the Environmental Science Research Institute. [http://hosting.uaa.alaska.edu/afjnd/courses/biol485-gis/Using%20GIS%20to%20Evaluate%20Land%20Use%20Change.htm]. 1997.

Targ, N. "A Third Policy Avenue to Address Environmental Justice: Civil Rights and Environmental Quality and the Relevance of Social Capital Policy." *Tulane Environmental Law Journal,* 2002, *16,* 167–174.

Taylor, R. A. "Do Environmentalists Care About the Poor?" *U.S. News and World Report,* Apr. 2, 1982, pp. 51–55.

United Church of Christ, Commission for Racial Justice. *Toxic Wastes and Race in the United States: A National Study on the Racial and Socio-Economic Characteristics of Communities Surrounding Hazardous Waste Sites.* New York: United Church of Christ, 1987.

U.S. Environmental Protection Agency. *Environmental Equity: Reducing Risk for All Communities.* EPA230-R-92-008 (vol. II). Washington, D.C.: U.S. Environmental Protection Agency, June 1992.

U.S. Environmental Protection Agency. *Framework for Cumulative Risk Assessment.* EPA/630/P-02/001F. Washington, D.C.: U.S. Environmental Protection Agency, May 2003.

West, P. C., Fly, F., and Marans, R. "Minority Anglers and Toxic Fish Consumption: Evidence from a State-Wide Survey of Michigan." In B. Bryant and P. Mohai (eds.), *Race and the Incidence of Environmental Hazards: A Time for Discourse.* Boulder, Colo.: Westview Press, 1992.

Wondolleck, J. M., and Yaffee, S. L. *Making Collaboration Work: Lessons from Innovation in Natural Resource Management.* Washington, D.C.: Island Press, 2000.

For Further Information

Web Sites

EPA Office of Environmental Justice, Washington, D.C.: [www.epa.gov/compliance/environmentaljustice].

Environmental Justice Resource Center, Clark Atlanta University. Atlanta, Ga. [www.ejrc.cau.edu].

Southwest Network for Environmental and Economic Justice, Albuquerque, N.M. [www.sneej.org].

Dudley Street Neighborhood Initiative, Boston. [www.dsni.org].

West Harlem Environmental Action, New York. [www.weact.org].

Books and Journals

Bullard, R. D. *Dumping in Dixie: Race, Class, and Environmental Quality.* (3rd ed.) Boulder, Colo.: Westview, 2000.

One of the first books to chronicle the rise of the environmental justice movement, *Dumping in Dixie* analyzes the interplay between environmental and social justice concerns, particularly in the South.

Community, Research, and Environmental Justice, Environmental Health Perspectives, Special Issue, Apr. 2002, *110,* (suppl. 2), 139–334.

This special issue compiles research methods and projects involving communities and disproportionate environmental health impacts.

Cole, L., and Foster, S. *From the Ground Up: Environmental Racism and the Rise of the Environmental Justice Movement.* New York: New York University Press, 2001.

From the Ground Up presents the history of the environmental justice movement through the telling of individual stories of local communities; it also provides an annotated bibliography of empirical studies and articles that document and describe disproportionate impact of environmental hazards by race and income.

Gauna, E., and Rechtschaffen, C. *Environmental Justice: Law, Policy, and Regulation.* Durham, N.C.: Carolina Academic Press, 2002.

This book is an interdisciplinary examination of environmental justice through a variety of regulatory contexts, including program design, standard setting, permitting, enforcement, cleanup, and brownfield redevelopment.

CHAPTER NINE

RELIGIOUS APPROACHES TO ENVIRONMENTAL HEALTH

Daniel J. Swartz

In recent years diverse religious institutions and organizations have devoted considerable energy and resources to addressing environmental health concerns. The Catholic Hospital Association has undertaken a variety of initiatives designed to reduce emissions of concern, particularly dioxins and mercury, as well as to educate its health care providers and patients about environmental health. The California Interfaith Partnership for Children's Health and the Environment, led by the Women of Reform Judaism and the National Council of Catholic Women, helped sponsor a series of legislative hearings on legislative and regulatory remedies to environmental health problems. The National Association of Evangelicals is participating in an ongoing "healthy families" project to educate its members about environmental health hazards. And in a twist on the popular phrase "What Would Jesus Do?" religious activists across the country have held events asking, "What Would Jesus Drive?" bringing considerable media attention to the health consequences of fuel-inefficient vehicles (Figure 9.1).

What is responsible for this eclectic set of activities? More generally, what can religious communities and institutions contribute to efforts addressing environmental health hazards? What barriers keep such communities from doing more, and how can these obstacles be best addressed? A thoughtful examination of these and related questions may bring significant new resources to bear on improving environmental health conditions.

FIGURE 9.1. WHAT WOULD JESUS DRIVE?

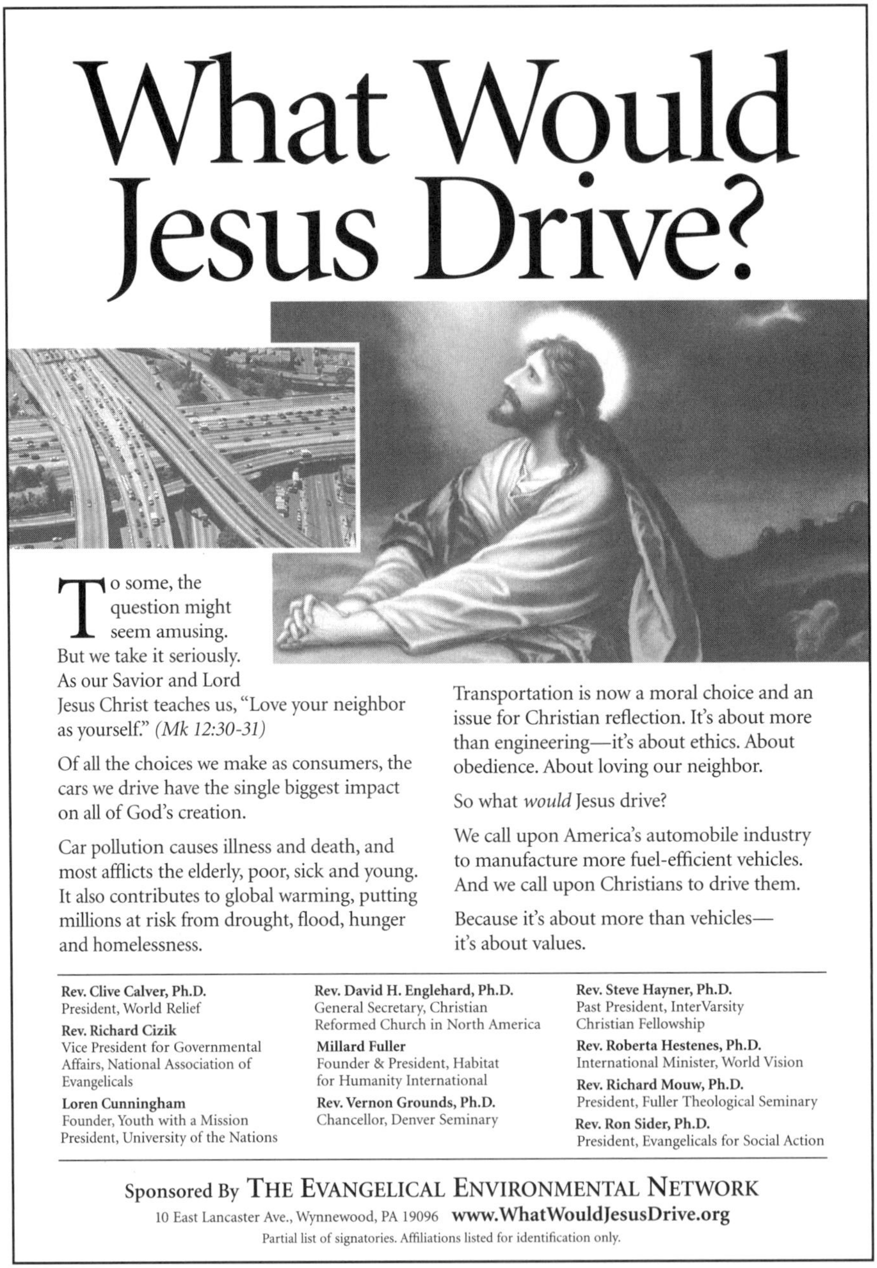
What Would Jesus Drive?
To some, the question might seem amusing. But we take it seriously. As our Savior and Lord Jesus Christ teaches us, "Love your neighbor as yourself." (Mk 12:30-31)
Of all the choices we make as consumers, the cars we drive have the single biggest impact on all of God's creation.
Car pollution causes illness and death, and most afflicts the elderly, poor, sick and young. It also contributes to global warming, putting millions at risk from drought, flood, hunger and homelessness.
Transportation is now a moral choice and an issue for Christian reflection. It's about more than engineering—it's about ethics. About obedience. About loving our neighbor.
So what would Jesus drive?
We call upon America's automobile industry to manufacture more fuel-efficient vehicles. And we call upon Christians to drive them.
Because it's about more than vehicles—it's about values.
Rev. Clive Calver, Ph.D.
President, World Relief
Rev. Richard Cizik
Vice President for Governmental Affairs, National Association of Evangelicals
Loren Cunningham
Founder, Youth with a Mission
President, University of the Nations
Rev. David H. Englehard, Ph.D.
General Secretary, Christian Reformed Church in North America
Millard Fuller
Founder & President, Habitat for Humanity International
Rev. Vernon Grounds, Ph.D.
Chancellor, Denver Seminary
Rev. Steve Hayner, Ph.D.
Past President, InterVarsity Christian Fellowship
Rev. Roberta Hestenes, Ph.D.
International Minister, World Vision
Rev. Richard Mouw, Ph.D.
President, Fuller Theological Seminary
Rev. Ron Sider, Ph.D.
President, Evangelicals for Social Action
Sponsored By THE EVANGELICAL ENVIRONMENTAL NETWORK
10 East Lancaster Ave., Wynnewood, PA 19096 www.WhatWouldJesusDrive.org
Partial list of signatories. Affiliations listed for identification only.

How Religious Communities May Understand Environmental Health

The actions that some religious communities and institutions have begun to take—and that many more in the future might begin to take—to address environmental health concerns have their foundation in religious understandings of environmental health. A full exploration of the ways in which various faith traditions view the environment, and health and the connections between them is far beyond the scope of this chapter (a "For Further Information" section at the end of the chapter cites some in-depth analyses). Even a brief summary, however, can highlight the potential power of religious approaches to environmental health.

In 1967, a landmark article by Lynn White Jr. (1967) sparked many scholarly and popular discussions of religious views of the role of the human in the environment. White argued that the Christian and Jewish views of this role were having negative environmental impacts and lay at the core of many environmentally harmful behaviors by individuals and societies. White wrote that based on his understanding of Genesis 1, the Christian and Jewish traditions placed the human at the center of the universe and gave humankind absolute dominion over every other living thing. (A "For Further Information" section at the end of the chapter describes the biblical and Talmudic sources cited here.) Since White wrote, hundreds of articles and, increasingly, full-length books have responded to these claims, offering a more nuanced understanding of these and other traditions.

This understanding focuses on three potentially "greener" elements of these faith traditions. First, these traditions generally place the divine, and not the human, at the center of the universe. Humankind is given absolute dominion over nothing—including itself—because it is subject to the will of the divine. Human wants and desires thus become secondary to the higher purposes of life. This can be seen in the Hebrew Bible through such institutions as the Sabbath, during which all work and profit taking must cease in order to honor the divine, and the Jubilee cycle, which proclaimed that God is the ultimate owner of the land and all property. In relation to the nonhuman elements of the environment, many religious traditions thus emphasize *stewardship* rather than *dominion*—that is to say, they emphasize long-term care for that which one does not own (because God is seen as the ultimate "owner") rather than despotic rule over chattel.

Second, one of those higher purposes of life is the celebration of the diversity of life. St. Thomas Aquinas wrote in his *Summa Theologica*, "The good of the species is greater than the good of the individual. Thus, a multiplicity of species adds more to the goodness of the universe than a multiplicity of individuals of one species. Because one single creature was not sufficiently representative of the divine goodness, God produced many and diverse creatures. Hence the whole universe together participates in the divine goodness more perfectly and represents it better than any single creature whatever" (sec. III B). The Talmud argues that "of all the Holy One, blessed be God, created, no species was created without purpose" (*Shabbat* 77b), and that "[h]umans were not created until the sixth day so that if our minds become too proud, we could be reminded, 'even the gnats preceded you in creation'" (*Sanhedrin* 38a). Teachings that value the nonhuman world can be found in abundance in many religions, from the Koran's praising of Allah's creative powers to indigenous traditions that declare various locations and creatures to be sacred.

Third, religious traditions also recognize that people are a part of, rather than apart from, the rest of the universe. Indeed, there is no word in the Hebrew Bible for *environment* because there was no notion of some separate realm. Properly understood, the environment is where we live, learn, work, grow, play and pray. A city is just as much a part of the environment as a remote wilderness retreat.

Such an understanding of the environment is fully consonant with, for example, the late chapters of Isaiah (45:6–7): "There is none but Me. I am the Lord and there is none else; I form light and create darkness; I make weal and create woe—I the Lord do all these things." Combating notions of separate gods of light and darkness, separate material and spiritual realms, Isaiah declared the absolute unity of God, a unity that, as the Jewish sage Maimonides would later teach, is more unified than a human mind can conceive. And as God is one, so too is God's universe one. This understanding presents a possible entry point for those concerned with environmental health; if the universe is unified, whatever we put out into the environment necessarily affects us, and thus any hazards produced can harm our health. In this view, NIMBY (not in my backyard) behaviors simply make no sense because there is nowhere that is not, in the broad view, our backyard.

This is expressed beautifully in the words of the eleventh-century Confucian teacher, Chang T'sai, in his *Western Inscription* (de Bary and others, 1960):

> Heaven is my father and earth is my mother, and even such a small creature as I finds an intimate place in their midst.
>
> Therefore, that which extends throughout the universe I regard as my body and that which directs the universe I consider as my nature.
>
> All people are my brothers and sisters, and all things are my companions.

In this unified environment the role of the human is often that portrayed in Genesis 2, rather than the interpretation of Genesis 1 highlighted by White: the first human was put in the Garden in order to *avad* and *shamar*. *Avad* has sometimes been translated as to "till" or to "work" the land—but its more basic meaning is to "serve." *Shamar* means to "guard," in particular to safeguard something that one does not own.

Most religious traditions do, however, also accord special worth to the human role, as White accurately pointed out. Rather than treating this as a barrier to involvement in environmental health, however, it could be understood as a simple recognition of the power of humans to affect the environment. Clearly, no other species on our planet can wreak as much ecological havoc, and no other species can take the steps necessary to protect all people from environmental health hazards.

Though religious institutions have traditionally been far more involved in health-related concerns than in environmental concerns, unique religious understandings of health have not been as broadly explicated as religious understandings of the environment. Perhaps this is due to an assumption that religious and secular views of health are in accord. Western medicine, however, has focused on the treatment of illness, and it often seems to regard health as merely the absence of pathology. In contrast the National Conference of Catholic Bishops (1981) noted in its pastoral letter on health and health care that "[h]ealth in the Christian perspective means wholeness—not only physical and emotional, but also spiritual and social" (p. 6). The bishops also show an understanding of the environmental factors that affect public health: "Inadequate housing, unemployment, lack of education, and a polluted environment are frequently causes of ill health. As church leaders, we will continue to seek social and institutional changes that deal with these underlying problems" (p. 9).

This broad view of health can be found in many religious traditions, going back thousands of years. The early rabbis considered matters of physical health and hygiene to be "Torah" of the highest and most important order, as is illustrated by this earthy anecdote:

> R. [that is, Rabbi] Huna asked his son Rabbah, "Why are you not to be found in the presence of Hisda, whose discourses on tradition are so keen?" Rabbah replied, "Why should I go to him? He speaks of unimportant matters. For example, he tells me that one who enters a privy should not sit down abruptly, nor strain overmuch, for the rectum is supported by three tooth-like glands and should these become dislocated [through the forcing], his health would be endangered." R. Huna replied, "R. Hisda discusses matters of health and you call them unimportant—all the more reason to go to him!" [*B. Shabbat* 82a].

Furthermore the traditional *mi-shebeyrach l'cholim* (Jewish prayer for the sick), indeed the very reference to God as *Rofey N'eyman* who bestows *refuah shleymah,* the

Faithful Healer bringing complete and whole health, shows a holistic understanding of health.

Perhaps not coincidentally, those involved with public health generally and environmental health more specifically have also begun to articulate a fuller, more positive definition of health. For example, the World Health Organization's definition of health, "A state of complete physical, mental, and social well-being and not merely the absence of disease or infirmity," closely matches these religious understandings.

However, such understandings have not yet translated into widespread involvement of religious communities and institutions with environmental health concerns. In part this is because religious communities, like most of the rest of the world, often overlook the connections between health and the environment. Consider the following exercise, which the author of this chapter has conducted hundreds of times. Ask an audience to close their eyes and think of the first image that comes to mind when they hear the word *environment.* Then ask people to raise their hands if there were any people in that image. No more than 10 percent of any audience, including religious audiences, has ever raised their hands.

This disconnect between consideration of the environment and consideration of health remains a significant barrier to religious involvement in environmental health concerns. Ironically, it has also been one of the barriers to broader religious involvement in environmental concerns more generally, because many faith-based organizations have seen them as "luxury" concerns, seemingly far less urgent than more traditional ministries to the poor and disenfranchised. This lack of connection also disconnects religious traditions from their own history, which is rich in examples of work addressing what we now understand as environmental health concerns. In the section of their pastoral letter that made recommendations for action, for example, the Catholic bishops wrote, "Emphasis should be placed on the promotion of health, the prevention of disease, and the protection against environmental and other hazards to physical and mental health" (National Conference of Catholic Bishops, 1981, p. 7). But such concerns long predate the term *environmental health.* For example, in his first ministries, eighteenth-century evangelist John Wesley not only provided free medical care to the poor of Bristol and London but also emphasized prevention of illness through the provision and maintenance of clean water (United Methodist Church, 1988).

Acting on the basis of such biblical teachings as that of Deuteronomy 23:13 to set up latrines outside war camps to ensure cleanliness, rabbinical authorities developed extensive public health regulations toward the beginning of the Common Era. They included, for example (from the Talmud, *Bava Batra*), extensive regulations on the siting of industries that might pollute the air, on the disposal of potentially hazardous waste, and the inspection of the safety and hygiene of wells.

Underlying such regulations was a commitment to try to prevent health problems, rather than merely to treat them once they occurred. Similar practices can be found in most major religions, such as the obligations of Muslims to provide clean water for travelers.

Guiding Principles of Environmental Health

There are rich, if currently unfulfilled, possibilities for religious communities and institutions to take actions addressing environmental health concerns. Even before such possibilities come fully to fruition, however, a number of religious teachings and values can serve as guiding principles not only for religious involvement but for the broader community as well. Indeed, the clear and forceful articulation of these principles may do as much as anything else to build public support for necessary environmental health measures. The following sections discuss a few of the many possible themes and principles that may be thus elucidated. These themes focus on children, as this subject has been found to be a compelling lens on the issue of environmental health for religious communities, both within themselves and when they enter into discussions with other groups. Jewish sources predominate, given the expertise of this chapter's author; nevertheless, they should prove helpful to people from many different faith backgrounds.

God Loves All People, Especially Children and Those the World Does Not Value

In the view of many religions, all people are created in the divine image and are connected to the realm of the divine. Many also teach that all children hold a special place in God's heart, as do all who are poor or otherwise vulnerable. For example, the Prophet Mohammed, himself an orphan, would, it is said, shorten his prayers anytime a child would cry in mosque, so that the child could more readily be comforted. In Exodus 22:20–22, we read, "You shall not wrong the stranger nor oppress them, for you were strangers in the land of Egypt. You shall not ill-treat any widow or orphan. If you do mistreat them, I will heed their outcry as soon as they cry out to me." Jesus taught, according to Matthew 18:2–5, "Whoever becomes humble like this child is the greatest in the kingdom of heaven. Whoever welcomes one such child in my name welcomes me." In the traditional Jewish naming ceremony, a passage from the prophet Ezekiel (16:6) is read that exemplifies God's profound connection to an abandoned child: "No eye pitied you, to have compassion on you, but instead you were cast into the open field, for you were abhorred and polluted on the day you were born. But when I passed over you, and saw you struggling in your birth-blood, I said unto you: 'In your blood live.' Yes, I said unto you, 'in your blood live.'"

Though such teachings obviously apply well beyond it, the implications for environmental health are profound. According to this view, for example, all children, equally beloved by God, deserve equal protection from environmental health hazards. But at present children of color and those living in low-income neighborhoods are far more likely than other children to be exposed to hazards that range from lead that poisons the brain to diesel exhaust that chokes young lungs. People of faith can and should be in the forefront of promoting environmental health for children, and holding society to account for not valuing and protecting every child.

Windows of Opportunity and Vulnerability

In the Talmud (*B. Bava Batra* 21a), Rabbi Joshua ben Gamla is celebrated with the following teaching: "the name of that man should always be mentioned on good occasion. But for him, the Torah would have been forgotten in Israel." The Talmud then presents a lengthy and instructive description of the action ben Gamla took that was so praiseworthy. Traditionally, teaching one's children was a *mitzvah* (commandment) incumbent upon the parent. Ben Gamla realized, however, that this condemned orphans or children with uneducated parents to endless generations of illiteracy. So he began to institute a public school system. His first attempt brought previously untaught teenagers to regional schools. Quickly, however, this effort failed. Indeed, the Talmud recounts that these teenagers beat and chased their teachers out of the classroom! Eventually, ben Gamla required that local, easily and safely accessible schools be built, with children beginning lessons at six and maximum teacher-pupil ratios specified.

Ben Gamla experienced one of the key lessons of children's environmental health, one that has all too frequently been ignored in health and safety laws and regulations: there are key developmental windows, windows of opportunity for healthy development and windows of vulnerability to disruptions of development. Irreversible damage can occur when an opportunity is missed or a vulnerability is exposed. Conversely, lasting good can come when health is protected and development promoted during those key windows.

Many sages understood this intimately, for they were first and foremost teachers. They expounded upon Proverbs 22:6: "Train children in the way they should go, and when they are old they will not depart from it." In *Midrash Proverbs* 22:6, Rabbi Joshua explained this verse as follows: the child may be compared to a heifer; if she is not taught to plow when young, it will be difficult for her to do so in the end. Or she may be compared to a wine branch; if you do not bend it when it is full of sap, once it hardens you can do nothing with it.

When viewed in the context of a culture that valued study above all else, Elisha ben Abuya's teaching in *Avot de Rabbi Nathan* (24) becomes especially poignant: "When people learn Torah in their youth, to what may they be compared? To ink written on a fresh sheet of parchment. When people learn in their old age, it is like ink written on a sheet that has been written on and erased, written on and erased."

Many other ancient traditions recognized these windows as well. For example, in the Confucian tradition it is taught that for the first three years of a child's life, parents are supposed to be completely devoted to their child, and a Hadith from the Prophet Mohammed teaches that it is "forbidden that any burden is put on children which would arrest or harm their natural development." These teachings imply a mandate to identify environmental health hazards that shut windows of opportunity and to prevent exposures to these hazards.

The Sacred Nature of Human Development

Why do windows of vulnerability and opportunity arise, and why should they matter to communities of faith? Clearly, the complicated interplay between the ongoing development of the child and positive or negative environmental factors should be of interest to researchers and policymakers who focus on children. But why is it a matter of import for faith communities in general?

Many religious traditions recognize stages in child development. The Yoruba tradition of Nigeria, for example, speaks of "robing a child with wisdom after robing him with clothes." Early Jewish sages paid particular attention to the stages of human development. For example, a sage who lived eighteen centuries ago wrote:

> Rabbi Simla would teach: what does a fetus resemble in the womb? Folded writing tablets. Its hands are against its temples; its elbows are on its legs; its heels are against its buttocks; and its head is between its knees. Its mouth is closed and its navel is open, and it eats and drinks what its mother eats and drinks. It produces no excrement, for if it did, it would kill its mother. When it comes out into the air of the world, what was closed becomes open and what was open becomes closed; if not, it would not be able to live a single hour [*B. Niddah* 30b].

The profound curiosity—and lack of judgment—of even young infants was also noted: "Come and observe: a goat-kid or a lamb, when it sees a pit, turns back. . . . But an infant places a hand on a serpent or a scorpion and is stung, or places a hand on hot coals and is burned" (*Avot de Rabbi Nathan* 16).

Ecclesiastes Rabbah 1:2 illustrates on the one hand recognition that different types of parental care are needed for different ages and on the other that some childhood behaviors put children at risk: "At the age of one, a child is like a king lounging in a canopied litter, being hugged and kissed by everyone. At two and three, a child is like a pig, sticking hands into the gutter and putting whatever is found into the child's mouth."

Some of this attention to children's development was for practical reasons, to understand what holy texts should be taught at which ages or to develop a timetable for children to assume the religious obligations of adults. But it also goes deeper, reflecting a belief that human development itself is a sacred process. The developmental process of children growing in knowledge, wisdom, and faith justified all of creation: "Resh Lakish said in the name of R. Judah the Patriarch: the world endures only for the sake of the breath of schoolchildren. Not even for the building of the Temple are children to be deprived of their study of Torah. Resh Lakish also said to R. Judah the Patriarch: 'I have a tradition from my forebears . . . that a city that has no children at school will be destroyed'" (*Shabbat* 119b).

There was also a recognition that the sacred goal of full human development was contingent. Both this goal and the recognition that if parents and society fail to live up to their obligations full development may not occur extend far back in the many religious traditions—back, for example, to the first chapter of Genesis. As creation progresses, all the other species are said to have the ability to reproduce *l'minahu*, "after their kind." A maple will automatically give birth to maples. Only for humans is this phrase omitted—because reaching full human potential is not automatic. On the other hand, although other acts of creation are seen as good, and creation as a whole is "very good," only to humans is the phrase "in the image of God" applied. This recognizes the profound potential of each person. But today it can also help us recognize that too many fall short of that potential, not through an act or omission of their own but rather because environmental toxicants have harmed their bodies and brains.

The Demands of Justice

Environmental health hazards are not equally distributed throughout society. Those who are economically or politically disadvantaged—especially low-income children of color—suffer from both higher exposures and fewer opportunities for amelioration of harm (see Chapter Eight). This stands in contradiction to the teachings of many world traditions promoting social justice and protecting the well-being of the most vulnerable.

The prophet Ezekiel (34:18–20) cast the treatment of the vulnerable by the powerful in terms of a God who is shepherd of all: "Is it not enough for you to graze on choice pasture, but you must also trample with your feet what is left from your grazing? And is it not enough for you to drink clear water, but you must also muddy with your feet what is left? And must My flock graze on what your feet have trampled and drink what your feet have muddied? Assuredly, thus said the Lord God to them, Here am I, I am going to decide between the stout animals and the lean."

The Gospels emphasize service to the "least of these," those ignored or cut off by society but welcomed into the community of the church. The Koran and the Hebrew Bible both speak often and forcefully on behalf of the widow, the orphan, and the stranger, all vulnerable and often exploited by society. The Hindu tradition teaches *daya,* "compassion," toward all, with a focus on those with the least power, and Swami Dayananda, following the teachings of King Ashoka, explained that this means that each day a person should make three sacrifices to promote justice and the common good. Buddhism teaches that parental love for children should be seen as an example of how all should be treated:

> Even as a mother protects with her life
> Her child, her only child,
> So with a boundless heart
> Should one cherish all living beings.
> [From the *Metta Sutta* (Salzberg, 1995, pp. vii–viii)

If we were to honor these priorities today, we would demonstrate our faith through policies that value all children equally and highly. We would place an emphasis on protecting the most vulnerable and most highly exposed children first and foremost. And we would ensure that every child is protected from environmental health hazards, especially those that inhibit the innate capacity of children to learn.

Parents' Societal Obligations to Child Development

Children are seen as both valued and vulnerable, worthy of and needing protection. But who should be doing the protecting, and from what should children be protected? A number of religious teachings shed interesting light on these questions. For example, the Talmud teaches that "[o]ur masters taught: with regard to their children, parents are obligated to . . . teach them Torah, to teach them a livelihood, and to get them married. Some say: also to teach them how to swim. R. Judah said: when parents do not teach their children a craft, it is as though they are teaching criminality. . . . R. Judah [also] said: 'A parent is also required to teach civic obligations'" (*B. Kiddushin* 29a).

Upon close examination, this list seems to cover most recognized developmental markers—fine and gross motor skills, language skills, social skills—as well as markers too often ignored, such as moral grounding and faith. The goal is not merely to avoid harm but also to raise a complete human being—which is by no means seen as an inevitable outcome.

Obligations fall first upon parents. But there is an underlying social responsibility that serves as a safety net. For example, in *B. Ketuba* 49b, the sages discuss how a man is obligated to maintain his young sons and daughters, even in cases of divorce. Were the man to fail in his obligations, he is to stand before all the people of the town and say, "even a raven craves to have young, but I do not care for children." If after this threat of public humiliation, he still does not maintain them, the town is obligated to do so. Recall as well the case of ben Gamla noted previously, where the parental duty to educate children became codified as a societal duty, in part in recognition of the looming creation of a permanent class division between the literate and illiterate.

These teachings are paralleled in many religious traditions. For example, an Igbo naming tradition from Nigeria puts it beautifully:

> Brothers and sisters, a new child is born.
> While in the womb, it was one woman's;
> Safely delivered, it is everybody's child.

Abdul Baha taught in the Baha'i tradition that it is incumbent upon all of society to expend all its forces on the education of the child. Traditional Javanese call this *gotong royong*, the mutual help due to all children.

Why are these societal obligations emphasized? Many religious traditions think of humanity throughout the world not as a loose collection of atomized individuals but rather as members of a community, placing at least some responsibility for all with all. For some, this reflects the unifying presence of God in the world, which means that everything is connected, and so all our actions affect each other, as in this often-quoted midrash: "Some people were sitting in a ship. One of them took a drill and began to bore a hole in the ship under where he was sitting. His companions said, what are you sitting and doing? He said, what has it to do with you? I am boring a hole under my part of the ship. They said, but the water is coming in and sinking the ship under us" (*Leviticus Rabbah* 4:5).

But our social obligations come from more than a sense of community and shared consequences. They also arise from the very nature of children. Children face unique threats not only because of their developing bodies and unique childhood behaviors but also for reasons that are social rather than medical. For the most part, young children lack the knowledge of what is and is not a hazard. And even when they do have that knowledge, they lack the power to rectify their situation. Sometimes, parents have that knowledge and power that their children lack. But often, especially in the case of environmental health hazards, parents simply cannot do it on their own.

No parent can by himself or herself clear the air of harmful pollutants or create transit alternatives to alleviate pollution from cars. Parents need help in ensuring that schools do not sicken students through poor indoor air quality, mercury spills, or excessive use of harmful pesticides. Parents cannot possibly do all the research or retain all the information about which consumer products and foods do what to children of all different ages. Thus there is a clear need for society to step in, to perform needed research, to set standards that protect all children, to set up programs making certain that standards are being vigorously and equitably enforced, and when exposures do occur, to help restore health to sickened children.

Preventing Harm

Public health emphasizes prevention of harm above amelioration after harm occurs. A similar emphasis is found in many religious traditions, as noted in the Catholic bishops' pastoral letter on health: "Emphasis should be placed on the promotion of health, the prevention of disease, and the protection against environmental and other hazards to physical and mental health" (National Conference of Catholic Bishops, 1981, p. 18). For example, in Deuteronomy 22:8 we read: "When you build a new house, you shall make a parapet for your roof, so that you do not bring bloodguilt on your house if anyone should fall from it." In other words, prevent someone from falling off a roof, because treatment afterward may well be too late. This "parapet principle," by the Middle Ages, becomes expanded to preventing "anything that is potentially dangerous" (*Shulchan Arukh, Hoshen Mishpat, Hilchot Shmirat HaNefesh* 427).

The Jewish tradition emphasizes prevention and precaution in response to general risks. In general, "regulations concerning danger to life are more stringent than ritual prohibitions" (*B. Hullin* 10a). The sages are quite explicit that there does not need to be a certainty of danger. Indeed, past safety is not considered a guarantee for the future: "R. Yannai said: 'A person should never stand in a place of danger and say that a miracle will be wrought.' . . . In Nehardea there was a dilapidated wall beside which Rav and Samuel would not walk, even though it had been standing this way for thirteen years" (*B. Ta'anit* 20b).

Prevention is also emphasized specifically in the realm of health: "Who is the most skilled physician? One who can prevent sickness" (*Sefer Hasidim* 17,22). Prevention is stressed especially in terms of one's own behavior. The rabbis rule that one may not injure another to prevent injury to oneself, even in commerce, where the general rule is that one person is not allowed to profit through something that causes harm to a neighbor. (See, for example, *Ribash, Responsa* 196.) Similar teachings are widespread throughout religious tradition. For example, precept 36 of *One Hundred and Eighty Precepts* (Schipper, 2001), a classical Daoist text, reads, "You should not throw poisonous substances into lakes, rivers, and seas" (pp. 81–82).

It would seem that a polluter that imposes risks on those who do not directly benefit, especially children, violates this standard. Meetings of clergy with corporate leaders might raise such ethical obligations, even in the light of a federal government that seems to moving away from protective regulations.

Finally, there are at least some indications that children were thought of as sensitive populations who need an extra measure of precaution and prevention built into their protections. For example: "It is told of R. Akiva that he never said 'it is time to leave the house of study,' except on the eves of Passover and Yom Kippur. On the eve of Passover, for the sake of children so that they would not fall asleep during the Seder. On the eve of Yom Kippur, so that his students could feed their children" (*B. Pesachim* 109a). If extra care is taken to ensure that children's meals are not delayed or to prevent the strain of striving to stay awake, how much more so should care be taken that no permanent physical and mental harm be inflicted upon them.

At present, however, many of our environmental health and safety laws respond to crises rather than trying to prevent them. Even more view children as merely small versions of adults, rather than as humans in a unique series of developmental stages that require extra protections. These religious teachings could make a strong case for designing protective programs that more actively seek to prevent harm and to forestall or eliminate crises, with extra measures of safety built in so that parents can sleep better, knowing that their children are protected.

Valuing the Future From Generation to Generation

Why, then, do children remain inadequately protected? In part this is due to the very social vulnerabilities noted previously. It is simply easier to exploit children; those with power can use it against children with far too much impunity. Furthermore, although "family values" may be bandied about in political campaigns, children do not make campaign contributions and do not vote. Thus it is too often politically expedient to ignore their needs when making policy decisions about where government resources will be expended. As the Talmud notes, "As with fish, so with people. The larger swallow the smaller" (*B. Avodah Zara* 4a).

But there is another, perhaps even more pervasive reason: our society today, especially our government, does not sufficiently value the future. Even as geologists, biologists, and astrophysicists explore further and further into deep time, most of society seems to have an ever-shrinking attention span. Sound bites dominate political discussion, complex problems receive fifteen minutes of fame or less, and policy decisions are timed to quarterly reports or election cycles. In contrast, despite being formulated in an era of shorter life spans and less penetrating glimpses into the depths of time, religious teachings have traditionally framed moral questions in the very long term.

Indeed, one of the great strengths of the faith community is its dedication to the long view (although this can also be a mixed blessing when it is used as a justification for moving slowly to address modern concerns). And there are valid religious reasons for thinking long term. For Confucians the moral elevation and well-being of the next generation was the primary goal of society. The Iroquois Nation made decisions in light of the consequences extending out to the seventh generation. In the Hebrew Bible, God makes pronouncements *l'olam,* forever, or even *l'olam va-ed,* "forever and further," over 400 times. Some 30 times God binds covenants *l'dor va-dor,* "from generation to generation."

Why this longer view? In part it is because we seek to live life through the lens of the Eternal One's vision, which, as Exodus 34:6 reminds us, is for the longest term of all: "The Lord, the Lord, a God compassionate and gracious, slow to anger, abounding in kindness and faithfulness, extending kindness to the thousandth generation."

In part, concerns for future generations are intimately connected to broader concerns for justice, particularly for protecting the weak and vulnerable. For example, the traditional Buddhist text *Metta Sutta* ("loving-kindness") states that those following the Buddhist way should treat all with justice (Salzberg, 1995, pp. vii–viii):

> Whether they are weak or strong, omitting none,
> The great or the mighty, medium, short or small,
> The seen and the unseen,
> Those living near and far away,
> Those born and to-be-born.
>
> . . . .
>
> Let none deceive another,
> Or despise any being in any state.
> Let none through anger or ill-will
> Wish harm upon another!

In part it is also because of the sense of community noted earlier. Communities, after all, have longer life spans than individuals. Thus, in the Talmudic parable of Honi's sleep (*Ta'anit* 23a) or the midrashic tale of Emperor Hadrian and the old man planting a fig tree (*Leviticus Rabbah* 25:5), the response of the elderly person planting to those mocking him is both simple and powerful: I plant for my descendants, as my ancestors planted for me. Similarly, the Dogon people of Mali hold that many different generations, including those that have died and those yet to be born, are all part of the same community.

This sense of generations linked together through love and intergenerational good deeds is reflected in a variety of sources. Proverbs 13:22 teaches, "A good person bequeaths to their children's children." According to a Hadith, the Prophet Mohammed said, "upon death, a person's deeds will stop—except for three: a charitable fund, knowledge left for people to benefit from, and a righteous child."

But more fundamental is a view, perhaps a human echo of God's farseeing vision, that there is no such thing as distant past or distant future—that it is all close, all indeed part of the present. Such a view of the past is not surprising in a text- and tradition-based system, where, for example, Rabbi Aha taught that "the casual conversations of the patriarch's slaves are more important than the religious laws of their present descendants" (*Genesis Rabbah* 60:8). But it extends with equal force into the future. Notice in this next story how Hanina ben Dosa and his wife refuse to put the present before the uncertain future:

> R. Hanina ben Dosa was very poor. One day his wife said to him, "How long must we suffer like this?" He replied, "What shall we do?" She replied, "Pray that you may be given something." He prayed, and a hand appeared that gave him a golden table leg. That night, a dream troubled his sleep. He heard a voice saying, "In the world to come, the righteous will eat at tables with three legs, but Hanina will eat at a table with only two legs." When he awoke, he spoke of this to his wife, and she said, "Are you content that the others will eat at tables with three legs and we will eat at a table with two legs?" He replied, "What shall we do?" She said, "Pray that the leg should be taken back again." He prayed and it was so. It was taught: the second miracle was greater than the first [*B. Ta'anit* 25a].

The obligation to treat the future as equal in value to the present is even stronger in cases of risks to health and well-being. For example, the following ruling reveals active consideration of consequences "until the end of time."

> In other cases, a man may pay money and effect expiation. But in capital cases, he is held responsible for the blood of the victim and for the blood of the

> posterity that would have been the victim's until the end of time. Thus we find that Cain, who slew his brother, was told, "The bloods of thy brother cry out unto Me" (Genesis 4:10), Not "the blood of thy brother" but "the bloods of thy brother"—his blood and the blood of the posterity [*B. Sanhedrin* 37a].

Nowhere are such views of the future more apt than when considering children's environmental health, which must be multigenerational. But neither our economic framework nor our political system fully considers the needs of today's children, let alone the needs of future generations. For example, the "future discount rate" that the federal Office of Management and Budget (OMB) requires the Environmental Protection Agency and other governmental agencies to use systemically devalues the future. According to the OMB's 7 percent discount rate, children lose half of their value every ten years—a policy that effectively puts the future on sale for half-price (just one decade out), amounting to institutional discrimination against children and reflecting ignorance about the long-term effects of persistent pollutants. Ensuring the full protection of future generations requires valuing them fully, as religious traditions call upon us to do.

Recognizing Limitations on Ownership

In U.S. law, property rights take precedence over many other rights. Most religious traditions, however, place limits on such rights, and in some cases evince a distinct suspicion about owning too much. Buddhism has developed extensive teachings on simplicity and the illusory nature of material wealth. Early Christian churches held property in common, so that none should become like the rich man portrayed in the Gospels as being less likely to reach salvation than a camel is to pass through the eye of a needle. The Jewish tradition teaches that no person is the ultimate owner of anything. Rather, "you and what you possess are God's" (*Avot* 3:7).

Because ownership is limited, so too are the uses of property. The Talmud (*B. Bava Kamma* 80b) teaches that Joshua placed ten limitations on property when he handed over the land of Israel as an inheritance. Some of these limitations were on behalf of the common good, such as allowing communal access to a new spring, should one arise. Some, such as avoiding a path that had become too hard and lumpy, were for comfort. And some were for health reasons, such as not delaying people from relieving themselves, for the rabbis believed that such delays caused a variety of illnesses. Even more dramatic are the traditions of the sabbatical and Jubilee years, which more directly assert God's ownership of the land.

Overall, God's ownership is seen as eternal, whereas human possession is seen not only as fleeting but also as far from absolute, even when it is at its most secure, as the *Midrash* humorously illustrates: "Why are certain coins called *zuzim*? Because they move themselves (*zazim*) from one to another. Why is money called *mammon*? Because what you count (*moneh*) so carefully is nothing at all" (*Numbers - Rabbah* 22:8).

What are the possible policy consequences of this view of property for children's environmental health? First of all, if God is the true owner, then any "discount rate" on the future should be from God's viewpoint—in other words, it should be zero. Second, society can and should regulate the use of property for reasons including but not limited to health. Finally, this view helps us move from thinking of "our children" to thinking of "all children." This earth and all in it and on it are ultimately "owned" by and beloved by God. The idea that we possess anything—including our children—is ultimately an illusion. The true bonds are those established by God, bonds that should bring all of humanity together. It is this common heritage, and our common duty to all children, that counts, not money.

Moving Toward the Fullness of Health

As noted previously, to people of faith, health is not merely the absence of disease but rather the tangible presence of wholeness and well-being. This too can become a guiding principle for action: "Members of the church follow the example of Jesus, therefore, when they carry out the work of healing—not only by providing care for the physically ill, but also by working to restore health and wholeness in all facets of the human person and the human community" (National Conference of Catholic Bishops, 1981, p. 4). Ideally, environmental health practices should help all people experience that wholeness.

In this context it is important to understand that for people of faith, God's creation all around us can be a potent source of that wholeness and well-being. All people should have positive interactions with their environments, to help them grow and develop in mind, body, and spirit. Such healthy environments range from healthy homes and schools to healthy green spaces. No one should be without opportunities to explore the wonders of creation for herself or himself.

Next Steps

This chapter has outlined a number of reasons why those working to address environmental health concerns might find it useful to build or strengthen partnerships with faith communities. What are some examples of successful partnerships, and what might be learned from these and other faith community experiences?

One key point is that religious institutions, like all institutions, may themselves take actions that aggravate or ameliorate environmental health concerns. Perhaps the most significant example to date of such institutions taking concrete steps to reduce environmental health hazards has been the partnership between the Catholic Hospital Association and Health Care Without Harm. Health Care Without Harm is an international coalition with a simple premise: those who seek to improve health should be the first to make sure that their institutional behaviors do not in fact harm health. Hospitals in the Catholic Health Association have worked to reduce their use and disposal of any products containing mercury and have also changed their usage of both procedures and products in order to avoid creating dioxins during waste incineration.

One of the most notable partnerships addressing environmental health on the policy level has been the National Religious Partnership for the Environment. The partnership is a joint project of the National Council of Churches of Christ, the U.S. Catholic Bishops Conference, the Coalition on the Environment and Jewish Life, and the Evangelical Environmental Network. Many partnership member groups have engaged in campaigns to highlight the possible consequences of global climate change and the policies that could prevent climate change. The "What Would Jesus Drive" campaign (Figure 9.1) is just one example of how the religious imagination can bring fresh voices and viewpoints to these concerns.

Partnerships have also been developed on local and state levels. The California Interfaith Partnership for Children's Health and the Environment (see Box 9.1) has, through the leadership of local chapters of the National Council of Catholic Women and the Women of Reform Judaism, made hundreds of presentations to congregations throughout the state to raise awareness of and concern about these issues. It has also been active in working for state-level legislation, providing backing for a number of progressive bills designed to reduce environmental health hazards.

Box 9.1. The California Interfaith Partnership for Children's Health and the Environment

Catholics, Jews, Protestants, and Orthodox Christians—since joined by other faith traditions—came together in late 2001 to form the California Interfaith Partnership for Children's Health and the Environment. The group spreads the word in religious communities about the impact of synthetic chemicals on health and gives people practical tips to reduce exposure in homes, schools, and houses of worship, says director Suellen Lowry. Members also encourage support for state legislation, such as a bill requiring more detailed labeling of personal care products—such as shampoos, nail polish, and lotions—that contain chemicals linked to cancer or birth defects. "As people of faith, we are called to care for the vulnerable," says Lowry, "and we ask our policymakers to heed this call, too." The partnership has held workshops in dozens of congregations across California and sponsored statewide hearings and conferences. It has received support especially from faith-based women's groups, who have a long history of working on social justice issues affecting children.

These partnerships, and the many others that have achieved similar successes, have grown slowly over a number of years. Public health and religious organizations and institutions often have vastly divergent backgrounds, staff, and missions—and perhaps most important of all, different cultures and languages. Success can be achieved only when groups take the time to learn about and from each other.

One important way that religious organizations, especially congregations, differ from public health groups is in the diversity of their agendas. A congregation's "social action" committee may be actively confronting world hunger, supporting international human rights, promoting economic justice, and so on. Environmental health will never be these committees' only focus. Furthermore, such committees are but one of the many activities in congregations, alongside prayer services, adult education, childhood education, life cycle celebrations, and so forth. Environmental health advocates need to be realistic about where on a congregation's overall list of priorities their concerns might be and also creative about demonstrating how existing congregational concerns (such as environmental justice concerns) tie in with environmental health.

Thought Questions

1. What place should *values* questions play in the practice of environmental health? What are possible advantages and drawbacks to using values language in a science-based discipline such as public health?
2. What common American attitudes have been barriers to greater investment in and greater priority given to public health in general and environmental health in particular? In what ways might various religious traditions help to reduce or eliminate such barriers?
3. How should individuals and organizations weigh future versus present risks and benefits?
4. Should public health professionals routinely consider questions of justice and equity in their work? Why or why not?

References

de Bary, W. T., and others. *Sources of Chinese Tradition.* (vol. 1) (p. 524). New York: Columbia University Press, 1960.

National Conference of Catholic Bishops. "Health and Health Care: A Pastoral Letter of the American Bishops." Washington D.C.: U.S. Catholic Conference, Nov. 19, 1981.

Salzberg, S. *Lovingkindness: The Revolutionary Art of Happiness.* Boston: Shambhala, 1995.

Schipper, K. (trans.). "Daoist Ecology: The Inner Transformation. A Study of the Precepts of the Early Daoist Ecclesia." In N. J. Girardot, J. Miller, and X. Liu (eds.), *Daoism and Ecology: Ways Within a Cosmic Landscape.* Cambridge, Mass.: Center for the Study of World Religions, Harvard Divinity School, 2001.

Thomas Aquinas. *Summa Theologica, Prima Pars.* Question 48, ad 2, In "Renewing the Earth: A Pastoral Statement of the United States Catholic Conference" (sec. III B). Nov. 14, 1991.

United Methodist Church, General Board of Church and Society. "Safety and Health in the Workplace and Community." Resolution 221. [http://www.umc-gbcs.org/issues/resolutions.php?resolutionid=65]. 1988.

White, L., Jr. "The Historical Roots of Our Ecologic Crisis." *Science,* 1967, *155,* 1203–1207.

For Further Information

Traditional Religious Texts

In this chapter, quotations from the Hebrew Bible (Genesis, Exodus, Deuteronomy, Isaiah, and Ezekiel) are taken from the Jewish Publication Society's *The Holy Scriptures According to the Masoretic Text,* and quotations from the New Testament (Matthew) are taken from *The Holy Bible: New Revised Standard Version. B. Shabbat, B. Pesachim, B. Kiddushin, B. Avodah Zara, Avot, Ta'anit, B. Ta'anit, B. Bava Kamma, Bava Batra, B. Bava Batra, Sanhedrin, B. Sanhedrin, B. Hullin, B. Niddah,* and *B. Ketuba* are tractates (major sections) of the Talmud; *Avot de Rabbi Nathan* ("The Fathers According to Rabbi Nathan") is also found in the Talmud. *Genesis Rabbah, Leviticus Rabbah, Numbers Rabbah,* and *Ecclesiastes Rabbah* are traditional collections of thought (traditionally called Midrash) on the ideas found in the respective books of the Bible. *Ribash* refers to a collection of *responsa* (answers to people's questions on many subjects) by a medieval Spanish rabbi. The medieval work *Sefer Hasidim* ("Book of the Pious") contains the ethical writings of members of a religiously strict medieval Germanic group. *Shulchan Arukh, Hoshen Mishpat, Hilchot Shmirat HaNefesh* refers to a section of the most authoritative Judaic legal code.

Other Publications

Hundreds of books addressing religious views on environmental issues are now available. For good surveys and reviews, see, for example:

Gottlieb, R. (ed.). *This Sacred Earth: Religion, Nature, Environment.* New York: Routledge, 1996.
Tucker, M. E., and Grim, J. (eds.). *Religions of the World and Ecology Series.* Cambridge, Mass. Harvard University Press, various dates.

The latter is a series of volumes from the Forum on Religion and Ecology, each looking at a specific faith tradition or group of traditions. For more information see the forum's Web site, probably the most comprehensive site addressing religion and the environment, with essays about a wide variety of religious traditions and environmental values and extensive bibliographies:

Forum on Religion and Ecology. [http://environment.harvard.edu/religion].

The National Religious Partnership for the Environment [http://www.nrpe.org] is the largest, most sustained effort to engage religious traditions in the United States in environmental concerns. Each of its four partnership groups has developed materials on environmental health:

Healthy Families, Healthy Environments, a project of the Evangelical Environmental Network [http://www.healthyfamiliesnow.org] and [http://www.creationcare.org].
Coalition on the Environment and Jewish Life [http://www.coejl.org].
National Council of Churches Eco-Justice program [http://www.nccecojustice.org].
U.S. Conference of Catholic Bishops, which has inaugurated a program on children's environmental health (http://www.nccbuscc.org/sdwp/ejp/children/index.html)

The Interfaith Power and Light movement works with diverse faith communities in sixteen states and regions across the country to address energy issues, including health concerns related to energy production and use. For materials and also links to Interfaith Power and Light projects, see

California Interfaith Power and Light [http://www.interfaithpower.org].
Greater Washington Interfaith Power and Light [http://www.gwipl.org].

The Biodiversity Project has developed several sets of materials to aid environmental groups in building partnerships with religious communities and institutions. See, for example:

The Biodiversity Project. *Building Partnerships with the Faith Community: A Resource Guide for Environmental Groups* [http://www.biodiversityproject.org/Building%20Partnerships.pdf].

PART TWO

ENVIRONMENTAL HEALTH ON THE GLOBAL SCALE

CHAPTER TEN

POPULATION PRESSURE

Don Hinrichsen

As the twenty-first century begins, population trends underlie much of the troubled relationship between humanity and the environment. The global population is growing, and much of this growth is in the poorest parts of the world. In addition, the world's population is redistributing from rural areas to cities. These changes place enormous pressure on resources and have broad implications for human health. This chapter introduces the basic principles of demography, the science that studies the size, density, and distribution of human populations; reviews global population trends and their impact on resources; and explores how these global trends link to human health.

Population, Resource Use, and the Environment

The number of people on earth is now 6.4 billion. Despite falling fertility rates in virtually every region of the world, the population continues to rise, by about 78 million per year. At this rate the world's population will increase by 1 billion every fourteen to fifteen years, until *replacement-level* fertility is reached, sometime later this century. Population growth will level off only if the global fertility rate reaches that replacement level (about 2.1 children per couple), but this will require a continued decline in fertility rates (United Nations Department of Economic and Social Affairs, Population Division, 2003).

According to the United Nations Department of Economic and Social Affairs, Population Division (2003), the global population is projected to continue rising, reaching 7.9 billion by 2025 and 9 billion by 2050 (using the midrange estimates). About 99 percent of this growth will occur in the world's poor, developing countries. Not surprisingly, the highest growth rates are found in the poorest countries, those the UN categorizes as least developed. These countries are found predominately in sub-Saharan Africa, the Middle East, and South Asia.

Even with the AIDS pandemic the population growth rates in the forty-four poorest developing countries are still above 2.5 percent per year, enough to double their populations over the next quarter century. Specifically, western Africa's population is increasing by an average of 2.7 percent per year, eastern Africa's by 2.5 percent, and middle Africa's by nearly 3 percent. Only southern Africa, which includes the relatively developed countries of South Africa, Botswana, Namibia, Lesotho, and Swaziland, has a lower collective growth rate, averaging 1 percent per year (Population Reference Bureau, 2003; World Health Organization, 2003).

In the past decade population growth has been slower than previously estimated. For example, the United Nations Department of Economic and Social Affairs, Population Division (2003) currently estimates that about 78 million people are being added to the world population every year, about 12 million fewer than previously estimated. In fact, annual world population growth fell from 2 percent in 1960 to 1.4 percent in 1999. Average fertility has fallen by about half, to three children per woman. At the same time, average life expectancy has risen, from forty-six years to sixty-six years, and the death rate has been cut in half, from 20 deaths per 1,000 people to 10 per 1,000 (UN Population Fund, 1999). Already, sixty-five countries, of which only nine are in the developing world, have fallen below replacement-level fertility, and if current trends continue, the populations of some developing countries will stabilize by the middle of the twenty-first century (UN Population Fund, 1999, 2003).

The rapid drop in fertility levels among women in the developed countries of Europe, Asia, and North America has, according to some analysts, given rise to a new demographic imperative. These analysts, who might be termed the "birth dearth promoters," have argued that the population problem is over and that now the world is facing depopulation. However, the birth dearth theory is undermined by the crucial fact that nearly half the planet's population is under the age of twenty-five. In fact, 1.2 billion people are between the ages of ten and nineteen, the largest cohort of young people in history (UN Population Fund, 2003). Because over 90 percent of them live in developing countries, their access to family planning and reproductive health, or lack of it, will determine to a great extent the future human numbers. Clearly, the future demographic profile of the planet will be written by the world's poorest countries, not its richest.

Although Africa's fertility rate has dropped on average across the entire continent (some countries remain exceptions), it is declining from a very high rate. A drop of half a percent—from 3 percent to 2.5 percent—will do little to stop the momentum of population growth. Poor populations will continue to grow in unsustainable fashion throughout much of Africa.

The drop in Africa's fertility levels is attributed in part to the AIDS pandemic. Currently, some 40 million people globally are HIV positive. Three-quarters of them can be found in sub-Saharan Africa. The main reason that populations are still growing in Africa is the continent's large population base, dominated by rising numbers of young people. Even with AIDS the momentum of numbers means that populations will continue to grow, especially if couples do not have the information and means to plan their families. Moreover, according to recent studies by UNAIDS (2004), the pandemic appears to be leveling off in many sub-Saharan countries, a result of advocacy efforts and prevention programs. Therefore the current trend in Africa continues to be toward a rising population. (See Box 10.1.)

Box 10.1. Measuring Population Impact

There is no easy way to measure the impact of human activities, including population growth, on the environment nor any single agreed-upon approach. Nevertheless several approaches have been developed that demonstrate the complex relationships involved (Cohen, 1995; Ehrlich and Holdren, 1971; Goodland, 1992).

One approach to measuring the impact of human use of natural resources is to place an economic value on *environmental goods and services.* These include such natural resources as unpolluted freshwater, clean air, ocean life, forests, and wetlands—resources that traditionally have been regarded as free goods or common resources. A recent study (Constanza, 1997) has estimated the total value of ecosystem services and products at $33 trillion per year—an amount that exceeds the total value of the global economy as traditionally measured ($29 trillion in 1998).

Although there is little agreement on how to value natural resources, some economists argue that environmental goods and services should be incorporated into estimates of gross domestic product (GDP), as are manufactured assets. Unlike manufactured capital, which depreciates in value over time, environmental capital (such as forests, fisheries, and unpolluted air and water) is currently not considered to depreciate, and no charge is made against current income as these resources are used up. "A country could exhaust its mineral resources, cut down its forests, erode its soils, pollute its aquifers, and hunt its wildlife and fisheries to extinction, but measured income would not be affected as these natural assets disappeared," as Robert Repetto of the World Resources Institute puts it (Hinrichsen, 1991, p. 3).

If natural resources were valued in the same way that manufactured assets are valued, it might help economies to use them more efficiently and to conserve them in order to ensure continued use in the future. Such valuations might help indicate the economic as well as ecological benefits of protecting the environment. In other terms, instead of drawing down their environmental capital, economies could begin to live on its interest (Goodland, 1992).

$$I = P \times A \times T.$$

This equation is one way of showing how developing countries with large and rapidly growing populations affect the environment, even at low levels of affluence and technology, and how developed countries with smaller populations also have a substantial impact, because their levels of affluence and technology are so high (UN Population Fund, 1991). In this equation, I is environmental impact, P is population (including size, growth, and distribution), A is the level of affluence (consumption per capita), and T is the technology used to provide the level of consumption.

The equation also helps to show the importance of slowing population growth as part of any strategy to reduce humanity's impact on the environment. For example, even if per capita resource consumption (A) declined or technologies (T) improved enough to reduce the environmental impact (I) of humanity by 10 percent, this gain would be eroded in less than a decade because global population (P) is growing at 1.4 percent per year (UN Population Fund, 1991).

At current levels of population and technology, the impact on the environment is considerable (Vitousek, Mooney, Lubchenco, and Melillo, 1997). Because consumption levels are rising and will continue to rise, using resources more efficiently and slowing population growth are essential to ease environmental impact and protect human health (Hinrichsen and Robey, 2000; Upadhyay and Robey, 1999).

Population and Urbanization

The world is also in the middle of an urban revolution. Currently, some 47 percent of the global population lives in towns and cities. Within a year or two of the publication of this book, 50 percent of all the people on earth will live in urban areas. By 2030, we will have reached the 60 percent mark (UN Department of Economic and Social Affairs, Population Division, 2002). The pace of urbanization in many developing countries is breathtaking. Big cities in Africa, for instance, are growing on average by around 4 percent per year, enough to double their populations in less than twenty years. (Conditions in these cities, and their health implications, are described in Chapter Sixteen.) This level of growth is unprecedented and for the most affected countries not sustainable. The infrastructure of most cities in developing countries cannot keep pace with such rapid and sustained urban population growth (Hinrichsen, Salem, and Blackburn, 2002).

The rapid urban growth in the developing world is being driven by people who are fleeing collapsing rural economies, lack of rural infrastructure and services, landlessness, and the lack of rural employment opportunities. These push and pull factors will continue to drive urbanization, especially in developing countries. Young people in particular are leading the flight to the cities.

Population and Environment

Population increases and rising per capita consumption levels are leading to environmental degradation and resource depletion at an unsustainable pace (Kasperson, Kasperson, and Turner, 1995, 1999). In fact the world's economies are currently overshooting the earth's capacity to regenerate natural resources by an estimated 37 percent, according to the 1997 Ecological Footprints of Nations study (Wackernagel and others, 1997).

Every individual has an environmental *footprint*—the person's effect on the surrounding environment. The aggregate impact of humanity on the environment varies in magnitude both with the number of people and with the amount of resources that they consume, waste, or pollute beyond use (Wackernagel and others, 1997). In some countries where population is growing rapidly and efficient technologies to protect the environment are lacking, there is little choice but to exploit natural resources to accommodate people's needs. In other countries, despite slower population growth and more efficient technologies, standards of living are so high that the population treads heavily upon nature.

In fact, if the entire world population were to have the same standard of living as the average American or Western European today, the equivalent of three worlds would be required to supply the needed resources at current rates of consumption and waste generation (UN Department of Economic and Social Affairs, 2003). In the United States, 293 million people—less than 5 percent of the world's total population—consume nearly 10 billion metric tons of resources a year—30 percent of total global consumption (Brown, Gardner, and Halweil, 1999). The average person in the United States uses the energy equivalent of fifty-five barrels of oil each year, compared to three barrels for the average person in Bangladesh.

When consumption levels are high, even slow rates of population growth mean dramatic increases in resource use (Box 10.2). In the United States in 1990, for example, population growth alone increased energy consumption by an estimated 110 million barrels of oil. The U.S. population was growing by around 1 percent per year in the early 1990s. That same year Bangladesh's population base was

130 million, growing by 2.5 percent per year but using only 9 million barrels of oil in total, a tiny amount compared to its size and rate of growth (UN Population Fund, 1991).

Box 10.2. Carrying Capacity

The term *carrying capacity* refers to the number of people the earth can support. Estimates of carrying capacity vary a great deal, depending on what is being included and how it is being measured. In 1976, for example, ecologist Roger Revelle said that the earth could support 40 billion people if everyone ate vegetarian diets of no more than 2,500 calories a day. Such a diet would necessitate the conversion of all farmland to the production of grains and vegetables (Cohen, 1995).

Another estimate is that the earth could support up to 10 billion people having meat diets (Cohen, 1995). Some have concluded that the earth's carrying capacity may have already been exceeded in the sense that many people live in poverty and that if people in low-income countries were to catch up with the living standards of people in the developed world the world could support only 2 billion people (Crenson, 1999).

Making calculations of how many people could exist on the earth under a variety of different scenarios probably is less important than determining how resources can be used wisely and managed sustainably to improve living standards without eventually destroying the natural environment that supports life itself. Environmentalists, economists, and demographers increasingly agree that efforts to protect the environment, achieve better living standards, and slow population growth tend to be "mutually reinforcing" (Roodman, 1998). The World Bank (1992) too has pointed out that reducing poverty, protecting the environment, and slowing population growth are closely linked.

Technology plays a mitigating role. Although the 20 percent of humanity in the most affluent countries consumes close to 60 percent of the world's energy, most industrialized countries use energy more efficiently and produce less pollution than developing countries do because the latter do not have the resources to invest in energy-saving technologies or pollution control (United Nations Development Programme [UNDP], 1997; World Health Organization, 1997). One of the greatest challenges posed by rising consumption and economic development is to use energy efficiently and to avoid pollution.

The Population-Environment Scorecard

In 1992, concerned about worsening environmental conditions, delegates to the United Nations Conference on Environment and Development (UNCED), held in Rio de Janeiro, Brazil, stressed the need for action. This Earth Summit, as it was also called, set specific goals for making environmental improvements. Five years later, however, in 1997, a special session of the UN General Assembly, known as the Rio Plus Five Conference, found that little progress had been made toward meeting any of the goals (UN Environment Programme, 2000). In each sector—arable land, freshwater, oceans, forests, biodiversity, and climate change—the 1997 UN assessment found that environmental trends either were no better than in 1992 or had worsened. The UN also found that poverty had increased, in part because of rapid population growth (UNDP, 1998).

Arable Land

At the beginning of the 1990s, about 560 million hectares (out of a total of 1.5 billion hectares) of prime cropland worldwide were degraded, meaning there were moderate to severe soil loss and depletion of soil nutrients, which reduced yields. At the end of that decade the number had risen by 10 percent to about 610 million hectares. In addition, about 1.2 billion hectares of grazing land now suffer from moderate to severe degradation, an increase of roughly 200 million over the number in 1990 (World Resources Institute [WRI], 1998). Around the world the total amount of cropland and grazing land that suffers from soil degradation equals an area the size of the United States and Mexico combined (WRI, 1998). Fertile topsoil is being depleted between 16 and 300 times faster than it can be replenished (Kendall and Pimental, 1994). The wide range of estimates is due to measurements covering markedly varied soil types and climatic conditions.

The Convention to Combat Desertification, negotiated at the 1992 Earth Summit, took effect in 1996 and by 1999 had been ratified by 145 countries. Nevertheless, donor countries have not committed the resources needed to tackle the problem of once productive land becoming desert, which is viewed as predominately a problem for the developing world (Agarwal, Narain, and Sharma, 1999).

Population growth has contributed to land degradation throughout the least developed countries. In many countries of Africa and Asia, sons inherit equal shares of land. Thus over the generations ever-growing families have meant ever-shrinking farmsteads, forcing many people onto the less productive, marginal farmland in hilly areas, drylands, and tropical forests (Doos, 1994; Brown and Mitchell, 1997).

As the rural environment deteriorates due to land degradation and shrinking farmsteads, small-scale farmers cannot produce enough food to feed their families. Women and girls, in particular, pay the price with poorer diets; they suffer increasingly from protein energy malnutrition and lack of vitamin A. The disease burden for poor rural families unable to coax a living from shrinking farmsteads is manifested in chronic anemia and respiratory infections along with greater susceptibility to malaria, dengue fever, and cholera.

Freshwater

A WRI study has reported that some 2 billion people, or one-third of the world's population, already live in areas experiencing moderate to severe water stress for at least part of the year. If trends continue this number will balloon to 4 billion by midcentury (Revenga and others, 2000). Chronic water shortages will be perhaps the most limiting factor on future economic development in these regions. Moreover, even though the *percentage* of the population without access to potable water declined during the 1990s, rapid population growth meant that in terms of actual numbers more people than before lacked clean water. At the close of the twentieth century an estimated 1.2 billion people lacked clean water, compared to about 1 billion in 1990. (The health implications of inadequate clean water are described in Chapter Eighteen.)

Oceans

During the 1990s, coastal wetlands—including mangrove forests, salt ponds, marshes, and brackish water estuaries—have deteriorated (Hinrichsen, 1998). Although global estimates of the extent of this degradation are not available, in 1995 the WRI found that the environments of as many as half of all coastal areas suffered from development pressures (Bryant, Rodenburg, Cox, and Nielsen, 1995).

Marine fisheries have declined dramatically over the course of the 1990s. Today, according to the Food and Agriculture Organization (FAO) of the United Nations (1999), 69 percent of major commercial fish stocks are either fully exploited, overfished, depleted, or are slowly recovering. Between 1990 and 1996, the amount of fish and shellfish hauled in by the world's distant water fleets fell sharply, from 5 million tons to 2 million, about the same level harvested in 1950. During the same period, however, aquaculture production soared from 16 million tons in 1990 to 35 million tons in 1996 (FAO, 1999). Marine pollution, coupled with the pressures of rising population densities and loss of coastal resources, threatens the livelihood of 200 million subsistence and small-scale fishing families and indirectly affects as many as 2 billion people in coastal areas (Hinrichsen, 1998).

A number of encouraging initiatives have been launched, but so far they have had little impact. An intergovernmental agreement to combat land-based sources of pollution was adopted in 1995, but its implementation is unclear and little progress has been made. Similarly, two international initiatives launched in 1995, although well intended, have yet to make an impact: the FAO Code of Conduct for Responsible Fisheries and the UN Agreement on Straddling Fish Stocks and Highly Migratory Fish Stocks.

Meanwhile, fisheries continue to be exploited at unsustainable rates. An estimated 2 billion people depend on seafood for their protein intake. The erosion of access to seafood has put the health of these 2 billion at risk. Most of them live in the Asia-Pacific region. Unless ways can be found to ensure access to edible fish and shellfish, the health of one-third of the plant's population is likely to deteriorate (FAO, 1995).

Forests

Since the 1992 Earth Summit, deforestation has increased in twenty countries with large forest resources. In the Amazon basin in Brazil, for instance, the deforestation rate has increased by some 34 percent since 1992, with about 1.5 million hectares of tropical forest a year being destroyed (World Wide Fund for Nature, 1996). Globally, about 16 million hectares of forest, an area roughly the size of Montana, are cut, bulldozed, or burned each year. Half the world's original (preindustrial) forest cover—over 3 billion hectares—has been lost, largely during the past four decades (WRI, 1997).

Attempts to advance an international forest convention date from 1990. But at the close of the decade, the international community shelved the idea as impractical—a move supported by many nongovernmental organizations on the grounds that a convention would only enshrine the standards of a weak consensus. The Earth Summit process did generate the Intergovernmental Panel on Forests in 1995, but in 1997, this group was transformed into the Intergovernmental Forum on Forests, with a secretariat established at the UN Division for Sustainable Development in New York. Owing to widespread opposition, no convention on forests is ever likely to get to the negotiating table. Instead, international action centers on getting countries to enforce existing legislation and forest conservation initiatives (Kendall and Pimental, 1994).

Healthy forest ecosystems are critical for maintaining the health and well-being of approximately half a billion people who depend on forests for all or part of their daily diets. With the forests gone, and biodiversity with them, subsistence cultures can no longer supplement diets dependent on one or two staples with fruits, nuts, berries, and bush meat harvested from the forests (WRI, 1997).

Biodiversity

Population growth exerts an inexorable pressure on ecosystems as resources are depleted and as human settlements alter and fragment habitats. One result is species loss, the only truly irreversible instance of environmental damage. The earth could be losing species at rates 100 to 10,000 times faster than natural background rates, but there is little agreement on the numbers lost over the past decade (Mace, 1998). It has been estimated, conservatively, that 27,000 plant and animal species were pushed into extinction every year during the 1990s (Eldredge, 1998). Moreover, the pace of extinction is expected to accelerate as more and more prime habitat is lost or degraded, in part by expanding populations and by rising consumer demand in the developed world for products from some of the most ecologically diverse countries (Myers, 1999). In addition, the FAO (1995) estimates that about three-quarters of the genetic diversity of domestic cultivars (cultivated crops) has been lost since 1900, with much of that destruction taking place over the past two decades.

Biodiversity has important implications for human health (Cincotta and Engelman, 2000; Grifo and Rosenthal, 1997). Many medications derive from plants, and medical research depends heavily on plant and animal species. Biodiversity is essential for world food production. Species loss may result in ecological imbalances, which may in turn promote the emergence and spread of human infectious diseases. The loss of biodiversity is therefore more than an environmental concern; it is a human health concern as well.

The Convention on Biological Diversity, which was opened for signature at Rio, entered into force in December 1993, and 175 countries have now ratified it. Unfortunately, the United States has not signed it. Without U.S. support, this convention is unlikely to fulfill its objectives (Kendall and Pimental, 1994).

Climate Change

Population growth and increasing prosperity together drive energy use. As described in Chapter Fifteen, the predominant sources of energy, such as biomass fuels and fossil fuels, release carbon dioxide when burned. The atmospheric concentration of carbon dioxide has reached about 380 parts per million, up from 280 before the industrial revolution. The rising levels of atmospheric carbon dioxide, in turn, contribute to climate change (see Chapter Eleven).

Climate change has become widely accepted as a growing global problem. Solving the problem will be more difficult than recognizing it. In 1997, delegates to the UN Framework Convention on Climate Change conference in Kyoto, Japan, adopted a global framework for addressing climate change. They agreed that developed countries should achieve a 5 percent reduction in emissions of greenhouse gases by 2008–2012 compared to their 1990 emission levels. The Kyoto Protocol was designed to enter into force when at least fifty-five nations, accounting for at least 55 percent of total 1990 carbon dioxide emissions, had ratified it, a landmark that was reached in February 2005. By mid-2005 149 nations had ratified or accepted the Kyoto protocol but these did not include the

United States, Australia, and other important emitters (see, for example, United Nations Framework Convention on Climate Change, 2004).

Population and Poverty

Rapid, unsustainable population growth is a principal contributor to poverty. Currently, between one in four and one in five of the earth's people live in absolute poverty, defined as earning less than one dollar per day. Each day, over a billion people in the world cannot satisfy their basic food needs. This level of poverty raises profound social justice concerns, and it also has obvious health implications. Each day, 35,000 children under the age of five die from starvation or from preventable infectious diseases aggravated by undernutrition.

Although the 1992 Earth Summit did not focus directly on slowing population growth or on improving living standards, Agenda 21, the summit's blueprint for action, discussed the scope and dimension of the problems caused by population growth and poverty. This document linked improvements to better resource management, identifying ecologically sensitive areas where heavy population pressures were stressing resources, and called for the empowerment of local communities so that people can have more opportunities to manage common resources upon which they depend for their survival. Equally important to achieving the goal of sustainable development are improving access to basic education for both boys and girls and advancing the status of women, among other recommendations (UN Foundation, 2000a). In 1994, two years after the Earth Summit in Rio, the United Nations International Conference on Population and Development (ICPD) was held in Cairo. Although the environment was not directly on the agenda, the important links between population, development, and the environment were covered in the ICPD Programme of Action. This document specifically mentions the important "inter-relationships between population, resources, the environment and development" (ICPD, 1994).

Lower fertility and slower population growth, however, have not brought an improved living standard for the average person. In 1990, about 2 billion people were living on the equivalent of $2 a day or less (Hinrichsen, 1997). In 2000, that number had risen to about 3 billion people, an increase of 1 billion in ten years (UN Foundation, 2000a). Although some of this increase reflects the economic problems of Southeast Asian economies in 1997, which drove millions from the lower-middle classes into poverty, it also reflects the fact that in many countries population growth has exceeded economic growth.

Partly due to differences in population growth, the gap between rich countries and poor countries has widened over the past decade. In 1990, the income gap between the world's richest and poorest countries was calculated at a ratio of 60 to 1 (in other words, the average income of a citizen of a developed country in Europe or North America was 60 times higher than the average income of a resident of a poor, developing country (Cohen, 1998). In 1999, the income gap was 74 to 1, and it could rise further to 100 to 1 before 2015, according to UN estimates (UN Foundation, 2000a). A disproportionate number of the world's poor are women and children. Since 1970, the number of rural women living in poverty has increased by 50 percent, compared to 30 percent for rural men (Power, 1992). Of particular concern is the fact that in sub-Saharan Africa and South Asia, countries with the world's highest fertility rates and fastest population growth also face the most poverty and the severest resource constraints. Chronic water shortages, widespread degradation of arable land, rampant deforestation, rapid urbanization, deteriorating health conditions, and other challenges confront these countries as they seek to develop their economies (Brown, Gardner, and Halweil, 1999; UN Foundation, 2000b; Munn, Whyte, and Timmerman, 1999; Chivian 2002).

Environmental Distress Syndrome

In recent years scientists have been becoming increasingly concerned about the health of the environment itself. "We are no longer talking only of an increased exposure to specific extraneous hazards as a cause of *bad* health. We are also recognizing the depletion or disruption of natural biophysical processes that are the basic source of sustained *good* health," as Tony McMichael (1997), professor of epidemiology at the London School of Hygiene and Tropical Medicine, has put it. At increasing risk, McMichael observes, are the ecosystems that determine the productivity of food-producing systems and such global systems as the hydrologic cycle and the stratospheric *ozone shield* that offers the earth protection from excessive solar ultraviolet radiation. Biologists recognize that human numbers and human actions are causing "rapid, novel, and substantial" changes to the environment (Vitousek, Mooney, Lubchenco, and Melillo, 1997). These changes include degrading soil and water supplies; altering nature's biogeochemical cycles, largely by releasing enormous amounts of carbon dioxide into the atmosphere; and destroying or altering biological resources.

Ecologists have begun to use the term *environmental distress syndrome* to describe the effects of deteriorating environmental conditions and growing threats to human health. Paul Epstein (1997), of Harvard University's Center for Health and the Global Environment, lists five symptoms of this syndrome:

1. The reemergence of infectious diseases, such as cholera, typhoid, and pneumonia, and the emergence of new diseases, such as drug-resistant tuberculosis and human reproductive disorders linked to industrial chemicals

2. The loss of biodiversity and the consequent loss of potential sources of new drugs and crops
3. The growing dominance of generalist species, such as crows and Canada geese
4. The decline in pollinators, such as bees, birds, bats, butterflies, and beetles, organisms that are indispensable for the preservation of flowering plants
5. The proliferation of harmful algal blooms along the world's coastlines, leading to more deadly outbreaks of diseases such as ciguatera poisoning and paralytic shellfish poisoning (see also UNDP, 1998)

Such trends pose a disturbing question: At what point might the depletion of the world's ecological and biophysical capital redound against the health of humanity? Evidence is mounting that we are already witnessing profound changes in ecosystem viability and a rise in both new and old infectious diseases. For example, the World Health Organization has reported that a recent epidemic of meningitis in sub-Saharan Africa coincided with an expansion of degraded agricultural and grazing land—a result of changes in land use patterns and regional climate change triggered by human activities (McMichael, 1997). Another study has linked more frequent and severe El Niño weather patterns to marked increases in diarrheal diseases in Peruvian children (Checkley and others, 2000).

Conclusion

The links between population, health, and the environment are not difficult to discern. As poverty deepens and environmental and human health conditions continue to deteriorate, scientists have been able to shed more light on the connections between the health of the environment and the health of vulnerable populations (Engelman, 1996). Having good health is not just a matter of having access to quality health services; it is more a matter of having access to a livable and healthy environment. Clearly, people cannot be healthy without an environment conducive to good health. Maintaining healthy ecosystems, which in turn support healthy human populations, remains one of the new millennium's critical challenges.

Unfortunately, the natural environment, upon which all human development rests, continues to deteriorate at alarming rates across virtually all resource sectors. The trends do not augur well for the future. The loss of biodiversity, water shortages and pollution, deforestation, desertification, the death of coastal zones—all these major trends are moving in the wrong direction. Population growth is a major driver of this movement. These trends compel us to ask some very fundamental questions. Can the gross depletion of essential life-support systems be halted in time? If not, is the earth headed for a sixth big extinction? Humanity's own? What will the future bring if climate change continues unabated and sea levels rise by one meter or more? What will happen as the world becomes predominately urban? Can we learn to live within our ecological constraints or boundaries? And can we reduce our ecological footprints so as to tread more lightly on the earth?

Thought Questions

1. Some environmental groups have focused on population control, or on limits to immigration, as central strategies. If you were on the board of an environmental group, would you support such an approach? Why or why not?
2. What can individuals do to reduce their ecological footprint?
3. Why is reducing fertility levels so important for poor developing countries; how does this affect health and how can it be done effectively?
4. Investing in and empowering women is considered one of the most cost effective investments a country can make toward economic and social development. Why is this the case?

References

Agarwal, A., Narain, S., and Sharma, A. (eds.). *Green Politics: Global Environmental Negotiations.* New Delhi: Centre for Science and Environment, 1999.

Brown, L., and Mitchell, J. *The Agricultural Link: How Environmental Deterioration Could Disrupt Economic Progress.* Worldwatch paper no. 136. Washington D.C.: Worldwatch Institute, Aug. 1997.

Brown, L., Gardner, G., and Halweil, B. *Beyond Malthus: Nineteen Dimensions of the Population Challenge.* New York: Norton, 1999.

Bryant, D., Rodenburg, E., Cox, T., and Nielsen, D. *Coastlines at Risk: An Index of Potential Development-Related Threats to Coastal Ecosystems.* Washington D.C.: World Resources Institute, 1995.

Checkley, W., and others. "Effects of El Nino and Ambient Temperature on Hospital Admissions for Diarrhoeal Diseases in Peruvian Children." *Lancet,* 2000, *355,* 442–450.

Chivian, E. (ed.). *Biodiversity: Its Importance to Human Health.* Center for Health and the Global Environment, Harvard Medical School. [http://www.med.harvard.edu/chge/Biodiversity_v2_screen.pdf]. 2002.

Cincotta, R. P., and Engelman, R. *Nature's Place: Human Population and the Future of Biological Diversity.* Washington D.C.: Population Action International, 2000.

Cohen, J. *How Many People Can the Earth Support?* New York: Norton, 1995.

Cohen, J. "How Many People Can the Earth Support?" *New York Review,* Oct. 8, 1998, pp. 29–31.

Constanza, R., and others. "The Value of the World's Ecosystem Services and Natural Capital." *Nature,* 1997, *387,* 253–260.

Crenson, M. "World Population Reaches 6 Billion." New York: Associated Press, Oct. 10, 1999.

Doos, B. "Environmental Degradation, Global Food Production and Risk for Large-Scale Migration." *Ambio,* 1994, *23*(3), 124–130.

Ehrlich, P., and Holdren, J. "Impact of Population Growth." *Science,* 1971, *171,* 1212–1217.

Eldredge, N. *Life in the Balance: Humanity and the Biodiversity Crisis.* Princeton, N.J.: Princeton University Press, 1998.

Engelman, R. "Population as a Scale Factor: Impacts on Environment and Development." Paper presented at the Conference on Population, Environment and Development, Washington, D.C., Mar. 13–14, 1996.

Epstein, P. "The Threatened Plague." *People & the Planet,* 1997, *6*(3), 14–17.

Food and Agriculture Organization of the United Nations. *Dimensions of Need: An Atlas of Food and Agriculture.* Rome: Food and Agriculture Organization of the United Nations, 1995.

Food and Agriculture Organization of the United Nations. *State of the World's Fisheries and Aquaculture 1998.* Rome: Food and Agriculture Organization of the United Nations, 1999.

Goodland, R. "The Case That the World Has Reached Limits." In R. Goodland, H. Daly, and S. Serafy (eds.), *Population, Technology and Lifestyle: The Transition to Sustainability.* Washington, D.C.: Island Press, 1992.

Grifo, F., and Rosenthal, J. (eds.). *Biodiversity and Human Health.* Washington, D.C.: Island Press, 1997.

Hinrichsen, D. "Economists' Shining Lie." *Amicus Journal,* 1991, *13*(2), 3–5.

Hinrichsen, D. "Rio + 5: Picking Up the Pieces." *People & the Planet,* 1997, *6*(4), 4–5.

Hinrichsen, D. *Coastal Waters of the World: Trends, Threats and Strategies.* Washington, D.C.: Island Press, 1998.

Hinrichsen, D., and Robey, B. *Population and the Environment: The Global Challenge.* Center for Communication Programs, Population Reports series M, no. 15. Baltimore, Md.: Johns Hopkins University School of Public Health, 2000.

Hinrichsen, D., Salem, R., and Blackburn, R. *Population Reports: Meeting the Urban Challenge.* Center for Communication Programs, Population Reports series M, no. 16. Baltimore, Md.: Johns Hopkins University, 2002.

International Conference on Population and Development. *Programme of Action of the International Conference on Population and Development.* [http://www.unfpa.org/icpd/icpd_poa.htm#ch1]. 1994.

Kasperson, J., Kasperson, R., and Turner, B. L. *Regions at Risk: Comparison of Threatened Environments.* UNU Studies of Critical Environmental Regions. Tokyo: United Nations University Press, Dec. 1995.

Kasperson, R., Kasperson, J., and Turner, B. L. "Risk and Criticality: Trajections of Regional Environmental Degradation." *Ambio,* 1999, *28*(6), 562–568.

Kendall, H., and Pimental, D. "Constraints on the Expansion of the Global Food Supply." *Ambio,* 1994, *23*(3), 200–206.

Mace, G. "Getting the Measure of Extinction." *People & the Planet,* 1998, *7*(4), 9.

McMichael, T. "Healthy World, Healthy People." *People & the Planet,* 1997, *6*(3), 6–9.

Munn, T., Whyte, A., and Timmerman, R. "Emerging Environmental Issues: A Global Perspective of SCOPE." *Ambio,* 1999, *28*(6), 464–471.

Myers, N. "What We Must Do to Counter the Biotic Holocaust." *International Wildlife,* 1999, *29*(2), 30–39.

Population Reference Bureau. "2003 World Population Data Sheet." Washington D.C.: Population Reference Bureau, 2003.

Power, J. *The Report on Rural Women Living in Poverty.* Rome: International Fund for Agricultural Development, 1992.

Revenga, C., and others. *Pilot Analysis of Global Ecosystems, Freshwater Systems.* Washington D.C.: World Resources Institute, 2000.

Roodman, D. *The Natural Wealth of Nations: Harnessing the Market for the Environment.* Worldwatch Environmental Alert Series. New York: Norton, 1998.

UNAIDS: The Joint United Nations Program on HIV/AIDS, United Nations Population Fund (UNFPA), and United Nations Development Fund for Women (UNIFEM). *Women and HIV/AIDS: Confronting the Crisis.* New York: United Nations, 2004.

United Nations Department of Economic and Social Affairs, Population Division. *World Urbanization Prospects: The 2001 Revision.* New York: United Nations, 2002.

United Nations Department of Economic and Social Affairs, Population Division. *World Population Prospects: The 2002 Revision.* New York: United Nations, 2003.

United Nations Development Programme. *Energy After Rio: Prospects and Challenges.* New York: United Nations, 1997.

United Nations Development Programme. *Human Development Report 1998.* New York: United Nations, 1998.

United Nations Environment Programme. *Global Environmental Outlook 2000.* London: Earthscan, 2000.

United Nations Foundation. "Globalization: Commentaries Probe Challenges of New Century." Press Release. Washington D.C.: UN Wire Service, Jan. 3, 2000a.

United Nations Foundation. "Water: Manila Meeting Highlights Southeast Asian Woes." Press Release. Washington D.C.: UN Wire Service, Jan. 21, 2000b.

United Nations Framework Convention on Climate Change. "Kyoto Protocol—What It Means: Status of Ratification." [http://unfccc.int]. 2004.

United Nations Population Fund. *Population and the Environment: The Challenges Ahead.* New York: United Nations Population Fund, 1991.

United Nations Population Fund. *The State of World Population 1999: Six Billion: A Time for Choices.* New York: United Nations Population Fund, 1999.

United Nations Population Fund. *The State of World Population 2003: Making 1 Billion Count.* New York: United Nations Population Fund, 2003.

Upadhyay, U. D., and Robey, B. *Why Family Planning Matters.* Population Reports, Series J., no. 49. Baltimore, Md.: Johns Hopkins University, Population Information Program, July 1999.

Vitousek, P. M., Mooney, H. A., Lubchenco, J., and Melillo, J. M. "Human Domination of Earth's Ecosystems." *Science,* 1997, *227,* 494–499.

Wackernagel, M., and others. *Ecological Footprints of Nations: How Much Nature Do They Use?* Xalapa, Mexico: Center for Sustainability Studies, Mar. 10, 1997.

World Bank. *World Development Report 1992: Development and the Environment.* New York: Oxford University Press, 1992.

World Health Organization. *Health and Environment in Sustainable Development: Five Years After the Earth Summit.* Geneva: World Health Organization, 1997.

World Health Organization. *HIV/AIDS Epidemiological Surveillance Update for the WHO African Region 2002.* [http://www.who.int/hiv/pub/epidemiology/pubafro2003/en/]. 2003.

World Resources Institute. *The Last Frontier Forests: Ecosystems and Economies on the Edge.* Washington, D.C.: World Resources Institute, 1997.

World Resources Institute. *World Resources 1998–99.* New York: Oxford University Press, 1998.
World Wide Fund for Nature. *Forests for Life.* Godalming, U.K.: World Wide Fund for Nature, 1996.

For Further Information

Peopleandplanet.net is a Web site that has information on issues of population, poverty, health, consumption, and the environment. It is maintained by Planet 21, a British nongovernmental organization, and sponsored by the United Nations Population Fund, the World Conservation Union, the World Wide Fund for Nature International, the International Planned Parenthood Federation, and the Swedish Development Co-operation Agency.

[www.peopleandplanet.net]

The United Nations Population Fund (UNFPA) maintains a useful Web site. Among other resources, it provides access to the *State of World Population Report,* an annual UNFPA report on various aspects of population, reproductive health, women's rights, and development.

[www.unfpa.org]

The Population Reference Bureau is a nongovernmental organization based in Washington that serves as an information resource about the population dimensions of important social, economic, and political issues.

[www.prb.org]

Our Ecological Footprint by Williams E. Rees and Mathis Wackernagel (Gabriola Island, BC: New Society Publishers, 1996) is an invaluable introduction to the effects of population and resource use on the environmental.

The following are annual or biannual reports that provide valuable information on population trends and related resource issues.

World Resources Report, published biannually by the World Resources Institute, Washington, D.C.
Global Environment Outlook, published by the UN Environment Programme.
State of the World Reports, published annually by Worldwatch Institute, Washington, D.C.

CHAPTER ELEVEN

CLIMATE CHANGE

Jonathan A. Patz

Climate change, whether due to natural variability or resulting from human activity, depends on the overall energy budget of the planet, the balance between incoming (solar) shortwave radiation and outgoing longwave radiation. This balance is affected by the earth's atmosphere, in much the same way that a glass greenhouse (or a car's windshield on a hot day) allows sunlight energy to penetrate through the glass and traps heat (infrared) energy inside. An atmosphere that retains more heat, because it has higher levels of so-called greenhouse gases, will result in higher average surface temperatures than will an atmosphere with lower levels of these gases.

The composition of the earth's atmosphere has changed since preindustrial times. Beginning approximately in the mid-1800s, the changes include increases in atmospheric levels of carbon dioxide (CO_2), methane (CH_4), and nitrous oxide (N_2O) that far exceed any changes occurring in the preceding 10,000 years. Historical levels of these greenhouse gases are known from analyses of air trapped in bubbles in Antarctic ice cores (Etheridge, Steele, Francey, and Langenfelds, 1998; Gulluck, Slemr, and Stauffer, 1998). For example, the concentration of CO_2, the major greenhouse gas, has risen by approximately 35 percent, from about 280 parts per million by volume (ppmv) in the late eighteenth century to about 380 ppmv at present. Higher greenhouse gas concentrations have contributed to warming of the earth—in an effect called *positive radiative forcing*—by absorbing and reemitting infrared radiation toward the lower atmosphere and Earth's surface (Figure 11.1; Table 11.1).

FIGURE 11.1. THE GREENHOUSE EFFECT.

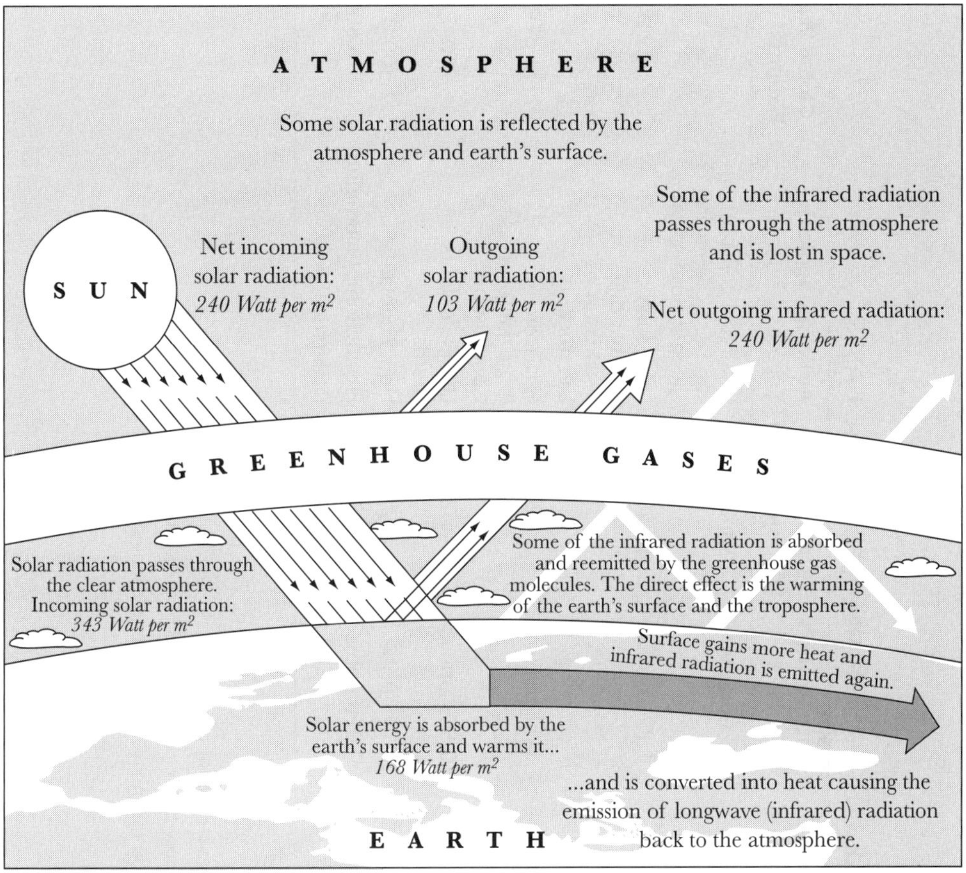

Source: United Nations Environment Program, Vital Climate Graphics collection.

Although the average effect across the earth's surface is a warming, there is more to the story than that. Warmer air holds more moisture, resulting in more precipitation (at least in some areas). Wind patterns change. Arctic and Antarctic ice melts, releasing vast amounts of water into the oceans, raising ocean levels and potentially altering the flows of ocean currents. The weather patterns that result from these and other changes vary greatly from place to place. Although many places become warmer, others become colder. Although some become wetter, others become drier. For these reasons the term *climate change* is more accurate than *global warming* and is the accepted term for this set of changes.

TABLE 11.1. THE MAIN GREENHOUSE GASES.

Greenhouse Gases	Chemical Formula	Preindustrial Concentration	Concentration in 1994	Atmospheric Lifetime (years)	Anthropogenic Sources	Global Warming Potential (GWP)[a]
Carbon dioxide	CO_2	278,000 ppbv	358,000 ppbv	Variable[c]	Fossil fuel combustion Land-use conversion Cement production	1
Methane	CH_4	700 ppbv	1,721 ppbv	12.2 ± 3	Fossil fuels Rice paddies Waste dumps Livestock	21[b]
Nitrous oxide	N_2O	275 ppbv	311 ppbv	120	Fertilizer Industrial processes Combustion	310
CFC-12	CCl_2F_2	0	0.503 ppbv	102	Liquid coolants Foams	6,200–7,100[d]
HCFC-22	$CHClF_2$	0	0.105 ppbv	12.1	Liquid coolants	1,300–1,400[d]
Perfluoromethane	CF_4	0	0.070 ppbv	50,000	Production of aluminum	6,500
Sulfur hexafluoride	SF_6	0	0.032 ppbv	3,200	Dielectric fluid	23,900

Note: ppbv = 1 part per billion by volume.

[a]GWP for 100-year time horizon.

[b]Includes indirect effects of tropospericozone water vapor production.

[c]No single lifetime for CO_2 can be defined because of the different rates of uptake by different sink processes.

[d]Net global warming potential (that is, including the indirect effect due to ozone depletion).

Source: Houghton and others, 2001.

Long-term climate change, whether from natural sources or due to human activity, can be observed as a signal against a background of natural climate variability (see Figure 11.2). To help us detect the meaning of this signal, we need historical climate data to estimate natural variability. Because instrument records are

FIGURE 11.2. VARIATIONS OF THE EARTH'S SURFACE TEMPERATURE ACROSS TWO TIME FRAMES.

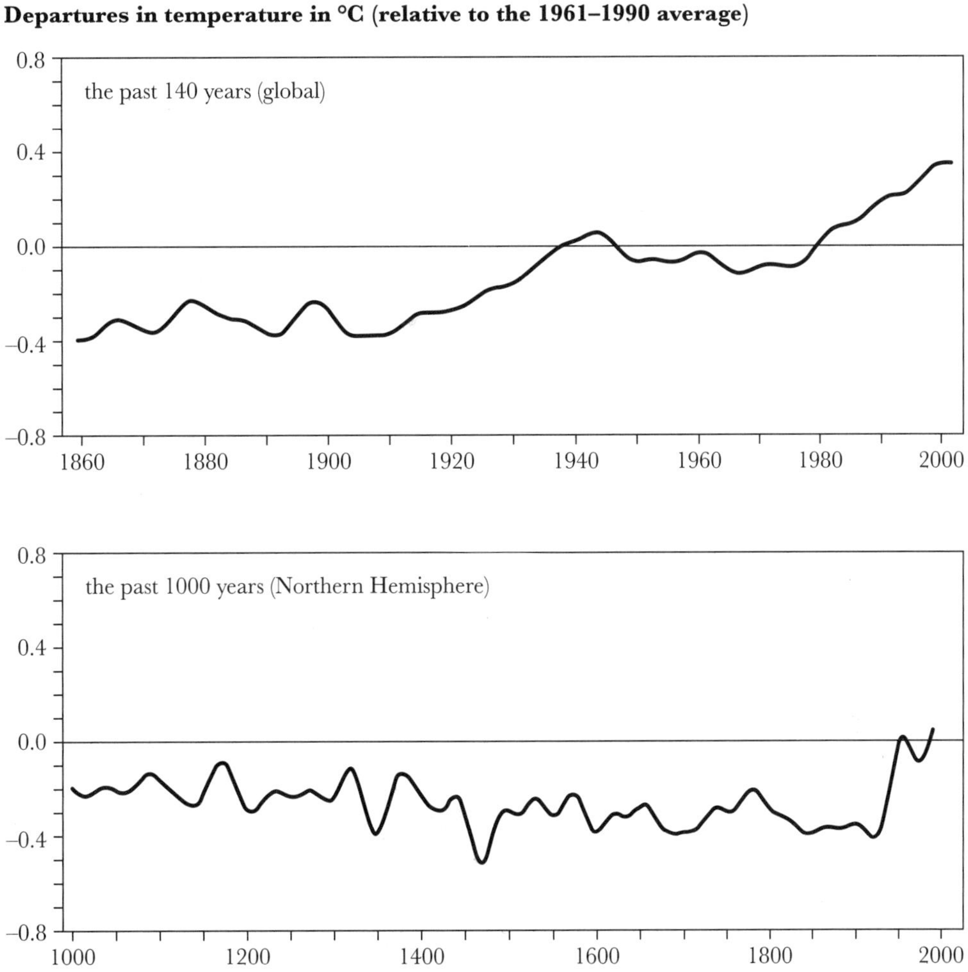

Data since the mid-1800s based on direct thermometer readings and data from prior years based on indirect sources (tree rings, corals, ice cores, and historical records). The line represents an average of variable readings at each point in time.

Source: Adapted from Watson and the Core Writing Team, 2001.

available only for the recent past (a period of less than 150 years), previous climates must be deduced from paleoclimatic records, including tree rings, pollen series, faunal and floral abundances in deep-sea cores, isotope analyses of coral and ice cores, and diaries and other documentary evidence. Results of these analyses show that surface temperatures in the mid to late twentieth century appear to have been warmer than they were during any similar period in the last 600 years in most regions and in at least some regions warmer than in any other century for several thousand years (Nicholls and others, 1996).

Since the late 1950s, global average surface temperature has increased by 0.6°C and snow cover and ice extent have diminished, sea level has risen on average by 10 to 20 cm during the past century, and ocean heat content has increased since the late 1950s (Houghton and others, 2001).

Projected Climate Change and Sea-Level Rise

A major source of information on climate change is the work of the United Nations Intergovernmental Panel on Climate Change (IPCC), which was established by the World Meteorological Organization (WMO) and the United Nations Environment Programme (UNEP) in 1988. Approximately every five years since 1990, the IPCC has conducted international assessments of the current scientific work on climate change, the potential impacts of this change, and various prevention options. This international body includes many outstanding scientists, representing multiple sectors, and its reports are viewed as the most authoritative assessments on the subject.

The IPCC predicts that over the next century, average global temperatures will increase between 1.8°C and 5.8°C and sea level will rise between 9 and 88 centimeters (Houghton and others, 2001), with midrange estimates of a global mean warming of 3°C and a sea-level rise of 45 cm (see Figure 11.3). Increased variability in the hydrologic cycle (more floods and droughts) is expected to accompany global warming trends. The rate of change in climate is faster now than it has been in any period in the last thousand years, with warming greater at the poles than at the equator.

Regional changes in climate, particularly increases in temperature, have already affected diverse physical and biological systems in many parts of the world. For example, river and lake ice is breaking up earlier in the year, and plant and animal ranges are moving to higher altitudes. Alpine species, such as certain wildflowers, will have no further terrain to which to migrate and could go extinct. Also, if Arctic sea ice continues to disappear at the current rapid rate, polar bears will be endangered by midcentury (Arctic Climate Impact Assessment, 2004).

The potential also exists for large-scale and potentially irreversible changes in the earth's systems, such as slowing of the ocean circulation that transports warm water

FIGURE 11.3. PROJECTED CHANGES IN GLOBAL TEMPERATURE: GLOBAL AVERAGE 1856–1999 AND PROJECTION ESTIMATES TO 2100.

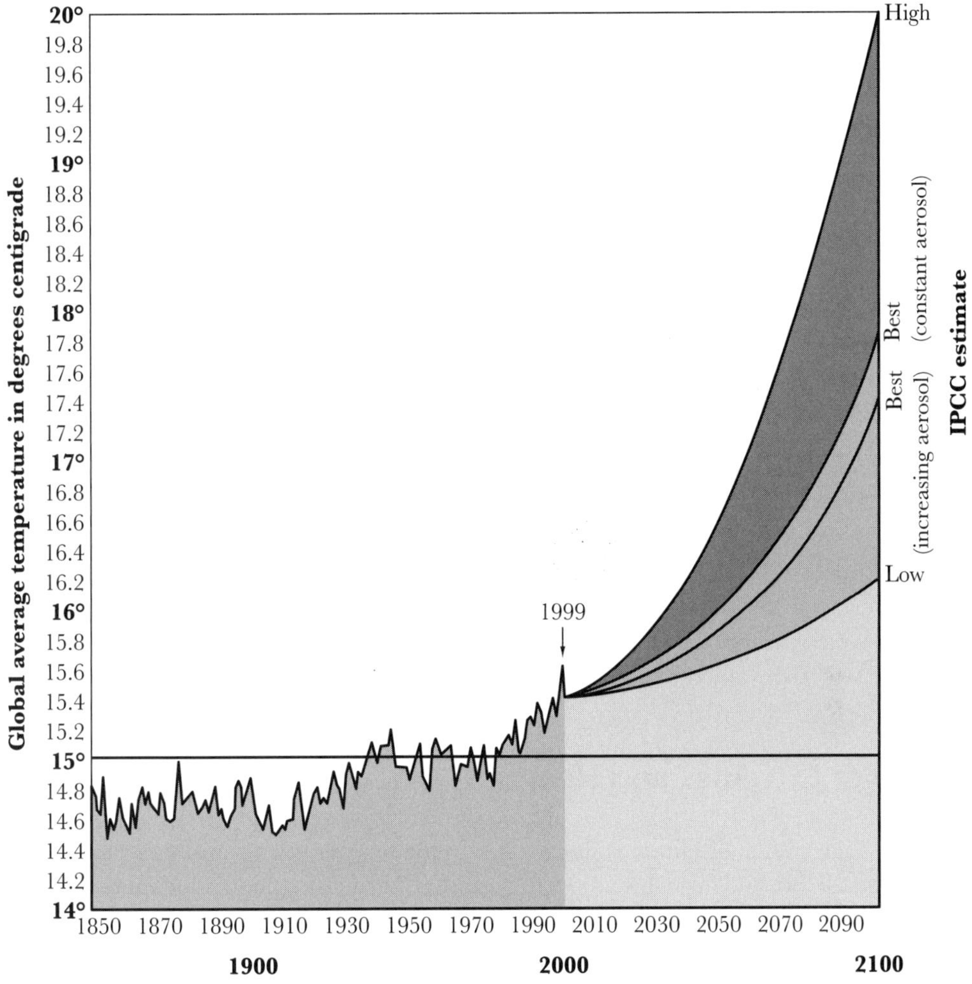

Source: Adapted from Watson and the Core Writing Team, 2001.

to the North Atlantic, large-scale melting of the Greenland and west Antarctic ice sheets, and accelerated global warming due to the positive feedbacks of the carbon cycle (such as the release of methane from thawing Arctic tundra). The probability of these events is unknown, but it is likely to be affected by how rapidly climate change evolves and its duration.

Particularly Vulnerable Regions

According to the IPCC certain regions and populations are more vulnerable than others to the health impacts of climate change:

- Areas or populations within or bordering regions with a high endemicity of climate-sensitive diseases (for example, malaria)
- Areas with an observed association between epidemic disease and weather extremes (for example, El Niño–linked epidemics)
- Areas at risk from combined climate impacts relevant to health (for example, stress on food and water supplies or risk of coastal flooding)
- Areas at risk from concurrent environmental or socioeconomic stresses (for example, local stresses from land-use practices or an impoverished or undeveloped health infrastructure) and with little capacity to adapt

Changes in seasonal river flows, increases in floods and droughts, decreased food security, and biodiversity loss are special concerns for parts of Africa, Latin America, and Asia. Low-lying coastal and delta regions (such as coastal China, Bangladesh, and Egypt and especially densely populated, low-lying, small island states such as coral reef atolls throughout Polynesia) and arid regions (such as eastern Africa and central Asia that already suffer from drought) are at special risk even without climate change and at elevated risk as the global climate warms (McCarthy and others, 2001).

Weather Extremes and Health

Such results of climate change as extreme temperatures, severe storms, rising sea levels, and droughts all put the health of the earth's populations at risk (NRC, 2001). And while slightly above average blood pressure or cholesterol in a population can impose a health risk, in the case of climate, it is the extremes of temperature and the water cycle that pose direct threats to human health.

Thermal Stress

Extremes of both hot and cold temperatures are associated with rates of morbidity and mortality higher than the rates in the intermediate, or *comfortable,* temperature range (Kilbourne, 1998). The relationship between temperature and morbidity and mortality is J-shaped, indicating asymmetry, with a steeper slope at higher temperatures (Curriero, Patz, Rose, and Lele, 2000). In the United States, heat waves are more deadly than hurricanes, floods, and tornadoes combined. However, the extent of temperature-related mortality also seems to vary according to geography.

The body's thermoregulatory mechanisms can cope with a certain amount of temperature rise through control of perspiration and vasodilation of cutaneous vessels (Horowitz and Samueloff, 1987). The ability to respond to heat stress is thus limited by the capacity to increase cardiac output as required for greater cutaneous blood flow. People can, however, adapt to high temperatures over time by increasing their ability to dissipate heat through these mechanisms.

On average about 175 Americans succumb to extremes of summer heat each year. An estimated 20,000 people were killed in the United States from 1936 through 1975 by the effects of heat and solar radiation (National Oceanic and Atmospheric Administration, 2001). However, the extreme 2003 European heat wave is estimated to have killed even more people (over 22,000) in just two weeks (Kovats, Wolf, and Menne, 2004). Table 11.2 shows the mortality during this heat wave, with numbers from Spain and Germany still pending. Note that generally very few deaths are attributed to "heat stroke" because the immediate cause of death for most victims of heat stress is cardiovascular or respiratory failure. In 1995, a weeklong heat wave in Chicago caused over 700 heat-related deaths (Whitman and others, 1997). Much of the excess mortality from heat waves is concentrated in the elderly and people with preexisting illness. That is, susceptible people who were likely to have died in the near future from other causes account for a proportion of these deaths (an outcome known as *harvesting*), but truly preventable excess deaths occur during heat waves as well.

TABLE 11.2. MORTALITY FROM THE 2003 HEAT WAVE IN EUROPE.

Country	Heat-Stroke Deaths	Excess Deaths (%)	Time Period	Method for Estimating Baseline Mortality
England/ Wales	1	2,045 (16%)	August 4 to 13	Deaths in same period in years 1998 to 2002
France	n.a.	14,802 (60%)	August 1 to 20	Average of deaths in same period in years 2000 to 2002
Italy	n.a.	3,134 (15%)	June 1 to August 15	Deaths in same period in year 2002
Portugal	7	2,099 (26%)	August 1 to 31	Deaths in same period in years 1997 to 2001
Spain	59	?		

Source: Kovats, Wolf, and Menne, 2004.

The *threshold* temperature above which mortality sharply increases is location specific (Kalkstein and Tan, 1996). The risk of death increases substantially during heat waves, when thermal stress persists for several consecutive days coupled with high overnight temperatures (Ramlow and Kuller, 1990). This suggests that there might be a critical load of heat stress, above which physiological coping mechanisms become inadequate. Vulnerability to heat waves is driven by socioeconomic factors such as poor housing. Therefore people in cities in developing countries may be more vulnerable to morbidity and mortality during heat waves.

An *urban heat island* is an urban area that generates and retains heat as a result of buildings, human and industrial activities, and other factors. Black asphalt and other dark surfaces (on roads, parking lots, and roofs) reduce albedo (reflectivity) and are dense, heat-retaining surfaces. In addition, urban areas are relatively lacking in trees, so they receive less of the cooling effect associated with evapotranspiration. Global warming is expected to increase both heat and humidity, aggravating the effect of heat islands and increasing heat stress on urban populations (Kattenberg and others, 1996). Urban nighttime heat retention can also be a factor in the greater number of heat-related deaths in urban compared to rural areas (Buechley, Van Bruggen, and Truppi, 1972). During heat waves, when stagnant atmospheric conditions may persist, air pollution often compounds the effects of these hot temperatures (Rooney, McMichael, Kovats, and Coleman, 1998; Bernard and others, 2001).

A recent study (Kalnay and Cai, 2003) estimates the mean surface warming due to urban sprawl and land-use change to be 0.27°C (0.49°F) for the continental United States. Urban areas may therefore face a compounded problem as they experience both global warming and localized warming from the heat island effect (Figure 11.4).

Severe Storms and Sea-level Rise

Floods, droughts, and extreme storms have claimed millions of lives during the past twenty years and have adversely affected the lives of many more millions of people and caused billions of dollars in property damage (Noji, 1997). On average, disasters killed 123,000 people worldwide each year between 1972 and 1996. Africa suffers the highest rate of disaster-related deaths (Loretti and Tegegn, 1996), although 80 percent of the people affected by natural disasters are in Asia. For every 1 person killed in a natural disaster, an estimated 1,000 people are affected (International Federation of Red Cross and Red Crescent Societies, 1998), either physically or through loss of property or livelihood. Mental disorders such as posttraumatic stress disorder (PTSD) may substantially affect population well-being, depending on the unexpectedness of the impact, the

FIGURE 11.4. URBAN HEAT ISLAND PROFILE.

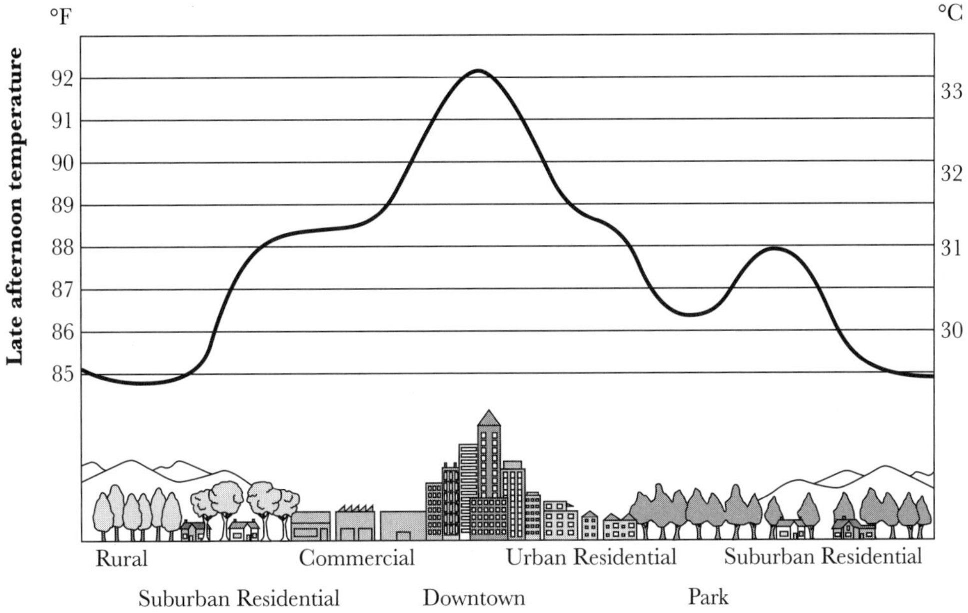

intensity of the experience, the degree of personal and community disruption, and long-term exposure to the visual signs of the disaster (Green, 1982).

Population concentration in high-risk areas such as floodplains and coastal zones increases vulnerability. Degradation of the local environment can also contribute significantly to vulnerability. For example, Hurricane Mitch, the most deadly hurricane to strike the Western Hemisphere in the last two centuries, caused 11,000 deaths in Central America, with thousands of other people still recorded as missing. Many fatalities occurred during mudslides in deforested areas (National Climatic Data Center, 1999). (Figure 11.5 shows where multiple landslides occurred in California following storms in 1998).

Hurricanes form only in regions where sea surface temperatures are above 26°C (Gray, 1979). Knutson, Tuleya, and Kurihara (1998) found that a sea surface warming of slightly over 2°C would intensify hurricane wind speeds by three to seven meters per second (or 5 to 12 percent). (However, predicting the number of hurricanes that will make landfall is currently not possible.)

In addition, sea surface warming will necessarily cause a rise in sea level. One expected effect will be an increase in flooding and coastal erosion in low-lying coastal areas. Under midrange climate change scenarios of a 40 cm sea-level

FIGURE 11.5. LANDSLIDES IN CALIFORNIA REPORTED FROM 1998 STORMS.

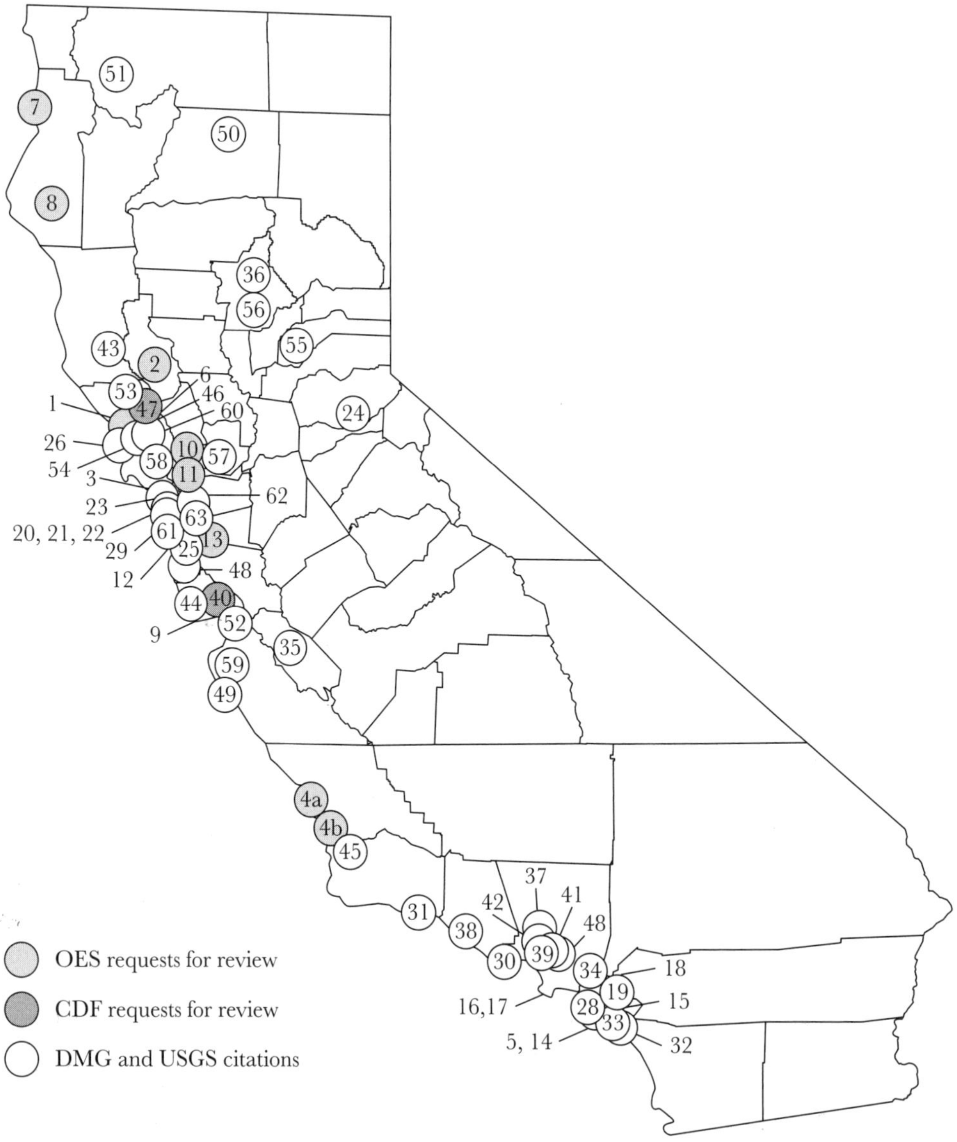

Note: OES = Office of Emergency Services; CDF = California Department of Forestry and Fire Protection.
Source: California Department of Conservation, Division of Mines and Geology, 1998.

FIGURE 11.6. POTENTIAL IMPACT OF SEA-LEVEL RISE ON BANGLADESH.

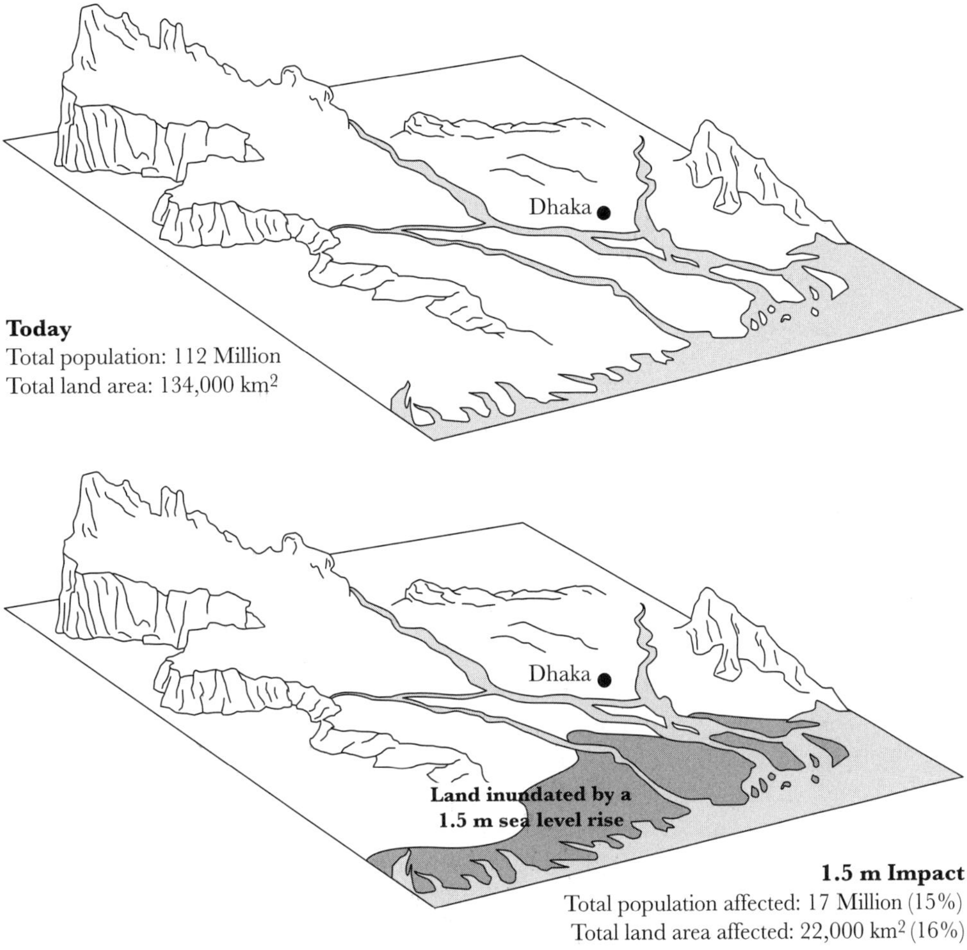

Source: Adapted from United Nations Environment Programme, 2002.

rise by the 2080s, the coastal regions at risk of storm surges are projected to expand and the population at risk to increase from the current 75 million to 200 million (McCarthy and others, 2001). Thirteen of the world's twenty current megacities are situated at sea level. Nicholls and Leatherman (1995) showed that the extreme case of a 1 meter rise in sea level could inundate numerous low-lying areas, affecting 18.6 million people in China, 13 million in Bangladesh (Figure 11.6), 3.5 million in Egypt, and 3.3 million in Indonesia. Countries such as Egypt,

Vietnam, Bangladesh, and small island nations are especially vulnerable, for several reasons. Coastal Egypt is already subsiding due to extensive groundwater withdrawal, and Vietnam and Bangladesh have heavily populated low-lying deltas along their coasts.

Rising sea levels may affect human health and well-being in other ways. Rising seas could result in salination of coastal freshwater aquifers and disrupt stormwater drainage and sewage disposal. These phenomena, with or without flooding, could force coastal communities to migrate (Myers and Kent, 1995). Refugees suffer substantial health burdens, overcrowding, lack of shelter, and competition for resources. Conflict may be one of the worst results emerging from such forced population migrations (Patz and Kovats, 2002).

Drought

Drought is also projected to be an increasing problem with climate change. As discussed in Chapter Eighteen, approximately 1.7 billion people, one-third of the world's population, currently live in water-stressed countries, and that number is projected to increase to 5 billion people by the year 2025. Decreases in average annual stream flow are anticipated in central Asia and southern Africa, where the food supply may be affected.

Food production depends on weather conditions, despite technological advances such as improved crop varieties and irrigation systems. According to the Food and Agriculture Organization (FAO) of the United Nations 790 million people in developing countries are malnourished, with Africa especially hard hit (FAO, 1999). In addition, diarrhea and diseases such as scabies, conjunctivitis, and trachoma are associated with poor hygiene and can result from a breakdown in sanitation when water resources become depleted (Patz, 2001).

Drought can also induce wildfires that threaten health both directly and through reducing air quality. Fire smoke carries a large amount of fine particles that exacerbate cardiac or respiratory problems, such as asthma and chronic obstructive pulmonary disease (COPD). For example, drought-induced fires in Florida in 1998 were associated with increased hospital emergency room visits for asthma, bronchitis, and chest pain (Centers for Disease Control and Prevention, 1999). Fire and climate change modeling for California has shown that the most severe effects of global climate change would occur in the Sierra foothills, where potentially catastrophic fires would increase by 143 percent in grassland and 121 percent in chaparral (Torn, Mills, and Fried, 1998). The same study showed that greater burn intensity resulted from a predicted change in fuel moisture and wind speeds.

Weather, Air Pollution, and Health

Climate change may affect exposure to air pollutants in many ways because it can influence both the levels of pollutants that are formed and the ways these pollutants are dispersed. If the climate becomes warmer and more variable, air quality is likely to suffer (Bernard and others, 2001).

Ozone is an example of a pollutant whose concentration may increase with a warmer climate. As explained in Chapter Fourteen, many species of trees emit volatile organic compounds (VOCs) such as isoprenes, which are precursors of ozone. Isoprene production is controlled primarily by leaf temperature and light. Biogenic VOC emissions are so sensitive to temperature that an increase of as little as 2°C could cause a 25 percent increase in these emissions (Guenther, 2002). Under the right circumstances, higher levels of isoprenes result in higher levels of ozone.

Moreover, higher temperatures increase ozone formation when precursors are present. As explained in Chapter Fourteen, the *ozone season* in affected cities occurs during summer months, when warmer temperatures promote ozone formation. This relationship is nonlinear, with a stronger correlation seen at temperatures above 32°C. (Particulate matter formation can also increase at higher temperature, due to increased gas-phase reaction rates.) One study showed that temperature variability can change peak ozone levels and twenty-four-hour average levels of particulate matter of 2.5 micrometers or less ($PM_{2.5}$) by 16 percent and 25 percent, respectively, when other meteorological variables and emission patterns are held constant (Aw and Kleeman, 2003). Another study, which modeled the impact of climate conditions fifty years in the future on air pollution (Hogrefe and others, 2004), predicted an increase in daily average ozone levels of 3.7 parts per billion. Moreover, there was substantial variation, with today's most polluted cities projected to experience the greatest increase in temperature-related ozone pollution. For fifteen cities in the eastern United States, the average number of days exceeding the health-based eight-hour ozone standard was found to increase by 60 percent—from twelve to almost twenty days per summer—by the 2050s because of global warming (see Figure 11.7) (Patz and others, 2004).

Another air contaminant that may increase with climate change is pollen. Higher levels of carbon dioxide promote growth and reproduction by many plants, including those that produce allergens. For example, ragweed plants experimentally exposed to high levels of carbon dioxide can increase their pollen production several-fold, perhaps part of the reason for rising ragweed pollen levels in recent decades (Ziska and Caulfield, 2000; Wayne and others, 2002). In a study

FIGURE 11.7. THE PROJECTED INCREASE IN OZONE EXCEEDANCE DAYS ASSOCIATED WITH GLOBAL WARMING.

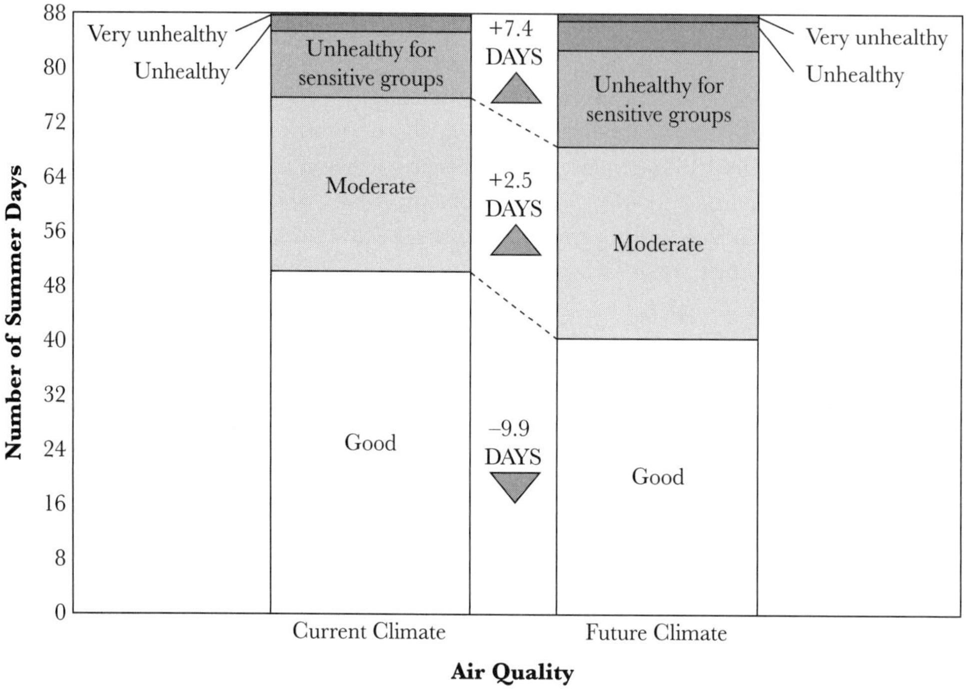

Source: Patz and others, 2004. © NRDC.

comparing urban and rural parts of Baltimore, ragweed grew faster, flowered earlier, and produced more pollen at urban locations than at rural locations, presumably because air temperature and CO_2 levels are significantly higher in urban areas (Ziska and others, 2003). This prompted the investigators to dub cities "harbingers of climate change." People who suffer from hay fever and seasonal allergies would be especially susceptible to these changes.

Once pollutants are formed, climate change may affect how much people are exposed. Weather influences the dispersal and ambient concentrations of many pollutants. For example, large high-pressure systems often create a temperature inversion, trapping pollutants in the boundary layer at the earth's surface. Similarly, increased wind accompanying warmer air may distribute pollutants over broad areas. It has been suggested that climate change should be expected to increase the frequency of occasions that combine very hot weather with increases in air pollutant concentrations (McMichael and others, 2001).

The relationship between climate change and air pollution is complex. Many feedback loops may operate, some helpful and others harmful. On the one hand, for example, some particles in the air reflect radiant energy and can help to cool the atmosphere; the best-known example is the cooling that follows major volcanic eruptions. On the other hand a warmer climate will mean more demand for energy to power air conditioners, resulting in more air pollution. Overall, for air pollution as for many other aspects of climate change, the impacts are not fully understood, but potential impacts on public health deserve careful attention.

Waterborne Diseases

Waterborne diseases are likely to become a greater problem as climate change continues and affects both freshwater and marine ecosystems. In freshwater systems, both water quantity and water quality can be affected by climate change. In marine waters, changes in temperature and salinity will affect coastal ecosystems in ways that may increase the risk of certain diseases.

Freshwater Ecosystems

Waterborne diseases are particularly sensitive to changes in the hydrologic cycle. As discussed in Chapter Eighteen, both water quantity and water quality play a role in waterborne disease.

The impact of climate change on water quantity is relatively straightforward. In some regions precipitation is expected to increase, whereas in others decreased precipitation, even to the point of ongoing drought, is predicted. Water shortages contribute to poor hygiene and that in turn contributes to diarrheal disease, especially in poor countries. At the other extreme, flooding can contaminate drinking water with runoff from sewage lines, containment lagoons (such as those used in animal feeding operations), or conventional nonpoint source pollution across watersheds.

Climate change, and associated severe weather events, can affect water quality in complex ways. One example is provided by cryptosporidiosis, one of the most prevalent diarrheal diseases in the world. Cryptosporidium is a protozoan associated with domestic livestock that can contaminate drinking water (where the oocyst is resistant to chlorine treatment) during periods of heavy precipitation. The 1993 cryptosporidiosis outbreak in Milwaukee, which resulted in 403,000 reported cases, coincided with unusually heavy spring rains and runoff from melting snow (MacKenzie and others, 1994). Similarly, studies of the Delaware River have shown that *Giardia* and cryptosporidium oocyst counts correlate with the amount of rainfall (Atherholt, LeChevallier, Norton, and Rosen, 1998). In fact a review of waterborne disease outbreaks in the United States from all causes over nearly fifty years demonstrated a distinct seasonality, a spatial clustering in key watersheds and an association with heavy precipitation (Curriero, Patz, Rose, and Lele, 2001). Certain watersheds, by virtue of associated land-use patterns and the presence of human and animal fecal contaminants, are at high risk of surface water contamination after heavy rains, and this has serious implications for drinking-water purity.

Heavy runoff after severe rainfall can also contaminate recreational waters and increase the risk of human illness. For example, heavy runoff leads to higher bacterial counts in rivers in coastal areas and at beaches along the coast; this association is strongest at the beaches closest to rivers (Dwight, Semenza, Baker, and Olson, 2002). This suggests that the public health risk of swimming at beaches increases with heavy rainfall, a predicted consequence of climate change.

Marine Ecosystems

Warm water and nitrogen favor blooms of marine algae, including two groups, dinoflagellates and diatoms, that can release toxins into the marine environment. These blooms—previously called *red tides*—can cause acute paralytic, diarrheic, and amnesic poisoning in humans, as well as extensive die-offs of fish, shellfish, and marine mammals and birds that depend on the marine food web. Over the past three decades the frequency and global distribution of toxic algal incidents appear to have increased, and more human intoxication from algal sources has occurred (Van Dolah, 2000). For example, during the 1987 El Niño, a bloom of *Gymnodinium breve,* previously confined to the Gulf of Mexico, extended northward after warm Gulf Stream water reached far up the U.S. east coast, resulting in human neurological poisonings from shellfish and in substantial fish kills (Tester and others, 1991). Similarly that year, an outbreak of amnesic shellfish poisoning occurred on Prince Edward Island when warm eddies of the Gulf Stream neared the shore and heavy rains increased nutrient-rich runoff (Hallegraeff, 1993).

Some bacteria, especially *Vibrio* species, also proliferate in warm marine waters. Copepods (or zooplankton), which feed on algae, can serve as reservoirs for *Vibrio cholerae* and other enteric pathogens. For example, in Bangladesh cholera follows seasonal warming of sea surface temperatures, which can enhance plankton blooms (Colwell, 1996). Similarly, during the 1997 and 1998 El Niño event, winter temperatures in Lima, Peru, increased more than 5°C above normal, and the number of daily hospital admissions for diarrhea increased by more than 200 percent compared to expected levels based on admissions over the prior five years (Checkley and others, 2000). Long-term studies of the El Niño Southern Oscillation, or ENSO, have confirmed this pattern. ENSO refers to natural year-to-year variations in sea surface temperatures, surface air pressure, rainfall, and atmospheric circulation across the equatorial Pacific Ocean. This cycle provides a model for observing climate-related changes in many ecosystems. ENSO has had an increasing role in explaining cholera outbreaks in recent years, perhaps because of concurrent climate change (Rodo, Pascual, Fuchs, and Faruque, 2002). Overall there is increasing evidence that climate change can contribute to the risk of waterborne diseases in both marine and freshwater ecosystems.

Vector-Borne Diseases

The life cycle of vector-borne pathogens (for example, protozoa, bacteria, and viruses) involves much time outside the human host and therefore much exposure to and influence from environmental conditions. The range of climatic conditions in which each infective or vector species can survive and reproduce is limited. The incubation time of a vector-borne infective agent within its vector organism is typically very sensitive to changes in temperature and humidity (Patz and others, 2003) (Box 11.1).

Box 11.1. Some Effects of Weather and Climate on Vector- and Rodent-Borne Diseases

Vector-borne pathogens spend part of their life cycle in cold-blooded arthropods that are subject to many environmental factors. Changes in weather and climate that can affect transmission of vector-borne diseases include temperature, rainfall, wind, extreme flooding or drought, and sea-level rise. Rodent-borne pathogens can be affected indirectly by ecological determinants of food sources affecting rodent population size, and floods can displace and lead them to seek food and refuge.

Temperature effects on selected vectors and vector-borne pathogens

Vector

Survival can decrease or increase depending on the species

Some vectors have higher survival at higher latitudes and altitudes with higher temperatures

Changes in the susceptibility of vectors to some pathogens (e.g., higher temperatures reduce the size of some vectors but reduce the activity of others)

Changes in the rate of vector population growth

Changes in feeding rate and host contact (which may alter the survival rate)

Changes in the seasonality of populations

Pathogen

Decreased extrinsic incubation period of pathogen in vector at higher temperatures

Changes in the transmission season

Changes in distribution

Decreased viral replication

Effects of changes in precipitation on selected vector-borne pathogens

Vector

Increased rain may increase larval habitat and vector population size by creating a new habitat

Excess rain or snowpack can eliminate habitat by flooding, thus decreasing the vector population size

Low rainfall can create habitat by causing rivers to dry into pools (dry season malaria)

Decreased rain can increase container-breeding mosquitoes by forcing increased water storage

Epic rainfall events can synchronize vector host-seeking and virus transmission

Increased humidity increases vector survival; decreased humidity decreases vector survival

Pathogen

Few direct effects but some data on humidity effects on malarial parasite development in the anopheline mosquito host.

Vertebrate Host

Increased rain can increase vegetation, food availability, and population size

Increased rain can also cause flooding and decrease population size but increase contact with humans

Decreased rain can eliminate food and force rodents into housing areas, increasing human contact, but it can also decrease population size

Increased Sea Level

Alter estuary flow and change existing salt marshes and associated mosquito species, decreasing or eliminating selected mosquito breeding sites (e.g., reduced habitat for *Culiseta melanura*)

Source: Gubler and others, 2001.

Mosquito-Borne Diseases

Malaria and arboviruses are transmitted to humans by mosquitoes. Because insects are cold-blooded, climate change can shift the distribution of mosquito populations, affect mosquito biting rates and survival, and shorten or lengthen pathogen development time inside the mosquito, which ultimately determines infectivity.

Malaria. Malaria is a temperature-sensitive disease. According to the World Health Organization (1996), malaria is the vector-borne disease most sensitive to long-term climate change. The incidence of malaria varies seasonally in highly endemic areas, and malaria transmission has been associated with temperature anomalies in some African highland areas (Githeko and Ndegwa, 2001). In the Punjab region of India excessive monsoon rainfall and resultant high humidity have been recognized for years as major factors in the occurrence of malaria epidemics. More recently in that region, malaria epidemics have increased approximately fivefold during the year following an El Niño year (Bouma and van der Kaay, 1996).

Arboviruses. The rate of dengue virus replication in *Aedes aegypti* mosquitoes in the laboratory increases directly with temperature. Biological-based models have been developed to explore the influence of projected temperature change on the incidence of dengue fever. When linked to future climate change projections, these models suggest that relatively small increases in temperature in temperate regions, given viral introduction into a susceptible human population, are likely to increase the potential for epidemics (Patz, Martens, Focks, and Jetten, 1998).

Certain arboviruses, such as Saint Louis encephalitis virus (SLEV), are associated with climatic factors. Using a hydrology model to simulate water table depth (WTD) and SLEV incidence in "sentinel" chickens, Shaman and colleagues (2002) estimated human transmission risk. The transmission cycle can be divided into four categories: *maintenance,* occurring between January and March; *amplification,* occurring between April and June; *early transmission,* occurring between July and September; and *late transmission,* occurring between October and December. Mosquito vectors interact with avian hosts during the period of amplification. The authors found that each episode in which sentinel chickens turned positive for SLEV was preceded by a wet period followed by a drought. The following sequence of events is hypothesized: spring drought forces the mosquito vector, *Culex nigripalpus,* to converge with immature and adult wild birds in restrictive, densely vegetated, hammock habitats. This forced interaction of mosquito vectors and avian hosts creates an ideal setting for rapid transmission and amplification of SLEV. Once the drought ends and water sources are restored, the infected vectors and hosts disperse and transmit SLEV throughout a much broader geographic area. This study suggests that similar drought-induced amplification might occur in other arboviruses.

Climate variability may also have an effect on West Nile virus (WNV), a disease only recently introduced into the New World. Like SLEV, WNV is a vector-borne zoonotic disease (that is, it can migrate from animals to humans), which is normally transmitted between birds by the *Culex pipiens* mosquito. This mosquito tends to breed in foul standing water. In drought conditions, standing water pools become even more concentrated with organic material. Birds may circulate around small water holes, so interaction with mosquitoes is likely increased. In 1999, these climatic conditions existed in the mid-Atlantic states. These weather events, together with urban and suburban environments suitable for avian species, may explain the U.S. epidemic of West Nile virus (Epstein, 2001).

Rodent-Borne Diseases

Hantavirus infections are transmitted largely by exposure to infectious excreta from rodents and may cause serious disease and a high fatality rate in humans. For hantavirus pulmonary syndrome, which newly emerged in the Southwest United States in 1993, weather conditions led to a growth in rodent populations and subsequent disease transmission followed by El Niño–driven heavy rainfall (Glass and others, 2000).

Extreme flooding or hurricanes can lead to outbreaks of leptospirosis. An epidemic of leptospirosis in Nicaragua followed heavy flooding in 1995. In one case-control study, a fifteenfold risk of disease was associated with walking through flooded waters (Trevejo and others, 1998).

Box 11.2. El Niño and Predictive Models for Early Warning Systems

The extreme climate variability brought on by the El Niño phenomenon can be used to predict disease outbreaks. The ENSO events themselves can be anticipated months in advance, so early warning systems (EWSs) for associated diseases are feasible.

Several studies have found strong ENSO-disease associations, and these associations are either already being used for early warning (as the findings of Glass and others, 2000, are) or have good potential for use in a weather-based disease early warning system.

Glass and others (2000) found that ENSO-related heavy rainfall, with subsequent increase in the rodent population, preceded human cases of hantavirus pulmonary syndrome (HPS) in the American Southwest. Landsat Thematic Mapper satellite imagery, collected the year before the outbreak, was used to estimate HPS risk by logistic regression analysis. Satellite and topographic elevation data showed a strong association between environmental conditions and HPS risk during the following year. Repeated analysis using satellite imagery from a non-ENSO year (1995) showed substantial decreases in HPS in medium- to high-risk areas. The U.S. Indian Health Service now uses this ENSO-based predictive model in a regional hantavirus early warming system.

Linthicum and others (1999) discovered a strong relationship between Rift Valley fever and ENSO-driven rainfall in East Africa. Rift Valley fever virus outbreaks in East Africa from 1950 to May 1998 followed periods of unusually high rainfall. Using Pacific and Indian Ocean sea surface temperature anomalies, coupled with Normalized Difference Vegetation Index (NDVI) satellite data, Rift Valley fever outbreaks could be predicted up to five months before they occurred in East Africa. Near-real-time monitoring with satellite images could pinpoint actual affected areas, with good prospects of becoming a useful disease EWS for targeting livestock vaccination efforts to protect both animals and humans.

Pascual and colleagues (Pascual and others, 2000; Rodo and others, 2002) analyzed ENSO-cholera relationships in Bangladesh. Results from nonlinear time series analysis supported an important role for ENSO in predicting disease epidemics. Considering a possible threshold effect, it may be feasible to develop a cholera EWS for this region.

Source: Adapted from Patz and others, 2003.

Land-Use Change, Microclimate, and Vector-Borne Diseases

Intact ecosystems, which preserve landscape integrity and biodiversity, form the basis of many essential ecosystem services (see Chapter One). However, global vegetation cover is changing far more rapidly than is global climate. Land cover is disrupted by such forces as deforestation, human settlement sprawl, industrial development, road construction (causing linear disturbances, for example), large water control projects (such as dams, canals, irrigation systems, and reservoirs), and climate change. Natural landscapes are being destroyed both incrementally and on a very large scale. A global pattern of landscape fragmentation has emerged.

These changes can affect human and wildlife health by altering both habitat and microclimate. The World Health Organization has recorded over thirty-six new, emerging infectious diseases since 1976; many of these are the direct result of landscape influence on disease ecology. In fact it is estimated that 75 percent of all emerging diseases derive from animal zoonoses (Taylor, Latham, and Woolhouse, 2001). A similar pattern is seen with reemerging diseases such as malaria and dengue fever; landscape changes have been accompanied by the spread of pathogens into new areas (Patz, 2001). For example, the various species of anopheline mosquitoes differ in their competence to transmit malaria. Because these species occupy a variety of ecological niches, habitat alterations may favor the spread of mosquitoes more likely to transit malaria. The recognition of these apparent links gave rise to the Millennium Ecosystem Assessment, an international effort to document the effect of degraded ecosystems on human health and well-being (http://www.millenniumassessment.org/).

Food Productivity and Malnutrition

Climate change is likely to have major effects on crop and livestock production. Some changes will be positive and others negative, and the net impact on food production will likely vary from place to place. Changes in food production will depend on several key factors. First are the direct effects of temperature, precipitation, CO_2 levels (relating to, for example, the CO_2 fertilization effect), and extreme climate variability and sea-level rise (Reilly, 1996). Next are the indirect effects of climate-induced changes in soil quality, incidence of plant diseases, and weed and insect populations. Greater heat and humidity will also increase food spoilage. In the U.K., researchers have found a strong relation between the incidence of food-borne disease and the temperature in the month preceding the illness (Bentham and Langford, 1995), suggesting food poisoning or spoilage. The last two decades have seen a continuing deterioration of food production in Africa, caused in part by persistent drought. Finally, the extent to which adaptive responses are available to farmers must be considered.

Poorer countries already struggle with large and growing populations and malnutrition and are particularly vulnerable to changes in food production. Some regions, such as arid and subhumid areas in Africa, are expected to experience marked reductions in crop yield, decreases in production, and increases in the risk of hunger as a result of climate change. One analysis indicates that by the year 2060, an additional 40 to 300 million people—relative to a projected baseline of 640 million people—could be at risk of malnutrition due to anthropogenic warming (Rosenzweig, Parry, Fischer, and Frohberg, 1993).

An interesting aspect of agricultural changes is the possibility of increased pesticide exposure. According to the National Agriculture Assessment Group (NAAG, 2002), climate change is expected to bring an increase in pest problems for most locations and most crops studied. Agricultural pesticide use poses risks not only for farmers and farmworkers but also for the population at large (see Chapter Twenty). In addition to affecting those exposed occupationally, pesticide aerosols can drift to nearby communities and pesticide-laden agricultural runoff can find its way into groundwater. Increased pesticide demand may unfold as yet another indirect health consequence of climate change.

Conclusion

The links between human health and climate change are diverse and occur via multiple pathways of exposure. Moreover, some of the long-term and complex problems posed by climate change may not be readily discernible over short time spans. Accordingly, we need expanded efforts in both classical and scenario-based risk assessment to anticipate these problems. In addition, the many health impacts of climate change must be studied in the context of many other environmental and behavioral determinants of disease.

Climate and health studies, for example, must consider key variables such as poverty, sanitation, land-use changes, and public health surveillance and mitigation programs. Paramount to a proper approach in this field is interdisciplinary cooperation. Increased disease surveillance, integrated modeling, and use of geographically based data systems will improve the ability of the medical community to take anticipatory measures.

The Public Health Approach to Climate Change

Two kinds of strategies, both familiar to public health professionals, are available for responding to climate change. The first, known as *mitigation,* corresponds to primary prevention, and the second, known as *adaptation* or *accommodation,* corresponds to secondary prevention.

Primary prevention refers to efforts to stabilize or reduce the production of greenhouse gases, that is, to address the anthropogenic cause of climate change. This goal can be achieved through policies and technologies that result in more efficient energy production and reduced energy demand. For example, sustainable energy sources such as wind and solar energy do not contribute to greenhouse gas emissions (see Chapter Fifteen). Similarly, transportation policies that rely on walking, bicycling, mass transit, and fuel-efficient automobiles result in fewer greenhouse gas emissions than are produced by the current U.S. reliance on large, fuel-inefficient automobiles for most transportation (see Chapter Seventeen). Much energy use occurs in buildings, and *green buildings* that emphasize energy efficiency, together with electrical appliances that conserve energy, also play a role in reducing greenhouse gas emissions. A final aspect of mitigation aims not to reduce the production of greenhouse gases, but to accelerate their removal. Carbon dioxide sinks such as forests are effective in this regard, so land-use policies that preserve and expand forests are an important tool in mitigating global climate change.

Accommodation refers to efforts to lessen the public health impact of climate change. For example, if we anticipate severe weather events such as hurricanes, then preparation by emergency management authorities and medical facilities can minimize morbidity and mortality. Similarly, public health surveillance systems can detect outbreaks of infectious diseases in vulnerable areas, a prerequisite to early control.

Ethical and Political Considerations

At this time the United Nations Framework Convention on Climate Change (FCCC) is the only international agreement under which national governments are responsible for reducing greenhouse gas emissions, the goal of course being to avoid, postpone, or reduce the environmental, economic, and social impacts of climate change. The Kyoto Protocol was negotiated within the FCCC in 1997 as the legal instrument to curb emissions of greenhouse gases. To be ratified, fifty-five countries were required to sign and participate, with the goal being an overall reduction of 55 percent of greenhouse gas emissions from industrial countries. Russia signed the treaty in 2004, joining Japan, Canada, and previously participating nations in Europe, clearing the way for the treaty to enter into force early in 2005. The United States and Australia have refused to ratify it from the outset, arguing that the scientific uncertainties were too large, the costs of compliance prohibitive, and the protocol's impact too marginal without the participation of the largest of the developing countries (for example, China and India). However, these developing countries are expected to sign onto the treaty once the richer countries have shown commitment and initiated greenhouse emissions mitigation.

It is true that stabilizing greenhouse gases at any level below 700 ppm (compared to a preindustrial level of 280 ppm and today's level of about 380 ppm) will require significantly deeper greenhouse gas reductions than called for by the Kyoto Protocol. However, objections from a developed country like the United States on the basis of fairness and efficacy require serious examination. The United States has 5 percent of the total world population yet produces 25 percent of the total annual greenhouse gas emissions. This discrepancy exemplifies the ethical implications posed by climate change. The capacity to cope with climate change impacts varies with a nation's wealth, technology, and general infrastructure. Poor populations in the developing world have little by way of industry, transportation, or intensive agriculture, they contribute only a fraction of the greenhouse gases per capita that the developed countries produce, and their capacity to protect themselves against the adverse consequences of what are mostly others' greenhouse gases is quite limited. Thus climate change is one of the largest environmental and health equity challenges of our times. Of course, if developing nations do not choose development pathways using more efficient energy technology, global climate change trends will intensify even as the imbalance of equity decreases (Patz and Kovats, 2002).

The potential impacts of climate change on the health of future human generations and the difficulty of reversing ecosystem changes once they have occurred warrant increased efforts by many scientific and development policy disciplines. Considering the broad array of impacts reviewed in this chapter, primary preventive measures to avert climate change, including reduction of greenhouse gas emissions and preservation of greenhouse gas sinks through appropriate land-use policies, are likely necessary in view of the scale of health impacts and the time frame in which confirming information may emerge. Understanding the linkages between climatological and ecological changes as determinants of disease will ultimately help us in constructing predictive models to guide effective disease prevention.

Thought Questions

1. Climate change is the major environmental health challenge of the twenty-first century. Agree or disagree, and explain your reasoning.
2. Consider a broad range of *current* environmental health problems that would be exacerbated by climate change. How might existing public health practices be altered to anticipate the effects of climate change?
3. What are some of the key driving forces behind both the risks of climate change and our vulnerabilities to that change? Which scientific experts would be best able to assemble a comprehensive assessment of climate change risks? What types of policymakers should be involved and at what levels (local, regional, international)?

References

Arctic Climate Impact Assessment. *Impacts of a Warming Arctic.* New York: Cambridge University Press, 2004.

Atherholt, T. B., LeChevallier, M. W., Norton, W. D., and Rosen, J. S. "Effect of Rainfall on Giardia and Crypto." *Journal of the American Water Works Association,* 1998, *90*(9), 66–80.

Aw, J., and Kleeman, M. J. "Evaluating the First-Order Effect of Inter-Annual Temperature Variability on Urban Air Pollution." *Journal of Geophysical Research—Atmospheres,* 2003, *108,* D12.

Bentham, G., and Langford, I. H. "Climate Change and the Incidence of Food Poisoning in England and Wales." *International Journal of Biometeorology,* 1995, *39,* 81–86.

Bernard, S. M., and others. "The Potential Impacts of Climate Variability and Change on Air Pollution-Related Health Effects in the United States." *Environmental Health Perspectives,* 2001, *109* (suppl. 2), 199–209.

Bouma, M., and van der Kaay, H. "The El Niño Southern Oscillation and the Historic Malaria Epidemics on the Indian Subcontinent and Sri Lanka: An Early Warning System for Future Epidemics?" *Tropical Medicine and International Health,* 1996, *1*(1), 86–96.

Buechley, R. W., Van Bruggen, J., and Truppi, L. E. "Heat Island Equals Death Island?" *Environmental Research,* 1972, *5*(1), 85–92.

California Department of Conservation, Division of Mines and Geology. "1998 Landslide Inventory." [http://anaheim-landslide.com/landslide98.htm]. 1998.

Centers for Disease Control and Prevention. "Surveillance of Morbidity During Wildfires:—Central Florida, 1998." *Morbidity and Mortality Weekly Report,* 1999, *48*(4), 78–79.

Checkley, W., and others. "Effects of El Nino and Ambient Temperature on Hospital Admissions for Diarrhoeal Diseases in Peruvian Children." *Lancet,* 2000, *355,* 442–450.

Colwell, R. R. "Global Climate and Infectious Disease: The Cholera Paradigm." *Science,* 1996, *274,* 2025–2031.

Curriero, F., Patz, J. A., Rose, J., and Lele, S. "The Association Between Extreme Precipitation and Waterborne Disease Outbreaks in the United States, 1948–1994." *American Journal of Public Health,* 2001, *91,* 1194–1199.

Dwight, R. H., Semenza, J. C., Baker, D. B., and Olson, B. H. "Association of Urban Runoff with Coastal Water Quality in Orange County, California." *Water Environment Research,* 2002, *74*(1), 82–90.

Epstein, P. R. "West Nile Virus and the Climate." *Journal of Urban Health,* 2001, *78*(2), 367–371.

Etheridge, D. M., Steele, L. P., Francey, R. J., and Langenfelds, R. L. "Atmospheric Methane Between 1000 A.D. and Present: Evidence of Anthropogenic Emissions and Climatic Variability." *Journal of Geophysical Research,* 1998, *103*(15), 979–993.

Food and Agriculture Organization of the United Nations. *The State of Food Insecurity in the World 1999.* Rome: Food and Agriculture Organization of the United Nations, 1999.

Githeko, A., and Ndegwa, W. "Predicting Malaria Epidemics in the Kenyan Highlands Using Climate Data: A Tool for Decision Makers." *Global Change & Human Health,* 2001, *2,* 54–63.

Glass, G. E., and others. "Using Remotely Sensed Data to Identify Areas of Risk for Hantavirus Pulmonary Syndrome." *Emerging Infectious Diseases,* 2000, *63*(3), 238–247.

Gray, W. "Hurricanes: Their Formation, Structure and Likely Role in the Tropical Circulation." In D. B. Shaw (ed.), *Meteorology over the Tropical Oceans.* London: Royal Meteorology Society, 1979.

Green, B. L. "Assessing Levels of Psychological Impairment Following Disaster: Consideration of Actual and Methodological Dimensions." *Journal of Nervous and Mental Disease,* 1982, *170,* 544–548.

Gubler, D. J., and others. "Climate Variability and Change in the United States: Potential Impacts on Vector- and Rodent-Borne Diseases." *Environmental Health Perspectives,* 2001, *109* (suppl. 2), 223–233.

Guenther, A. "The Contribution of Reactive Carbon Emissions from Vegetation to the Carbon Balance of Terrestrial Ecosystems." *Chemosphere,* 2002, *49*(8), 837–844.

Gulluk, T., Slemr, F., and Stauffer, B. "Simultaneous Measurements of CO_2, CH_4, and N_2O in Air Extracted by Sublimation from Antarctica Ice Cores: Confirmation of the Data Obtained Using Other Extraction Techniques." *Journal of Geophysical Research,* 1998, *103*(15), 971–978.

Hallegraeff, G. M. "PA Review of Harmful Algal Blooms and Their Apparent Global Increase." *Phycologia,* 1993, *32*(2), 79–99.

Hogrefe, C., and others. "Simulating Changes in Regional Air Pollution over the Eastern United States Due to Changes in Global and Regional Climate and Emissions." *Journal of Geophysical Research-Atmospheres,* 2004, *109,* D22301.

Horowitz, M., and Samueloff, S. "Circulation Under Extreme Heat Load." In P. Dejours (ed.), *Comparative Physiology of Environmental Adaptations.* Vol. 2. Basel: Karger, 1987.

Houghton, J. T., and others (eds.). *Climate Change 2001: The Scientific Basis.* Contribution of Working Group I to the Third Assessment Report of the Intergovernmental Panel on Climate Change (IPCC). Cambridge, England: Cambridge University Press, 2001.

International Federation of Red Cross and Red Crescent Societies. *World Disaster Report 1997.* New York: Oxford University Press, 1998.

Kalkstein, L. S., and Tan, G. "Human Health." In K. M. Strzepek and J. B. Smith (eds.), *As Climate Changes: International Impacts and Implications.* New York: Cambridge University Press, 1996.

Kalnay, E., and Cai, M. "Impact of Urbanization and Land-Use Change on Climate." *Nature,* 2003, *423,* 528–531.

Kattenberg, A., and others. "Climate Models: Projections of Future Climate." In J. Houghton and others (eds.), *Climate Change 1995: The Science of Climate Change.* Contribution of Working Group I to the Second Assessment Report of the Intergovernmental Panel on Climate Change. New York: Cambridge University Press, 1996.

Kilbourne, E. M. "Illness Due to Thermal Extremes." In R. B. Wallace (ed.), *Maxcy-Rosenau-Last Public Health and Preventive Medicine.* (14th ed.) Stamford, Conn.: Appleton & Lang, 1998.

Knutson, T. R., Tuleya, R. E., and Kurihara, Y. "Simulated Increase of Hurricane Intensities in a CO2-Warmed Climate." *Science,* 1998, *279*(5353), 1018–1020.

Kovats, S., Wolf, T., and Menne, B. "Heatwave of August 2003 in Europe: Provisional Estimates of the Impact on Mortality." *Euroserveillance Weekly.* [http://www.eurosurveillance.org/ew/2004/040311.asp#7]. 2004.

Linthicum, K. J., and others. "Climate and Satellite Indicators to Forecast Rift Valley Fever Epidemics in Kenya. *Science,* 1999, *285,* 397–400.

Loretti, A., and Tegegn, Y. "Disasters in Africa: Old and New Hazards and Growing Vulnerability." *World Health Statistics Quarterly,* 1996, *49,* 179–184.

MacKenzie, W. R., and others. "A Massive Outbreak in Milwaukee of Cryptosporidium Infection Transmitted Through the Public Water Supply." *New England Journal of Medicine,* 1994, *331*(3), 161–167.

Mann M. E., Bradley R. S., and Hughes M. K. "Global-Scale Temperature Patterns and Climate Forcing over the Past Six Centuries." *Nature,* 1998, *392,* 779–787.

McCarthy, J., and others (eds.). *Climate Change 2001: Impacts, Adaptation, and Vulnerability.* Contribution of Working Group II to the Third Assessment Report of the Intergovernmental Panel on Climate Change. New York: Cambridge University Press, 2001.

McMichael, A., and others. "Human Health." In J. McCarthy and others (eds.), *Climate Change 2001: Impacts, Adaptation, and Vulnerability.* Contribution of Working Group II to the Third Assessment Report of the Intergovernmental Panel on Climate Change. New York: Cambridge University Press, 2001.

Myers, N., and Kent, J. *Environmental Exodus: An Emergent Crisis in the Global Arena.* Washington, D.C.: Climate Institute, 1995.

National Agriculture Assessment Group. *Agriculture: The Potential Consequences of Climate Variability and Change for the United States.* New York: Cambridge University Press, 2002.

National Climatic Data Center. "Mitch: The Deadliest Atlantic Hurricane Since 1780." [http://www.ncdc.noaa.gov/ol/reports/mitch/mitch.html]. 1999.

National Oceanic & Atmospheric Administration. *Climate and Weather: Backgrounder Series.* Environmental Health Center of the National Safety Council. [http://www.nsc.org/ehc/climate.htm]. 2001.

National Research Council. *Under the Weather: Climate, Ecosystems, and Infectious Disease.* Washington, D.C.: National Academies Press, 2001.

Nicholls R., and Leatherman S. "Global Sea-Level Rise." In K. Strzepek and J. Smith (eds.), *As Climate Changes: International Impacts and Implications* (pp. 92–123). New York: Cambridge University Press, 1995.

Nicholls, N., and others. "Observed Climate Variability and Change." In J. Houghton and others (eds.), *Climate Change 1995: The Science of Climate Change.* Contribution of Working Group I to the Second Assessment Report of the Intergovernmental Panel on Climate Change. New York: Cambridge University Press, 1996.

Noji, E. K. "The Nature of Disaster: General Characteristics and Public Health Effects." In E. K. Noji (ed.), *The Public Health Consequences of Disasters.* New York: Oxford University Press, 1997.

Pascual, M., and others. "Cholera Dynamics and El Nino-Southern Oscillation." *Science,* 2000, *289,* 1766–1769.

Patz, J. A. "Public Health Risk Assessment Linked to Climatic and Ecological Change." *Human and Ecological Risk Assessment,* 2001, *7*(5), 1317–1327.

Patz, J. A., and Kovats, R. S. "Hotspots in Climate Change and Human Health." *British Medical Journal,* 2002, *325,* 1094–1098.

Patz, J. A., Martens, W.J.M., Focks, D. A., and Jetten, T. H. "Dengue Fever Epidemic Potential as Projected by General Circulating Models of Global Climate Change." *Environmental Health Perspectives,* 1998, *106,* 147–153.

Patz, J. A., and others. "Climate Change and Infectious Diseases." In A. J. McMichael and others (eds.), *Climate Change and Human Health: Risks and Responses.* Geneva: World Health Organization, 2003.

Patz, J. A., and others. "Heat Advisory: How Global Warming Causes More Bad Air Days." NRDC Report. New York: Natural Resources Defense Council, 2004.

Ramlow, J. M., and Kuller, L. H. "Effects of the Summer Heat Wave of 1988 on Daily Mortality in Allegheny County, PA." *Public Health Reports,* 1990, *105,* 283–289.

Reilly, J. (ed.). "Agriculture in a Changing Climate: Impacts and Adaptations." In R. T. Watson, M. C. Zinyowera, and R. H. Moss (eds.), *Climate Change 1995: Impacts, Adaptations, and Mitigation of Climate Change: Scientific-Technical Analyses.* Contribution of Working Group II to the Second Assessment Report of the Intergovernmental Panel on Climate Change. New York: Cambridge University Press, 1996.

Rodo, X., Pascual, M., Fuchs, G., and Faruque, A. S. "ENSO and Cholera: A Nonstationary Link Related to Climate Change? *Proceedings of the National Academy of Sciences of the United States of America,* 2002, *99*(20), 12901–12906.

Rooney, C., McMichael, A. J., Kovats, R. S., and Coleman, M. P. "Excess Mortality in England and Wales, and in Greater London, During the 1995 Heatwave." *Journal of Epidemiology and Community Health,* 1998, *52,* 482–486.

Rosenzweig, C., Parry, M. L., Fischer, G., and Frohberg, K. *Climate Change and World Food Supply.* Research Report no. 3. Oxford, U.K.: Environmental Change Unit, Oxford University, 1993.

Shaman, J., and others. "Using a Dynamic Hydrology Model to Predict Mosquito Abundances in Flood and Swamp Water." *Emerging Infectious Diseases,* 2002, *8*(1), 6–13.

Taylor, L. H., Latham, S. M., and Woolhouse, M. E. "Risk Factors for Human Disease Emergence." *Philosophical Transactions of the Royal Society of London Part B: Biological Sciences,* 2001, *356,* 983–989.

Tester, P. A., and others. "An Expatriate Red Tide Bloom, Transport, Distribution, and Persistence." *Limnology and Oceanography,* 1991, *36,* 1053–1061.

Torn, M. S., Mills, E., and Fried, J. *Will Climate Change Spark More Wildfire Damage?* LBNL Report no. 42592. Lawrence, Calif.: Lawrence Berkeley National Laboratory, 1998.

Trevejo, R. T., and others. "Epidemic Leptospirosis Associated with Pulmonary Hemorrhage: Nicaragua, 1995. *Journal of Infectious Diseases,* 1998, *178,* 1457–1463.

United Nations Environment Programme. "Potential Impact of Sea-Level Rise on Bangladesh." Vital Climate Graphics. [http://www.unep.net/explorer/gne_content.cfm?DataID=9160&mode=GNE]. 2002.

U.S. Environmental Protection Agency. *The Ozone Report: Measuring Progress Through 2003.* Washington, D.C.: U.S. Environmental Protection Agency, 2004.

Van Dolah, F. M. "Marine Algal Toxins: Origins, Health Effects, and Their Increased Occurrence." *Environmental Health Perspectives,* 2000, *108*(suppl. 1):133–141.

Watson, R. T., and the Core Writing Team. *Climate Change 2001: Synthesis Report.* Cambridge, England: IPCC and Cambridge University Press, 2001.

Wayne, P., and others. "Production of Allergenic Pollen by Ragweed (*Ambrosia artemisiifolia L.*) Is Increased in CO_2-Enriched Atmospheres." *Annals of Allergy, Asthma & Immunology,* 2002, *88*(3), 279–282.

Whitman, S., and others. "Mortality in Chicago Attributed to the July 1995 Heat Wave." *American Journal of Public Health,* 1997, *87,* 1515–1518.

World Health Organization. *World Health Report 1996: Fighting Disease, Fostering Development.* Geneva: World Health Organization, 1996.

Ziska, L., and Caulfield, F. "The Potential Influence of Rising Atmospheric Carbon Dioxide (CO_2) on Public Health: Pollen Production of the Common Ragweed as a Test Case." *World Resources Review,* 2000, *12,* 449–457.

Ziska, L. H., and others. "Cities as Harbingers of Climate Change: Common Ragweed, Urbanization, and Public Health." *Journal of Allergy and Clinical Immunology,* 2003, *111*(2), 290–295.

For Further Information

Several additional major reports and review papers on the health effects of climate change are available. The reports of the UN Intergovernmental Panel on Climate Change (IPCC) represent some of the most authoritative and exhaustive. The latest report was published in 2001, and the next assessment is due in 2006.

Intergovernmental Panel on Climate Change, key summary reports and official graphs and figures [http://www.ipcc.ch].

United Nations Environment Programme (UNEP), materials for educators and the public [http://www.grida.no].

Ecohealth, useful information and student exercises for middle and high school teachers and students [http://ecohealth101.org].

The United States, the United Kingdom, The Netherlands, Portugal, Japan, and several other countries have conducted risk assessments of climate change. For the health findings of the U.S. National Assessment see

Johns Hopkins Bloomberg School of Public Health [http://www.jhsph.edu/nationalassessment-health].

A new international assessment on the effects of degraded ecosystems worldwide on human health and well-being has just been released. The report can be found at

The Millennium Ecosystem Assessment [http://www.millenniumassessment.org].

For information on global climate and land-use change impacts on ecosystems and human health see

Center for Sustainability and the Global Environment (SAGE) [http://www.sage.wisc.edu].

CHAPTER TWELVE

WAR

Barry S. Levy
Victor W. Sidel

War is conventionally defined as armed conflict between, or among, nation-states. The term is also used to denote armed conflicts *within* nations (*civil wars* or *wars of liberation*) and armed actions by clandestine or rebel groups against governments or occupying forces (*guerilla wars, insurgencies,* or *intifadas*) (Sidel and Levy, 2003). War has both immediate and long-term profound impacts on human health (Levy and Sidel, 2000).

Direct and Indirect Impacts of War on Human Health

Today armed conflicts are primarily civil wars (conflicts within countries, to which other countries sometimes contribute military troops) that continue to rage in many parts of the world. For example, a total of twenty-one major armed conflicts occurred in nineteen different locations during 2002, and during the post–Cold War period of 1990 to 2001, there were fifty-seven major armed conflicts in forty-five locations, all but three of which were civil wars (Stockholm International Peace Research Institute, 2002, 2003). War accounts for many deaths as well as many nonfatal injuries and illnesses, many of which have long-term sequelae, ranging from disabling injuries to posttraumatic stress disorder. During the twentieth century, 191 million people died during wars, and many more suffered both the immediate and long-term health consequences of physical and psychological trauma. A particularly disturbing trend has been the increasing percentage of civilian deaths as a proportion of all deaths during war; during World War I, 14 percent of all deaths were among civilians, whereas during some wars in the 1990s, 90 percent of all deaths were among civilians (Garfield and Neugut, 2000).

Much of the morbidity and mortality during war, especially among civilians, has been the result of indirect impacts, including destruction of societal infrastructure, including food and water supply systems, health care facilities and public health services, sewage disposal systems, power plants and electric grids, and transportation and communication systems. Destruction of infrastructure has led to food shortages and resultant malnutrition, contamination of food and of drinking water and resultant foodborne and waterborne illness, and health care and public health deficiencies and resultant disease. War also makes many people refugees and internally displaced persons, whose basic human needs may not be met; a substantial number of the 12 to 20 million refugees and 22 to 25 million internally displaced persons in the world today have been uprooted from their homes as a result of war or the threat of war (Worldwatch Institute, 2003). In addition, war diverts resources, promotes violence as a means of settling disputes, and adversely affects the environment—the focus of this chapter.

Impacts of Other Military Activities, Including Preparation for War, on Human Health

Other military activities, including preparation for war, can also adversely affect human health. Some of the impacts are direct, such as injuries and deaths during training exercises; others are indirect. Like war itself, preparation for war can divert human, financial, and other resources that otherwise might be used for health and human services. Governments' and societies' preoccupation with preparation for war often known as *militarism,* may lead to massive diversion and subversion of efforts to promote human welfare. Diversion of resources is a problem worldwide but especially acute in developing countries. Many developing countries have substantially higher military expenditures than health-related expenditures; for example, in 1990, Ethiopia spent the equivalent of $16 per capita for military expenditures and only $1 per capita for health, and Sudan spent $25 per capita for military expenditures as opposed to $1 per capita for health (Foege, 2000).

This diversion may be exacerbated by policies that lead to *preemptive war* (when an attack is allegedly imminent) and *preventive war* (when an attack may allegedly occur some time in the future). Such policies, in addition to being illegal under international law, may increase the number of military interventions, increase the diversion of resources to war, and increase environmental damage.

In addition, war and preparation for war can promote violence as a means for settling disputes. Familiarity with use of weapons through military training and war, especially assault weapons, may lead to their use in civilian life afterward. Furthermore, war often glorifies violence. The glorification of war is so pervasive that, generation after generation, young males have been drawn into proving their manhood by going to battle. Now women too are assuming combatant roles. Familiarity with the use of weapons and an acceptance of violence as a means of settling disputes may be a factor contributing to the high rate of gun-related deaths in the United States, by far the highest rate among developed countries.

Impacts of War and Other Military Activities on the Environment

The following section of this chapter focuses on the impacts of war and the preparation for war and other military activities on the environment. We consider the impacts of various types of weapons and other environmental contaminants and also the use of nonrenewable fuels and other materials by the military.

Conventional Weapons

Arms generally known as *conventional weapons,* consisting of explosives, incendiaries, and guns of various sizes, range from small arms and light weapons to artillery. Conventional weapons have accounted for the overwhelming majority of adverse environmental consequences due to war. During World War II, for example, both sides engaged in extensive *carpet bombing* of cities. This not only accounted for many deaths and injuries in Europe and Japan but also caused widespread devastation of urban environments. Another example is the bombing of mangrove forests during the Vietnam War, which led to the destruction of these forests. The resultant bomb craters remain several decades afterward, often filling with stagnant water that is a breeding ground for mosquitoes that transmit malaria and other mosquito-borne diseases. Yet another example is the more than 600 oil fires in Kuwait during Gulf War I, which accounted for widespread environmental devastation as well as respiratory symptoms among people who were exposed to their smoke (Box 12.1).

Box 12.1. The Kuwait Oil Fires

In February 1991, at the end of Gulf War I, retreating Iraqi troops detonated with dynamite more than 600 oil wells in Kuwait, leading to fires that created extensive air pollution. Over 4 million barrels of oil burned a day, and it is estimated that 3,400 metric tons of soot were introduced into the environment of the Persian Gulf between February and November 1991 (Petruccelli and others, 1999).

A study of 1,599 U.S. soldiers after their return from Kuwait found that they experienced eye and upper respiratory tract irritation, shortness of breath, cough, rashes, and fatigue more frequently than other soldiers did during a baseline period. These symptoms were associated with reported proximity to the oil fires, and their occurrence declined after the soldiers departed from Kuwait (Petruccelli and others, 1999).

Another study of 1,560 veterans who served in this war demonstrated that self-reported exposure was associated with asthma, bronchitis, and major depression but did not find an association between these health problems and modeled exposures. The study authors therefore concluded that their findings did not support the idea that the veterans' respiratory symptoms were caused by exposure to oil-fire smoke (Lange and others, 2002). A study of feral cats collected from Kuwait concluded that the oil fires had had little or no long-term effect on the animals examined (Moeller and others, 1994). Another study, on the genotoxicity of soot obtained from the Kuwait oil fires, found dose-dependent increases for both sister chromatid exchanges in human peripheral blood lymphocytes and mutations at the hprt locus in a human lymphoblast cell line; however, similar responses were seen in these two assays when an air particulate sample from the Washington, D.C., area was similarly tested (Kelsey and others, 1994).

The Kuwait oil fires stand as an enduring example of the environmental devastation that occurs in war. In this case, the "fog of war" extended from the fires to the subsequent understanding of the health effects of this exposure. The fact that self-reported exposure was more closely linked to symptoms than was modeled exposure may reflect deficiencies in modeling, may indicate that the exposure was not hazardous, or may suggest that cumulative exposures to smoke, stressful situations, and other wartime conditions act together to adversely affect health. Public health professionals have a responsibility to evaluate the impact of environmental hazards during war and the preparation for war and to work toward the control and prevention of these hazards.

Nuclear Weapons

Nuclear weapons have been increasingly widespread among nations since their development in the 1940s. There are now an estimated 28,000 nuclear warheads in at least eight nations (the United States, Russia, the United Kingdom, France,

China, Israel, India, Pakistan, and possibly North Korea). (In the United States the nuclear stockpile reached a peak in 1967 with approximately 32,000 nuclear warheads of thirty different types. The peak in explosive capacity was reached in 1960 with an explosive capacity equivalent to 20,000 megatons [20 billion tons, or 40 trillion pounds] of TNT, equivalent to 1,400,000 of the nuclear bombs dropped on Hiroshima.) In 2003, the total in the U.S. stockpile was about 10,400 warheads, totaling about 2,000 megatons, equivalent to 140,000 Hiroshima-size bombs. Five thousand of the nuclear weapons in the United States and Russia and possibly more in other countries are on "hair-trigger" alert, ready to fire on a few minutes' notice.

Small nuclear devices have also been produced. The United States once built more than 300 *special atomic demolition munitions* (SADMs, or *backpack nukes*) but dismantled them in the late 1980s and early 1990s because they represented a potential security threat if stolen. Each SADM weighed 163 pounds and could be carried in a backpack. Its explosive power ranged up to 1 kiloton, equal to 1,000 tons of TNT, enough to destroy the center of a city (Windrem, 1997).

The detonation of nuclear bombs over Hiroshima and Nagasaki in August 1945 during World War II led to the immediate deaths of approximately 200,000 people, primarily civilians; brought lasting injury and later death to many others; and caused massive devastation—and widespread radioactive contamination—of the environment in these two cities (Figure 12.1) (Yokoro and Kamada, 2000). Today, in addition to the potential for the further use of nuclear weapons by national armed forces, such as that described in the recent U.S. Nuclear Posture Review, which threatened use of nuclear weapons under a wider range of circumstances than previously specified, the threat that they may be used by individuals and groups is increasing.

From 1945 to 1990, the United States produced approximately 70,000 nuclear weapons; other nations also produced large numbers of these weapons. This production of nuclear weapons has led to major environmental contamination. For example, the area around Chelyabinsk in Russia has been heavily contaminated with radioactive materials from a nearby nuclear weapons production facility. The level of ambient radiation in and near the Techa River in that area has been documented up to twenty-eight times the normal background radiation level (Keller, 1989). Similarly, leakage of radioactive materials from storage of wastes from nuclear weapons production at Hanford, along the Columbia River in Washington State, has led to extensive radioactive contamination. Open-air testing of nuclear weapons by the United States, the Soviet Union, and other countries has also led to environmental contamination, with increased rates of leukemia and other cancers among populations who were downwind from these tests (Box 12.2).

FIGURE 12.1. NAGASAKI AFTER DETONATION OF A NUCLEAR BOMB, AUGUST, 1945.

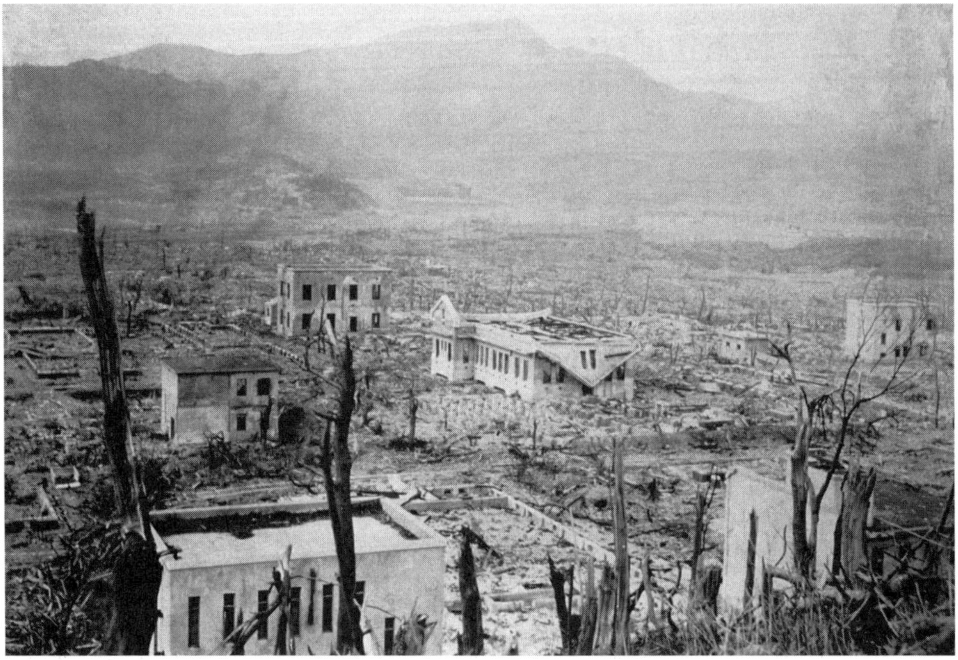

Source: © CORBIS.

Box 12.2. Malignancies Associated with Radioactive Fallout

The world's population has been exposed to low levels of fission products from the testing of nuclear weapons in the atmosphere. Epidemiological associations have been demonstrated between leukemia and nuclear fallout in the general population, especially among people living in areas downwind from open-air testing locations. The strongest association has been with acute and myeloid types of leukemia among children. In addition, the entire U.S. population had increased leukemia rates during and for several years after open-air nuclear testing took place; the rates fell sharply afterward (Archer, 1987). Veterans who received high gamma radiation doses, while participating as military personnel in the U.S. atmospheric nuclear weapons testing program from 1945 to 1962, have had higher mortality from lymphopoietic cancers (relative risk: 3.72; 95% confidence interval [CI]: 1.27–10.83) (Dalager, Kang, and Mahan, 2000). U.S. Navy veterans who participated in atmospheric nuclear testing in

1958 in the Pacific have had increased mortality from cancer (relative risk: 1.42; 95% CI: 1.03–1.97), and specifically from liver cancer (relative risk: 6.42; 95% CI: 1.17–35.3), but no increase in leukemia or lymphoma mortality (Watanabe, Kang, and Dalager, 1995). Servicemen and male civilians from the United Kingdom who participated in the U.K.'s atmospheric nuclear weapons tests and experimental programs in the 1950s and early 1960s have had an increased risk of leukemia, excluding chronic lymphatic leukemia (relative risk: 1.83; 90% CI: 1.15–2.93) (Muirhead and others, 2003).

A weak association has been found between bone marrow dose of radiation from radioactive fallout from the Nevada nuclear test site and all types of leukemia in Utah. The greatest risk of developing acute leukemia was found in people in the high-dose group who were younger than twenty years of age at the time of exposure and who died before 1964 (Stevens and others, 1990). People exposed to more than 2.0 sieverts (Sv) of ionizing radiation from nuclear weapons tests in Kazakhstan from 1949 to 1963 had an almost doubled increased risk of leukemia (odds ratio: 1.91; 95% CI: 0.38–9.67). There was also an excess relative risk for leukemia of 10 percent per 1 Sv of additional exposure (Abylkassimova and others, 2000). People in Norway and Sweden exposed to radioactive fallout from nuclear testing in northwest Russia had an increased risk of thyroid cancer during childhood and adolescence (Lund and Galanti, 1999). The populations of both the United States and the Marshall Islands exposed to radiation from U.S. nuclear weapons testing have had, as a result, an increased occurrence of thyroid cancer that increased with radiation dose to the thyroid (Institute of Medicine, 1999; Takahashi and others, 2003).

Populations were also exposed to radiation after the April 1986 accident at Chernobyl, Ukraine. Populations in Europe most highly exposed to Chernobyl fallout had a slightly higher leukemia incidence and an increasing leukemia risk with estimated cumulative excess radiation dose (Hoffmann, 2002). Children under ten who lived within 150 kilometers (approximately 90 miles) of Chernobyl had an increase in thyroid cancers, likely caused by direct external or internal exposure to short-lived radioactive isotopes, such as iodine-131 and iodine-133 (Shibata and others, 2001).

Public health professionals have a responsibility to help ensure that testing of nuclear weapons, especially in the atmosphere, does not resume.

The dismantling and disposal of nuclear weapons has also led to environmental contamination. The primary site for the disassembly of U.S. nuclear weapons is the Pantex Plant, located seventeen miles northeast of Amarillo in the Texas panhandle. Overall the United States has dismantled about 60,000 nuclear warheads since the 1940s; during the 1990s, 11,751 warheads were dismantled. More than 12,000 plutonium pits (hollow shells of plutonium encased in steel or other metal that are essential components of nuclear weapons) are stored in containers at Pantex. Plans are underway to produce as many as 80 new pits annually at Los Alamos National Laboratory, and the Bush administration advocates building a modern pit facility capable of producing 250 to 900 pits annually by 2018.

Plutonium, an element first produced in the Manhattan Project in 1942, has a half-life of 24,000 years. This new element brings with it extremely long-lasting ionizing radiation risks to health. There has been vigorous debate on methods, such as vitrification, for preventing contamination of the environment by this human-made element, which is also produced by nuclear power plants. However, none of the suggested methods has yet been widely implemented. Merely burying plutonium carries the risk of later leaks as a result of earthquakes or other disasters.

Radiological Weapons

So-called *dirty bombs* (conventional explosive devices mixed with radioactive material) or attacks on nuclear power plants with explosive weapons could scatter highly radioactive material over a wide area. Another example of a radiological weapon is depleted uranium (DU) employed as a casing for armor-penetrating shells. DU is uranium from which the uranium isotope usable in nuclear weapons or in fuel rods for nuclear power plants has been removed. Uranium is an extremely dense material, and a DU casing increases the ability of a shell to penetrate the armor of tanks; uranium is also pyrophoric and bursts into flame on impact. DU-encased shells were used by the United States during Gulf War I and Gulf War II and the war in Kosovo; similar shells were used by the U.K. in Gulf War II. DU, which is both radioactive and extremely toxic, has been demonstrated to cause environmental contamination when used as a weapon. When DU enters the body through ingestion, inhalation, or other means, it is known to affect health through alpha particle irradiation, but there is as yet no clear evidence that environmental contamination by DU weapons has affected health. Use of DU as a weapon is considered "conventional" and legal by the nations using it, but is considered by others to be illegal under the Geneva Conventions and other international treaties.

Chemical Agents

A variety of chemical weapons and related materials have the potential to contaminate the environment during war and the preparation for war. The potential for exposure exists not only for military and civilian populations exposed in wartime but also for workers involved in the development, production, transport, or storage of these weapons and for community residents living near facilities where these weapons are developed, produced, transported, or stored. In addition, disposal of these weapons, involving disassembly and incineration, can represent hazards.

During the Vietnam War the U.S. military used defoliants on mangrove forests and other vegetation, which not only defoliated and killed trees and other plants but may also have led to excessive numbers of birth defects and cases of cancer among nearby residents. In addition, development and production of conventional weapons involves the use of many chemicals that are toxic and can contaminate the environment. Furthermore, there is now a plausible threat that agents other than nation-states may use chemical weapons. For example, a Japanese cult, Aum Shinrikyo, released sarin, a volatile nerve agent, in the subway systems of two Japanese cities in the mid-1990s, resulting in the deaths of nineteen people and injuries to thousands (Spanjaard and Khabib, 2003).

The Chemical Weapons Convention (CWC), which went into effect in 1997, prohibits all development, production, acquisition, stockpiling, transfer, and use of chemical weapons. It requires each nation to destroy its chemical weapons, its chemical weapons production facilities, and any chemical weapons it may have abandoned on the territory of another nation. The verification provisions of the CWC affect not only the military sector but also the civilian chemical industry worldwide through certain restrictions and obligations regarding the production, processing, and consumption of chemicals that are considered relevant to the objectives of the convention. These provisions are to be verified through a combination of reporting requirements, routine on-site inspection of declared sites, and short-notice challenge inspections. The Organization for the Prohibition of Chemical Weapons (OPCW) (established by the CWC and located in The Hague) ensures the implementation of the provisions of the CWC.

This required disposal of chemical weapons has raised a controversy about the safety of the two methods of disposal planned: incineration and chemical neutralization. The United States, on the one hand, has planned to use incineration as the means of demilitarizing its chemical weapons. This method has already been used at Johnston Island in the Pacific to demilitarize nerve agents shipped there from Okinawa and from NATO forces in Europe. Facilities have been constructed for the incineration of chemical weapons stockpiles at sites in the United States. Russia, on the other hand, plans to use chemical neutralization to dispose of its chemical weapons. The debate over safety concerns the fact that incineration leads to the decomposition of the chemical agents into small particles, which are released into the atmosphere through small smokestacks. Some contend that chemical neutralization provides a safer means of disposal, but the Russian process creates a complex organic "soup" that must be mixed with bitumen, a tar-like substance, before disposal in landfills. Scientific and political differences the use of these two methods must be resolved quickly if the United States, Russia, and other countries are to proceed with timely disposal and meet the deadlines imposed by the CWC. Exposure to chemicals or to medications designed to protect against chemical weapons is among the potential causes of Gulf War syndrome that have been investigated (Box 12.3).

Box 12.3. Gulf War Syndrome

Among the approximately 700,000 U.S. military personnel involved in the Persian Gulf War from August 1990 to June 1991, at least 40,000, and perhaps considerably more, have complained of a variety of neurological and other symptoms that are collectively referred to as Gulf War syndrome (GWS). Symptoms have included fatigue, muscle discomfort, joint pain, skin disorders, loss of balance, sensory symptoms, neurobehavioral manifestations, and other disturbances. Potential explanations have included exposures to air contaminants from burning oil wells (see Box 12.1); organophosphate nerve agents; pyridostigmine bromide and other acetylcholine esterase (AChE) inhibitors that were used to protect against potential nerve gas exposure; the insect repellent DEET; pesticides, including permethrin, an insecticide extensively sprayed on military uniforms to protect against insect-borne diseases; depleted uranium; various vaccines; and stress. However, no single causative factor has been identified, and it is probable that this syndrome represents a number of different disorders caused by a complex interaction of multiple factors (Ismail, 2001; Albers and Berent, 2000; Shapiro, Lasarev, and McCauley, 2002; Plapp, 1999). Nevertheless, investigation has shown that many Gulf War veterans are seriously impaired by brain illnesses or injuries that were sustained during this war (Haley, Maddrey, and Gershenfeld, 2002).

An international, multidisciplinary project has summarized current knowledge on unexplained symptoms after terrorism and war. It concluded that in situations involving illness without objective signs or valid laboratory evidence of structural pathology on clinical examination, epidemiological and scientific evidence needs to be carefully scrutinized to determine whether a new and unique illness has occurred or whether this illness can be explained by existing diagnostic entities, such as fibromyalgia, chronic fatigue syndrome, and chronic multisystem illness (Clauw and others, 2003).

Public health professionals have a responsibility to promote further study of Gulf War syndrome and other illnesses among military personnel so that ways to reduce exposure of these individuals to environmental hazards can be found, and to advocate for improved treatment and support of those who are injured or made ill during war.

Biological Agents

Biological agents consist of bacteria, viruses, other microorganisms, and their toxins, which can not only produce illness in humans but can also lead to long-term contamination of the environment that may affect humans, other animals, and plants. For example, Gruinard Island, off the coast of Scotland, was contaminated by a test use of anthrax spores by the U.K. and the United States in 1942. During the 1950s and 1960s, secret, large-scale, open-air tests at the U.S. Army Dugway Proving Ground may have introduced the microorganisms that cause Q fever and Venezuelan equine encephalitis into the deserts of western Utah. In 1979, the accidental release of anthrax spores near Sverdlovsk, in the Soviet Union, resulted in at least seventy-seven cases of inhalation anthrax and at least sixty-six deaths (Meselson and others, 1994).

Antipersonnel Landmines

Antipersonnel landmines are explosives planted on or under the ground by military personnel. They have been termed "weapons of mass destruction, one person at a time." Approximately 100 million landmines are still deployed worldwide in approximately 60 countries. An estimated 230 to 245 million landmines are stockpiled by about 100 countries. Landmines have often been placed in rural areas, posing a threat to residents of these areas and often disrupting farming, herding livestock, and other activities and making large areas uninhabitable. Civilians are the ones most likely to be injured or killed by landmines, which continue to injure and kill 15,000 to 20,000 people annually (Figure 12.2) (International Campaign to Ban Landmines, 2000; Stover, Cobey, and Fine, 2000). (Box 12.4 describes the Anti-Personnel Landmine Convention.)

Box 12.4. Anti-Personnel Landmine Convention

In 1997, the Convention on the Prohibition of the Use, Stockpiling, Production, and Transfer of Anti-Personnel Mines and on Their Destruction (also known as the Ottawa Convention and as the Mine Ban Treaty) was opened for signature; it entered into force in 1999. For developing and leading the International Campaign to Ban Landmines, Jody Williams received the Nobel Peace Prize in 1997. As of January 2005, 152 nations had signed the Mine Ban Treaty, including all nations in the Western Hemisphere except the United States and Cuba and all nations in the North Atlantic Treaty Organization (NATO) except the United States. The other forty-two nations that had not signed the treaty at that time were Russia, most of the former Soviet republics, most nations in the Middle East, and many Asian nations, including China, India, and Pakistan. As a result of this treaty there has been less use of antipersonnel mines, a dramatic decrease in production of landmines, an almost complete end to trade in mines, rapid destruction of mines that have been stockpiled, fewer mine victims in critically affected countries, and more land demined, although an enormous amount of expensive and dangerous demining remains to be done. (More information can be obtained from a number of sources, including the home page of the International Campaign to Ban Landmines, 2005).

Public health professionals have a responsibility to promote the Mine Ban Treaty and to advocate for the abolition of all landmines, complete demining of all mined land, and the treatment and support of those who have been injured by landmines.

FIGURE 12.2. THIS GIRL, AT THE INDIRA GANDHI CHILDREN'S HOSPITAL IN KABUL, AFGHANISTAN, LOST BOTH HER LEGS AFTER STEPPING ON A LANDMINE NEAR HER VILLAGE OUTSIDE KABUL IN 1989.

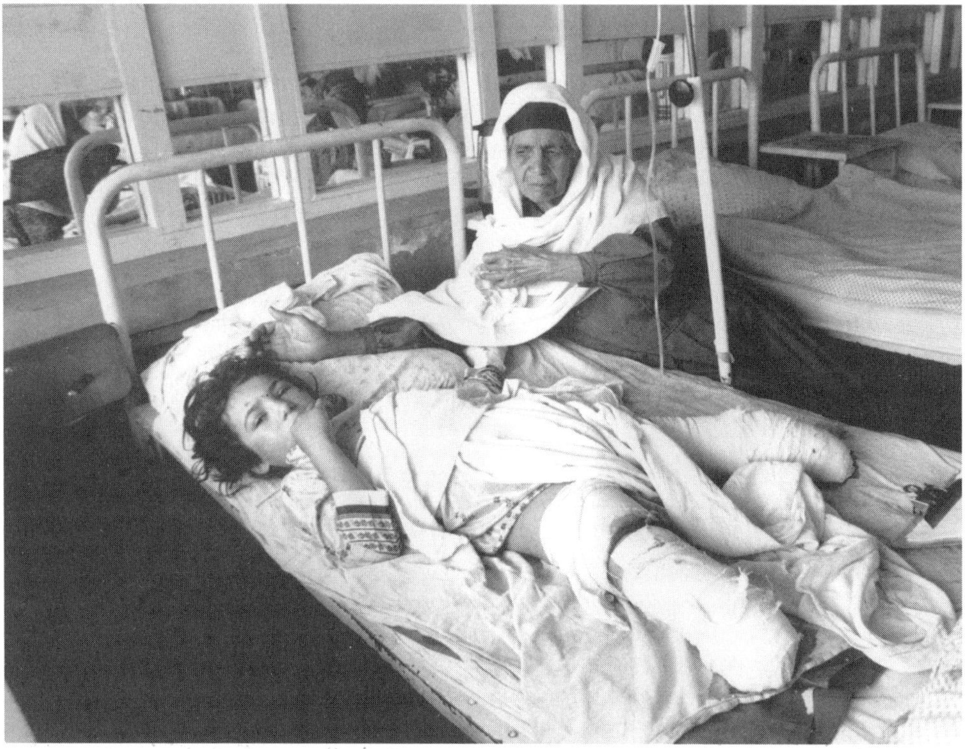

Source: © Howard Davies/CORBIS.

Hazardous Wastes

Hazardous wastes from military operations are potential contaminants of air, water, and soil. Consider these illustrative examples of military hazardous waste sites. At Otis Air Force Base, in Massachusetts, groundwater was contaminated with trichloroethylene (TCE), classified by the International Agency for Research on Cancer as a probable carcinogen, and other toxins. In adjacent towns, lung cancer and leukemia rates have been 80 percent above the state average. At the Rocky Mountain Arsenal, in Colorado, 125 chemicals were dumped over thirty years of nerve gas and pesticide production, "the most contaminated square mile on earth" according to the Army Corps of Engineers. At McChord Air Force Base, in Washington State, benzene, classified as a definite human carcinogen by the

International Agency for Research on Cancer, was found on the base in concentrations as high as 503 parts per billion (ppb), nearly 1,000 times the state's limit of 0.6 ppb (Renner, 1991).

Use of Nonrenewable Fuels and Other Materials by the Military

Both during war and the preparation for war the military forces of many nations consume huge amounts of fossil fuels and other nonrenewable materials. Energy consumption by military equipment can be substantial. For example, an armored division of 348 battle tanks operating for one day consumes more than 2.2 million liters of fuel, and a carrier battle group operating for one day consumes more than 1.5 million liters of fuel. In the late 1980s, the U.S. military annually consumed 18.6 million tons of fuel (more than 44 percent of the world's total), and emitted 381,000 tons of carbon monoxide, 157,000 tons of oxides of nitrogen, 78,000 tons of hydrocarbons, and 17,900 tons of sulfur dioxide (Renner, 2000).

What Can Be Done

The environmental problems created by war and the preparation for war can appear overwhelming. However, standard public health principles and implementation measures can be successfully applied in addressing these problems. The following section of this chapter highlights three of these public health approaches: surveillance and documentation, education and awareness raising, and advocacy for sound policies and programs. Avoiding or mitigating the environmental health consequences of war is only one of the reasons to try to avoid war, and probably not the most compelling reason at that. This is common in environmental health; we often do things for many reasons, of which environmental health is only one.

Surveillance and Documentation

Much can be accomplished by undertaking surveillance and other activities to document environmental problems arising from war and the preparation for war. Surveillance can consist of producing both technical and nontechnical reports that identify potential environmental problems. Technical approaches to surveillance can involve both environmental monitoring and biological monitoring, the latter to document and assess the human burden of environmental contaminants and their adverse health consequences. Nontechnical approaches to surveillance can involve obtaining information from such diverse sources as physician reports, government agency assessments, and reports in the mass media.

Education and Awareness Raising

Much can also be accomplished by educating and by raising the awareness of health professionals, policymakers, and the general public about these environmental problems. In order to disseminate information effectively, a multifaceted approach is often necessary, incorporating use of the mass media, publications by professional organizations and citizens' groups, and personal communications of various types. In the current age of information most people are deluged with communications from many different sources, and it is important to help them distinguish accurate from inaccurate information and set priorities among competing needs.

Advocacy for Sound Policies and Programs

Finally, much can also be accomplished by advocating for improved policies and programs to minimize the impact of war on the environment and to prevent war itself. Here are several policies and programs that environmental health professionals and others can support to achieve these goals:

Strengthening the Nuclear Weapons Treaties. Although treaties now exist that ban chemical weapons and biological weapons, there is no comprehensive treaty banning the use or mandating the destruction of nuclear weapons. Instead, a series of overlapping incomplete treaties has been negotiated. The Partial Test Ban Treaty (PTBT) of 1963, prompted in part by concerns about radioactive contamination, banned nuclear tests in the atmosphere, under water, and in outer space. The expansion of the PTBT, the Comprehensive Nuclear-Test-Ban Treaty (CTBT), a key step toward nuclear disarmament and preventing proliferation, was opened for signature in 1996 and has not yet entered into force. It bans nuclear explosions, for either military or civilian purposes, but does not ban computer simulations and subcritical tests, which some nations rely on to maintain the option of developing new nuclear weapons. As of early 2005, the CTBT had been signed by 175 nations and ratified by 120. Entry into force requires ratification by all 44 nuclear-capable nations (those with nuclear reactors), of which 33 had ratified it by early 2005 (Progress can be tracked at the Web site of the Preparatory Commission for the Comprehensive Nuclear-Test-Ban Treaty Organization [http://www.ctbto.org/]).

The Treaty on the Non-Proliferation of Nuclear Weapons (also called the Non-Proliferation Treaty, or NPT) was opened for signature in 1968 and entered into force in 1970. By early 2005, a total of 188 nations had ratified this treaty. The five nuclear weapon states recognized under the NPT—China, France, Russia, the United Kingdom, and the United States—are parties to it, although

India, Pakistan, Israel, and North Korea are not. The NPT attempts to prevent the spread of nuclear weapons by restricting transfer of certain technologies. It relies on a control system carried out by the International Atomic Energy Agency (IAEA), which also promotes nuclear energy. In exchange for the commitment of the non-nuclear weapon states not to develop or otherwise acquire nuclear weapons, the NPT commits the nuclear weapon states to good-faith negotiations on nuclear disarmament. Every five years since 1970 the parties have held a review conference to assess implementation of the treaty. The review conference in 2000 identified and approved practical steps toward the total elimination of nuclear arsenals, but no concrete steps were taken. The 2005 NPT review conference similarly did not produce any concrete results.

The Anti-Ballistic Missile (ABM) Treaty between the United States and the Soviet Union was signed and entered into force in 1972. Because it limits defensive systems that would otherwise spur an offensive arms race, this treaty has been seen as the foundation for the strategic nuclear arms reduction treaties. In late 2001, U.S. president George W. Bush announced that the United States would withdraw from the ABM Treaty within six months and gave formal notice, stating that the treaty "hinders our government's ability to develop ways to protect our people from future terrorist or rogue-state missile attacks."

The United States should help stop the spread of nuclear weapons by actively supporting and adhering to treaties such as the Nuclear Non-Proliferation Treaty and by setting an example for the rest of the world by renouncing the first use of nuclear weapons and the development of new nuclear weapons. It should work with Russia to dismantle nuclear warheads and increase funding for programs to secure nuclear materials so they will not be misused.

Strengthening the Chemical Weapons Convention. The Chemical Weapons Convention (CWC) is the strongest of the arms control treaties outlawing a single class of weapons. As described earlier, inspection and verification of compliance with its provisions lies in the hands of the Organization for the Prohibition of Chemical Weapons (OPCW). Controversies about safety and protection of the environment during the CWC-required disposal of chemical weapons have delayed completion of this disposal, and large stockpiles still remain in a number of nations, posing a continuing threat to health and to the environment. The United States has failed to fully support the OPCW in its difficult tasks of inspection and in urging nations to comply with CWC.

Strengthening the Biologic and Toxin Weapons Convention. Although the development, production, transfer, or use of biological weapons was prohibited by the 1975 Biologic and Toxin Weapons Convention (BWC), several nations are believed to retain stockpiles of such weapons. The verification measures included in the BWC are weak, and attempts to strengthen them have been unsuccessful. During 2002, the United States blocked attempts to strengthen the verification measures of the BWC, announcing that such measures might lead to disclosure of U.S. industrial or military secrets. The United States must be urged to reverse its rejection of the international community's attempts to develop strong inspection and verification protocols for the BWC. Efforts must be made to convince all nations to support strengthening of the BWC, and all nations must refrain from secret activities, often termed "defensive," that may fuel a biological arms race.

Perhaps even more important, global public health capacity to deal with all infectious diseases must be strengthened. The best individual and collective efforts at diagnosing and treating disease outbreaks can be overwhelmed by any natural or intentionally induced epidemic. Consequently, support for strong global preventive public health capabilities provides the best ultimate defense against ever-evolving threats. Without this support, significant vulnerabilities will remain in impoverished and underserved populations.

Promoting the Anti-Personnel Landmine Convention Forty-two nations, as of January 2005, had neither signed nor ratified the Mine Ban Treaty, including China, India, Iran, Iraq, Israel, Russia, and the United States. Resources are desperately needed to clear the landmines currently deployed. All nations must be urged to contribute more resources to this task.

Conclusion

Traditionally, public health has played a major role in war. Much of this, like the clinical work of military medicine, has been designed to maintain the fighting ability of soldiers, for example, with immunizations against anthrax and smallpox. In recent years, however, public health professionals outside the armed forces have advocated a broader public health approach—the primary prevention of war. We encourage health professionals not only to undertake the specific measures to address the environmental problems created by war and the preparation for war that are described in this chapter but also to work toward the prevention of war.

Thought Questions

1. A military base has contaminated the groundwater in a rural community with organic solvents and other chemicals. If you were the public health officer for this community, what measures would you take to address this problem?

2. What international actions should be taken to limit the spread of nuclear weapons and ultimately to ban them? In considering a ban on nuclear weapons, what lessons might be learned from the Chemical Weapons Convention and the Biologic and Toxin Weapons Convention?
3. How can health professionals advocate for more nations, including the United States, to sign the treaty that bans antipersonnel landmines, and for more resources to be made available for removal of landmines that have previously been deployed?
4. What priorities should be established to improve global defenses against biological agents (regardless of their mode of transmission)?

References

Abylkassimova, Z., and others. "Nested Case-Control Study of Leukemia Among a Cohort of Persons Exposed to Ionizing Radiation from Nuclear Weapon Tests in Kazakhstan (1949–1963)." *Annals of Epidemiology,* 2000, *10,* 479.

Albers, J. W., and Berent, S. "Controversies in Neurotoxicology." *Neurology Clinics,* 2000, *18,* 741–764.

Archer, V. E. "Association of Nuclear Fallout with Leukemia in the United States." *Archives of Environmental Health,* 1987, *42,* 263–271.

Clauw, D. J., and others. "Unexplained Symptoms after Terrorism and War: An Expert Consensus Statement." *Journal of Occupational and Environmental Medicine,* 2003, *45,* 1040–1048.

Dalager, N. A., Kang, H. K., and Mahan, C. M. "Cancer Mortality Among the Highest Exposed US Atmospheric Nuclear Test Participants." *Journal of Occupational and Environmental Medicine,* 2000, *42,* 798–805.

Foege, W. H. "Arms and Public Health: A Global Perspective." In B. S. Levy and V. W. Sidel (eds.), *War and Public Health.* (Updated ed.) Washington, D.C.: American Public Health Association, 2000.

Garfield, R. M., and Neugut, A. I. "The Human Consequences of War." In B. S. Levy and V. W. Sidel (eds.), *War and Public Health.* (Updated ed.) Washington, D.C.: American Public Health Association, 2000.

Haley, R., Maddrey, A. M., and Gershenfeld, H. K. "Severely Reduced Functional Status in Veterans Fitting a Case Definition of Gulf War Syndrome." *American Journal of Public Health,* 2002, *92,* 46–47.

Hoffmann, W. "Has Fallout from the Chernobyl Accident Caused Childhood Leukaemia in Europe? A Commentary on the Epidemiologic Evidence." *European Journal of Public Health,* 2002, *12,* 72–76.

Institute of Medicine and National Research Council. *Exposure of the American People to Iodine-131 from Nevada Nuclear Tests: Review of the National Cancer Institute Report and Public Health Implications.* Washington, D.C.: National Academics Press, 1999, p. 6.

International Campaign to Ban Landmines. *Landmine Monitor Report 2000: Toward a Mine-Free World.* New York: Human Rights Watch, 2000.

International Campaign to Ban Landmines. Home page. [www.icbl.org]. 2005.

Ismail, K. "A Review of the Evidence for a 'Gulf War Syndrome.'" *Occupational and Environmental Medicine,* 2001, *58,* 754–760.

Keller, B. "Soviet City, Home of the A-Bomb, Is Haunted by Its Past and Future." *New York Times,* July 10, 1989, pp A1–A2.

Kelsey, K. T., and others. "Genotoxicity to Human Cells Induced by Air Particulates Isolated During the Kuwait Oil Fires." *Environmental Research,* 1994, *64,* 18–25.

Lange, J. L., and others. "Exposures to the Kuwait Oil Fires and Their Association with Asthma and Bronchitis Among Gulf War Veterans." *Environmental Health Perspectives,* 2002, *110,* 1141–1146.

Levy, B. S., and Sidel, V. W. (eds.). *War and Public Health.* (Updated ed.) Washington, D.C.: American Public Health Association, 2000.

Lund, E., and Galanti, M. R. "Incidence of Thyroid Cancer in Scandinavia Following Fallout from Atomic Bomb Testing: An Analysis of Birth Cohorts." *Cancer Causes & Control,* 1999, *10,* 181–187.

Meselson, M., and others. "The Sverdlovsk Anthrax Outbreak of 1979." *Science,* 1994, *266,* 1202–1208.

Moeller, R. B., Jr., and others. "Assessment of the Histopathological Lesions and Chemical Analysis of Feral Cats to the Smoke from the Kuwait Oil Fires." *Journal of Environmental Pathology, Toxicology and Oncology,* 1994, *13,* 137–149.

Muirhead, C. B., and others. "Follow Up of Mortality and Incidence of Cancer 1952–98 in Men from the UK Who Participated in the UK's Atmospheric Nuclear Weapon Tests and Experimental Programmes." *Occupational and Environmental Medicine,* 2003, *60,* 165–172.

Petruccelli, B. P., and others. "Health Effects of the 1991 Kuwait Oil Fires: A Survey of US Army Troops." *Journal of Occupational and Environmental Medicine,* 1999, *41,* 433–439.

Plapp, F. W., Jr. "Permethrin and the Gulf War Syndrome." *Archives of Environmental Health,* 1999, *54,* 312.

Renner, M. "Assessing the Military's War on the Environment." In L. R. Brown and others (eds.), *State of the World 1991.* New York: Norton, 1991.

Renner, M. "Environmental and Health Effects of Weapons: Production, Testing, and Maintenance." In B. S. Levy and V. W. Sidel (eds.), *War and Public Health.* (Updated ed.) Washington, D.C.: American Public Health Association, 2000.

Shapiro, S. E., Lasarev, M. R., and McCauley, L. "Factor Analysis of Gulf War Illness: What Does It Add to Our Understanding of Possible Health Effects of Deployment?" *American Journal of Epidemiology,* 2002, *156,* 578–585.

Shibata, Y., and others. "15 Years After Chernobyl: New Evidence of Thyroid Cancer." *Lancet,* 2001, *358,* 1965–1966.

Sidel, V. W., and Levy, B. S. "War, Terrorism, and Public Health." *Journal of Law, Medicine & Ethics,* 2003, *31,* 516–523.

Spanjaard, H., and Khabib, O. "Chemical Weapons." In B. S. Levy and V. W. Sidel (eds.), *Terrorism and Public Health: A Balanced Approach to Strengthening Systems and Protecting People.* New York: Oxford University Press, 2003.

Stevens, W., and others. "Leukemia in Utah and Radioactive Fallout from the Nevada Test Site: A Case-Control Study." *Journal of the American Medical Association,* 1990, *264,* 585–591.

Stockholm International Peace Research Institute. *SIPRI Yearbook 2002: Armaments, Disarmament and International Security.* New York: Oxford University Press, 2002.

Stockholm International Peace Research Institute. *SIPRI Yearbook 2003: Armaments, Disarmament and International Security.* New York: Oxford University Press, 2003.

Stover, E., Cobey, J. C., and Fine, J. "The Public Health Effects of Land Mines: Long-Term Consequences for Civilians." In B. S. Levy and V. W. Sidel (eds.), *War and Public Health.* (Updated ed.) Washington, D.C.: American Public Health Association, 2000.

Takahashi, T., and others. "The Relationship of Thyroid Cancer with Radiation Exposure from Nuclear Weapon Testing in the Marshall Islands." *Journal of Epidemiology,* 2003, *13,* 99–107.

Watanabe, K. K., Kang, H. K., and Dalager, N. A. "Cancer Mortality Risk Among Military Participants of a 1958 Atmospheric Nuclear Weapons Test." *American Journal of Public Health,* 1995, *85,* 523–527.

Windrem, R. "Did Soviets Build Mini A-Bombs? A Look at What Happened to Miniature Atomic Weapons." [http://www.msnbc.com/news/113675.asp]. Sept. 1997.

Worldwatch Institute. *Vital Signs.* Washington, D.C.: Worldwatch Institute, 2003.

Yokoro, K., and Kamada, N. "The Public Health Effects of the Use of Nuclear Weapons." In B. S. Levy and V. W. Sidel (eds.), *War and Public Health.* (Updated ed.) Washington, D.C.: American Public Health Association, 2000.

For Further Information

Levy, B. S., Shahi, G. S., and Lee, C. "The Environmental Consequences of War." In B. S. Levy and V. W. Sidel (eds.), *War and Public Health.* (Updated ed.) Washington, D.C.: American Public Health Association, 2000.

Sidel, V. W. "The Impact of Military Preparedness and Militarism on Health and the Environment." In J. E. Austin and C. E. Bruch (eds.), *The Environmental Consequences of War: Legal, Economic, and Scientific Perspectives.* New York: Cambridge University Press, 2000.

Sidel V. W., and Shahi, G. S. "The Impact of Military Activities on Development, Environment, and Health." In G. S. Shahi and others (eds.), *International Perspectives on Environment, Development, and Health: Toward a Sustainable World.* New York: Springer, 1997.

CHAPTER THIRTEEN

DEVELOPING NATIONS

Jerome Nriagu
Jaymie Meliker
Mary Johnson

The health and disease patterns of societies and communities evolve in response to environmental, technological, biotic, demographic, social, economic, and cultural stimuli. The twenty-first century has dawned with the human population distributed into three distinct worlds: the First World (developed countries, "Upper Earth," or developed economies), Second World (high-income developing countries, "Middle Earth," or developing economies) and Third World (low-income developing countries, "Lower Earth," or underdeveloped economies).

One Earth, Three Worlds

The postindustrial countries of the First World are immersed in high technology, with glittering advances in electronics, medical research, genomic manipulation, fiber optics, synthetic materials, alloys, and fabrication processes. In this world, people's lives revolve around virtual entertainment, cash-free and Internet shopping, mobile phones, rapid transportation, and on-demand mass production. This is a culture of smart bombs and automobiles, cloned animals and human parts, space exploration, robotics, weapons of mass destruction, and an impressive computerization of most business and home life—but diminished connection to the natural environment (Meister, 2001). In this setting health statistics are dominated by "degenerative and man-made diseases," such as hyperlipidemias, obesity, diabetes, cardiovascular diseases, and neuropsychiatric disorders. The Second World countries are consumed by the desire to attain First World status. These countries feature rapid industrial, technological and social change, with little concern for the attendant environmental pollution. For the Third World countries, most things are going wrong. They have limited or poor management of natural resources, high infant and maternal mortality rates, low literacy and education, political instability, corrupt political leaders and government institutions, untrained manpower and flight of capital, vandalism by military and law enforcement officers, civil strife, famine, deteriorated educational, medical service, and business infrastructures, depleted agricultural soils, and a high burden of endemic and communicable disease morbidity and mortality (Meister, 2001). How to reconcile these disparities into a cooperative framework, in which the three worlds coexist and in which the planetary ecosystem is protected, is currently under intense discussion.

The dawn of the new millennium also reflects a major transition in the health of human populations, marked by disturbing evidence of widening gaps in health among the three worlds. Over the past fifty years average life expectancy at birth has increased globally by almost 20 years, from about 46.5 years in the period from 1950 to 1955 to 65.2 years in 2002. This gain is not uniformly distributed; in 2002, life expectancy ranged from 78 years for women in developed countries to less than 46 years for men in sub-Saharan Africa (World Health Organization [WHO], 2003). For millions of children in Africa, the biggest health challenge today is to survive until their fifth birthday and their chances of doing so are less than they were a decade ago. In many Third World countries, local and regional environmental problems are major contributors to disease and death. Inadequate supplies of clean water, poor sanitation, smoky cooking fuels, waste accumulation in neighborhoods, disease-carrying pests, improper use of pesticides, food poisoning exacerbated by poor handling and preservation techniques, and poor housing and overcrowded conditions are closely interrelated environmental processes. Virtually anyone living, working, and socializing in many Third World neighborhoods is exposed to environmental hazards, with children, women, and the elderly being particularly vulnerable (Thomas, Seager, and Mathee, 2002).

People in most countries of the Third World are disproportionately exposed to the so-called traditional hazards (generally associated with lack of development), which differ from the *modern* (Second World) hazards of uncontrolled industrial development and the *postmodern* (First World) hazards of sedentary lifestyles and material excess. As countries or regions shift from one world to another, the change in patterns of exposure and in health risks that accompanies that shift from one level of economic activity to another can be described as a *risk transition* (Sims and

Butter, 2000). In many countries of the Second and Third Worlds, the processes of globalization and industrialization often result in simultaneous exposure to both traditional and modern environmental risks, a double jeopardy known as *risk overlap*. Squalid urban areas exemplify the mixed environmental hazards faced in many developing countries. In addition, *ecological risk traps* may arise, that is, major polluting industries may be located in a fairly isolated, nonadaptive traditional community. In these situations the overlay of the toxic effects of industrial emissions on the traditional risks may overwhelm a population's coping capacity, with catastrophic consequences.

The Changing Disease Burden in the Third World

Of the 57 million people who died in 2002, almost 20 percent (10.5 million) were children less than five years old. Nearly 98 percent of the child deaths occurred in the developing countries (WHO, 2003). Of the twenty countries in the world with the highest child mortality, nineteen are in Africa, the exception being Afghanistan. A baby born in Sierra Leone is 100 times more likely than a child born in Singapore or Iceland to die before the age of five (WHO, 2003). On the other end of the demographic spectrum, over 60 percent of deaths in developed countries involved people over the age of seventy, compared to 10 percent in African countries (WHO, 2003). The probability of death is remarkably different in the three worlds, with the death rates in Third World countries being much higher and occurring at younger ages.

A demographic revolution is clearly underway throughout the world (see Chapter Ten). There are now about 600 million people aged sixty years and over in the world, and this total is expected to reach 2 billion by 2050, with the vast majority being in the developing countries (WHO, 2003). It is projected that older people will comprise more than 15 percent of the total population in countries like Brazil, China, and Thailand by 2025, and in Colombia, Indonesia, and Kenya the number will increase up to fourfold during the next twenty-five years (WHO, 2003). Population aging is propelled by two overlapping factors: a decline in fertility rates of the overall population, resulting in a reduction in the proportion of children, and an increase in the proportion of older people as mortality rates decline. The effect of the environment on this demographic transition, in terms of the health of elderly population, needs more attention than it is currently getting. In developed countries aging populations have an increased prevalence of chronic diseases and disability. This trend will likely be different in Third World countries, where a compounding of risk factors for communicable disease and age-related chronic diseases will present an unpredictable but challenging set of health problems.

The disparity between the First and Third World countries in adult mortality risk continues to widen. Almost 75 percent of the 45 million deaths in 2002 involving adults aged fifteen years and over were caused by noncommunicable diseases (WHO, 2003). Communicable diseases and maternal, perinatal, and nutritional conditions accounted for 8.2 million adult deaths (representing about 18 percent of all deaths), whereas injuries killed 4.5 million adults in 2002 (WHO, 2003). As shown in Table 13.1, the principal attributable causes of death in developing countries are childhood and maternal undernutrition, exposure to environmental risks, and unsafe sexual practices, whereas diet-related risks are the leading cause of death in the developed countries.

Although mortality statistics are generally the simplest measure of population health status, they fail to estimate the true disease burden because they do not account for morbidity and disability. Some effort has therefore been made to derive composite measures that can better describe the health status of populations. One such approach is the *disability-adjusted life years* (DALYs) concept (Murray and Lopez, 1996), which combines *years of life lost* (YLL) through premature death with *years lived with disability* (YLD). One DALY can be thought of as one lost year of healthy life, and the measured disease burden is the gap between the health status of a given population and that of a normative global reference population with high life expectancy lived in full health. The DALY figures for different regions provide a guide to the relative distribution of disease burdens; the higher the DALYs, the greater the burden. The leading risk factors for the global burden of disease are shown in Table 13.2. Most of the disease and disability categories have direct or indirect environmental components, although in different ways and to different degrees. Among the leading environmentally related risk factors are being underweight or having nutritional insufficiencies (undernutrition is the leading single risk factor, accounting for over 9 percent of global DALYs) and experiencing inadequate water supply and sanitation (sixth-ranked), indoor air pollution, lead pollution, outdoor air pollution, and climate change. It has been estimated that 25 to 30 percent of the global disease burden is attributable to environmental factors (Smith, Corvalan, and Kjellstrom, 1999), and this estimate does not include the confounding effects of the environment on the etiology of other diseases.

Estimated DALYs for children and young adults for 2002 show a disproportionate burden of disease in Third World countries compared to the developed countries. About 40 percent of the lost years of healthy life in Third World countries in 2002 resulted from diseases in children younger than five, compared to only 6 percent for the same age group in developed countries (WHO, 2003).

There are large disparities in the environmentally related disease burden for various segments of the population. For instance, children less than five years old make up only 12 percent of the global population but account for about

TABLE 13.1. ATTRIBUTABLE MORTALITY BY RISK FACTOR, LEVEL OF DEVELOPMENT, AND GENDER, 2000.

	High Mortality Developing		*Low Mortality Developing*		*Developed*	
Risk Factor	**Male**	**Female**	**Male**	**Female**	**Male**	**Female**
Total deaths (in thousands)	13,758	12,654	8,584	7,373	6,890	6,601
Childhood and maternal undernutrition						
Underweight	12.6%	13.4%	1.8%	1.9%	0.1%	0.1%
Iron deficiency	2.2	3.0	0.8	1.0	0.1	0.2
Vitamin A deficiency	2.3	3.3	0.2	0.4	<0.1	<0.1
Zinc deficiency	2.8	3.0	0.2	0.2	<0.1	<0.1
Other diet-related risks and physical inactivity						
Blood pressure	7.4	7.5	12.7	15.1	20.1	23.9
Cholesterol	5.0	5.7	5.1	5.6	14.5	17.6
Body mass index	1.1	2.0	4.2	5.6	9.6	11.5
Low fruit and vegetable intake	3.6	3.5	5.0	4.8	7.6	7.4
Physical inactivity	2.3	2.3	2.8	3.2	6.0	6.7
Sexual and reproductive health risks						
Unsafe sex	9.3	10.9	0.8	1.3	0.2	0.6
Lack of contraception	NA	1.1	NA	0.2	NA	0.0
Addictive substances						
Smoking and oral tobacco	7.5	1.5	12.2	2.9	26.3	9.3
Alcohol	2.6	0.6	8.5	1.6	8.0	−0.3
Illicit drugs	0.5	0.1	0.6	0.1	0.6	0.3
Environmental risks						
Unsafe water, sanitation, and hygiene	5.8	5.9	1.1	1.1	0.2	0.2
Urban air pollution	0.9	0.8	2.5	2.9	1.1	1.2
Indoor smoke from solid fuels	3.6	4.3	1.9	5.4	0.1	0.2
Lead exposure	0.4	0.3	0.5	0.3	0.7	0.4
Climate change	0.5	0.6	<0.1	<0.1	<0.1	<0.1
Occupational risks						
Risk factors for injury	1.0	0.1	1.4	0.1	0.4	0.0
Carcinogens	0.1	<0.1	0.5	0.2	0.8	0.2
Airborne particulates	0.3	<0.1	1.6	0.2	0.6	0.1
Ergonomic stressors	0.0	0.0	0.0	0.0	0.0	0.0
Noise	0.0	0.0	0.0	0.0	0.0	0.0
Other selected risks to health						
Unsafe health care injections	1.1	0.9	1.8	0.9	0.1	0.1
Childhood sexual abuse	0.1	0.2	0.1	0.2	0.1	0.1

Source: WHO, 2002.

TABLE 13.2. ATTRIBUTABLE DALYS BY RISK FACTOR, LEVEL OF DEVELOPMENT, AND SEX, 2000.

	High Mortality Developing		*Low Mortality Developing*		*Developed*	
Risk Factors	**Male**	**Female**	**Male**	**Female**	**Male**	**Female**
Total DALYs (in thousands)	420,711	412,052	223,181	185,316	117,670	96,543
Childhood and maternal undernutrition						
Underweight	14.9%	15.0%	3.0%	3.3%	0.4%	0.4%
Iron deficiency	2.8	3.5	1.5	2.2	0.5	1.0
Vitamin A deficiency	2.6	3.5	0.3	0.4	<0.1	<0.1
Zinc deficiency	3.2	3.2	0.3	0.3	0.1	0.1
Other diet-related risks and physical inactivity						
Blood pressure	2.6	2.4	4.9	5.1	11.2	10.6
Cholesterol	1.9	1.9	2.2	2.0	8.0	7.0
Body mass index	0.6	1.0	2.3	3.2	6.9	8.1
Low fruit and vegetable intake	1.3	1.2	2.0	1.8	4.3	3.4
Physical inactivity	0.9	0.8	1.2	1.3	3.3	3.2
Sexual and reproductive health risks						
Unsafe sex	9.4	11.0	1.2	1.6	0.5	1.1
Lack of contraception	NA	1.8	NA	0.6	NA	0.1
Addictive substances						
Smoking and oral tobacco	3.4	0.6	6.2	1.3	17.1	6.2
Alcohol	2.6	0.5	9.8	2.0	14.0	3.3
Illicit drugs	0.8	0.2	1.2	0.3	2.3	1.2
Environmental risks						
Unsafe water, sanitation, and hygiene	5.5	5.6	1.7	1.8	0.4	0.4
Urban air pollution	0.4	0.3	1.0	0.9	0.6	0.5
Indoor smoke from solid fuels	3.7	3.6	1.5	2.3	0.2	0.3
Lead exposure	0.8	0.7	1.4	1.4	0.8	0.5
Climate change	0.6	0.7	0.1	0.1	<0.1	<0.1
Occupational risks						
Risk factors for injury	1.5	0.1	2.1	0.3	1.0	0.1
Carcinogens	0.1	<0.1	0.2	0.1	0.4	0.1
Airborne particulates	0.1	0.0	0.8	0.1	0.4	0.1
Ergonomic stressors	0.0	0.0	0.1	0.1	0.1	0.1
Noise	0.3	0.1	0.5	0.3	0.4	0.3
Other selected risks to health						
Unsafe health care injections	0.9	0.8	1.1	0.5	0.1	0.1
Childhood sexual abuse	0.3	0.7	0.5	0.8	0.3	1.0

Source: WHO, 2003.

FIGURE 13.1. AGE-STANDARDIZED RATES OF YEARS LIVED WITH DISABILITY (YLDS), DEVELOPED AND DEVELOPING COUNTRIES, 2002.

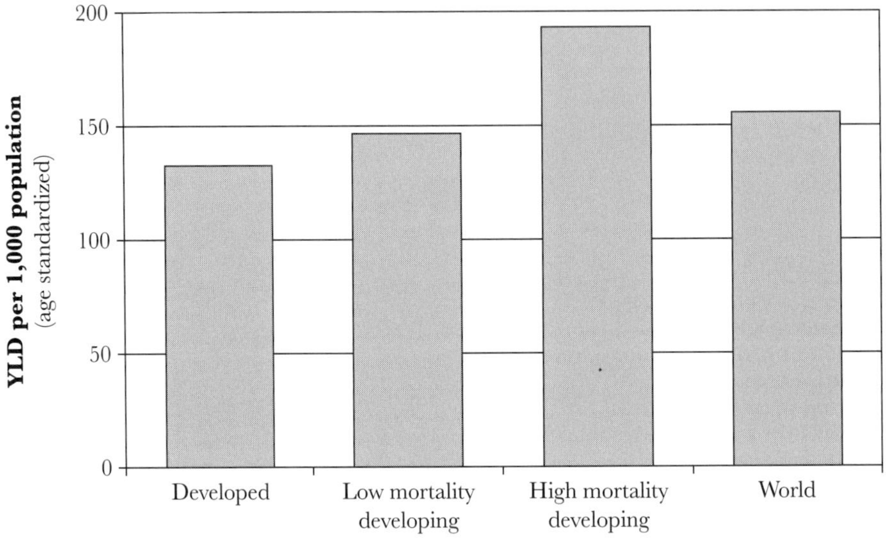

Source: WHO, 2003.

43 percent of the total disease burden, due to environmental risks (Smith, 2002; Smith, Corvalan, and Kjellstrom, 1999). Even when the DALY is standardized with respect to age, there are still significant differences in morbidity burden between developing and developed countries (Figure 13.1). As a result of demographic trends, lifestyle transitions, and changes in the distribution of environmental risk factors (associated primarily with migration to overcrowded urban areas), there has been a rapid increase in the incidence of noncommunicable diseases (such as asthma, food-related chronic diseases, and neuropsychiatric conditions) in Third World communities. Most developing countries now face a double burden made up of both communicable and noncommunicable diseases. Furthermore, disabilities tend to be more prevalent and more severe in developing countries because risks cluster among highly vulnerable subpopulations and accumulate over time (WHO, 2003). As a result of the risk overlap, the Third World populations may confront more complex and more diverse patterns of disease than populations in developed countries do; they not only face a higher risk of premature death but also live a higher proportion of their lives with poor health.

Globalization: Bad Medicine for Developing Countries

The twenty-first century is a time of tumultuous change in which economic interdependence is increasing rapidly, information technology is accelerating the spread of ideas, human influence on natural cycles and processes has become evident on a global scale, and the spread of an infectious disease around the globe is only a plane ride away. This process of interlocking economic, social, technological, political, and cultural changes emerging around the world has been called *globalization,* a phenomenon that is shrinking space and increasing the speed of interaction, changing our views of the world and of ourselves, and breaking down national and cultural barriers. An unmistakable outcome of the globalization phenomenon so far is that as the economies grow, people in the First World get richer, some in the Second World escape poverty, and disparities with the Third World widen. The wealth and health in one world are increasingly being created at the cost of development in the other two worlds, and the imbalance is marginalizing a majority of the people on the planet. This scenario has led to a divergence of opinion on the likely effects of globalization on the environment-health interface.

On the one hand, proponents of globalization argue that health is a crucial resource because it is linked to the stability and security that foreign investors seek. A healthy population is a critical asset for the development of a country, and business companies are more likely to invest in communities where the health risks are manageable. Proponents see globalization as providing economic, technological, and social opportunities for renewed commitments to the environment and community health. Free enterprise on a global economic playing field, leveled by international agreements to reduce market barriers, should, they argue, usher in an age of affluence for all and lift everyone to a new height of well-being. Cuts in agricultural subsidies and the opening of trade in agricultural products should increase efficiency and raise the income of farmers.

Proponents also point to the promise of technological diffusion. Agriculture, they maintain, will benefit from progress in biotechnology, which will increase yields and reduce the pressure on natural resources in many countries. Improvements in irrigation techniques will minimize the health effects of water resource developments. Advances in technology and structural changes in economies will produce social and environmental benefits by reducing production and delivery costs. The development and spread of more efficient vehicles that run on cleaner fuels will reduce the consumption of fossil fuels and the emission of pollutants from this source. Deregulation will open up micropower development, especially in rural areas of Third World countries, where the power supply has been limited by the high cost of electrical grids (United Nations Environment Programme [UNEP], 2002). Advances in nanotechnology should improve material use efficiency and biotechnology can have positive effects on wastewater treatment and remediation of contaminated sites. Supporters thus trust globalization and liberalization to generate corporate wealth, spur new technologies, and create new enterprises that improve people's livelihoods and help communities pay for social and health programs and abate environmental problems.

On the other hand, there is growing concern over the damaging effects of global markets on the distribution of health risks. Critics note the accumulation of wealth and power in just a few transnational corporations and countries, far removed from areas where the wastes of unbridled economic growth accumulate. They see unequal expansion of modern production methods around the world with a disproportionate number of highly polluting industries being located in Third World countries. They worry about two-track, market-driven global development that divides humanity into privileged and excluded, North and South, and modernist and traditionalist factions. They perceive manipulative and one-sided (selfish) approaches to global negotiations and unfair international agreements on sustainable development. Too often the focus of international health agreements has been on technological fixes that originate in First World countries rather than on indigenous interventions to improve the health of local communities. Many are apprehensive that globalization's legacy to their children will be an impoverished, toxified, and fragile world that is economically, ecologically, and socially depleted. Critics consider the emerging global consumer culture that encourages lifestyles based on individualism and greed to be a fundamental threat to the social fabric of many communities in Third World countries.

Globalization clearly produces major driving forces that can change environmental health risks at the global, regional, and local scales. The transnational forces of globalization, especially the massive movements of goods and people, alter the risk and susceptibility of local populations to ill health and disease. The movement of health hazards from the First World to the Second and Third Worlds (including the export of firearms, industrial wastes, and pollution), the heavy and inefficient use of energy, the production of greenhouse gases leading to global warming, and the plundering of natural resources and spoliation of the environment add to existing environmental risk factors. Table 13.3 shows some likely direct and indirect effects of globalization on environmental health risks in developing countries. It is clear that the effect of globalization on health involves many diffuse determinants and overlapping risks and that the critical determinants of health in many developing countries are increasingly global and cannot simply be attributed to individual nations. Many of the transnational factors noted in Table 13.3, driven by privatization-oriented policies of international institutions, seem to be at odds with the sociocultural constructs and community risk-sharing traditions in many developing countries. Notions of justice, social

TABLE 13.3. EFFECTS OF GLOBALIZATION ON THE HEALTH OF PEOPLE IN DEVELOPING COUNTRIES.

Global Transnational Factor	Consequence and Probable Impact on Health Risks in Developing Countries
Environmental degradation and unsustainable consumption patterns	
Resource depletion (arable land, freshwater, and forestry products)	Reduced standard of living leading to hunger, undernutrition, unsafe water, poor sanitation and hygiene; higher indoor pollution from burning wood substitutes; potential violence between countries
Water and air pollution	Regional and local environmental health impacts; exacerbation of existing endemic diseases
Ozone depletion and increased ultraviolet radiation	Changes in composition of local fauna and flora leading to malnutrition; toxification of human food chain; increased prevalence of systemic disorders (skin and eye)
Accumulation of greenhouse gases and global warming	Major shifts in infectious disease patterns and vector distribution; increased trauma due to frequent weather disasters (such as storms and floods) and worsening food shortages; reduced soil productivity in tropical countries; increased exposure to thermal extremes (cardiovascular and respiratory mortality)
Food security	
Increased export of cash crops to developed countries	Shortage of staple local foods as manpower and resources go into producing export crops; higher prices for locally produced foods, making them unaffordable to the poor
Increased global food trade and a decline in food aid	Food shortages in marginalized countries; increased migration and civil unrest
Overfishing to meet growing demand for seafood	Reduced supply of fish protein in coastal communities; destruction of traditional lifestyles
Increased use of pesticides and fertilizers	Exposure to toxic residues in foods; toxic metals introduced into food chain with fertilizers
Import of protein-rich and sugared foods	Increased overnutrition-related health problems (such as high blood pressure, high cholesterol, and obesity)
Macroeconomics	
Structural adjustment policies and downsizing	Marginalization; poverty; inadequate social support nets
Structural and chronic unemployment	Higher morbidity and mortality; increased violence
Trade	
Marketing of tobacco	Increased morbidity and mortality due to lung cancer, cardiovascular, and chronic respiratory diseases
Dumping of unsafe and ineffective drugs by multinationals	Harmful or ineffective therapy
Import of contaminated foodstuffs and feed	Spread of infectious diseases across borders
Global redistribution of polluting industries	Increased risk of occupational and environmental exposure to toxic chemicals from disproportionate siting of these industries

(*Continued*)

TABLE 13.3. EFFECTS OF GLOBALIZATION ON THE HEALTH OF PEOPLE IN DEVELOPING COUNTRIES. (*Continued*)

Global Transnational Factor	Consequence and Probable Impact on Health Risks in Developing Countries
Travel	
Cross-border movements of large masses for business or pleasure	Infectious disease transmission; export of harmful lifestyles (such as smoking and high-risk sexual behavior)
Migration and demographic changes	
Increased refugee population	Environmental degradation; incubation of infectious pathogens
Brain drain	Loss of trained manpower and intellectual resources, leading to poor health systems management; economic loss
Technology	
Patent protection of new technologies under trade-related intellectual property rights agreements	Benefits of new health-related technologies developed in global market unaffordable for the poor; marginalization of poor countries in research and development
Patent drugs	Traditional healing practices discouraged; new drugs from local plants unaffordable to the poor
Communications and media	
Global marketing of harmful commodities such as tobacco	Active promotion of health-damaging practices
Risk communication	Inappropriate or misunderstood in poor communities
Foreign policies	
Policies based on national self-interest, xenophobia, or protectionism	Threat to multinationalism and global cooperation required to address shared transnational health concerns
Global security	Increased number of firearms, which can lead to increased violence; restriction on export of goods and services from some countries; reduction of investments in poor countries where health risks are unmanageable
Privatization-oriented policies	Reduced and inappropriate quality of health care for the poor; promotion of international commodification and trade in human organs
Human rights	Withholding of emergency and humanitarian assistance

Source: Adapted from Kickbusch and Buse, 2001.

responsibility, and human rights, key to the development of sustainable health systems, are antithetical to the continued plundering of global resources.

Despite the extraordinary advances of the twentieth century, huge disparities persist in the morbidity and mortality experienced in the First and Third Worlds, and this is due primarily to the ill effects of poverty. Environmental risks and poverty are closely interwoven. Poverty hinders the development of clean water supplies and proper sanitation, drives the migration into overcrowded cities with substandard housing and high air pollution levels, is related to indoor air pollution from the burning of biofuels or urban solid wastes, increases exposure to intentional and unintentional injuries and the risk of lead poisoning, and is primarily responsible for undernutrition with far-reaching effects. Globalization has been a bad medicine for developing countries where more than half of the population still lives on less than $2 per day, and it will likely remain so for the foreseeable future.

Current environmental challenges and human vulnerabilities in sub-Saharan Africa show the limitations and difficulties of globalizing health in Third World regions (Thomas, Seager, and Mathee, 2002). Both the poverty of most sub-Saharan African countries and their total dependence on natural resources for people's livelihoods increase their vulnerability to environmental change and risk overlaps. The changes that began in the 1960s seem to have worsened their poverty, and their environments and human capital have continued on a downward spiral, making the population more susceptible to environmental health risk factors. Over 60 percent of the population lives in ecologically vulnerable areas characterized by a high degree of sensitivity and low degree of resilience (UNEP, 2002). Rapid population growth and overexploitation of natural resources, deepening poverty, and increasing food insecurity have brought about environmental changes that have taken a toll on the public's health. Mismanagement of natural resources, the impacts of disasters and civil strife, and response to external pressures (such as economic adjustment plans) have exacerbated environmental health risks in the region. Other factors such as weak institutional and legal frameworks, corruption, and poor economic performance have left most sub-Saharan countries with limited choices and low coping capacity. It is easy to see why the distinction between globalization and exploitation is blurred for many people in this part of our earth.

The remainder of this chapter deals with recent trends in environmental risk factors that have contributed to health disparities in the three worlds. It addresses five arenas: agriculture, nutrition, air quality, urbanization, and water. Each is a primary domain of environmental health, and each poses particular health challenges to the people of developing nations.

Agriculture

Agriculture, forestry, and fishing furnish not only the food and natural resources on which societies depend but also provide the livelihood of about half of the world's population. In many Third World countries, subsistence farming accounts for over 75 percent of the gross domestic product. The output of the world's food-producing systems has greatly increased and changed over recent decades to meet the rising demand of a rapidly growing population. In spite of degradation of land and water resources, there is as yet no global shortage of food or the capacity to produce it. However, due to social, political, and economic constraints and lack of education, undernutrition remains a leading risk factor for ill health and premature death in most Third World countries.

As agriculture is integrated into the global economy, agricultural systems must be intensified, marginal lands brought into use, and new crops and farming practices developed. At the same time, arable land is being threatened by soil erosion, overgrazing, soil depletion in clear-cut areas, salinization, and other types of land degradation and also by the expansion of urban, industrial, and other developments. The development of agro-ecosystems needed to feed the local population and grow cash crops for the export market invariably involves environmental changes. Health and its environmental determinants are closely related to land use and land tenure, and the recent phenomenon of the *green revolution* in the developing countries has been accompanied by significant shifts in environmental health risk factors, a matter that has not received much scientific enquiry. An important element of the green revolution is an increasing reliance on pesticides, which has led to untold numbers of poisonings in many developing countries (see Box 13.1).

Box 13.1. Pesticide Hazards in Developing Countries

Chemical pesticides are used throughout the world to protect crops, forests, and plantations (for example, cotton plantations) from pests and to combat insect-borne endemic diseases, such as malaria. In developing countries hundreds of thousands of tons of pesticides are applied annually, with applications increasing each year. Access to expensive, safer pesticides is limited in developing countries, whereas less expensive, more acutely toxic pesticides are more readily available. Although the use of many of these pesticides has been banned or curtailed in more developed countries, these chemicals are widely available on the world market.

In addition, more than 500,000 tons of obsolete pesticides are stockpiled in developing countries. These stockpiles accumulated when the governments of developing countries prohibited the use of some pesticides, after quantities of them had been imported. The list of banned pesticides includes the persistent organic pollutants (POPs) aldrin, chlordane, DDT, dieldrin, endrin, and heptachlor. Many of these stockpiles receive no attention, even though over time pesticides deteriorate and form by-products; occasionally these by-products are more toxic than the original substances. Pesticides and their by-products frequently leak into soil, contaminating groundwater or volatilizing into the atmosphere.

Reliable estimates of pesticide exposures and poisonings are not widely available because of inadequate surveillance systems. However, surveys suggest that pesticides poison approximately 25 million agricultural workers in developing countries each year. For example, about 7 percent of agricultural workers in Malaysia suffer pesticide poisoning, compared to 4.5 percent in Costa Rica, and 3 percent in Sri Lanka. Aside from acute poisonings, the long-term effects of persistent exposure to pesticides include reproductive dysfunction, neurological disease, and cancer.

Pesticide poisoning in developing countries is frequently attributed to lack of personal protective equipment or protective clothing suitable for tropical climates, poor knowledge and understanding of safety procedures, application of pesticides in concentrations exceeding guidelines, and poor maintenance facilities for spray equipment and container disposal. For instance, training programs for agricultural workers to learn how to apply, store, and dispose of pesticides are rarely available. Similarly, legislation to manage pesticide use is patchy and seldom enforced. Enforcement of legislation and implementation of training programs could prevent numerous pesticide poisonings and result in immediate health benefits.

Sources: London and others, 2002; Ecobichon, 2001; Koh and Jeyaratnam, 1996.

Expected shifts in environmental determinants of health related to agricultural development programs are shown in Table 13.4. The impacts of the risk factors may be moderated by simultaneous demographic and socioeconomic shifts. All agricultural developments must be contextualized, however—considered in terms of their local ecological and human impacts. For instance, changes in land-use patterns can have varying impacts on environmental health in different parts of the world (WHO, 1997). The expansion of irrigation in Senegal following the construction of the Diama Dam at the mouth of the Senegal River caused a massive epidemic of intestinal schistosomiasis. However, deforestation in Southeast Asia destroyed the habitat of the most important local malaria vector, *Anopheles dirus,* and caused a sharp decline in malarial transmission. Subsequent afforestation (commercial tree planting, usually on grasslands), reforestation, and the development of plantation agro-ecosystems (with fruit, rubber, and palm trees) are reversing this trend and sometimes leading to higher malarial transmission rates than occurred in the primary forest environment (WHO, 1997). Another example may be found in irrigation projects in Sri Lanka that have led to major biodiversity loss, leaving the malarial vector, *Anopheles culicifacies,* as the sole representative of a previously rich mosquito fauna. Insect disease-vector densities, biting patterns, and associated transmission risks can also be influenced by the presence or absence of livestock in agro-ecosystems. The risk burden attributable to the change in agrobusiness from simple agrarian to modern methods has not been quantified. However, the potential for adverse impacts is enormous; a recent report (Mascie-Taylor and Karim, 2003) showed that soil-transmitted helminth

TABLE 13.4. CHANGES IN ENVIRONMENTAL HEALTH RISK FACTORS ASSOCIATED WITH AGRICULTURAL DEVELOPMENT.

Development Program	Direct Environmental Changes	Secondary Environmental Changes	Environmental Health Risk Factors
Irrigation development	Waterlogging Hydrological changes Salinization Increased water surface area Increased relative humidity	Increased weed densities; possible loss of diversity Increased insect populations Greater chemical inputs Magnet for urban and industrial developments Increased erosion	Introduction of new vector species Increased vector densities Chemical poisoning Changed composition of vector population Prolonged transmission season Exposure of villagers to new pathogens
Land-use changes	Reduced biodiversity or habitat Deforestation	Changed composition of fauna and flora Increased erosion and loss of soil fertility	Changed vector longevity Changed composition of vector population
Cropping patterns	High-yield varieties Shift from subsistence to cash crops Accelerated cropping cycle Plantation agriculture	Greater chemical inputs Greater densities of insect populations Spread of opportunistic and invasive species Increased water pollution	Chemical poisoning Reduced predator insect densities Increased pests and disease-vector densities Mycotoxins

Livestock management	Changes in livestock densities and distribution New breeds of livestock Contaminated animal wastes	Changed densities of blood-sucking pests Soil pollution	Changed disease transmission potential Hormones, antibiotics, and pesticides used in animal husbandry
Mechanization	Changes in livestock densities Loss of ecological features Increased loss of soil quality	Changed densities of blood-sucking insects Reduced refuge areas for predator insects Air and water pollution	Changed disease transmission potential
Chemical inputs	Increased levels of herbicides, pesticides, and fungicides Increased fertilizer application	Chemical contamination Eutrophication of water bodies Expansion of aquatic weeds Soil contamination with toxic metals (cadmium)	Chemical poisoning Introduction of new vector species Development of insect resistance in vector populations

Source: Adapted from Bradley and Narayan, 1987.

infections and schistosomiasis (both of which can be aggravated by large-scale agricultural development) account for 43.5 million DALYs, second only to tuberculosis (46.5 million) and well ahead of malaria (34.1 million).

Nutrition

Traditional lifestyles remain part of the ancient heritage of peoples in most Third World countries. Methods of gathering, preparing, and using native foods and medicines have evolved in ways that promote health. Unlike practices in the developed countries, every element of traditional meals is intertwined with the environment through medicinal, religious, educational, or social customs and beliefs. Traditional duties in the provision and service of meals and traditional exposure patterns are often gender and age specific. Although many factors are involved in what and how people choose to eat, people generally prefer the foods they grow up eating. Every region in the world has its own staple crops and sources of animal protein, and local communities have developed their own ways of combining foods to make meals.

Environmental factors, including water availability, the physical and chemical properties of soils, and prevailing climatic conditions, control local food patterns. These factors also determine the bioavailable forms of essential microelements in soils and hence their concentrations in foods. Under wet tropical conditions, weathering processes preferentially leach out key essential micronutrients (such as zinc, copper, cobalt, and selenium) from the characteristic pisolitic, bauxitic, and "red" soils found in many developing countries. Foods in many developing countries thus tend to be naturally deficient in some essential microelements, as exemplified by the epidemic of Keshan-Beck disease due to selenium deficiency in some regions of China. Undernutrition, often driven by deficiencies of essential micronutrients, involves a complex interplay between the physical environment and social, political, cultural, and economic elements. Because work on hunger and malnutrition has been dominated by social and political scientists, the underlying environmental determinants of the problem have often been overlooked.

The Impact of Undernutrition

Hunger and undernutrition remain the most pervasive risk factors for human morbidity and mortality, especially in the developing countries (Tables 13.1 and 13.2). Many people associate food shortages and malnutrition with famines caused by wars and political upheavals, environmental disasters (such as floods and earthquakes), and environmental catastrophes (such as overgrazing). However, the problem in developing countries often relates to complex ongoing socioecological factors such as poor resource management and economic adjustment plans; these limit food choices, increase local food prices, and reduce people's buying power. Factors that can influence the availability and equitable distribution of safe, nutritious, and affordable foods in developing countries include

- Traditions and beliefs that constrain an individual's food choices. In many African cultures, pregnant and postpartum women are limited to certain foods and other foods (including eggs, onions, certain seafood, and many green, leafy vegetables) are strictly forbidden. Restriction of food choices increases the risk of inadequate consumption of essential microelements.
- Reduced capacity for local food production owing to unfavorable land titles that debar a majority of the population from owning land.
- Declining investments in agricultural research, irrigation, and rural infrastructure.
- Uneducated farmers who cannot adopt advanced technologies and crop management techniques to achieve higher rates of return on their lands.
- Conversion of forests to cropping and grazing lands, leading to loss of hunting grounds (game is an important source of animal protein in traditional diets) and reducing the availability of wild fruits and vegetables that used to be traditional food staples.
- Urbanization and associated roadways that destroy arable lands and suck away the able-bodied workers while placing excessive demand on food supply from rural communities.
- Inadequate food-handling and distribution systems, which result in massive preharvest and postharvest losses.
- Lack of food storage and preservation capacity, making some critical dietary sources of essential microelements seasonal commodities.

These changes in land-use and agriculture in developing nations have had a major impact on health and its environmental determinants. Over generations, many small farmers had developed sophisticated knowledge of how to sustain yields from their farms under difficult circumstances. In recent years, drivers of environmental degradation have left large numbers of poor farmers with only poor-quality land. The impact of the impoverishment of peasant farmers on disease burden is dramatic.

It is estimated that undernutrition (and especially underweight) caused 3.7 million deaths, about 1 in 15 deaths globally, in 2000 (Table 13.1). Almost

1.8 million deaths from this cause occurred in Africa and accounted for about 20 percent of deaths in that region (Table 13.1). About 138 million DALYs (9.5 percent of the global total) were attributed to underweight in 2002; the high loss of healthy life years reflecting the fact that undernutrition results in high mortality among young children (WHO, 2002). Underweight accounts for about 15 percent of the DALYs in sub-Saharan Africa, compared to <1 percent in many developed countries. The synergy between undernutrition and infectious diseases is well documented. Diarrhea, pneumonia, acute upper respiratory infections, measles, and other infections are more severe in undernourished children and carry a higher risk of mortality (Pelletier, 1994). At the same time, some of the most common infectious diseases in children (including diarrhea, respiratory infections, measles, intestinal helminth infections, and malaria) have long been recognized to influence rates of physical growth and of malnutrition among children in developing countries (West, Caballero, and Black, 2001). Analyses of underweight-morbidity relationships suggest that 50 to 70 percent of the burden of diarrheal diseases, measles, malaria, and lower respiratory infections in children is attributable to undernutrition (WHO, 2002). An estimated 56 percent of all childhood deaths may be explained by the potentiating effects of undernutrition on the burden of infectious diseases (Pelletier, 1994). Complications accompanying malnutrition are believed to claim nearly half of the 10 million annual deaths among children under the age of five in the developing countries (West, Caballero, and Black, 2001).

Elderly people must be considered to be at high risk of undernutrition, especially those living in impoverished settings in developing countries. Results from a limited number of surveys suggest that 25 to 35 percent of older people in low-income populations may be in a chronic state of acute undernutrition (Chilima and Ismail, 1998). This is not surprising because poverty is a strong risk factor for undernutrition. Specific age-related disorders that may be potentiated by undernutrition include sarcopenia with attendant muscle weakness, impaired mobility and body function; various dementias likely of nutritional origin; and osteoporosis with resultant bone fracture (West, Caballero, and Black, 2001). The aging-environment-disease interface remains unexplored, but a number of perspectives can be mentioned. Higher susceptibility of the elderly to indoor air pollution from biofuels has been reported (Mishra, 2003). Aging brings to the fore the cumulative environmental insults, which gradually reduce the resiliency of cellular and body functions below the threshold for diseases. Aging is an inevitable and programmed cellular degradation process that can be potentiated by exposure to environmental and nutritional stressors. Irrespective of the exact mechanisms of aging-environment interactions, undernutrition among the elderly population is an immense and growing public health problem in the developing countries that needs considerably more attention than it is currently getting.

The Risk Transition to Overnutrition

On the other end of the nutrition spectrum in developing countries lies the problem of overnutrition. The globalization of production and marketing, along with changes in the social and economic status of the upper and middle classes, is rapidly increasing the consumption of alcohol, tobacco, and processed and fast foods in developing countries. Policies regarding local production and processing, import regulations, and subsidies have also altered the relative balance between the kind and cost of imported foods and the kind and cost of locally grown foods. The shift in diet toward a higher fat content (meats and fat-rich foods are considered status symbols of economic advancement), more refined carbohydrates, less fiber, more salt, and more diversity leads to overnutrition. This Westernization process also involves changes in living and working patterns as people shift to less physical activity and less labor and also to smoking cigarettes. This changing pattern in dietary habits and physical inactivity has given rise to overnutrition, with attendant hypertension, hyperlipidemias, overweight, and obesity, which are in turn risk factors for chronic diseases such as cancers, heart disease, stroke, diabetes, and mental illness, especially in rapidly growing urban populations. At the same time, parasitic infections associated with diarrhea, impaired growth and development, bladder cancers, micronutrient deficiency anemia, decreased physical fitness and work capacity, and impaired cognitive function remain pandemic in most of these urban and rural communities. The arrival of a whole group of noncommunicable diseases on top of persistent communicable diseases has resulted in a dramatic increase in the burden of diseases in Third World countries, the so-called double jeopardy phenomenon.

Cardiovascular diseases (CVDs) (including heart disease and stroke), often caused by tobacco use, overnutrition and physical inactivity, have recently emerged as a major public health problem in most Third World countries (WHO, 2003). CVDs have become the first and second causes of adult death in many developing countries, accounting for about one-third of all deaths. Twice as many deaths from CVDs occur in developing countries as in developed countries. For example, stroke mortality rates in rural and urban areas of Tanzania are higher than those for England and Wales (WHO, 2003). In terms of DALYs, CVDs rank third in disease burden (after injuries and neuropsychiatric disorders) in developing countries (WHO, 2003) and have reached epidemic proportion.

Air Pollution

From a global perspective, there is a clear dichotomy in air pollution trends. In First World countries levels of many pollutants have declined markedly, the combined result of technological, legislative, and community interventions. In most developing countries, in contrast, levels of air pollution continue to rise, reflecting growing fossil fuel consumption and intensification of manufacturing activities (Krzyzanowski and Schwela, 1999). Urban population growth in developing countries has been relentless, and Third World cities now boast some of the highest levels of air pollution in the world. Combustion processes generate a complex mixture of substances that may be primary pollutants (such as particulates) or that may form in subsequent atmospheric reactions (as ozone and sulfate aerosols do). Although attention is generally focused on a few *priority* pollutants (sulfur oxides [SO_x], nitrogen oxides [NO_x], particulate matter, ozone, carbon monoxide [CO], and lead), thousands of toxic substances are released to the atmosphere. Our knowledge of the chemical composition, speciation, and toxicity of many air pollutants has serious gaps. A detailed discussion of air pollution and its health effects appears in Chapter Fourteen.

It is estimated that as many as 1.4 billion urban residents, many of them in developing countries, breathe air with contaminant levels that exceed WHO air quality guidelines. Ambient air pollution has been linked to a variety of chronic and acute health effects. For instance, as described in Chapter Fourteen, exposure to fine particulate matter (PM) is associated with respiratory disease, cardiovascular mortality, and lung cancer (Samet and Cohen, 1999; WHO, 2002). Pollutants such as ozone and lead are associated with other serious health effects, and the bioaerosols may be a vector for a number of infectious pathogens. Urban air pollution plays a major role in childhood respiratory infections (Romieu, Samet, Smith, and Bruce, 2002). It has been estimated that fine particulate matter is responsible for 5 percent of global tracheal, bronchus, and lung cancer incidence as well as 2 percent of cardiovascular deaths and 1 percent of mortality from respiratory infections, corresponding to about 800,000 deaths (1.4 percent of total) and 7.9 million DALYs (0.8 percent of total) annually. This burden occurred predominantly in developing countries, especially the Western Pacific and Southeast Asian regions. Because of limitations in data, reliable air pollution morbidity estimates are not available; when a proper assessment is done, the burden of disease attributed to all ambient air pollution will likely be very high.

Indoor Air Pollution

Anthropogenic air pollution began when humans discovered and tamed the wildfire. Fire (or combustion) is a "dirty" process that releases a variety of pollutants that threaten human health. The major sources of indoor air pollution in developing countries remain the use of biomass and coal for cooking and heating, and of liquid fuel (heating oil and kerosene or paraffin) for heating and lighting, with significant contributions as well from environmental tobacco smoke, pesticide sprays and mosquito coils, and household furnishings and products (Smith and Mehta, 2003). These sources emit a host of pollutants including PM, carbon monoxide, toxic organic compounds such as polycyclic aromatic hydrocarbons (PAHs, an important component of fire smoke), and volatile organic compounds (VOCs). Indoor air quality is also affected by outdoor pollution sources. A significant fraction of the load of indoor pollutants is deposited as house dust or trapped by rugs, furniture, furry pets, and stuffed animals. Contaminated house dust is a major health hazard to children, who readily ingest it through hand-to-mouth activities, and thus it must be included in any discussion of indoor risk factors.

By far the bulk of indoor air pollution in developing countries results from burning biofuels such as charcoal, crop wastes, and animal dung. According to some estimates, more than half of the world's population still relies on biofuels for cooking and heating (Bruce, Perez-Padilla, and Albalak, 2000), and in many sub-Saharan countries, biofuels supply up to 95 percent of domestic energy (Ezzati and Kammen, 2002). These fuels typically are burned indoors in simple household devices such as a pit, three-stone hearth, or U-shaped brick enclosure. These highly inefficient burners bring about incomplete combustion, and they are typically located in small rooms without adequate ventilation. Under these conditions, high volumes of toxic air pollutants are generated, including SO_x (primarily from coal), NO_x, PM, CO, PAHs, heavy metals, and dozens of other organic compounds. Specific cooking styles release other types of toxic fumes to the indoor environment. Stir-frying, deep-frying in oil, and preheating oil before food is added often release cooking oil fumes containing a complex mixture of compounds including aldehydes (malonyldialdehyde, 4-hydroxy-2,3-nonenal, and 4-hydroxy-2,3-alkenals of different chain lengths), PAHs, aromatic amines, and nitro-PAHs, which are common in tobacco smoke (Wu and others, 2004). Because cooking occurs for several hours each day at times when people are present indoors, the potential exposure to cookfire emissions is high. Recent studies show that typical indoor concentrations of PM, CO, and PAHs often exceed the WHO-recommended safe levels (Ezzati and Kammen, 2002), with fine PM concentrations in excess of 2,000 μ/m^3 reported in some biofuel-using households (Balakrishnan and others, 2002). Indoor use of biofuels is also responsible for some of the highest levels of ambient air pollution recorded in rural communities (Smith, 1987; Roy, Bruce, and Dalgado, 2002). In cities in China the burning of biomass (mostly coal) in individual homes contributes about 30 percent of the outdoor particulate and sulfur dioxide pollution (Moore, Gould, and Keary, 2003).

Exposure to indoor air pollution from biofuel combustion has been linked, with varying degrees of robustness, to a number of health outcomes, including acute respiratory infection (ARI), middle ear infection (otitis media), chronic obstructive pulmonary disease (COPD), lung cancer (mainly from coal smoke), asthma, cancer of the nasopharynx and larynx, tuberculosis, perinatal conditions, low birthweight, and diseases of the eye such as cataract and blindness (Bruce, Perez-Padilla, and Albalak, 2000; Roy, Bruce, and Dalgado, 2002; Ezzati and Kammen, 2002; Balakrishnan and others, 2002). Cooking oil fumes have been associated with lung cancer among nonsmoking women in some areas of China (Tung and others, 2001) and are known to be genotoxic (Wu and others, 2004). Indoor smoke from biofuels accounts for an estimated 36 percent of lower respiratory infections, 22 percent of the COPD, and 1.5 percent of trachea, bronchus, and lung cancer worldwide (WHO, 2002). About 2.7 percent of DALYs worldwide have been attributed to indoor smoke, with 32 percent of this DALY burden occurring in Africa and 37 percent Southeast Asia. Global mortality due to indoor air pollution from biofuels is estimated to range from 1.5 to 2 million in 2002, about 4 to 5 percent of total deaths worldwide (Ezzati and Kammen, 2002).

In most developing countries women are mainly responsible for gathering, carrying, and cooking with fuel wood (Golshan, Faghihi, and Marandi, 2002; Sims and Butter, 2000) and thus are disproportionately exposed to risk from these sources. Each element of the biofuel cycle (gathering, carrying, burning) carries its own health risks for women. Besides exposure to heat, sun, and rain, women wood gatherers can suffer falls, bruises, cuts, fractures, and insect and snake bites and are exposed to infectious disease pathogens (such as mosquito and tsetse fly bites) and even to land mines. Fuel wood typically is transported by headloading, which can result in fatigue, headaches, joint and chest pain, musculoskeletal disorders, increased risk of prolapsed uterus, and weakened resistance to infections (Smith, 1987). The risks of exposure to biofuel emissions were noted earlier. Children, especially girls, usually stay with their mothers while food is being prepared and thus also experience extended exposure to biofuel emissions.

Smoking and drying are common, age-old food preservation technique in developing countries. In most cases, the foods (fish, meat, or vegetables) are dried or smoked indoors by placing them above the biofuel-burning, nonvented cookstoves. During the drying or smoking the toxic chemicals in the biofuel emissions (especially PAHs, aldehydes, and toxic metals) coat and permeate the foods being processed. The health risks of the dried fish and meats sold widely in African countries have not been well studied. The black, smoky exterior of these foods likely contains carcinogens and may represent a human health hazard. A recent study found high concentrations of arsenic (30 to 70 percent higher than those in normal food) in chili peppers and corn dried over coal-burning cookstoves; consumption of these dried foods was responsible for widespread chronic arsenic poisoning in the Guizhou Province of China (Liu and others, 2002). In urban areas the food-drying smoke may be generated by burning plastic, newspapers, wrapping papers, preserved wood, and other types of household wastes, which would change the concentrations and types of toxic substances in the dried foods.

Lead Poisoning

Lead poisoning remains one of the most preventable diseases of environmental origin in the world today. The sources of lead in the environments of developing countries are legion: base metal smelters, iron and steel production, secondary lead smelters, leaded house paints, lead pipes in water distribution systems, automobile parts (from solders to wheel-balancing weights), ammunition, batteries, cable shields, pigments, laboratory chemicals, and various alloys (Agency for Toxic Substances and Disease Registry, 2000). The environmental lead source of greatest concern is the automobile tailpipe. Most developed countries have removed lead from gasoline. By 2002, over 100 countries representing about 90 percent of global gasoline sales had phased lead out of their gasoline, leading to substantial decreases in population blood lead (PbB) levels (Meyer, McGeehin, and Falk, 2003). In contrast, the lead content of gasoline sold in Africa has been increased, typically to 0.4 to 0.8 g/L, to meet the octane requirement of the large fleet of old (used) vehicles imported from the developed countries (Nriagu, Jinabhai, Naidoo, and Coutsoundis, 1997). The continued sale of leaded gasoline by multinational corporations in the face of mounting evidence that millions of children in urban areas of African and other developing countries are poisoned by lead raises compelling ethical and moral questions.

Emission of lead from smelting operations in developing countries is an ongoing concern. These smelters generally employ outdated technology or are equipped with inefficient pollution control devices. Secondary smelters, involved in recycling the lead in car batteries, are being disproportionately sited in developing countries because they cannot meet pollution control regulations in the developed countries. Cottage industries, including such service and repair businesses as appliance repair, battery repair or reprocessing to take out the lead, welding, paint finishing, auto bodywork, carburetor repair, oil change services, and processing of metal scraps, are a growing source of lead pollution in urban areas of developing countries. Environmental risks from cottage industries are highest in the home environment, where children live and play. Deteriorating lead paint on walls of older buildings, improperly glazed pottery and ceremonial glasses, traditional and herbal medicines, and beauty aids can become significant sources of lead exposure in some countries as well.

Worldwide, about 120 million people have PbBs in the range of 5 to 10 μg/dL; levels for 50 to 100 million people are believed to exceed 10 μg/dL. About 10 to 30 percent of all children have PbB levels above 5 μg/dL, with over 90 percent of these afflicted children being in the developing countries (WHO, 2002). Most countries in the world currently accept a PbB value above 10 μg/dL to be a level of concern. About 234,000 deaths worldwide and 12.9 million (0.9 percent) DALYs are attributable to lead poisoning (WHO, 2002). Young children in developing countries are particularly susceptible to lead poisoning. They accompany their mothers, often tied to their mothers' backs, when their mothers go to crowded marketplaces or vend foods or small goods at roadside stalls. Many of the common endemic diseases (including malaria, schistosomiasis, and dengue fever) can affect the absorption of lead or development of systemic lead poisoning. More important, significant inverse associations have been demonstrated between blood lead levels and the dietary intake of a number of micronutrients, including iron, zinc, calcium, and vitamins C and D (Gallicchio, Scherer, and Sexton, 2002). In addition, total fat and caloric intakes have been positively associated with blood lead levels. The fact that nutrient intake in young children is a risk factor for elevated blood lead levels is of concern in view of the epidemic of undernutrition and underweight in developing countries. The health effects of lead at various exposure doses are summarized in Box 13.2.

Box 13.2. Health Effects of Environmental Lead Exposure

The literature on human toxicity of lead is voluminous. At high doses of exposure, no human organ is immune to lead toxicity, and the domino effect may progress to coma and even death. At the moderately elevated and low levels of exposure typical in environmental media, lead can damage the central nervous, renal, cardiovascular, hematological, and reproductive systems. Infants are particularly susceptible to lead poisoning because they absorb lead more readily than adults and their developing nervous and immune systems are more vulnerable to the effects of lead than those of adults. Epidemiological studies have found that childhood lead exposure is associated with neuropsychiatric disorders including lowered IQ, impaired mental and physical development, hyperactivity, hearing loss, reduced attention span, aggression, somatic complaints, and antisocial and delinquent behavior. A significant association between elevated blood lead at relatively low levels and delayed pubertal development in girls has recently been reported (Wu, Buck, and Mendola, 2003). There does not appear to be a safe threshold of lead exposure. Even exposures to picomolar concentrations of lead have been shown to stimulate kinase C, a calcium- and phospholipid-dependent enzyme that can mediate cellular proliferation, differentiation, and function and is critical to signal transduction. The effects of such cellular change on the viability of organ systems and the wellness of an individual are unknown.

A weak association between long-term, low-level exposure to lead and development of hypertension has been reported for men and women. Past exposure to lead may result in decreased reserve capacity of the brain and detrimental effects on neuropsychological functions, which may become manifest in old age. More than 90 percent of the body burden of lead is located in the bone, where it has an average half-life of about ten years. During periods of increased bone turnover, such as during pregnancy, lactation, and menopause, these skeletal bone stores can be mobilized, long after the external exposure, posing a hazard to the fetus at critical times in its organ development and to the nursing child. The bone loss during menopause, mediated by decreased estrogen production, may release enough lead to constitute a hazard to women in old age. Lead exerts both direct and indirect effects on bone turnover and has been implicated as a risk factor for osteoporosis, which is increasing rapidly in developing countries, especially among women (Vahter, Berglund, Akesson, and Linden, 2002).

Urbanization

According to a recent report, 48 percent of the world's population currently lives in an urban environment; by the year 2030, 5 billion people will live in cities (United Nations Department of Economic and Social Affairs, Population Division, 2004). Most of this rapid urbanization is expected to occur in the developing world, where urban migration, urbanicity, and the growth of megacities have already shaped the public health landscape (United Nations Department of Economic and Social Affairs, 2004). Chapter Sixteen presents a detailed review of urbanization; this chapter reviews the impacts of environmental health risks in densely populated, low-income cities in Third World countries.

With few exceptions, urban growth in many Third World countries has outstripped the capacity of municipal and local governments to provide even basic health and other services. Among the numerous megaslums that have formed in the outskirts of Third World cities, lack of reliable access to electricity limits the use of cleaner fuels for cooking. Even among urban residents with access to electricity, many continue to rely on coal, kerosene, and biomass burning for heating and cooking. In a study of fuel smoke pollution and health in Hanoi, 96 percent of respondents were connected to the electrical grid, but only 35 percent used electricity for cooking (Ellegard, 1996). A similar study in Maputo found that although 30 percent were connected, less than a third of that number used electricity in cooking (Ellegard, 1996). Overcrowding in urban areas, especially in conditions of extreme poverty, can lead to increased exposure to indoor pollutants. For example, crowding may require household members to sleep in closer proximity to indoor pollution sources such as the stove or fireplace.

Crowding also produces high volumes of human waste. Unplanned land-use development typical of urban slums in Third World countries may lead to contamination of water and food supplies with biological wastes and interfere with personal hygiene practices. These conditions foster communicable disease transmission among the urban poor. In some crowded cities people may also keep livestock, a practice that contributes to microbial pollution, contamination of food and water, and transmission of pathogens from animals to humans (zoonoses).

The health impacts of low-income settlements result from two critical drivers: physiological responses to physical aspects of the environment, such as air pollution, and behavioral responses to the slum environment. In developing countries these health impacts are exacerbated by the rapid, unplanned manner in which urbanization occurs and by the relative absence of adequate resources and infrastructure to mitigate the adverse effects of urbanicity. Another factor is the tendency for polluting industries, waste dumps, and waste management facilities to be located near low-income neighborhoods, with no clear demarcation between residential and industrial areas. Bad sanitation may lead to contaminated water supplies and human wastes finding their way into the local food chain. Solid wastes may clog drains, resulting in accumulation of water in which mosquitoes breed; use of mosquito coils and pesticides to combat these pests may add to air pollution and chemical hazards. Flies that thrive on wastes contaminate foods with pathogens, and the lack of education on food safety can lead to a high incidence of food poisoning. In low-income settlements local environmental problems are generally major contributors to disease and death.

Although many of the health impacts of urbanicity are similar across the middle classes in both developed and developing countries, low-income settlements create a vastly different environment with different health impacts for the urban poor in developing countries compared with their counterparts in developed countries. Urbanization was historically driven by the existence of urban job opportunities in the manufacturing sector. In the Third World today, urbanization is primarily driven by rural deprivation rather than by economic growth or industrialization. Urban migration is often preceded by natural disaster such as drought or flooding. Following the loss of agrarian livelihood, the displaced rural population migrates to the city in search of job opportunities, typically overwhelming the available urban employment. Rural migrants who make it to the city alive usually wind up among the masses of urban slum dwellers and urban poor when the hoped-for opportunities for economic advancement fail to materialize. In their struggle to secure a livelihood, they may accept low-wage jobs that expose them and their families to environmental hazards. They have limited resources to cope with illness or injury when they occur. Some become street vendors, exposed to high levels of vehicular pollution, and a few become waste pickers, exposed to hazardous materials.

Movement in the Third World from a traditional rural area to an urban one changes the social environment and lifestyle of the newly urbanized population. The permissive social environment, relative anonymity, and lack of traditional mores in the cities produce an environment conducive to sexual promiscuity, smoking, drinking, and drug use. The combination of crowding and relative anonymity in the city also gives rise to increased violence. The relaxation of formerly strict sexual taboos among young, affluent city dwellers in the developing world can have many negative consequences, ranging from unwanted pregnancies to the spread of sexually transmitted diseases such as AIDS. The anonymity and lack of social support, in addition to the appalling conditions faced by many urban dwellers in the Third World, has also given rise to an epidemic of mental health problems to among these men and women, and even among their children (World Health Organization, 2001).

The increasing asthma burden among urban residents in the developing countries demonstrates the impact of and the intersection of behavioral and traditional environmental risk factors in these populations. The prevalence of asthma is currently highest in the First World countries (Beasley and others 2000). However, with the transition away from traditional practices, customs and land use, the prevalence of asthma has increased among Third World populations that have become increasingly Westernized. An increase in asthma prevalence has also been reported among immigrant populations that relocate to Australia and the United States (Johnson and others, 2005; Powell and others, 1999). Immigrant populations tend to adopt the asthma prevalence in the country to which they move, suggesting that immigrants from developing countries with low asthma prevalence who relocate in Westernized countries with high prevalence are at increased risk for asthma (Leung, Carlin, Burdon, and Czarny, 1994). Comparisons of urban and rural communities in the developing world consistently report higher asthma prevalence among urban populations.

Epidemiological studies have reported that people who grow up on a farm have a lower risk of developing asthma, suggesting that agrarian exposures may be a protective aspect of a traditional lifestyle (Alm and others, 1999). Obesity, an emblematic disease of Westernization, is another risk factor for asthma in the developed countries. An association between high dietary fat and asthma has also been found in the developing countries (Huang and Pan, 2001), suggesting that changes in traditional diet and lifestyle such as increased fast-food consumption and reduced exercise may contribute to asthma risk in addition to risks for other chronic diseases among transitioning populations. The level of ambient air pollution is an obvious difference between urban and rural communities; however, it is unclear whether ambient air pollution plays a causal or exacerbatory role in asthma etiology. It has also been suggested that the disparity between urban and rural asthma prevalence can be explained by characteristics of urban lifestyle such as carpets, indoor pets, and crowding that increase indoor allergen concentrations in urban environments (Ng'ang'a and others, 1998, Woodcock and others, 2001). The explanation for the increase in asthma in transitioning populations remains elusive and likely involves a complex interaction between behavioral and environmental risk factors.

Water

Water is essential for life. Access to clean water has been designated a human right by the United Nations Committee on Economic, Cultural and Social Rights. Nevertheless, approximately 1.1 billion people live in developing countries without continuous access to safe drinking water. In low-income developing countries, less than 50 percent of the population has access to safe drinking water, as compared to 75 to 90 percent in high-income developing countries and more than 90 percent in developed countries. Rural populations in low-income developing countries have considerably less access to safe drinking water than do those living in urban areas (Table 13.5). In parts of sub-Saharan Africa, Latin America, and

TABLE 13.5. POPULATION WITH AND WITHOUT ACCESS TO SAFE DRINKING WATER (FREE OF DISEASE-CAUSING MICROBES), 2000.

Region	Urban Population with Access (%)	Rural Population with Access (%)	Population Without Access (in millions)
Africa	85	47	300
Asia	93	75	693
Oceania	98	63	3
Latin America and the Caribbean (including Mexico)	93	62	78
Europe	100	87	26
North America	100	100	0
World	94	71	1,100

Source: WHO, 2000.

the Caribbean, less than 40 percent of the rural population have access to safe drinking water. Furthermore, the availability of safe drinking water in rural areas often depends on the labor of women and young girls, who spend hours each day fetching water for the home.

Safe drinking water generally refers to water that is free of disease-causing microbes, including bacteria, viruses, protozoa, and small animals such as worms. These biota can be considered *traditional* health hazards in drinking water supplies. In addition to traditional hazards, water may carry high concentrations of chemical contaminants that can cause health problems. In developing countries, concentrations of anthropogenic chemical contaminants are on the rise and can be designated *modern* health hazards. Examples are pesticides, nitrates, industrial pollutants, and disinfection by-products. In addition to anthropogenic contaminants, elevated concentrations of natural environmental contaminants may be found in drinking water supplies. Though these natural contaminants are difficult to categorize in a traditional-modern framework, the presence in drinking water of naturally occurring contaminants, such as arsenic and fluoride, causes unwanted health effects. Natural contaminants are most prevalent in groundwater supplies and are a growing concern in developing countries, due to their increasing reliance on groundwater. A detailed overview of water and health is provided in Chapter Eighteen; this chapter focuses on health hazards associated with traditional, modern, and natural environmental contaminants of particular concern in Third World countries.

Microbial contamination of source water, lack of sanitation services, and inadequate personal hygiene form a triad that gives rise to communicable diseases. Extensive volumes have been written on communicable diseases transmitted through unsafe drinking water (Hunter, Waite, and Ronchi, 2002; WHO, 2000). Because these diseases are detailed in Chapter Eighteen, they are discussed only briefly here. Approximately 2.6 million people, mostly children, die annually from water-related communicable diseases in developing countries. In contrast just 3,500 deaths from this cause befall citizens of developed countries (Murray and Lopez, 1996). Shigella, a bacterium that causes dysentery, or bloody diarrhea, is responsible for approximately 2.2 million deaths each year. Intestinal worms infect about 10 percent of the population in developing regions, leading to malnutrition, anemia, and retarded growth. Trachoma, caused by the bacterium *Chlamydia trachomatis,* is the leading cause of preventable blindness, leading to 6 million cases worldwide. These microbial diseases can largely be prevented by providing access to microbial-free drinking water, adequate disposal systems for human excrement, and information about appropriate personal hygiene.

Concerted efforts have been made during recent decades to increase access to safe drinking water in Third World countries. They have resulted in increased distribution of disinfected surface water in many urban areas and in more access to groundwater supplies through the drilling of community wells in rural communities. More recently, increasing attention is being given to inexpensive point-of-use disinfection systems for household water treatment, especially in rural areas where groundwater is not available. One such device, known as the Safe Water System (SWS), consists of locally produced and bottled sodium hypochlorite solution, a 5 to 10 mL measuring cap on each bottle to monitor dosage, a plastic container to store disinfected water and prevent recontamination, and educational and social marketing materials to encourage changes in personal hygiene. The inexpensive SWS has been shown to be effective in reducing rates of diarrhea in periurban and rural communities of Bolivia and Zambia, and some effort is being made to export it to other countries (Suk and others, 2003). Few countries in the Third World can afford the capital investment needed to pipe safe water to most citizens, and inexpensive household-level interventions are increasingly being viewed as worthwhile alternatives.

Modern health hazards from anthropogenic contaminants are also beginning to receive attention in developing countries. Centralized chlorination of drinking water leads to the formation of disinfection by-products that may be carcinogenic to humans (International Agency for Research on Cancer, 1987). Industrial discharges of toxic chemicals taint groundwater and surface water supplies. Estimates suggest that approximately 60 percent of smelting and 50 percent of lead mining operations are located in developing countries (Yanez and others, 2002), causing trace metal pollution (for example, cadmium, nickel, and lead) in aquatic systems (Nriagu and Pacyna, 1988). In most cases water is consumed without treatment. Millions of people in developing countries drink rainwater collected from rooftops, stem flows, or other systems. In many urban areas this source of drinking water becomes contaminated through scavenging of airborne pollutants and leaching of air toxics deposited on the roof surfaces.

Nonpoint source water pollution from agricultural activity is also a concern in developing countries. Pesticides and nitrates are applied heavily to farmland in developing countries and infiltrate well water supplies. For instance, in the Philippines, concentrations of nitrates and pesticides (DDT, butachlor, endosulfan, and carbofuran) exceeding safe drinking-water limit standards have been detected in shallow groundwater supplies (Bouman, Castaneda, and Bhuiyan, 2002). Exposure to elevated nitrate levels in well water supplies can cause methemoglobinemia, a disease characterized by insufficient oxygen reaching the brain, turning babies, who are especially vulnerable, a faint bluish color. A wide variety of diseases, from cancer to neurodegenerative disorders, are associated with exposure to nitrates and pesticides, but the contribution of this exposure pathway to the disease burden in developing countries has yet to be assessed.

Finally, elevated concentrations of natural elements also cause numerous health problems for populations around the world. Specific elements of concern in water include arsenic, fluoride, radon, sodium, and uranium. Excessive levels of these natural contaminants are commonly detected in groundwater supplies. For example, high fluoride concentrations have been documented in groundwater in large parts of Africa, the Middle East, China, and southern and western Asia. Low concentrations of fluoride (for example, 0.8 to 1.2 mg/L) can prevent tooth decay and strengthen bones. At slightly higher concentrations, however, dental and skeletal fluorosis can result, with attrition of tooth enamel and fluoride deposits in bone, respectively. The total number of people drinking water with fluoride concentrations above WHO's guideline (1.5 mg/L) is not known. However, estimates suggest that tens of millions of individuals are suffering from fluorosis, with high prevalences in China and India.

Elevated levels of arsenic have been reported in groundwater in many parts of the world. To date, high levels of arsenic have been identified in groundwater from twenty-three countries on six continents, and additional contaminated aquifers are continually being discovered. Globally, 45 million people are estimated to be exposed to levels of arsenic in drinking water exceeding 50 μg/L, the maximum contaminant limit (MCL) allowable in many countries (Table 13.6). More than 100 million people are exposed to levels of arsenic exceeding the WHO's MCL of 10 μg/L.

Health effects that have been associated with ingestion of groundwater high in arsenic include peripheral vascular diseases (such as blackfoot disease, which presents with numbness of one or more extremities, progressing to black discoloration, ulceration, and gangrene), skin lesions, diabetes mellitus, cerebrovascular disease, and cancer. More recent studies have linked high levels

TABLE 13.6. ESTIMATED POPULATION EXPOSED TO ARSENIC IN DRINKING WATER AT CONCENTRATIONS >50 μg/L, THE MCL IN MANY COUNTRIES.

Country	Population Exposed
Bangladesh	30,000,000
West Bengal, India	6,000,000
Taiwan	900,000
Mainland China	5,600,000
Vietnam	1,000,000
Argentina	270,000
Chile	500,000
Mexico	400,000
United States	350,000
Hungary	29,000
Total	45,000,000

Source: Adapted from Smedley and Kinniburgh, 2002.

of arsenic in drinking water with health effects ranging from infant mortality to cancers of the skin, lungs, bladder, and kidney. Arsenic poisoning has become an epidemic and a major public health problem in some developing countries (see Box 13.3), and investigators continue to explore affordable methods to reduce arsenic concentrations in water to safe levels.

Box 13.3. Arsenic Poisoning in Bangladesh

Historically, surface water in Bangladesh has been contaminated with microorganisms, causing significant morbidity in infants and children. In the 1970s and '80s, the United Nations Children's Fund (UNICEF), working with the Bangladesh Department of Public Health Engineering, installed tube wells as a putative source of safe drinking water for the Bangladeshi people. Tube wells are about 5 cm in diameter, inserted into the ground at shallow depths less than 50 m, and capped with a cast-iron or steel hand pump. It is estimated that more than 11 million tube wells have been dug in Bangladesh. In the early 1990s, the well water, which had seemingly provided a solution to the country's water problems, was discovered to have high concentrations of arsenic. Standard water testing procedures did not check for arsenic during initial well installation.

The maximum concentration of arsenic permitted in drinking water in Bangladesh is 50 μg/L, whereas the WHO recommended standard is 10 μg/L. The scale of the arsenic contamination has not been fully documented, and precise estimates of the population at risk are unavailable. However, an estimated 25 to 35 million people are exposed to arsenic in drinking water at levels exceeding 50 μg/L, and 50 to 60 million people are exposed to concentrations exceeding 10 μg/L. The effects mentioned earlier, skin lesions, peripheral vascular diseases, diabetes mellitus, cerebrovascular disease, and cancer, have been linked to this arsenic exposure and are estimated to affect more than 100,000 people in Bangladesh. Arsenic contamination of water in Bangladesh is one of the worst environmental health disasters in history, and more health problems are expected in coming years.

Despite the unimaginable scale of arsenic-related health problems in Bangladesh, there is hope. More than 50 percent of tube wells in Bangladesh have arsenic concentrations below 10 μg/L. Efforts are ongoing to identify tube wells that have water with low arsenic content and to discover simple, inexpensive, effective arsenic treatment strategies for tube wells with high arsenic concentrations (see, for example, Massachusetts Institute of Technology, 2001). (For further information on chronic arsenic poisoning, see Arsenic Project, 2005.)

People in developing countries face triple and sometimes quadruple jeopardy when attempting to manage environmental risks from unsafe water supplies. Traditional health hazards of microbial contamination, modern hazards of anthropogenic pollutants, and hazards of natural environmental contaminants have been discussed. In addition, *postmodern* water quality hazards, such as endocrine disruptors, are a growing problem around the world. Endocrine disruptors are widespread in water supplies in developed countries due to extensive use of human and veterinary pharmaceuticals and reproductive hormones. Endocrine disruptors are likely to be a concern in water supplies of developing countries in the future, as personal care products and industrial pharmaceuticals are more broadly adopted.

Injuries

Most injuries are associated directly or indirectly with environmental risk factors and are thus preventable. Examples of environmental factors that drive injuries include poorly designed cookstoves that carry a risk of burns (especially to children) and house fires; poorly designed roadways; substandard housing at risk of collapse, especially in slum areas; inadequate land-use planning that places people in the path of flooding and landslides; accidental poisonings by pesticides needed to deal with effects of newly created breeding grounds or of building next to pest-infested habitats such as a stream; and festering domestic and interpersonal violence, especially in urban slums. It is estimated that about 30 percent of the global burden of unintentional injuries is attributable to environmental risk factors (WHO, 1997). A general review of injuries as an environmental health problem is presented in Chapter Twenty-Five. This chapter focuses on the effects of the environmental risk transition on injuries in developing countries, with special emphasis on roadway injuries.

Although injuries are major contributors to global morbidity and mortality in both developing and developed countries, a clear transition in injury risks occurs with a change in level of development. Injuries from fires, agricultural injuries, drownings, wood-acquisition injuries, and war-related violence dominate the early stages of development, and road traffic, intentional, and industrial injuries appear to increase with economic development (WHO, 1997). Because injuries disproportionately affect young adults, their economic impact can be profound; the resulting long-term disability affects productivity, especially among low-income groups, whose earning capacity is often based on physical ability. Injuries can be divided into two broad categories: *intentional injuries,* such as rape, battery, child and spousal abuse, suicide, police or military brutality, and war-related violence, and *unintentional injuries,* such as road traffic injuries, harm from fires, drownings, falls, poisonings, injuries resulting from natural disasters, and workplace injuries. Together, injuries from these sources constitute a hidden epidemic among young

TABLE 13.7. GLOBAL DALYS DUE TO INJURIES, 2002.

	Global (%)	Male (%)	Female (%)	Africa (%)	Africa (% all injuries)[b]
All injuries[a]	12.2 (182.6)	15.5 (120.4)	8.7 (62.2)	8.5 (31.0)	
Unintentional injuries[a]	8.9 (133.5)	10.9 (84.4)	6.8 (49.0)	5.9 (21.5)	69.5
Road traffic accidents	2.6	3.5	1.6	2.0	23.2
Poisonings	0.5	0.6	0.4	0.3	3.4
Falls	1.1	1.3	0.9	0.3	0.0
Fires	0.8	0.6	1.0	0.5	6.4
Drownings	0.7	1.0	0.5	0.5	6.2
Other	3.3	3.9	2.6	2.3	26.8
Intentional injuries[a]	3.3 (49.1)	4.6 (36.0)	1 (13.1)	2.6 (9.5)	30.5
Self-inflicted	1.4	1.6	1.2	0.2	2.9
Violence	1.4	2.3	0.5	1.5	17.1
War	0.4	0.7	0.1	0.9	10.6
Other	0.0	0.0	0.0	0.0	0.0

[a]The number of DALYs (in millions) is shown in parentheses.

[b]The contribution (as a percentage) of each risk factor to the total injury burden for Africa.

Source: WHO, 2003.

adults in the developing countries. They were among the major causes of healthy life years lost, accounting for 182.6 million DALYs in 2002, or 12.2 percent of the global total (15.5 percent among men and 8.7 percent among women) (Table 13.7). In Africa, injuries accounted for 31 million DALYs, or 8.5 percent of the total. In parts of South America, Eastern Europe, and the eastern Mediterranean, more than 30 percent of the disease burden among male adults fourteen to forty-four years old can be attributed to injuries (WHO, 2003). Worldwide, intentional injuries accounted for 3.3 percent of DALYs, and unintentional injuries for 8.9 percent (Table 13.7).

Road traffic injuries are among the leading causes of disease burden, especially in the fourteen- to forty-four-year-old age group (WHO, 2003). Traffic crashes kill or severely injure more than 20 million drivers, passengers, and pedestrians each year, with the burden falling most heavily on developing countries (WHO, 2003). Developing countries bear 90 percent of the DALYs lost to traffic injuries and death, and this epidemic is rising rapidly especially in Asia. It is projected that by 2020, vehicular deaths will increase by nearly 150 percent in China and by 80 percent or more in many developing countries (Kopits and Cropper, 2003). Injuries due mostly to traffic crashes account for up to one-third of the acute patient cases in many Third World hospitals and 30 to 86 percent of trauma admissions (Odero, Garner, and Zwi, 1997). Besides the human toll, the economic cost of road crashes in developing countries has been estimated at about $65 billion, a heavy burden on economic development and a financial drain on national health care systems (WHO, 2003).

Road infrastructure in developing countries rarely keeps pace with the sharp rise in the number of vehicles on the roads, resulting in unsafe driving conditions, massive traffic jams, road rage, vehicular crashes, and harm to pedestrians. Vehicles in developing countries are more likely to be involved in fatal crashes (by as much as 200-fold in some cases) than are vehicles in more developed countries (Jacobs, Aaron-Thomas, and Astrop, 2000). The face of traffic death is different in the three worlds. In developed countries, driver and passenger deaths generally account for 50 to 60 percent of traffic fatalities, with the majority of deaths occurring on rural roads (WHO, 2003). In developing countries, in contrast, a large fraction of the fatalities occur among vulnerable road users in urban areas, including pedestrians, bicyclists, carts, rickshaws, motorcyclists, moped and scooter riders, and among passengers on trucks and buses (WHO, 2003). The urban poor in developing countries are disproportionately exposed to vehicular injuries because they tend to live in overcrowded areas with narrow streets and no speed controls, operate businesses from roadside stalls, often walk to destinations on the streets, and have their children play on streets. WHO (2003) estimates that a large fraction (about 44 percent) of the vehicular mortality and morbidity can be prevented by environmental intervention strategies.

Conclusion

Environmental health exists against a complex backdrop of environmental, technological, demographic, political, economic, and cultural factors. For much of the world's population, living in Third World countries, these factors seem to conspire to threaten health. People are exposed to traditional environmental hazards, such as contaminated water and biofuel smoke, and at the same time to modern environmental hazards, such as chemical toxins. Globalization has accelerated change throughout the world; one result has been migration of hazards from developed nations to developing nations, concentrating hazardous environmental exposures and creating a risk overlap by superimposing modern on traditional exposures. In combination with poverty, undernutrition, and rapid urbanization, the toll on health can be enormous.

This chapter has discussed five areas of environmental health: agriculture, nutrition, air quality, urbanization, and water. (A sixth area, occupational health, also has special relevance in developing nations and is discussed in

Chapter Twenty-Three; also see Frumkin, 1999.) Much of the discussion in this chapter reprised material presented elsewhere in this book, but with a focus on developing nation settings, where exposure levels are often higher, populations more susceptible, and public health responses less effective than they are in developed nations. As the twenty-first century proceeds, achieving environmental health for all remains a pressing challenge and a moral necessity.

Thought Questions

1. What is environmental risk transition? What are the impacts of this phenomenon on the health of people in Third World countries?
2. What are the risks and benefits of globalization on the health of people in (a) developed countries and (b) developing countries?
3. Describe the diseases commonly associated with (a) traditional lifestyles and (b) Westernized lifestyles.
4. Discuss how a safe drinking-water supply, sanitary disposal of human waste, and good behavioral hygiene practices can limit water-based microbial diseases. Discuss why, despite tremendous efforts by WHO and UNICEF, billions of people currently live without safe drinking-water or sanitation services.
5. How might climate change (such as global warming) affect the availability and quality of water supplies?
6. What might be responsible for the fact that most countries in Africa are still using leaded gasoline, which has been banned in many other countries of the world?
7. What might be responsible for the rising incidence of asthma in developing countries? To what extent might this be a result of the confluence of lifestyles?

References

Agency for Toxic Substances and Disease Registry. "Toxicological Profile for Lead (Update)." Atlanta, Ga.: Agency for Toxic Substances and Disease Registry, 2000.

Alm, J., and others. "Atopy in Children of Families with an Anthroposophic Lifestyle." *Lancet,* 1999, *353,* 1485–1488.

Arsenic Project. "Introduction." [http://phys4.harvard.edu/~wilson/arsenic/arsenic_project_introduction.html]. 2005.

Balakrishnan, K., and others. "Daily Average Exposures to Respiratory Particulate Matter from Combustion of Biomass Fuels in Rural Households of Southern India." *Environmental Health Perspectives,* 2002, *110,* 1069–1075.

Beasley, R., Crane, J., Lai, C., and Pearce, N. "Prevalence and Etiology of Asthma." *Journal of Allergy and Clinical Immunology,* 2000, *105*(2), 466–472.

Bouman, B.A.M., Castaneda, A. R., and Bhuiyan, S. I. "Nitrate and Pesticide Contamination of Groundwater Under Rice-Based Cropping Systems: Past and Current Evidence from the Philippines." *Agriculture, Ecosystems and Environment,* 2002, *92,* 185–199.

Bradley, D. J., and Narayan, R. "Epidemiological Patterns Associated with Agricultural Activities in the Tropics with Special Reference to Vector-Borne Diseases." In *Effects of Agricultural Development on Vector-borne Diseases.* Rome, Food and Agriculture Organization of the United Nations, 1987.

Bruce, N., Perez-Padilla, R., and Albalak, R. "Indoor Air Pollution in Developing Countries: A Major Environmental Health Challenge." *Bulletin of the World Health Organization,* 2000, *78,* 1080–1092.

Chilima, D. M., and Ismail, S. J. "Anthropometric Characteristics of Older People in Malawi." *European Journal of Clinical Nutrition,* 1998, *52,* 643–649.

Ecobichon, D. J. "Pesticide Use in Developing Countries." *Toxicology,* 2001, *160,* 27–33.

Ellegard, A. "Cooking Fuel Smoke and Respiratory Symptoms Among Women in Low-Income Areas in Maputo." *Environmental Health Perspectives,* 1996, *104,* 980–985.

Ezzati, M., and Kammen, D. M. "The Health Impacts of Exposure to Indoor Air Pollution from Solid Fuels in Developing Countries: Knowledge, Gaps and Data Needs." *Environmental Health Perspectives,* 2002, *110,* 1057–1066.

Frumkin, H. "Across the Water and Down the Ladder: Occupational Health in the Global Economy." *Occupational Medicine,* 1999, *14*(3), 637–663.

Gallicchio, L., Scherer, R., and Sexton, M. "Influence of Nutrition Intake on Blood Lead Levels of Young Children at Risk for Lead Poisoning." *Environmental Health Perspectives,* 2002, *110,* A767–A771.

Golshan, M., Faghihi, M., and Marandi, M. "Indoor Women Jobs and Pulmonary Risks in Rural Areas of Isfahan, Iran, 2000." *Respiratory Medicine,* 2002, *96*(6), 382–388.

Huang, S., and Pan, W. "Dietary Fats and Asthma in Teenagers: Analyses of the First Nutrition and Health Survey in Taiwan (NAHSIT)." *Clinical and Experimental Allergy,* 2001, *31,* 1875–1880.

Hunter, P. R., Waite, M., and Ronchi, E. (eds.). (2002). *Drinking Water and Infectious Disease: Establishing the Links.* London: IWA Publishing, 2002.

International Agency for Research on Cancer. "Overall Evaluations of Carcinogenicity: An Updating of IARC Monographs, Volumes 1 to 42." *IARC Monographs on the Evaluation of Carcinogenic Risk to Humans,* 1987, (suppl. 7) 1–440.

Jacobs, G., Aaron-Thomas, A., and Astrop, A. *Estimating Global Road Fatalities.* Report no. 445. London: Transport Research Laboratory, 2000.

Johnson, M., and others. "Asthma Prevalence and Severity in Arab American Communities in the Detroit Area, Michigan." *Journal of Immigrant Health,* 2005, *7*(3), 165–178.

Kickbusch, I., and Buse, K. "Global Influences and Global Responses: International Health at the Turn of the Twenty-First Century." In M. H. Merson, R. E. Black, and A. J. Mills (eds.), *International Public Health.* Gaithersburg, Md.: Aspen, 2001.

Koh, D., and Jeyaratnam, J. "Pesticide Hazards in Developing Countries." *Science of the Total Environment,* 1996, *188* (suppl. 1), S78–S85.

Kopits, E., and Cropper, M. "Traffic Fatalities and Economic Growth." Policy Research Working Paper no. 3035. Washington, D.C.: World Bank, 2003.

Krzyzanowski, M., and Schwela, D. "Patterns of Air Pollution in Developing Countries." In S. T. Holgate, H. S. Koren, J. M. Samet, and R. L. Maynard (eds.), *Air Pollution and Health.* New York: Academic Press, 1999.

Leung, R. C., Carlin, J. B., Burdon, J. G., and Czarny, D. "Asthma, Allergy and Atopy in Asian Immigrants in Melbourne." *Medical Journal of Australia,* 1994, *161*(7), 418–425.

Liu, J., and others. "Chronic Arsenic Poisoning from Burning of High-Arsenic-Containing Coal in Guizhou, China." *Environmental Health Perspectives,* 2002, *110,* 119–122.

London, L., and others. "Pesticide Usage and Health Consequences for Women in Developing Countries: Out of Sight, Out of Mind?" *International Journal of Occupational and Environmental Health,* 2002, *8,* 46–59.

Mascie-Taylor, C.G.N., and Karim, E. "The Burden of Chronic Disease." *Science,* 2003, *302,* 1921–1922.

Massachusetts Institute of Technology. "Arsenic Remediation Technologies: Online Informational Database." [http://web.mit.edu/murcott/www/arsenic]. 2001.

Meister, E. A. "Global Environmental Health." In R. W. Buckingham (ed.), *A Primer on International Health.* Needham Heights, Mass.: Allyn & Bacon, 2001.

Meyer, P. A., McGeehin, M. A., and Falk, H. "A Global Approach to Childhood Lead Poisoning Prevention." *International Journal of Hygiene and Environmental Health,* 2003, *206,* 363–369.

Mishra, V. "Effect of Indoor Air Pollution from Biomass Combustion on Prevalence of Asthma in the Elderly." *Environmental Health Perspectives,* 2003, *111,* 71–76.

Moore, M., Gould, P., and Keary, B. S. "Global Urbanization and Impact on Health." *International Journal of Hygiene and Environmental Health,* 2003, *206,* 269–278.

Murray, C.J.L., and Lopez, A. D. (eds.). *The Global Burden of Disease, Global Health Statistics: A Compendium of Incidence, Prevalence and Mortality Estimates for over 200 conditions.* Global Burden of Disease and Injury Series, Vol. 2. Cambridge, Mass.: Harvard School of Public Health on behalf of the World Health Organization and the World Bank, 1996.

Ng'ang'a, L. W., and others. "Prevalence of Exercise Induced Bronchospasm in Kenyan School Children: An Urban-Rural Comparison." *Thorax,* 1998, *53*(11), 919–926.

Nriagu, J. O., Jinabhai, C. C., Naidoo, R., and Coutsoundis, A. "Lead Poisoning of Children in Africa, II: Kwazulu/Natal, South Africa." *Science of the Total Environment,* 1997, *197,* 1–11.

Nriagu, J. O., and Pacyna, J. M. "Quantitative Assessment of Worldwide Contamination of Air, Water and Soils by Trace Metals." *Nature,* 1988, *333,* 134–140.

Odero, W., Garner, P., and Zwi, A. "Road Traffic Injuries in Developing Countries: A Comprehensive Review of Epidemiological Studies." *Tropical Medicine and International Health,* 1997, *2,* 445–460.

Pelletier, D. L. "The Potentiating Effects of Malnutrition on Child Mortality: Epidemiologic Evidence and Policy Implications." *Nutrition Reviews,* 1994, *52,* 409–415.

Powell, C. V., and others. "Respiratory Symptoms and Duration of Residence in Immigrant Teenagers Living in Melbourne, Australia." *Archives of Disease in Childhood,* 1999, *81*(2), 159–162.

Romieu, I., Samet, J. M., Smith, K. R., and Bruce, N. "Outdoor Air Pollution and Acute Respiratory Infections Among Children in Developing Countries." *Journal of Occupational and Environmental Medicine,* 2002, *44,* 640–649.

Roy, E., Bruce, N., and Dalgado, H. "Birth Weight and Exposure to Kitchen Wood Smoke During Pregnancy in Rural Guatemala." *Environmental Health Perspectives,* 2002, *110,* 109–114.

Samet, J. M., and Cohen, A. J. "Air Pollution and Lung Cancer." In S. T. Holgate, H. S. Koren, J. M. Samet, and R. L. Maynard (eds.), *Air Pollution and Health.* New York: Academic Press, 1999.

Sims, J., and Butter, M. E. *Gender Equity and Environmental Health.* Harvard Center for Population and Development Studies, Working Paper Series vol.10, no. 5, June 2000. [http://www.hsph.Harvard.edu/organizatons/healthnet/HUpapers/gender/simsbutter.html]. 2000.

Smedley, P. L., and Kinniburgh, D. G. "A Review of the Source, Behavior and Distribution of Arsenic in Natural Waters." *Applied Geochemistry,* 2002, *17,* 517–568.

Smith, K. R. *Biomass Fuels, Air Pollution and Health: A Global Perspective.* New York: Plenum, 1987.

Smith, K. R. "Indoor Air Pollution in Developing Countries: Recommendations for Research." *Indoor Air,* 2002, *12,* 198–207.

Smith, K. R., Corvalan, C., and Kjellstrom, T. "How Much Global Ill-Health Is Attributable to Environmental Factors?" *Epidemiology,* 1999, *10,* 573–574.

Smith, K. R., and Mehta, S. "The Burden of Disease from Indoor Air Pollution in Developing Countries: Comparison of Estimates." *International Journal of Hygiene and Environmental Health,* 2003, *206,* 279–289.

Suk, W. A., and others. "Environmental Threats to Children's Health in Southeast Asia and the Western Pacific." *Environmental Health Perspectives,* 2003, *111,* 1340–1347.

Thomas, E. P., Seager, J. R., and Mathee, A. "Environmental Health Challenges in South Africa: Policy Lessons from Case Studies." *Health & Place,* 2002, *8,* 251–261.

Tung, Y. H., and others. "Cooking Oil Fume-Induced Cytokine Expression and Oxidative Stress in Human Lung Epithelial Cells." *Environmental Research,* 2001, *87*(1), 47–54.

United Nations Department of Economic and Social Affairs, Population Division. *World Urbanization Prospects: The 2003 Revision.* [http://www.un.org/esa/population/publications/wup2003/WUP2003Report.pdf]. 2004.

United Nations Environment Programme. *Africa Environmental Outlook.* Nairobi: United Nations Environment Programme, 2002.

Vahter, M., Berglund, M., Akesson, A., and Linden, C. "Metals and Women's Health." *Environmental Research,* 2002, *A88,* 145–155.

West, K. P., Caballero, B., and Black, R. E. "Nutrition." In M. H. Merson, R. E. Black, and A. J. Mills (eds.), *International Public Health.* Gaithersburg, Md.: Aspen, 2001.

Woodcock, A., and others. "Pet Allergen Levels in Homes in Ghana and the United Kingdom." *Journal of Clinical Immunology,* 2001, *108*(3), 463–465.

World Health Organization. *Health and Environment in Sustainable Development: Five Years After the Earth Summit.* Geneva: World Health Organization, 1997.

World Health Organization. WHO/UNICEF Joint Monitoring Programme for Water Supply and Sanitation. *Global Water Supply and Sanitation Assessment 2000 Report.* Geneva: World Health Organization, 2000.

World Health Organization. *The World Health Report 2001: Mental Health: New Understanding, New Hope.* Geneva: World Health Organization, 2001.

World Health Organization. *The World Health Report 2002: Reducing Risks, Promoting Healthy Life.* Geneva: World Health Organization, 2002.

World Health Organization. *The World Health Report 2003: Shaping the Future.* Geneva: World Health Organization, 2003.

Wu, T., Buck, G. M., and Mendola, P. "Blood Lead Levels and Sexual Maturation in U.S. Girls: The Third National Health and Nutrition Examination Survey, 1988–1994." *Environmental Health Perspectives,* 2003, *111,* 737–740.

Wu, M. T., and others. "Environmental Exposure to Cooking Oil Fumes and Cervical Intraepithelial Neoplasm." *Environmental Research,* 2004, *94,* 25–32.

Yanez, L., and others. "Overview of Human Health and Chemical Mixtures: Problems Facing Developing Countries." *Environmental Health Perspectives,* 2002, *110*(suppl. 6), 901–909.

For Further Information

Aron, J. L., and Patz, J. A. (eds.). *Ecosystem Change and Public Health: A Global Perspective.* Baltimore, Md.: Johns Hopkins University Press, 2001.

The International Society for Urban Health (ISUH). *Urban Health Literature Review.* [http://www.isuh.org/resources/resources.html].

IRC International Water and Sanitation Centre. *World Water Day Report, 2001.* [http://www.worldwaterday.org/2001/report/index.html]. 2001.

Kasperson, J. X., and Kasperson, R. E. (eds.). *The Global Environmental Risk.* Tokyo: United Nations University Press, 2001.

Merson, M. H., Black, R. E., and Mills, A. J. (eds.). *International Public Health.* Gaithersburg, Md.: Aspen, 2001.

United Nations. "Johannesburg Summit 2002: World Summit on Sustainable Development." [http://www.johannesburgsummit.org]. 2002.

United Nations Department of Economic and Social Affairs, Population Division. *World Urbanization Prospects: The 2003 Revision.* [http://www.un.org/esa/population/publications/wup2003/WUP2003Report.pdf]. 2003.

United Nations Health and Development Section, Emerging Social Issues Division (UNESCAP). *Urbanization and Health.* [www.unescap.org/esid/hds/issues/UrbanizationHealth.pdf]. n.d.

World Health Organization. The World Health *Report 2002: Reducing Risks, Promoting Healthy Life.* [www.who.int/whr/2002/en]. 2002.

PART THREE

ENVIRONMENTAL HEALTH ON THE REGIONAL SCALE

CHAPTER FOURTEEN

AIR POLLUTION

Michelle L. Bell
Jonathan M. Samet

Air pollution has long been a contributor to ill health. With the discovery of fire, humans began to pollute both the air in the places they lived and the air outside. As urban areas developed, pollution sources, such as chimneys and industrial processes, became concentrated in those areas, leading to visible and damaging pollution dominated by smoke. The harmful effects of air pollution were recognized early. In "On Air, Water, and Places," written nearly 2,500 years ago, Hippocrates (1849) noted that people's health could be affected by the air they breathe and that the quality of the air differed by area. In thirteenth-century London, air pollution was so severe that a commission was established to address the problem and abatement strategies followed (Brimblecombe, 1986). At that time air pollution was generally a local matter, generated from kilns, hearths, and furnaces; since then, with growing populations, industrialization, and fossil fuel–based transportation, the characteristics of air pollution have changed. The transport of air pollution across large distances means that damaging effects often occur far from the pollution source. Air pollution problems now range from the local to the global scale and occur on a variety of timescales. Chapters Eleven and Twenty-Two address climate change and indoor air pollution, respectively. This chapter focuses on major ambient, or outdoor, air pollutants, which today generally cause harm to health and the environment on local and regional scales.

Modern-day recognition of the dangers of ambient air pollution can be traced to several extreme episodes during the last century. In 1930, in the Meuse

FIGURE 14.1. MORTALITY AND AIR POLLUTION LEVELS DURING 1952 LONDON FOG.

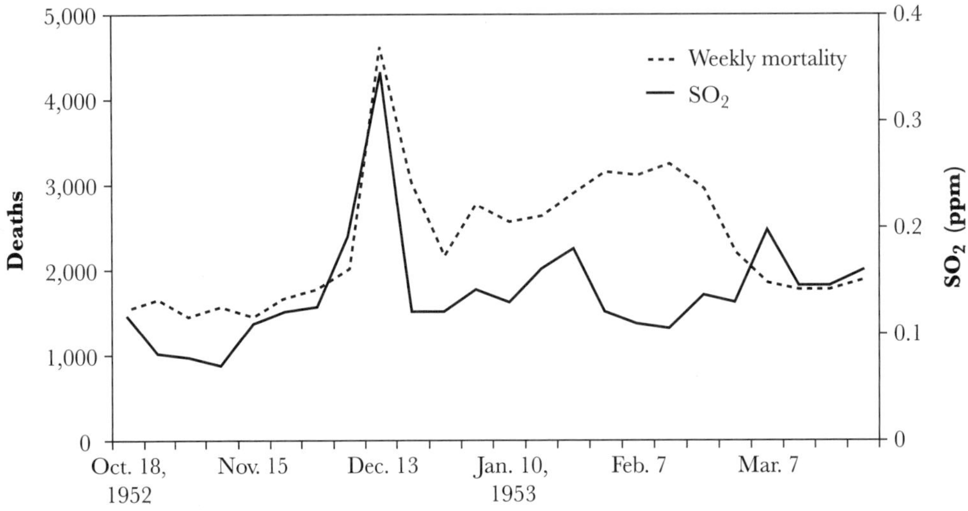

Source: Adapted from Bell and Davis, 2001.

Valley in Belgium, more than sixty people died during an episode of severe air pollution, over ten times the usual mortality rate (Firket, 1936; Nemery, Hoet, and Nemmar, 2001). In describing the event the original investigators warned that should such an air pollution episode occur in a city with a larger population, such as London, thousands would die. In late October 1948, industrial pollution settled on Donora, a small town in southwestern Pennsylvania (Davis, 2002; Schrenk and others, 1949). Twenty people died during and shortly after this event, or about six times the typical mortality rate. Perhaps the most severe such event took place in London in December 1952 (see Figures 14.1 and 14.2 and Box 14.1). In these and similar episodes, pollution levels and subsequent health effects were so severe that the connection between air pollution and health was readily apparent.

Box 14.1. London 1952: One of the World's Worst Air Pollution Disasters

By the 1950s, high concentrations of air pollutants in London were common, with levels far above modern-day regulatory standards. In fact dirty air and London's characteristic "pea souper" fogs were long known as a "London particular," noted by

FIGURE 14.2. CARDIAC EMERGENCY BED SERVICE APPLICATIONS AND SO_2 LEVELS DURING THE 1952 LONDON FOG.

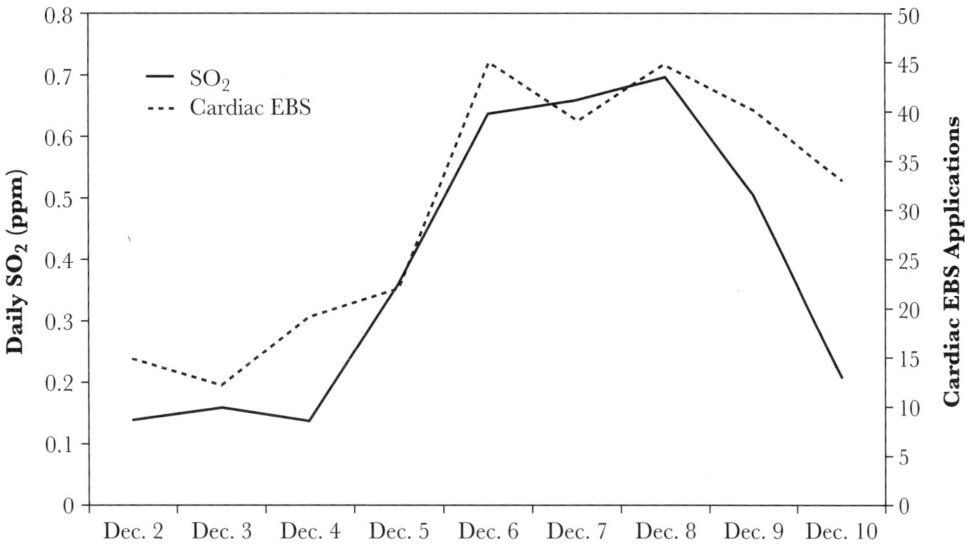

Source: Adapted from Bell and Davis, 2001.

tourists, authors such as Charles Dickens, and painters such as Claude Monet. However from December 5 to 9, 1952, an unprecedented air pollution event took place, so severe that it warranted attention from the general public, scientists, the media, and the government.

Several factors contributed to the high pollution levels in London. Coal was a primary method of home heating at the time. A particularly cold winter meant that even more coal was burned. Stagnant atmospheric conditions prevented pollution from dispersing, allowing it to accumulate in the city. Levels of sulfur dioxide (SO_2) and total particulate matter rose to dangerous heights, far above even the prevailing British standards. Pollution became so thick that visibility was reduced to near zero. Some longtime residents became disoriented, finding their way home by feeling along the sides of buildings. A theater performance was stopped because pollution seeped into the auditorium, and the audience could not see the stage. Traffic came to a near standstill.

The association between health and air pollution during this episode was evident, as the strong rise in air pollution was immediately followed by a sharp increase in sickness and death. Mortality rates rose to three times their normal levels. As the death toll mounted, mortuaries did not have enough room for the bodies, undertakers ran out of coffins, and florists ran out of flowers. Hospital admissions and insurance claims for new illnesses also rose. Applications to the Emergency Bed Service (EBS), which occurred when a patient could not be admitted to a particular hospital, reached a record high. Increases in these indicators of morbidity mirrored increases in air pollution concentrations. For example, Figure 14.2 depicts the applications for EBS for cardiac disease and the daily levels of SO_2 in Greater London over the days of the 1952 episode. Later analysis of archived autopsy lung tissue found soot and an excess of other particles (Hunt, Abraham, Judson, and Berry, 2003).

Mortality rates did not return to normal levels until several months after the fog. The initial government report of this episode, released in 1954, hypothesized that an influenza epidemic accounted for the extra deaths during these months (U.K. Ministry of Health, 1954). However, more recent analysis showed that only a fraction of the excess mortality could be attributed to influenza (Bell and Davis, 2001; Bell, Davis, and Fletcher, 2004), which indicates that the true death toll from this pollution is 10,000 to 12,000, rather than the 3,000 to 4,000 typically reported.

This air pollution disaster, along with others, including the 1948 episode in Donora, Pennsylvania (Davis, 2002), acted as a catalyst for the study of air pollution epidemiology and for government intervention. The U.K. Clean Air Act was enacted in 1956, followed by the U.S. Clean Air Act in 1963. This and similar episodes serve as reminders of the dangers of air pollution.

In response to episodes such as those in Donora and London, many governments, particularly those of the United States and the United Kingdom, enacted legislation to improve air quality and initiated research to increase the understanding of risks to health. Today most of the industrialized world rarely experiences air pollution concentrations on the scale of the London fog of 1952, yet exceedingly high levels still exist in many developing regions. Despite regulatory control measures that have lowered allowable concentrations, air pollution continues to harm health in the industrialized world as well. In 2002, the World Health Organization's Global Burden of Disease Initiative estimated that each year ambient air pollution causes 800,000 premature deaths (Ezzati and others, 2002).

Types of Ambient Air Pollution

The ambient concentration of an air pollutant in a particular location depends on many factors, including emissions sources, weather (for example, temperature, wind speed and direction, and precipitation), and land patterns. Under conditions of stagnant winds and a temperature inversion, air pollution does not disperse, leading to higher pollutant concentrations; this is a relatively common occurrence in valleys and areas lacking open spaces. A temperature inversion occurs when, contrary to normal conditions, temperature increases with altitude, creating a layer of warmer air above a layer of cooler air on the earth's surface. Inversions typically occur in the morning or when air descends from higher altitudes. Pollutant concentrations for a given area can vary on a seasonal or daily basis, depending on weather and sources of emissions, such as traffic patterns and wood burning. Some pollutants, such as tropospheric ozone (O_3) and small particles that have long residence times in the atmosphere, can travel large distances, resulting in damaging effects that can extend far beyond the sources.

Air pollutants may be categorized by source or by physical and chemical characteristics. Table 14.1 lists several major air pollutants and provides examples of their sources, their health effects, and relevant U.S. regulations and guidelines from the World Health Organization (WHO, 2000). An air pollutant may be either directly emitted (*primary*) or formed in the atmosphere through the physical and chemical conversion of precursors (*secondary*). For example, emissions of carbon monoxide (CO) from car tailpipes are primary emissions; however, ozone, a secondary pollutant, is formed in the atmosphere through the chemical conversion of other pollutants. Another important distinction between air pollution sources is whether the emissions are natural or the result of human activity. Naturally occurring pollutants include biogenic volatile organic compounds (VOCs) from vegetation, pollens, volcanic gases, and dust from deserts.

A further way in which air pollutants differ is in their physical form; they may be gases or particles (small solids or liquids suspended in air). *Aerosols* are small solid or liquid particles suspended in air. Physical form and chemical characteristics (for example, the solubility of a gas) affect the pollutant's ability to penetrate into the respiratory system. Other factors that affect respiratory penetration are a pollutant's ambient concentration and an individual's ventilation rate (number of breaths per minute). For example, exercise increases the depth and rate of ventilation. Route of breathing is also relevant: nasal breathing results in the removal of some pollutants in the nasal passage, while this filtering is bypassed with oral breathing. Gaseous pollutants that are highly soluble in water, such as SO_2, are largely removed by the upper airway, whereas less water soluble gases, such as O_3, and particles can penetrate deeper into the lungs.

A final way of classifying air pollutants relates to the way they are regulated legally. One commonly used term is *criteria pollutants.* This category includes several major pollutants (carbon monoxide, lead, nitrogen dioxide, ozone, particulates, and sulfur dioxide) for which the U.S. Environmental Protection Agency (EPA) has promulgated National Ambient Air Quality Standards (NAAQS) under the Clean Air Act. A second regulatory category is *hazardous air pollutants.* This category, established by the Clean Air Act Amendments of 1990, includes a number of volatile organic chemicals, pesticides, herbicides, and radionuclides. The name *hazardous pollutants* is somewhat confusing because this category does

TABLE 14.1. MAJOR AMBIENT AIR POLLUTANTS: SOURCES, HEALTH EFFECTS, AND REGULATIONS.

Pollutant	Source Types and Major Sources[a]	Health Effects[a]	Regulations and Guidelines[b]
Lead	Primary Anthropogenic: leaded fuel (phased out in some locations such as the U.S.), lead batteries, metal processing	Accumulates in organs and tissues Learning disabilities, cancer, damage to the nervous system	*U.S. NAAQS*[c] Quarterly average: 1.5 $\mu g/m^3$ *WHO Guidelines*[d] Annual: 0.50 $\mu g/m^3$
Sulfur dioxide	Primary Anthropogenic: combustion of fossil fuel (power plants), industrial boilers, household coal use, oil refineries Biogenic: decomposition of organic matter, sea spray, volcanic eruptions	Lung impairment, respiratory symptoms Precursor to PM Contributes to acid precipitation	*U.S. NAAQS* Annual arithmetic mean: 0.03 ppm (80 $\mu g/m^3$) 24-hour average: 0.14 ppm (365 $\mu g/m^3$) *WHO Guidelines* 10-minute average: 500 $\mu g/m^3$ 24-hour average: 125 $\mu g/m^3$ Annual: 50 $\mu g/m^3$
Carbon monoxide	Primary Anthropogenic: combustion of fossil fuels (motor vehicles, boilers, furnaces) Biogenic: forest fires	Interferes with delivery of oxygen Fatigue, headache, neurological damage, dizziness	*U.S. NAAQS* 1-hour average: 35 ppm (40 mg/m^3) 8-hour average: 9 ppm (10 mg/m^3) *WHO Guidelines* 15-minute average: 100 mg/m^3 30-minute average: 60 mg/m^3 1-hour average: 30 mg/m^3

Particulate matter[e]	Primary and secondary Anthropogenic: burning of fossil fuel, wood burning, natural sources (for example, pollen), conversion of precursors (NO_x, SO_x, VOCs) Biogenic: dust storms, forest fires, dirt roads	Respiratory symptoms, decline in lung function, exacerbation of respiratory and cardiovascular disease (for example, asthma), mortality	*U.S. NAAQS* PM_{10} Annual arithmetic mean: 50 $\mu g/m^3$ 24-hour average 150 $\mu g/m^3$ $PM_{2.5}$ Annual arithmetic mean: 15 $\mu g/m^3$ 24-hour average: $\mu g/m^3$ *WHO Guidelines* No guideline specified; recommendation based on dose-response
Nitrogen oxides	Primary and secondary Anthropogenic: fossil fuel combustion (vehicles, electric utilities, industry), kerosene heaters Biogenic: biological processes in soil, lightning	Decreased lung function, increased respiratory infection Precursor to ozone Contributes to PM and acid precipitation	*U.S. NAAQS* Annual arithmetic mean: 0.053 ppm (100 $\mu g/m^3$) Related to compliance with NAAQS for ozone *WHO Guidelines* 1-hour average: 200 $\mu g/m^3$ Annual: 40 $\mu g/m^3$
Tropospheric ozone	Secondary Formed through chemical reactions of anthropogenic and biogenic precursors (VOCs and NO_x) in the presence of sunlight	Decreased lung function, increased respiratory symptoms, eye irritation, bronchoconstriction	*U.S. NAAQS* 1-hour average: 0.12 ppm (235 $\mu g/m^3$) 8-hour average: 0.08 ppm (157 $\mu g/m^3$) *WHO Guidelines* 8-hour average: 120 $\mu g/m^3$
"Toxic" ("hazardous") pollutants (such as asbestos, mercury, dioxin, some VOCs)	Primary and secondary Anthropogenic: industrial processes, solvents, paint thinners, fuel	Cancer, reproductive effects, neurological damage, respiratory effects	EPA rules on emissions for more than 80 industrial source categories (for example, dry cleaners, oil refineries, chemical plants) EPA and state rules on vehicle emissions

(*Continued*)

TABLE 14.1. MAJOR AMBIENT AIR POLLUTANTS: SOURCES, HEALTH EFFECTS, AND REGULATIONS. (*Continued*)

Pollutant	Source Types and Major Sources[a]	Health Effects[a]	Regulations and Guidelines[b]
Volatile organic compounds (such as benzene, terpenes, toluene)	Primary and secondary Anthropogenic: solvents, glues, smoking, fuel combustion Biogenic: vegetation, forest fires	Range of effects, depending on the compound Irritation of respiratory tract, nausea, cancer Precursor to ozone Contributes to PM	EPA limits on emissions EPA toxic air pollutant rules Related to compliance with NAAQS for ozone
Biological pollutants (such as pollen, mold, mildew)	Primary Biogenic: trees, grasses, ragweed, animals, debris Anthropogenic systems, such as central air-conditioning, can create conditions that encourage production of biological pollutants	Allergic reactions, respiratory symptoms, fatigue, asthma	

[a]This table lists only a sample of the sources and health effects associated with each pollutant. Additionally, health effects may be the result of characteristics of a pollutant mixture rather than the result of a single pollutant.

[b]Additional legal requirements often apply, such as state regulations.

[c]U.S. NAAQS = U.S. National Ambient Air Quality Standards.

[d]WHO Guidelines = WHO Air Quality Guidelines (WHO, 2000).

[e]Sources and effects of particulate matter can differ by size.

not include all known hazardous air pollutants (for example, it does not include carbon monoxide), and it does include some pollutants for which the hazard level is unknown.

Studies of Air Pollution and Health

The health effects of air pollution have been studied extensively through diverse research methods, including epidemiological, human exposure, and animal and other toxicological studies. Each approach has strengths and weakness, and drawing a complete picture of the ways in which air pollution affects health requires an examination of results from complementary research designs.

Epidemiological studies investigate the relationship between air pollutant concentrations and health outcomes under real-world conditions of exposure, typically in large populations in community settings (Gordis, 2004). Air pollution monitoring data are often used as surrogates for individual exposure, although people's activity patterns (that is, time spent in different environments such as work and home) determine their individual exposures. Health outcomes are generally assessed through public health databases, questionnaires, or tests of pulmonary functions. For example, a landmark study of air pollution and mortality in six U.S. cities enrolled schoolchildren and adults, using outdoor monitors in each city to estimate exposure to air pollution. People in the city with the highest air pollution levels had a 26 percent higher mortality rate than those in the least polluted city (Dockery and others, 1993). Another epidemiological study, the American Cancer Society's Cancer Prevention Study (CPS) II, followed about 500,000 adults in 151 U.S. metropolitan areas. This investigation also used aggregate-level (that is, monitor measurements) exposure data and individual-level health information. The investigators found that participants in the most polluted areas had a 17 percent higher mortality rate than those in the least polluted areas (Pope and others, 1995, 2002).

A key advantage of epidemiological studies is the use of real-world populations and air pollution concentrations. However, epidemiological studies may be limited by their inability to control fully for confounding factors, such as temperature, weather, population characteristics, the presence of pollutants, and the difficulty of estimating personal exposure accurately. In general, random error in the estimation of exposure tends to reduce the sensitivity of epidemiological studies in detecting effects. Confounding may falsely increase or decrease the apparent effect of air pollution.

Controlled human exposure studies expose volunteers to a specified concentration of a particular air pollutant or pollutant mixture in a laboratory setting and measure their health responses (Sandstrom, 1995). Unlike epidemiological research, exposure studies can control for potential confounding factors, deliver a carefully characterized exposure, and incorporate relatively invasive and complex methods for outcome assessment. To protect participants' safety, such research examines health effects that are mild, acute, and reversible. For example, human exposure studies may investigate heart rate variability and lung function changes (Devlin and others, 2003) and the fraction of particles that are deposited in the lung (Daigle and others, 2003). Exposures are typically of short duration and at low concentrations. Human exposure studies are not suitable for research on chronic health effects or more severe health outcomes. These studies are, however, particularly useful for characterizing mechanisms of injury in order to bridge from animal to human studies and for assessing threshold concentrations for short-term effects.

Animal studies involve short- or long-term exposures to a pollutant mixture under well-characterized conditions. Animals are sometimes exposed to outdoor pollution and even placed at sites of particular interest, such as along roadways. Generally, rodents are used for such experiments, but dogs and primates have also been studied. Like human exposure studies, animal studies in the laboratory have the strength of well-defined pollution exposures; thus exposure-response relationships can be addressed. For example, animal exposure studies of air pollution have been used to research respiratory and heart rates in rats (Nadziejko and others, 2002), DNA damage in mice (Soares and others, 2003), brain damage in dogs (Calderón-Garcidueñas and others, 2002), and myocardial ischemia in dogs (Wellenius and others, 2003).

Animal studies sometimes incorporate invasive assessment procedures, such as lung biopsies. Biological samples can be collected for detailed study of a mechanism of injury. However, evidence from animal studies may be subject to uncertainty when extrapolated to people, and responses sometimes vary even among animal species.

Sources and Health Effects of Major Outdoor Pollutants

The health consequences of air pollution are wide-ranging, extending from effects on comfort and well-being to respiratory symptoms and even to premature death. This section reviews the sources and health impacts of the common outdoor air pollutants (summarized in Table 14.1). Much human health research aims to investigate a particular pollutant, while controlling for potential confounding by other pollutants, just as Table 14.1 presents information one pollutant at a time. Indeed, some pollutants, such as CO, appear to have individual, specific health effects. However, air pollution is actually a complex mixture of multiple pollutants, such as SO_2 and O_3, and damage from air pollution may result from the combined effects (interaction) of several pollutants. Synergistic interactions may produce effects larger than anticipated from studies of the individual pollutants. Air pollution regulatory programs generally provide individual standards for each pollutant, even though the health effects may be related and pollutants may share similar sources.

Particulate Matter

Particulate matter (PM) refers to a generic class of pollution rather than to a particular, individual pollutant with a specified chemical structure, such as SO_2. *PM* is the term applied to solid or liquid particles suspended in air, regardless of their chemical composition. This pollutant can either be primary (directly emitted) or secondary (formed in the atmosphere through physical and chemical conversion of gaseous precursors such as nitrogen oxides [NO_x], sulfur oxides [SO_x], and VOCs). PM results from the burning of fuel (for example, emissions from power plants), unpaved roads, industry, and wood-burning stoves and from natural sources such as pollen, dust, salt spray, erosion, and mold. PM concentrations can vary within a region or even a city according to proximity to various PM sources (for example, sites near major highways may have comparatively high PM levels).

The composition of particulate matter differs by geographic area and can also vary with season, source, and meteorology. In the eastern United States, PM often has a substantial sulfate component, reflecting the contributions of emissions from power plants. In the western United States, transportation emissions contribute a larger fraction of PM, often creating a substantial nitrate component. In the U.S. Northwest, wood burning may be a dominant source of PM during colder seasons. Windblown dust can be an important source of PM in desert climates such as are found in the southwestern United States.

Particles are generally categorized according to their size, using a measure called the *aerodynamic diameter.* This is the diameter of a uniform sphere of unit density that would attain the same terminal settling velocity as the particle of interest. Aerodynamic diameter is determined by a particle's shape and density, and this measure permits comparison of particles having irregular shapes and different sizes and densities. Thus PM_{10} refers to particles with an aerodynamic diameter of 10 microns or less, $PM_{2.5}$, or *fine* PM, has an aerodynamic diameter of up to 2.5 microns, and *ultrafine* particles have a diameter of up to 0.1 microns. *Total suspended particles* (TSP) refers to almost all particles in the air and is typically measured as PM mass up to particles of about 45 microns in diameter. Figure 14.3 depicts the typical mass distribution of particles in an urban area, showing

FIGURE 14.3. PARTICULATE MATTER MASS DISTRIBUTION.

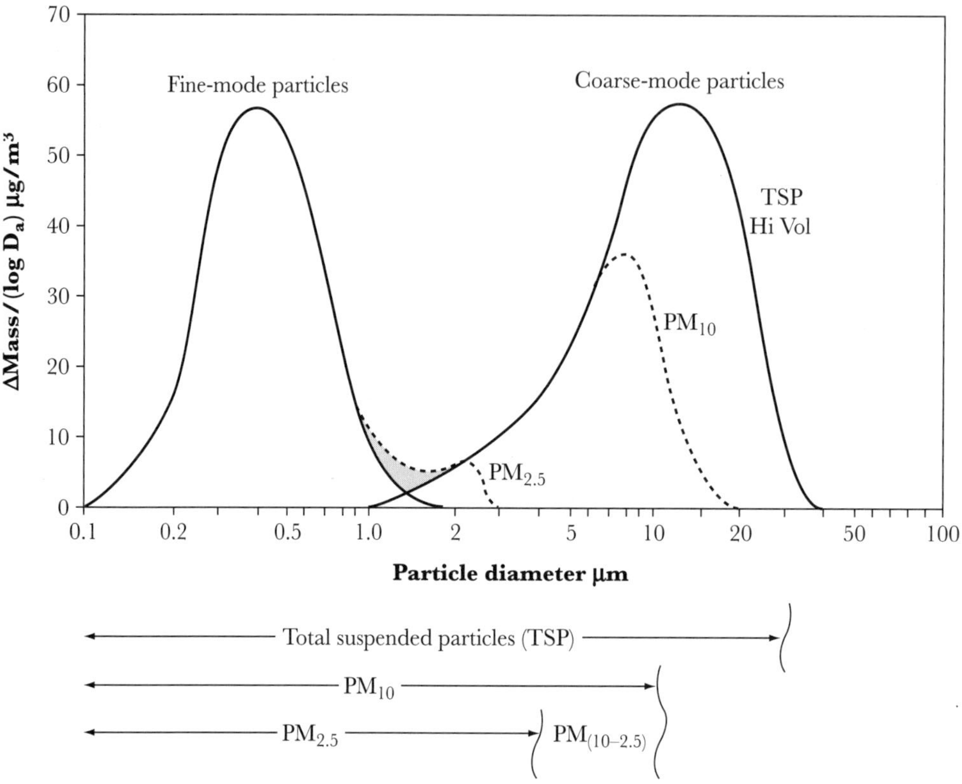

two modes, one of fine particles, which tend to be of secondary origin, and the other of *coarse* particles, which are more likely to be primary.

A particle's size is related to its source. The size determines how it is transported in the atmosphere, where it is deposited in the environment, and where it is deposited in the respiratory system. Smaller particles are of special health concern because they penetrate more deeply into the lung. Such particles are typically generated through combustion processes. Diesel exhaust, a combination of gases and particles, is of particular concern because of widespread diesel use and because these particles are extremely small (<1 micron) (Kagawa, 2002). In addition, the gas phase of diesel contains numerous hazardous air pollutants such as benzene, formaldehyde, and polycyclic aromatic hydrocarbons.

Ambient levels of particulate matter, as indicated by PM_{10}, $PM_{2.5}$, or other measures, have been associated with health effects such as increased hospital and emergency room admissions, respiratory symptoms, decline in pulmonary function, exacerbation of chronic respiratory and cardiovascular diseases, and premature mortality (EPA, 2003). Laboratory animals exposed to PM experienced a range of responses, including inflammation and pulmonary injury (Broeckaert and others, 1997; Dye and others, 2001). Time series studies, which track day-to-day variation in PM levels and in mortality, have shown that acute PM exposure is associated with increased mortality, which peaks within a few days of exposure, reminiscent of the London and Donora episodes described earlier but occurring even at today's lower levels of PM exposure (see, for example, Health Effects Institute [HEI], 2003; Samet and others, 2000a, 2000b; Schwartz, 2000). Longitudinal studies such as the Six Cities study and CPS II (described earlier) also demonstrate a link between long-term PM exposure and mortality (see, for example, Dockery and others, 1993; Krewski and others, 2000; Pope and others, 1995, 2002). A National Research Council committee recently reviewed the status of this evidence (National Research Council, 2004).

Regulations for PM have evolved in response to a greater understanding of how PM affects human health. When the original National Ambient Air Quality Standard on particulate matter was established in 1971, it addressed total suspended particles (TSP), but this standard was replaced with one for PM_{10} when it became clear that these smaller particles were more closely associated with health effects. Later evidence demonstrated that even smaller particles, $PM_{2.5}$, were responsible for adverse health effects, and a $PM_{2.5}$ standard was added in 1997.

Although PM and health have been studied extensively, much remains unknown. For example, the health risk of particle exposure may depend on characteristics of the PM, such as its content of metals, acidity, organics, or sulfates or combinations of these components (HEI, 2002). Determining the harmful aspects of PM is a critical research need (National Research Council, 2004). Similarly, the biological mechanisms by which PM causes premature mortality are not well understood. Leading hypotheses focus on reflexes in the lung that lead to autonomic nervous systems changes, perhaps predisposing individuals to arrhythmias, and on inflammation that in turn predisposes to thrombosis or related changes (Brook and others, 2004). Further research will clarify the effects of PM and will likely have an impact on regulation as well.

Sulfur Dioxide

SO_2 is a water-soluble gas that was a primary component of the 1952 London fog. Sulfur oxides are produced from the combustion of sulfur-containing fuels and materials, such as coal and metal ores. Some coal, such as that from the eastern United States, has a particularly high sulfur content. Power plants are the main source of SO_2 emissions. Other sources are industrial boilers, trains, ships, and metal processing facilities. Household use of coal can contribute significant amounts of SO_2 as well. In some regions, such as parts of China, coal is the primary fuel for cooking and heating and causes high levels of SO_2 indoors. Natural sources of SO_2 include volcanoes.

SO_2 can be converted to sulfuric acid (Seinfeld and Pandis, 1998), and therefore contributes to acid deposition, which harms vegetation, materials, and wildlife. SO_2 also contributes to the formation of particulate matter. Sulfate aerosols, a major component of fine particulate matter, can travel far from their sources. The tall stacks of power plants often release pollution above the inversion layer, which reduces local pollution but allows emitted pollutants to migrate long distances.

Because SO_2 is highly soluble in water, most inhaled SO_2 is absorbed by the mucous membranes of the upper airways, with little reaching the lung; however, increased ventilation and oral breathing, for example, during exercise, can raise the dose delivered to the lung (Schlesinger, 1999). SO_2 exposure has been associated with reduced lung function, bronchoconstriction (increased airway resistance), respiratory symptoms, hospitalizations due to cardiovascular and respiratory symptoms, eye irritation, adverse pregnancy outcomes, and mortality. However, it is difficult to attribute these reported associations to SO_2 alone, because SO_2 is a precursor to particulate matter and generally exists as a component of a complex, combustion-related pollutant mixture. Experimental studies suggest that some persons with asthma may be particularly sensitive to SO_2 itself. Controlled exposure studies have shown that effects can occur after very short exposures (for example, ten minutes) in some people with asthma, whereas epidemiological research has shown effects associated with long-term exposure (for example, yearly levels).

Nitrogen Oxides

Nitrogen oxides (NO_x) make up a category of highly reactive gases containing nitrogen and oxygen, such as nitrogen dioxide (NO_2) and nitric oxide (NO). These pollutants react in the atmosphere to form additional pollutants and toxic compounds, including nitroarenes. NO_x is produced through combustion, including fossil fuel combustion, when the nitrogen that comprises almost 80 percent of air is oxidized. The sources of NO_x therefore include car and truck engines, electric utilities, and industries. Indoor air pollution can also contribute to NO_2 through kerosene heaters, unvented gas stoves and heaters, and tobacco smoke. Natural sources of NO_x include stratospheric intrusion (when NO_x enters the troposphere from the stratosphere), biological processes in the soil, forest fires, and lightning, but the principal sources today are power plants and motor vehicles. In the United States, motor vehicles currently account for half of all NO_x emissions.

Like ozone, NO_2 is nearly insoluble in water and can reach the lower respiratory tract. Health effects of NO_2 include irritation of the eyes, nose, and throat at higher concentrations, short-term decreases in lung function, and possibly increased respiratory infections and symptoms among children. It is difficult to separate the effects of NO_x from related air pollution components such as ozone and particulate matter (Ackermann-Liebrich and Rapp, 1999). Both NO and NO_2 are toxic gases, and NO_2 is regulated as a criteria pollutant under the Clean Air Act. Nitrogen oxides also have indirect but important roles as precursors. NO_x is a precursor of tropospheric ozone and secondary particulate matter and plays a crucial role in the formation of acid precipitation. Nitrous oxide (N_2O) is a greenhouse gas, which contributes to global warming (see Chapter Eleven). NO_x and the pollutant species formed as it undergoes chemical reactions can travel long distances, so health effects may take place far from the source. Although emissions have declined in recent decades, by approximately 15 percent between 1983 and 2002, emissions from some sources, such as off-road vehicle engines, are rising (EPA, Office of Air Quality Planning and Standards, 2003).

Volatile Organic Compounds (VOCs)

VOCs are a category of organic chemicals with a high vapor pressure that readily evaporate at normal temperature and pressure. They include benzene, chloroform, formaldehyde, isoprene, methanol, and monoterpenes, along with hundreds of additional compounds. VOCs originate from natural sources including such vegetation as oak and maple trees; power plants and industrial processes such as those involving chemicals and solvents; and transportation, including motor vehicles and off-road transportation such as aircraft, construction equipment, and lawn mowers. Motor vehicle emissions account for about 75 percent of transportation-related VOC emissions, with most of these emissions originating from the approximately 20 percent of vehicles that are older and poorly maintained (EPA, 1996). In many locations biogenic sources contribute more to VOCs than anthropogenic emissions. For example, in 1990, 77 percent of VOC emissions in the mid-Atlantic region were biogenic (Mid-Atlantic Regional Air Management Association, 1997). In fact the natural appearance that gives the Blue Ridge Mountains and the Great Smoky Mountains their names results from biogenic VOCs (mostly isoprene) that form aerosols. VOCs are precursors of ozone but also have such independent health effects as irritation of the respiratory tract, headaches, and carcinogenicity.

Tropospheric Ozone

Ozone is present in the troposphere, the lowest atmospheric layer, which extends to approximately 10 to 15 km above the earth's surface, and in the stratosphere, which extends from the troposphere to about 45 to 55 km above the earth's surface. Stratospheric ozone forms the naturally occurring *ozone layer* that protects the earth's surface from ultraviolet radiation, whereas tropospheric ozone, sometimes called *ground level ozone,* is a harmful pollutant. To communicate the difference between stratospheric and tropospheric ozone, the EPA has introduced the slogan "Good up high—bad nearby."

Tropospheric ozone is a colorless gas and a photochemical oxidant formed through complex, nonlinear chemical reactions involving the precursors VOCs and NO_x in the presence of sunlight. As a result, pollution involving ozone is sometimes referred to as *photochemical smog.* Stratospheric ozone can also intrude into the troposphere. The basic photochemical cycle of NO_x and O_3, which is driven by solar radiation, is shown below, although ozone formation involves numerous other chemical reactions (Seinfeld and Pandis, 1998):

$$
\begin{aligned}
NO_2 + h\nu &\rightarrow NO + O \\
O + O_2 + M &\rightarrow O_3 + M \\
O_3 + NO &\rightarrow NO_2 + O_2
\end{aligned}
$$

where $h\nu$ represents light energy, and M represents N_2, O_2, or another molecule that absorbs excess energy, which stabilizes O_3.

Due to the complex chemistry that generates ozone, controlling ozone levels is a difficult challenge. Decreased emissions of either NO_x or VOCs could potentially result in higher ozone levels, depending on the initial concentrations of the two main categories of precursors among other factors (Seinfeld and Pandis, 1998). In some areas, referred to as NO_x-limited, reductions of NO_x may be the most effective way to reduce ozone levels, whereas in VOC-limited areas, reducing VOC emissions may be more effective.

Concentrations of ozone are highly seasonal, with higher levels appearing during the hotter months; they also show strong diurnal patterns, following sunlight and transportation emissions patterns. Urban areas tend to have higher ozone concentrations owing to proximity to emissions of ozone precursors. After ozone precursors are emitted they can travel downwind in an expanding plume and contribute to the formation of ozone, which itself can travel with wind patterns. Thus, elevated concentrations can result from the transport of ozone and its precursors up to hundreds of miles away. Ozone problems tend to be regional, rather than localized. Ozone levels are generally lower indoors than outdoors, because ozone adsorbs to indoor surfaces and rapidly breaks down.

Ozone is not highly soluble in water, a characteristic that helps it to reach the lower respiratory tract. Because of its oxidant properties, ozone can break molecular bonds and rapidly damage human tissue. Short-term exposure to ozone for healthy adults has been associated with temporarily decreased lung function, increased airway resistance, and increased respiratory symptoms, such as coughing and wheezing. These changes are reflected by increases in clinic visits, emergency room visits, school absenteeism, and hospitalizations following high-ozone days. Ozone has also been associated with premature death (Bell and others, 2004).

People with asthma are especially susceptible to the effects of ozone, because ozone inflames the airway linings and can trigger asthmatic attacks. However, healthy nonasthmatics can also be affected (EPA, 1996; Lippmann, 1989). Children, having narrow caliber airways, are also especially susceptible (see Chapter Twenty-Eight). People who spend time outdoors, such as those who exercise or work outdoors, are susceptible because of their greater ozone exposure. Long-term ozone exposure may contribute to the development of chronic lung diseases, such as asthma and bronchitis, and may accelerate aging of the lungs. Ozone concentrations have also been associated with impaired lung development in children (Gauderman and others, 2002).

Carbon Monoxide

Carbon monoxide is a colorless, odorless gas formed by incomplete combustion of carbonaceous material, such as gasoline, natural gas, oil, coal, tobacco, and other organic materials. Motor vehicles contribute the majority of CO emissions to outdoor air, and consequently CO concentrations tend to be higher in areas with high traffic density and during times of high traffic volume. Carbon monoxide levels may also be high in congested urban areas with slow-moving traffic. Automobiles emit more CO during colder weather and while idling or moving slowly. Other sources include off-road vehicles and wildfires. Wood burning also produces significant CO emissions in some areas. Elevated CO levels typically occur during colder periods because of increased vehicular emissions and inversion conditions that prevent pollution from dispersing.

When CO is inhaled, it binds to hemoglobin, with over 200 times the affinity of oxygen, to form carboxyhemoglobin (COHb). An increased level of COHb reduces the transport of oxygen to tissues and inhibits the release of oxygen (EPA, 2000). The brain and heart are sensitive to low-oxygen conditions and are especially vulnerable to the effects of COHb on oxygen transport and delivery to tissues. Thus persons with cardiovascular and respiratory disease are particularly susceptible to the adverse health effects resulting from CO exposure. Health responses to CO include visual impairment, fatigue, decreased dexterity, dizziness, and nausea. Severe neurological damage or mortality can result from extremely high CO levels such as CO poisoning from exposures indoors.

Lead

Lead (Pb) has been used in pipes, paint, solder in food cans, and batteries; however, historically, lead in ambient air came largely from lead added to fuel as an antiknock agent. As described in Box 14.2, the rise and fall of leaded gasoline use in the United States coincided with a rise and fall in population blood lead levels, demonstrating the effectiveness of air pollutants at reaching much of the population.

Box 14.2. Leaded Gasoline and Blood Lead Levels in the United States

The phasing out of lead from gasoline is one of the single most important and successful environmental health initiatives of the twentieth century and illustrates the successful motivation of regulation and policy by epidemiological evidence in order to improve human health. In December 1921, three General Motors engineers reported that the addition of tetraethyl lead (TEL) to motor vehicle fuel both enhanced the performance of internal combustion engines and reduced engine knock, and TEL-spiked gasoline was introduced into the American fuel market in 1923. Within a year of the widespread use of leaded gasoline, the lethal potential of TEL surfaced when workers involved in production of the additive fell sick and died at several refineries in New Jersey and Ohio. This epidemic of lead poisoning prompted the U.S. Surgeon General to suspend the production and sale of leaded gasoline temporarily in 1925; he then appointed a panel of experts to investigate the recent fatalities and to assess the possible danger that might arise from the widespread distribution of lead via its sale as a gasoline additive. The panel ruled that there was no justification for the prohibition of leaded gasoline, provided that its distribution and use were regulated. However, the development of such regulations was not of the highest priority during the ensuing decades of depression, war, and postwar boom. It was not until the implementation of the Clean Air Act of 1970, in the early 1970s, that the U.S. Environmental Protection Agency moved to lower lead levels in U.S. gasoline to accommodate catalytic converters, which were fouled by the lead. By this time evidence had been growing on the adverse health effects of chronic, low-level lead exposure as well.

The Clean Air Act of 1970 required that the EPA establish National Ambient Air Quality Standards (NAAQS) to reduce ambient air levels of several major air pollutants, including airborne lead. Further, the law specifically required the phasing out of leaded gasoline by the mid-1980s. Although these mandatory reductions were controversial, their issuance coincided with the introduction of the catalytic converter, a device introduced by General Motors to reduce exhaust emissions of NO_x, CO, and hydrocarbons. The converters themselves would not lower lead emissions, but their use made leaded gasoline impossible because the lead would deactivate the main catalytic element, platinum. After the implementation of the Clean Air Act and the introduction of the catalytic converter, steps were taken quickly to shift the country's vehicle fleet to unleaded gasoline, which was introduced in the U.S. in 1975. The total market share of unleaded gasoline increased over the following decades as lead additives were phased out; on January 1, 1996, leaded gasoline was prohibited for use in highway vehicles in the United States. The consequent reduction in air lead particulate concentrations measured at monitoring sites across the United States from 1977 to 1996 is shown in Figure 14.4.

As the use of leaded gasoline decreased, so did human exposure to inhaled lead, a result that has been documented through the analysis of human blood samples collected across the United States. The second National Health and Nutrition Examination Survey (NHANES II) began in 1976, just after the introduction of unleaded gasoline in the United States, and the blood lead levels of 9,832 participants aged one to seventy-four years were measured. The mean blood lead level of all participants from

FIGURE 14.4. U.S. AIR LEAD CONCENTRATIONS, 1977–1996.

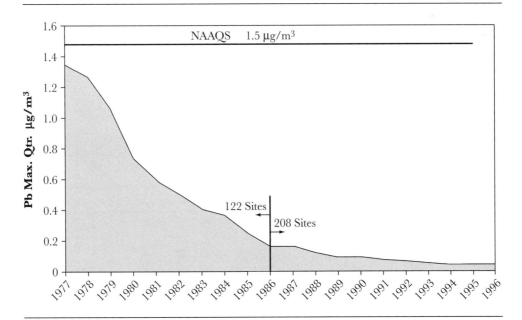

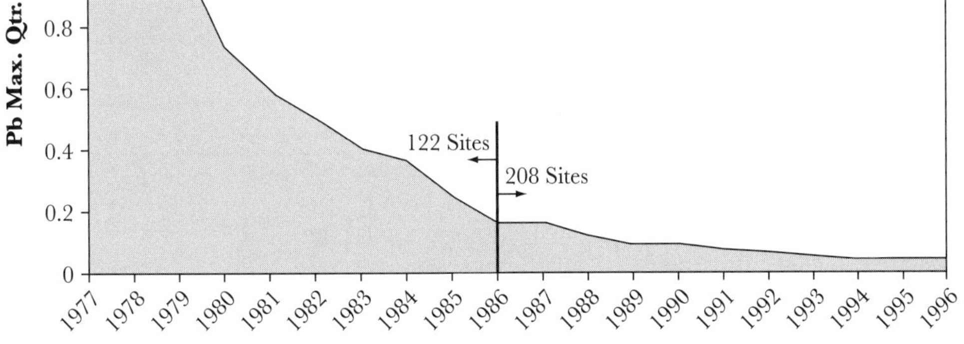

1976 to 1980 was 12.8 to 13.9 μg/dL (geometric mean 12.8 μg/dL). When Mahaffey, Annest, Roberts, and Murphy published these results in 1982, 1.9 percent of the study population met the definition established by the Centers for Disease Control and Prevention (CDC) for "elevated" blood lead levels, which at the time was ≥30 μg/dL, and 77.8 percent of the participants had blood lead levels ≥10 μg/dL. During the first phase of the third National Health and Nutrition Examination Survey (NHANES III), blood samples from 12,119 participants were collected from 1988 to 1991. The geometric mean blood lead level had dropped 78 percent, to 2.8 μg/dL, in NHANES III participants, and the decrease was observed across all age, racial, and ethnic groups. Further, the proportion of the study population with blood lead levels ≥30 μg/dL decreased to 0.2 percent, and the proportion with a concentration ≥10 μg/dL (the new CDC definition of an "elevated" blood lead level) was 4.3 percent. Pirkle and colleagues (1994) attributed the observed decline in blood lead levels to the removal of lead from gasoline and also the removal of lead from the solder used on food cans. In 1997, the CDC updated this information with data from Phase II of NHANES III (covering the years 1991 to 1994), reporting a further drop in the overall mean blood level to 2.3 μg/dL. Preliminary data on blood lead levels obtained from 1999 to 2000 for the subsequent NHANES IV study revealed that blood lead levels continued to decline; the mean blood lead concentration of the study participants greater than one year of age was 1.66 μg/dL (CDC, 2003). This followed the 1996 ban on leaded gasoline sales in the United States. Figure 14.5 illustrates the change in blood lead levels in the U.S. since 1976.

FIGURE 14.5. CHANGE IN U.S. BLOOD LEAD LEVELS, 1976–2000.

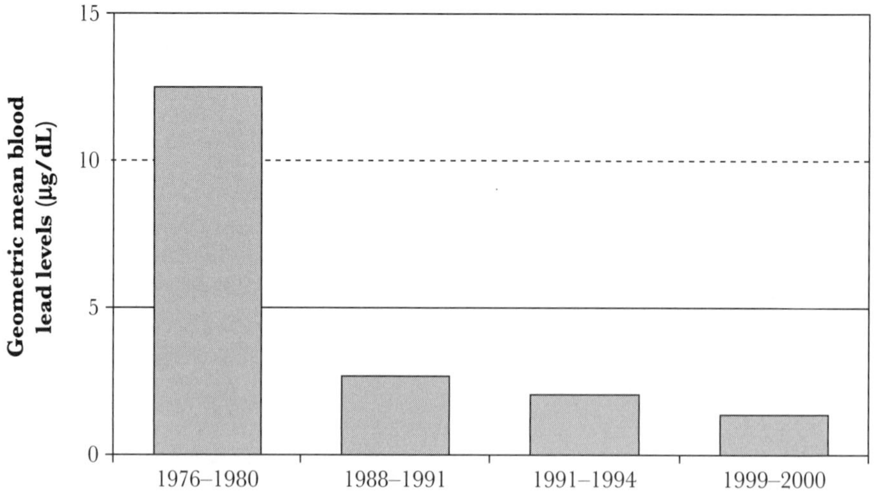

In 1994, the United Nations Commission on Sustainable Development called for elimination of leaded gasoline worldwide. Blood levels of lead have been shown to decline with the elimination of lead additives in fuel. Many countries, such as Canada, Argentina, the United States, and Japan, have already phased out leaded gasoline or have plans to do so. In these countries nonairborne sources of lead, such as ingestion of leaded paint, are a larger health concern than airborne lead. However, lead additives are still common elsewhere, for example, in many African countries. Metal processing, lead smelters, waste incineration, and the manufacture and reclamation of lead batteries are also sources of atmospheric lead.

Lead can be harmful even at low doses because it accumulates in the body, mostly in the bones, which then function as ongoing internal sources of exposures. The absorption of lead depends on physiological characteristics such as health status, age, and nutritional status. The health effects of lead have been studied extensively. Exposure to lead can cause damage to the nervous system and kidneys and can interfere with red blood cell formation, reproductive function, and gastrointestinal function. Children and pregnant women are particularly vulnerable because the developing nervous system is a target of lead toxicity.

Air Toxics

Hundreds of other ambient air pollutants exist in addition to those already described. They include hydrochloric acid, captan, parathion, naphthalene, biphenyl, vinyl bromide, methyl bromide, dioxin, and cadmium, to name a few. Exposure to these pollutants can occur through inhalation, but they also enter other environmental media such as water and food. Therefore exposure can occur through eating foods, drinking water, or coming in contact with soil that has been contaminated by atmospheric deposition. Health effects of these air toxics include damage to the neurological, immune, respiratory, and reproductive (for example, reduced fertility) systems, as well as developmental problems and some cancers. Like humans, animals may experience health problems if exposed to sufficient quantities of air toxics. Some air toxics accumulate in tissues, so that the concentrations in aquatic or marine animals can rise to levels far above those in the surrounding air and water. Polychlorinated biphenyls (PCBs) are one example of such a pollutant. The increase in concentrations occurs higher in the food chain—for example, as larger fish eat contaminated smaller fish. This can result in human exposures to elevated levels of PCBs through eating seafood.

Mercury

Mercury is naturally occurring but can be released into the atmosphere, soil, or water through human activities. Because mercury commonly contaminates coal,

coal-fired power plants are the largest source of airborne mercury in the United States, contributing approximately 40 percent. Mercury exposure can occur through inhalation, skin contact, or ingestion. The health effects of mercury depend on its chemical form. For example, elemental mercury is more toxic to the kidney, whereas methylmercury is more toxic to the brain.

Elemental mercury in the atmosphere can be deposited into water bodies, converted into methylmercury by microorganisms, and then consumed by fish. Because mercury accumulates in tissues, fish can have high concentrations of mercury, especially those fish higher in the food chain, such as shark, swordfish, and king mackerel. When people consume these fish, the mercury can then be passed on to them. The U.S. Food and Drug Administration (2001) issued an advisory recommending that nursing women, pregnant women, and women of childbearing age who may become pregnant avoid eating shark, swordfish, king mackerel, and tilefish and that they eat no more than an average of twelve ounces a week of other types of fish. The nutritional benefits of seafood must be weighed against the health dangers of consuming mercury (Egeland and Middaugh, 1997). Mercury targets the nervous system, causing impaired vision and coordination, memory loss, personality disturbances, and occasionally death, and it targets the kidneys as well. Children and fetuses are at special risk for mercury poisoning.

Air Pollution Prevention and Control

The pathway from ambient air pollution to human health involves several steps:

1. Release of the pollutant or precursors from the source
2. Transport of the pollutant or precursors (in this case, by air), and possible chemical and physical transformation
3. Exposure (via inhalation or in some cases through other media) after atmospheric deposition of the pollutant
4. Health responses (for example, asthma attack or death)

Mitigation of the health effects of air pollution can take place at any of these steps.

With air pollution, as with many other areas of environmental health, the preferred approach to controlling the health effects is primary prevention (see Chapter Twenty-Nine). For air pollutants this means reducing the emissions of a pollutant or its precursors at the source. For power plants, this approach might consist of installing scrubbers to remove SO_2 from gaseous emissions, reducing the demand for power, burning low- rather than high-sulfur coal, or making a switch to cleaner fuel sources altogether and producing electricity from the energy in wind, sun, or water. For vehicle emissions, primary prevention efforts include reducing the number of miles traveled (through so-called transportation demand management, such as telecommuting and carpooling; see Chapter Seventeen), driving cleaner, more efficient vehicles, using cleaner fuels (for example, unleaded gasoline), promoting public transportation, and implementing inspection and maintenance programs.

Regulatory Approaches

Regulation of air pollution is primarily a federal responsibility, through the Clean Air Act, and several major approaches to regulation have evolved. First, limits are set on the ambient levels of pollutants allowable in particular areas. Second, limits are set on emissions from sources such as factories and power plants. Third, polluters may be required to use certain technologies designed to limit their emissions. Fourth, market-based incentives can be implemented to induce polluters to decrease their emissions. Finally, regulations can require public disclosure of information about emissions, in an effort to motivate reduction. The Clean Air Act and related legislation use all these methods in a complex regulatory framework.

Ambient standards are limits on the concentration of specific pollutants in outdoor air, which in turn may require emissions reductions in areas with higher pollution levels. The prime example of limits on ambient air pollution levels is the set of National Ambient Air Quality Standards (NAAQS). Ambient standards are established for the criteria pollutants: O_3, SO_2, PM, lead, NO_2, and CO. The criteria pollutants are so named because EPA is required to review the NAAQS and relevant scientific evidence at least every five years and, if necessary, to revise the standards. The agency prepares a *criteria document* as part of this review.

There are two types of NAAQS for criteria pollutants: *primary* standards, established to protect human health with an adequate margin of safety, not only for the general population but for sensitive populations such as children and the elderly; and *secondary* standards, meant to protect welfare concerns such as the environment, visibility, and property damage. States with areas that do not meet the NAAQS—known as *nonattainment areas*—must develop and submit for EPA approval a *state implementation plan* (SIP) outlining how the state proposes to come into compliance.

An important feature of ambient standards is that they cannot protect everyone because of the range of susceptibility. Despite the intent to protect public health with a margin of safety, standard setting is a political process that involves compromises. Moreover, emerging scientific evidence sometimes reveals that levels of exposure previously considered safe may actually carry some risk. For example, ozone exposure has been shown to affect lung function in some people at levels as low as forty parts per billion, well within "safe" exposures permitted by EPA standards.

Emissions standards are used for many pollutants and sources. Emissions standards limit the amount of air pollution that can be emitted from a specific source, placing limits on CO emitted from motor vehicles, for example, and requiring permits for major stationary sources. This is the principal approach to pollutants labeled *hazardous* or *toxic,* pollutants that are not criteria pollutants but that cause serious health and environmental damage. The present listing of 188 such pollutants includes VOCs, pesticides, herbicides, and radionuclides. Some, such as benzene, vinyl chloride, toluene, and chloroform, are carcinogens. Although hazardous pollutants have diverse sources, they originate mainly from industries and waste products. Hazardous pollutants are regulated through specific standards for the different types of sources, such as chemical plants and oil refineries. (Table 14.1 displays the regulatory standards and guidelines for several pollutants.)

Technology requirements are a further approach to regulation. In this approach the EPA tells a polluter not only how much it may emit but also what techniques it must use to limit emissions. These requirements have names such as *best available control technology* (BACT) and *maximum achievable control technology* (MACT). Such approaches are typically used in combination with emissions standards. For example, the National Emissions Standards for Hazardous Air Pollutants (NESHAP) are set at a level intended to provide an ample margin of safety to protect public health, given the maximum achievable control technology and consideration of cost and nonhealth impacts. The MACT is defined as the technology that will result in the largest achievable reduction of emissions. A specific example of a technology requirement is that for catalytic converters on automobiles.

Market-based regulatory approaches have increasingly come to supplement, and in some cases supplant, traditional command-and-control regulations. For example, emissions-trading programs set a cap on the total amount of a pollutant that can be emitted but allow different polluters to trade permits (or the right to pollute). The intent is to achieve the most economically efficient distribution of emissions reductions by allowing facilities the flexibility to choose their equipment and design and by creating financial incentives for better performance than traditional emissions regulations would require. By turning low emissions into a financial asset, this so-called cap-and-trade approach could encourage the development of new technology that provides better air quality control. Two prominent cap-and-trade programs are the SO_2 allowances system in the EPA's Acid Rain Program and the Regional Clean Air Incentives Market (RECLAIM).

The sulfur allowance trading portion of the Acid Rain Program lowers nationwide SO_2 emissions in two phases. In the first phase, begun in 1995, an SO_2

emissions cap was set for the heaviest polluters among electric power generators. In 2000, the second phase lowered the allowable emissions on these large facilities and established limits for smaller, cleaner sources and new generators. Each source has a number of *allowances*, representing the amount of SO_2 it is allowed to emit. Unused allowances can be sold to other facilities or banked for future use.

RECLAIM was adopted by the South Coast Air Quality Management District in 1993 to lower ozone and particulate matter levels in southern California through reduced emissions of NO_x and SO_x. Facilities that reduce annual emissions below their reduction targets can sell their unused right to pollute to other facilities. Additionally, in calculating emissions the *bubble* approach is used, which means that all emissions from a facility are considered together, in contrast to the command-and-control approach, which regulates each piece of equipment and process individually. Another example of a cap-and-trade program is the regional NO_x program in the northeastern United States, designed to address ozone.

Cap-and-trade programs can be problematic when the pollution's damaging effects are localized or cumulative. Transferring emissions from one area to another could lead to *hot spots* of damage near sources with higher emissions. An additional consideration with regard to emissions trading approaches is the cost of transactions, which if high can lower the economic efficiency of the overall program and hinder trading.

Finally, *information requirements* represent yet another regulatory approach. The EPA's Toxics Release Inventory (TRI) is an annual public report on toxic chemical releases and related activities for certain industries and federal facilities. Members of the public can access this information and learn about air pollution emissions from their local facilities.

States are free to promulgate requirements that are stricter than federal regulations. For example, the State of New York requires power plants and large stationary sources to reduce emissions of NO_x below what is federally required, and many states have specific requirements for vehicle emissions, such as the California Low Emission Vehicle program. Over thirty states and the District of Columbia currently have vehicle inspection and maintenance programs, which vary in their required frequency and stringency.

Technological Controls

Reduction of ambient air pollution levels can be achieved through changes in technology, that is, through the use of alternative technology (for example, using public transportation instead of individual automobiles), the modification of existing technology (for example, switching to low-sulfur coal), or the development of new, cleaner technologies (for example, advances in fuel efficiency). Such technological advances are primary prevention strategies in environmental health (see Chapter Twenty-Nine). An example of a technological air quality control is the catalytic converter. In the 1970s, car manufacturers began installing catalytic converters, which convert CO, hydrocarbons, and NO_x into less harmful by-products and thereby reduce emissions. The use of the catalytic converter and advances in its design caused ambient levels of CO to plunge in spite of an increase in the number of vehicle miles traveled. In the United States, CO emissions dropped by nearly half between 1970 and 1990. However, areas with traffic congestion can still reach elevated CO levels. The use of coal as a household heating source has declined in many countries, such as Great Britain, also causing CO levels to decline. Other examples of technological developments that reduce air pollution are emulsified fuels, dust suppression, and soil stabilization products that prevent particulate matter from becoming airborne, diesel engine emission controls, baghouse filtration products, and scrubbers.

Many air pollution control technologies remove impurities in air by trapping them or converting them to another compound or medium. Examples are dust collectors and filters that trap small particles in the gas stream. Absorption technologies remove impurities by trapping them in an aqueous solution containing chemicals that absorb the pollution. In adsorption equipment, gaseous pollutants are transferred to the surface of a solid adsorbent, such as activated carbon. Condenser processors convert gaseous pollution to a liquid, and electrostatic precipitators give particle pollutants a positive or negative charge and collect them on oppositely charged collection plates. The efficiency of air pollution removal technologies depends on such factors as performance (for example, how rapidly filters become clogged), temperature, design features, and the nature of the pollutant. Even equipment with 99 percent removal efficiency permits some pollution to enter the atmosphere. Moreover, such controls reduce air pollution but create another challenge: the disposal of the solid or liquid waste they produce (see Chapter Nineteen).

Other Approaches to Protecting Public Health

Although most air pollution control strategies are aimed at lowering emissions, efforts are also directed at changing the transport of air pollutants, exposure to pollutants, and the health response. The transport of air pollutants is affected by the location of polluting facilities, how the land lies and the wind blows in a region, and the height and design of pollution stacks. Tall smokestacks, an early approach to controlling air pollution locally, function to disperse pollutants over larger areas. Lowering personal exposure to pollutants can also reduce air pollution's adverse health effects. An example of this latter strategy is the use of the ozone alert day: when unhealthy ozone levels are anticipated, the public is notified so that susceptible people (for example, children, people with asthma, and the elderly) can modify their exposure by staying indoors. Finally, the health impacts of air pollution can be affected by people's access to health care systems and the quality of those systems, available treatment options, and communication among agencies. For instance, should an industrial release of air pollutants occur, a physician would likely be able to treat patients more effectively if he or she knew what harmful pollutant was involved.

Regional Air Pollution and Other Environmental Problems

Many atmospheric pollutants affect air quality and human health through multiple pathways. For example, NO_2 affects health directly but also contributes to the formation of ozone, and SO_2 contributes to the formation of particulate matter. Ambient air pollutants also figure into many other environmental problems. NO_x and SO_x are the primary causes of acid precipitation. Indoor air pollution levels are related to both indoor sources and the penetration of outdoor air. PM and ozone affect visibility. The same fossil fuel burning processes that generate ambient air pollutants also produce greenhouse gases such as CO_2 and methane (CH_4), which contribute to global climate change. Many technologies and policies to mitigate ambient air pollution could also reduce production of greenhouse gases, and vice versa (Cifuentes and others, 2001). Thus the control of regional air pollution and of related health consequences is intertwined with ecological health and climate change.

Thought Questions

1. What are the primary air pollution problems in your community? What are the main sources of air pollution?
2. How do your everyday activities contribute to air pollution?
3. How is regional air pollution related to other health and environmental issues?
4. Air pollution is a complex mixture of multiple contaminants, however air pollutants are often regulated and studied individually. Why is this the case? What are the consequences of this approach? How can the difficulties this raises be addressed?
5. What actions can be taken to lower air pollution emissions? Consider possibilities at multiple levels: the individual, the community, the government, and so forth.

References

Ackermann-Liebrich, U., and Rapp, R. "Epidemiological Effects of Oxides of Nitrogen, Especially NO_2." In S. T. Holgate, J. M. Samet, H. S. Koren, and R. L. Maynard (eds.), *Air Pollution and Health.* New York: Academic Press, 1999.

Bell, M. L., and Davis, D. L. "Reassessment of the Lethal London Fog of 1952: Novel Indicators of Acute and Chronic Consequences of Acute Exposure to Air Pollution." *Environmental Health Perspectives,* 2001, *109* (suppl. 3), 389–394.

Bell, M. L., Davis, D. L., and Fletcher, T. "A Retrospective Assessment of Mortality from the London Smog Episode of 1952: The Role of Influenza and Pollution." *Environmental Health Perspectives,* 2004, *112,* 6–8.

Bell, M. L., and others. "Ozone and Mortality in 95 U.S. Urban Communities, 1987 to 2000." *Journal of the American Medical Association,* 2004, *292,* 2372–2378.

Brimblecombe, P. *The Big Smoke: A History of Air Pollution in London Since Medieval Times.* New York: Methuen, 1986.

Broeckaert, F., and others. "Reduction of the Ex Vivo Production of Tumor Necrosis Factor Alpha by Alveolar Phagocytes After Administration of Coal Fly Ash and Copper Smelter Dust." *Journal of Toxicology and Environmental Health,* 1997, *51,* 189–202.

Brook, R. D., and others. "Air Pollution and Cardiovascular Disease: A Statement for Healthcare Professionals from the Expert Panel on Population and Prevention Science of the American Heart Association." *Circulation,* 2004, *109,* 2655–2671.

Calderón-Garcidueñas, L., and others. "Air Pollution and Brain Damage." *Toxicologic Pathology,* 2002, *30,* 373–389.

Centers for Disease Control and Prevention. "Update: Blood Lead Levels—United States, 1991–1994." *Morbidity and Mortality Weekly Report,* 1997, *46,* 141–146.

Centers for Disease Control and Prevention. *Second National Report on Human Exposure to Environmental Chemicals.* Atlanta, Ga.: Centers for Disease Control and Prevention, 2003.

Cifuentes, L., and others. "Climate Change: Hidden Health Benefits of Greenhouse Gas Mitigation." *Science,* 2001, *293,* 1257–1259.

Daigle, C. C., and others. "Ultrafine Particle Deposition in Humans During Rest and Exercise." *Inhalation Toxicology,* 2003, *15,* 539–552.

Davis, D. L. *When Smoke Ran Like Water: Tales of Environmental Deception and the Battle Against Pollution.* New York: Basic Books, 2002.

Devlin, R. B., and others." Elderly Humans Exposed to Concentrated Air Pollution Particles Have Decreased Heart Rate Variability." *European Respiratory Journal,* 2003, *40* (suppl.), S76–S80.

Dockery, D. W., and others. "An Association Between Air Pollution and Mortality in Six U.S. Cities." *New England Journal of Medicine,* 1993, *329,* 1753–1759.

Dye, J. A., and others. "Acute Pulmonary Toxicity of Particulate Matter Filter Extracts in Rats: Coherence with Epidemiological Studies in Utah Valley Residents." *Environmental Health Perspectives,* 2001, *109* (suppl. 3), 395–403.

Egeland, G. M., and Middaugh, J. P. "Balancing Fish Consumption Benefits with Mercury Exposure." *Science,* 1997, *278,* 1904–1905.

Ezzati, M., and others. "Selected Major Risk Factors and Global and Regional Burden of Disease." *Lancet,* 2002, *360,* 1347–1360.

Firket, J. "Fog Along the Meuse Valley." *Transactions of the Faraday Society,* 1936, *32,* 1192–1197.

Gauderman, W. J., and others. "Association Between Air Pollution and Lung Function Growth in Southern California Children: Results from a Second Cohort." *American Journal of Respiratory and Critical Care Medicine,* 2002, *166,* 76–84.

Gordis, L. *Epidemiology.* (3rd ed.) Philadelphia: Saunders, 2004.

Health Effects Institute. *Understanding the Health Effects of Components of the Particulate Matter Mix: Progress and Next Steps.* Cambridge, Mass.: Health Effects Institute, 2002.

Health Effects Institute. *Revised Analyses of Time-Series Studies of Air Pollution and Health.* Cambridge, Mass.: Health Effects Institute, 2003.

Hippocrates. "On Air, Water, and Places." In *The Genuine Works of Hippocrates* (F. Adams, trans.). London: Sydenham Society, 1849.

Hunt, A., Abraham, J. L., Judson, B., and Berry, C. L. "Toxicologic and Epidemiologic Clues from the Characterization of the 1952 London Smog Fine Particulate Matter in Archival Autopsy Lung Tissues." *Environmental Health Perspectives,* 2003, *111,* 1209–1214.

Kagawa, J. "Health Effects of Diesel Exhaust Emissions: A Mixture of Air Pollutants of Worldwide Concern." *Toxicology,* 2002, *181-182,* 349–353.

Krewski, D., and others. *Reanalysis of the Harvard Six Cities Study and the American Cancer Society Study of Particulate Air Pollution and Mortality.* Special Report of the Institute's Particle Epidemiology Reanalysis Project. Cambridge, Mass.: Health Effects Institute, 2000.

Lippmann, M. "Health Effects of Ozone: A Critical Review." *Journal of the Air Pollution Control Association,* 1989, *39,* 672–695.

Mahaffey, K. R., Annest, J. L., Roberts, J., and Murphy, R. S. "National Estimates of Blood Lead Levels, United States, 1976–1980: Association with Selected Demographic and Socioeconomic Factors." *New England Journal of Medicine,* 1982, *307,* 573–579.

Mid-Atlantic Regional Air Management Association. *1995 Ozone Atlas for the Mid-Atlantic Region.* Baltimore, Md.: Mid-Atlantic Regional Air Management Association, 1997.

Nadziejko, C., and others. "Immediate Effects of Particulate Air Pollutants on Heart Rate and Respiratory Rate in Hypertensive Rats." *Cardiovascular Toxicology,* 2002, *2,* 245–252.

National Research Council, Committee on Research Priorities for Airborne Particulate Matter. *Research Priorities for Airborne Particulate Matter: IV. Continuing Research Progress.* Washington, D.C.: National Academies Press, 2004.

Nemery, B., Hoet, P.H.M., and Nemmar, A. "The Meuse Valley Fog of 1930: An Air Pollution Disaster." *Lancet,* 2001, *357,* 704–708.

Pirkle, J. L., and others. "The Decline in Blood Lead Levels in the United States: The National Health and Nutrition Examination Surveys (NHANES)." *Journal of the American Medical Association,* 1994, *272,* 284–291.

Pope, C. A., III, and others. "Particulate Air Pollution as a Predictor of Mortality in a Prospective Study of U.S. Adults." *American Journal of Respiratory and Critical Care Medicine,* 1995, *151,* 669–674.

Pope, C. A., III, and others. "Lung Cancer, Cardiopulmonary Mortality, and Long-Term Exposure to Fine Particulate Air Pollution." *Journal of the American Medical Association,* 2002, *287,* 1132–1141.

Samet, J. M., and others. *The National Morbidity, Mortality, and Air Pollution Study, Part I: Methods and Methodologic Issues.* Cambridge, Mass.: Health Effects Institute, 2000a.

Samet, J. M., and others. *The National Morbidity, Mortality, and Air Pollution Study, Part II:. Morbidity and Mortality from Air Pollution in the United States.* Cambridge, Mass.: Health Effects Institute, 2000b.

Sandstrom, T. "Respiratory Effects of Air Pollutants: Experimental Studies in Humans." *European Respiratory Journal,* 1995, *8,* 976–995.

Schlesinger, R. B. "Toxicology of Sulfur Oxides." In S. T. Holgate, J. M. Samet, H. S. Koren, and R. L. Maynard (eds.), *Air Pollution and Health.* New York: Academic Press, 1999.

Schrenk, H. H., and others. "Air Pollution in Donora, PA: Epidemiology of the Unusual Smog Episode of October 1948, Preliminary Report." Public Health Bulletin no. 306. Washington, D.C.: U.S. Public Health Service, 1949.

Schwartz, J. "The Distributed Lag Between Air Pollution and Daily Deaths." *Epidemiology,* 2000, *11,* 320–326.

Seinfeld, J. H., and Pandis, S. N. *Atmospheric Chemistry and Physics: From Air Pollution to Climate Change.* New York: Wiley, 1998.

Soares, S. R., and others. "Urban Air Pollution Induces Micronuclei in Peripheral Erythrocytes of Mice in Vivo." *Environmental Research,* 2003, *92,* 191–196.

U.K. Ministry of Health. *Mortality and Morbidity During the London Fog of December 1952.* Reports on Public Health and Medical Subjects no 95. London: U.K. Ministry of Health, 1954.

U.S. Environmental Protection Agency. *Air Quality Criteria for Ozone and Related Photochemical Oxidants.* EPA/600/P-93/004a-cF. Washington, D.C.: U.S. Environmental Protection Agency, Office of Research and Development, National Center for Environmental Assessment, 1996.

U.S. Environmental Protection Agency. *Air Quality Criteria for Carbon Monoxide.* EPA 600/P-99/001F. Washington, D.C.: Environmental Protection Agency, Office of Research and Development, 2000.

U.S. Environmental Protection Agency. *Fourth External Review Draft of Air Quality Criteria for Particulate Matter (June 2003).* EPA/600/P-99/002aD. Research Triangle Park, N.C.: U.S. Environmental Protection Agency, National Center for Environmental Assessment, 2003.

U.S. Environmental Protection Agency, Office of Air Quality Planning and Standards. *Latest Findings on National Air Quality: 2002 Status and Trends.* EPA 454/K-03-001. Research Triangle Park, N.C.: Environmental Protection Agency, 2003.

U.S. Food and Drug Administration. "An Important Message for Pregnant Women and Women of Childbearing Age Who May Become Pregnant About the Risks of Mercury in Fish." Consumer Advisory. College Park, Md.: U.S. Food and Drug Administration, Center for Food Safety and Applied Nutrition, 2001.

Wellenius, G. A., and others. "Inhalation of Concentrated Ambient Particles Exacerbates Myocardial Ischemia in Conscious Dogs." *Environmental Health Perspectives,* 2003, *111,* 402–408.

Wilson, W. E., and Suh, H. H. "Fine Particles and Coarse Particles: Concentration Relationships Relevant to Epidemiologic Studies." *Journal of the Air and Waste Management Association,* 1997, *47,* 1238–1249.

World Health Organization. *WHO Air Quality Guidelines.* (2nd ed.) Copenhagen: World Health Organization, Regional Office for Europe, 2000.

For Further Information

The U.S. Environmental Protection Agency maintains several useful Web pages on air pollution and health.

[www.epa.gov]

The Plain English Guide to the Clean Air Act (EPA-400-K-93-001) gives a brief introduction the CAA, including how its associated regulations aim to protect human health.

[www.epa.gov/oar/oaqps/peg_caa/pegcaain.html]

EPA's Air Pollutants Web site contains links to information on specific air pollutants, as well as monitoring, emissions and sources, and the damaging effects of air pollution including health impacts.

[www.epa.gov/ebtpages/airairpollutants.html]

The World Health Organization (WHO) provides several Web sites on air quality, with links to the health-based WHO Air Quality Guidelines.

[www.euro.who.int/air/www.who.int/phe/health_topics/air/en/]

EPA periodically reviews scientific evidence relating to the criteria pollutants and summarizes this information in their "Criteria Documents." The criteria documents for ozone, carbon monoxide, and particulate matter are listed in the References Section. Interested readers should refer to EPA for the most recent criteria documents. For example, at the time of this writing EPA is preparing a new criteria document for ozone.

CHAPTER FIFTEEN

ENERGY PRODUCTION

Richard Rheingans

Energy is an essential input to most human activities, from household activities like cooking and heating to transportation to economic production. Energy use promotes health and well-being in innumerable ways. Petroleum used for land, sea, and air transportation allows people and goods to move more freely. Household heating, cooling, and cooking, whether provided by electricity, gas, or biomass, protect individuals from health risks associated with hot and cold weather and from foodborne and waterborne diseases. Electricity is essential for public health services, including water treatment and hospitals. Energy used for industrial production can provide jobs and increased household income, which tend to result in improved health. In fact energy use is closely linked to economic development on a global scale in a two-way relationship: energy helps boost productivity and improve standards of living, and higher standards of living in turn lead to greater energy demand.

But energy generation and use can also threaten public health. Mining coal places miners at risk, and burning coal releases air pollutants. Building dams to produce hydroelectric energy can alter local ecosystems, increasing the risk of waterborne diseases. Nuclear energy plants pose risks of catastrophic releases, as exemplified by incidents at the Three Mile Island and Chernobyl nuclear reactors, and long-term risks from the nuclear wastes generated. These health hazards typically operate as environmental exposures, so the health implications of energy use are very much an environmental health concern.

Clearly, energy choices can have positive and negative impacts on health. Individuals, governments, and private firms routinely make a wide range of decisions regarding their energy use—how much to use, what type to use, and how to acquire it. These decisions typically turn on matters of cost and availability, and decision makers often overlook the far-reaching public health consequences of their decisions.

This chapter describes the patterns of energy use throughout the world, including the sources, amounts, and purposes of energy used. It also describes the health consequences of various forms of energy. Lastly, the chapter explores some of the key challenges individuals and nations face in their energy decision making, with an emphasis on public health consequences.

Patterns of Human Energy Use

Energy use varies widely across the globe. Two general patterns are evident. First, the people of wealthier nations use substantially more energy per capita than the people of poor nations use. Second, the sources of energy vary with level of affluence.

In the developed countries (defined in this chapter as members of the Organization for Economic Cooperation and Development), per capita energy use is approximately 4,600 kilogram-oil-equivalents (kgoe) per year, compared to 828 kgoe/year in developing countries (Table 15.1). The contrast is even greater when we compare the United States, with a use of 7,921 kgoe/year, to sub-Saharan African countries such as Tanzania, with a use of only 391 kgoe/year. Although developed countries account for only 22 percent of the global population, they consume 61 percent of the energy used annually (World Resources Institute [WRI], 2004).

The relative distribution of energy use also differs between regions (Table 15.1). Industry accounts for 25 to 40 percent of total energy use in every region (International Energy Agency, 2002). Transportation accounts for a large portion of energy use in regions with lower population densities, such as North America and Oceania. Residential use accounts for a larger fraction of total energy use in developing country regions, although actual per capita residential use is less.

Energy use is expected to continue to grow rapidly over coming decades. The International Energy Agency (IEA) estimates that global primary energy demand will increase by 1.7 percent annually between 2000 and 2030, reaching a total of 15.3 million ton equivalents of oil. This is a slightly slower rate than the rate between 1970 and 2000. The rate of growth in energy demand is expected to be greatest in low- and middle-income countries, increasing from 30 percent of total energy demand in 2000 to 43 percent in 2030 (IEA, 2002). The projected increases in energy use will be driven by increases in population, expanded industrial and agricultural production, and increased household energy use

TABLE 15.1. PER CAPITA ENERGY USE BY SECTOR AND REGION, 1999.

Region	Per Capita Energy Use (kgoe)	Sector (% of Total) Industry	Transportation	Agriculture	Service	Residential
World	1,631.3	35.6	26	2.5	7.6	27.3
Asia	890.1	41.8	16	3.1	4.8	35.2
Europe	3,621.3	36.7	25	2.9	8.7	26.7
Middle East and North Africa	1487.1	34.1	25	2.2	3.9	19.8
Sub-Saharan Africa	NA	NA	NA	NA	NA	NA
North America	7,928.5	27.6	40	1.1	12.5	17.1
Central America and Caribbean	1,265.4	41.2	35	2.5	3.8	21.6
South America	1,088.8	43.4	32	4.4	5.2	17.3
Oceania	NA	NA	NA	NA	NA	NA
Developed	4,600.1	33.9	31	2.2	10.4	21
Developing	827.9	38.5	18	2.9	3.4	35.8

Source: WRI, 2004.

associated with increasing incomes. Growth in energy consumption in developing countries is expected to occur across all these sectors (IEA, 2002). Economic growth, urbanization, and industrialization are predicted to result in increased energy use in industry, agriculture, and services. Some of the largest expected changes relate to household energy use resulting from increased numbers of personal vehicles and increased access to electricity (Box 15.1).

Box 15.1. Household Energy Demand and Electricity in Developing Countries

Household energy demand and fuel choice are closely related to income level (IEA, 2002). The poorest households often can afford only traditional biomass fuels for basic needs such as heating and cooking. As household incomes rise, energy use increases and energy sources change. Electricity is used to power household appliances, and petroleum products are used for personal vehicles. In addition, kerosene and propane often become more common sources for cooking and heating. As income increases further, electricity demand increases still more to power air conditioners, computers, and other appliances. Household heating and cooking become more dependent on electricity and natural gas.

Increasing household access to electricity is seen as an important component of economic development and is essential for reducing the environmental and health impacts associated with collecting and using biomass fuels. Approximately 1.6 billion people do not have access to electricity. The majority live in rural areas of developing countries, in particular in sub-Saharan Africa (509 million) and South Asia (801 million) (IEA, 2002). As populations continue to grow (primarily in urban areas), the number of people lacking access is expected to decline slightly, assuming that governments can provide reliable electricity services to rapidly growing urban areas.

Access to electricity has expanded rapidly over the past three decades, with electrification rates increasing from 25 percent of developing country households in 1970 to 64 percent in 2000 (IEA, 2002). Although electrification is a necessary step for households to transition to cleaner energy sources, it is not a guarantee that they will change. Between 1980 and 2000, China achieved electricity access for 98 percent of its population, extending access to over 700 million people (IEA, 2002). However many households in China continue to rely on locally available coal for household cooking and heating, due to price and habit.

Energy Sources and Associated Health Risks

Although there is great heterogeneity in the amounts and types of energy used across the globe (Table 15.2), individuals and governments confront several common challenges. How can they best provide the energy services needed to meet daily household needs and economic production with the resources available to them and at the same time control the negative health and environmental consequences?

For each source of energy it is useful to consider the entire *fuel cycle:* fuel extraction or collection, processing or refinement, direct use for energy (as in gasoline combustion in an automobile engine or coal combustion in steel manufacturing) or transformation into another energy form (as in electricity generation), and disposal of any waste material. Throughout the fuel cycle there are *upstream* and *downstream* environmental and health effects, often far removed from the point where the energy services are consumed.

A wide range of fuels is used to meet household and national energy needs (Table 15.3). Most energy available for human use comes from the sun, either directly as solar energy or (much more typically) indirectly. Fossil fuels such as oil, natural gas, and coal were formed over millions of years from plants that sequestered solar energy through photosynthesis. Biomass fuels such as wood, peat, and crop residues also form from plants that sequester solar energy, although biomass fuels form on a human rather than a geological timescale and are therefore considered renewable. Wind, hydroelectric, wave, and tidal energy derive from the movement of air and water, a movement driven by solar energy. Geothermal energy exploits the heat within the earth's crust, and nuclear energy exploits the energy within atoms of uranium.

TABLE 15.2. OVERALL ENERGY USE AND SOURCE BY REGION, CURRENT AND PROJECTED, MILLION OIL-TON EQUIVALENTS.

Region	2000	2030
World	6,032	10,080
OECD economies	3,593	4,942
North America	1,778	2,526
Europe	1,254	1,635
Pacific	561	781
Transition economies	683	1,019
Developing economies	1,756	4,119
China	577	1,254
East Asia	280	668
South Asia	205	590
Latin America	290	695
Middle East	256	499
Africa	149	403

Source: IEA, 2002.

TABLE 15.3. ELECTRICITY GENERATION SOURCES BY REGION (IN TERAWATT HOURS, TWH), 2000.

	Source						
Region	Total	Coal	Oil	Gas	Nuclear	Hydro	Other (renewables)
World	15,391	5,989	1,241	2,676	2,586	2,650	249
OECD economies	9,598	3,733	601	1,515	2,230	1,311	208
North America	4,813	2,247	237	704	881	640	104
Europe	3,164	943	178	508	918	538	79
Pacific	1,622	542	186	304	431	133	26
Transition economies	1,484	340	82	509	255	295	3
Developing economies	4,308	1,916	557	652	100	1,044	38
China	1,387	1,081	46	19	17	222	2
East Asia	585	151	126	171	38	82	16
South Asia	635	420	32	58	19	104	2
Latin America	804	33	94	98	13	550	15
Middle East	462	24	195	228	0	16	0
Africa	435	207	63	78	13	71	2

Source: IEA, 2002.

These sources of energy may be classified in many ways, such as in terms of renewability, cost or efficiency. An approach with great relevance to public health is the *energy ladder* (sometimes called the *fuel ladder*). The energy ladder classifies fuels according to several related criteria: from traditional to modern, dirtier to cleaner, less expensive to more expensive, less commercial to more commercial, and exposed point-of-use combustion to more distant combustion (Reddy, 1982; Hosier and Dowd, 1987; Leach, 1992; Smith and others, 1994; Barnes and Floor, 1996; Saatkamp, Masera, and Kammen, 2000). As families gain socioeconomic status they opt out of inefficient, inexpensive, and dirty sources of household energy such as dung, fuel wood, and charcoal, and move up the energy ladder. Although this concept arose in the context of residential fuel use in developing nations, it can be generalized to global fuel patterns (Figure 15.1).

The decision about which fuel to use often depends on purpose, costs, availability, and environmental and health consequences. Individuals and nations with the fewest resources typically have the fewest choices. This forces them to consume less energy and to choose sources that are less costly but often especially harmful to the environment and human health. Examples include the reliance on burning wood for household energy and low-grade coal for

FIGURE 15.1. THE ENERGY LADDER.

Solar, wind, hydrogen cells
Electricity generated at a distant power station and delivered to homes through wires
Kerosene or natural gas burned in relatively clean, well-ventilated devices (for example, stoves, water heaters)
Coal burned in enclosed, well-ventilated stoves
Biomass fuels burned in efficient stoves
Coal burned in open hearths or similar arrangements
Biomass fuels (crop residues, dung, wood) burned in open hearths or similar arrangements

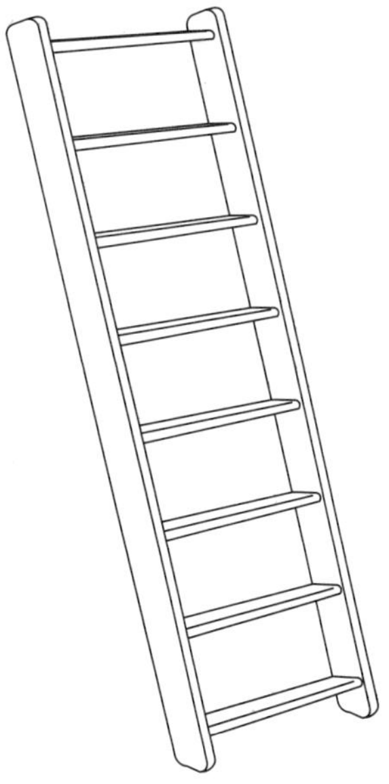

Note: Energy sources closer to the top are generally cleaner, more technology-dependent, and more expensive, and combustion occurs farther from the end user.

industrial production in many developing countries. As more resources become available, cleaner (but more costly) alternatives can be chosen (such as liquefied petroleum gas for household energy and natural gas for industrial production).

Fossil Fuels

Fossil fuels formed over millions of years through the transformation of ancient organic matter under pressure and heat. Depending on the organic matter and the exact conditions this can produce coal, petroleum, natural gas, or other substances such as tars. Table 15.4 summarizes forms of fossil fuels and their common uses. Fossil fuels account for 80 percent of the global primary energy supply.

TABLE 15.4. FOSSIL FUEL TYPES AND USES.

Fuel	Origin	Uses
Oil	Liquid formed from ancient organic deposits under heat and pressure	Refined and transformed into various liquid fuels such as gasoline and kerosene; also used directly in electricity generation.
Coal	Solid mineral deposits formed from ancient organic deposits under pressure	Used for electricity production, industrial power generation, home heating and cooking
Natural gas	Gaseous deposits formed from ancient organic deposits; often found in combination with oil or coal deposits	Used for electricity production, industrial power generation, home heating and cooking
Butane	Gaseous hydrocarbon present in natural gas and can be refined from oil; pressurized and liquefied for transportation	Household heating and cooking
Propane	Gaseous hydrocarbon present in natural gas and can be refined from oil; pressurized and liquefied for transportation.	Household heating and cooking
Liquified petroleum gas	Combination of propane and butane pressurized to form a liquid	Household heating and cooking, especially in developing countries
Gasoline	Derived from crude oil	Vehicles and other small combustion engines
Kerosene	Derived from crude oil	Heating and lighting

This supply includes coal (23 percent), oil (36 percent), and natural gas (21 percent). In developed countries, fossil fuels account for the majority of the total energy consumed (83 percent); in developing countries they represent a smaller fraction of total energy (72 percent).

The consumption of fossil fuels is expected to continue to increase (IEA, 2002). Increasing demand for electricity production is predicted to result in significant increases in coal and natural gas use, and increases in ownership of personal vehicles will continue to increase demand for petroleum. Fossil fuel use is theoretically finite, because petroleum, gas, and coal are being consumed at a far faster rate than they are being replenished. In fact, application of the Hubbert peak—a method of predicting when petroleum extraction will peak and then decline—suggests that global demand will exceed supply early in the twenty-first century, and the disparity between supply and demand will continue to increase indefinitely (Deffeyes, 2001; Goodstein, 2004). Coal, however, appears plentiful for at least decades and possibly longer, although world demand is growing rapidly.

The use of fossil fuels for energy creates environmental health risks throughout the fuel cycle, from extraction and refining to combustion.

Coal. Coal is used directly in electric power generation and in heavy industrial operations such as steel and cement production. It accounts for 48 percent of electricity generation in the United States and Canada, 78 percent in China, and 39 percent globally (IEA, 2002). In countries such as China, where it is locally available, it is also used for household heating and cooking needs.

The use of coal as an energy source creates environmental and health impacts throughout the fuel cycle (Freese, 2003). Underground coal deposits are extracted through underground or open-pit mining. In the former, miners use tunnels to extract coal from under the overlying material. In the latter, material above the coal is completely removed to gain access to the coal. Coal mining can pose significant environmental and health risks to workers and nearby communities. Coal miners are exposed to airborne coal dust that can lead to pneumoconiosis, or black lung disease, and can increase the risk of developing other conditions, such as tuberculosis. They are also at risk of injuries due to cave-ins and explosions. Coal mining can result in significant pollution of nearby aquatic systems, particularly when significant amounts of overlying material and debris are dumped into local streams during open-pit mining. This dumping releases impurities in the coal (including sulfur and heavy metals) into the waterways, disrupting aquatic ecosystems and potentially contaminating drinking water supplies.

Box 15.2. Growing Energy Demand in China and the Challenge of Balancing Economic Growth and Public Health

With over 1 billion inhabitants and one of the fastest growing economies in the world, China's energy situation highlights the environmental and health challenges faced across the globe. With approximately 20 percent of the world's population, China accounts for 28 percent of global coal demand and produces 14 percent of anthropogenic CO_2 emissions (IEA, 2002). Between 1990 and 2000, the country achieved rapid economic growth, with the per capita GDP rising 8.7 percent annnually, more than four times the global average. This growth was accompanied by increases in per capita energy consumption (2.3 percent annually) and CO_2 emissions (2.9 percent) (IEA, 2002).

Even though China's economic growth may not remain at the same high levels, the country's economy is expected to continue to boom. Growth in industry, services, and residential demand may result in an energy demand that more than doubles between 2000 and 2030 (IEA, 2002). How this energy need is met will have important health consequences for the population of China and the globe.

In 2000, coal accounted for 69 percent of China's primary energy demand. The International Energy Agency estimates that although China's use of coal is expected to rise (by 2.2 percent per year), other energy sources are expected to grow more rapidly, including natural gas (5.5 percent per year), nuclear (9 percent per year), and hydroelectric (3.5 percent per year). As the number of private vehicles increases, oil consumption will also continue to rise (3 percent per year). This decreasing relative reliance on coal will be the product of changes in the structure of the industrial sector (mergers and closure of inefficient plants, particularly in the steel and cement industries), energy conservation measures, and reduced coal consumption by residential users. In spite of greater use of cleaner alternatives, coal will continue to provide the majority (60 percent) of the nation's primary energy demand due to its local availability and price. Recent environmental regulations have, however, resulted in the closure of highly polluting coal mines and lower emissions from coal-using industries.

China provides a snapshot of the health challenges posed by energy and economic development. As the economy continues to grow and household incomes rise, energy use will continue to grow, due in particular to increases in industrial production, consumption of electricity, and transportation. Such increases in energy use can result in significant increases in emissions of CO_2, CO, particulates, sulfur oxides, nitrogen oxides, and other pollutants. At the same time, economic growth itself provides some opportunities to reduce the environmental and health impact of the energy used. The transition from coal to electricity for basic residential needs reduces indoor and outdoor air pollution. Economic growth can make government resources available for improved regulation of factory and electricity generation emissions and can also increase the use of improved technologies to reduce emissions and improve energy efficiency.

Perhaps the most significant consequences of coal use are the downstream consequences associated with coal combustion. The burning of coal results in the release of carbon monoxide, carbon dioxide, particulate matter, polycyclic aromatic hydrocarbons, and other organic chemicals. Oxides of nitrogen (NO_x) are released as a by-product of oxidation of air, and other pollutants are created from impurities contained in the organic material from which the coal was formed. The most notable of these other pollutants are sulfur oxides (SO_x, from sulfur contained in the coal) and metals such as mercury and vanadium. The concentration of sulfur and mercury in coal can vary greatly, depending on the original organic material.

These released chemicals pose significant health risks related to where and how they are used. When coal is used for household heating and cooking, as is common in many developing countries, improper ventilation can result in significant indoor exposure to these contaminants. In particular, exposures to carbon monoxide and particulates are associated with respiratory and cardiovascular health effects. These same pollutants, released from household and industrial coal sources, can result in locally high levels of contamination, especially under specific weather and geographic conditions.

As detailed in Chapter Fourteen, exposures to NO_x (and the resulting ozone), SO_x, particulates, and polycyclic aromatic hydrocarbons create a wide range of health risks including eye and airway irritation, respiratory infections, asthma, cardiopulmonary disease, and cancer. These tend to occur at the local and regional scale where the contaminants remain concentrated.

Heavy metals, mercury in particular, are also released during the combustion of coal, resulting in local and regional exposures. Downwind communities can be exposed to airborne mercury. After the mercury is deposited, whether on land or water, it eventually enters aquatic systems. It is then taken up by aquatic organisms and accumulates in fish, particularly those at the top of the food chain. Coal combustion contributes 48 percent of the annual mercury emissions in the United States (U.S. Environmental Protection Agency [EPA], 1997). Mercury exposure can result in neurological and developmental effects.

The combustion of all fossil fuels results in the release of carbon dioxide, an important greenhouse gas (see Chapter Eleven). Coal combustion accounts for 40 percent of the annual anthropogenic CO_2 emissions (WRI, 2004). Increasing combustion of fossil fuels, especially coal, is expected to be a major contributor to climate change in coming decades.

Petroleum. The use and health impacts of petroleum, or oil, share many common features with the impacts of coal. However, as a liquid, petroleum is more portable and denser in energy than coal. This makes it particularly appropriate for use in the transportation sector, where petroleum products power motor vehicles, aircraft, and boats. Forty-seven percent of global petroleum use is for transportation (IEA, 2002). Petroleum is also used in electricity generation, in industrial and agricultural operations, and for residential needs.

As with other fossil fuels, there are upstream environmental and health threats (those associated with petroleum extraction, processing, and transportation) as well as downstream effects (those associated with combustion). Petroleum is extracted through drilling into underground reservoirs, where it has been trapped by layers of bedrock. These reservoirs can be found below land or sea. Exploration and drilling can result in occupational injuries associated with explosions and fires. In order to be used, petroleum must be refined into products such as gasoline. This process results in the release of carcinogenic hydrocarbons, such as benzene, that can affect workers and nearby communities.

Direct health effects associated with the combustion of petroleum result from the release of particulate matter, carbon monoxide, carbon dioxide, nitrogen and sulfur oxides, and polycyclic aromatic hydrocarbons. Vehicle emissions of particulates and ozone-forming nitrogen oxides are an important cause of air pollution in large urban areas and along major truck transportation routes (see Chapter Seventeen).

In many countries lead is added to gasoline as an octane enhancer (to improve the efficiency of the gasoline combustion in motor vehicles). When the leaded gasoline is burned, lead is released into the air as part of the vehicle exhaust. Once in the air, lead can be directly inhaled or ingested as dust that settles near high-traffic areas. Even low levels of prenatal and early childhood lead exposures are associated with developmental and neurological effects. Eliminating lead from gasoline has been an effective measure for reducing childhood lead poisoning in the United States and other developed countries. However, in many developing countries, lead is still added to gasoline (Institute of Medicine, 1996).

In addition to these local and regional health impacts, petroleum combustion releases carbon dioxide, contributing to the greenhouse effect. Annual CO_2 emissions from petroleum contribute 42 percent of the global anthropogenic releases each year (WRI, 2004). Finally, impending petroleum scarcity may trigger armed conflict (Klare, 2001, 2004); such *resource wars* are a direct threat to public health (Chapter Twelve).

Natural Gas. Natural gas was produced along with other fossils fuels during the transformation of ancient organic material. It is used for electricity generation (35 percent of total global use) as well as to meet industrial and residential energy needs (IEA, 2002). The use of natural gas is expected to continue to rise as a fraction of total energy use as new reservoirs are identified and brought into production and as the infrastructure for transporting natural gas is improved.

Natural gas burns cleaner and has a greater energy yield than other fossil fuels do. Upstream health effects include fire and explosion risks during the process of exploration, drilling, and transportation. The downstream impacts are similar to those associated with other fossil fuels, although often less severe. In particular, emission levels of sulfur oxides, nitrogen oxides, and heavy metals are much lower for natural gas compared to levels from coal or oil combustion.

Reducing Fossil Fuel Impacts. A number of approaches can be taken to reduce the environmental health consequences of fossil fuel use. Upstream consequences can be reduced through improved extraction and processing technologies and the establishment and enforcement of occupational safety and health regulations.

Downstream consequences associated with particulates, CO, SO_x, NO_x, and other contaminants can be reduced by a combination of measures, such as switching to cleaner fossil fuels or to renewables. For example, switching from coal to natural gas for electricity generation can reduce SO_2 emissions. Similarly, switching from coal to liquefied petroleum gas for household heating and cooking in developing countries can reduce emissions of particulates. Using a cleaner grade of a particular fuel type (for example, switching from high-sulfur to low-sulfur coal) can have a similar effect. These strategies are not necessarily effective in reducing CO_2 emissions, however.

Changes in technologies can also reduce emissions and exposures. Potential technological changes include improvements in efficiency, for example, improved automobile fuel mileage or more efficient electricity generation. Such changes mean that less fuel is required to provide a given energy yield; thus all the related health hazards are reduced also. Improvements in emission control technologies can also reduce the levels of some contaminants being released into the environment, but not levels of CO_2. The primary obstacle to many of these changes is the short-term cost of switching to more expensive fuels or new technologies.

A final strategy for reducing the health effects associated with fossil fuel use is to reduce the level of energy use for nonessential activities. Conservation offers the benefits of economic efficiency as well as health and environmental improvements.

Biomass

Biomass fuels are combustible organic materials produced by plants on a timescale of months to years; examples include wood, peat, crop residues (such as corn husks and coconut shells), and animal dung (which derives from nondigestible plant components in the animal diet). Although biomass fuel has been used for thousands of years and is a traditional energy source in many cultures, there is a renewed interest in biomass as an environmentally sound, renewable source of energy, using crops grown for this purpose, such as alfalfa, grasses, corn, and fast-growing trees. Biomass can be burned directly, or in modern processes, it can be converted first into other combustible materials, such as ethanol or methanol, or even gasified. In fact the conversion of biomass into more convenient forms is not new; wood has been converted to charcoal through oxygen-poor combustion for many centuries.

It has been estimated that 2.4 billion people rely on burning fuelwood, agricultural residues, or animal dung as their primary source of residential energy (IEA, 2002). Biomass fuels are particularly important in sub-Saharan Africa and South Asia, where they account for over 90 percent and 80 percent of residential energy use, respectively (IEA, 2002). In rural areas biomass fuels typically come from crop residues, animal dung, and collected fuelwood. In urban areas charcoal, which is lighter and more efficient, is often more common. Biomass fuels are also used for industrial operations in some developing and developed countries where such fuels are readily available. Biomass will continue to be an important source of household energy in developing countries (IEA, 2002). Even in countries where access to electricity in both urban and rural areas has been expanded greatly, traditional fuels continue to be an important and sometimes preferred energy source.

The health effects associated with biomass fuel use occur both upstream (during collection) and downstream (during their actual use). The collection of fuelwood can be a time- and labor-intensive task, especially in areas where overcollection has resulted in reduced availability. Traveling long distances with heavy loads exposes women and children (who typically do most of the collecting) to musculoskeletal injuries and to vector-borne diseases and is a significant drain on caloric resources. In addition, the time required for fuel collecting can reduce the time available for health-promoting behaviors, such as those focused on hygiene, child care, and education. Moreover, biomass fuel use can place pressure on forest and agricultural resources. Fuelwood collection is not considered a major cause of deforestation on a global scale (Matthews, Payne, Rohweder, and Murray, 2000). However, in areas with high population densities or fragile forest ecosystems, fuelwood collection can devastate local forests, leading to erosion and reduced water quality and availability.

The burning of tradition biomass fuels for household energy needs is a major cause of indoor air pollution in developing countries (WHO, 1992). Incomplete burning results in the release of particulates and CO, along with CO_2 and other contaminants. Often fuels are burned in open fires or poorly vented stoves, allowing the contaminants to build up in the home. As a result the concentration of particulates and CO in homes with open burning of biomass fuels can be much higher than outdoor concentrations are in heavily polluted cities. The highest levels of exposures occur among the women in these households, who spend more time than the men near the fire and cooking, among the infants strapped to their mothers' backs, and among small children who may spend time indoors. The health effects associated with indoor air pollution from biomass use include chronic obstructive pulmonary disease, acute respiratory infections, low birthweight, infant and perinatal mortality, pulmonary tuberculosis, cancer, and cataracts (Bruce, Neufeld, Boy, and West, 1998; Bruce, Perez-Padilla, and Albalak, 2000; Ezzati and Kammen, 2001). In addition to the hazards associated with indoor air pollution, biomass fuel use (especially in open stoves or fires) also poses an injury risk to children and others who are working or playing in proximity to these fires.

Biomass fuel offers the prospect of affordable, renewable, and clean fuel, and considerable effort is being invested to develop innovative biomass sources. Several approaches are available for reducing the health hazards associated with biomass fuel use. Some of the environmental and health consequences associated with fuelwood collection can be reduced through proper community forest management and woodlots designed and managed to produce wood sustainably. These approaches can reduce the time and energy required for collection as well as the environmental damage associated with overharvesting. One approach to reducing the health consequences associated with indoor air pollution is the promotion of improved cookstoves. The various designs have two common features. First, they contain and enclose the fire, resulting in a more efficient burning that reduces the emission of particulates and the total amount of fuel required. Second, the fumes from the fire are vented outside the home to prevent them from concentrating indoors. Although the improved stoves can effectively reduce emissions, initial costs and cultural preferences for traditional cooking practices have limited their adoption in some settings.

Hydroelectric

Hydroelectric power is generated when falling water passes turbines and turns them, generating electricity. Electricity generated by small and large dams contributes only 17 percent to global electricity generation (IEA, 2002). However, in regions such as Latin America, abundant water resources (and a relative scarcity of other resources such as coal) make hydroelectric energy a more cost-effective alternative. In Latin America, hydroelectric power contributes 68 percent to the total regional electricity supply (IEA, 2002). Hydroelectric power is also a cost-effective alternative in China, where the famous Three Gorges dam has increased the share of hydroelectric power in the country.

Hydroelectric power offers important advantages. It creates no combustion products and does not contribute to climate change (although greenhouse gases can be emitted from reservoirs). Although the initial capital costs of dam construction are very high, energy production costs very little thereafter. However, recent decades have seen increasing awareness of the environmental and social costs of large dam projects (Rosenberg and others, 1997). These costs include the displacement of populations and loss of cultural artifacts in the flooded areas upstream of the dams, decreased fish catches downstream, major disruption of local ecosystems, and in many cases increased human health risks. In some specific dam projects, such infectious diseases as malaria, Rift Valley fever, and filariasis have increased following dam construction. For example, when the Porto Primavera hydroelectric power station flooded an area of 2,200 square kilometers at the border of the São Paulo and Mato Grosso do Sul states in Brazil, tick infestation on deer in the area increased dramatically, increasing the risk of tickborne diseases for local residents (Szabo, Labruna, Pereira, and Duarte, 2003). Similarly, before-after studies of two large hydroelectric dams in Côte d'Ivoire showed a large increase in the prevalence of *Schistosoma mansoni* (but not of *S. haematobium*) in local populations (N'Goran, Diabate, Utzinger, and Sellin, 1997). Another health risk is increased methylation of mercury in the relatively anaerobic conditions deep in reservoirs; the methylmercury concentrates in the aquatic food chain and poses a risk of toxicity to humans. The rapid expansion of hydroelectric power seen over the past three decades is not likely to continue in the future, as concerns over environmental and social consequences of large dam projects increase.

Nuclear

Nuclear fission uses uranium as a fuel. The uranium atoms are split and the controlled chain reaction produces heat and radioactive material. The heat is used to generate steam that turns turbines that generate electricity. Nuclear energy provides approximately 17 percent of global electricity generation, with the majority of that (86 percent) occurring in OECD countries. This production capacity is concentrated in countries where the regulatory climate is more accepting of nuclear power, such as France. The International Energy Agency estimates that nuclear power generation will decline in developed countries over the next three decades but increase 300 percent in developing countries (IEA, 2002).

Several features make nuclear power an attractive alternative for developing countries trying to meet the expanding electricity demand for residential and industrial uses. Unlike fossil fuel power production, nuclear power production does not produce CO_2 or contribute to climate change. Nor does it affect local or regional air pollution as coal-fired electricity does. Economically, its use is less dependent on constant imports of raw materials that may not be locally available. However, expansion is limited by the local availability of technology and by public concerns over the health risks.

The primary health risks of nuclear power are associated with the disposal of radioactive waste material and the possibility of radioactive releases as a result of accidents, as happened at Chernobyl. The splitting of uranium-235 atoms in the nuclear fission process produces plutonium and also lighter elements such as strontium-90 and cesium-137. These by-products are classified as high-level waste that can produce a variety of health effects or death in humans (see Chapter Twenty-Four). The lighter elements produce more damaging, penetrating radiation but have a shorter half-life (approximately 35 years), whereas plutonium has a much longer half-life (around 24,000 years). These waste products present significant challenges, in that they must be transported to and stored in carefully designed waste facilities for extremely long periods. Public opposition to these facilities poses a significant obstacle to nuclear power in developed countries. In developing countries, risks from nuclear waste may be greater if the country lacks the necessary regulatory and enforcement capacity to ensure that such waste is safely transported and stored.

The disaster at the Chernobyl nuclear reactor, located near Kiev, demonstrated the significant health risks associated with inadequate safety and operational controls in nuclear power facilities. In April 1986, during a cleaning operation, an uncontrolled reaction occurred, resulting in an explosion and fire in one of the four reactors at the facility. The initial explosion killed over 30 people and caused the evacuation of over 100,000 people. The explosion and fire released iodine-131 into the environment. Subsequent studies documented significant increases in childhood thyroid cancers and increases in cancer-related mortality, leukemia, other thyroid disease, and psychological effects (United Nations Scientific Committee on the Effects of Atomic Radiation, 2000). Although nuclear power will remain an attractive option to developing countries with growing energy needs, the storage and transportation of radioactive materials and the potential for accidental release of these materials pose a significant public health threat.

New Renewable Energy Sources

Over the past three decades a number of new renewable energy technologies have been developed and improved to the point where they are economically viable, at least in some settings. They include means of producing solar, wind, and geothermal power. Others, involving fuel cells and hydrogen, for example, may become more important in coming decades. Combined, these sources currently account for less than 1 percent of global electricity production and are projected to increase tenfold and to account for 3 percent of production by 2030. They will continue to be important in settings where natural conditions make them more cost effective (settings with high, sustained winds or high solar radiation) and for off-grid applications.

These new renewable energy sources have significantly fewer associated health risks than do the fossil fuel sources they are likely to replace. Nevertheless there are some important risks and negative externalities that must be considered. Commercial production of electricity from wind requires large open areas with high, sustained winds. The concentration of windmills in a single location can produce a visual and auditory impact on local residents that may threaten well-being or quality of life. The manufacture of photovoltaic cells for use in solar energy operations produces small quantities of hazardous materials. If not properly managed and disposed of they can pose a health risk to workers or nearby communities. Opportunities for managing these risks include identifying less hazardous substitutes for the chemicals involved, reducing the concentrations or quantities of chemicals used, or improving waste management.

Energy Decision Making

Making decisions about energy sources involves considering many externalities (or negative impacts), weighing trade-offs in cost and quality, evaluating the larger economic issues, and assessing health impacts.

Externalities

Every energy source is associated with various types and levels of negative environmental, health, and social impacts. Among these impacts, for example, are the occupational hazards associated with coal mining, the effect of dams on levels of some infectious diseases, and the health effects associated with burning traditional and fossil fuels. The people placed at risk often are not the same people who benefit from the energy services, and the costs associated with these impacts are often not included in the price paid by the end user. Negative impacts that are not incorporated in the market price of energy are referred to as *externalities*.

The economic value of these externalities can be significant. A European Commission study estimated the economic cost of externalities from transportation and electricity production (using coal, oil, gas, nuclear fission, and renewables), including the impacts on morbidity and mortality (from air pollution and traffic crashes), damage to buildings and crops, and ecosystem disruption (including climate change). The external costs of electric power derived from coal in the different EU countries ranged from 2 to 10 eurocents/kWh, compared to a market price of 3 to 4 eurocents (European Commission, 2003). This cost compared to externality costs of 1 to 4 eurocents/kWh for power from gas and less than 1 eurocent/kWh for hydroelectric, nuclear, solar, and wind power. These externality costs distort decision making by providing implied subsidies, whose cost is borne by the general public. If these costs were added to the market price charged by providers and paid by consumers, coal and other fossil fuels would become relatively more expensive, compared to cleaner alternatives.

Several regulatory and institutional approaches can partially address the distortions in decision making that result from externalities. Emission reductions through technology changes or more stringent regulation can reduce the externality costs associated with some energy sources. Externality costs can also be internalized by including them in the price of specific energy sources by means of taxes. This would make market prices better reflect the true social costs of different energy sources but would increase overall energy costs. Alternatively, direct subsidies could be provided to support the use of cleaner sources, potentially equalizing the level of subsidy without increasing energy costs.

Energy Ladder: Cost and Quality Trade-Offs

Globally, over 2 billion people rely on traditional fuel sources for the cooking, heating, and other residential needs. The combustion of charcoal, wood, crop residues, animal dung, and low-quality coal inside the home poses a direct threat to the health of the family (see the examples in Table 15.5). In spite of the health risks,

TABLE 15.5. AIR EMISSIONS FROM TRADITIONAL FUELS USED IN COOKSTOVES IN INDIA.

Fuel	Carbon Dioxide (g/MJ)	Nitrous Oxide (g/MJ)
Propane	126	0.002
Biogas	144	0.002
Kerosene	138	0.002
Wood	305	0.018
Crop residues	565	0.028
Charcoal	710	0.018
Dung	876	0.022

Note: g/MJ = grams per megajoule.

Source: Smith and others, 2000.

families choose these fuel sources due to their low cost and greater availability compared to improved alternatives. As household incomes rise, fuel consumption patterns start to change. Additional income makes it possible to switch to alternatives that are less polluting, such as kerosene, liquefied petroleum gas (LPG), and electricity. This move up the energy ladder can have important health benefits for household members.

However, rising incomes do not automatically result in climbing the energy ladder. Traditional fuel sources require little if any infrastructure to obtain them, as long as they are locally available. In contrast, improved sources such as kerosene and LPG require distribution networks, and electricity requires a significant infrastructure investment by governments or private providers. Even when these alternatives are available and households can afford them, they are not always used, especially if there is a cultural preference for cooking with wood or if fuelwood is considered "free."

A similar phenomenon exists on the industrial and national scale. The choice of fuels for electricity production presents power providers and regulators with a set of trade-offs between energy cost and environmental and health quality. Table 15.6 shows the levels of CO_2, SO_2, and nitrogen oxide emissions from electricity production using coal and natural gas in the United States. For every unit of electricity produced, coal results in 1,000 times the SO_2 and 8 times the nitrogen oxide releases compared to natural gas. However natural gas is more costly per kilowatt hour. As a result, moving from coal to gas production presents a trade-off between cost and environmental emissions. Renewable sources such as wind and solar result in even lower emission levels but at still higher costs. These trade-offs are similar to those faced by developing country households. However, one important difference is that

TABLE 15.6. U.S. EMISSIONS AND COSTS OF ELECTRICITY PRODUCTION BY FUEL TYPE, 2000.

	Generation	*Carbon Dioxide*		*Sulfur Dioxide*		*Nitrogen Oxides*		*Cost*
	Billion kWh	**Total (tons)**	**Tons/ Million kWh**	**Total (tons)**	**Tons/ Million kWh**	**Total (tons)**	**Tons/ Million kWh**	**Cents per Million Btu**
Coal	1,966	1,915	974	10,952	5,570	4,799	2,441	120
Petroleum	111	95	851	744	6,691	178	1,601	418
Natural gas	601	315	524	3	5	661	1,100	430

Source: Energy Information Administration, 2003.

households using biomass fuels would directly benefit from the reduced emissions associated with moving up the energy ladder. In contrast, electricity producers do not have a direct incentive to move up the energy ladder in the absence of regulatory or customer pressure.

Economics

Household and national decisions regarding energy use are closely tied to economics. The income level of a household or country affects the energy choices that are realistically available, and the availability of affordable energy can have an important impact on a household's or country's economic level. Economic development is highly energy intensive. Industrial development requires access to affordable energy for factories, offices, and infrastructure. Agricultural intensification also requires affordable energy for farm machinery, fertilizer production, irrigation, and processing. National governments see obtaining and maintaining inexpensive energy as essential to attracting investment and maintaining economic growth. However, this can undermine regulatory efforts to internalize negative externalities or to encourage households or industries to move up the energy ladder. This perceived tension between growth and energy decisions operates in both developed and developing countries. However, consumers in developed countries may be more able to pay for improvements in environmental quality without jeopardizing economic growth.

In developing countries, access to affordable and convenient energy, including propane for heating and cooking and electricity for lighting, can greatly benefit household productivity. Propane for cooking can make more time available to women and children by reducing the need to collect fuelwood. A household electricity connection expands the available daylight hours and enables many types of household enterprises.

Health Impact Assessment

Decisions regarding energy policies and programs have implications that reach beyond public health to issues of economic growth, environmental quality, dependence on other nations, and social effects. As a result, at times it is difficult for decision makers to see and weigh the public health impacts of their decisions. This poses a challenge to public health professionals concerned with ensuring that these impacts are adequately considered. *Health impact assessment* (HIA) is a method for identifying, quantifying, and communicating these effects to decision makers. (Box 15.3 lists some energy policies that have important implications for health.)

Box 15.3. Energy Policy as Public Health Policy

Energy policy decisions are driven by a wide range of objectives, including economic development, national security, personal convenience, and conservation goals. In this complex mix, it is often difficult to see the direct impact these decisions have on public health. Nevertheless, in many ways energy decisions are public health decisions, even if they are not discussed and debated in those terms. Here are some of the ways in which energy and related policy decisions can directly influence public health:

- Gasoline taxes are much higher in Europe than in the United States, resulting in reduced private automobile use and emissions in Europe.
- The lack of incentives (tax breaks or direct investment) for research and development of alternative energy sources is likely to reduce the contribution alternative sources can make to national and global electricity production.
- Efforts to protect or promote domestically available energy sources (such as coal in the United States) in order to reduce reliance on imported sources can result in the continued use of a more polluting source.
- Electrification projects in developing countries can increase household energy use but also often change the primary energy source being used (for example, from biomass to coal or natural gas).

Health impact assessment is a structured approach to estimating the impact of a program or policy—both positive and negative—on the health of specific population. Its purpose is to provide decision makers with reliable information on the effects in order to improve their decision making (Banken, 1999; European Centre for Health Policy, 1999; Kemm, Parry, and Palmer, 2004). The methodology has been applied to a wide range of projects including roadways (Fehr, 1999), transit projects (Kjellstrom, van Kerkhoff, Bammer, and McMichael, 2003; Dora and Racioppi, 2003), waste site expansions (Fehr, 1999), urban renewal plans (Cave and Curtis, 2001), housing policy (Douglas and others, 2001; den Broeder, Penris, and Put, 2003), and water privatization plans (Fehr, Mekel, Lacombe, and Wolf, 2003), as well as to energy projects such as the Chad pipeline (Leonard, 2003) and the Ouagadougou Water Supply Project (Mercier, 2003). The approach has also been used to examine energy projects ranging from hydroelectric power to energy conservation to infrastructure investments.

Lerer and Scudder (1999) describe the potential impacts of the Lesotho Highlands Water Project, one of the world's largest dams, providing electricity for Lesotho and South Africa. A health impact assessment of the project includes all the potential positive and adverse effects on health. The potential negative impacts include increased HIV as a result of migration related to construction and increased sexual activity, increases in parasitic diseases due to changing habitat for vectors such as mosquitoes, occupational injuries during construction, and diminished food security among the displaced population. The potential benefits include reduced reliance on biomass fuels among the beneficiaries; increased food security, due to expanded irrigation; and reduced injuries and illnesses, an outcome related to improved flood control.

Conclusion

Energy is essential for everyday activities from heating and cooking in our homes to industrial and agricultural economic activities. Households, companies, and nations are constantly making decisions about energy use, including the amount and type to use to satisfy their basic needs. In addition to providing these energy services, the decisions can have a direct impact on public health issues ranging from indoor and outdoor air pollution to climate change and infectious diseases. In some cases, such as household use of traditional biomass fuels, the impacts are concentrated at a local level. In other cases, such as the construction of a hydroelectric dam or electricity generation from coal, the impacts are regional or global in scale. Energy decisions, whether made in developed or developing countries and whether made by households or governments, often link economic and health issues. Both rich and poor countries weigh the advantages of cleaner energy sources against the potential increases in costs. Similarly, households consider costs, health, and convenience in deciding what type of personal transportation to use or fuel to use for home cooking and heating.

Thought Questions

1. Identify three major sources of energy you use on a typical day. Where are they produced or processed? What are the hazards associated with them, and whom do those hazards affect?
2. What energy ladders do you face in your decisions regarding energy use? What are the health consequences of your decisions (for you or others)? How do the energy ladder decisions faced by others potentially affect you?
3. How can developing countries balance the demand for low-cost energy and the need to protect public health?
4. In many ways energy decisions are hidden public health decisions. Identify an energy policy issue currently in the news, describe its implications for public health and assess whether those impacts are being considered.

References

Banken, R. "From Concept to Practice: Including the Social Determinants of Health in Environmental Assessments." *Canadian Journal of Public Health,* 1999, 90 (suppl. 1), S27–S30.

Barnes, D. F., and Floor, W. M. "Rural Energy in Developing Countries: A Challenge for Economic Development." Annual Review of Energy and Environment, 1996, 21, 497–530.

Bruce, N., Neufeld, L., Boy, E., and West, C. "Indoor Biofuel Air Pollution and Respiratory Health: The Role of Confounding Factors Among Women in Highland Guatemala." *International Journal of Epidemiology,* 1998, *27,* 454–458.

Bruce, N., Perez-Padilla, R., and Albalak, R. "Indoor Air Pollution in Developing Countries: A Major Environmental and Public Health Challenge." *Bulletin of the World Health Organization,* 2000, *78*(9), 1078–1092.

Cave, B., and Curtis, S. "Developing a Practical Guide to Assess the Potential Health Impact of Urban Regeneration Schemes." *Promotion and Education,* 2001, *8*(1), 12–16.

Deffeyes, K. S. *Hubbert's Peak: The Impending World Oil Shortage.* Princeton, N.J.: Princeton University Press, 2001.

den Broeder, L., Penris, M., and Put, G. V. "Soft Data, Hard Effects: Strategies for Effective Policy on Health Impact Assessment—An Example from the Netherlands." *Bulletin of the World Health Organization,* 2003, *81*(6), 404–407.

Dora, C., and Racioppi, F. "Including Health in Transport Policy Agendas: The Role of Health Impact Assessment Analyses and Procedures in the European Experience." *Bulletin of the World Health Organization,* 2003, *81*(6), 399–403.

Douglas, M. J., and others. "Developing Principles for Health Impact Assessment." *Journal of Public Health Medicine,* 2001, *23*(2), 148–154.

Energy Information Administration. *Annual Energy Review 2002.* Washington D.C.: Energy Information Administration, 2003.

European Centre for Health Policy. *Gothenburg Consensus Paper: Health Impact Assessment: Main Concepts and Suggested Approach.* [http://www.who.dk/document/PAE/Gothenburgpaper.pdf]. 1999.

European Commission. *External Costs: Research Results on Socio-Environmental Damages Due to Electricity and Transport.* Luxembourg: Office for Official Publications of the European Communities, 2003.

Ezzati, M., and Kammen, D. M. "Quantifying the Effects of Exposure to Indoor Air Pollution from Biomass Combustion on Acute Respiratory Infections in Developing Countries." *Environmental Health Perspectives,* 2001, *109,* 481–488.

Fehr, R. "Environmental Health Impact Assessment: Evaluation of a Ten-Step Model." *Epidemiology,* 1999, *10,* 618–625.

Fehr, R., Mekel, O., Lacombe, M., and Wolf, U. "Towards Health Impact Assessment of Drinking-Water Privatization:—The Example of Waterborne Carcinogens in North Rhine-Westphalia (Germany). *Bulletin of the World Health Organization,* 2003, *81*(6), 408–414.

Freese, B. *Coal: A Human History.* Cambridge, Mass.: Perseus Books, 2003.

Goodstein, D. *Out of Gas: The End of the Age of Oil.* New York: Norton, 2004.

Hosier, R. H., and Dowd, J. "Household Fuel Choice in Zimbabwe: An Empirical Test of the Energy Ladder Hypothesis." *Resources and Energy,* 1987, *9,* 347–361.

Institute of Medicine, Board on International Health, Committee to Reduce Lead Exposure in the Americas. *Lead in the Americas: A Call for Action.* Washington, D.C.: National Academies Press, 1996.

International Energy Agency. *World Energy Outlook.* Paris: International Energy Agency, 2002.

Kemm, J., Parry, J., and Palmer, S. *Health Impact Assessment: Concepts, Theory, Techniques, and Applications.* New York: Oxford University Press, 2004.

Kjellstrom, T., van Kerkhoff, L., Bammer, G., and McMichael, T. "Comparative Assessment of Transport Risks: How It Can Contribute to Health Impact Assessment of Transport Policies." *Bulletin of the World Health Organization,* 2003, *81*(6), 451–457.

Klare, M. *Resource Wars: The New Landscape of Global Conflict.* New York: Henry Holt, 2001.

Klare, M. *Blood and Oil: The Dangers and Consequences of America's Growing Dependency on Imported Petroleum.* New York: Henry Holt, 2004.

Leach, G. "The Energy Transition." *Energy Policy,* 1992, *20,* 116–123.

Leonard, L. "Possible Illnesses: Assessing the Health Impacts of the Chad Pipeline Project." *Bulletin of the World Health Organization,* 2003, *81,* 427–433.

Lerer, L., and Scudder, T. "Health Impacts of Large Dams." *Environmental Impact Assessment Review,* 1999, *19,* 113–123.

Matthews, E., Payne, R., Rohweder, M., and Murray, S. *Pilot Analysis of Global Ecosystems: Forest Ecosystems.* Washington D.C.: World Resources Institute, 2000.

Mercier, J.-R. "Health Impact Assessment in International Development Assistance: The World Bank Experience." *Bulletin of the World Health Organization,* 2003, *81,* 461–462.

N'Goran, E. K., Diabate, S., Utzinger, J., and Sellin, B. "Changes in Human Schistosomiasis Levels After the Construction of Two Large Hydroelectric Dams in Central Côte d'Ivoire. *Bulletin of the World Health Organization,* 1997, *75*(6), 541–545.

Reddy, A.K.N. "Rural Energy Consumption Patterns: A Field Study." *Biomass,* 1982, *2,* 255–280.

Rosenberg, D. M., and others. "Large-Scale Impacts of Hydroelectric Development." *Environmental Reviews,* 1997, *5*(1), 27–54.

Saatkamp, B. D., Masera, O. R., and Kammen, D. M. "Energy and Health Transitions in Development: Fuel Use, Stove Technology, and Morbidity in Jarácuaro, México." *Energy for Sustainable Development,* 2000, *4,* 7–16.

Smith, K. R., and others. "Air Pollution and the Energy Ladder in Asian Cities." *Energy,* 1994, *19,* 587–600.

Smith, K. R., and others. *Greenhouse Gases from Small-Scale Combustion Devices in Developing Countries, Phase IIA: Household Stoves in India.* Research Triangle Park, N.C.: U.S. Environmental Protection Agency, 2000.

Szabo, M. P., Labruna, M. B., Pereira, M. C., and Duarte, J. M. "Ticks (Acari: Ixodidae) on Wild Marsh-Deer (*Blastocerus dichotomus*) from Southeast Brazil: Infestations Before and After Habitat Loss." *Journal of Medical Entomology,* 2003, *40*(3), 268–274.

United Nations Scientific Committee on the Effects of Atomic Radiation. *2000 Report to the General Assembly.* [http://www.unscear.org/reports/2000_2.html]. 2000.

U.S. Environmental Protection Agency. *Mercury Study Report to Congress, Vol. II: An Inventory of Anthropogenic Mercury Emissions in the United States.* EPA-452/R-97-004, Washington, D.C.: U.S. Environmental Protection Agency, 1997.

World Health Organization. *Indoor Air Pollution from Biomass Fuel.* WHO/PEP/92-3-A. Geneva: World Health Organization, 1992.

World Resources Institute. *EarthTrends: The Environmental Information Portal.* [http://earthtrends.wri.org]. 2004.

For Further Information

London Health Commission. *Energy and Health: Making the Link.* London: London Health Commission, 2003.

United Nations Development Programme, "Energy for Sustainable Development" [http://www.undp.org/energy].

United Nations Development Programme, "World Energy Assessment" [http://www.undp.org/seed/eap/activities/wea].

National Renewable Energy Laboratory [http://www.nrel.gov].

International Energy Initiative [http://www.ieiglobal.org].

World Resources Institute [http://www.wri.org].

International Energy Agency [http://www.iea.org].

World Energy Council [http://www.worldenergy.org].

United Nations Development Programme. *World Resources 2002–2004: Decisions for the Earth: Balance, Voice, and Power.* Washington, D.C.: World Resources Institute, 2003.

United Nations Development Programme. *World Energy Assessment Overview: 2004 Update.* New York: United Nations Development Programme, 2004.

CHAPTER SIXTEEN

URBANIZATION

Sandro Galea
David Vlahov

The world is an increasingly urban place. At the beginning of the nineteenth century only 5 percent of the world's population lived in urban areas. By the end of the twentieth century that proportion had risen to about 46 percent. Current projections suggest that more than half the world's population will be living in urban areas by 2007 and that nearly two-thirds of the world's population will live in cities by 2030. Overall global population growth in coming decades will be primarily in cities.

The pace of increase in urban areas is projected to differ by region of the world and by initial city size. In particular, most global population growth will occur in the less wealthy regions of the world, with the most rapid growth expected in Asia and Africa. Even though North America and Europe are currently the most urbanized regions, the number of urban dwellers in the least urbanized region, Asia, was in 2000 already greater than the urban populations in North America and Europe combined.

Some of the most dramatic examples of this growth have been in megacities (cities with populations greater than 10 million, such as New York and Los Angeles; Mexico City, São Paulo, and Buenos Aires; Calcutta, Delhi, Mumbai, Dhaka, and Karachi; Jakarta and Manila; Lagos, London, Paris, and Tokyo). The proportion of people living in megacities is expected to rise from 4.3 percent of the global population in 2000 to 5.2 percent in 2015, with considerably faster growth in the developing world. For example, Calcutta's population is projected

FIGURE 16.1. GLOBAL URBAN POPULATION GROWTH IN WEALTHY VERSUS LESS WEALTHY COUNTRIES.

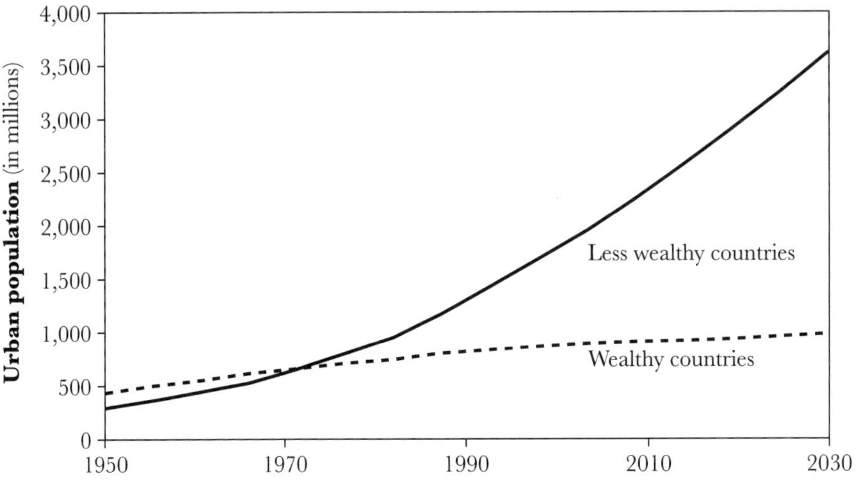

Source: United Nations Department of Economic and Social Affairs, Population Division. 2002.

to grow by 1.9 percent per year between 2000 and 2015, compared to 0.4 percent for New York City.

Although megacities attract much attention, most of the world's population growth will occur in smaller cities. Large cities in developing countries will account for approximately a fifth of the world's population growth, but small cities will account for almost half the growth. Therefore a growing number of relatively small cities throughout the world will contain most of the world's population in the twenty-first century. Figure 16.1 shows trends in the global urban population, comparing urban populations in the wealthy and less wealthy countries of the world. Figure 16.2 focuses on the less wealthy countries, showing their changing urban and rural populations. The references at the end of this chapter provide sources of further information on global urbanization demographic trends.

Urbanization is probably the most important contemporary global demographic trend. It also represents a shift in the human environment—a profound alteration of thousands of years of human ecology. It is therefore important to consider the implications of urbanization for population health. This chapter offers a primer on urbanization and its role in shaping population health. We first discuss some methodological issues, primarily problems with defining and measuring cities and urbanization itself. Next we discuss why urbanization matters for human health on the global level, focusing on four mechanisms: population factors,

FIGURE 16.2. URBAN VERSUS RURAL POPULATIONS IN LESS WEALTHY COUNTRIES.

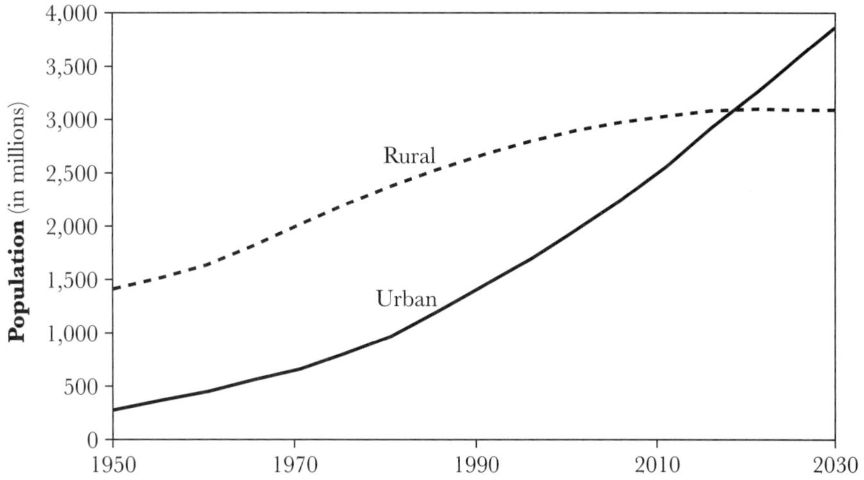

Source: United Nations Department of Economic and Social Affairs, Population Division. 2002.

service provision, the social environment, and the physical environment. We then offer a historical overview of thinking about cities and health and discuss ways to consider the evidence linking urbanization, city living, and health. We conclude with comments about building healthy cities and about the ways in which urban planning and environmental design may contribute to improved population health.

What Is a City?

It is likely that each of us has a different working definition of *city*, derived from our background and experience, and that each of us carries a different image of city. We are in good company. Novelist and Nobel laureate Saul Bellow (1970) suggested that asking how Americans view New York City "is perhaps like asking how Scotsmen feel about the Loch Ness monster. It is our legendary phenomenon, our great thing, our world-famous impossibility. New York is stirring, insupportable, agitated, ungovernable, demonic. No single individual can judge it adequately." Indeed, cities can defy definition and challenge the imagination. Cities are elegant, sophisticated places—think of Fifth Avenue, the Champs Elysée, Copacabana. Cities are also dense, teeming, and dangerous places—think of the squatter colonies of Rio de Janeiro and Lagos and the abandoned streets of the South

Bronx. Cities can be distinctive (there is only one Paris) or can look monotonous and interchangeable (think of most North American midsize cities). Cities can be small, compact areas that are easily navigated on foot, and they can be vast, sprawling, automobile-dependent metropolises that are pedestrian hostile. In short, cities, and by extension urban experiences, represent profoundly diverse human habitats, a fact that highlights some of the challenges inherent in considering how cities may affect health.

It therefore comes as no surprise that there are multiple and inconsistent definitions of both *urban* and *urbanization* (Goldstein, 1994). An appreciation of this complexity is essential in seeking an understanding of how cities and urbanization may affect human health.

No definition of urban places has been universally adopted by national governments, and the working definition of *urban* varies widely among countries. Among the 228 countries on which the United Nations has data, about half use administrative definitions of *urban* (for example, living in the capital city), 51 use size and density, 39 use functional characteristics (for example, economic activity), 22 have no definition of *urban,* and 8 define all (for example, Singapore) or none (for example, Polynesian countries) of their population as *urban.* Official statistics of bodies such as governmental agencies and the United Nations rely on country-specific designations and do not use a uniform definition of *urban.* In some instances, definitions of *urban* in adjacent countries vary tremendously. For example, *urban* places in Bolivia include localities with 2,000 or more inhabitants. In neighboring Peru, populated centers with 100 or more dwellings grouped contiguously and administrative centers of districts are designated *urban.* Global statistics on urbanization therefore embody international definitional differences, the results of statistical or historical precedent, and in some cases, political expedience.

Compounding these difficulties, definitions of *urban* have changed over time, and in different ways in different countries (Box 16.1 discusses the U.S. Census Bureau definition), and these differences are frequently embedded in calculations about changing urban proportions. For example, Box 16.2 highlights some of the changing definitions of *urban* in China over the past century.

Box 16.1. The Census Bureau Definition of *Urban*

The U.S. Bureau of the Census (2002) defines an urbanized area as "a place and the adjacent densely settled surrounding territory that together comprise a minimum population of 50,000 people. . . . The 'densely settled surrounding territory' adjacent to the place consists of territory made up of one or more contiguous blocks having a population density of at least 1,000 people per square mile." But this definition raises a further question; places outside the specific size and density parameters are designated nonurban. But is the issue that simple? Although it is tempting to classify urban versus nonurban dichotomously, a more nuanced appreciation of gradations of urbanicity may also be helpful. There are relatively few cities like Las Vegas, isolated from other urban areas by vast underpopulated spaces. Most cities (think, for example, of New York City) are part of a far-reaching, densely populated area that continues uninterrupted for miles beyond the city center, transitioning gradually into *suburban* and *exurban* areas. Thus a dichotomous definition of *urban* fails to recognize the periurban areas that may share some characteristics of cities and may have "typically urban" health conditions.

The Census definition also raises questions about absolute size and density parameters. Although defining a *threshold* population size facilitates demographic analyses, it is conceivable that areas with fewer than 50,000 people, particularly in sparsely populated areas, may also share many characteristics of cities. For example, fewer than 30,000 people live in Whitehorse, the capital of Canada's Yukon Territory. However, Whitehorse has the greatest density of people for hundreds of miles and as such functions like a city for the surrounding area, sharing with cities issues of population density and heterogeneity.

Box 16.2. Changing Definitions of *Urban* in China

China's definitions of *urban* have changed substantially during the last two decades, reflecting changes in urbanization policy, political ideology, and stage of economic development. Currently, the urban population size depends on four factors: the criteria for designating a settlement as urban, the boundaries of designated places, the household registration system, and urban status among the unregistered population. The definition of *city* in China is relatively straightforward, because cities are established with the approval of the federal government. However, official urban statistics also include some people living in towns, the definitions for which have changed substantially over the years. In 1964 and 1984, revisions in urban classification effectively increased the number of Chinese cities and the size of the urban population. Prior to 1964, a *town* was an area with more than 2,000 permanent residents of whom 50 percent or more were nonagricultural. After the 1964 revision, a *town* was a place with more than 3,000 permanent residents of whom at least 70 percent were nonagricultural or a place with between 2,500 and 3,000 permanent residents of whom 85 percent or more were nonagricultural. After the 1984 revision, a *town* was the location of a county-level government agency; a place with fewer than 20,000 people of whom at least 2,000 were nonagricultural; a place with more than 20,000 people of whom at least 10 percent were nonagricultural; or a remote area, mountainous area, small-sized mining area, small harbor, tourism area, or border area with a nonagricultural population less than 2,000. Therefore, the size of the urban population in China, as it appears in official statistics, depends on how nonagricultural population is defined. Because this distinction is made by local residents and village committees, there is substantial uncertainty about the usefulness of some of these statistics.

Source: International Institute for Applied Systems Analysis, 1999.

Another change in urban form, especially in wealthy countries where automobile travel has become the norm, is the expansion of cities into periurban, or fringe, areas—the phenomenon known as suburban sprawl. Box 16.3 describes this process.

Box 16.3. Urban Sprawl

A prominent feature of urbanization in recent decades, especially in North America, has been *urban sprawl.* Changes in both *land use* and *transportation* have combined to produce this shift in the traditional form of cities, in which cities expand over large geographic distances and farmland and forest are converted to residential use (Figure 6.3). Land is used at a low density, in the range of one household per acre, instead of the traditional urban densities of five or ten households per acre. Land-use mix is

FIGURE 16.3. URBAN SPRAWL IN THE NEW YORK METROPOLITAN AREA.

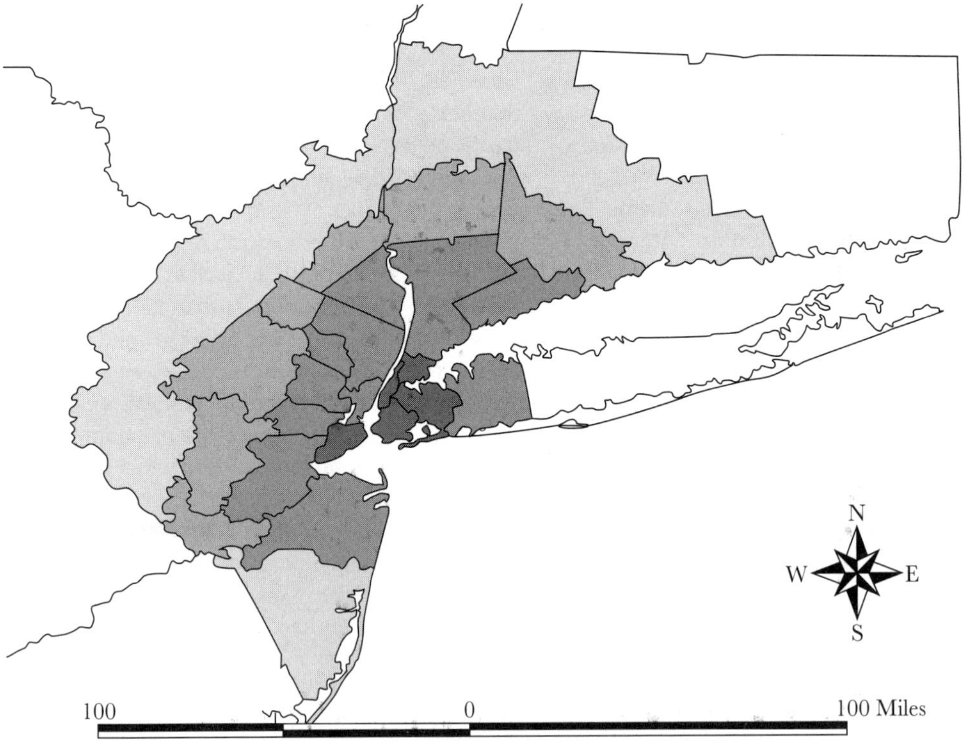

Note: New York City is home to about 8 million people, and the concentric areas, indicated by shaded bands, contain 7.6 million, 3.3 million, and 2.4 million, for a total metropolitan population of approximately 21 million.

also low; instead of residential, commercial, office, recreational, educational, and other uses being contiguous, each is separated from the other, a separation often enforced by zoning laws.

As a result of the low density and the separation of land uses, the distances between destinations—say, from home to school, home to work, or home to the store—are typically long, well beyond walking or bicycling distance. Moreover, mass transit is impractical in low-density development, where not enough people are clustered near trip origins and trip destinations to enable siting of transit stations. As a result the predominant form of travel is driving. Extensive road networks are built, running from the *loop and lollipop* networks of residential subdivisions (which replace the gridlike arrangements of traditional cities and towns) to secondary *feeder* roads to massive highway systems (Figure 16.4). Nevertheless, connectivity is often low; a trip from home to school of half a mile as the crow flies may take two miles on surface roads that meander their way out of residential subdivisions and onto feeder roads. By the early twenty-first century, about half the U.S. population—a majority of those in metropolitan areas—lived in the suburbs.

In recent years researchers have studied the possible effects of sprawl on health. One effect became apparent early in central cities, where poverty concentrated upon the migration of more affluent residents, jobs, and economic activity to the suburbs (Wilson, 1996; Jargowsky, 2002). This concentrated poverty has disastrous consequences for health (Adler, Marmot, McEwen, and Stewart, 1999). Other effects manifest in the suburbs. As people drive more, they walk less and are less physically active overall; these sedentary lifestyles contribute to overweight, cardiovascular disease, cancers, and other conditions (see Chapter Seventeen). The reliance on driving also adds to air pollution and increases the risk of motor vehicle crashes. The land-use patterns of sprawling metropolitan areas can threaten water supplies and contribute to the urban heat island effect. And the social aspects of sprawl may threaten mental health in various ways (think of road rage) and undermine social capital (Frumkin, Frank, and Jackson, 2004).

To study the effects of sprawl researchers need to measure it. The most common approach has been to use the Sprawl Index, developed by planner Reid Ewing and colleagues (Ewing, Pendall, and Chen, 2002). These researchers focused on both land use and transportation and identified four categories for measurement: the strength or vibrancy of activity centers and downtown areas (a measure of sense of place and consolidation of commercial and recreational activities); accessibility of the street network (reflecting connectivity); residential density; and land-use mix (the mix of homes, jobs, and services at the neighborhood level). The Sprawl Index combines twenty-two specific measures grouped under these four categories. It has shown the most sprawling U.S. metropolitan areas to be in the South and Southeast, with a few in California as well. The least sprawling areas are in the Northeast, in California (San Francisco), and in Hawaii (Honolulu).

Using the Sprawl Index, researchers have studied the effects of sprawl on physical activity levels, injury levels, and markers of cardiovascular health such as blood pressure, among other outcomes (Ewing, Schieber, and Zegeer, 2003; Ewing and others,

FIGURE 16.4. URBAN SPRAWL: IN THE TOP PHOTO DENVER SPREADS TO THE FOOT OF THE ROCKY MOUNTAINS; IN THE BOTTOM PHOTO A SUBURBAN RESIDENTIAL SUBDIVISION ADOPTS A TYPICAL LOOP AND LOLLIPOP PATTERN.

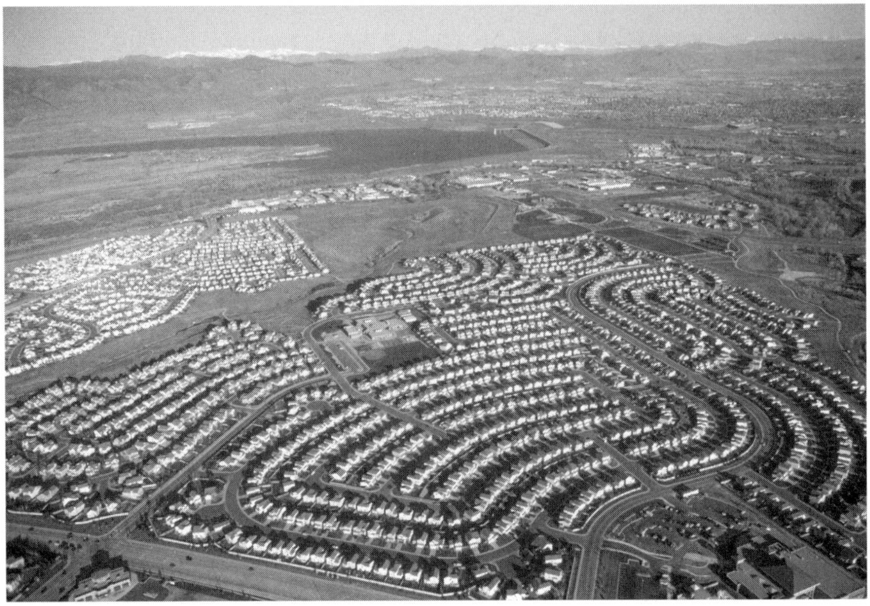

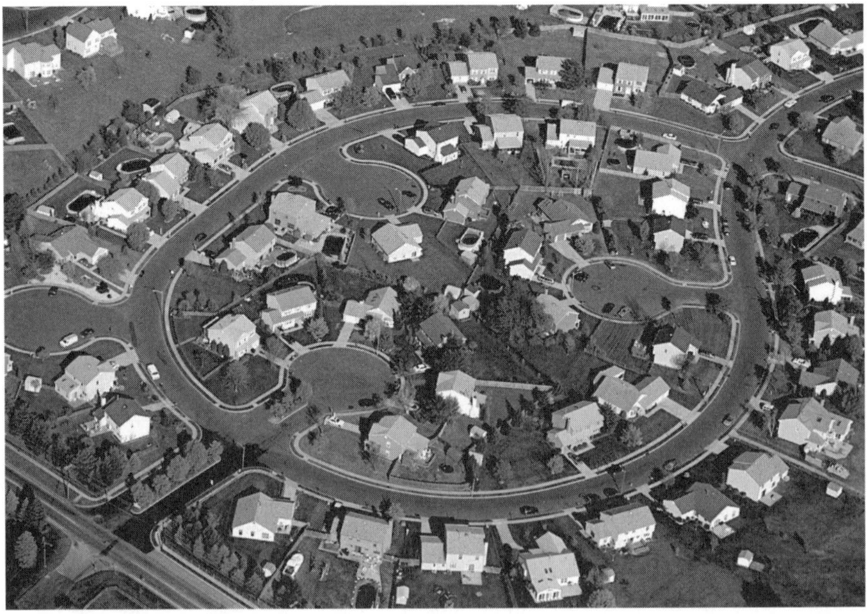

2003; Sturm and Cohen, 2004; Lopez, 2004; Vandegrift and Yoked, 2004; Kelly-Schwartz, Stockard, Doyle, and Schlossberg, 2004). Although the results are not entirely consistent, they generally support the hypotheses that sprawl is associated with less physical activity, more injuries, more weight gain, and perhaps higher blood pressure, after controlling for other important variables.

But cities are not static. They form and change over time, in a process called *urbanization,* and this process of change may also affect health. Most authorities identify urbanization with population growth, through natural population increase or migration, or both. However, population growth in cities is a complex idea. Metrics of urbanization may include the absolute annual increase in urban population size, the rate of urban population growth, the level of urbanization, and the rate of urbanization. Other elements of urbanization include changing urban age and gender structures, among others. Box 16.4 discusses the implications of these different measures of urbanization.

Box 16.4. Measuring Urbanization: An International Example

Tanzania and Bhutan were two of the most rapidly urbanizing countries during the 1990s. However, the population of Tanzania is four times larger than that of Bhutan (Tanzania had 25.5 million people in 1990 and 33.7 million in 2000; Bhutan had 6 million people in 1990 and 8 million in 2000), and the percentage of the Tanzanian population that was living in urban areas (21.7 percent in 1990 and 32.3 percent in 2000) was also four times larger than Bhutan's (5.2 percent in 1990 and 7.1 percent in 1990 in 2000). Therefore, by the end of 2000, although the two countries had had comparable percentage increases in population size, the urban population growth was approximately six times larger in Tanzania than it was in Bhutan (64.9 percent and 13 percent, respectively). In addition to these considerations, mathematical representations of urbanization are, of course, fundamentally simplifications of overall urban population dynamics.

Why Cities Matter

Why concern ourselves with cities in a textbook on environmental health? If cities are the predominant human environment of the twenty-first century, then it is difficult to consider any aspect of environmental health without thinking of the role of cities. Urban issues are embedded in many academic disciplines, although sometimes so deeply that they are barely acknowledged. For example, epidemiological research into the health of homeless populations rarely dwells on urban conditions as a determinant of either homelessness or of the health of the homeless, but urbanism and urbanization are undoubtedly primary determinants both of homelessness and of the conditions of homeless persons in different cities. Research that treats urban conditions simply as background and fails to consider them as determinants of health can shed little light on *how* cities may affect health. In order to understand better the relationships among features of the urban environment and health we must identify the features of cities that may have implications for health. The diversity of cities worldwide means, naturally, that there is no single form of *urban living* but rather a range of conditions with some shared features. By considering these shared features we can understand the role that urbanization may play in shaping population health.

Population Factors

Fundamentally, cities are places where large numbers of people live in close proximity. For these city dwellers, urban contexts shape the resources available to them, their interpersonal contacts, and their lifestyle choices. Accordingly, population factors are among the principal factors that shape urban population health. City dwellers routinely come into close contact with people of disparate socioeconomic status and with racially and ethnically diverse groups. Several considerations arise from this observation. First, although interacting with socioeconomically and ethnically diverse groups may be enlightening, it may also introduce significant stress. Stress, in turn, can shape health in general and mental health in particular (see, for example, Pearlin, Lieberman, Menaghan, and Mullan, 1981; Scheck, Kinicki, and Davy, 1995). Although much research in this area has considered individual-level stressors, contextual factors are increasingly recognized as sources of stressors and as mediators of the impact of stressors on individual health (Elliott, 2000). An important additional factor is that persons of different socioeconomic status may confront stressors such as violence or pollution differently and have unequal access to resources for coping with stressors. Second, the close proximity of large numbers of people introduces the risk of contagion, both of infectious diseases but also of ideas and behaviors. Although contagion is well recognized with respect to communicable disease, contagion of ideas, behaviors, and social examples is a relatively new concept. In epidemiology it is understood that all things being equal, the risk of disease transmission is higher among people in close proximity than in dispersed groups. Social learning theory suggests that the same may hold for ideas and behavior; such phenomena as unhealthy behaviors or panic in the context of a disaster may be more likely to spread in dense urban areas. Because of these factors urban populations may start from a disadvantaged position compared to nonurban populations.

Services and Resources

The role of urban areas in shaping health is tied to the availability of services and resources for urban populations. In the wealthier countries, cities offer a rich array of health and social services and even the poorest urban neighborhood often has dozens of social service agencies, each with a distinct mission and portfolio. Even in less wealthy countries, cities are more likely than are nonurban areas to offer social and health services. These services may complement and enhance positive health behaviors or provide health care to the ill. However, services are frequently available only in limited ways to low-income urban residents. In the United States, for example, low-income people and people of color, who are overrepresented in urban areas, are those most likely to lack health insurance coverage (Williams and Rucker, 2000). Uninsured people face barriers to care, receive poorer quality care, and are more likely to rely on emergency systems (Merzel, 2000). Recent immigrants, homeless people, and inmates released from jail or prison, all of whom are also disproportionately represented in urban areas, also face specific obstacles in obtaining health care. These groups then put a burden on health systems not adequately funded or prepared to care for them. Many cities display a substantial disparity in the quality of care provided to persons living in wealthier neighborhoods and to persons in less wealthy neighborhoods (Andrulis, 2000). The well-equipped, lucrative medical practice opportunities in a city draw service providers from the lower-paid public service clinics, particularly when these latter facilities face limited resources and wavering political commitment.

Social Environments

The population density in cities and the unique living conditions that frequently arise are important shapers of cities' social environments that may also have substantial implications for health. The social environment is described by the structure and characteristics of relationships among people in a community. Components of the social environment include social networks, social capital, segregation, and the social support that interpersonal interactions provide. (Comprehensive definitions of many of these factors are given elsewhere; see, for example, Berkman and Kawachi, 2000.) Social environments can both support and damage health through a variety of pathways. For example, social norms in densely populated urban areas can support health-related behaviors involving smoking, diet, exercise, and sexual behavior (King and others, 2003). Social supports can buffer the impact of daily stressors and provide access to goods and services that promote health (for example, housing, food, informal health care) (Berkman, Glass, Brissette, and Seeman, 2000). Social segregation, commonly along racial or ethnic and socioeconomic lines, has been shown to be associated with poorer health in cities. Numerous theories explain the reciprocal relationship between the urban social environment and health. For example, social learning theory suggests that people look to their social networks, peer groups, and role models to help them set behavior and make personal choices (see, for example, Montgomery and Casterline, 1993). This has substantial implications in the urban context, where social networks can be dense and either beneficial or detrimental to health. Also, residents of cities share in multiple *common goods,* ranging from physical assets such as parks to social assets such as collective efficacy and social capital. *Social capital* refers to resources that support collective action, enforce norms, and generate reciprocity. It provides a structure for individual social networks and assumes substantial importance in densely populated urban areas, where the behavior of others may affect the norms of daily life far more than in sparsely populated areas. Empirical studies (for example, Kawachi, Kennedy, Lochner, and Prothrow-Stith, 1997) have shown that social capital is associated with health; in the dense social environments of cities this may be especially salient.

Social comparison theory, which describes how people routinely measure themselves against others (Festinger, 1954), is also relevant to urban life. This comparison might lead people to strive to emulate others, to abandon the "competition" altogether, or to other responses. In cities, comparison with other reference groups is relatively easy. Jencks and Mayer (1990) have suggested that in the urban context, adolescents who perform social comparisons and recognize limited opportunities may respond by forming gangs that perpetuate violence.

Physical Environments

Cities also are characterized by distinct physical environmental features that may affect health (Box 16.5). These features resonate with the traditional concerns of environmental health.

Box 16.5. Features of the Urban Physical Environment and Their Health Implications

Features of the Physical Environment	Potential Health and Social Problems
Inadequate water and sanitation	Infectious diseases (for example, malaria, dengue, tuberculosis)
Crowding	Infectious diseases, stress, mental health problems, intentional and unintentional injuries
Inadequate land to grow food	Costly and/or scarce fresh foods
Inadequate garbage disposal	Infectious disease, demoralization
Noise pollution	Hearing problems, stress
Air pollution	Respiratory and cardiovascular disease, early mortality
Traffic	Injuries
Inadequate housing	Homelessness

Urban areas typically feature a heavily built environment, reliance on human-made systems for water and food provision, and reliance on housing that, not infrequently in less wealthy countries, is substandard. McNeill (2000) has argued that the primary feature distinguishing the twentieth century from previous centuries and cities from nonurban areas is the degree to which humans have become the primary influence on the physical environment. As cities grow, the features of the physical environment that can affect health also grow. Highways and streets can pollute water through runoff, destroy green space, influence motor vehicle use and injury rates, and contribute to the urban heat island effect (see Chapter Eleven). The urban infrastructure is also part of the physical environment and determines how a city provides water, disposes of garbage, and provides energy. As this expensive infrastructure ages in a period of declining municipal resources, breakdowns may increase, causing health problems related to water, sewage, or disposal of solid waste. Depending on their construction, city structures such as bridges and skyscrapers may be vulnerable to natural or human-made disasters, as the September 11, 2001, terrorist attacks on New York City demonstrated. Other threats to health include hazardous waste landfills, often located in or near urban areas, which may be associated with risks of low birthweight, birth defects, and cancers. Noise exposure, a common urban problem, may contribute to hearing impairment, hypertension, and ischemic heart disease. Ultimately, urban design may also influence crime and violence rates, demonstrating the close interactions among urban physical and social environments (Sampson, Raudenbush, and Earls, 1997).

This potential of the urban physical environment to shape health may differ fundamentally from city to city. In a city in a less wealthy country the key features of the physical environment relevant to health are likely to be water and sanitation. In the most recent global burden of disease assessment, unsafe water and poor sanitation and hygiene were shown to account for almost 6 percent of the burden of disease in high-mortality developing regions (primarily via infectious diseases), exceeding all but two other risk factors (Ezzati and others, 2002). In light of this finding, developing effective water and sanitation systems in cities in less wealthy countries is the clear public health priority that if implemented effectively could save millions of lives annually. However, developing effective water and sanitation systems takes time and resources. In addition, motor vehicle mortality is generally much higher in low-income than in high-income regions, usually as a direct reflection of rapidly growing vehicular transportation, poor road conditions, and lax driving standards (Nantulya and Reich, 2003; see also Chapters Thirteen and Twenty-Five). Investment in road infrastructure is then critical in low-income urban areas, but it is an investment that frequently does not take place in cities already under substantial financial strain.

In cities in wealthy countries the urban physical environment may affect health via air quality, noise pollution, or inadequate housing. In many densely populated, relatively small cities, issues of inadequate housing are paramount. Inadequate housing may be associated with exposure to lead paint, molds, or hazardous structural defects. Housing shortages are frequently associated with homelessness, which implies a range of health problems, including substantial early mortality. In contrast, in cities (or parts of cities) characterized by suburban sprawl, such features of the physical environment as inadequate public transportation, absent opportunities for physical activity, and scarce common green space may be important health risks. Inadequate public transportation can significantly limit the mobility and health behaviors of the elderly, absent sidewalks and a lack of nearby destinations can preclude walking, and limited park space can contribute to an erosion of social capital, all with adverse effects on health (see Box 16.3). Understanding the impact of the physical environment requires an understanding of each city's particular circumstances. (Figures 16.5 and 16.6 display diverse urban scenes.)

FIGURE 16.5. CARACAS: A GLITTERING MODERN BUSINESS DISTRICT IN THE BACKGROUND AND SUBSTANDARD HOUSING IN THE FOREGROUND REFLECT RAPID RURAL-URBAN MIGRATION THAT STRAINS URBAN SERVICES.

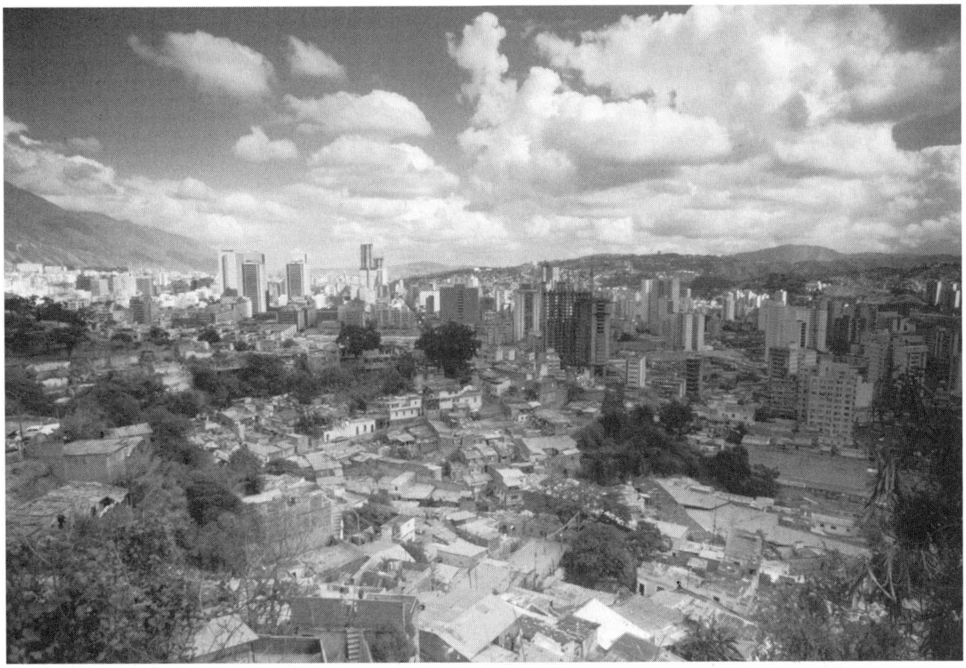

The effect of cities on health is not all negative; cities also represent tremendous opportunities to enhance health. For example, the urban physical environment offers economies of scale in implementing effective safe water and sanitation systems, improving transportation, reducing the risks from disasters, and siting medical services. Satterthwaite (2000) has argued that the fundamental problem in many world cities is not the rapid pace of urbanization but the failure of urban government to take creative advantage of opportunities to improve public health. In addition, as discussed earlier, cities can afford to develop a wealth of social resources (for example, schools) that far surpass what is possible in smaller communities.

FIGURE 16.6. MANILA: SUBSTANDARD HOUSING NEAR CONTAMINATED WATER IS EVIDENT BUT SO ARE SIGNS OF ELECTRICITY AND TELEVISIONS IN HOMES.

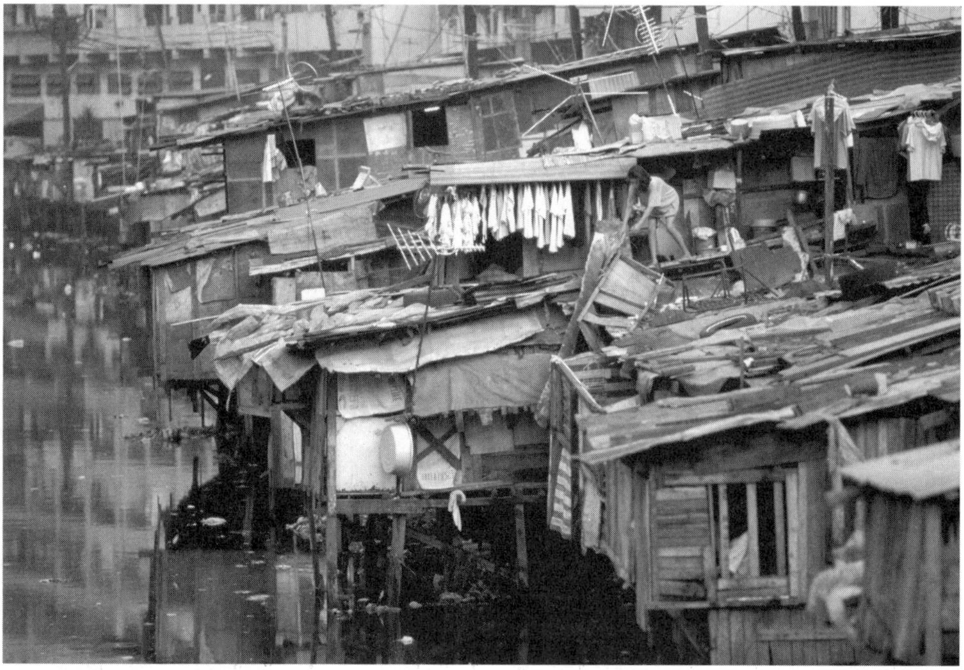

Physical Environment and Health: Are Cities Good (or Bad) for Our Health?

Now that we have established that cities *may* be important determinants of health, what does the evidence show? Interest in urban health is not new; it has been a focus of research and discussion for centuries. Writers from several eras in Western European and North American history considered cities unwholesome and unhealthy, and in many ways they were correct. Early urbanization in Europe featured extremely high population densities and concentrations of marginalized populations, pollution, and crime, and rural populations enjoyed better health than urban populations. Observations during the seventeenth, eighteenth, and nineteenth centuries fed a growing recognition of the role of physical and social environments in shaping health and well-being. Chief among these, Jean-Jacques Rousseau's work was influential in introducing to Western thought an appreciation of the role of place and institutions in shaping well-being. Subsequent writers and social theorists specifically postulated that urban living was detrimental to health. Notably, Émile Durkheim provided seminal insights about the role of norms and societal disintegration, and several theorists adapted many of these concepts in considering how the etiology and distribution of pathology unfold in cities.

Poets and novelists provide some of the most eloquent historical testaments to the impact of nineteenth-century cities on health. The English romantic poet Percy Bysshe Shelley observed in 1819 that

> Hell is a city much like London—
> A populous and a smoky city;
> There are all sorts of people undone,
> And there is little or no fun done;
> Small justice shown, and still less pity.

Charles Dickens's novels recount the tribulations of nineteenth-century city life. It is worth noting, however, that other literary figures, notably Walt Whitman, expressed equally adamant appreciation of cities, with Whitman considering visits to Manhattan in particular to be "the best and most effective medicine" for his soul. Indeed, the urban environment in many Western cities improved dramatically at the turn of the twentieth century, and coincident with this improvement the health of urban populations also improved. For example, one analysis at the time showed that although for much of the nineteenth century infant mortality rates were higher in urban areas in Imperial Germany than they were in nonurban areas, a dramatic reduction in urban infant mortality started in the 1870s, in advance of a comparable decline in the rest of the country (Vogele, 1994). This analysis suggested that urban environmental improvements led to the rapid improvement in infant health in Imperial Germany and that a similar pattern was typical of many European industrialized societies.

Modern research methods have allowed more careful empirical study of the effects of city living on health. These studies have differed, with some showing health benefits and others suggesting the opposite. For example, studies have shown both a higher prevalence and lower prevalence of mental health problems in cities compared to nonurban areas (Dohrenwend and Dohrenwend, 1974; Kessler and others, 1994; Paykel and others, 2000). Such comparisons, however, suffer from the oversimplification of what likely is a complicated relationship. Cities may affect health, but the net relationship between cities and health is likely to reflect the range of factors—population factors and features of the social and physical environment—discussed earlier. Living in a particular city may entail exposures and experiences that threaten health—say, violence and air pollution—but may also offer important health benefits such as better social supports and social services. Clearly, then, asking how a "city" affects overall "health" is a simple approach to a larger, more complicated question.

In order to analyze how cities affect health, we propose three key questions:

1. Are specific features of urban living causally related to health?
2. Are these features differentially distributed between urban and nonurban areas and within urban areas (for example, between urban neighborhoods)?
3. To what extent are these features unique to a particular city or different among cities?

Two health issues, injuries and infectious diseases, illustrate the application of these questions to urban health.

Injuries

Injuries are a major worldwide cause of lost years of healthy life; also see Chapters Thirteen and Twenty-Five). Globally, intentional injuries (including suicide, homicide, and war) account for the same number of lost DALYs as does tuberculosis, whereas unintentional injuries result in more lost DALYs than do cardiovascular disease or cancer. In developing countries, in 1990, injuries accounted for over one-third of all DALYs lost among men aged fifteen to forty-four (Murray and Lopez, 1996).

Many features of urban environments may affect injury morbidity and mortality. With respect to intentional injury, violence is one of the major causes, and in most parts of the world violence is more prevalent in large cities than in nonurban areas. In cities, violence is concentrated among young men in low-income neighborhoods. In São Paulo, for example, among men aged fifteen to twenty-four, those in low-income areas are over five times more likely than those in high-income areas to be homicide victims (Grant and others, 1999). In New York City, homicide rates for young men have for several decades been higher in neighborhoods with low socioeconomic status (Karpati and others, 2003). Social theorists have proposed explanations for the higher prevalence of violence in urban areas. Social disorganization theory has suggested that signs of physical disorder in cities ("broken windows") encourage acts of violence and unsafe sex (Cohen and others, 2000, 2003). Although empirical research in the area is scarce, new work has shown that collective efficacy, or residents' capacity and inclination to act to limit deviant behavior, protects against neighborhood violence (Sampson, Raudenbush, and Earls, 1997). This suggests that neighborhood-level social factors may account for some of the observed differences in homicide rates among different cities and between cities and nonurban areas.

To understand the possible association between urban living and intentional violence, then, we must consider many aspects of the city. Population factors, including population density and racial or ethnic segregation, may affect the likelihood of intergroup tensions and related violence. The social environment, including collective efficacy, and the physical environment, including building and street design, the presence or absence of settings for safe recreation, and the availability of social services including medical treatment for victims of violence, may all be important. The relative balance of these factors likely differs from city to city, and public health professionals must identify the aspects of urban living that influence intentional injury risk in each setting.

With respect to unintentional injury, urban residents may be at higher risk than rural residents, although the evidence in this regard is conflicting (Odero, Garner, and Zwi, 1997). The factors that operate here may differ from those important to intentional injuries. Worldwide, the vast majority of unintentional injuries and about half of all trauma-related hospital admissions result from motor vehicle crashes. Many factors play a role in these injuries, including the presence and quality of roads, the enforcement of driving regulations, and the use of alcohol when driving, all of which may differ from city to city and between urban and nonurban areas. In addition, the morbidity from unintentional injury may well differ by gender and racial or ethnic group, depending on the social norms that influence driving in each region.

Another example of unintentional injury is fatal drug overdose. Evidence from New York City suggests that characteristics of urban neighborhoods are associated with the risk of overdose in cities (Galea and others, 2003). Once again, multiple features of the urban environment may be associated with risk. These may include population factors such as the spread of drug use through social networks, which may make available the means to injure oneself; social norms affecting drug use; and physical environments such as boarded up buildings and empty lots that present opportunities for illicit drug use.

The urban conditions that affect injury risk are not static. The process of becoming urban may in and of itself be an important determinant of injury. For example, rapid urbanization may bring a dramatic increase in road traffic as workers travel back and forth from suburbs to city centers. If the existing road network cannot accommodate the traffic volume, it is the rapid urban growth (and the resulting demands on infrastructure) that is itself a key factor in urban motor vehicle crashes. Therefore, both the features of the city at various points in time and the characteristics of urbanization can determine population health.

Infectious Disease Transmission

Each category of potential urban health determinant may affect the transmission of infectious disease. First, population density is unequivocally associated with the likelihood of infectious disease; higher density increases the risk of disease transmission, whether by sexual contact, fecal-oral spread, or respiratory spread. Therefore, dense cities may well be expected to have higher transmission rates of infectious disease. Second, available health and social resources may play a tangible role in the control of infectious disease morbidity and mortality. For example, widely available antiretroviral therapy has resulted in a dramatic decline in HIV-related mortality in North America. Less dramatically, widely available confidential testing and treatment for sexually transmitted disease has the potential to reduce complications and transmission. Third, many aspects of the urban social environment facilitate, or hinder, the transmission of infectious disease. Social learning theory, discussed earlier, provides a framework for considering how individuals' social networks influence their health risk behaviors. For example, the density of one's social networks and the norms in those networks are associated with risky sexual behavior and with use of injected drugs, both of which increase the risk of infectious disease transmission (Latkin, Hua, and Forman, 2003). Finally, several features of the physical environment, such as the degree of disrepair, may affect transmission of infectious disease (Cohen and others, 2000). Neighborhoods with markedly deprived built environments may facilitate or even encourage deviant or high-risk behavior. Conversely, water and sanitation infrastructures are clearly components of a city's built environment that reduce morbidity and mortality, particularly in children in less wealthy countries (Cutler and Miller, 2005). Other, perhaps less obvious features of the urban built environment that may affect infectious disease transmission include building ventilation systems, which may harbor infectious diseases such as Legionnaires' disease.

Again, urbanization—the process of change—may play an important role. Population density may increase precipitously during rapid urbanization, straining the public health infrastructure. The influx of mobile populations may be accompanied by new infectious agents, rapidly changing social network structures, and degradation of the built environment, all of which may elevate infectious disease transmission above baseline. However, as with injuries, urbanization also presents opportunities to reduce infectious disease. For example, in low-income regions of the world, urbanization is frequently associated with improved education and potentially with greater health awareness and less health risk behavior.

In summary, in considering the relation between city living and health outcomes such as injury and infectious disease, we need to identify the network of urban features that may play a role, including population factors, service delivery, the social environment, and the built environment, understand their interrelationships, and consider the extent to which interventions that address these factors may improve population health.

Building Healthy Cities in an Urban Future

The scale of current urbanization suggests that the world of the twenty-first century will emerge as substantially different from the world we know today. By 2025, more than 5.5 billion people, out of a world population of 8.5 billion, will live in urban places; this can be compared to a total world population of about 6 billion at the dawn of this century. Some 4.4 billion people will be living in towns and cities in developing countries, including some 1 billion in China's and 750 million in India's urban areas. In most of the Americas, more than 80 percent of the population will live in urban areas, whereas in Africa and Asia, levels of urbanism will vary considerably among countries. Although there will probably be more than fifty megacities by 2025, most of the world's urban population will live in smaller cities, with a growing number of small (having fewer than a million people) urban centers, particularly in Africa and Asia. As the world becomes more urban the challenge will be to ensure sustainability of population health in cities and perhaps even to take advantage of urbanization to improve health.

Cities are not static, and urban change is frequently associated with changes in urban health. The challenge is to understand the features of cities that affect health, and to improve upon cities to protect the health of their residents.

Undoubtedly, the greatest potential for impact lies in cities in less wealthy countries. In many African and Asian cities, given current resource scarcity and projected urban growth, substantial social, ecological, or economic problems may be inevitable (Haughton and Hunter, 1994; Johnson, 1993). Service provision, including the provision of drinking water, is a pressing issue in almost all less wealthy countries (Hardoy, Mitlin, and Satterthwaite, 1990). For example, in cities such as Bangkok, Dar es Salaam, and Kinshasa, fewer than half of all households have access to piped water, and most rely on water from private water connections and vendors. Garbage collection and sewage disposal are plagued by similar problems; most cities in Africa have no sewers at all, and the existing sewage systems serve only the rich in these cities. However, these problems do not necessarily suggest that the future urbanized world is headed for a catastrophe. There is a long history of doomsaying in the academic literature, most of it tied to population growth, and by and large social, economic, and technological innovations have averted the predicted disasters (Meadows, Meadows, Randers, and Behrens, 1972; Meadows, Meadows, and Randers, 1993). Most cities in both wealthy and less wealthy countries are cleaner today and the residents in general have a better quality of life and more amenities than was the case a quarter of a century ago (McMichael, 1993). This suggests that with appropriate intervention we can exploit trends in urbanization to effect vast improvements in the health of populations.

What are the best strategies for improving cities and protecting the health of urban populations? The standard public health approach—identifying risk factors based on data, intervening to interrupt the risk factors, evaluating the results, and correcting course as necessary—can be illustrated by two examples: Moving to Opportunity for Fair Housing, a project in the United States, and the World Health Organization's worldwide Healthy Cities program.

Moving to Opportunity for Fair Housing (MTO) is a ten-year research demonstration project in five U.S. cities (Baltimore, Boston, Chicago, Los Angeles, and New York City), sponsored by the U.S. Department of Housing and Urban Development (1999). Its goals are to develop more effective strategies to improve housing for recipients of housing assistance in urban areas and to assess whether changes in families' physical environments, specifically in their housing, will improve family members' health (among other outcomes). This program combines tenant-based rental assistance with housing counseling to help very low income families move from poverty-stricken urban areas to low-poverty neighborhoods. In each of the cities, low-income households are randomly selected to receive housing vouchers that must be used in areas with less than 10 percent poverty. These families receive assistance that helps pay their rent as well as housing counseling to help them find and successfully use housing in low-poverty areas. In order to evaluate the efficacy of moving families to housing in better neighborhoods, control families are also selected and monitored in the same cities. Early results from the MTO program have been encouraging. At the three-year follow-up of the New York site, parents who moved to low-poverty neighborhoods reported significantly less distress than parents who remained in high-poverty neighborhoods. Boys who moved to less poor neighborhoods reported significantly fewer anxiety or depression and dependency problems than did boys who stayed in public housing, suggesting that improving housing could have substantially beneficial health effects (Leventhal and Brooks-Gunn, 2003). Although this program design is clearly unique and impossible to replicate on a large scale, it provides convincing evidence of the value of improving housing as a means of improving health, even in cities in wealthy countries.

The Healthy Cities movement is an international project sponsored by the World Health Organization (n.d.) that works directly with local government to promote health in cities. The program is intended to provide national and local governments with ways of dealing with the urban determinants of health discussed in this chapter, including pollution, housing, transportation, and other aspects of the physical environment; social support and features of the social environment; and improved health and social resources. As part of its work with local governments, the Healthy Cities movement measures the local urban health burden and makes health issues relevant and understandable to local agencies through analysis and policy advocacy. A Municipal Health Plan is developed as a template for improving awareness of environmental and health problems in schools, workplaces, and marketplaces, and among health services and other organizations, and this encourages local governments to act to improve these determinants of health. Most of the work of the Healthy Cities movement thus far has been in higher-income countries, although from 1995 to 1999, the WHO supported Healthy City Projects (HCPs) in Cox's Bazar (Bangladesh), Dar es Salaam (Tanzania), Fayoum (Egypt), Managua (Nicaragua), and Quetta (Pakistan). In the first evaluation of these projects, there was evidence that key stakeholders had an improved understanding of the role of the urban environment in shaping health but limited political will to act on this awareness (Harpham, Burton, and Blue, 2001). Although the success of the Healthy Cities movement remains difficult to assess, it represents a worldwide effort to raise awareness among key decision makers about the role of cities in shaping health, potentially setting the stage for local interventions such as the MTO program described previously. In addition, this program exemplifies the potential for a synergy among multiple sectors, including public health agencies, environmental movements, and municipal governments, that will ultimately be essential to improving health in complex urban areas.

In an increasingly urbanizing world, the features of cities that affect health may, even when their role is limited, have a tremendous aggregate impact on large numbers of people. It is therefore very much a public health mandate to identify urban characteristics at multiple levels—features of population, the physical environment, the social environment, and urban service provision—and to determine how these characteristics interact to affect health and disease. Building healthier cities has the potential to improve population health dramatically in the coming century.

Thought Questions

1. Select a common health problem. How might characteristics of urban living affect population distribution of this disease? How might these relationships be different in wealthy and less wealthy countries?

2. How might differences within cities affect population distribution of a particular disease? What are the characteristics of urban communities that might be consistently associated with particular health outcomes in different cities?
3. Given limitless resources, what intervention would you implement to improve the health of urban populations in wealthy countries? In less wealthy countries?
4. What might the implications of our increasing technological capacities be for the world's cities? For population health?

References

Adler, N. E., Marmot, M., McEwen, B. S., and Stewart, J. *Socioeconomic Status and Health in Industrial Nations: Social, Psychological, and Biological Pathways.* Annals of the New York Academy of Sciences, no. 896. New York: New York Academy of Sciences, 1999.

Andrulis, D. P. "Community, Service, and Policy Strategies to Improve Health Care Access in the Changing Urban Environment." *American Journal of Public Health,* 2000, *90,* 858–862.

Bellow, S. "World Famous Impossibility." *New York Times,* p. 115, Dec. 6, 1970.

Berkman, L. F., Glass, T., Brissette, I., and Seeman, T. E. "From Social Integration to Health: Durkheim in the New Millennium." *Social Science & Medicine,* 2000, *51,* 843–857.

Berkman, L. F., and Kawachi, I. (eds.). *Social Epidemiology.* New York: Oxford University Press, 2000.

Cohen, D., and others. "'Broken Windows' and the Risk of Gonorrhea." *American Journal of Public Health,* 2000, *90,* 230–236.

Cohen, D. A., and others. "Neighborhood Physical Conditions and Health." *American Journal of Public Health,* 2003, *93,* 467–471.

Cutler, D., and Miller, G. "The Role of Public Health Improvements in Health Advances: The Twentieth-Century United States." *Demography,* 2005,*42,* 1–22.

Dohrenwend, B. P., and Dohrenwend, B. S. "Psychiatric Disorders in Urban Settings." In S. Arieti (ed.), *American Handbook of Psychiatry.* Vol. 11. New York: Basic Books, 1974.

Elliott, M. "The Stress Process in Neighborhood Context." *Health & Place,* 2000, *6,* 287–299.

Ewing, R., Pendall, R., and Chen, D. *Measuring Sprawl and Its Impact.* [http://www.smartgrowthamerica.com/sprawlindex/MeasuringSprawl.pdf]. 2002.

Ewing, R., Schieber, R. A., and Zegeer, C. V. "Urban Sprawl as a Risk Factor in Motor Vehicle Occupant and Pedestrian Fatalities." *American Journal of Public Health,* 2003, *93,* 1541–1545.

Ewing, R., and others. "Relationship Between Urban Sprawl and Physical Activity, Obesity, and Morbidity." *American Journal of Health Promotion,* 2003, *18*(1), 47–57.

Ezzati, M., and others (Comparative Risk Assessment Collaborating Group). Selected Major Risk Factors and Global and Regional Burden of Disease. *Lancet,* 2002, *360,* 1347–1360.

Festinger, L. "A Theory of Social Comparison Processes." *Human Relations,* 1954, *7,* 117–140.

Frumkin, H., Frank, L., and Jackson, R. *Urban Sprawl and Public Health: Designing, Planning and Building for Healthy Communities.* Washington, D.C.: Island Press, 2004.

Galea, S., and others. "Income Distribution and Risk of Fatal Drug Overdose in New York City Neighborhoods." *Drug and Alcohol Dependence,* 2003, *70*(2), 139–148.

Goldstein, S. "Demographic Issues and Data Needs for Mega-City Research." In R. J. Fuchs and others (eds.), *Mega-City Growth and the Future.* New York: United Nations University Press, 1994.

Grant, E. and others. *State of the Art of Urban Health in Latin America.* London: South Bank University, 1999.

Hardoy, J. E., Mitlin, D., and Satterthwaite, D. "Urban Change in the Third World: Are Recent Trends a Useful Pointer to the Urban Future?" In D. Cadman and G. Payne (eds.), *The Living City.* New York: Routledge, 1990.

Harpham, T., Burton, S., and Blue, I. "Healthy City Projects in Developing Countries: The First Evaluation." *Health Promotion International,* 2001, *16*(2), 111–125.

Haughton, G., and Hunter, C. *Sustainable Cities.* London: Regional Studies Association, 1994.

International Institute for Applied Systems Analysis. "Data—Urbanization." [http://www.iiasa.ac.at/Research/LUC/ChinaFood/data/urban/urban_8.htm]. 1999.

Jargowsky, P. "Sprawl, Concentration of Poverty, and Urban Inequality." In G. D. Squires (ed.), *Urban Sprawl: Causes, Consequences, and Policy Responses.* Washington, D.C.: Urban Institute Press, 2002.

Jencks, C., and Mayer, S. E. "The Social Consequences of Growing Up in a Poor Neighborhood." In L. E. Lynn and M.G.H. McGeary (eds.), *Inner-City Poverty in the United States.* Washington, D.C.: National Academies Press, 1990.

Johnson, S. P. *The Earth Summit: The United Nations Conference on Environment and Development.* London: Graham and Trotman, 1993.

Karpati, A., and others. *New York City Community Health Profiles.* New York: New York Department of Health and Mental Hygiene, 2003.

Kawachi, I., Kennedy, B. P., Lochner, K., and Prothrow-Stith, D. "Social Capital, Income Inequality, and Mortality." *American Journal of Public Health,* 1997, *87,* 1491–1498.

Kelly-Schwartz, A. C., Stockard, J., Doyle, S., and Schlossberg, M. "Is Sprawl Unhealthy? A Multilevel Analysis of the Relationship of Metropolitan Sprawl to the Health of Individuals." *Journal of Planning Education and Research,* 2004, *24*(2), 184–196.

Kessler, R. C., and others. "Lifetime and 12-Month Prevalence of DSM-III-R Psychiatric Disorders in the United States." *Archives of General Psychiatry,* 1994, *41,* 8–19.

King, G., and others. "Smoking in Cape Town: Community Influences on Adolescent Tobacco Use." *Preventive Medicine,* 2003, *36,* 114–123.

Latkin, C. A., Hua, W., and Forman, V. L. "The Relationship Between Social Network Characteristics and Exchanging Sex for Drugs or Money Among Drug Users in Baltimore, MD, USA." *International Journal of STD & AIDS,* 2003, *14*(11), 770–775.

Leventhal, T., and Brooks-Gunn, J. "Moving to Opportunity: An Experimental Study of Neighborhood Effects on Mental Health." *American Journal of Public Health,* 2003, *93,* 1576–1582.

Lopez, R. "Urban Sprawl and Risk for Being Overweight or Obese." *American Journal of Public Health,* 2004, *94,* 1574–1579.

McMichael, M. *Planetary Overload: Global Environmental Change and the Health of the Human Species.* New York: Cambridge University Press, 1993.

McNeill, J. R. *Something New Under the Sun: An Environmental History of the Twentieth Century.* New York: Norton, 2000.

Meadows, D. H., Meadows, D. L., Randers, J., and Behrens, W. W. *The Limits to Growth.* New York: University Books, 1972.

Meadows, D. H., Meadows, D. L., and Randers, J. *Beyond the Limits: Confronting Global Collapse, Envisioning a Sustainable Future.* White River Junction, Vt.: Chelsea Green, 1993.

Merzel, C. "Gender Differences in Health Care Access Indicators in an Urban, Low-Income Community." *American Journal of Public Health,* 2000, *90,* 909–916.

Montgomery, M. R., and Casterline, J. B. "The Diffusion of Fertility Control in Taiwan: Estimates from Pooled Cross-Section, Time-Series Models." *Population Studies,* 1993, *47*(3), 457–479.

Murray, C.J.L., and Lopez, A. D. (eds.). *The Global Burden of Disease: A Comprehensive Assessment of Mortality and Disability from Diseases, Injuries and Risk Factors from 1990 and Projected to 2020.* Global Burden of Disease and Injury Series, Vol. 1. Cambridge, Mass.: Harvard School of Public Health on Behalf of the World Health Organization and the World Bank, 1996.

Nantulya, V. M., and Reich, M. R. "Equity Dimensions of Road Traffic Injuries in Low- and Middle-Income Countries." *Injury Control and Safety Promotion,* 2003, *10,* 13–20.

Odero, W., Garner, P., and Zwi, A. "Road Traffic Injuries in Developing Countries: A Comprehensive Review of Epidemiological Studies." *Tropical Medicine and International Health,* 1997, *2,* 445–460.

Paykel, E. S., and others. "Urban-Rural Mental Health Differences in Great Britain: Findings from the National Morbidity Survey." *Psychological Medicine,* 2000, *30,* 269–280.

Pearlin, L., Lieberman, M., Menaghan, E., and Mullan, J. "The Stress Process." *Journal of Health and Social Behavior,* 1981, *22,* 337–356.

Sampson, R. J., Raudenbush, S. W., and Earls, F. "Neighborhoods and Violent Crime: A Multilevel Study of Collective Efficacy." *Science,* 1997, *277,* 918–924.

Satterthwaite, D. "Will Most People Live in Cities?" *British Medical Journal,* 2000, *321,* 1143–1145.

Scheck, C., Kinicki, A., and Davy, J. "A Longitudinal Study of a Multivariate Model of the Stress Process Using Structural Equations Modeling." *Human Relations,* 1995, *48,* 1481–1510.

Sturm, R., and Cohen, D. A. "Suburban Sprawl and Physical and Mental Health." *Public Health,* 2004, *118,* 448–496.

United Nations Department of Economic and Social Affairs, Population Division. *World Urbanization Prospects: The 2001 Revision.* New York: United Nations, 2002.

U.S. Bureau of the Census. "Census 2000 Urban and Rural Classification." [http://www.census.gov/geo/www/ua/ua_2k.html]. 2002.

U.S. Department of Housing and Urban Development. "Moving to Opportunity for Fair Housing Demonstration Program: Current Status and Initial Findings." [www.huduser.org/publications/fairhsg/mto.html]. 1999.

Vandegrift, D., and Yoked, T. "Obesity Rates, Income, and Suburban Sprawl: An Analysis of US States." *Health & Place,* 2004, *10*(3), 221–229.

Vogele, J. P. "Urban Infant Mortality in Imperial Germany." *Social History of Medicine,* 1994, *7*(3), 401–425.

Williams, D. R., and Rucker, T. D. "Understanding and Addressing Racial Disparities in Health Care." *Health Care Financing Review,* 2000, *21*(4), 75–90.

Wilson, W. J. *When Work Disappears: The World of the Urban Poor.* New York: Knopf, 1996.

World Health Organization. "Healthy Cities Makes a Difference." [www.who.dk/document/hcp/hcpwebuk.pdf]. n.d.

For Further Information

Numerous books provide good introductions to urban history and urban form. Two sweeping overviews are

Hall, P. *Cities in Civilization.* New York: Pantheon Books, 1998.

Mumford, L. *The City in History: Its Origins, Its Transformations, and Its Prospects.* Orlando: Harcourt Brace, 1961.

A third introduction to this topic focuses on U.S. cities:

Glaab, C. N., and Brown, A. T. *A History of Urban America.* (3rd ed.) New York: Macmillan, 1983.

Excellent sources on cities in the developing world are

Hardoy, J. E., Mitlin, D., and Satterthwaite, D. *Environmental Problems in an Urbanizing World: Finding Solutions in Africa, Asia, and Latin America.* London: Earthscan, 2001.

Panel on Urban Population Dynamics, Committee on Population, and National Research Council of the National Academies. *Cities Transformed: Demographic Change and Its Implications in the Developing World.* Washington, D.C.: National Academies Press, 2003.

For a focus on urban health in the developing world, see

Harpham, T., and Tanner, M. (eds.). *Urban Health in Developing Countries: Progress and Prospects.* New York: St. Martin's Press, 1995.

Academic journals have increasingly turned their attention to urban health topics. Special issues on the built environment, including much that is relevant to urban health, have been published by the *American Journal of Public Health,* 2003, *93*(9), and the *Journal of Urban Health,* 2003, *80*(4).

For additional urban health information and bibliographies, literature reviews, and Internet links see

International Society for Urban Health [http://www.isuh.org].

CHAPTER SEVENTEEN

TRANSPORTATION AND HEALTH

John Balbus
Dushana Yoganathan Triola

Perhaps no other feature so defines modern society as mobility. Two hundred years ago no human could travel faster than the wind while on water or faster than another animal could carry him or her on land. Now, in the twenty-first century, a growing number of people on the planet have access to transportation technologies that can carry them from continent to continent in a matter of hours, and they own personal vehicles that can move them great distances at speeds more than ten times faster than horse-drawn vehicles (Box 17.1). With increased speed and mobility have come great societal benefits. Transport of goods, people, and ideas has led to greater wealth and technological advances, and the increased ability to transport food has led to better protection from famine and malnutrition. But there have also been significant costs to the environment, to public health, and to quality of life. Large groups of indigenous peoples have succumbed to unfamiliar diseases brought by travelers from other cultures, transportation systems pollute the air and make large amounts of land unfit for habitat or other natural purposes, and the speed and heavy machinery of transportation contribute to nearly a million deaths around the world each year due to crashes (Box 17.2). The benefits and harms of transportation can be examined on a global scale, but public health professionals are more likely to encounter transportation policies and plans on the community level. This chapter examines the associations between community health and transportation, with added detail on motor vehicle crashes, how transportation impacts air quality, and the implications for physical activity and health from reliance on motorized travel.

Box 17.1. The Evolution of Transportation

3500 BCE	Fixed wheels on carts are invented.
2000 BCE	Horses are domesticated and used for transportation.
181–234	The wheelbarrow is invented.
1662	In France, Blaise Pascal invents the first public, horse-drawn bus.
1769	In France, Nicolas Joseph Cugnot invents the first self-propelled, steam-powered road vehicle.
1790	The modern bicycle is invented.
1807	Robert Fulton designs the first steamboat and tests it on the Hudson River; regular passenger service soon begins.
1814	In England, George Stephenson invents the first steam-powered railroad locomotive.
1862	In France, Jean Lenoir makes an automobile with a petroleum-powered engine.
1869	The first transcontinental railroad is completed when the Central Pacific and Union Pacific Railroads meet in Promontory, Utah.
1871	The first cable car is invented.
1885	In Germany, Karl Benz builds the world's first automobile powered by an internal combustion engine.
1895	In Germany, Rudolf Diesel invents an engine that comes to be known as the diesel engine.
1895	The world's first omnibus, built by Karl Benz, goes into scheduled service between Deuz and Siegen, Germany.
1903	The Wright brothers invent and fly the first motorized airplane.
1908	The first production Model T Ford is assembled in Detroit; Henry Ford improves the assembly line for automobile manufacturing.
1920s	Lead is added to gasoline to boost octane levels and improve engine performance.
1935	The first successful passenger airline flight.
1947	The first supersonic jet flight.
1940s–'50s	The contribution of motor vehicles to urban smog begins to be recognized.
1956	The Interstate Highway Act introduces the divided highway.

1959	California becomes the first state to set tailpipe emissions standards.
1965	The Motor Vehicle Air Pollution Control Act amends the Clean Air Act of 1963; first federal controls on motor vehicle emissions.
1974	The Clean Air Act Amendments lead to rules requiring unleaded gasoline in new cars.
1997	The first gasoline-electric hybrid automobile is offered to the public, by Japan's Toyota.

Sources: Data from About, Inc., 2005; American Meteorological Society, 2005.

Box 17.2. Transportation: Moving Goods, People, and . . . Germs?

The English word and public health concept of *quarantine* is based on the Italian practice of isolating ships arriving from areas with dangerous diseases for forty days (*quaranta giorni* in Italian, shortened to *quarantina*). What was clear, even long before the discovery of bacteria and viruses, was that increased travel and contact among people from far-flung nations resulted in the carriage and spread of devastating diseases. Here are some examples:

- Smallpox carried by European explorers devastated New World populations in places like Santo Domingo and Mexico, killing one-third to one-half of the people in the initial epidemics.
- Plague, carried for centuries along trade routes in the Old World, reached California at the start of the twentieth century, where it caused an epidemic, became established among rodents in the area, and persists today as an endemic zoonotic focus.
- Disease-carrying mosquitoes constantly hitch rides in long-distance vessels. The *Aedes albopictus* mosquito, a competent carrier of many diseases, including West Nile virus and dengue, arrived in the United States in a shipment of used tires and has since established itself in twenty-one states. Mosquitoes are also common free-loaders on international airplane flights: one survey found living mosquitoes in twelve of sixty-seven airplanes arriving from tropical countries.

In addition to spreading disease-causing agents such as microbes and vectors, global travel has also resulted in the transfer of invasive, nonnative species that may cause severe ecological damage by dominating their new ecosystems. Examples range from zebra mussels in the Great Lakes, imported from the Caspian Sea via ships' ballast (Great Lakes Information Network, 2005), to the infamous Africanized bees (the so-called killer bees), which migrated northward into the United States from Mexico after being imported into South America from Africa.

Transportation Terminology and Trends

The language of transportation planners includes terms not commonly used in the language of public health professionals. To work at the interface, public health students and professionals need to acquire some key terms used in the transportation world:

Mode share is the proportion of trips made using a particular mode of transportation (for example, private automobile, walking, public bus).

Vehicle miles traveled (VMT) is a measure of the cumulative distance traveled using a particular travel mode.

Proximity refers to the distances between trip origins and destinations. An important aspect of proximity is land use. For example, mixed-use development, which places residential, office, retail, and recreational uses near each other, increases proximity.

Connectivity refers to the ease of moving directly from trip origin to destination. It is determined by such things as land-use patterns, the configuration of the street network, and the presence or absence of pedestrian facilities such as sidewalks.

Mode shares for the various modes of transportation vary widely over time (Figure 17.1), between developed and developing countries, and even between developed countries (Figure 17.2 and Table 17.1). U.S. mode shares are skewed toward personal automobile use: nearly 90 percent of trips in the United States are made by automobile, and less than 7 percent of trips in urban areas are made by walking or bicycling. This automobile mode share is among the world's highest. In urban areas in The Netherlands, for example, more than 45 percent of trips are made on foot or bicycle. Additionally, Americans use their cars for two-thirds of all trips shorter than a mile and 89 percent of trips between one and two miles long (Pucher and Dijkstra, 2003). This has serious implications for public health in each of the three main areas of focus: because pollution emissions are highest when automobiles are first started, more miles spent on short trips means more pollutants per mile driven; increased automobile use for short trips around the home may also be expected to increase rates of crash-related injuries and fatalities; and as the car replaces walking and bicycling for short trips, levels of physical activity decline further.

FIGURE 17.1. MODE SHARE OF COMMUTING TO WORK IN THE UNITED STATES, 1960–2000.

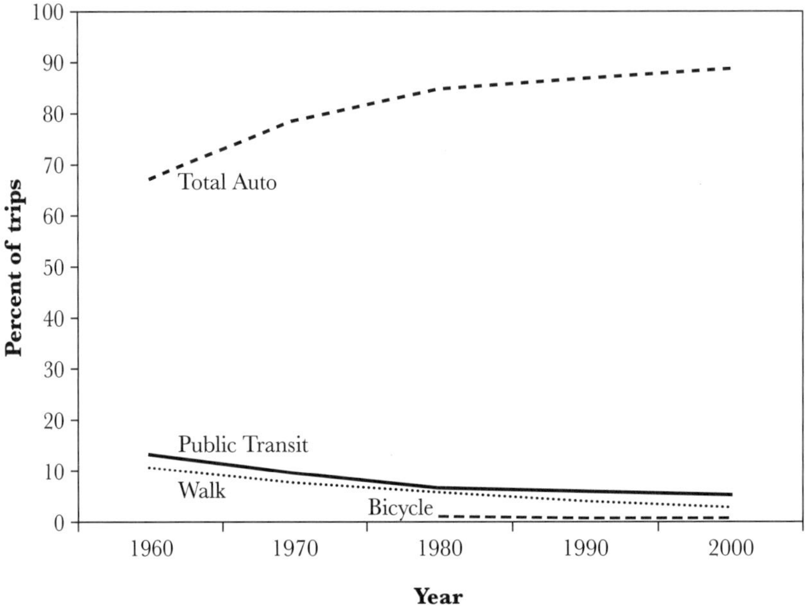

Note: Observe the steady increase in the use of automobiles and the concomitant decrease in walking and transit riding.

Source: Adapted from Pucher and Renne, 2003, table 1.

TABLE 17.1. MODE SHARE OF TRIPS IN URBAN AREAS BY COUNTRY (PROPORTION OF TOTAL), 1990.

Country	Car	Public Transport	Bicycling	Walking	Walking Plus Bicycling	Other
Austria	39	13	9	31	40	8
Canada	74	14	1	10	11	1
Denmark	42	14	20	21	41	3
France	54	12	4	30	34	0
Germany	52	11	10	27	37	0
Italy	25	21	NA	NA	54	NA
The Netherlands	44	8	27	19	46	2
Norway	68	7	NA	NA	25	NA
Sweden	36	11	10	39	49	4
Switzerland	38	20	10	29	39	3
England and Wales	62	14	8	12	20	4
United States	84	3	1	9	10	3
Mean (rounded)	52	12	10	23	34	3

Source: Adapted from Pucher and Lefevre, 1996, table 2.4; data primarily from national transport ministries.

FIGURE 17.2. PERCENTAGE OF TRIPS IN URBAN AREAS MADE BY BICYCLING AND WALKING, SELECTED COUNTRIES OF NORTH AMERICA AND EUROPE, 1995.

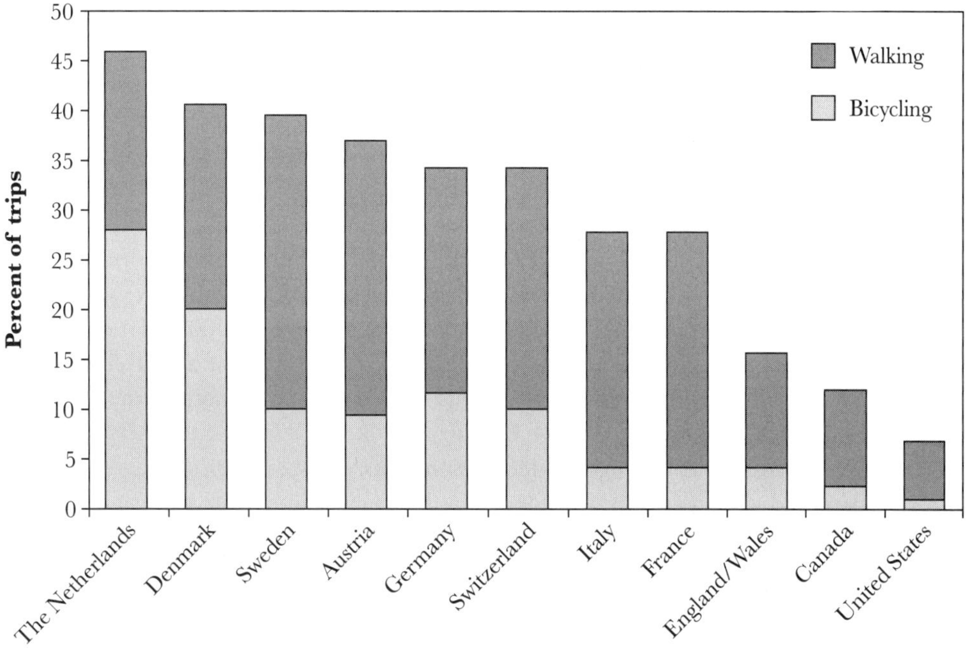

Note: Distributions are intended to shown approximate differences.
Source: Pucher and Dijkstra, 2003.

Benefits of Transportation

Before turning to health risks associated with transportation, we will first outline the public health benefits associated with today's improvements in transportation infrastructure and facilities. The current transportation system, which relies heavily on polluting motorized vehicles and consumes massive amounts of energy, has been developed to meet human needs and aspirations. Some have hypothesized that humans see travel as an end unto itself, but more basic human needs, such as access to food, employment, education, and health care, are also more effectively met through improved mobility. In addition to moving humans to and from important resources, transportation systems have been developed to move goods over large distances. Our global economy has become dependent on long-distance transport of foods, raw materials, and manufactured goods. Public health disparities arise locally and globally when either the distribution of the benefits or the distribution of the pollution and other harms from improved transportation systems is unequal among population groups. We explore some of these equity issues in the various sections of this chapter.

One of the outcomes of a highly developed transportation system in the United States is the widespread distribution of food. This enables access to fresh fruits and vegetables in locations that otherwise would be without these health-promoting foodstuffs. The widespread distribution of food also leads to more efficient production of foods, as those regions best suited to growing certain types of foods are able to deliver their produce to a larger market and to benefit from economies of scale (U.S. Department of Agriculture [USDA], Agricultural Marketing Service, 2004). The link between food production and transportation is far from trivial; in the United States agriculture accounts for roughly one-third of all freight transport (USDA, Agricultural Marketing Service, 2004). Trucks are increasingly used for this purpose, accounting for 45 percent of all trips devoted to transporting food. Another 32 percent of trips that carry food, primarily heavy bulk items like grains, are made by railroad.

In addition to bringing food to communities, transportation systems must bring people to sources of nutritious food. This is especially important in areas of poverty and disadvantage, where local food stores may offer limited selections of nutritious food and where people are more likely to rely on public transportation for food shopping (Kaufman, MacDonald, Lutz, and Smallwood, 1997). Studies have shown that people receiving food stamps cite transportation barriers as a reason for infrequent shopping trips and food insecurity (Cohen and others, 1999) and that the absence of nearby sources of healthy foods results in diets lower in fruits and vegetables (Morland and others, 2003). Although the selection and prices of nutritious foods in disadvantaged areas may depend primarily on social factors other than transportation, access to convenient and safe public transit in these areas may be a critical factor in people's nutrition and health.

Adequate transportation systems allow people to access opportunities for employment; greater mobility affords greater flexibility in job opportunities and places to live. Yet the ability to travel greater distances has also led to disparities in access to employment. As job growth has shifted from the inner cities to outlying suburban areas, access to employment has become more and more dependent on automobile ownership. Less than 50 percent of jobs in major metropolitan areas are accessible by public transit, yet nearly half of workers with incomes under $10,000 do not own a car (Federal Transit Administration, 2002). The problem is even worse for those with disabilities, who are disproportionately represented in low-income groups. For those who cannot afford cars, the generally poor public transportation services in the outlying suburbs create a significant barrier to employment. Programs like the Job Access Reverse Commute (JARC) initiative, created by federal transportation legislation, aim to lower that barrier by subsidizing improved public transit from the inner cities to employment centers outside the cities.

The last benefit to be considered is access to health care. Clearly, the ability to speed people quickly over great distances has saved countless lives through the development of surface and air transportation systems for acutely ill and injured people. For less serious situations, however, the presence or absence of transportation options is a key determinant of whether many people, particularly those with disabilities or those unable to afford private automobiles, can receive ongoing care for chronic conditions. One survey found that 9 percent of children from families earning less than $50,000 missed doctor's appointments due to lack of transportation. The problem was more severe for those with incomes below the poverty line and those in rural areas (Children's Health Fund, 2001). Thus, even when governments provide medical insurance to low-income families with children, access to health care may still be limited due to lack of adequate transportation systems to get those children to checkups and ongoing medical care appointments.

Transportation and Injuries

One consequence of high speeds and heavy vehicles is that motor vehicle crashes involve significant transfers of energy, and human beings involved in crashes are highly vulnerable to traumatic injuries. As described in Chapter Twenty-Five, motor vehicle crashes are the leading cause of death in people between the ages of one and thirty-four, and the rate of motor vehicle fatalities is highest among those first learning to drive (young adults ages sixteen to twenty-four) and the elderly (those over seventy-four) (U.S. Department of Transportation [DOT], 2002a). People can be killed or injured as operators or passengers of motor vehicles; however, a significant proportion of people are also harmed as pedestrians or bicyclists struck by motor vehicles. To a certain extent the involvement of pedestrians and bicyclists in motor vehicle crashes is a function of how many pedestrians and bicyclists are on or near the roads relative to cars. The first recorded motor vehicle collision in U.S. history occurred in 1896 in New York City and involved a bicycle (DOT, 2002b). During the twentieth century, cars took over the roadways, leading to ever-increasing numbers of crashes and fatalities, which peaked in the 1970s and '80s. The public health approach to reducing injuries and deaths due to motor vehicle crashes has grown in sophistication and effectiveness over the past thirty years, helping to lower the numbers of crashes and fatalities. Additional details on this approach appear in Chapter Twenty-Five.

Motor Vehicle Crashes

The burden of injuries and fatalities from motor vehicle crashes is staggering. In the United States in 2002, 42,815 people were killed and another 2,926,000 injured in motor vehicle crashes (DOT, 2002a). According to the National Highway Traffic Safety Administration (NHTSA), the economic cost of motor vehicle crashes in the United States in fiscal year 2000 was more than $230 billion (NHTSA, 2001), which is 2.3 percent of the U.S. gross national product (NHTSA, 2000). This figure includes not only medical costs but also costs arising from lost productivity, legal fees, insurance administration, travel delay, property damage, and workplace losses. Although the current public health and economic burdens from motor vehicle crashes are huge, they would be even larger were it not for the concerted efforts of the transportation and public health communities to make driving safer. With the aid of the Haddon matrix (see Chapter Twenty-Five), improvements have been made to vehicles (air bags, steel door guard beams), driver behaviors (seat belt laws, efforts to reduce drunken driving), and the driving environment (improvements in road markings and designs). As a result the motor vehicle fatality rate has had a striking decline, from 5.50 fatalities per 100 million miles traveled in 1966 to 1.50 fatalities per 100 million miles traveled in 2002 (DOT, 2002a). Detailed statistics on nonfatal crashes have been collected only since 1988, but they show a slight decline in the total number of crashes and the proportion of crashes resulting in injuries and fatalities (DOT, 2002a). Focused efforts to reduce drunken driving have led to a significant decline in rates of alcohol-related fatalities since 1988 (DOT, 2002a). Over the past ten years, however, modest improvements in transportation safety have failed to reduce the burden of traffic crashes. This is because the use of cars (measured as total vehicle miles traveled, or VMT) has grown faster than the fatality rate has declined. Between 1992 and 2002, for example, the rate of fatalities per 100 million miles traveled dropped from 1.75 to 1.5, but the number of fatalities actually rose by over 3,000. During the same time frame, VMT increased by over 27 percent. It is clear that further progress in reducing fatalities from motor vehicle crashes will require either a new breakthrough in safety technology, a decline in motor vehicle use, or some combination of both.

Pedestrian Crashes

More than 10 percent of those killed in motor vehicle crashes are pedestrians. In 2002, 4,808 pedestrians were killed by motor vehicles, and over 70,000 were injured (DOT, 2002a). The fatality rate for pedestrians tends to increase with age, with those over seventy-four having a rate of 3.62 per 100,000 people. Male pedestrians are more than twice as likely as female pedestrians to be killed. Fatal pedestrian crashes are more likely to occur at night, in urban areas, during normal weather conditions, and away from intersections and crosswalks. Alcohol intoxication also plays a role in nearly half (46 percent) of fatalities, with the pedestrian victim more frequently intoxicated than the vehicle operator (34 percent versus 13 percent) (DOT, 2002c). Fatality and injury rates have been declining steadily over the past thirty years, although the rate of walking, as measured by the percentage of people walking to work, has also declined steadily during that time. It is not clear whether the decline in pedestrian fatalities is due to improved safety or simply decreased exposure to the risks of walking (Surface Transportation Policy Project [STPP], 2002).

Pedestrian fatality rates are higher for nonwhite ethnic minorities than for whites in the United States. Surveys conducted in Atlanta, Washington, D.C., and Los Angeles have shown fatality rates among Latinos to be up to six times higher than rates among whites. Rates are higher among African Americans as well. Although African Americans make up 12 percent of the U.S. population, they account for 20 percent of all pedestrian fatalities. The reasons for these disparities have not been well-studied, but lower rates of car ownership and higher rates of walking to work, among Latinos in particular, have been cited as one cause (STPP, 2002).

Urban form appears to be associated with pedestrian fatality rates. When pedestrian fatality rates are compared across U.S. cities after adjusting for the proportion of people who walk to work, a pattern emerges. The highest adjusted pedestrian fatality rates are in the newer, more sprawling cities of the Southeast and Southwest, like Orlando, Houston, and Phoenix. Older cities that tend to have higher walking rates and more compact designs, such as New York and Boston, have far lower adjusted pedestrian fatality rates (STPP, 2002). Availability of crosswalks is an important factor: 45 percent of fatalities whose locations were characterized, occurred in locations with no crosswalks. Despite the fact that pedestrians account for over 10 percent of total motor vehicle–related fatalities and walking is the mode of 5.4 percent of all trips made, pedestrian infrastructure receives less than 1 percent of the federal spending on transportation (STPP, 2002).

Although children under fifteen do not have the highest pedestrian fatality rates, they account for nearly 10 percent of all pedestrian fatalities, and nearly 24 percent of all pedestrian injuries (DOT, 2002a). Fatal pedestrian crashes are the second leading cause of death in children between the ages of five and fourteen years old (STPP, 2002). Child pedestrians are uniquely at risk due to engaging in play activities around their homes. Forty percent of child pedestrian injuries occur after school hours (between 5:00 and 9:00 P.M.), and nearly half occur over the weekend (Friday afternoon through Sunday). Among older children the majority of pedestrian fatalities are due to *dart-outs* into traffic, with the child being struck by an oncoming car (Brison, Wicklund, and Mueller, 1988). In 2002, 79 percent of child pedestrian fatalities occurred outside marked intersections. A British study of fatal head injuries in children noted that 80 percent of fatal pedestrian head injuries occurred within 1 mile of home (Sharples, Storey, Aynsley-Green, and Eyre, 1990), and a study in Oakland, California, found that nearly two-thirds of child pedestrian fatalities occurred within 0.25 miles of home (Tester, Rutherford, Wald, and Rutherford, 2004). In the Oakland study, installing speed bumps as traffic calming devices reduced fatality risks to children living on those streets by over 50 percent.

Bicyclist Crashes

Bicyclists account for roughly 2 percent of motor vehicle crash fatalities and injuries. As with pedestrian fatalities, bicyclist fatalities are more likely in nonintersection locations, in urban areas, and between the hours of 5:00 and 9:00 P.M. The fatality rate for children between the ages of five and fourteen is about 40 percent higher than the overall rate (3.2 versus 2.3 per million population) (DOT, 2002b). In 2002, males were eight times more likely to be killed riding a bicycle than females, and in nearly one in four fatal bicycle crashes, the bicyclist was intoxicated with alcohol.

Comparing Risks Among Modes of Travel

If people shift their travel modes from motorized forms to nonmotorized forms, there are important public health benefits, including reduced air pollution and increased physical activity. But does a shift from motor vehicles to walking and bicycling increase the risk of injury and death, offsetting any health gains? Comparative risk studies tend to rank travel by mass transit (air, rail, and bus) as safest, followed by personal motor vehicles, with walking, bicycling, and motorcycle riding being the most dangerous. For example, a recent study by the National Academy of Sciences (NAS) that focused on school travel found that children were at highest risk of dying (per 100 million miles) when bicycling and walking (Transportation Research Board of the National Academies, 2002). But the relative ranking of these risks changes significantly, depending on the measure of risk used. Using miles traveled as the denominator favors modes that are faster, such as airplanes and automobiles. When risks in the NAS study were measured in terms of trips, the most dangerous mode turned out to be a personal automobile driven

TABLE 17.2. FATALITY RATES PER MILLION PASSENGERS BY TRAVEL MODE, GREAT BRITAIN, 1992.

	Fatalities per Km	Fatalities per Trip	Fatalities per Hour of Travel
Motorcycle or moped	9.7	100	300
Foot	5.3	5.1	20
Bicycle	4.3	12	60
Water	0.6	25	12
Car	0.4	4.5	15
Van	0.2	2.7	6.6
Rail	0.1	2.7	4.8
Bus	0.04	0.3	0.1
Air	0.03	55	15

Note: Relative crash risk depends on the unit of measure. Faster modes rank low in crash rates when measured on a per unit of distance basis but do not rank low when measured on a per trip or per hour of travel basis.

Source: Litman, 2002.

by a teenager. The difference in risks depending on measure used can be seen in Table 17.2.

Measuring risk per trip taken may be most appropriate when considering replacing short car trips with nonmotorized trips. There are additional reasons to believe that fatality statistics may be misleading. Nonmotorized trips tend to be shorter than motorized ones, thus lowering exposure, and the risks from walking and bicycling tend to be overestimated due to higher risk groups (young children and the elderly) disproportionately using these modes (Victoria Transport Policy Institute [VTPI], 2004). Some studies have suggested that the health benefits of increased activity outweigh any increase in risk from being struck by a vehicle (Frank and Engelke, 2000; Andersen, Schnohr, Schroll, and Hein, 2000). Most important, improvements in pedestrian and bicycle facilities, sidewalks, and roadways can lead to a substantial reduction in pedestrian and bicyclist risk (Pucher and Dijkstra, 2003).

Transportation And Air Quality

Official recognition of the significant contribution of motorized vehicles to air pollution dates to the late 1950s, when the state of California passed the first regulations on motor vehicle emissions. Since then, air pollution from cars and trucks has continued to be a focus of regulations as well as an ongoing subject of public health research. With recent technological advances the emission of air pollutants from individual cars and trucks has decreased dramatically. Compared to their emissions of thirty years ago, cars now emit less than 10 percent as much of many pollutants per mile driven, but because miles driven have risen threefold during that time, the benefits of reduced emissions have been partially offset. Air pollutants from the transportation sector can be broadly divided into three categories: greenhouse gases (primarily carbon dioxide, a topic discussed in Chapter Eleven); criteria air pollutants (six major ubiquitous air pollutants, including ozone and particulate matter, as described in Chapter Fourteen); and air toxics (a larger number of additional pollutants dispersed into the air by transportation and having known toxic health effects). What comes out of a tailpipe depends largely on the composition of the fuel that goes into the engine and the types of control devices and filters in the exhaust system. So long as carbon-based fossil fuels are used for transportation, combustion will always produce carbon dioxide. Similarly, the combustion of fuels mixed with nitrogen-rich air leads to the formation of nitrogen oxides. Air toxics and volatile organic compounds can result either from partial combustion of fuel or fuel additives or from components that pass through the engine uncombusted. Volatile organic compounds also enter the air through evaporation during fueling. This section outlines the relative contribution of the transportation sector to overall levels of these three categories of pollutants, special considerations for exposures to air pollutants from the transportation sector, and studies of health effects related to transportation sources of air pollution.

The trends over time of transportation-related emissions of criteria air pollutants and the relative contributions of on-road, nonroad (or off-road), and stationary sources of the Environmental Protection Agency's six priority mobile source air toxics are shown in Figures 17.3 and 17.4. The transportation sector currently accounts for 30 to 50 percent of important criteria air pollutants such as carbon monoxide and the ozone precursors nitrogen oxides and volatile organic compounds (VOCs). Relative contributions differ over time and in different places. For example, in 1982, motor vehicles in the United States emitted over 70 percent of all lead pollution into the air. By 2002, lead had been eliminated from gasoline, and motor vehicles were emitting negligible amounts of lead, contributing to the 93 percent reduction in overall lead emissions (Environmental Protection Agency [EPA] 2004). But even though lead air pollution from motor vehicles is no longer a problem in the United States or other countries that have banned lead in gasoline, it remains a significant cause of low-level lead poisoning in other countries throughout the world. For pollutants other than lead, the transportation sector has assumed greater relative importance in the United States, as cleaner manufacturing technologies and the migration of polluting industries have diminished the relative emissions from manufacturing.

FIGURE 17.3. TRENDS IN EMISSIONS OF CRITERIA AIR POLLUTANTS FROM TRANSPORTATION-RELATED SOURCES, 1970–1997.

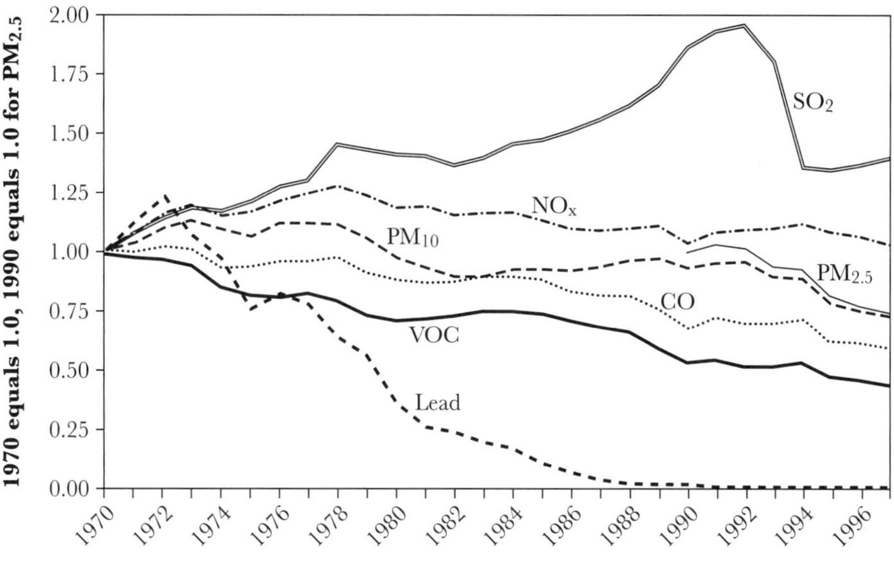

Source: EPA, 1998.

FIGURE 17.4. RELATIVE CONTRIBUTION OF ON-ROAD, NONROAD, AND STATIONARY SOURCES TO SIX PRIORITY MOBILE SOURCE AIR TOXICS, IN CALIFORNIA'S SOUTH COAST AIR BASIN, 1999.

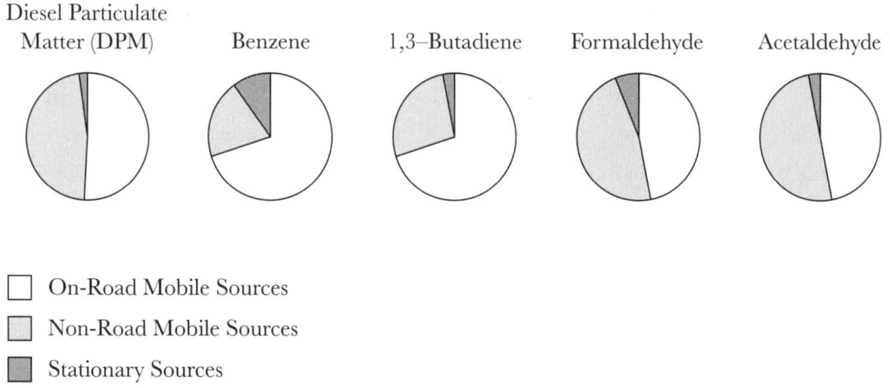

Source: Federal Highway Administration, 2003; data from the South Coast Air Quality Management District's MATES-II study.

Where Do Transportation-Related Exposures to Air Pollutants Occur?

Regulators divide air pollution sources into three broad categories: *stationary sources,* which are usually major emitters like large manufacturing facilities and power plants; *area sources,* which are smaller stationary emitters, such as dry cleaners or auto body shops; and *mobile sources,* including on-road vehicles such as cars and trucks and nonroad vehicles such as construction equipment, locomotives, farm equipment, and even ferries and boats. Transportation sources are generally mobile sources of pollution. Because of this, they have traditionally been dealt with through emissions and fuel technologies that reduce emissions per vehicle, with little consideration given to the locations of those vehicles. Because U.S. land-use and development patterns have involved the creation of huge multilane roadways, however, it has become increasingly clear that transportation sources are not randomly distributed geographically but instead can be thought of as *linear* sources, with the roadways themselves becoming the *sources,* even though the pollution is produced by the vehicles on each roadway. Some roadways, such as those between major ports and urban or distribution centers, are used most heavily by large trucks. Because virtually all large trucks burn diesel fuel, these roadways are particularly concentrated areas of diesel exhaust emissions. The location of residential areas adjacent to these heavily used highways creates the potential for *hot spots,* small areas with particularly high air pollution exposures.

The impact of these hot spots on human health is a subject of active investigation. Concerns have been raised that many of these hot spots are low-income neighborhoods that face other environmental as well as social threats to health (see Chapter Eight). Some of these neighborhoods may have disproportionately high rates of asthma, for instance, which would increase the numbers of those most susceptible to harm from elevated air pollution levels. For example, studies in the Harlem section of New York City have documented widespread exposure to diesel particulates among adolescents (Northridge and others, 1999) and high levels of elemental carbon associated with local truck traffic (Kinney and others, 2000). In the Roxbury section of Boston, local community groups have teamed up with the Harvard School of Public Health to educate community members about asthma and air pollution and to document exposure levels at hot spots in their community (Loh and others, 2002). These communities face exposures not just from the location of major roadways but also from the local siting of other parts of the transportation infrastructure (such as bus and subway terminals) or other facilities (such as trash transfer stations).

The interiors of motor vehicles may have higher concentrations of traffic-related air pollutants than the ambient air. A study conducted on Sacramento and

Los Angeles roadways revealed higher levels of gaseous air pollutants inside cars on freeways than in the ambient air near the freeways. Having a highly polluting car in front of the test car had a large effect on the interior air quality (Rodes and others, 1998). Several studies conducted in school buses have demonstrated that exposures to particulate air pollution are far greater inside the school buses, especially when the windows are closed, than ambient concentrations would predict (Natural Resources Defense Council, 2001; California Air Resources Board, 2003).

Asthma, Respiratory Health, and Transportation-Related Air Pollution

Asthma is a disease characterized by chronic inflammation of the small airways of the lungs and heightened reactivity of the smooth muscles of those airways to irritants and allergens, resulting in episodes of wheezing, coughing, and difficulty breathing. For reasons that are not well understood, the number of people with asthma has been increasing dramatically in the United States and in many other parts of the world. Between 1980 and 1996, for example, the prevalence of asthma in children under four increased 160 percent (Mannino and others, 1998). Transportation-related air pollutants, including fine particulates, ozone, nitrogen oxides, and air toxics, are all capable of irritating the lungs and airways and triggering asthma attacks (see Chapter Fourteen). Although attributing the health effects of any specific air pollutant to a particular source of that pollutant is difficult, a number of studies have assessed the associations between living near roadways and various measures of asthma and respiratory health.

Transportation sources of air pollution are a well-established threat to children's respiratory health (Venn and others, 2001; Ciccone and others, 1998; Brauer and others, 2002). Studies have shown associations between living near roads with high traffic and being diagnosed with asthma (Edwards, Walters, and Griffiths, 1994), being hospitalized for asthma (Lin and others, 2002), and having outpatient visits for asthma (English and others, 1997). Of note, studies have found that heavy truck traffic increases the respiratory health risk of a nearby highway. For example, truck traffic is associated with asthma diagnoses (Van Vliet and others, 1997), asthma symptoms (Duhme and others, 1996), and reduced lung function (Brunekreef, 1997).

Transportation-Related Air Pollution and Mortality

In addition to associations with asthma and respiratory health, fine particulates are associated with increased mortality from cardiovascular causes (Pope and others, 2002; Samet and others, 2000; Dockery and others, 1993). Several studies have specifically investigated deaths from cardiovascular and other causes and traffic-related air pollutant exposures. One study from Amsterdam found that 100 $\mu g/m^3$ traffic-related increases in black smoke and nitrogen dioxide were associated with increased relative risks of dying (Roemer and van Wijnen, 2001), and another study showed a nearly twofold increase in risk of cardiovascular mortality associated with living near a roadway (Hoek and others, 2002). Using a different methodology, other researchers classified sources of fine particles, using marker elements for crustal particles (silicon), coal combustion particles (selenium), and motor vehicle fuel combustion particles (lead). Particles associated with motor vehicle fuels had the strongest association with mortality, whereas particles of crustal origin did not have an association with mortality (Laden, Neas, Dockery, and Schwartz, 2000).

Transportation-Related Air Pollution and Cancer

Lastly, there is concern that air toxics and particulates from transportation sources increase the cancer risk among people who live near roadways. Several sources indicate that the primary source of cancer risk from air toxics is diesel particulates (South Coast Air Quality Management District, 2004; Environmental Defense, 2004) which can come from either on-road sources such as trucks and buses or nonroad sources such as construction equipment. A study in Stockholm (Nyberg and others, 2000) found a 40 percent increase in lung cancer risk for people in the highest category of average traffic-related nitrogen dioxide (NO_2) exposure. Little association was observed between sulfur dioxide (SO_2, a surrogate for indoor heating fuel combustion products) and lung cancer. The study authors concluded that urban air pollution increases lung cancer risk and that vehicle emissions may be particularly important. Two studies investigating the association between traffic-related exposures and childhood leukemia had conflicting results. A study in Denver (Pearson, 2000), on the one hand, found that children residing within 750 feet of roads with the highest traffic density (more than 20,000 vehicles per day) faced more than a sixfold increase in the risk of all cancers and more than an eightfold increase in the risk of leukemia compared to children with the lowest traffic density exposures. A case-control study conducted in Los Angeles of children with leukemia (Langholz and others, 2002), on the other hand, using methodology similar to that of the Denver study, found no association between traffic density and leukemia after controlling for the type and amount of electrical wiring in the home. The Los Angeles study relied on more recent traffic measurements for exposure assessment. The authors, however, were unable to explain the difference in outcomes between their study and the Denver study.

Solutions for Transportation-Related Air Pollution

As previously noted, technological advances have dramatically reduced the emissions of air pollutants per car. Changes in fuel composition, including the removal of lead and the addition of fuel additives like oxygenates, changes in engine design, and the addition of catalytic converters in car exhaust systems have all led to reductions in air pollutant emissions. The one notable exception to this trend is the greenhouse gas carbon dioxide, which is directly related to fuel consumption and automobile use. Because both of these have continued to climb steadily so too have transportation-related carbon dioxide emissions (see Chapter Eleven).

In the United States, cars, light trucks, and other passenger vehicles sold after 2004 must comply with a new set of standards known as *Tier 2* (EPA, 2000c). These standards limit vehicle emissions for a number of pollutants including nitrogen oxides (NO_x), particulates, and nonmethane organic gases. Along with establishing limits on vehicle emissions, the Tier 2 standards also set lower caps (eventually 30 parts per million) on the amount of sulfur in gasoline, thereby reducing formation of secondary particulate matter. These strict new emissions standards were recognized as being necessary to offset the air pollution implications of the ongoing growth in the nation's VMTs. Stricter emission control standards will also be implemented for diesel trucks beginning in 2007. Table 17.3 summarizes the

TABLE 17.3. REPRESENTATIVE FEDERAL EMISSIONS STANDARDS FOR AUTOMOBILES AND TRUCKS, 1970–2010.

Pollutant (units)	1970	1980	1990	2000	2010
Automobile[a]					
NO_x (g/mi)	3.0	2.0	1.0	0.6	0.07
Hydrocarbons (g/mi)	3.4	1.5	0.41	0.31	0.09
Carbon monoxide (g/mi)	NA	7.0	3.4	4.2	4.2
Particulate matter (g/mi)	NA	NA	0.20	0.1	0.01
Heavy-duty trucks[b]					
NO_x (g/bhp-hr)	NA	NA	6.0	4.0	0.2
Hydrocarbons (g/bhp-hr)	NA	NA	1.3	1.3	0.14
Carbon monoxide (g/bhp-hr)	NA	NA	15.5	15.5	
Particulate matter (g/bhp-hr)	NA	NA	0.6	0.1	0.01

Note: g/mi = grams per mile; g/bhp-hr = grams per brake horsepower hour. The standard changed from total volatile organic compounds (VOCs) to nonmethane hydrocarbons (NMHCs) between 1990 and 2000.

[a] Data from EPA, 2000b, tables 3.10 and 3.12. The basis for the 2010 data is EPA's Tier 2, bin 5, which is similar to required fleet averages; see EPA, 2000c.

[b] EPA, 1997; EPA, 2000a.

increasingly strict emission standards for automobiles and trucks. Once these new standards are fully implemented, after 2010, further controls on transportation-related air pollutants will be most readily achieved by reducing production of the more polluting vehicle types or reducing vehicle miles traveled. And as indicated, the only way to reduce carbon dioxide emissions from cars will be to substitute higher efficiency cars in existing fleets or reduce miles driven.

Transportation and Physical Inactivity

As transportation technology has advanced, the need for the traveler to expend physical energy has decreased. With people spending more and more of their waking hours as drivers or passengers of automobiles, more and more hours of relative physical inactivity result. Table 17.4 compares the energy expenditure required for different forms of transportation. Walking, at 2.8 *metabolic equivalents* (METS), consumes roughly 75 percent more calories than driving a car does, at 1.6 METS. A national survey conducted to document personal energy expenditure found that although driving a car required little energy, it was the top-ranked category of personal energy expenditure, accounting for 10.9 percent of the daily total (Dong, Block, and Mandel, 2004).

The relatively large amount of time spent in automobiles is also demonstrated by the decline in trips taken by walking or bicycling. In the 1960s, more than 10 percent of trips in the U.S. were *nonmotorized* (VTPI, 2003). Currently, it is estimated that only 6 percent of all trips of U.S. adults and children are made

TABLE 17.4. ENERGY EXPENDITURE (IN METS) DURING VARIOUS MODES OF TRAVEL.

Activity	Energy Expenditure
Driving car	1.6
Walking	2.0–4.0
Hiking (exercise)	6.0
Jogging	8.7
Bicycling	3.0–9.0

Note: One MET (metabolic equivalent) is the energy expended while sitting quietly. A MET level greater than 1 signifies more intense activities. A level of 3 to 6 METs indicates moderate intensity activity, and a MET level greater than 6 indicates vigorous intensity activity. The values listed here are for an average adult, weighing 70 kg.

Source: Data from Family Practice Notebook, 2004; National Center for Chronic Disease Prevention and Health Promotion, 2005.

on foot or on bicycle (STPP, 2003). Members of lower-income households tend to make more trips by foot or bicycle, due to a lower prevalence of automobile ownership. As income rises, the proportion of trips made by personal automobile tends to rise as well.

This decline in nonmotorized travel is part of a growing public health crisis of physical inactivity. Only 25 percent of Americans aged eighteen and older engage in the recommended level of physical activity (U.S. Department of Health and Human Services [DHHS], 2003), which is thirty minutes of moderate intensity activity, such as walking or slow biking, performed at least five days per week, or twenty minutes of vigorous activity performed at least three days per week (Centers for Disease Control and Prevention [CDC], 2001).

Children in particular seem to be less and less physically active. Only about half of those aged twelve to twenty-one engage in regular, vigorous physical activity, and preschool children spend the majority of their playtime in sedentary activities (DHHS, 1996; Strauss, 1999). Less than two-thirds of high school students achieve at least moderate intensity physical activity (DHHS, 2003). Between 1977 and 1996, children's trips on foot decreased from 16 percent to 9 percent of their total trips. This shift away from walking and bicycling has been especially noticeable in trips made to school. A recent survey found that children living within a mile of school, made only 14 percent of their trips to school by foot or bicycle (Dellinger, 2002).

Health Impacts of Physical Inactivity

The adverse health effects of decreased physical activity include cardiovascular disease, diabetes, colon cancer, obesity, and increased overall mortality. Mortality is particularly notable. In a cohort of 10,000 men and 3,000 women followed for over eight years, physical activity was analyzed as a risk factor for all-cause and cause-specific mortality. Age-adjusted all-cause mortality rates increased from 18.6 per 10,000 person-years in the most fit men to 64 per 10,000 in the least fit men, and from 8.5 to 39.5 per 10,000 person-years between the most fit and least fit women (Blair and others, 1989). The leading cause of mortality in the United States is cardiovascular disease, for which sedentary lifestyle is a significant risk factor. Many studies have confirmed the association between physical inactivity and cardiovascular disease. Men with reduced physical activity are three to five times more likely to die from cardiovascular disease than are men who are physically fit (Wei and others, 1999). Compared with women who do not exercise, women who walk at least ten blocks per day have a 33 percent lower risk of cardiovascular disease (Blair and others, 1996). It has been estimated that approximately 35 percent of excess cardiovascular disease could be eliminated with increased physical activity (Hahn, Teutsch, Rothenberg, and Marks, 1990; CDC, 1993).

Cardiovascular disease is linked with high blood pressure and diabetes, both of which have been shown to increase as participation in physical activity drops. A twelve-year cohort study of 4,800 men and women showed that low levels of physical fitness increased relative risk for the development of hypertension, after adjustment for age, sex, baseline BMI (or body mass index, which is a measure of weight in proportion to height that is associated with body fat and health risk), and baseline blood pressure (Blair, Goodyear, Gibbons, and Cooper, 1984). Non-insulin-dependent diabetes mellitus has been shown to decline as energy expenditure increases (Helmrich, Ragland, Leung, and Paffenbarger, 1991). The 70,102 women participating in the Nurses' Health Study were disease-free at baseline and evaluated for risk of type 2 diabetes. Over the eight years of follow-up, there were 1,419 new cases of type 2 diabetes. After adjusting for age, smoking, alcohol use, history of hypertension, and history of hypercholesterolemia, faster usual walking pace was noted to be independently associated with decreased risk (Hu and others, 1999). Physical inactivity also contributes to the growing epidemic of obesity, which is itself independently associated with poorer health outcomes and increased mortality. Levels of daily energy expenditure are currently lower than they were in preindustrial society (Hill and Melanson, 1999). According to the recently conducted National Health and Nutrition Examination Survey III, 39.4 percent of men and 24.7 percent of women are overweight, with a BMI above 25 and below 29.9, and 19.9 percent of men and 24.9 percent of women are obese, with a BMI of 30 or more (Flegal, Carroll, Ogden, and Johnson, 2002).

Children's health is also dependent on adequate physical activity. The Committee on Atherosclerosis, Hypertension, and Obesity in the Young and the American Heart Association have agreed that atherosclerosis commences in childhood. These groups propose that children should participate in regular activities, ideally generating energy expenditures at 50 to 60 percent of maximal exertion, in order to reap the benefits associated with a physically active lifestyle, such as weight control, lower blood pressure, improved psychological well-being, and a predisposition to increased physical activity in adulthood (Ressel, 2003). Many of the negative health effects of physical inactivity in children stem from obesity. Rates of obesity doubled in U.S. children from the 1970s to the 1990s (Troiano and Flegal, 1998), with 13 percent of six- to eleven-year-olds and 14 percent of twelve- to seventeen-year-olds being overweight in 1999 (Wang and Dietz, 2002). Childhood obesity is associated with diabetes (Rocchini, 2002), asthma, sleep apnea, and gallbladder disease (Barlow and Dietz, 1998). A study that examined changes in hospital discharge rates for obesity-associated diseases over twenty years found that the number of discharges for diabetes doubled, from 1.43 percent in

1981 to 2.36 percent in 1997, and the discharges for gall bladder diseases tripled, from 0.18 percent to 0.59 percent. Sleep apnea discharges also increased, from 0.14 percent to 0.75 percent (Wang and Dietz, 2002). Although these percentages cannot be equated with disease prevalence, they raise the possibility that rates for these conditions are increasing.

Other benefits of physical activity include decreased risk of colon cancer and decreased symptoms of depression and other mental illness. The highest level of physical activity is associated with a 30 to 50 percent reduced risk of colon cancer, as shown in numerous studies that used different measures of occupational or leisure-time activity and controlled for diet and other risk factors (Colditz, Cannuscio, and Frazier, 1997; Lee, 2003). For healthy individuals, twenty to forty minutes of one-time aerobic-type activity reduces anxiety and improves mood (Raglin, 1990).

The economic costs resulting from the health complications of physical inactivity and obesity among Americans run quite high. Of the total cost of cardiovascular disease, $31 billion is attributable to obesity and overweight (American Heart Association, 2003). Hospital costs for treating obesity-related disorders among children rose threefold between 1979 and 1999, from $35 million to $127 million (Paluska, 2002). According to the American Heart Association, increasing physical activity among inactive Americans over the age of fifteen could reduce annual national medical costs by $76 billion (Ressel, 2003).

Links Between Transportation and Physical Activity

From the previous discussion it is clear that physical activity levels are declining in the United States at the same time as people are relying less on their own power to get around and more on personal motorized vehicles. But determining which specific factors are driving these trends, and the extent to which declines in walking and bicycling affect general levels of physical activity is more difficult. This is in part due to the fact that the government does not collect as many statistics about nonmotorized travel as about motorized travel, so data on nonmotorized trips and who is taking them are less available. In addition, researchers have not reached consensus on how to define and measure, for the purposes of studying personal transportation habits, the different factors related to urban and transportation planning and land-use patterns. Despite these difficulties some conclusions can be drawn from the existing literature, and the recent increased research interest in this area should bring a greater understanding of these issues in the near future.

Many factors contribute to people's choices for getting around. Some of these factors are personal, such as health status, fatigue, perceptions of risk and safety, and pure personal preference. Some are cultural, as suggested by differences among countries and even among cities within the United States. But some are structural or environmental; they are determined by the way communities are designed and built. These factors include the presence of sidewalks, trails, crosswalks, pedestrian bridges, and other pedestrian and bicycle facilities (Nelson and Allen, 1997; Pucher, 1997). As mentioned earlier, community design factors such as proximity and connectivity of commercial destinations to residential areas also influence both actual and perceived abilities of people to walk or bicycle for short trips. This has been demonstrated in several studies that compared the transportation mode choices of people in neighborhoods that differed in design. Several studies have shown that residents of neighborhoods with more traditional designs (greater connectivity, access to transit) used nonmotorized and public transportation far more than did residents of neighborhoods with newer designs that reduced connectivity (Friedman, Gordon, and Peers, 1994; Handy, 1992; Shriver, 1997). More work is needed to define the specific factors responsible for these differences in transportation behavior.

Mental Health

Transportation has long been associated with both positive and negative impacts on mental well-being. Travel, especially solo travel, is used as a metaphor for personal development and enlightenment in world literature, and modern advertising certainly capitalizes on images of serene, solitary, mood-enhancing travel, particularly in automobiles. At the same time, travel can be extremely stressful. State-of-the-art, long-distance transportation prior to the nineteenth century (that is, on horseback or in horse-drawn coaches) was not only physically uncomfortable but stressful, due to risks of robbery, injuries, being stranded, and so forth. With the advent of motorized transportation, the physical comfort of long-distance travel has improved markedly, but travel still can bring considerable mental stress, whether that travel is for daily commuting or simply for pleasure.

A number of studies document an association between travel and physiological markers of stress. These studies have examined both driving automobiles and traveling by mass transit, including trains. Travel is associated not only with physiological markers of stress (Bellet, Roman, and Kostis, 1969; Singer, Lundberg, and Frankenhaeuser, 1978) but also with stress-related health effects, including cardiovascular illness and back and neck pain (LeCount and Rukstinat, 1929; Kelsey and Hardy, 1975). As with many other environmental health problems, rich insights into the stress-related impacts of driving come from occupational studies—in this case, studies of professional drivers. Studies of bus, taxi, and truck drivers consistently show increased risk of cardiovascular disease and back pain

(Belkić and others, 1994; Hedberg, Jacobsson, Langendoen, and Nystrom, 1991). It is likely that factors other than psychological stress play a role in causing these health problems. Exposure to carbon monoxide and other air pollutants is likely to influence heart disease, and prolonged sitting and whole body vibration are likely to influence back and neck pain. Nonetheless, the fact that driving elevates physiological markers of stress makes this mechanism a plausible contributor to driving-associated health problems.

Another manifestation of driving-related stress is aggressive behavior. The term *road rage* has been coined to describe extreme, uncontrolled acts of aggression by automobile drivers. In addition to being a sign of mental distress, road rage is also a risk factor for more serious injuries and fatalities. One survey of injuries and fatalities associated with aggressive driving behavior recorded 218 deaths and 12,610 injuries in 10,037 incidents reported to the police or the press between January 1990 and September 1996 (Mizell, 1997). These deaths and injuries resulted not only from automobile crashes directly related to aggressive driving but also from personal assaults by drivers and passengers involved in these incidents. These most serious events, however, are the tip of the iceberg. Aggressive driving behaviors, ranging from gesturing or yelling at other drivers to keeping another car from changing lanes, have been shown in many surveys to be surprisingly common. A 1995 survey found that 90 percent of drivers had experienced aggressive driving and that 60 percent of drivers had committed some act of aggressive driving behavior, the most common being flashing their headlights (45 percent) or making rude gestures (22 percent) (Joint, 1997). Predictors of aggressive driving, in addition to male gender, young age, and particular personality types, include traffic congestion and urban sprawl (Hennessy and Wiesenthal, 1997; Shinar, 1998; STPP, 1999). To the extent that traffic congestion and sprawl-like patterns of development contribute to these dysfunctional behaviors, public health professionals have an opportunity to work with transportation and planning professionals to mitigate these factors.

Noise and Transportation

Noise can be defined as unpleasant or unwanted sounds or as sounds that are damaging to health (Wallace and Doebbeling, 1998). Ambient noise levels vary depending on the nature of noise sources in the environment and the distance from them. According to the Federal Highway Administration (2000), at a distance of 50 feet and traveling at 50 mph, a pickup truck emits 70 decibels (dB) of noise, a medium truck emits 80 dB of noise, and a modified motorcycle emits 90 dB of noise (DOT, 2004). The noise level produced by roadways is affected directly by traffic speed, traffic density, and the types of vehicles traveling. Greater numbers of vehicles, faster speeds, and larger vehicles tend to create more noise (DOT, 2004). At a distance of 100 feet, light traffic emits approximately 50 dB of noise, and heavy traffic can exceed 90 dB. Aircraft are substantial noise sources as well. For people living within two miles of a major airport, overhead airplane flights result in noise levels over 80 dB. Some planes actually emit more than 100 dB of sound.

Numerous health effects are associated with noise, including hearing loss, increased blood pressure, heart disease, changes in hormonal levels, and circulatory problems (Ising and Kruppa, 2004; Stansfeld and Matheson, 2003). Exposure to impulse sounds, such as fireworks or loud motorcycles (National Institute on Deafness and Other Communication Disorders, 2002), puts people at a greater risk for hearing loss than exposure to continuous noise does (Wallace and Doebbling, 1998). Noise-induced hearing loss begins to occur with exposure to noise levels over 70 dB (World Health Organization, 2004), while the U.S. Occupational Safety and Health Administration has established its upper permissible limit at 85 dB over eight hours. Levels between 70 and 85 dB may place more susceptible populations, especially those with concomitant diseases that affect the inner ear, at risk. It is unlikely that residential exposures exceed 85 dB continuously, but residents and workers exposed to urban traffic noise have been shown to suffer varying degrees of hearing loss (Leong and Laortanakul, 2003).

Noise exposure is associated with cardiovascular health effects ranging from hypertension to myocardial infarction. These associations have been strongest in occupational settings where noise exposure has been correlated with significantly higher diastolic blood pressures in the exposed workers (Talbott and others, 1999). Noise exposure has long been known to increase levels of adrenergic hormones, which may be a primary mechanism for chronic cardiovascular effects (Spreng, 2000). The associations between noise and cardiovascular health in communities exposed to transportation-related noise have been less consistent. A meta-analysis of literature primarily from Europe associated hypertension with exposures to airplane noise and myocardial infarction with roadway noise, but the authors noted that these findings could have been affected by uncontrolled confounding (van Kempen and others, 2002). A more recent study found that men living in a home with over 70 dB sound levels for more than ten years had an 80 percent increase in risk of myocardial infarction (Babisch and others, 2005).

Noise exposure has been associated with adverse psychological and developmental impacts as well. Both aircraft and roadway noise have been associated with increases in psychological symptoms and medication use but not with increased incidence of psychiatric illness (Stansfeld, Haines, and Brown, 2000). Other important effects from noise include poor classroom behavior (Lercher, Evans, Meis, and Kofler, 2002), "noise annoyance," or subjective disruption or irritation attributed to noise, and decreased reading comprehension (Haines and others, 2001a). Reading ability has been shown to be impaired in schools located in areas of high aircraft noise (Haines and others, 2001b;Hygge, Evans, and Bullinger, 2002). However, socioeconomic factors may confound the association between noise and reading comprehension (Haines, Stansfeld, Head, and Job, 2002).

There are several ways to reduce community exposure to traffic noise: reduce the amount of noise produced per vehicle, reduce the number or the speed (or both) of vehicles driving past communities, construct sound barriers around large highways, and route new or expanded highways through less densely populated areas. A 1988 EPA noise standard for medium- and heavy-duty trucks sets a limit of 80 dB at a distance of fifteen meters. Most roadways are under state or local jurisdiction, however, leading to a variety of practices in different areas. In many urban areas, residential neighborhoods have instituted restrictions on truck traffic, at all times or during certain hours, to reduce noise exposures. The Federal Highway Administration (2000) has set maximum outdoor noise levels for different types of land use, ranging from 57 dB in areas requiring serenity and quiet (for example, memorials) to 72 dB in developed areas without hospitals, schools, and the like nearby. Many new highway projects now require the construction of sound barriers alongside the roadways to ensure that sound levels in adjacent residential areas do not exceed these limits. Aircraft noise in communities near airports can similarly be reduced by engineering quieter engines, altering use of the airport according to the time of day and specific type of aircraft, and setting land-use policies. The Federal Aviation Administration estimates that federal efforts at noise reduction since 1970 have reduced the number of people exposed to excessive aircraft noise from 7 million in 1975 to 600,000 in 2000 (U.S. General Accounting Office, 2000). This has been accomplished primarily through restrictions on the noisier turbojet engines but also by requiring sound barriers around runways and taxiways and setting tougher soundproofing standards for buildings near airports.

Integrated Solutions to Transportation-Related Health Problems

Transportation policy is often debated in purely economic or engineering terms, but as this chapter shows, transportation has far-reaching effects on public health. Because transportation is *upstream* in the causal chains that affect human health, it is more easily ignored than, for example, air and water quality. Yet because it is an upstream determinant, changes in transportation policies and behaviors can have numerous downstream effects on public health. And because transportation constitutes such a huge portion of the economic activity of developed countries, the degree to which transportation policies and behaviors are designed to mitigate health impacts can make a great difference in the ultimate effects on public health. Public health needs to be part of the transportation planning process, and transportation hazards and healthy solutions need to be understood by public health professionals.

Interventions for transportation problems tend to have synergistic effects. For example, expansion of public transit systems improves traveler safety, reduces emissions of toxic air pollutants and greenhouse gases, and promotes greater physical activity (as people walk to and from stops and stations for trip destinations and origins). In addition, increased ridership of public transit lessens traffic congestion, with concomitant economic and psychosocial benefits, and if expanded public transit is linked with transit-oriented development, additional social benefits of community building and decreased travel times accrue. Similarly, measures that improve the safety of bicyclists and pedestrians encourage walking and bicycling for trips that might otherwise be taken with a personal automobile, leading to decreased air emissions, increased physical activity, and other benefits.

Ultimately, a suite of changes in community planning and transportation system design is needed to mitigate the adverse health impacts of transportation. Conventional transportation planning tends to favor automobile transport at the expense of nonmotorized transport. Data collection and analysis methods systematically ignore or undercount walking and bicycling trips, leading to underinvestment in those modes. And an emphasis on lane widening, increasing parking spaces and traffic speeds, and developing new commercial centers far from denser residential neighborhoods makes communities increasingly inhospitable to nonmotorized transport (Litman, 2003). Technological advances in cars, trucks, and buses have provided most of the risk reductions related to air pollutants and vehicle crashes up until now. But technological advances in emissions reduction and vehicle safety ultimately have limits. Moreover, they do not address some of the larger societal issues related to transportation, such as equity of access and mobility, time wasted and stress induced on congested roadways, obsolescence and decay of dense urban neighborhoods, and physical inactivity.

Legislative Solutions

Federal funding drives transportation policies. In the United States, federal transportation spending underwent a significant reorganization in 1991 with the passage of the Intermodal Surface Transportation Efficiency Act (ISTEA). This bill, and the successor bill that reauthorized federal transportation spending in 1997

(TEA-21), introduced new flexibility, public involvement, and accountability into the transportation planning process. One key change was ensuring that transportation projects would not lead to air pollution emissions that exceeded limits set in state air quality improvement plans. In addition, two new programs (Congestion Mitigation and Air Quality, or CMAQ, and Transportation Enhancements) brought needed federal dollars to support transportation investments that are less polluting and that can reduce traffic congestion. These programs have helped expand public transit, have greatly increased the mileage of bicycle paths throughout the United States, and have paid for the installation of traffic calming devices and other safety enhancements. Transportation spending bills come up for reauthorization every six years or so, and these occasions are critical opportunities for public health professionals to promote more healthy transportation policies.

Health Impact Assessments

One tool for ensuring that public health is considered in transportation plans is a transportation-specific health impact assessment. Current federal regulations require that large road-building and other infrastructure projects complete an environmental impact statement (EIS) that examines the environmental consequences of the project and likely alternatives. Although federal highway officials are required to assess and mitigate the adverse effects of air pollution from highway projects, these provisions often remain unenforced. Health impact assessments could either be incorporated into the environmental impact statements, or be added as a separate element in the transportation planning process. The form of health impact assessments might range from a simple checklist to a resource-intensive quantitative risk assessment. The United States has not incorporated health impact assessments into policy decisions at present, but numerous European countries, Canada, and Australia have committed to do so. The formal introduction of health impact assessments offers the promise that policy decisions will be influenced by public health concerns, but it may have adverse consequences if the format of the health impact assessment is too vague or too burdensome to be effective (Krieger and others, 2003).

Roadway Design

Along with improvements in the safety features of motor vehicles, there have been significant investments over the past several decades in roadway *improvements* designed to improve safety. Where those improvements have included widening and straightening roadways, however, safety may unexpectedly decline, due to the higher speeds that wider, straighter roadways enable (VTPI, 2004). In contrast, traffic calming devices such as speed bumps and tables, narrowed roadways with high sidewalks, and traffic circles have not only led to improved safety outcomes but have also reduced motorized vehicle use in some communities. A study of traffic calming in the United States reported an average 7 mph decline in vehicle speed, and a volume-adjusted 4 percent decline in crashes, but international studies have shown better results, with an average 11 mph decline in vehicle speed in Europe and an 8 to 100 percent decrease in crashes (depending on the specific type of device) (Institute of Transportation Engineers and Federal Highway Administration, 1999). The reason for superior results outside the United States is not clear, but may be partly due to more intensive traffic calming using multiple interventions. Along with these improvements in safety, traffic calming has been noted to reduce total miles traveled by motorized vehicle because of reduced travel speeds and the increased safety and convenience of walking and bicycling (VTPI, 2004). In addition to devices designed specifically for traffic calming, roadway design features such as widened sidewalks, bike lanes, improved crosswalks, and curb cutouts that facilitate bicycling and walking also serve a traffic calming function. Designing roadways to be safe for all modes of travel is essential public health policy (see, for example, Box 17.3).

Box 17.3. Safe Routes to School

An example of an intervention that provides multiple public health benefits is the Safe Routes to School program. This program combines social interventions with improvements in pedestrian and bicycle infrastructure. Enforcement of local traffic laws is promoted, educational programs are created in the schools and communities, and special events like Walk to School Days are initiated. One innovative idea in the Safe Routes to School toolkit (NHTSA, 2002) is Walking School Buses, a project that organizes parents and children into walking groups with predetermined "stops" to encourage participation and enhance pedestrian safety. With additional funding these programs can provide a number of safety enhancements, including sidewalk and trail building, improved crosswalks, and traffic calming. By changing personal travel habits among children and parents from driving to walking and providing the needed safety infrastructure to do so without increasing risk of injuries, these programs safely increase physical activity, reduce air pollution emissions, and increase social interactions. These programs are funded on a state or local level, but legislation to establish a federal funding source is currently pending.

Incentives to Change Transportation Behavior

Policies and practices that aim to change transportation behavior in order to achieve societal and health-related goals such as decreased traffic congestion, reduced traffic crashes, and reduced air pollution, are collectively called *transportation demand management,* or TDM (see VTPI, n.d.). These policies and practices include economic or travel incentives, innovative community and transportation planning, and improvements in nonmotorized and public transit facilities and services. Many people are now familiar with one such practice, the creation of *high-occupancy vehicle* (HOV) lanes on crowded highways. These lanes encourage carpooling and ride sharing by enabling higher speeds for cars with multiple passengers. Economic incentives to reduce congestion and unnecessary vehicle use (and hence air pollution, primarily) include charging higher tolls during peak travel times (*congestion pricing*) and *pay as you drive* insurance, which scales automobile insurance rates according to one's actual amount of driving. A summary of various TDM strategies and their potential health benefits is shown in Table 17.5.

TABLE 17.5. SAFETY BENEFITS OF VARIOUS TRANSPORTATION DEMAND MANAGEMENT (TDM) STRATEGIES.

Goals	TDM Strategies	Safety Impacts
Traffic speed reductions	Traffic calming; vehicle restrictions	Can increase safety by reducing crash frequency and severity and reducing total vehicle mileage; can increase nonmotorized travel.
Access management	Access management	Impacts depend on details. Can reduce per-mile vehicle crash rates, but can increase traffic volumes and speeds; can support more efficient land use and mode shifts.
Time and route shifts	Flextime; congestion pricing	Impacts are mixed. Reducing congestion tends to reduce crashes but may increase severity of crashes that do occur.
Shifts to transit	Transit improvements; HOV priority; park & ride	Can increase safety due to greater safety for transit passengers and reduced vehicle traffic; can increase safety and health if transit travel leads to reductions in total person-miles or increases walking.
Shifts to ride sharing	Ride sharing; HOV priority	Can produce modest safety benefits; potential increased safety due to reduced vehicle traffic.
Shifts to nonmotorized modes	Walking and cycling improvements; traffic calming	Impacts are mixed. Can increase crash risk to participants, but can reduce risk to other road users, reduce total person-miles, and improve aerobic health.

(*Continued*)

TABLE 17.5. SAFETY BENEFITS OF VARIOUS TRANSPORTATION DEMAND MANAGEMENT (TDM) STRATEGIES. (*Continued*)

Goals	TDM Strategies	Safety Impacts
Vehicle mileage reductions	Various pricing or TDM programs; other TDM strategies	Can increase safety by reducing the risks of causing a crash and of being hit (each 1 percent reduction in vehicle-miles tends to reduce crash costs by about 1.6 percent).
Distance-based insurance	PAYD insurance; distance-based pricing	Can reduce total traffic, with anticipated safety increases; can give high-risk motorists an extra incentive to reduce mileage.
Improved vehicle availability	Car sharing; taxi improvements	May increase automobile use by some drivers, but can usually reduce overall vehicle traffic.
Vehicle fuel efficiency	Fuel price increases; fuel efficiency standards	Impacts are mixed. Shifts to smaller vehicles may increase risk to some occupants but reduce risk to other road users.
Mobility substitutes	Telework; delivery services	Can increase safety by reducing vehicle mileage, but rebound effects often offset a portion of the benefits.
Land-use and transport system changes	Various land-use management and planning reforms	Can increase safety by reducing personal travel and encouraging shifts to alternative modes; can increase walking and cycling, providing aerobic exercise.
Improved personal security	Address security concerns; GRH; new urbanism	Can directly improve personal security; can reduce crashes and improve health if this supports shifts to walking, cycling, and public transit.
Safety education	Marketing; encouragement of bicycling	Can reduce bicycle crash rates; can encourage shifts to cycling.

Note: HOV = high-occupancy vehicle; PAYD = pay as you drive; GRH = guaranteed ride home.

Source: Victoria Transport Policy Institute, 2004.

Conclusion

Few economic sectors are as visible a part of people's daily lives as transportation. Every day, every individual makes multiple decisions about how and when to travel. These personal decisions are in turn influenced by other decisions made at many levels, from the family to the local, state, and federal governments. Although the technological demands of transportation have meant that transportation policy decisions have in the past been made largely by transportation engineers and urban planners, the many health ramifications of these decisions make it essential that public health professionals play a stronger role in forming transportation policy. This chapter has summarized the most significant ways in which these decisions about transportation affect public health. With this introduction, students are urged to deepen their understanding and to work to ensure that transportation systems and policies enhance the public's well-being rather than harm it.

Thought Questions

1. You have been requested to perform a health impact assessment for a highway expansion project in an urban community. What information about the community and about the project would you request? What health end points would you include in your assessment?
2. *Transportation policy is health policy.* Agree or disagree with this statement, and justify your answer.
3. You have been asked by local officials to increase schoolchildren's walking to school in your community. How would you go about this project?

References

About, Inc. "Inventors: The History of Transportation." [http://inventors.about.com/library/inventors/bl_history_of_transportation.htm]. 2005.

American Heart Association. "Heart and Stroke Statistical Update—2003." [http://www.americanheart.org/downloadable/heart/10461207852142003HDSStatsBook.pdf]. 2003.

American Meteorological Society. "Legislation: A Look at U.S. Air Pollution Laws and Their Amendments." [http://www.ametsoc.org/sloan/cleanair/cleanairlegisl.html]. 2005.

Andersen, L. B., Schnohr, P., Schroll, M., and Hein, H. O. "All-Cause Mortality Associated with Physical Activity During Leisure Time, Work, Sports and Cycling to Work." *Archives of Internal Medicine,* 2000, *160*(11), 501–506.

Babisch, W., Beule, B., Schust, M., Kersten, N., Ising, H. "Traffic Noise and Risk of Myocardial Infarction." *Epidemiology,* 2005, *16*(1), 33–40.

Barlow, S. E., and Dietz, W. H. "Obesity Evaluation and Treatment: Expert Committee Recommendations." *Pediatrics,* 1998, *102,* e29.

Belkić, K., and others. "Mechanisms of Cardiac Risk Among Professional Drivers." *Scandinavian Journal of Work, Environment & Health,* 1994, *20*(2), 73–86.

Bellet, S., Roman, L., and Kostis, J. "The Effects of Automobile Driving on Catecholamine and Adrenocortical Excretion." *American Journal of Cardiology,* 1969, *24,* 365–368.

Blair, S. N., Goodyear, N. N., Gibbons, L. W., and Cooper, K. H. "Physical Fitness and Incidence of Hypertension in Healthy Normotensive Men and Women." *Journal of the American Medical Association,* 1984, *252,* 487–490.

Blair, S. N., and others. "Physical Fitness and All-Cause Mortality: A Prospective Study of Healthy Men and Women." *Journal of the American Medical Association,* 1989, *262,* 2395–2401.

Blair, S. N., and others. "Influences of Cardiorespiratory Fitness and Other Precursors on Cardiovascular Disease and All-Cause Mortality in Men and Women." *Journal of the American Medical Association,* 1996, *276,* 205–210.

Brauer, M., and others. "Air Pollution from Traffic and the Development of Respiratory Infections and Asthmatic and Allergic Symptoms in Children." *American Journal of Respiratory and Critical Care Medicine,* 2002, *166*(8), 1092–1098.

Brison, R. J., Wicklund, K., and Mueller, B. A. "Fatal Pedestrian Injuries to Young Children: A Different Pattern of Injury." *American Journal of Public Health,* 1988, *78,* 793–795.

Brunekreef, B., and others. "Air Pollution from Truck Traffic and Lung Function in Children Living Near Motorways." *Epidemiology,* 1997, 8, *8,* 298–303.

California Air Resources Board. "Characterizing the Range of Children's Pollutant Exposure During School Bus Commutes." [http://ftp.arb.ca.gov/carbis/research/schoolbus/report.pdf]. 2003.

Centers for Disease Control and Prevention. "Public Health Focus: Physical Activity and Prevention of Coronary Heart Disease." *Morbidity and Mortality Weekly Report,* 1993, *42*(35), 669–672.

Centers for Disease Control and Prevention. *Increasing Physical Activity: A Report on Recommendations of the Task Force on Community Preventive Services.* [http://www.cdc.gov/mmwr/preview/mmwrhtml/rr5018a1.htm]. 2001.

Children's Health Fund. "Survey Reveals Millions of U.S. Children Unable to Access Health Care Due to Lack of Transportation." [http://www.childrenshealthfund.org/release071201.html]. 2001.

Ciccone, G., and others. "Road Traffic and Adverse Respiratory Effects in Children." SIDRIA Collaborative Group. *Occupational and Environmental Medicine,* 1998, *55*(11), 771–778.

Cohen, B., and others. *Food Stamps Participants' Food Security and Nutrient Availability: Final Report 1999.* Contract no. 53-3198-4-025, MPR Reference no. 8243-140. [http://www.fns.usda.gov/oane/MENU/Published/NutritionEducation/Files/nutrient.pdf]. 1999.

Colditz, G. A., Cannuscio, C. C., and Frazier, A. L. "Physical Activity and Reduced Risk of Colon Cancer: Implications for Prevention." Cancer Causes & Control, 1997, *8*(4), 649–667.

Dellinger, A. M. "Barriers to Children Walking and Biking to School." Centers for Disease Control and Prevention. [http://www.cdc.gov/mmwr/preview/mmwrhtml/mm5132a1.htm]. 2002.

Dockery, D. W., and others. "An Association Between Air Pollution and Mortality in Six U.S. Cities." *New England Journal of Medicine,* 1993, *329,* 1753–1759.

Dong, L., Block, G., and Mandel, S. "Activities Contributing to Total Energy Expenditure in the United States: Results from the NHAPS Study." *International Journal of Behavioral Nutrition and Physical Activity.* [http://www.ijbnpa.org/content/1/1/4]. 2004.

Duhme, H., and others. "The Association Between Self-Reported Symptoms of Asthma and Allergic Rhinitis and Self-Reported Traffic Density on Street of Residence in Adolescents." *Epidemiology,* 1996, *7,* 578–582.

Edwards, J., Walters, S., and Griffiths, R. K. "Hospital Admissions for Asthma in Preschool Children: Relationship to Major Roads in Birmingham, United Kingdom." *Archives of Environmental Health,* 1994, *49*(4), 223–227.

English, P., and others. "Examining Associations Between Childhood Asthma and Traffic Flow Using a Geographic Information System." *Environmental Health Perspectives,* 1999, *107,* 761–767.

Environmental Defense. "Chemicals Contributing to Estimated Cancer Risk." [http://www.scorecard.org/env-releases/hap/cancer-risk.tcl?geo_area_type=us&geo_area_id=us]. 2004.

Family Practice Notebook. "Exercise Energy Expenditure." [http://www.fpnotebook.com/SPO32.htm]. 2004.

Federal Highway Administration. "Highway Traffic Noise in the United States: Problem and Response." [http://www.fhwa.dot.gov/environment/probresp.htm]. 2000.

Federal Highway Administration. *Transportation-Related Air Toxics: Case Study Materials Related to US 95 in Nevada.* Revised Final White Paper STI-902370-2308-RFWP. [http://www.fhwa.dot.gov/environment/airtoxic/casesty1.htm#toc]. 2003.

Federal Transit Administration. "Job Access and Reverse Commute Program Grants." *Federal Register* 67, no. 67 (Apr. 8, 2002), 16790–16799.

Flegal, K. M., Carroll, M. D., Ogden, C. L., and Johnson, C. L. "Prevalence and Trends in Obesity Among US Adults, 1999–2000." *Journal of the American Medical Association,* 2002, *288,* 1723–1727.

Frank, L., and Engelke, P. "How Land Use and Transportation Systems Impact Public Health." Centers for Disease Control and Prevention. [http://www.cdc.gov/nccdphp/dnpa/pdf/aces-workingpaper1.pdf]. 2000.

Friedman, B., Gordon, S., and Peers, J. "Effect of Neotraditional Neighborhood Design on Travel Characteristics." *Transportation Research Record,* 1994, *1466,* 63–70.

Great Lakes Information Network. "Zebra Mussels in the Great Lakes Region." [http://www.great-lakes.net/envt/flora-fauna/invasive/zebra.html#overview]. 2005.

Hahn, R. A., Teutsch, S. M., Rothenberg, R. B., and Marks, J. S. "Excess Deaths from Nine Chronic Diseases in the United States, 1986." *Journal of the American Medical Association,* 1990, *264*(20), 2654–2659.

Haines, M., Stansfeld, S., Head, J., and Job, R. F. "Multilevel Modeling of Aircraft Noise on Performance Tests in Schools Around Heathrow Airport London." *British Medical Journal,* 2002, *56,* 139–144.

Haines M., and others. "Chronic Aircraft Noise Exposure, Stress Responses, Mental Health and Cognitive Performance in School Children." *Psychological Medicine,* 2001a, *31,* 265–277.

Haines, M., and others. "The West London Schools Study: The Effects of Chronic Aircraft Noise Exposure on Child Health." *Psychological Medicine,* 2001b, *38,* 1385–1396.

Handy, S. "Regional Versus Local Accessibility: Neo-Traditional Development and Its Implications for Non-Work Travel." *Built Environment,* 1992, *18*(4), 253–267.

Hedberg, G., Jacobsson, K. A., Langendoen, S., and Nystrom, L. "Mortality in Circulatory Diseases, Especially Ischaemic Heart Disease, Among Swedish Professional Drivers: A Retrospective Cohort Study." *Journal of Human Ergology,* 1991, *20*(1), 1–5.

Helmrich, S. P., Ragland, D. R., Leung, R. W., and Paffenbarger, R. S., Jr. "Physical Activity and Reduced Occurrence of Non-Insulin-Dependent Diabetes Mellitus." *New England Journal of Medicine,* 1991, *325,* 147–152.

Hennessy, D. A., and Wiesenthal, D. L. "The Relationship Between Traffic Congestion, Driver Stress, and Direct Versus Indirect Coping Behaviours." *Ergonomics,* 1997, *40,* 348–361.

Hill, J. O., and Melanson, E. L. "Overview of the Determinants of Overweight and Obesity: Current Evidence and Research Issues." *Medicine and Science in Sports and Exercise,* 1999, *31*(11), S515–S521.

Hoek, G., and others. "Association Between Mortality and Indicators of Traffic-Related Air Pollution in The Netherlands: A Cohort Study." *Lancet,* 2002, *360,* 1203–1209.

Hu, F. B., and others. "Walking Compared with Vigorous Physical Activity and Risk of Type 2 Diabetes in Women: A Prospective Study." *Journal of the American Medical Association,* 1999, *282,* 1433–1439.

Hygge, S., Evans, G. W., and Bullinger, M. "A Prospective Study of Some Effects of Aircraft Noise on Cognitive Performance in Schoolchildren." *Psychological Sciences,* 2002, 469–474.

Institute of Transportation Engineers and Federal Highway Administration. *Traffic Calming: State of the Practice.* [http://www.ite.org/traffic/tcstate.htm#tcsop]. Aug. 1999.

Ising, H., and Kruppa, B. "Health Effects Caused by Noise: Evidence in the Literature from the Past 25 Years." *Noise & Health,* 2004, *6*(22), 5–13.

Joint, M. "Road Rage." In AAA Foundation for Traffic Safety, *Aggressive Driving: Three Studies.* [http://www.aaafoundation.org/pdf/agdr3study.pdf]. Mar. 1997.

Kaufman, P. R., MacDonald, J. M., Lutz, S. M., and Smallwood, S. M. *Do the Poor Pay More for Food? Item Selection and Price Differences Affect Low-Income Household Food Costs.* U.S. Department of Agriculture. Agricultural Economic Report no. 759. [http://jan.mannlib.cornell.edu/reports/general/aer/AER759.pdf]. Nov. 1997.

Kelsey, J. L., and Hardy, R. J. "Driving of Motor Vehicles as a Risk Factor for Acute Herniated Lumbar Intervertebral Disc." *American Journal of Epidemiology,* 1975, *102,* 63–73.

Kinney, P. L., and others. "Airborne Concentrations of PM(2.5) and Diesel Exhaust Particles on Harlem Sidewalks: A Community-Based Pilot Study." *Environmental Health Perspectives,* 2000, *108,* 213–218.

Krieger, N., and others. "Assessing Health Impact Assessment: Multidisciplinary and International Perspectives." *Journal of Epidemiology and Community Health,* 2003, *57,* 659–662.

Laden, F., Neas, L. M., Dockery, D. W., and Schwartz, J. "Association of Fine Particulate Matter from Different Sources with Daily Mortality in Six U.S. Cities." *Environmental Health Perspectives,* 2000, *108,* 941–947.

Langholz, B., and others. "Traffic Density and the Risk of Childhood Leukemia in a Los Angeles Case-Control Study." *Annals of Epidemiology,* 2002, *12,* 482–487.

LeCount, E. R., and Rukstinat, G. J. "Sudden Death from Heart Disease While Motoring." *Journal of the American Medical Association,* 1929, *92,* 1347–1348.

Lee, I. M. "Physical Activity and Cancer Prevention: Data from Epidemiologic Studies." *Medicine and Science in Sports and Exercise,* 2003, *35*(11), 1823–1827.

Leong, S. T., and Laortanakul, P. "Monitoring and Assessment of Daily Exposure of Roadside Workers to Traffic Noise Levels in an Asian City: A Case Study of Bangkok Streets." *Environmental Monitoring and Assessment,* 2003, *85*(1), 69–85.

Lercher, P., Evans, G. W., Meis, M., and Kofler, W. W. "Ambient Neighbourhood Noise and Children's Mental Health." *Occupational and Environmental Medicine,* 2002, *59,* 380–386.

Lin, S., and others. "Childhood Asthma Hospitalization and Residential Exposure to State Route Traffic." *Environmental Research,* 2002, *88*(2), 73–81.

Litman, T. "If Health Matters." Victoria Transport Policy Institute. [http://www.vtpi.org/tdm/tdm58.htm]. 2002.

Litman, T. "Integrating Public Health Objectives in Transportation Decision-Making." *American Journal of Health Promotion,* 2003, *18*(1), 103–108.

Loh, P., and others. "From Asthma to AirBeat: Community-Driven Monitoring of Fine Particles and Black Carbon in Roxbury, Massachusetts." *Environmental Health Perspectives,* 2002, *110* (suppl. 2), 297–301.

Mannino, D. M., and others. "Surveillance for Asthma—United States, 1960–1995." *Morbidity and Mortality Weekly Report: CDC Surveillance Summaries,* 1998, *47*(1), 1–27.

Mizell, L. "Aggressive Driving." In AAA Foundation for Traffic Safety, *Aggressive Driving: Three Studies.* [http://www.aaafoundation.org/pdf/agdr3study.pdf]. Mar. 1997.

Morland, K., Wing, S., and Diez Roux, A. "The Contextual Effect of the Local Food Environment on Residents' Diets: The Atherosclerosis Risk in Communities study." *American Journal of Public Health,* 2002, *92,* 1761–1767.

National Center for Chronic Disease Prevention and Health Promotion. "Physical Activity for Everyone: Home." [http://www.cdc.gov/nccdphp/dnpa/physical]. 2005.

National Highway Traffic Safety Administration. "The Economic Impact of Motor Vehicle Crashes 2000." [http://www.nhtsa.dot.gov/people/economic/econimpact2000/EconomicImpact.pdf]. 2000.

National Highway Traffic Safety Administration. "District of Columbia Toll of Motor Vehicle Crashes, 2001." [http://www.nhtsa.dot.gov/STSI/State_Info.cfm?Year=2001&State=D.C.]. 2001.

National Highway Traffic Safety Administration. "Safe Routes to School." [http://www.nhtsa.dot.gov/people/injury/pedbimot/bike/Safe-Routes-2002/toc.html]. 2002. National Institute on Deafness and Other Communication Disorders. "Noise-Induced Hearing Loss." [http://www.nidcd.nih.gov/health/hearing/noise.asp]. 2002.

Natural Resources Defense Council. "No Breathing in the Aisles: Diesel Exhaust Inside School Buses." [http://www.nrdc.org/air/transportation/schoolbus/sbusinx.asp]. 2001.

Nelson, A. C., and Allen, D. "If You Build Them, Commuters Will Use Them: Association Between Bicycle Facilities and Bicycle Commuting." *Transportation Research Record,* 1997, *1578,* 79–82.

Northridge, M. E., and others. "Diesel Exhaust Exposure Among Adolescents in Harlem: A Community-Driven Study." *American Journal of Public Health,* 1999, *89,* 998–1002.

Nyberg, F., and others. "Urban Air Pollution and Lung Cancer in Stockholm." *Epidemiology,* 2000, *11,* 487–495.

Paluska, S. "The Role of Physical Activity in Obesity Management." *Clinics in Family Practice,* 2002, *4,* 369.

Pearson, R. L. "Distance-Weighted Traffic Density in Proximity to a Home is a Risk Factor for Leukemia and Other Childhood Cancers." *Journal of the Air and Waste Management Association,* 2000, *50*(2), 175–180.

Pope, C. A., III, and others. "Lung Cancer, Cardiopulmonary Mortality, and Long-Term Exposure to Fine Particulate Air Pollution." *Journal of the American Medical Association,* 2002, *287,* 1132–1141.

Pucher, J. "Bicycling Boom in Germany: A Revival Engineered by Public Policy." *Transportation Quarterly,* 1997, *51*(4), 31–46.

Pucher, J., and Dijkstra, L. "Promoting Safe Walking and Cycling to Improve Public Health: Lessons from The Netherlands and Germany." *American Journal of Public Health,* 2003, *93,* 1509–1516.

Pucher, J. R., and Lefevre, C. *The Urban Transport Crisis in Europe and North America.* London: Macmillan, 1996.

Pucher, J., and Renne, J. L, "Socioeconomics of Urban Travel: Evidence from the 2001 NHTS." *Transportation Quarterly,* 2003, *57*(3), 49–77.

Raglin, J. S. "Exercise and Mental Health: Beneficial and Detrimental Effects." *Sports Medicine,* 1990, *9*(6), 323–329.

Ressel, G. W. "AHA Releases Scientific Statement on Cardiovascular Health in Childhood." *American Family Physician,* 2003, *67*(3), 645–646.

Rocchini, A. P. "Childhood Obesity and a Diabetes Epidemic." *New England Journal of Medicine,* 2002, *346,* 854–855.

Rodes, C., and others. "Measuring Concentrations of Selected Air Pollutants Inside California Vehicles." Sacramento: California Air Resources Board, 1998.

Roemer, W. H., and van Wijnen, J. H. "Daily Mortality and Air Pollution Along Busy Streets in Amsterdam, 1987–1998." *Epidemiology,* 2001, *12,* 649–653.

Samet, J. M., and others. "Fine Particulate Air Pollution and Mortality in 20 U.S. Cities, 1987–1994." *New England Journal of Medicine,* 2000, *343,* 1742–1749.

Sharples, P. M., Storey, A., Aynsley-Green, A., and Eyre, J. A. "Causes of Fatal Childhood Accidents Involving Head Injury in Northern Region, 1979–86." *British Medical Journal,* 1990, *301,* 1193–1197.

Shinar, D. "Aggressive Driving: The Contribution of the Drivers and the Situation." *Transportation Research Part F: Traffic Psychology and Behaviour,* 1998, *1,* 137–160.

Shriver, K. "Influence of Environmental Design on Pedestrian Travel Behavior in Four Austin Neighborhoods." *Transportation Research Record,* 1997, *1578,* 64–75.

Singer, J., Lundberg, U., and Frankenhaeuser, M. "Stress on the Train: A Study of Urban Commuting." In A. Baum, J. E. Singer, and S. Valins (eds.), *Advances in Environmental Psychology,* Vol. 1: *The Urban Environment.* New York: Wiley, 1978.

South Coast Air Quality Management District. *The Multiple Air Toxics Exposure Study (MATES-II).* [http://www.aqmd.gov/matesiidf/matestoc.htm]. 2004.

Spreng, M. "Possible Health Effects of Noise Induced Cortisol Increase." *Noise & Health,* 2000, *2*(7), 59–64.

Stansfeld, S., Haines, M., and Brown, B. "Noise and Health in the Urban Environment." *Reviews on Environmental Health,* 2000, *15*(1–2), 43–82.

Stansfeld, S. A., and Matheson, M. P. "Noise Pollution: Non-Auditory Effects on Health." *British Medical Bulletin,* 2003, *68,* 243–257.

Strauss, R. S. "Self-Reported Weight Status and Dieting in a Cross-Sectional Sample of Young Adolescents: National Health and Nutrition Examination Survey III." *Archives of Pediatrics & Adolescent Medicine,* 1999, *153*(7), 741–747.

Surface Transportation Policy Project. *Aggressive Driving: Are You at Risk?* [http://www.transact.org/report.asp?id=56]. 1999.

Surface Transportation Policy Project. *Mean Streets 2002.* [http://www.transact.org/PDFs/ms2002/MeanStreets2002.pdf]. 2002.

Surface Transportation Policy Project. "American Attitudes Toward Walking and Creating Better Walking Communities." [http://www.transact.org/library/factsheets/health.htm]. 2003.

Talbott, E. O., and others. "Evidence for a Dose-Response Relationship Between Occupational Noise and Blood Pressure." *Archives of Environmental Health,* 1999, *54,* 71–78.

Tester, J. M., Rutherford, G. W., Wald, Z., and Rutherford, M. W. "A Matched Case-Control Study Evaluating the Effectiveness of Speed Humps in Reducing Child Pedestrian Injuries." *American Journal of Public Health,* 2004, *94,* 646–650.

Transportation Research Board of the National Academies. *The Relative Risks of School Travel.* [http://www.nap.edu/html/SR269/SR269.pdf]. 2002.

Troiano, R. P., and Flegal, K. M. "Overweight Children and Adolescents: Description, Epidemiology, and Demographics." *Pediatrics,* 1998, *101*(3), 497–504.

U.S. Department of Agriculture, Agricultural Marketing Service. "Transportation, Trade, and U.S. Agriculture." In *Agricultural Transportation Challenges for the 21st Century: A Framework for Discussion.* [http://www.ams.usda.gov/tmd/summit/chap2.pdf]. 2004.

U.S. Department of Health and Human Services. *Physical Activity and Health: A Report of the Surgeon General.* Atlanta, Ga.: Centers for Disease Control and Prevention, National Center for Chronic Disease Prevention and Health Promotion, 1996.

U.S. Department of Health and Human Services. *Healthy People 2010: Understanding and Improving Health.* [http://www.healthypeople.gov/Document/pdf/uih/uih.pdf]. 2003.

U.S. Department of Transportation. *Traffic Safety Facts 2002.* [http://www-nrd.nhtsa.dot.gov/pdf/nrd-30/NCSA/TSFAnn/TSF2002Final.pdf]. 2002a.

U.S. Department of Transportation. *Traffic Safety Facts 2002: Pedalcyclists.* [http://www-nrd.nhtsa.dot.gov/pdf/nrd-30/NCSA/TSF2002/2002pcyfacts.pdf]. 2002b.

U.S. Department of Transportation. *Traffic Safety Facts 2002: Pedestrians.* [http://www-nrd.nhtsa.dot.gov/pdf/nrd-30/NCSA/TSF2002/2002pedfacts.pdf]. 2002c.

U.S. Department of Transportation. *Highway Traffic Noise.* [http://www.fhwa.dot.gov/environment/htnoise.htm]. 2004.

U.S. Environmental Protection Agency. *Emissions Standards Reference Guide for Heavy-Duty and Non-Road Engines.* EPA420-F-97-014. [http://www.epa.gov/otaq/cert/hd-cert/stds-eng.pdf]. Sept. 1997.

U.S. Environmental Protection Agency. *National Air Pollutant Emission Trends, 1900–1997.* Washington, D.C.: U.S. Environmental Protection Agency, 1998.

U.S. Environmental Protection Agency. *Indicators of the Environmental Impact of Transportation.* EPA 230-R-99-001. [http://www.epa.gov/otaq/transp/99indict.pdf]. 1999.

U.S. Environmental Protection Agency. *Heavy-Duty Engine and Vehicle Standards and Highway Diesel Fuel Sulfur Control Standards.* EPA420-F-00-057. [http://www.epa.gov/otaq/regs/hd2007/frm/f00057.pdf]. Dec. 2000a.

U.S. Environmental Protection Agency. *National Air Emissions Trends, 1900–1998.* [http://www.epa.gov/ttn/chief/trends/trends98/chapter3.pdf]. 2000b.

U.S. Environmental Protection Agency. *Tier 2 Standards.* [http://www.epa.gov/otaq/regs/ld-hwy/tier-2/frm/fr-t2reg.pdf]. 2000c.

U.S. Environmental Protection Agency. "EPA Lead Trends." [http://www.epa.gov/airtrends/lead.html]. 2004.

U.S. General Accounting Office. *Aviation and the Environment: FAA's Role in Major Airport Noise Programs.* [http://www.netvista.net/~hpb/rc00098.pdf]. 2000.

van Kempen, E. E., and others. "The Association Between Noise Exposure and Blood Pressure and Ischemic Heart Disease: A Meta-Analysis." *Environmental Health Perspectives,* 2002, *110,* 307–317.

Van Vliet, P., and others. "Motor Vehicle Exhaust and Chronic Respiratory Symptoms in Children Living Near Freeways." *Environmental Research,* 1997, *74*(2), 122–132.

Venn, A. J., and others. "Living Near a Main Road and the Risk of Wheezing Illness in Children." *American Journal of Respiratory and Critical Care Medicine,* 2001, *164*(12), 2177–2180.

Victoria Transport Policy Institute. "Socioeconomics of Urban Travel: Evidence from the 2001 NHTS." *Transportation Quarterly,* 2003, *57,* 49–77.

Victoria Transport Policy Institute. "Evaluating Safety and Health Impacts TDM Impacts on Road Safety, Personal Security and Public Health." [http://www.vtpi.org/tdm/tdm58.htm]. 2004.

Victoria Transport Policy Institute. "About This Encyclopedia." *Online TDM Encyclopedia.* [http://www.vtpi.org/tdm/tdm12.htm]. n.d.

Wallace, R. B., and Doebbeling, B. N. "Effects of the Physical Environment: Noise as a Health Hazard." In R. B. Wallace (ed.), *Maxcy-Rosenau-Last Public Health and Preventive Medicine.* (14th ed.) Stamford, Conn.: Appleton & Lang, 1998.

Wang, G., and Dietz, W. H. "Economic Burden of Obesity in Youths Aged 6 to 17 Years: 1979–1999." *Pediatrics,* 2002, *109*(5), e81.

Wei, M., and others. "Relationship Between Low Cardiorespiratory Fitness and Mortality in Normal-Weight, Overweight, and Obese Men." *Journal of the American Medical Association,* 1999, *282,* 1547–1553.

World Health Organization. "Adverse Health Effects of Noise." [http://www.who.int/docstore/peh/noise/Comnoise3.htm]. 2004.

For Further Information

Here are selected additional resources for students interested in more details on public health impacts of transportation.

National Highway Traffic Safety Administration [www.nhtsa.gov].

The National Highway Traffic Safety Administration collects and publishes federal data on traffic crashes, injuries, and mortality.

Surface Transportation Policy Project [www.transact.org].

The Surface Transportation Policy Project is a diverse, nationwide coalition working to ensure safer communities and smarter transportation choices that enhance the economy, improve public health, promote social equity, and protect the environment. They periodically publish reports on traffic and pedestrian safety.

The Victoria Transportation Policy Institute [http://www.vtpi.org/].

The Victoria Transport Policy Institute is an independent research organization dedicated to developing innovative and practical solutions to transportation problems. They publish a useful online encyclopedia describing these solutions.

United States Environmental Protection Agency, Office of Transportation and Air Quality (OTAQ) [http://www.epa.gov/otaq/].

The EPA Office of Transportation and Air Quality provides information on linkages between transportation planning and air quality as well as the regulations that pertain to this topic.

Texas Transportation Institute (TTI) [http://tti.tamu.edu/].

TTI is an official research agency for the Texas Department of Transportation and the Texas Railroad Commission. TTI works closely with many state and federal agencies as well as the private sector to improve the safety and efficiency of the transportation system.

Environmental Defense [http://www.environmentaldefense.org/go/traffic].

Environmental Defense is a leading national nonprofit organization that links science, economics, and law to create innovative, equitable, and cost-effective solutions to society's most urgent environmental problems. The organization's Web site provides background information on linkages among land use, transportation, and health and outlines a number of solutions.

These two books provide further information about the effects of transportation on health.

British Medical Association. *Road Transport and Health.* London: British Medical Association, 1997.
Frumkin, H., Frank, L., and Jackson, R.J. *Urban Sprawl and Public Health.* Washington: Island Press, 2004.

CHAPTER EIGHTEEN

WATER AND HEALTH

Timothy Ford

The existence of life, whether human, animal, avian, reptilian, amphibian, plant, or microbe, depends on water. The search for life (as we understand it) on other planets is always predicated on the search for evidence of water. Humans are approximately 60 percent water, and we cannot survive for more than a few days without it. It is therefore not surprising that human culture has been defined by water over the centuries. One has only to look at development along the major river systems of the world to realize how the water environment has dominated, and continues to dominate, human cultures.

The Hydrologic Cycle

Our planet would appear to have a surfeit of water, but most water is unavailable for human use. Over 97 percent of the world's water is salty, found in the oceans and (to a much lower extent) in inland seas and saltwater lakes. What remains is freshwater, but over two-thirds of this is locked in the Antarctic and Arctic ice caps. The freshwater that remains, in rivers and lakes, in the atmosphere, and within the ground, makes up less than 1 percent of the world's water. This is the supply potentially available for drinking, irrigating crops, and other uses.

Water is in continuous motion among these various locations, in a so-called hydrologic cycle that dominates the health of the planet. Without continuous

FIGURE 18.1. THE HYDROLOGIC CYCLE.

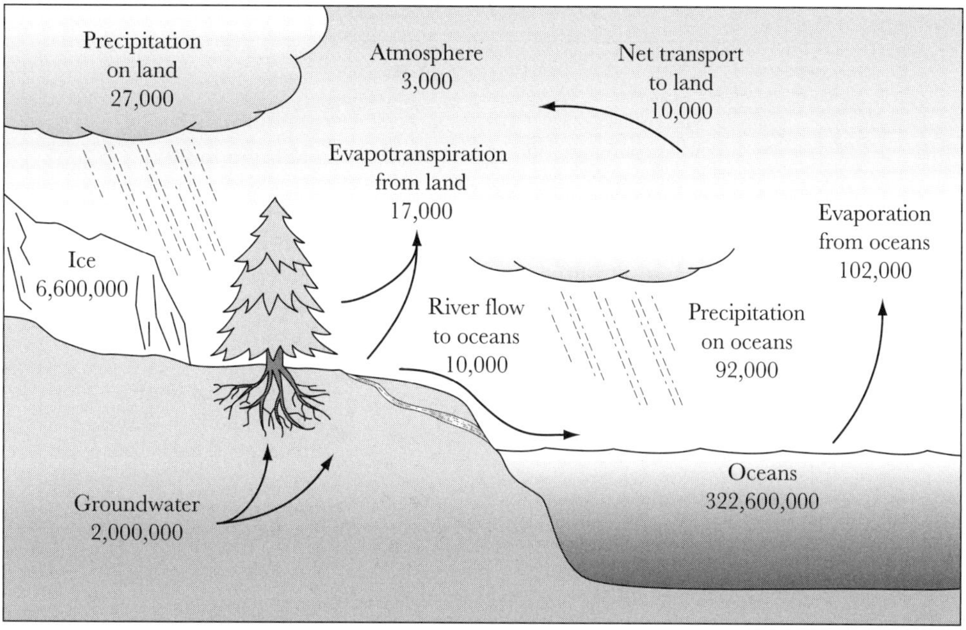

Note: Pools are in cubic miles; fluxes are in cubic miles per year.

Source: Redrawn from Winter, Harvey, Franke, and Alley, 2001. Originally modified from Schlesinger, W. H. *Biogeochemistry-An Analysis of Global Change.* San Diego: Academic Press, 1991, with permission from Elsevier.

evaporation from the oceans, precipitation on land, and runoff back to the oceans, no surface or groundwater recharge can take place, and we would eventually exhaust our available freshwater supplies. Figure 18.1 provides a diagrammatic overview of the hydrologic cycle—the dominant flows, or fluxes, and the critical reservoirs, or pools.

The hydrologic cycle teaches us to view water and health with a holistic perspective. The compartments of the hydrologic cycle are either directly or indirectly connected, and perturbation of one compartment is likely to affect all other compartments and therefore both human and ecological health. These interconnections are diagrammatically illustrated in Figure 18.2. This chapter explores these interconnections. It describes several processes that are crucially important to humans, including water consumption, waste production, waste treatment and discharge, and treatment for reuse, and outlines the multitude of health concerns at each step.

FIGURE 18.2. SCHEMATIC OF THE INTERCONNECTIONS BETWEEN WATER AND HEALTH.

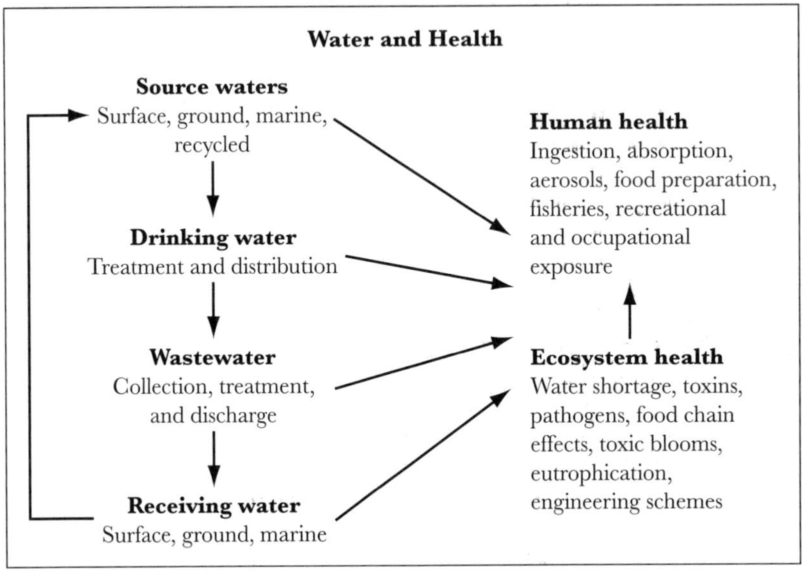

Important Definitions

Available freshwater supplies are often conceptually divided into surface water and groundwater. The U.S. Environmental Protection Agency (EPA, 2004) defines these terms as follows:

- *Surface water:* all water naturally open to the atmosphere (rivers, lakes, reservoirs, ponds, streams, impoundments, seas, estuaries, and so forth)
- *Groundwater:* the supply of freshwater found beneath the earth's surface, usually in aquifers, which supplies wells and springs

Because surface water and groundwater are not independent of each other, an overlap category is also recognized. The EPA defines this as

- *Groundwater under the direct influence of surface water:* any water beneath the surface of the ground with: (1) significant occurrence of insects or other microorganisms, algae, or large-diameter pathogens; (2) significant and relatively rapid shifts in water characteristics such as turbidity, temperature, conductivity, or pH which closely correlate to climatological or surface water conditions

These distinctions are important because they directly affect how we view the quality of a water resource and how we manage that resource. Ideally, water used as a drinking-water source (often called *source water*) should be of the highest quality, reducing the cost of water treatment and the risk of contamination. Groundwater has traditionally been considered a high-quality resource, because as rainfall and other surface waters percolate through soil into groundwater, they are cleaned by physical, chemical, and microbiological processes in the soil. However, the traditional confidence in groundwater may not always be well placed, as human activities such as land management practices can influence even relatively deep aquifers. Surface water, or groundwater under the direct influence of surface water (GWUDI), has traditionally been less favored as a source for drinking water. However, groundwater is not always available, and municipalities may have no choice but to implement extensive and costly surface water treatment. At present, just over half of Americans get their drinking water from surface sources.

Surface and GWUDI water may be considered suitable for agricultural, industrial, or recreational uses with no or limited treatment. Different criteria are therefore developed and applied to source waters, depending on their ultimate use. Surface waters that are used as drinking-water sources are regulated by far stricter criteria, for example, than are waters used to irrigate crops. A fuller discussion of water regulations appears later in this chapter.

Water Use and Water Scarcity

Water scarcity may be one of the most critical health threats to human society today. In the long term, societies can survive only on renewable resources. When a resource is nonrenewable then it is available only in finite quantities, and when a resource is extracted faster than it can be renewed then eventually supply will not meet demand. Either pattern of use is nonsustainable. The most familiar examples of finite resources are fossil fuels. As explained in Chapter Fifteen, fossil fuel use is nonsustainable in the long term, leading to considerable pressure to develop alternative energy sources. Just as fossil fuels are mined, so is water. Technology has allowed us to extract more and more of the water trapped within the earth's crust. This has allowed human habitation, and agricultural and industrial development, to spread to arid areas of the planet that are poorly suited to sustain human life. Unfortunately, in arid regions aquifer recharge rates are low, and the deep aquifers laid down by countless ice ages are being gradually depleted. (Several books provide informative discussions of water use and water scarcity; see, for example, Gleick, 1993, 1998, 2000, 2002; Clarke, 1993; Postel, 1997.)

Figure 18.3 shows the Ogallala Aquifer, a groundwater resource so well known that it was highlighted in *National Geographic* magazine (Zwingle, 1993). This vast

FIGURE 18.3. THE OGALLALA AQUIFER.

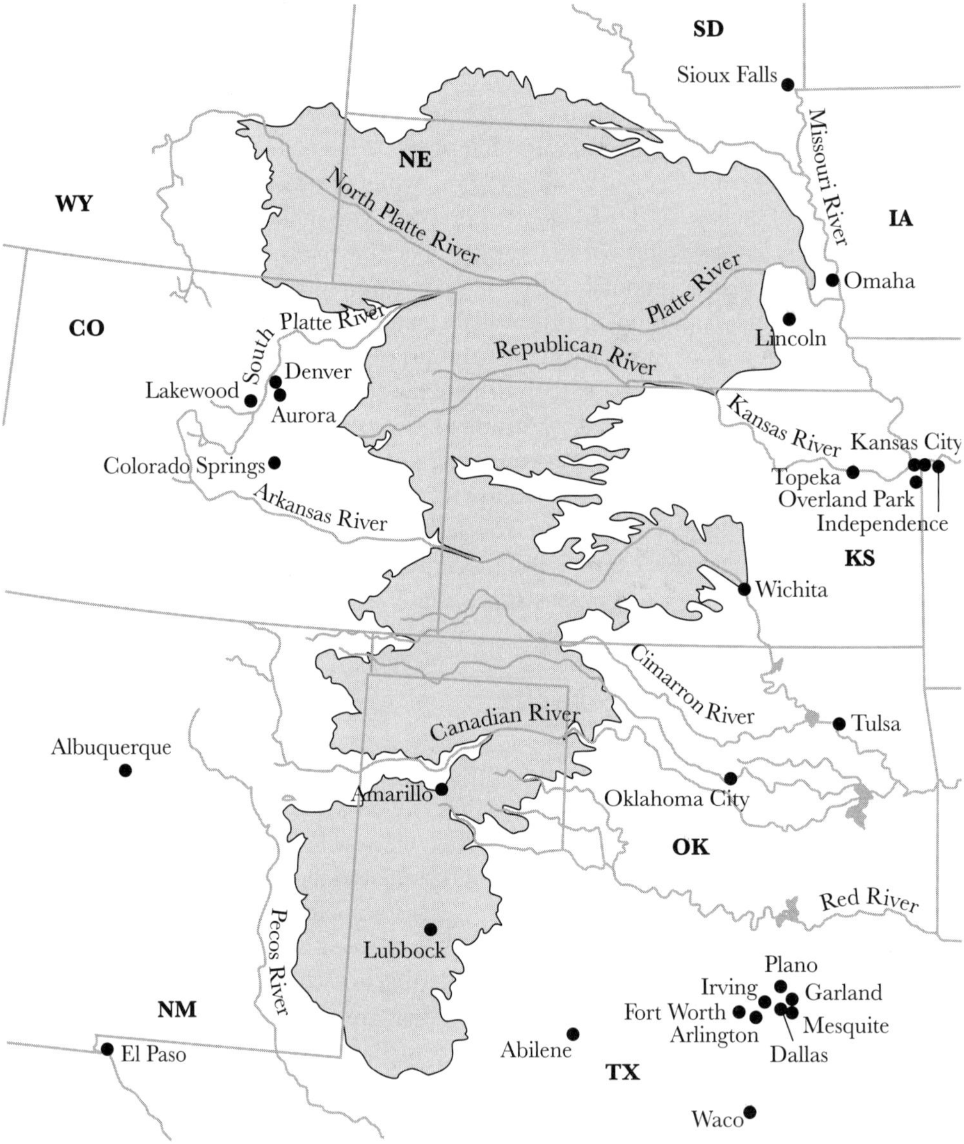

Source: USGS High Plains Regional Ground-Water Quality Study (USGS, 2004).

aquifer underlies 174,000 square miles in parts of eight states from South Dakota to Texas, and provides an estimated 30 percent of all groundwater used for irrigation in the United States (U.S. Geological Survey [USGS], 2004). It was water from the Ogallala that helped convert the central plains of North America from a dust bowl to an agriculturally rich region. However, the Ogallala is a finite resource. It consists of *fossil water,* water sequestered underground for thousands of years, and the current rate of water extraction far exceeds the rate at which it is replenished. For some states, groundwater supplies are expected to be depleted in the next twenty to thirty years. Already, farmers in the region are having to drill much deeper wells or rely on surface water instead, which has lowered farm yield in the region substantially. In addition to water scarcity, water quality in parts of the aquifer may have been compromised by agricultural practices.

Population and Water Scarcity

The adequacy of the water supply reflects a balance among water availability, population, and the ways in which people use water. In many parts of the world, as described in Chapter Ten, population pressure places a severe strain on water resources. According to the U.S.-based Population Action International, by 2025 27 percent of nations will face *water stress* (defined as a water supply at or below 1,700 m^3 per person per year), and an additional 11 percent of nations will face *water scarcity* (defined as a water supply at or below 1,000 m^3 per person per year) (Engelman and others, 2004). These numbers reflect all domestic, industrial, and agricultural water use for a region. They are based on conservative projections of population growth; if population growth is higher than anticipated, then water will be relatively more scarce. Although some countries have enormous supplies of water (Greenland, the world's leader, has more than 10 million m^3 per capita per year), others are arid. At the extreme limit of water availability, the West Bank and the Seychelles have zero per capita water availability and are entirely dependent on other countries for their water supply.

Water use varies not only with population but with level of development and affluence. At one extreme, people in wealthy countries with ample water supplies are relatively profligate users of water. In the United States, for example, where the supply of renewable freshwater is estimated to be 10,800 m^3 per person per year (not including Alaska or Hawaii) (United Nations Educational, Cultural and Scientific Organization [UNESCO], 2003), the estimated annual per capita withdrawal is 1,688 m^3. Of this, 12 percent is used in homes, 46 percent in industry, and 42 percent in agriculture (Pacific Institute, 2003). The 12 percent used in homes represents 555 liters per person per day, of which less than 0.2 percent is required for drinking (based on EPA's estimated daily water consumption of 927 ml per person per day (EPA, 2000). Advanced sanitation (including flush toilets) is the norm in the United States and requires large amounts of domestic water use.

In contrast, Somalia's supply of renewable freshwater is far lower, an estimated 1,538 m^3 per person per year. The per capita withdrawal is also far lower than that in the United States, an estimated 70 m^3 per year, of which 3 percent is used in homes, a negligible amount is used in industry, and 97 percent is used for agriculture. In this case, domestic water use represents 5.75 liters per person per day, of which close to 20 percent is required for consumption. There is little margin of safety in this situation, and a temporary disruption of the water supply, such as a drought, can be devastating.

Agriculture and Water Scarcity

The division of water use in Somalia is typical for many of the less developed countries and reflects the enormous amount of water that is needed to grow food. In fact, on a global scale, agriculture accounts for almost 70 percent of water withdrawal (UNESCO, 2003). Many Web sites list water-related facts, and one much-quoted figure, taken from the Web site of Brita (2005), a major manufacturer of household drinking water filters, is that approximately 6,800 gallons of water are required to grow a day's food for a family of four. Another oft-quoted figure is that 1,000 tons of water are required to produce 1 ton of wheat (Postel, 1999). Nonedible crops such as cotton also require large amounts of water; the decimation of the Aral Sea is attributed to cotton irrigation (Ellis, 1990). As a result, it is not surprising that agricultural uses of water are the greatest global contributors to water scarcity and to depletion of aquifers. Considerable efforts have been made over the past decade to replace conventional irrigation with methods that minimize water wastage, such as drip or other micro-irrigation techniques. (The irrigation "crisis" is described in detail in Postel, 1999.)

Political Implications

The dependence of food production on irrigation links freshwater use with food security and therefore with human nutrition and well-being. Accordingly, the political implications of water scarcity are enormous. Most of the major rivers and aquifers of the world cross international or at least state borders. Any use of water by one nation or state affects all downstream users. Impoundments (dams) are particularly damaging to downstream users, as they dramatically reduce water flow for these communities, particularly during dry seasons. There are numerous examples of national and international crises emerging from shared water resources (as shown in Table 18.1). In the extreme, these crises may erupt into

TABLE 18.1. HOT SPOTS: PAST AND POTENTIAL FUTURE WATER RESOURCE CONFLICTS.

River Basin	Length (km)	Countries	Source of Conflict
Nile	6,693	Tanzania, Kenya, Zaire, Burundi, Rwanda, Ethiopia, Uganda, Sudan, and Egypt	Irrigation
Tigris/Euphrates	1,840/2,700	Turkey, Syria, Iraq, and Iran	Hydroelectric projects; irrigation
Indus/Beas/Sutlej/Ravi	2,896 (Indus)	India, Pakistan, and Tibet	Diversions; Sikh versus Hindu
Ganges/Brahmaputra	2,414/2,896	India, Bangladesh, Nepal, and Bhutan	Deforestation and siltation; diversions
Jordan	93	Israel, Jordan, Lebanon, and Syria	Diversions (arguably the underlying cause of Arab-Israeli conflicts)
Parana/Paraguay	3,998 (Parana)	Brazil, Paraguay, Bolivia, Argentina, and Uruguay	Dams (hydroelectric)
Rio Grande	3,057	United States and Mexico	Development; irrigation
Colorado	2,336	United States and Mexico	Development; irrigation

what has been called *resource wars* (Klare, 2001). (More detailed discussions can be found in Chapter Twelve of this volume; Clarke, 1993; Gleick, 1993, 1998.)

Climate Change and Water

Global climate change is discussed in detail in Chapter Eleven. Here, we consider the effect of climate change on water. Warming global temperatures will result in increased evaporation from the oceans, an increase in water vapor in the atmosphere, and increasing precipitation, including more severe weather events (Easterling and others, 2000). There is also a positive feedback loop involved, because more water vapor in the atmosphere will exacerbate the greenhouse effect. Weather changes are expected to be complex, with precipitation increasing in some regions and decreasing in others. The burden of water scarcity may shift. For example, on the one hand, increases in rainfall could benefit arid regions.

On the other hand, mountainous regions that depend primarily on snowpack for their water may experience shortages if warmer temperatures prevent snow accumulation. Although climate models are filled with uncertainty and predictions must be viewed with extreme caution, it appears likely that the hydrologic cycle as we now know it will change in coming decades and that in some regions water scarcity may substantially worsen.

Human Impacts on Aquatic Systems

Not only do water quantity and quality affect human health but human activities affect every aspect of aquatic ecosystems. Hydrodynamics—the way water moves—is dramatically altered by projects such as dams, levies, canals, channelization, concretization, and extraction. In turn, fundamental nutrient cycles are altered in ways that completely change the biology and chemistry of a system. In extreme cases this can lead to eutrophication (when high nutrient loads stimulate blooms of algae in the water, in turn stimulating microbial activity). Oxygen is used up and massive fish kills may result. As shown in Table 18.2,

TABLE 18.2. EXAMPLES OF HEALTH CONSEQUENCES OF ENGINEERING SCHEMES.

Engineering Scheme	Examples	Environmental Consequences	Health Effects
Dams and irrigation projects	Aswan High Dam, Egypt; Sennâr Dam, Sudan; Akosombo Dam, West Africa	Created habitat for snails that carry the schistosome parasite	Dramatic increases in schistosomiasis
Hydroelectric projects	James Bay	Conditions created for methylation of mercury in sediments and subsequent accumulation through the food chain	Levels of mercury in Inuit that exceed WHO health guidelines
Channelization	Mississippi River	Exacerbated extreme Midwest flooding events	Huge economic consequences, loss of property, and loss of livestock; depression
Channelization, intensive draining, diking, and developing	Florida's Kissimmee River, Lake Okeechobee, and the Everglades	Destroyed habitat for wildfowl and fish nurseries; caused lake eutrophication, algal blooms, and fish kills; reduced groundwater recharge, and dramatically changed the Everglades ecosystem	Primarily ecological and economic; long-term effects on human health of changes to Florida's hydrological cycle as yet unknown

changes such as these can directly affect health, completing a cycle of humans to water to humans.

Water contaminants fall into two general categories, chemical and biological. Chemical contaminants, such as arsenic, may occur naturally or may be discharged into water through industrial, agricultural, municipal, and recreational activity. Biological contaminants include bacteria, viruses, and protozoans; these originate from many sources, including human and animal wastes. The next two sections of this chapter present information on these two categories of contaminants.

Chemical Contaminants

A wide variety of chemicals can contaminate water, as shown in Table 18.3. These contaminants may originate from either point sources or nonpoint sources, which are defined as follows (EPA, 2004).

- *Point source:* a stationary location or fixed facility from which pollutants are discharged; any single identifiable source of pollution; for example, a pipe, ditch, ship, ore pit, factory smokestack.
- *Nonpoint sources:* diffuse pollution sources (that is, the pollutants do not have a single point of origin or are not introduced into a receiving stream from a specific outlet; for example, they are pollutants carried off the land by stormwater). Common nonpoint sources are agriculture, forestry, urban, mining, construction, dams, channels, land disposal, saltwater intrusion, and city streets.

Examples of point source chemical releases include discharges of mercury, solvents, or polychlorinated biphenyls (PCBs) from industrial drainpipes, and leakage of MTBE and petrochemicals from corroding underground gasoline tanks. A major example of a nonpoint source is agricultural runoff containing pesticides and nutrients. City streets and parking lots are important nonpoint sources; these sources can result in massive contamination of surface and groundwaters, as the impermeable surfaces accumulate high concentrations of street contaminants such as oils and household wastes that then run off during heavy rainfall. Some contaminants, such as toxic metals and acidity in mine drainage, can arise from both point and nonpoint sources. Other sources of anthropogenic contaminants include deep injection of wastes into groundwater, lead leaching from older drinking-water distribution pipes, and the vast quantities of pharmaceuticals that are released in human sewage and from agriculture and aquaculture.

TABLE 18.3. CLASSES OF CHEMICAL CONTAMINANTS IN WATER.

	Classes	Examples
Petroleum and coal hydrocarbons	Crude oil	Alkanes, heterocyclics, aromatics
	Refined oil	Gasoline, diesel, heating fuels
	Combustion or conversion products	Polycyclic aromatic hydrocarbon (PAHs), synfuels, by-products
Synthetic organics	Halogenated hydrocarbons	Polychlorinated biphenyls (PCBs), chlorofluorocarbons (CFCs), pesticides, solvents
	Plasticizers, phthalic acid esters	Polyvinyl chloride (PVC), DEHP
	Others	Surfactants, organophosphate pesticides, synthetic pyrethrinoids, fuel additives (MBTE)
Metals	Cadmium, mercury, lead, silver, zinc, copper, chromium, nickel, arsenic	
Radionuclides	Transuranics	Plutonium, americium, curium
	Fission products	Cesium-137, strontium-90
	Activation products	Cobalt-60, manganese-54, zinc-65, chromium-51
	Natural	U-Th decay series
Disinfection by-products	Chlorination, chloramination, and ozonation by-products	Chloroform, trichloroacetic acids, chlorinated furanones, bromate
Industrial wastes	Process by-products, from mining, dredging, and other resource extraction processes	Many of the chemicals already named, plus acids, ash, desalination brines, heat (from cooling water), anticorrosion chemicals, cyanide, and so forth
Municipal and agricultural wastes (not including pathogens)	Nutrients, range of household and agricultural chemicals, including those suspected to cause endocrine disruption	Phosphorus, nitrogen, carbon, silicon, antibiotics, disinfectants, pesticides, fluoride, nonylphenol ethoxylates,[a] and so forth

[a]Of recent concern are the nonylphenol ethoxylates, chemicals that have been used extensively—as detergents, emulsifiers, wetting agents and dispersing agents—in a wide range of industrial processes and consumer products. These compounds and their degradation products are thought to have estrogenic properties with profound consequences for aquatic biota (disrupting or preventing reproduction) and may also be a human health concern.

Source: Adapted in part from Capone and Bauer, 1992.

Naturally Occurring Chemical Contaminants

Many naturally occurring chemicals are toxic to humans. In most cases these result from nonpoint sources. Chemicals that naturally occur in the earth's soils and rocks, for example, can readily diffuse into ground or surface waters. As a result, water may be naturally enriched with fluoride, selenium, arsenic, and a variety of other chemicals. Nitrogen contamination of ground and surface waters is often attributed to wastewater discharge or excessive addition of fertilizers. However, leguminous plants, such as soybeans and alfalfa, which have a symbiotic relationship with bacteria that fix atmospheric nitrogen, may also contribute to nitrate enrichment of ground and surface waters (Cox and Kahle, 1999).

Arsenic is an important example of a naturally occurring toxic contaminant of water. Very high levels of arsenic exist in groundwater in Bangladesh and West Bengal. To reduce risks of epidemic cholera and other diarrheal diseases, the United Nations Children's Fund (UNICEF) began a program in the 1970s to install tube wells throughout these regions. The consequent exposure to arsenic in drinking water (described in greater detail in Chapter Thirteen, Box 13.3), is considered one of the greatest environmental disasters in history. However, even lower levels of arsenic contamination, as occur in many parts of the United States, are cause for concern, as there is strong evidence linking these exposures to skin disease and cancer. Stricter regulations have met political barriers due to the fact that arsenic is a naturally occurring compound that is expensive to remove from drinking water. Many medium, small, and very small water systems (defined as serving 3,301 to 10,000, 501 to 3,300, and 25 to 500 people, respectively) use source water contaminated with arsenic, at concentrations that barely met the old standard of 50 $\mu g/l$. To meet the new recommended standard of 10 $\mu g/l$, many of these systems require technologies far beyond their limited operating budgets (Ford and others, 2005). For some water systems, meeting these standards may result in generation of large volumes of arsenic-contaminated wastes. This in itself could present an environmental health risk, as disposal practices have not yet been fully established or their safety tested.

An increasingly recognized natural source of chemical contaminants is toxins produced primarily by algae and cyanobacteria. Human activity can promote the production of these toxins through nutrient loading and resulting eutrophication. From the perspective of drinking water and recreational use of freshwaters, cyanobacterial blooms are of particular concern.

Cyanobacteria, sometimes imprecisely called *blue-green algae,* are simple photosynthetic organisms closely related to bacteria, found in water bodies throughout the world. Water bodies that are rich in nutrients, such as eutrophic lakes, agricultural ponds, or catch basins, may support proliferation of cyanobacteria. In some cases a body of clear water can become turbid, discolored (green, blue-green, or reddish-brown) and covered with a film, or scum, in just a few days. Several genera of cyanobacteria, including *Microcystis, Anabaena,* and *Aphanizomenon,* release a wide range of low molecular weight chemicals that include neurotoxins, hepatotoxins, skin and gastrointestinal irritants, enzyme inhibitors, and compounds that create taste and odor problems, such as geosmin. People who drink or swim in contaminated waters may be at risk, as are livestock and wildlife. Numerous fatalities have been reported (Bartram and Chorus, 1999; Metcalf and Codd, 2004).

In addition to the cyanobacteria, many species of planktonic algae produce toxins that accumulate in shellfish or finfish, resulting in poisonings. These include paralytic shellfish poisoning (PSP, caused by saxitoxins), diarrheic shellfish poisoning (DSP, caused by okadaic acid), amnesic shellfish poisoning (ASP, caused by domoic acid), neurotoxic shellfish poisoning (NSP, caused by brevetoxins), and ciguatera fish poisoning (CFP, caused by ciguatoxin or maitotoxin). A number of these poisonings are life threatening and constitute major public health threats worldwide, with enormous economic implications due to fisheries closures. (Many resources on this topic are available through the Woods Hole Oceanographic Institution, 2005.)

Anthropogenic Chemical Contaminants

Industrialization has left an enormous legacy of contamination. Exploitation of the earth's resources has resulted in ground and surface waters contaminated with heavy metals and hydrocarbons. Uncontrolled industrial discharges, military activities, landfills, leaking underground storage tanks, agricultural activities, and many other human activities have and continue to contaminate ground and surface waters.

Anthropogenic chemicals can be divided into a number of classes, as described in Table 18.3. However, in terms of broad categories, they can be thought of as organic, inorganic, or a combination of the two, as in the case of methylmercury. The environmental fate and transport of a contaminant chemical is a direct function of its chemistry (discussed later in this section). For example, the organic contaminants popularly known as persistent organic pollutants (POPs) are so named because their chemistry dictates that they are degraded at negligible or only very slow rates by naturally occurring microbes, are rapidly partitioned into soils or sediments, and consequently are present in the environment for very long periods of time. PCBs, the classic example of a POP, persist for decades at multiple hazardous waste sites throughout the United States and globally (see the section on environmental reservoirs later in this chapter).

It is sobering to think about the number of chemicals dispersed into the environment. The USGS (2000) estimates that about 1 billion pounds of pesticides are used in the United States every year, with about 80 percent used in agriculture. As part of its National Water Quality Assessment Program (NAWQA), the USGS is conducting the Pesticide National Synthesis Project to obtain an assessment of pesticides in the streams, rivers, and groundwater of the United States. For a wealth of information on pesticide contamination, see USGS, 2000; for discussion of a variety of additional water quality issues in the United States, see NAWQA, 2005.) (An interesting example of this information is a report on the pesticides used on golf courses and detected in groundwater beneath those sites (USGS, 1998), which lists no fewer than thirty-nine herbicides, thirty insecticides, thirty-two fungicides, four nematicides, three adjuvants (chemicals added to pesticide formulations to increase efficiency), and seven growth hormones. Golf courses in New Jersey alone are credited with twenty-eight herbicides, fifteen insecticides, twenty-five fungicides, one nematicide, and seven growth hormones. Very few of these chemicals have been rigorously tested for aquatic toxicity but may be considered POPs that will remain in sediments and soils for many years, decades, or even centuries (see the section on storage later in this chapter).

Transformations

Once contaminants are released into the aquatic environment, they have considerable potential for both chemical and biological transformation to more or less toxic forms, analogous to the human biotransformation described in Chapter Two. As a result, although water may contain parent molecules such as pesticides and herbicides, a range of degradation products may also be present. Remediation, whether chemical or biological, attempts to replicate some of these changes, reducing toxic chemicals to nontoxic degradation products such as CO_2, CH_4, H_2O, or, in the case of metals, insoluble or otherwise nonbioavailable forms. Unfortunately, transformations in the natural environment frequently result in more toxic or increasingly bioavailable forms. For example, in the presence of oxygen (aerobic conditions), many groups of organisms are capable of breaking down trichloroethylene, a commonly used solvent that frequently ends up in groundwater. One end product is vinyl chloride, a known carcinogen that cannot be further degraded under aerobic conditions.

Biological Transformations. For almost every organic contaminant released to the aquatic environment, there appears to be a microbe that can employ the compound as an energy or carbon source, or simply assist in its degradation through the process of cometabolism, where enzymes that evolved for another substrate fortuitously degrade the contaminant with no benefit to the microbe. As with organic contaminants, reduced forms of certain metals can be used as energy sources (electron donors) and oxidized forms can be used as energy sinks (electron acceptors). (Many textbooks discuss microbial metabolism and pollutant interactions, for example, Mitchell, 1992; Madigan, Martinko, and Parker, 2004.)

One other major interaction between microbes and contaminants results from detoxification mechanisms. The methylation of mercury may be one such mechanism, although the specific benefits of this process to the microbe are currently unknown. The case of the James Bay poisonings mentioned in Table 18.2 provides a good example of the process. Impoundments built for hydroelectricity in the James Bay region of Quebec resulted in extensive flooding of forested lands. Organic matter degradation by microbes resulted in consumption of oxygen, anoxic conditions at the sediment water interface, and ideal conditions for growth of anaerobic sulfate-reducing bacteria (SRB). SRB are known to convert inorganic mercury, either naturally occurring in soils or from atmospheric deposition, to methylmercury, which is highly lipid soluble and rapidly accumulates through the food chain. Contaminated fish were then eaten by Inuit communities, resulting in concentrations of mercury in people that exceeded World Health Organization (WHO) guidelines (Calow and Petts, 1992).

Chemical Transformations. A leading example of chemical transformations is the formation of disinfection by-products (DBPs). When chlorine is added to drinking water as part of the disinfection process, it reacts with naturally occurring organic compounds present in source and distributed waters. The result is potentially toxic chlorinated-by-products. Examples of these compounds include halomethanes such as chloroform, bromoform, dichloromethane, and dibromomethane. Similarly, ozone reacts with naturally occurring bromine to form toxic bromates. DBPs are discussed in more detail later in this chapter.

Deposition, Storage, and Bioconcentration

For many years it was thought that chemicals discharged into receiving waters would simply be diluted to the point that they could be ignored. In recent years it has become abundantly clear that dilution is no longer sufficient. Chapter Two described how chemicals move through the body in predictable ways, a keystone of toxicology; the same is true for chemicals in ecosystems, including hydrologic cycles, as demonstrated in Figure 18.4.

The fate of a given chemical in receiving waters is a function of both its physical and chemical nature. The degree to which a chemical may partition into sediments or into the biota depends to some degree on its partition coefficient, a measure of its relative affinity for an organic solvent (octanol) and water. This in turn depends to some degree on measures of solubility and hydrophobicity.

FIGURE 18.4. PESTICIDE MOVEMENT IN THE HYDROLOGIC CYCLE, INCLUDING PESTICIDE MOVEMENT TO AND FROM SEDIMENT AND AQUATIC BIOTA WITHIN THE STREAM.

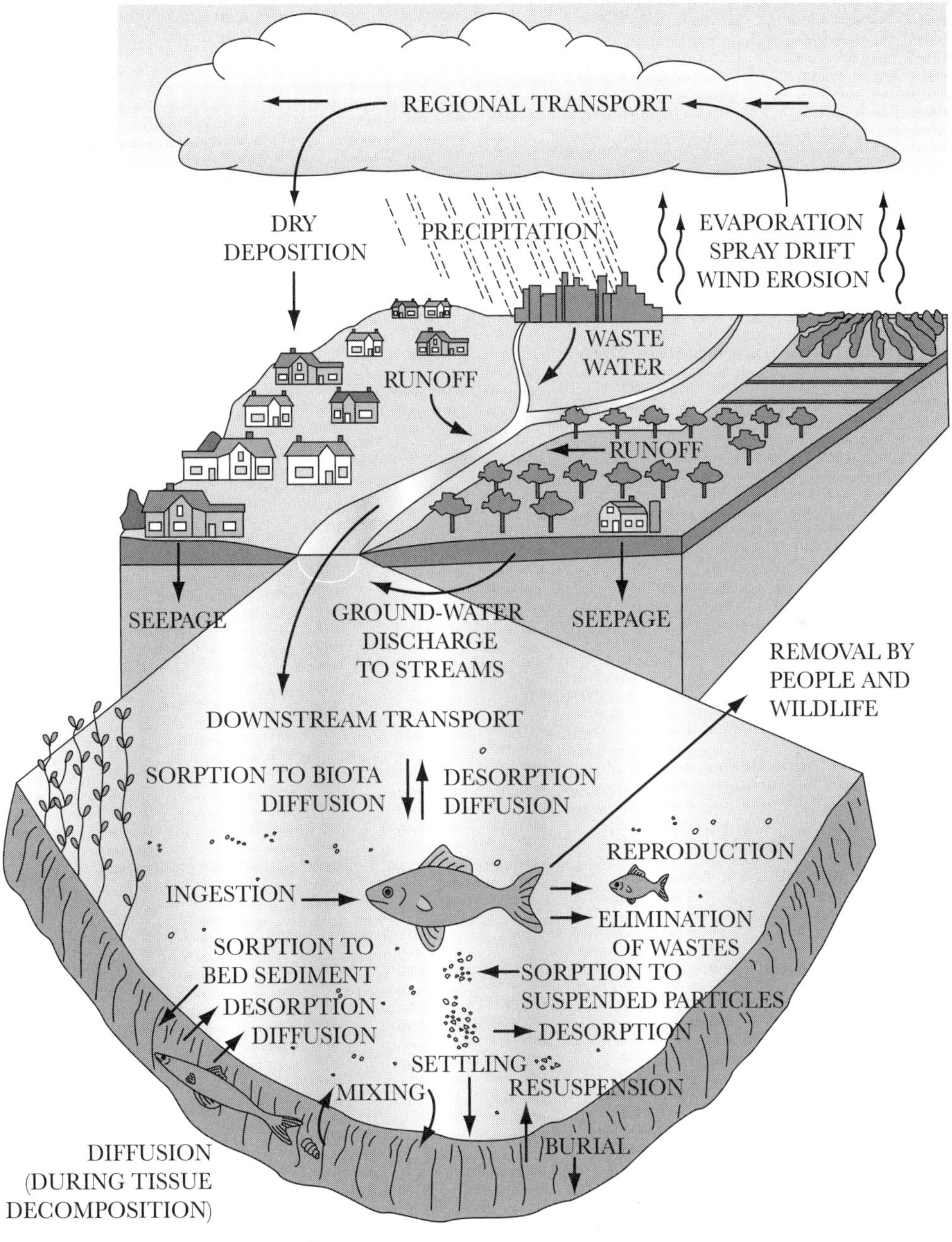

Source: USGS, 2000, as modified from Majewski and Capel, 1995.

In turn, each of these parameters affects the bioavailability and subsequent toxicity of a given chemical.

Bioavailability. An insoluble metal salt such as cadmium, lead, or copper sulfide, or an organic contaminant that is tightly adsorbed to sediment particles, is unlikely to be taken up by an organism. Conversely, other substances are physically and chemically available to be taken up, and they are known as *bioavailable.* This concept requires careful definition. Although contaminants resting in undisturbed sediments may not pose an immediate health threat, their chemical characteristics may predispose them to accumulate in biological tissues. Such organic or organometallic compounds are generally nonpolar (*hydrophobic,* or water fearing) as opposed to polar (*hydrophilic,* or water-loving). They are relatively insoluble in water, but once ingested—for example, by benthic invertebrates that burrow in the sediments—they may accumulate through the food chain, as they are readily soluble in lipids. (Excellent textbooks are available to further an understanding of the complexities of chemical partitioning in sediments, water, and the biota, for example, Schwarzenbach, Gschwend, and Imboden, 1993; Morel and Hering, 1993; Stumm and Morgan, 1996.)

Environmental Reservoirs. Many environments therefore represent potential reservoirs of contaminants. The group of organic compounds that degrade slowly in the environment, known as persistent organic pollutants (POPs), includes many of the synthetic organic chemicals mentioned in Table 18.3. Because they generally have low solubility, they tend to partition to sediments, particulate material, or the biota in aquatic systems, where they have been considered no longer bioavailable. One group of POPs that has received attention over the last two decades has been the polychlorinated biphenyls (PCBs). Originally considered inert, PCBs were used extensively in the electronics industry as dielectric material in capacitors and transformers and as binding or insulating materials for a wide range of applications, including building materials. As a result of past disposal practices, numerous sites now exist in the United States and globally where concentrations of PCBs reach levels in the tens of thousands of parts per million. The Hudson River in New York and New Bedford Harbor in Massachusetts are two of the better-known PCB-contaminated Superfund sites in the United States.

Unfortunately, evidence is now accruing that PCBs cause cancer and other health effects in animals (Agency for Toxic Substances and Disease Registry, 2000) and are therefore potentially of concern to human health. PCBs are broken down at extremely slow rates by sediment bacteria. Anaerobic organisms can initially remove chlorine atoms from highly chlorinated PCBs, but the resulting molecules resist further degradation unless exposed to aerobic conditions where other groups of bacteria continue the degradation process. Although considerable research has been undertaken to find ways to accelerate biodegradation *in situ,* to date these biological processes are so slow that several decades to centuries may be needed to demonstrate substantial levels of degradation. Short of extensive dredging, sediments remain reservoirs of PCBs and sources of exposure through the food chain for the foreseeable future.

Health Effects

A vast number of potentially toxic chemicals have been discharged into or formed in waterways and can potentially end up in surface water and groundwater. Evidence suggests multiple health effects, ranging from birth defects to cancer (Table 18.4). However, the links between waterborne chemical exposures and

TABLE 18.4. EXAMPLES OF STUDIES LINKING EXPOSURE TO CHEMICALS IN DRINKING WATER WITH INCREASED HEALTH RISK.

Place	Contaminant	Source	Health Effect	Certainty?	Useful Reference
Cape Cod, Massachusetts	Perchloroethylene (PCE)	Leachate from vinyl lining of water pipes	Breast cancer	Small to moderate increased risk	Aschengrau, Rogers, and Ozonoff, 2003
Churchill County, Nevada	Tungsten and arsenic	Unknown	Leukemia	Speculative	CDC, 2003
Woburn, Massachusetts	Solvents including trichloroethylene (TCE)	Chemical manufacturing wastes	Childhood leukemia	Probable, with caution	Costas, Knorr, and Condon, 2002
Bergen, Essex, Morris, and Passaic Counties, New Jersey	TCE and PCE	Not specified	Leukemia and non-Hodgkins lymphoma	Link with exposure suggested	Cohn and others, 1994
Gassim Region, Saudi Arabia	Petroleum oils	Refineries?	Carcinoma of the esophagus	Speculative	Amer, El-Yazigi, Hannan, and Mohamed, 1990
Northwestern Illinois	TCE, PCE, and other solvents	Landfill?	Bladder cancer	Speculative	Mallin, 1990

health outcomes have been difficult to prove conclusively. Epidemiological studies face several challenges: exposures that are relatively low and difficult to measure, exposures to the chemicals of concern through routes other than water, and confounding by competing causes of diseases of interest. These challenges are more fully explained in Chapter Three.

Microbiological Contaminants

After considering the sources of microbiological contaminants and how they may be used to indicate water quality, this section describes some specific environmental pathogens of concern and the transformation, deposition, storage, and bioconcentration of microbiological contaminants in the water supply.

Sources

Since ancient times, people have recognized that human and animal wastes can contaminate water and threaten health. A great many pathogenic organisms can be found in water. Many of these are shown in Table 18.5, together with their infectious dose and the diseases they cause. Like chemical contaminants, biological contaminants can come from point sources such as leaking septic systems or nonpoint sources such as runoff from city streets.

Because most (but not all) biological contaminants result from human or animal wastes, waste treatment practices play a major role in water contamination. Sewage is managed in many ways, from the primitive to the highly technical, as illustrated in Figure 18.5. Human waste can be discharged directly to receiving waters through surface water runoff from open defecation sites, a common occurrence in many developing countries, or processed in ways ranging from a simple shallow pit to a larger community sewage system. These latter systems require large volumes of water for efficient operation, so large amounts of wastewater are generated, requiring subsequent treatment before release to receiving waters. Wastewater treatment and discharge can place a heavy burden on receiving waters in terms of pathogens, nutrients, and toxic chemicals. For some river systems, wastewater makes up the primary flow during dry seasons. Groundwater can also be contaminated with human pathogens from leaking septic systems, contaminated runoff infiltrating wellheads, and seepage from animal feedlots.

An idealized wastewater treatment process is shown in Figure 18.6, which is loosely based on Boston's Deer Island treatment plant (Massachusetts Water

TABLE 18.5. PATHOGENS IN DRINKING WATER: INFECTIOUS DOSES, DISEASES, AND ADDITIONAL COMMENTS.

Pathogen	Infectious Dose[a]	Disease(s)	Comments
Bacteria			
Vibrio cholerae	10^8	Cholera	New toxigenic serogroups with antibiotic resistance
Salmonella spp.	10^{6-7}	Salmonellosis	Antibiotic resistance
Shigella spp.	10^2	Shigellosis	Antibiotic resistance
Toxigenic *E. coli*	10^{2-9}	Diarrheal diseases	Major identified cause of diarrheal disease
For example, *E. coli* O157		Hemolytic-uremic syndrome	Enteropathogenic, enterotoxigenic, and enterohemorrhagic strains identified including multiple antibiotic resistant strains
Campylobacter spp.	10^6	Campylobacteriosis	Antibiotic resistance
Leptospira spp.	3	Leptospirosis	Increases with flooding events
Francisella tularensis	10	Tularemia	Significance in drinking water unknown
Yersinia enterocolitica	10^9	Yersiniosis	Significance in drinking water unknown
Aeromonas spp.	10^8	Skin and respiratory infections	Gastritis?
Helicobacter pylori	?	Gastric ulcers or cancer	Exposure route unknown
Legionella pneumophila	>10	Legionellosis, Pontiac fever	Underestimated cause of pneumonia
Mycobacterium avium	?	Disseminated infections	Increasing in healthy populations
Protozoa			
Giardia lamblia	1–10	Giardiasis	Underdiagnosed
Cryptosporidium parvum	1–30	Cryptosporidiosis	Underdiagnosed, extreme chlorine resistance
Naegleria fowleri	High?	Primary amoebic meningoencephalitis	Disease very rare, yet exposures common
Acanthamoeba spp.	?	Encephalitis and others	Transmission of bacterial pathogens?
Entamoeba histolica	10–100	Dysentery	High rates of infection and associated mortality
Cyclospora cayetanensis	?	Cyclosporidiosis	Most outbreaks associated with contaminated produce
Isospora belli	?		Significance in drinking water unknown
Microsporidia	?	Microsporidiosis	May be widespread
Balantidium coli	25–100		Significance in drinking water unknown
Toxoplasma gondii	?	Toxoplasmosis	Significance in drinking water unknown
Viruses[b]	1–10	Diarrheal disease, meningitis, heart disease, liver disease, and so forth	Incidence probably dramatically underestimated; many viruses may remain to be discovered

Note: Data compiled from WHO, 1993; Hazen and Toranzos, 1990; Geldreich, 1996.

[a]Infectious dose is the number of infectious agents that produce infection (asymptomatic or symptomatic) in 50 percent of tested volunteers and is therefore not useful for risk estimates for disease.

[b]Viruses include caliciviruses (especially Norovirus), Poliovirus, Coxsachievirus, Echovirus, Reovirus, Adenovirus, Hepatitis A, Hepatitis E, Rotavirus, Astrovirus, Coronavirus, and others to be identified.

Source: Reproduced from Ford, 2004.

FIGURE 18.5. SANITATION OPTIONS.

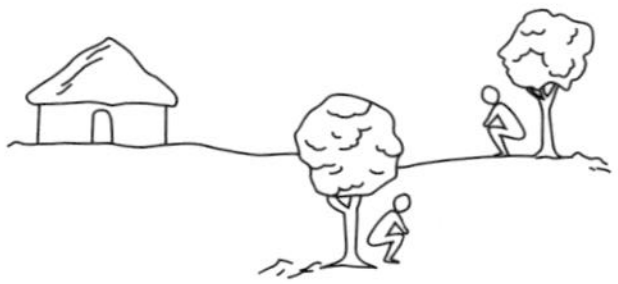

Open defecation — obvious health risks, particularly in built-up areas.

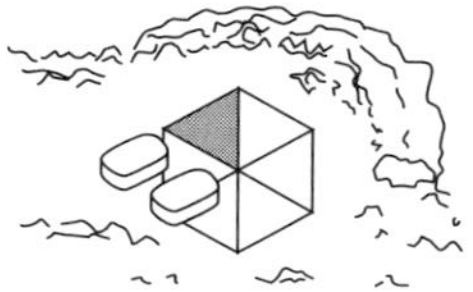

Shallow pit — flies and hookworm problems.

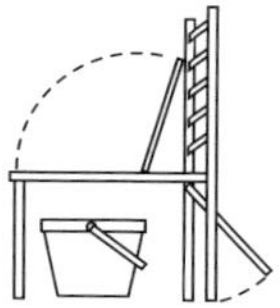

Bucket latrine — odor, flies, excreta disposal (known as "nightsoil").

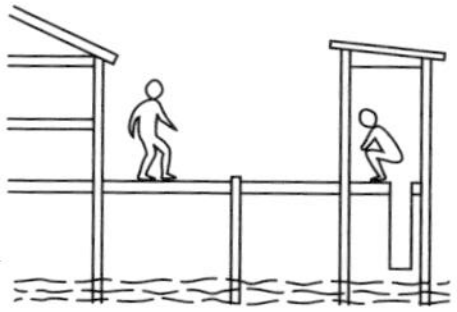

Overhung latrine — severe health risks, particularly for downstream users.

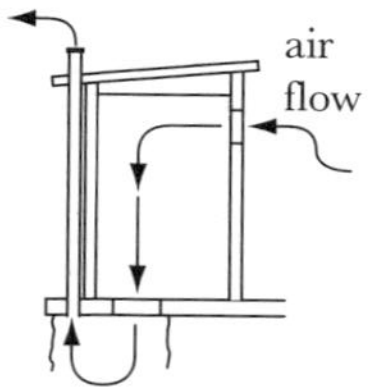

Pit latrine. There are many versions of the pit latrine: simple, borehole, ventilated (shown here), double-pit, pour-flush and off-set pour-flush (both have water traps to prevent flies and odor); each has its own set of advantages and disadvantages, detailed in Franceys, Pickford, and Reed, 1992.

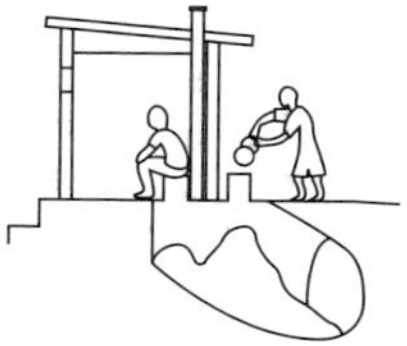

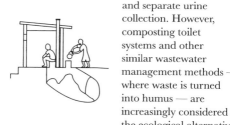

Composting latrine — needs careful operation and separate urine collection. However, composting toilet systems and other similar wastewater management methods — where waste is turned into humus — are increasingly considered the ecological alternative; see Del Porto and Steinfeld, 2000.

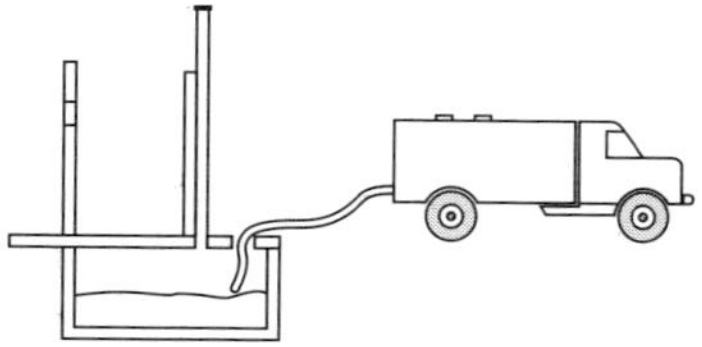

Vaults and cesspits — high cost and need for reliable collection service.

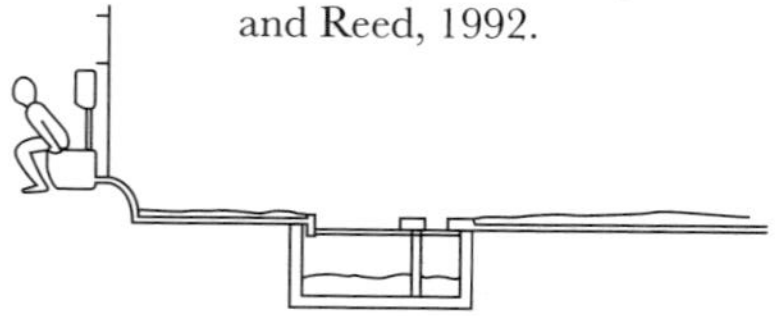

Septic tank – the septic tank (and its smaller version the Aqua-privy) relies on separation of solids (sludge), liquid, and scum. The liquid and scum flow out to an absorption field, and the sludge requires regular mechanical removal. A major concern is the soil type and siting of the absorption field, particularly in relation to drinking-water wells.

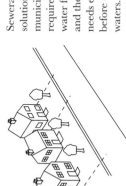

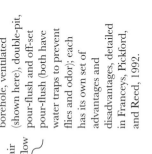

Sewerage — although the solution of choice for most municipalities, the system requires large volumes of water for efficient operation and the collected wastewater needs extensive treatment before discharge to receiving waters.

Source: Diagrams reproduced from Franceys and others, 1992. © World Health Organization.

FIGURE 18.6. AN IDEALIZED WASTEWATER TREATMENT SYSTEM, BASED ON BOSTON'S DEER ISLAND SYSTEM.

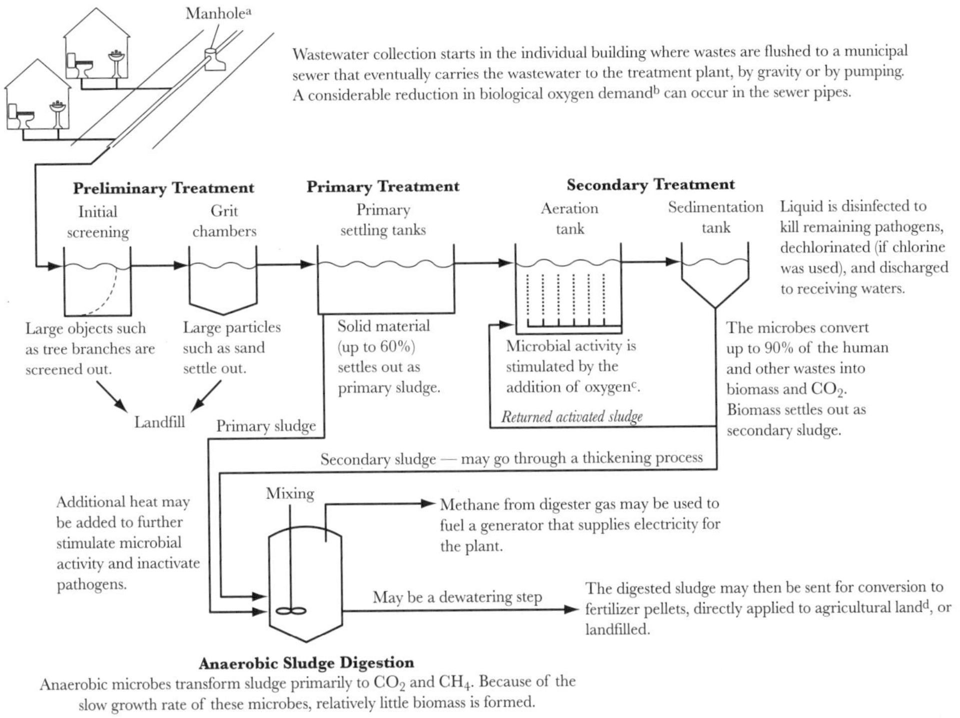
Manhole[a]
Wastewater collection starts in the individual building where wastes are flushed to a municipal sewer that eventually carries the wastewater to the treatment plant, by gravity or by pumping. A considerable reduction in biological oxygen demand[b] can occur in the sewer pipes.
Preliminary Treatment
Initial screening
Grit chambers
Primary Treatment
Primary settling tanks
Secondary Treatment
Aeration tank
Sedimentation tank
Liquid is disinfected to kill remaining pathogens, dechlorinated (if chlorine was used), and discharged to receiving waters.
Large objects such as tree branches are screened out.
Large particles such as sand settle out.
Landfill
Solid material (up to 60%) settles out as primary sludge.
Primary sludge
Microbial activity is stimulated by the addition of oxygen[c].
Returned activated sludge
The microbes convert up to 90% of the human and other wastes into biomass and CO_2. Biomass settles out as secondary sludge.
Secondary sludge — may go through a thickening process
Additional heat may be added to further stimulate microbial activity and inactivate pathogens.
Mixing
Methane from digester gas may be used to fuel a generator that supplies electricity for the plant.
May be a dewatering step
The digested sludge may then be sent for conversion to fertilizer pellets, directly applied to agricultural land[d], or landfilled.
Anaerobic Sludge Digestion
Anaerobic microbes transform sludge primarily to CO_2 and CH_4. Because of the slow growth rate of these microbes, relatively little biomass is formed.

Note: Most municipal wastewater can be treated using this or a similar treatment train. However, if industrial or other sources of toxic chemicals are present, wastes may need to undergo far more technologically sophisticated and expensive tertiary treatment. Further discussion of wastewater treatment is beyond the scope of this chapter and many excellent texts are available to the reader (for example, Bitton, 1999).

[a]Manholes give access from the street to the main sewer for maintenance. However, there may also be direct connections to street drains in the case of a combined sewer system. This may dramatically increase the volume of wastewater that the treatment plant has to process, often overwhelming the system and allowing untreated wastewater to be released to receiving waters.

[b]*Biological oxygen demand,* or BOD, is a measure of the readily assimilable organic carbon present in wastewater. BOD is defined as the amount of oxygen used by microorganisms in the aerobic degradation of organic wastes over a set time period and temperature (usually five days at 20°C).

[c]Secondary treatment can range from an energy-intensive activated sludge system, where oxygen is added to accelerate microbial activity, to simple aeration ponds, which rely on the action of wind, algae, and macrophytes to facilitate oxygen transfer.

[d]Land application of sewage sludge is facing increasingly stringent regulations due to concerns about pathogens and toxic chemicals in the food chain and about potential contamination of ground and surface waters.

Resources Authority, n.d.). Systems such as this are expensive to build and maintain, and in general only the wealthiest municipalities can afford such extensive systems.

In recent years waterborne disease outbreaks in North America have been linked to exceptionally heavy rainfall and resultant flooding. This is not surprising given the increased emphasis on high-density farming practices and their proximity to water supplies. Two outbreaks are illustrative: the outbreak of cryptosporidiosis in Milwaukee in 1993 and the outbreak of *E. coli* O157 in Walkerton, Ontario, in 2000. (These and other outbreaks are discussed in detail by Hrudey and Hrudey, 2004.)

The Milwaukee outbreak was the largest documented waterborne disease outbreak in the United States. An estimated 400,000 people became ill, and there were more than 50 associated deaths. In this outbreak, water underwent complete treatment (coagulation, sedimentation, rapid sand filtration, and chlorination), disinfection (1.5 mg/L chlorine) was not deficient or interrupted, and standards for coliforms (<1/100 ml) and turbidity (<1 NTU [nephelometric turbidity unit]) were met. Operational lapses were identified, including poor mixing during coagulation and restarting of dirty filters without backwashing. However, the root cause was presumably massive numbers of *C. parvum* oocysts being washed into Milwaukee's source water, Lake Michigan, close to the city's water intakes. A number of sources of contamination were suspected, including runoff from farms, sewage treatment, or other unidentified sources during the heavy rainfalls that preceded the outbreak (Mac Kenzie and others, 1994). Archived stool samples subsequently showed that the *C. parvum* were all the human genotype (type 1), strongly suggesting that human sewage was in fact the source (Sulaiman and others, 1998).

The 2000 outbreak of *E. coli* O157 in Walkerton, Ontario, sickened hundreds of people and caused seven deaths. In this case the indicator organism, *E. coli,* was measured in drinking water, but no action was immediately taken. The root cause was presumably *E. coli* O157 and other pathogens, such as *Campylobacter,* contaminating a shallow well that was sited inappropriately close to an adjacent cattle farm. Retrospective studies established *E. coli* O157:H7 and *Campylobacter* as the primary agents of the outbreak, with strains matched between stool samples, water samples, and manure samples by molecular typing methods (discussed in Hrudey and Hrudey, 2004). Box 18.1 provides a chronology of the outbreak. However, the reader is also referred to the Report of the Walkerton Commission of Inquiry (O'Connor, 2002) for fascinating insights into this tragic event, the lessons learned, and the political ramifications from waterborne disease deaths that few would think could happen in developed countries.

Box 18.1. Chronology of Events During the Walkerton, Ontario, *E. coli* O157 Outbreak in 2000

Preamble. The town of Walkerton, Ontario, was taking part of its source water from a well adjacent to a local farming operation. Problems began around May 2000.

- May 12: Heavy rains sustained for several days are thought to have caused pathogens in cattle manure either to infiltrate the wellhead or to contaminate the aquifer through seepage.
- May 17: Tests of the drinking water indicate the presence of coliforms and *E. coli* in samples taken on May 15. However, the general manager of the Public Utilities Commission fails to notify appropriate health officials.
- May 18: Walkerton residents begin to report symptoms of gastrointestinal illness; two children with bloody diarrhea are hospitalized.
- May 19: Health officials contact the Public Utilities Commission and are assured that the water is safe.
- May 20–21: The number of illnesses continues to rise. The government health officer orders a "boil water" advisory, despite continued assurances from the utility personnel.
- May 22: First person dies.
- May 23: Independent tests show that *E. coli* O157:H7 is present in the drinking water. Hundreds of people complain of symptoms, more than 150 people seek hospital treatment, and a two-year-old girl dies.
- May 24: Two more deaths.
- May 25: Fifth death, and four children listed as critical.
- May 29: Sixth death.
- May 30: Seventh death.
- May 31: Public inquiry ordered.

Outcome. The utility had been falsifying records for some time, and the chlorination system had not been working properly. The utility operator "did not like the taste of chlorine." Class action suits and criminal investigations have followed, but the real outcome of this tragedy is the implementation of far stricter regulations for Ontario's drinking water—and the realization that proper operator training is critical.

Source: Adapted from Ford and others, 2005.

The Indicator Concept

To monitor the microbiological quality of water, measurable indicators are needed. Although many microbial species could be chosen for this purpose (see Table 18.6), the traditional indicator has been the coliform group. The premise has been that the concentration of coliform organisms reflects the overall microbial quality of water.

TABLE 18.6. THE INDICATOR APPROACH.

Indicator	What Does It Indicate	Limitations
Coliforms	Presence of the coliform group of bacteria, many of which are present in human or animal fecal material.	Certain coliforms grow naturally in drinking water biofilms, particularly at warmer temperatures. Not indicative of protozoa or viruses.
E. coli	Presence of *E. coli*; strong indication of fecal contamination.	Inactivated more rapidly than other pathogens. Not indicative of protozoa or viruses.
Coliphage	Indicative of the presence of viruses specific to *E. coli*	May or may not be indicative of viral pathogens. Not indicative of protozoa or bacteria.
Enterococci	May be indicative of presence of animal wastes as well as human waste.	Not indicative of protozoa or viruses.
Clostridium	Spore-forming bacteria; anaerobes; protozoa.	Not indicative of viruses.
Pseudomonas	Survives in drinking water biofilms; may indicate presence of bacterial pathogens that are more persistent than the coliforms.	Not indicative of protozoa or viruses.
Aeromonads	Survives in drinking water biofilms; may indicate presence of bacterial pathogens that are more persistent than the coliforms.	Not indicative of protozoa or viruses.
Human-specific *Bacteroides fragilis* bacteriophage	Indicative of the presence of viruses specific to *B. fragilis*; may be present when coliphage is absent.	May or may not be indicative of viral pathogens. Not indicative of protozoa or bacteria.
Turbidity	May indicate that the water exceeds turbidity regulations. Some studies show increased risk for waterborne disease at high turbidity (pathogens adhere to particles).	Only measures turbidity; cannot be directly correlated to pathogen loading.
Residual chlorine	Measures the disinfectant residual at the tap. Absence of residual chlorine has been shown in some studies to be consistent with waterborne disease.	Only measures residual chlorine; cannot be directly correlated to pathogen loading.

Methods to detect and quantify coliform counts have become increasingly sophisticated. In the early 1900s, growth of bacteria on a nutrient agar plate at ~37°C was thought to be indicative of possible contamination by enteric organisms (reviewed in Payment, Sartory, and Reasoner, 2003). In more recent decades, coliform bacteria were enumerated in selective liquid culture media, using a technique known as the *most probable number* method. The *membrane filtration* technique has now gained in popularity, and currently, *enzyme-specific assays*, which are accurate and can be easily conducted by water utility personnel, have gained favor. (Geldreich, 1996, provides a good discussion of these tests.)

However, the indicator concept with its reliance on total coliform counts has recently been challenged. Once human pathogens have contaminated ground and surface waters, their fate is very much organism specific. In fact, the coliform group is inactivated relatively rapidly, whereas other human pathogens can survive for extended periods. This is particularly true for the pathogenic protozoa that form highly resistant cysts or oocysts and the viruses that appear to survive adsorbed to particulate material. As a result, a reassuringly low coliform count could belie a dangerous level of other organisms. Alternative approaches to monitoring water quality might include measuring *E. coli* rather than total coliforms as the primary indicator of fecal contamination and using additional indicators of viral and protozoan contamination. (The advantages and shortcomings of the indicator approach have been discussed extensively in the literature; useful references are available on the American Academy for Microbiology Web site: Ford and Colwell, 1995; Rose and Grimes, 2001.)

Environmental Pathogens

There is also a wide range of environmental pathogens—organisms that although they may be discharged in human sewage are distinguished by their ability not only to persist in the environment but also to grow and proliferate. Two of the better-known examples of this type of pathogen are *Legionella pneumophila* and the environmental mycobacteria.

As with exposure to chemicals, exposure to waterborne pathogens can occur through multiple transmission routes. Some are obvious, such as ingestion of contaminated water or exposure through recreational use, either through unintended ingestion or through skin abrasions or alternative *portals of entry* (eye, ear, anal, urogenital). Other, perhaps less obvious, routes of exposure include breathing contaminated aerosols from showers, toilet flushing, dish washing, garden hoses, fountains, waterfalls, and cooling towers and from air conditioner, humidifier, and refrigerator drip pans. Many infectious agents are also transmitted through the use of hot tubs and whirlpool spas (see Box 18.2).

Box 18.2. The Hidden Hazards of Hot Tubs

When you next decide to bathe in a hot tub, indoor swimming pool, or even your shower, you will not be alone! Many bacteria find these environments ideal for survival and proliferation. In particular the environmental mycobacteria have been implicated in a number of outbreaks of the pulmonary disease known as *hot tub lung. Legionella pneumophila* has caused outbreaks of legionellosis and Pontiac fever and *Pseudomonas aeruginosa* has been implicated in outbreaks of folliculitis. In addition, *lifeguard lung,* a form of hypersensitivity pneumonitis, is associated with frequent exposure to pool aerosols containing endotoxin, a cell wall component of gram-negative bacteria. In fact bacteria thrive in these environments, particularly in piping systems where water remains stagnant for much of the time, and are probably associated with biofilms (discussed under *storage*).

Transformations

Like chemical contaminants, microbial contaminants can be transformed once they are discharged into receiving waters. Often these changes result in less risk to humans. Environmental stress can rapidly inactivate a number of pathogenic organisms, or at least create a viable but nonculturable (Colwell and others, 1985) or *injured* (Singh and McFeters, 1990) state. However, those same stress factors might also increase an organism's virulence. One way in which this could occur is through adaptation to intracellular survival and growth. Recent research suggests that some pathogens can survive, resist chlorine, and even grow within protozoan *hosts.* Examples include species of *Escherichia, Citrobacter, Enterobacter, Klebsiella, Salmonella, Yersinia, Shigella, Legionella,* and *Campylobacter* (King, Shotts, Wooley, and Porter, 1988). More recently, some environmental mycobacteria have been shown to survive in protozoan hosts (reviewed in Pedley and others, 2004). At least in the case of *Legionella* and the mycobacteria, adaptation to the protozoan host may be a mechanism that allows the pathogens to elude the human immune system through intracellular survival and growth in macrophages (reviewed in Samrakandi, Ridenour, Yan, and Cirillo, 2002).

Vibrio cholerae, the organism that causes cholera, presents a special case of an interaction between a pathogen and plankton, one that can be viewed as an environmental transformation. The *Vibrio* associates with plankton, particularly zooplankton such as copepods, a strategy that appears to allow it to multiply and concentrate to infectious doses. Although this may not directly increase virulence, it seems to play a role in initiating the cycle of epidemic cholera transmission (Colwell, 1996).

Large quantities of antibiotics are discharged to receiving waters through wastewater discharge, agriculture, and aquaculture practices. The likely consequence of these discharges is increased antibiotic resistance among naturally occurring microbes, with the potential for transfer of resistance factors to human pathogens (Levy, 1998). This transformation can lead to increasing numbers of pathogens in the environment that resist antibiotic treatment, and therefore represent an increased threat to human health (Levy, 1998; Shea, 2003).

Deposition, Storage, and Bioconcentration

Just as chemicals may accumulate in higher organisms, a number of different pathogens can become concentrated in organisms. The best-known example is filter feeding shellfish, such as oysters and clams. Outbreaks of food poisoning often occur as the result of consumption of shellfish that have concentrated planktonic algae, viruses, bacteria, or even protozoa. Infectious disease outcomes from eating contaminated shellfish, crustacea, and fish that have concentrated fecal wastes include hepatitis A, norovirus, campylobacteriosis, salmonellosis, cryptosporidiosis, and *Vibrio*-related diseases including cholera. In fact any infectious disease agent transmissible by water could potentially be concentrated in aquatic organisms.

What about storage reservoirs for pathogens? Early studies showed that the fecal coliform indicator organisms (Table 18.6) were concentrated 100- to 1,000-fold more in bottom sediments than they were in overlying waters (Van Donsel and Geldreich, 1971). Similarly, *Salmonella* and other pathogens have been shown to survive in sediments for extended periods. Recent research suggests that *Salmonella* may even be transmitted from contaminated sediments via chironomid (midge) larvae (Moore, Martinez, Gay, and Rice, 2003).

Biofilms. An important *storage area* is the biofilm, or slime, that forms on any surface in contact with water but is of particular concern in drinking-water pipes. Biofilms provide protective environments that may allow microbes to survive chemical stressors such as disinfectants in the overlying water and may even allow certain pathogens to proliferate (for example, *Legionella,* the mycobacteria, and others). Biofilms are also known to contribute to pipeline degradation, "dirty water," odor, and blockage (Ford, 1993). They are also nutrient-rich environments that potentially provide ideal conditions for gene transfer (virulence factors, antibiotic resistance factors) between microbes that are in close proximity to each other.

Wildlife and Wildfowl. Another major environmental reservoir for pathogens is wildlife and wildfowl. Many enteric pathogens such as *Salmonella* species are natural inhabitants of the intestinal tracts of both warm- and cold-bloodied animals. Others may be fortuitously carried through the intestinal tracts of wildlife and wildfowl due to their presence in human and animal garbage. Wildfowl have emerged as a particular concern for protected watersheds. However well the perimeter of a surface water is fenced, only the smallest areas can be effectively covered. Scavenger birds such as gulls may be a particular problem, as they are attracted to human garbage. A recent USGS report (Converse, Wolcott, Docherty, and Cole, 2001) reviewed studies that showed that *Campylobacter, Listeria, Salmonella, Escherichia coli, Cryptosporidium, Chlamydia,* Rotavirus, and other potentially pathogenic microbes have been isolated from feces of wildfowl, including gulls, Canada Geese, and ducks.

The Global Burden of Waterborne Disease

The primary source of information on the global burden of disease is the World Health Organization. Each year, WHO publishes the World Health Report (see, for example, WHO, 2003c), with a series of annexes that describe mortality and morbidity (reported as disability-adjusted life years, or DALYs, to express both the severity of disease and years lost through premature death). This information is reported for the preceding year through national registries that are estimated to represent about 30 percent of the global burden of disease. Although waterborne disease is not specifically identified, the category *diarrheal disease* is always included, as are malaria and a number of other tropical diseases related to water. In the case of diarrheal disease, multiple routes of exposure to infectious (and chemical) causes exist, including water, food, and person-to-person transmission. However, it is virtually impossible to distinguish these routes clearly, as the spread of diarrheal disease within a population can be dominated by *secondary transmission.* In other words, an initial infection caused by consumption of contaminated drinking water may then rapidly spread through person-to-person transmission or through food contaminated by the water itself or by the infected individual.

A commonly quoted estimate of the impact of waterborne diseases is between 2 and 3 million deaths in children under the age of five each year (for example, Ford and Colwell, 1995). The official WHO figures for morbidity and mortality from diarrheal diseases for 2002 are approximately 1.8 million deaths and 61.1 million DALYs (WHO, 2003b). This burden is comparable to the mortality and morbidity figures for other leading infectious diseases: 2.8 million deaths and 86.1 million DALYs for HIV/AIDS; 1.6 million deaths and 35.4 million DALYs for tuberculosis; and 1.2 million deaths and 44.7 million DALYs for malaria. When examining the global burden of waterborne disease, several considerations are important:

- WHO figures are based on numbers reported by individual member states and undoubtedly underestimate the burden of diarrheal disease. Questionnaire-based studies to examine community incidence of gastrointestinal disease suggest that officially reported figures may underestimate actual incidence by several hundredfold (reviewed in Ford, 1999).

- *The World Health Report for 1996* suggests that 70 percent of diarrheal episodes are caused by contaminated foods (WHO, 1996). However, water may play a role in this pathway, as contaminated water may have been used in food preparation.
- Diarrheal disease is not the only outcome from waterborne disease (discussed in Ford and Colwell, 1995).
- WHO figures may understate the importance of waterborne diseases. Patients with HIV/AIDs often die of opportunistic infections, including waterborne diseases such as cryptosporidiosis and disseminated infections from environmental mycobacteria. Therefore, some deaths attributed to HIV/AIDS may also be attributable to waterborne diseases.
- Malaria is considered a water-related disease, and anthropogenic changes to the watershed may increase the habitat for mosquitoes that carry the protozoan pathogen.

Vector-Borne Diseases

Some of the most prevalent and deadly infectious diseases in the world are transmitted by vectors that are related to water (see Table 18.7). In fact, water plays a critical role in vector-borne disease transmission. The 2003 WHO mortality and morbidity figures for malaria reflect a slight increase from 2001. Clearly, the global burden of suffering from malaria remains vast. Other major vector-borne diseases whose life cycles are associated with water include those caused by blood, liver, lung, and gastrointestinal flukes, hemorrhagic viruses, hemoflagellate protozoa, blood and tissue nematodes, and tapeworms. Their vectors include mosquitoes, blackflies, crustacea, and fish.

Waterborne diseases may be controlled, and in some cases eliminated, through changes in water sources, water quality, and human behavior, offering enormous prospects for public health advances. The effort to control dracunculiasis is perhaps the best example of a successful eradication program (aside from the program that eradicated smallpox). Dracunculiasis is an extremely debilitating disease caused by ingestion of copepods carrying the guinea worm. The disease causes extraordinary suffering to people in poorer nations who depend on poor-quality water sources. Essentially through hygiene education and water source protection, a disease that previously infected millions of people every year was reduced to about 75,000 cases in 2000, with 73 percent in the Sudan and the remainder in sub-Saharan Africa. (For further information on dracunculiasis and the eradication program, see WHO, 2004.) Box 18.3 illustrates the rapid decline in dracunculiasis cases and the measures that are currently being undertaken to eradicate this disease.

TABLE 18.7. EXAMPLES OF VECTOR-BORNE DISEASES WITH RISK FACTORS ASSOCIATED WITH WATER.

Disease	Pathogen	Vector	Risk Factors	Control Strategies
Malaria	*Plasmodium falciparum, P. vivax, P. malariae,* and *P. ovale* (protozoa)	Anopheles mosquitoes	Standing water (mosquito breeding sites); being outdoors in malaria endemic areas, particularly in the evenings; no prior exposures	Removal of standing water; chemoprophylaxis; bed nets; behavior modification; insecticide sprays
Onchocerciasis (river blindness)	*Onchocerca volvulus* (nematode)	*Simulium* spp. (blackflies)	Flowing streams with vegetation	Avoid endemic areas
Schistosomiasis	*Schistosoma mansoni, S. japonicum,* and *S. haematobium* (trematodes)	Snails	Flooding; damming; creation of irrigation ditches	Destruction of snails or habitat; avoiding contact with water in endemic areas; proper disposal of human waste
Dracunculiasis	*Dracunculus medinensis* (Guinea worm—nematode)	Copepod	Contaminated drinking water	Provision of disinfected drinking water; prevention of source water contamination
West Nile encephalitis	West Nile Virus (flavivirus)	Culex mosquitoes	Standing water; vegetation; discarded tires (hold stagnant water)	Removal of standing water; screens; behavior modification; insecticide sprays
Fish tapeworm	*Diphyllobothrium* spp. (cestoda)	Copepods and fish	Ingestion of undercooked or raw fish	Thorough cooking

Box 18.3. Dracunculiasis Eradication

In the 1980s, millions of people were infected with dracunculiasis (guinea worm disease), and hundreds of millions were considered at risk from contaminated water. The guinea worm's larvae live in copepods in water. When a person drinks the contaminated water, the ingested larvae begin to burrow into surrounding tissues and mate. The males die, but the females may grow to a meter in length and contain millions of embryos. The female eventually migrates to the skin surface and breaks through, causing intense pain and high risk of secondary infection of the ulcerated tissue. Before the female breaks through the skin, approximately one year after initial infection, the victim may be unaware of the infection. He or she typically bathes the infected ulcer in water, and this releases larvae, which subsequently mature in the copepod host to complete the cycle. In 1986 and again in 1991, the World Health Organization established the Dracunculiasis Eradication Program, effectively reducing incidence of the disease by 95 percent (WHO data reported in Spearman, 1998) Since then, progress has been continuing, and each year new countries report the successful elimination of the disease. Today, dracunculiasis remains in the poorest countries, where people lack access to clean water. The Sudan has clearly been one of the major problem areas.

In fact, eradication of the disease is relatively straightforward—stopping the transmission cycle. Since there is no treatment for the disease, programs focus first on identifying infected individuals and preventing them from recontaminating water sources and, second on educating people to filter or boil drinking water (relatively coarse filtration material can remove the copepods) or treating selected water sources to kill the copepods.

Together with UNICEF, CDC, and Global 2000, WHO has adopted the following strategy (WHO, 2004):

- implement effective case containment measures in all endemic villages,
- establish a community-based surveillance system in every known endemic village with monthly reporting of cases, supervision, and integration of surveillance for other major preventable diseases,
- target specific interventions (provision of safe water, health education, community mobilization, filter distribution, and treatment of selected water sources with temephos (Abate®),
- map all endemic villages and maintain global and national dracunculiasis databases for monitoring of the epidemiological situation,
- sustain advocacy for eradication of the disease, and
- certify dracunculiasis eradication country by country world-wide.

Waterborne Diseases

Although a wide range of diseases is caused by waterborne pathogens (Table 18.6), the most common outcome, and the one that most frequently remains undiagnosed, is acute gastrointestinal infection (AGI). AGI can be caused by viruses, bacteria, or protozoa. In addition, symptoms similar to AGI may be caused by chemical contaminants. The etiology of waterborne disease is strongly affected by the sources of the infectious agents. For example, *Shigella* species are primarily human pathogens, and shigellosis outbreaks can usually be associated with contamination from human sewage. *E. coli, Campylobacter, Salmonella,* and many of the protozoan and viral pathogens are zoonotic. In other words, they are also associated with livestock, wildlife, and wildfowl. Hence fecal contamination of water from any of these sources can result in a waterborne disease outbreak, which is why there is increasing concern about high-density animal husbandry practices, particularly in areas prone to flooding (Wing, Freedman, and Band, 2002).

Viral Diseases. Viruses are increasingly implicated as major causative agents of AGI. In the United States alone, it has been estimated that 80 percent of the 38.6 million annual cases of gastroenteritis are caused by viruses (Mead and others, 1999). Of well over 100 known viruses that can potentially be transmitted in drinking water, the caliciviruses and rotaviruses are most commonly diagnosed. However, types of Poliovirus, Coxsachievirus, Echovirus, Reovirus, Adenovirus, Hepatitis A, Astrovirus, Coronavirus, and Hepatitis E have been implicated in waterborne outbreaks, and there may be many further, as yet uncharacterized, groups of viruses that could cause AGI and other disease manifestations.

Scientific understanding of the role of viruses in waterborne diarrhea has been limited by the difficulties inherent both in their specific diagnosis and in measurement of the agents in drinking water and food. For example, the caliciviruses are now thought to be the major causes of both food and waterborne illness worldwide, but research has been limited by the fact that they cannot be cultured. This fascinating family of viruses first came to light in 1972 after electron microscopists identified small round particles in samples from an outbreak of AGI that had occurred in Norwalk, Ohio, four years earlier, when 50 percent of children and teachers at an elementary school became sick. Analysis of surveillance data between 1995 and 2000 in Europe suggested that this specific group of caliciviruses (one of potentially four different Calicivirus genera), now known as noroviruses, accounts for more than 85 percent of all nonbacterial outbreaks of gastroenteritis (Lopman and others, 2003). In the United States, Mead and others (1999) estimated that noroviruses caused 23 million cases of gastroenteritis each year.

A recent review describes three distinct groups pathogenic to humans that have now been identified using molecular epidemiology techniques (Lopman, Brown, and Koopmans, 2002). This approach amplifies and "fingerprints" genetic material (in this case RNA), so researchers can compare potential sources of infection with clinical samples. Using these techniques it has been shown that caliciviruses are transmitted through drinking water, shellfish, uncooked foods such as salads and fruits, food handling, environmental exposures (bathing, contaminated surfaces, and so forth), and person to person. In fact, person to person transmission is thought to be the major route of infection, including infection through aerosol formation caused by the *projectile vomiting* characteristic of these infections. Further advances in molecular epidemiology may also show that animals are a source of infection, as they have been shown to be infected by strains of Calicivirus that are quite similar to the three human pathogen groups. The clinical and public health significance of human caliciviruses is considerable, particularly as there appears to be no long-term immunity to these agents in humans.

Bacterial Diseases. Of the bacterial diseases, campylobacteriosis remains the most common form of bacterial dysentery, followed by pathogenic *E. coli,* salmonellosis, and shigellosis. The global incidence of these diseases is difficult to estimate. In the United States, Morris and Levin (1995) estimated that water causes 35,000 case of shigellosis, 59,000 cases of salmonellosis, 150,000 cases of *E. coli* infection, and 320,000 cases of campylobacteriosis each year. These diseases are of course prevalent worldwide, but many other infectious agents that are relatively under control in developed countries remain epidemic in other countries. Cholera (caused by *Vibrio cholerae*) and typhoid (caused by *Salmonella typhi*) are perhaps the best-known examples of waterborne disease that have caused global pandemics in the past. Typhoid tends to emerge in less developed countries in epidemic proportions where sanitation is compromised. This happened in Chile during the 1980s and was attributed, at least in part, to irrigation of vegetables with wastewater, increased rainfall, inadequate water treatment, and a deteriorating economy (Cabello and Springer, 1997).

On a global basis morbidity and mortality from *E. coli* infections are today thought to exceed those of cholera and other identified waterborne disease. The *E. coli* strains that produce enterotoxin (enterotoxigenic *E. coli,* or ETEC), can also be enteropathogenic or enterohemorrhagic, as in the notorius *E. coli* O157-H7 outbreak in Walkerton (Box 18.1). Estimates of morbidity and mortality from cholera are in the tens of thousands per year. In contrast, ETEC are estimated to cause approximatly 400 million diarreal episodes, with 700,000 deaths among children less than five years old each year (reported in Chakraborty and others, 2001).

Many opportunistic pathogens can also be transmitted through water. These include species of *Aeromonas, Pseudomonas, Klebsiella,* and others. It is extremely difficult to estimate the contributions of these agents to morbidity and mortality through consumption of drinking water. Certainly they are a major cause of hospital-acquired infections with high associated mortality risks. Other opportunistic pathogens of interest include *Legionella,* the nontuberculous mycobacteria, and

Helicobacter pylori. Legionella and the nontuberculous mycobacteria occupy a unique niche in their ability to proliferate in hot-water systems, their environmental ubiquity, and their resistance to disinfection. In the case of *Legionella,* the global burden of disease is thought to exceed reported numbers by a wide margin. In the United States it has been estimated that *Legionella* causes at least 13,000 cases of bacterial pneumonia per year (Breiman and Butler, 1998). Researchers are divided on whether water is a significant route for dissemination of *Helicobacter pylori.*

Cholera remains both epidemic and pandemic (affecting multiple countries) due in part to its ability to survive and multiply in the environment associated with plankton and other aquatic organisms (Colwell, 1996). There have now been seven pandemics of cholera since 1817, the most recent of which reached South America in 1991 and had reportedly caused more than a million cases and 10,000 deaths by 1994 (Pan American Health Organization, 1995). There are several possible theories to account for cholera's arrival in South America, including transport in a ship's bilge water (associated with plankton), transport in infected individuals, or transport in imported foods. Alternatively, it could have been endemic, surviving in the environment and only emerging with compromised sanitation after the continent had been free of epidemic cholera for more than 100 years. The truth may never be known. Cholera may emerge when sanitation practices break down, but blooms of aquatic organisms have also been associated with cholera outbreaks in Bangladesh (Colwell and Huq, 1994). The ecological linkages are fascinating, and the reader is encouraged to examine the growing literature on this topic.

Cholera is of particular interest because there is evidence that it is beginning to change. The causative agent of the past seven pandemics has been *V. cholerae,* serogroup O1. In the early 1990s, *V. cholerae,* serogroup O139, emerged in India in epidemic form, the first time that a non-O1 serogroup of *V. cholerae* was shown to cause epidemic cholera. There is now molecular evidence that O139 strains were derived from O1 strains through genetic modification (Faruque, Albert, and Mekalanos, 1998). It is important to learn more about the conditions that resulted in emergence of the toxigenic O139 serogroups and that could therefore result in many more, perhaps environmentally hardier, serogroups of this pathogen. The emergence of epidemic strains could occur through mutation of existing strains or through gene transfer. This is diagramatically represented in Figure 18.7. Although the example is *V. cholerae,* the principle illustrated could apply equally to other pathogens, such as the toxigenic *E. coli.* In the case of gene transfer, virulence factors could also be transferred between species. Both mutation and gene transfer would appear possible within the drinking-water distribution system, where organisms are likely to be exposed to a variety of stressors such as chlorine and metal ions (Ford, 1993).

FIGURE 18.7. EMERGENCE OF NEW EPIDEMIC SEROGROUPS OF *VIBRIO CHOLERAE*.

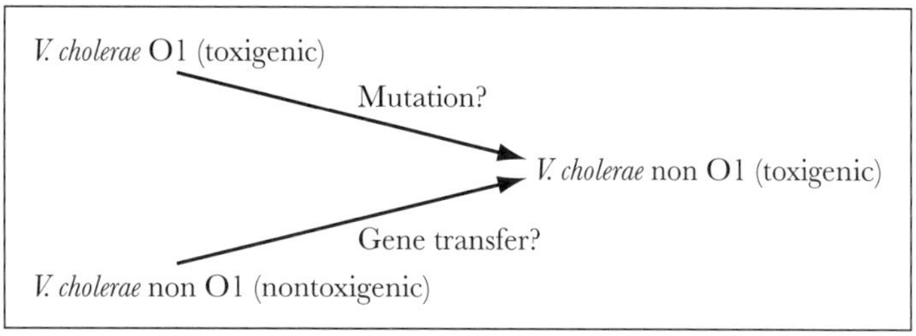

Source: Reproduced from Ford, 2005.

Protozoal Diseases. Protozoa receive considerable media attention due to the size of recent outbreaks, which are partially due to low infectious doses and high resistance to water treatment. *Cryptosporidium parvum* has attracted most attention, with *C. parvum* replacing *Giardia lamblia* as the most common cause of waterborne disease outbreaks in the U.K., and the second most common cause in the United States. In the case of *Cryptosporidium,* its global distribution is far broader than reported, due in part to misdiagnosis. For example, in Russia where monitoring for the pathogen has been introduced only in the last few years, recent seroprevalence studies (studies that examine the presence of antibodies to a specific pathogen in blood samples) suggest that almost 90 percent of the population sampled had been exposed to *Cryptosporidium* infection (Egorov and others, 2004). Studies by the same authors found *Cryptosporidium* oocysts in most source waters tested and in stool samples of approximately 7 percent of people with diarrhea (Egorov and others, 2002).

Additional protozoa of current interest include *Cyclospora* and *Toxoplasma,* although a waterborne route of transmission is far from proven. A third group of protozoans, the microsporidia, are smaller than other protozoans and are increasingly recognized as causative agents of both human and animal diseases. They are also more likely to penetrate filtration systems than the larger protozoa are, so it is reasonable to suspect a waterborne route of exposure. (A number of publications provide useful in-depth reviews of the protozoan pathogens; see, for example, Marshall, Naumovitz, Ortega, and Sterling, 1997; Hunter, 1997.)

Fungal Diseases. Recent studies have suggested that fungal species, including *Aspergillus, Cladosporium, Epicoccum, Penicillium,* and *Trichoderma,* are frequently isolated from treated drinking water (Arvanitidou, Kanellou, Constantinides, and Katsouyannopoulos, 1999). *Candida* yeasts are also occasionally isolated from drinking water and apparently correlate with the indicator organisms, total and fecal coliforms. A number of fungi and yeasts isolated from drinking water are potential pathogens, or at least can produce toxic metabolites and readily spoil foods.

Viroids and Prions. To date there is no direct evidence of transmission of viroids through water. Viroids, single stranded RNA, are thought to cause only plant diseases. Like similar infectious agents known as satellite RNAs, which are dependent on a helper virus for replication, these agents are unlikely to pose a serious threat to human health through drinking water. Of course the absence of any information linking these agents to human disease does not mean that in future linkages will not emerge. For example, the Hepatitis Delta agent is essentially a viroid encapsulated in a hepatitis B coat.

In contrast, prions, infectious proteinaceous material, have risen to prominence following the devastating economic threat and perceived human health threat from the bovine spongiform encephalopathy (BSE) outbreak in the U.K. (The BSE Inquiry, 2000). Although prions have not been isolated from drinking waters, it is reasonable to consider the risks of contamination from, for example, rendering wastes, abattoirs, and landfills.

Safe Drinking Water

Ensuring the safety of drinking water extends from the source to the faucet: protection of water sources from contamination, water treatment to remove contaminants, and protection of water from recontamination during distribution.

Source Protection

Probably the most important consideration for protection of human health in relation to potable water supplies is provision of high-quality source water. Watershed protection is critical to this process but often comes into direct conflict with development and with recreational uses of watersheds. In many metropolitan areas development has dramatically outstripped the availability of high-quality source water. Inevitably, many municipalities are dependent today on surface waters that may receive wastewaters, both treated and untreated. Protection of source waters involves maintaining generous buffers, limiting access for recreational purposes, and preventing agricultural and industrial uses. Many would argue that all wildlife and wildfowl should be prevented from accessing source water, however impractical this may be. New York City has gone to extraordinary lengths to protect upstate source water, as described in Box 18.4. This approach turned out to be more cost effective than treating water arriving from contaminated sources.

Box 18.4. Protecting Source Water for New York City

Early settlers in what is now New York obtained water from shallow wells. The chronology of subsequent water source development for New York City, adapted from the history of the New York City Water System (New York City Department of Environmental Protection, 2002), is presented in the following list:

1677	The first public well is dug.
1776	A local reservoir is constructed to serve a population of approximately 22,000. Water is distributed through hollow logs.
Early 1800s	Local wells and reservoirs become polluted and the supply is insufficient. The decision is made to extract water from the Croton River through construction of a reservoir and aqueduct (see Figure 18.8).
1842	The "old Croton Reservoir" and the "old Croton Aqueduct" are put in service. Water is conveyed to storage reservoirs in the city prior to distribution, primarily through cast-iron pipes.
1890	A second aqueduct (the "new Croton Aqueduct") is put in service to convey more water from the Croton watershed.
1905	The Board of Water Supply is created and the decision is taken to develop the Catskill watershed.
1915	The Ashokan Reservoir and Catskill Aqueduct are completed.
1928	Development of the Catskill system is completed, including the Schoharie Reservoir and the Shandaken Tunnel.
1927	Plans are submitted to develop the Rondout watershed and Delaware River tributaries within the State of New York.
1937	In spite of legal action brought by the State of New Jersey, construction of the "Delaware system" is begun.
1944	Completion of the Delaware Aqueduct; 1950, completion of the Rondout Reservoir; 1954, completion of the Neversink Reservoir; 1955, completion of the Pepacton Reservoir; 1964, completion of the Cannonsville Reservoir.

New York City's water supply is specifically designed so that reservoirs have interconnections that allow flexibility and virtually ensure that effects of localized droughts are minimized. The system delivers water to the city primarily by gravity and is therefore relatively economical. However, development of these watersheds is not without political implications. The Delaware River basin includes parts of Delaware, New Jersey, New York, and Pennsylvania. Each state relies in part on the basin for water for drinking or industrial uses. However, as the upstream user,

FIGURE 18.8. NEW YORK CITY'S WATER SUPPLY SYSTEM.

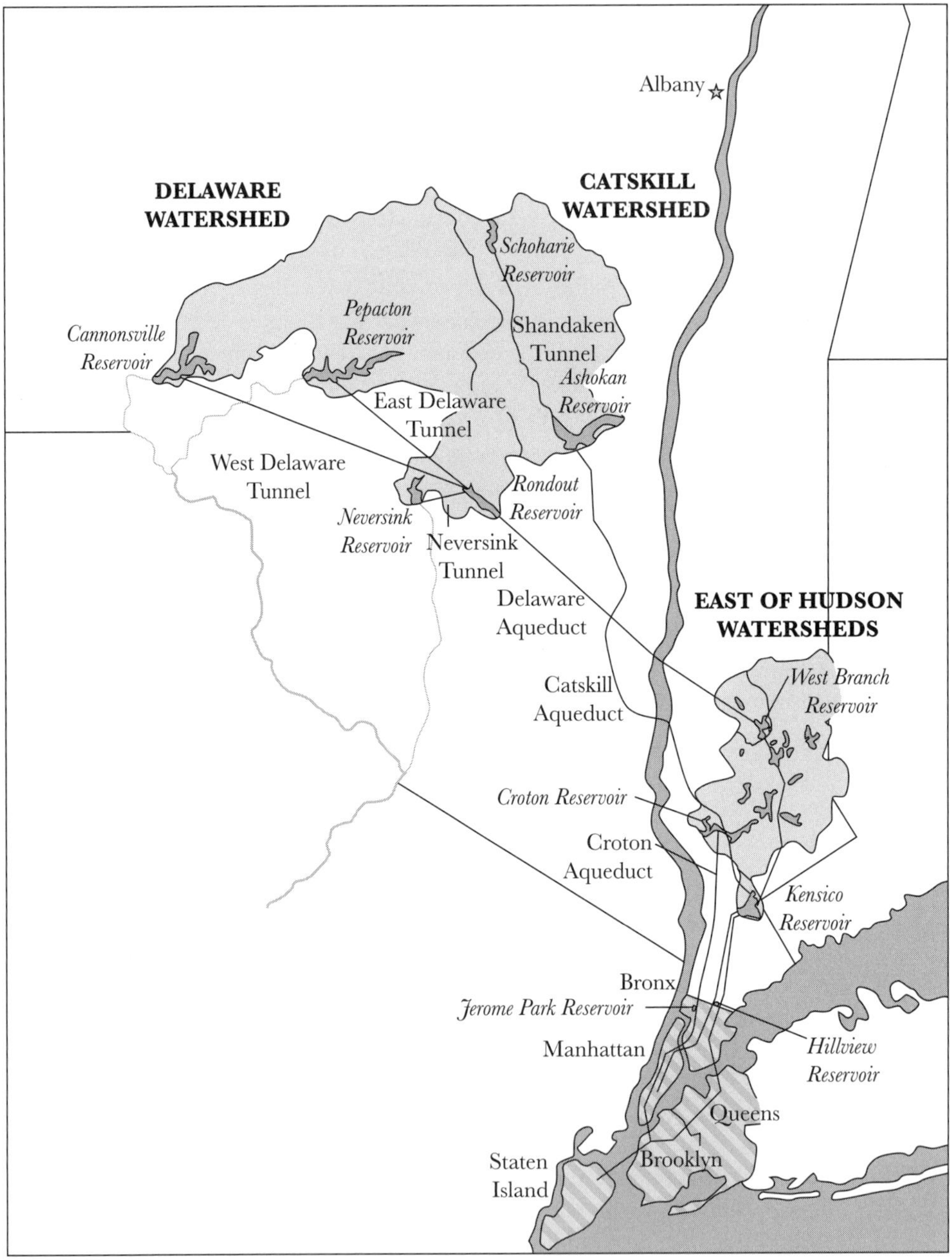

Source: The Catskill Center for Conservation and Development, n.d.

New York's development of this water supply can potentially affect the three downstream users. The Croton, Catskill, and Delaware watersheds include prime recreational and agricultural lands. In addition, the many upstream communities that have developed in these watersheds resent the fact that they cannot fully use these resources that must be protected to serve a population some 100 miles downstream.

For New York, as for other major municipalities in the United States without filtration (including Boston, Portland, and Seattle), the rules changed in 1989. As part of the Safe Drinking Water Act, in this year the EPA promulgated the Surface Water Treatment Rule (SWTR). The SWTR requires filtration of all public water supply systems supplied by unfiltered surface water unless a series of criteria, referred to as the *filtration avoidance criteria,* are met. New York City has published these criteria on its Web site (New York City Department of Environmental Protection, 1997):

- Objective Water Quality Criteria—the water supply must meet certain levels for specified constituents including coliforms, turbidity and disinfection by-products.
- Operational Criteria—a system must demonstrate compliance with certain disinfection requirements for inactivation of *Giardia* and viruses; maintain a minimum chlorine residual entering and throughout the distribution system; provide uninterrupted disinfection with redundancy; and undergo an annual on-site inspection by the primacy agency to review the condition of disinfection equipment.
- Watershed Control Criteria—a system must establish and maintain an effective watershed control program to minimize the potential for contamination of source waters by *Giardia* and viruses.

The City of New York faces billions of dollars in costs to implement filtration of its drinking water and hence has gone to exceptional lengths to prove that it can meet these criteria. In addition to programs to purchase land in the watersheds, the New York City Department of Environmental Protection published *Final Rules and Regulations for the Protection from Contamination, Degradation and Pollution of the New York City Water Supply and Its Sources* (1997). This 122-page document provides a regulatory framework for the following potential watershed contaminants: "hazardous substances and hazardous wastes, radioactive materials, petroleum products, human excreta, wastewater treatment plants, sewerage systems, service connections and discharges to sewerage systems, subsurface sewerage treatment systems, storm water pollution prevention plans and impervious surfaces, miscellaneous point sources, solid waste, agricultural activities, pesticides, fertilizers and snow disposal and storage and use of winter highway maintenance materials" (New York City Department of Environmental Protection, 1997).

Water Treatment

Given that many source waters are of poor quality, and that even high-quality source water can become contaminated, some level of water treatment is considered essential. Arguably, the water treatment train begins with conveyance of water from the source to the plant. Prevention of contamination during conveyance, which in certain cases could be hundreds of miles of pipeline, aqueduct, or even open ditches, is clearly important.

Water treatment consists of several sequential steps (see Figure 18.9). Water entering the treatment plant may undergo coarse filtration to remove vegetation, trash, dead animals, and other large solids. Chemicals may be added for specific purposes; for example, potassium permanganate may be added to oxidize soluble iron and manganese, making them easier to remove. (These metals, when present, discolor water and stain clothing and plumbing fixtures.) The next step is coagulation and precipitation. In this step a chemical such as aluminum sulfate is added, together with lime and sodium bicarbonate, which causes suspended solids, bacteria, and other particles to clump together into *floc*. The floc is then allowed to settle out, removing these materials from the water. Filtration comes next, although in some plants a disinfecting step, such as ozonation, is added to reduce microbial counts and prevent excessive microbial growth on filter materials. Filtration methods range from simple, time-honored techniques such as slow sand filtration to sophisticated technologies such as nanofiltration, depending on the resources available and the size of the population served.

The final step is postfiltration disinfection. Since the early twentieth century, chlorination has been the most widely used form of disinfection. Chlorine and chlorine compounds are thought to act as disinfectants by denaturing enzymes. Chlorine has the advantage of forming a residual in water as it flows from the treatment plant through the pipes of the distribution system to faucets. This helps prevent regrowth of microorganisms in the distribution system (although biofilms impede this goal). More recently, with concerns about the potential toxicity of chlorination by-products, alternative forms of disinfection such as ozonation and pulsed UV have been gaining popularity. Table 18.8 compares alternative forms of disinfection with chlorination.

Disinfection Resistance. One reason for exploring alternatives to chlorination is the growing realization that a number of microbes are apparently capable of surviving at the "safe" chlorination levels typically maintained in drinking water. Mechanisms of survival vary from a relatively resistant cell wall to intracellular survival. One of the most resistant microorganisms is the protozoan *Cryptosporidium parvum*, mentioned earlier. *C. parvum* forms extremely environmentally resistant oocysts that allow the organism to resist chlorine concentrations at levels that far

FIGURE 18.9. A MULTIBARRIER APPROACH TO MAXIMIZE THE MICROBIOLOGICAL QUALITY OF WATER.

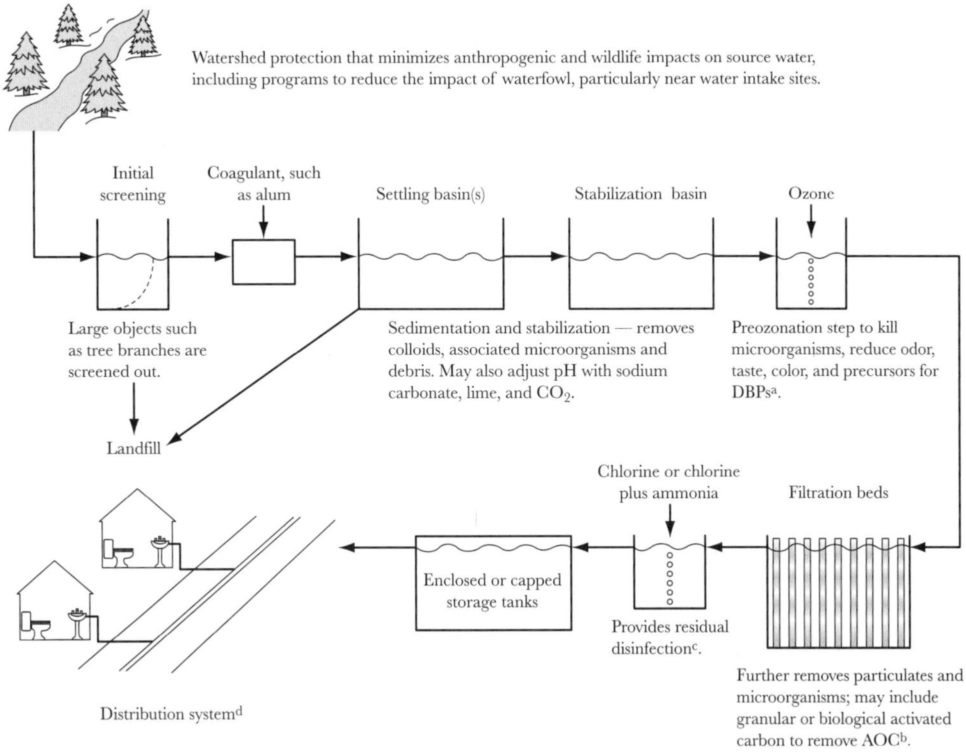

Note: This presumes a treatment system that has sufficient capacity to maintain adequate pressure throughout the distribution system for twenty-four hours per day and that minimizes opportunities for microbial colonization of the pipelines.

[a]Disinfection by-products are formed by ozonation of source waters, including aldehydes and brominated by-products (discussed in Boorman and others, 1999). UV disinfection, used extensively in wastewater treatment, is rapidly gaining acceptance as an alternative to ozonation.

[b]AOC = assimilable organic carbon—carbon that can be readily used by microorganisms and therefore stimulates their growth.

[c]Residual disinfection requires a chemical that will not be rapidly broken down in the distribution system so that it retains some disinfecting activity at point of use (the tap). To date the only practical chemicals appear to be chlorine or chloramines. Chloramination may be preferable to using chlorine, as it is believed that chloramines penetrate biofilms more effectively than chlorine alone. They also reduce DBP formation and are more effective at a high pH (a high pH is often necessary for corrosion control). Where chloramination is used, intermittent chlorination and system flushing is recommended, as chlorine is the more powerful oxidizing agent.

[d]A rigorous program is necessary to upgrade distribution system networks and to prevent interconnections through leakage, backflushing, improper hydrant use, and so forth.

TABLE 18.8. APPROACHES TO DISINFECTION.

Disinfectant	Benefits	Concerns	Cost
Chlorine	Retains a residual; strong disinfectant	Taste and odor; toxicity of by-products; some microbes are resistant; not effective at high pH	Moderate
Chloramination	Retains a residual; used for a wider range of pHs; may penetrate biofilms more effectively than free chlorine	Weaker disinfectant; some by-products formed but less than with free chlorine	Moderate
Chlorine dioxide	Powerful disinfectant; no by-products formed	Toxic; cannot be stored; chemically unstable; no residual	Expensive
Ozone	Powerful disinfectant; can be effective against chlorine-resistant microbes	Must be generated on site; can increase assimilable organic carbon; forms bromates	Expensive, but can be economical with a large operation
UV (pulsed)	Short contact time; no toxic by-products; not influenced by pH or temperature	No residual; not effective with high-turbidity water	Increasingly competitive and gaining in popularity

exceed those considered safe for drinking water treatment. Ozonation is thought to be marginally more effective against *C. parvum,* but does tend to be more expensive and does not provide a residual in the distribution system. There appears to be no alternative to chlorination for maintaining a residual, although addition of ammonia with chlorine to form chloramines is an alternative, particularly if a high pH is maintained as part of a corrosion control strategy. Disinfection resistant strategies can be summarized as follows (Ford, 1999):

- Cyst formation (protozoans); spore formation (for example, *Bacillus* sp.)
- Resistant cell wall (for example, mycobacteria)
- Viable but nonculturable (many bacterial species); injured (for example, indicator species); dwarf forms (for example, *Vibrio* sp.)
- Biofilm associated (for example, *Legionella pneumophila, Pseudomonas aeruginosa,* and many others); particle associated (for example, viruses)
- Intracellular survival (for example *Legionella pneumophila, Mycobacterium avium,* and so forth)

Disinfection By-Product Toxicity. Given the necessity for residual disinfection in distributed water, some chlorine (or chloramines) must be added posttreatment. However, chlorine compounds react with naturally occurring organic matter to form *disinfection by-products* (DBPs). The best-recognized DBPs are trihalomethanes such as chloroform and trichloroacetic acid. However, the range of disinfection by-products is enormous given the range of chemical precursors that can occur in source water. There has been some recent focus on a chlorinated furanone, 3-chloro-4-(dichloromethyl)-5-hydroxy-2(5H)-furanone, known as mutagen X. A laboratory in Finland has estimated that this compound may be greater than 100-fold more mutagenic than chloroform. However, it is present at much lower concentrations than chloroform (Boorman and others, 1999).

There is accumulating evidence that many of these chlorinated organic compounds are carcinogenic. Much of this evidence comes from animal experiments using high-dose exposures. Human exposures through drinking water are typically orders of magnitude lower, and the extent of risk to humans has been difficult to quantify. Moreover, although toxicological data are available for the trihalomethanes and haloacetates, little information is available on other DBPs. Hence, there is great uncertainty about the overall risk of DBPs. One estimate is that DBPs are responsible for 4,200 cases of bladder cancer and 6,500 cases of rectal cancer in the United States each year (Morris and others, 1992), and DBPs have been estimated to cause approximately three additional cancer deaths per 10,000 population in Taiwan (Yang, Chiu, Cheng, and Tsai, 1998).

The risk levels associated with DBPs are of concern, but they are substantially lower than the risks associated with contaminated water, especially in developing nations. In Africa, infant mortality rates from inadequate and unsafe water are between 2 and 5 percent annually (Taylor, 1993). In Latin America, in 1990, several million cases of diarrheal disease were reported, with an estimated 300,000 deaths (de Macedo, 1993). And in the United States, 5,000 deaths are attributed to foodborne illness each year (Mead and others, 1999), of which some proportion is very likely due to preparation of food with contaminated water.

In many settings, then, the risk of microbiological contamination of water eclipses the risk of DBPs. Many water experts conclude that the microbiological quality of drinking water should never be compromised for ill-defined health risks from DBPs. However, once tap water is confirmed to be free of infectious doses of pathogens, it is reasonable to explore ways to reduce the potential toxicity from DBPs. In the United States and other developed countries, this has involved examination of alternative forms of disinfection (Clark and Boutin, 2001). However, for many countries, economic reality makes these technologies and their continued maintenance an unrealistic solution and chlorine remains the most practical effective way to reduce waterborne disease.

Water Distribution

Water distribution is a critical step, and its failure has been implicated in many cases of drinking water contamination and waterborne disease outbreaks. Water, generally containing a disinfectant residual, may be distributed through hundreds of miles of pipeline throughout a major city. In addition to the major distribution lines, the water also flows through building pipelines. All these pipes are potential sites for cross-contamination through a variety of processes. Metal pipes are susceptible to corrosion and through time can develop holes that may cause external sources of water to enter the pipes during periods of low pressure. This happens, for example, when hydrants are extensively used during firefighting. Low pressure in the drinking water system can also cause back siphonage from pipes or tubing left hanging in sinks or other water or waste storage. This is a particular issue in high-rise buildings, where distribution system pressure may be insufficient to maintain supply to top floors throughout a twenty-four-hour period. Where this is the case, there is a tendency for residents to fill bathtubs and other vessels to provide a reserve. In the absence of external contamination, regrowth of microorganisms in distribution lines is a very real problem. This is particularly true at dead end sites such as fire hydrants. Water remains essentially stagnant at these sites, and any residual chlorine in the system is rapidly combined with organic matter, allowing microbes to grow and proliferate (Ford, 1993).

Point-of-Use Treatment and Bottled Water

An alternative to direct consumption of tap water that consumers increasingly consider is a point-of-use treatment device or bottled water for their potable water supply. These are certainly viable options, but it is necessary to maintain a point-of-use device properly to avoid exacerbating water quality problems by, in effect, providing a "biofilm reactor" that encourages microbial growth. Bottled water places the consumer at the mercy of the manufacturer, as bottled water is not currently as rigorously regulated as municipal water. In addition, there is a compelling argument that if the money people are willing to pay for point-of-use filters and bottled water were invested in municipal treatment and distribution, many current health risks (real and perceived) could be mitigated.

Regulatory Framework

Water quality monitoring regulations are well developed for a vast suite of chemicals, driven primarily by the increasingly sensitive technologies that can be used for measuring trace levels of contaminants. Unfortunately, the same is not true for microbial contaminants. The indicator approach (Table 18.6) remains the primary method for assessing microbiological quality of drinking water, despite the fact that many pathogens survive for extended periods in drinking water in the absence of these indicators. Indeed, a number of environmental pathogens may be present in drinking water in the complete absence of any contamination source.

The Safe Drinking Water Act

In the Safe Drinking Water Act (SDWA) (EPA, 2005), passed in 1974 and amended in 1986 and 1996, the U.S. Congress mandated the Environmental Protection Agency to regulate contaminants in drinking water that might pose a risk to human health. This complex piece of legislation has a number of important provisions.

A central strategy of the SDWA is to set permissible levels of contaminants in drinking water provided by public drinking-water utilities. EPA establishes two sets of benchmarks, one based on ideal health goals and the other based on feasibility. In the first set, known as Maximum Contaminant Level Goals (MCLGs), a goal is defined as the "level of a contaminant in drinking water below which there is no known or expected risk to health" after drinking two liters of water each day for seventy years. These levels are set to include a margin of safety. For many contaminants, such as carcinogens, lead, and some pathogens, MCLGs are set at zero. MCLGs are public health goals, not enforceable standards. In contrast, Maximum Contaminant Levels (MCLs) are legal limits. They are set as close to MCLGs as possible, taking into account both technological feasibility and cost.

The National Primary Drinking Water Regulations (NPDWR) promulgated by the EPA are based on these benchmarks. These regulations now extend to fifty-three organic compounds, sixteen inorganic compounds, four classes of radionuclides, four types of disinfection by-products, and three disinfectants. In terms of microbial contaminants, *Cryptosporidium, Giardia lamblia, Legionella,* and viruses are regulated, but only in terms of percentage of removal or inactivation by treatment. Heterotrophic plate counts (a measure of microbial load), turbidity, and total coliform levels (including fecal coliforms and *E. coli*) are also regulated and can be directly measured, but as discussed earlier, these indicators are imperfect markers of the presence of pathogens. The EPA also publishes National Secondary Drinking Water Regulations (NSDWR), which are nonenforceable guidelines for contaminants that cause cosmetic or aesthetic problems in drinking water.

The SDWA includes additional regulatory requirements. For example, EPA has established monitoring schedules, monitoring methods, and acceptable treatment technologies. Also, as discussed in Box 18.4, the Surface Water Treatment Rule governs filtration of public water supply systems.

As a requirement of the 1996 Amendment to the SDWA, EPA is required to publish, every five years, a list of contaminants that are not subject to regulation at the time of publication but that are anticipated to occur in drinking water and may require future regulation. Known as the Contaminant Candidate List (CCL), the latest iteration, CCL 2, includes forty-two chemical and nine microbiological contaminants. The CCL helps guide the EPA's research agenda. Chemicals on the list undergo extensive toxicity assessments, and risks of exposure through drinking water are characterized to the degree that current methodologies allow. The CCL 2 includes the following microbiological contaminants:

- Viruses:—adenoviruses, caliciviruses, coxsackieviruses, and echoviruses
- Bacteria: *Aeromonas hydrophila, Helicobacter pylori, Mycobacterium avium intracellulare* (MAC), cyanobacteria, and their toxins
- Protozoa:—*Microsporidia* (*Enterocytozoon* and *Septata*)
- Algae: freshwater algae and their toxins

With the possible exception of *A. hydrophila,* these contaminants are unlikely to be regulated in the near future. However, the CCL provides an important indication of contaminants that will receive growing public health attention.

Total Coliform Rule

In 1989, the EPA finalized the Total Coliform Rule. This rule is currently the driving force behind drinking water safety and frequently serves as the first indication (other than turbidity) of potential contamination. The rule requires a water system to establish a regular coliform sampling plan, with sample sites that accurately represent water quality throughout the distribution system. Any sample that is positive for total coliforms requires repeat samples and must be tested for fecal coliforms or *E. coli.* Specific requirements vary somewhat depending on the population served; however, for a large municipality, having more than 5 percent of samples test positive for total coliforms in a month constitutes a monthly Maximum Contaminant Level violation that must be reported to the municipality's respective state by the end of the next business day and the public must be notified within thirty days. Acute MCL violations result from any repeat fecal coliform or *E. coli* positive sample, or any routine fecal coliform or *E. coli* positive sample followed by a repeat total coliform sample. In the case of an acute violation the state must be notified by the end of the next business day and the public must be notified within twenty-four hours.

An additional component of the Total Coliform Rule that is designed to protect smaller public water systems is the Sanitary Survey. Every system collecting fewer than five samples per month is required to have regular Sanitary Surveys, usually every five years. This survey is designed to evaluate the entire water system, its operations, and its maintenance in order to ensure public health. (The EPA Web site provides numerous resources for conducting Sanitary Surveys, including a guidance manual; see EPA, 1999.)

Consumer Confidence Reports

An important outcome of the 1996 Amendment to the SDWA has been the requirement for utilities to provide Consumer Confidence Reports. The requirement was finalized in 1998 and is designed to "enable Americans to make practical, knowledgeable decisions about their health and their environment." In addition to carrying out rapid notification when coliform counts are high, water systems are required, at a minimum, to inform consumers annually of (EPA, 1998)

- the lake, river, aquifer, or other source of the drinking water;
- an explanation of the susceptibility to contamination of the local drinking water source;
- how to get a copy of the water system's complete source water assessment
- the level of any contaminant found in local drinking water, as well as EPA's MCL for comparison;
- the likely source of that contaminant;
- the potential health effects of any contaminant detected in violation of an EPA health standard;
- an explanation of the system's actions to address any contaminant and restore safe drinking water;
- the water system's compliance with other drinking water-related rules;
- an educational statement for vulnerable populations about avoiding *Cryptosporidium;*
- educational information on nitrate, arsenic, or lead in areas where these contaminants are detected above 50 percent of EPA's standard; and
- phone numbers of additional sources of information, including the water system and EPA's Safe Drinking Water Hotline (800-426-4791).

Recreational Water Standards

The EPA and state agencies also regulate recreational waters. For example, swimming advisories are posted where indicator organisms exceed recommended levels. For freshwater, current standards are 126 *E. coli* per 100 ml or 33 enterococci per 100 ml. The regulations state that only one of these two indicator organisms should be used. For seawater, the standard is set at 35 enterococci per 100 ml. (For further information on recreational water safety and on the rationale for standards, see EPA, 2003; Bartram and Rees, 2000; WHO, 2003a.)

Conclusion

Finally, a few new issues deserve some attention: How should we be assessing current water safety risks? How should we be dealing with the appearance of new diseases that may be transmitted by means of water? What use can we make of molecular epidemiology in assessing water quality? And what is the potential for wastewater reuse?

Risk Characterization for Water Contaminants

Risk assessment is the process used to prioritize interventions and to reduce human exposure to environmental sources of chemicals and pathogens, as described in Chapter Thirty-Two. However, microbiological risk assessment raises some additional considerations. These involve exposure assessment, variability, and complexity.

To identify microbial hazards, *spot* samples are generally taken from finished water at the treatment plant, and occasionally at conveniently accessible sites in the distribution system. However, distribution of pathogens is extremely heterogeneous in drinking water. Most consumers will not ingest an infectious dose of a pathogen, and measurements of water samples will frequently be zero. However, a few individuals may consume a large number of infectious microbes. Moreover, as previously discussed, most pathogens are poorly indicated by the presence of the routinely monitored coliform group. Utilities expect that major contamination events in a watershed will be recognized from turbidity spikes; however, this is not always the case. Turbidity spikes were not excessive for the contamination event in Milwaukee in 1993 (Mac Kenzie and others, 1994). An event of far smaller magnitude may not result in elevated turbidity, or minor spikes may be missed. Although a rare event, a *plug* of infectious oocysts, cysts, or viruses could enter the distribution system and be very easily missed by a spot sampling program, yet contain sufficient numbers to virtually ensure that ingestion will result in infection (Gale, 2001). Exposure assessment therefore remains a challenge in microbial risk assessment.

Similarly, variability is a key challenge. People vary in the doses of pathogens they sustain, an outcome related both to variation across the drinking-water system and to variation in individuals' consumption of water. People also vary in their responses to a specific infectious dose, depending on individual susceptibility (age, health, and other factors), prior exposure (immunity), and the degree of virulence of the pathogen itself (affected by numerous environmental factors).

Infectious agents themselves vary. Organisms may lose virulence and even infectivity in the distribution system or after exposure to disinfection. Conversely, organisms may increase or change in virulence and in their ability to resist antibiotics following environmental exposures.

Complexity arises in numerous ways. To begin with, water is a complex environment. It may be contaminated by both chemicals and microbes, and these two classes of contaminants interact. Some chemicals of concern are actually bacterial, fungal, or algal toxins. Some may be produced within the distribution system pipeline by the action of certain groups of organisms; the sulfate-reducing bacteria produce sulfides and other sulfur-containing chemicals, nitrifying bacteria produce nitrites and nitrates from ammonia compounds (either in source water or from chloramination). And some chemicals—the disinfection by-products—result from water treatment practices to minimize microbial contamination.

Partly for these reasons, the health risks associated with drinking water are still not fully defined and quantified. The World Health Organization publishes drinking water quality standards that are internationally recognized. In some cases, such as the WHO's current standard for arsenic, these standards are more stringent than those of the U.S. EPA. It is likely that health risks are minimal for individuals without predisposing factors—in developed nations individuals with predisposing factors would be the very young, the elderly, the pregnant, and those with compromised immune function. However, on the global scale, susceptible individuals may be as common as the nonsusceptible. Malnutrition, stress, concomitant diseases, and socioeconomic deprivation increase susceptibility. The global risk from contaminated water may be enormous.

Despite this risk, people in areas with contaminated water may, paradoxically, be protected by immunity resulting from multiple prior exposures. By all the criteria just mentioned, these populations are highly susceptible, yet immunity results in lower than expected incidence of many waterborne diseases. This immunity must come at some cost to the individual, but there is not yet a robust approach to estimate the burden of disease from exposure to multiple infectious agents (and toxins). This complexity—like the complexity within water itself—continues to challenge microbial risk assessment efforts (Gale, 2001; Fewtrell and Bartram, 2001).

The Phenomenon of New Disease

Many factors can promote the real or apparent emergence of a new disease. New ecological niches, such as the hot-water systems that support growth of *Legionella*, may contribute. Factors such as population density and increasing numbers of susceptible individuals (the very young, the elderly, pregnant women, and the immunocompromised) could provide an extensive human reservoir for opportunistic pathogens and promote changes in virulence patterns, even in developed countries. Increased adaptation to the human host might be responsible for increased infection rates in populations with no underlying susceptibility (for example, mycobacterial diseases).

Legionella pneumophila, E. coli O157, *Vibrio cholerae* O139, *Helicobacter pylori, Cryptosporidium parvum,* and *Hepatitis E,* are all examples of microorganisms categorized as "new" or "newly recognized" pathogens. Well-established pathogens should arguably be added to this list as they develop antibiotic resistance and can change virulence patterns (Ford, 1999). Research is clearly needed to understand better the ecology of the water environment that may promote new disease emergence. One research priority is biofilms, the microbial films that form on the surfaces of pipe material, which may provide an opportunity for horizontal gene transfer both within and between species. The biofilm environment may also promote expression of plasmids through exposure to chemical stressors such as metals. An increasing body of research links metal resistance with multiple antibiotic resistance determinants, presumably expressed on the same plasmids (discussed in Ford, 1993).

Molecular Epidemiology

Gene chips are tiny devices whose surfaces contain arrays of DNA or RNA fragments. When water comes into contact with the gene chip, biological materials in the sample could potentially be identified through fluorescent labeling This emerging technology may one day play a role in monitoring water quality. A recent American Academy for Microbiology report begins with the imagined scenario that a gene chip placed in the flow of water will one day detect each pathogen, with the fluorescence response triggering an alarm that prompts an appropriate treatment response (Rose and Grimes, 2001).

At present, however, the role of gene chip technology is limited by the inability to analyze and interpret accurately the vast amounts of data generated. There are also at least two major technical challenges. First, in order for a gene chip to be developed and its results understood, the target organisms must be characterized and a highly specific gene segment recognized. However, most organisms in drinking water have yet to be characterized. Second, the organism's genetic material must come in contact with the chip surface in order to hybridize to the probe. However, the heterogeneous distribution of microbes in drinking water and the need to lyse the cell are barriers that dramatically reduce the potential sensitivity of the technique. Nevertheless, gene chip technology is likely to play an increasing role in identifying water contaminants.

Wastewater Reuse

This discussion would not be complete without returning to the topic of wastewater. A vital step in providing adequate, safe drinking water is to understand that wastewater is a valuable resource. Today, water reuse programs are increasingly encouraged in the more arid states in the United States, primarily for nonpotable uses. This involves separate collection of black water (primarily toilet wastes, although it may also include other wastewater rich in organics, such as the effluent from a garbage disposal system) and gray water (other sources of wastewater such as bath and shower water). The gray water can then be used to irrigate nonedible plants and in some cases can also be used for toilet flushing.

The simplest use of gray water is direct discharge from the house to the landscape. However, there are understandable health concerns as bath and shower water may contain potential pathogens. A wide range of gray water treatment systems is available. These systems may be sufficiently sophisticated (and expensive) to remove both chemical and biological contaminants and essentially to mimic the water treatment process (Figure 18.9) on a small scale. The use of recycled wastewater to augment diminishing supplies of drinking water is just beginning. The barriers to wastewater recycling are probably issues of public perception more than cost. Just as many arid nations increasingly rely on desalination to supply drinking water, treatment technologies are more than capable of recycling wastewater to a potable quality. The predicted increase in the number of water-scarce countries during the twenty-first century makes education in this area critical. However, water recycling alone will not be sufficient without a concerted effort to conserve the available remaining resources. Figure 18.10 shows an idealized scheme for future provision of safe drinking water. Although this process would be expensive, it is increasingly recognized that water is dramatically undervalued and should be appropriately priced. It is often stated that water is a human right (WHO, 2003b). Certainly, like food, it is a human necessity. However, as mentioned earlier, people are willing to purchase bottled water at considerable expense because of their real and perceived concerns for the quality of water at the tap. There is no question that the true cost of water should be subsidized for those who cannot afford it, but realistic pricing for those who can afford to pay could dramatically improve the safety of drinking water for everyone.

However, a word of caution is necessary. How safe should our drinking water be? Arguably, for the immunocompromised it can never be too safe. Filtration technologies may one day provide water, at least at the level of the treatment plant, that is 100 percent free not only of infectious agents but also of all microorganisms.

FIGURE 18.10. IDEALIZED SCHEME FOR SAFE DRINKING WATER.

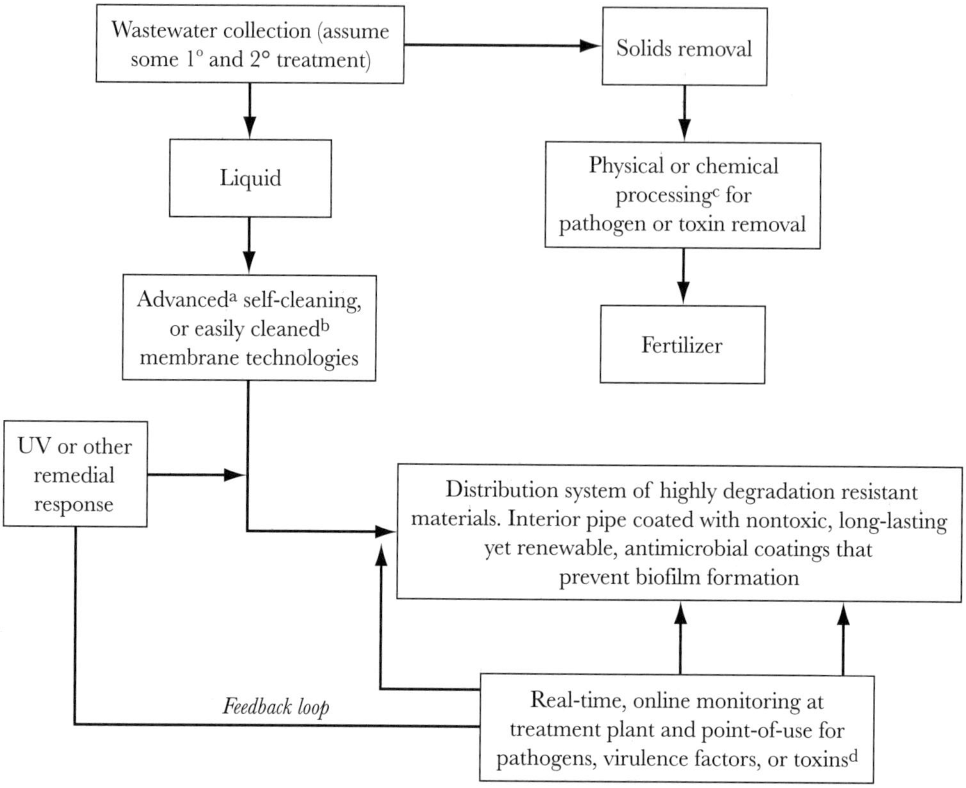

[a]Many companies now invest heavily in microfiltration, ultrafiltration, nanofiltration, and reverse osmosis membrane technologies. Hollow-fiber filtration technologies, for example, are allowing filtration capacities adequate for municipal water systems.
[b]For example, patented gas backwash systems for USFilter's Memcor® microfiltration systems.
[c]There is currently considerable debate on appropriate criteria for land application of sewage sludges, known as *biosolids.* Treatment produces biosolids that range from Class B biosolids, with a consequent risk to surface waters, to Class A biosolids, which are essentially pathogen free.
[d]The ideal monitoring tool depicted in a recent American Academy of Microbiology report (Rose and Grimes, 2001).

Source: Reproduced from Ford, 2005.

Perhaps distribution pipes will eventually be lined with materials that effectively prevent biofilm buildup. However, is this in fact optimal for the immunocompetent? Some waterborne exposure to microorganisms may be important in developing and maintaining healthy immune systems.

Thought Questions

1. Global warming may bring increasing temperatures over the next twenty years. What might be the potential consequences for waterborne and water-related diseases? Choose a specific disease, and discuss how it may be affected.
2. Almost every city has a deteriorating water distribution system. As a result, municipalities lose between 30 and 50 percent of distributed water. Imagine yourself to be the manager of a municipal water facility, and discuss options for reducing water loss. What are the alternatives, if any, to distributed water, and what would be the health risks associated with each alternative?
3. Given the number of options for water treatment available today, what would your recommendations need to take into account if you were involved in installing a new water treatment plant in a developing country with high rates of enteric diseases?
4. *The coliform group has been used for most of the past century as an indicator of fecal pollution. However, directly monitoring for pathogens such as* Vibrio cholerae *would be far more protective of public health.* Please agree or disagree with this statement, and give your reasons.
5. Describe the Aral Sea disaster. Discuss health consequences to the local communities and the long-term fate of this ecosystem.
6. *The answer to a waterborne disease outbreak is to "shock" chlorinate.* Explore this statement and the health risks that would be mitigated. What new health risks might emerge from the application of large doses of chlorine?
7. What health concerns arise from reuse of wastewater? What exposure pathways to pathogens might occur from land application of sewage sludge, reuse of wastewater for irrigation of garden plants, and toilet flushing?
8. *Relative to developing countries, waterborne disease in the United States is a nonissue. The CDC reports very few deaths from waterborne disease outbreaks, and we therefore have no reason to worry.* Identify and discuss the potential fallacies in this statement.

References

Agency for Toxic Substances and Disease Registry. "Toxicological Profile for Polychlorinated Biphenyls (PCBs)." [http://www.atsdr.cdc.gov/toxprofiles/tp17.html]. 2000.

Amer, M. H., El-Yazigi, A., Hannan, M. A., and Mohamed, M. E. "Water Contamination and Esophageal Cancer at Gassim Region, Saudi Arabia." *Gastroenterology,* 1990, *98,* 1141–1147.

Arvanitidou, M., Kanellou, K., Constantinides, T. C., and Katsouyannopoulos, V. "The Occurrence of Fungi in Hospital and Community Potable Waters." *Letters in Applied Microbiology,* 1999, *29,* 81–84.

Aschengrau, A., Rogers, S., and Ozonoff, D. "Perchloroethylene-Contaminated Drinking Water and the Risk of Breast Cancer: Additional Results from Cape Cod, Massachusetts, USA." *Environmental Health Perspectives,* 2003, *111,* 167–173.

Bartram, J., and Chorus, I. (eds.). *Toxic Cyanobacteria in Water: A Guide to Their Public Health Consequences, Monitoring and Management.* World Health Organization. [http://www.who.int/docstore/water_sanitation_health/toxicyanobact/begin.htm]. 1999.

Bartram, J., and Rees, G. (eds.). *Monitoring Bathing Waters: A Practical Guide to the Design and Implementation of Assessments and Monitoring Programs.* [http://www.who.int/water_sanitation_health/bathing/bathing3/en]. 2000.

Bitton, G. *Wastewater Microbiology.* (2nd ed.) Hoboken, N.J.: Wiley-Liss, 1999.

Brita. "Water Facts." [http://www.brita.com/life/waterfacts.shtml]. 2005.

Boorman, G. A., and others. "Drinking Water Disinfection Byproducts: Review and Approach to Toxicity Evaluation." *Environmental Health Perspectives,* 1999, *107,* 207–217.

Breiman, R. F., and Butler, J. C. "Legionnaires' Disease: Clinical, Epidemiological, and Public Health Perspectives." *Seminars in Respiratory Infections,* 1998, *13,* 84–89.

The BSE Inquiry. *The BSE Inquiry Report.* [http://www.bseinquiry.gov.uk/report/index.htm]. 2000.

Cabello, F., and Springer, A. D. "Typhoid Fever in Chile 1977–1990: An Emergent Disease." *Revista medica de Chile,* 1997, *125,* 474–482.

Calow, P., Petts, G. (eds.). *The Rivers Handbook: Hydrological and Ecological Principles.* Vol. 1. Oxford, UK: Blackwell Scientific, 1992.

Capone, D. G., and Bauer, J. E. "Microbial Processes in Coastal Pollution." In R. Mitchell (ed.), *Environmental Microbiology.* New York: Wiley, 1992.

The Catskill Center for Conservation and Development. "New York City's Water Supply System." [http://www.catskillcenter.org/programs/csp/H20/Lesson4/nycmap.gif]. n.d.

Centers for Disease Control and Prevention. "Cross-Sectional Exposure Assessment of Environmental Contaminants in Churchill County, Nevada." [http://www.cdc.gov/nceh/clusters/Fallon/study.htm]. 2003.

Chakraborty, S., and others. "Concomitant Infection of Enterotoxigenic *Escherichia coli* in an Outbreak of Cholera Caused by *Vibrio Cholerae* O1 and O139 in Ahmedabad, India." *Journal of Clinical Microbiology,* 2001, *39,* 3241–3246.

Clark, R. M., and Boutin, B. K. (eds.). *Controlling Disinfection By-Products and Microbial Contaminants in Drinking Water.* EPA/600/R-01/110. [http://www. epa.gov/ORD/NRMRL/Pubs/600R01110/600R01110.htm] 2001.

Clarke, R. *Water: The International Crisis.* Cambridge, Mass.: MIT Press, 1993.

Cohn, P., and others. "Drinking Water Contamination and the Incidence of Leukemia and Non-Hodgkin's Lymphoma." *Environmental Health Perspectives,* 1994, *102,* 556–561.

Colwell, R. R. "Global Climate and Infectious Disease: The Cholera Paradigm." *Science,* 1996, *274,* 2025–2031.

Colwell, R. R., and Huq, A. "Vibrios in the Environment: Viable but Non-Culturable *Vibrio Cholerae.*" In I. K. Wachsmuth, O. Olsvik, and P. A. Blake (eds.), *Vibrio Cholerae and Cholera: Molecular to Global Perspectives.* Washington, D.C.: ASM Press, 1994.

Colwell, R. R., and others. "Viable but Nonculturable *Vibrio Cholerae* and Related Pathogens in the Environment: Implications for Release of Genetically Engineered Microorganisms." *Biotechnology,* 1985, *3,* 817–820.

Converse, K., Wolcott, M., Docherty, D., and Cole, R. *Screening for Potential Human Pathogens in Fecal Material Deposited by Resident Canada Geese on Areas of Public Utility.* Madison, Wis.: U.S. Geological Service, National Animal Health Center, 2001.

Costas, K., Knorr, R. S., and Condon, S. K. "A Case-Control Study of Childhood Leukemia in Woburn, Massachusetts: The Relationship Between Leukemia Incidence and Exposure to Public Drinking Water." *Science of the Total Environment,* 2002, *300*(1–3), 23–35.

Cox, S. E., and Kahle, S. C. *Hydrogeology, Ground-Water Quality, and Sources of Nitrate in Lowland Glacial Aquifers of Whatcom County, Washington, and British Columbia, Canada.* USGS Water-Resources Investigations Report 98-4195. Washington, D.C.: U.S. Geological Survey, 1999.

de Macedo, C. G. "Balancing Microbial and Chemical Risks in Disinfection of Drinking Water: The Pan American Perspective." In G. F. Craun (ed.), *Safety of Water Disinfection: Balancing Chemical and Microbial Risks.* Washington: ILSI Press, 1993.

Del Porto, D., and Steinfeld, C. *The Composting Toilet System Book: A Practical Guide to Choosing, Planning and Maintaining Composting Toilet Systems, a Water-Saving, Pollution-Preventing Alternative.* Concord, Mass.: Center for Ecological Pollution Prevention, 2000.

Easterling, D. R., and others. "Climate Extremes: Observations, Modeling, and Impacts." *Science,* 2000, *289,* 2068–2074.

Egorov, A. I., and others. "Contamination of Water Supplies with *Cryptosporidium* and *Giardia Lamblia* and Diarrheal Illness in Selected Russian Cities. *International Journal of Hygiene and Environmental Health,* 2002, *205,* 281–289.

Egorov, A. I., and others. "Serological Evidence of *Cryptosporidium* Infections in a Russian City and Evaluation of Risk Factors for Infection." *Annals of Epidemiology,* 2004, *14,* 129–136.

Ellis, W. S. "A Soviet Sea Lies Dying." *National Geographic,* Feb. 1990, pp. 73–93.

Engelman, R., and others. *People in the Balance: Population and Natural Resources at the Turn of the Millennium.* Population Action International. [http://www.populationaction.org/resources/publications/peopleinthebalance/pb_water_freshwater.shtml]. 2004.

Faruque, S. M., Albert, M. J. and Mekalanos, J. J. "Epidemiology, Genetics, and Ecology of Toxigenic *Vibrio Cholerae.*" *Microbiology and Molecular Biology Reviews,* 1998, *62,* 1301–1314.

Fewtrell, L., and Bartram, J. (eds.). *Water Quality: Guidelines, Standards and Health: Assessment of Risk and Risk Management for Water-Related Infectious Disease.* [http://www.who.int/water_sanitation_health/dwq/whoiwa/en]. 2001.

Ford, T. E. "The Microbial Ecology of Water Distribution and Outfall Systems." In T. E. Ford (ed.), *Aquatic Microbiology: An Ecological Approach.* Malden, Mass.: Blackwell, 1993.

Ford, T. E. "Microbiological Safety of Drinking Water: United States and Global Perspectives." *Environmental Health Perspectives,* 1999, *107,* 191–206.

Ford, T. E. "Future Needs and Priorities." In Cloete, T. E., Rose, J., Nel, L. H., and Ford T. E. (eds.), *Microbial Waterborne Pathogens.* London: IWA, 2004.

Ford, T. E., and Colwell, R. R. "A Global Decline in Microbiological Safety of Water: A Call for Action." [http://www.asm.org/academy/index.asp?bid=2202]. 1995.

Ford, T. E., Rupp, G., Butterfield, P., and Camper, A. "Protecting Public Health in Small Water Systems: Report of an International Colloquium." Montana Water Center. [http://water.montana.edu/colloquium/]. 2005.

Franceys, R., Pickford, J., and Reed, R. *Guide to the Development of On-Site Sanitation.* [http://www.who.int/water_sanitation_health/hygiene/envsan/onsitesan/en]. 1992.

Gale, P. "Developments in Microbiological Risk Assessment for Drinking Water." *Journal of Applied Microbiology,* 2001, *91,* 191–205.

Geldreich, E. E. *Microbial Quality of Water Supply in Distribution Systems.* Boca Raton, Fla.: CRC Press, 1996.

Gleick, P. H. (ed.). *Water in Crisis: A Guide to the World's Fresh Water Resources.* New York: Oxford University Press, 1993.

Gleick, P. H. (ed.). *The World's Water: The Biennial Report on Freshwater Resources.* Washington, D.C.: Island Press, 1998, 2000, 2002.

Hazen, T. C., and Toranzos, G. A. "Tropical Source Waters." In G. A. McFeters (ed.), *Drinking Water Microbiology.* New York: Springer, 1990.

Hrudey, S. E., and Hrudey, E. J. *Safe Drinking Water: Lessons from Recent Outbreaks in Affluent Nations.* London: IWA, 2004.

Hunter, P. R. *Waterborne Disease: Epidemiology and Ecology.* Hoboken, N.J.: Wiley, 1997.

King, C. H., Shotts, E. B., Wooley, R. E., and Porter, K. G. "Survival of Coliforms and Bacterial Pathogens Within Protozoa During Chlorination." *Applied and Environmental Microbiology,* 1988, *54,* 3023–3033.

Klare, M. T. *Resource Wars: The New Landscape of Global Conflict.* New York: Henry Holt, 2001.

Levy, S. B. "The Challenge of Antibiotic Resistance." *Scientific American,* Mar. 1998, pp. 46–53.

Lopman, B. A., Brown, D. W., and Koopmans, M. "Human Caliciviruses in Europe." *Journal of Clinical Virology,* 2002, *24,* 137–160.

Lopman, B. A., and others. "Viral Gastroenteritis Outbreaks in Europe, 1995–2000." *Emerging Infectious Diseases,* 2003, *9,* 90–96.

Mac Kenzie, W. R., and others. "A Massive Outbreak in Milwaukee of *Cryptosporidium* Infection Transmitted Through the Public Water Supply." *New England Journal of Medicine,* 1994, *331,* 161–167.

Madigan, M. T., Martinko, J. M., and Parker, J. *Brock Biology of Microorganisms.* (10th ed.) Upper Saddle River, N.J.: Prentice Hall, 2004.

Majewski, M. S., and Capel, P. D. *Pesticides in the Atmosphere: Distribution, Trends, and Governing Factors.* Chelsea, Mich.: Ann Arbor Press, 1995.

Mallin, K. "Investigation of a Bladder Cancer Cluster in Northwestern Illinois." *American Journal of Epidemiology,* 1990, *132,* 96–106.

Marshall, M. M., Naumovitz, D., Ortega, Y., and Sterling, C. R. "Waterborne Protozoan Pathogens." *Clinical Microbiology Reviews,* 1997, *10,* 67–85.

Massachusetts Water Resources Authority. "The Deer Island Sewage Treatment Plant." [http://www.mwra.state.ma.us/03sewer/html/sewditp.htm]. n.d.

Mead, P. S., and others. "Food-Related Illness and Death in the United States." *Emerging Infectious Diseases,* 1999, *5,* 607–625.

Metcalf, J. S., and Codd, G. A. *Cyanobacterial Toxins in the Water Environment: A Review of Current Knowledge.* [http://www.fwr.org/cyanotox.pdf]. 2004.

Mitchell, R. (ed.). *Environmental Microbiology.* Hoboken, N.J.: Wiley-Liss, 1992.

Moore, B. C., Martinez, E., Gay, J. M., and Rice, D. H. "Survival of *Salmonella Enterica* in Freshwater and Sediments and Transmission by the Aquatic Midge *Chironomus Tentans* (*Chironomidae: Diptera*)." *Applied and Environmental Microbiology,* 2003, *69,* 4556–4560.

Morel, F.M.M., and Hering, J. G. *Principles and Applications of Aquatic Chemistry.* (2nd ed.) Hoboken, N.J.: Wiley, 1993.

Morris, R. D., and Levin, R. "Estimating the Incidence of Waterborne Infectious Disease Related to Drinking Water in the United States." In E. G. Reichard and G. A. Zapponi (eds.), *Assessing and Managing Health Risks from Contamination: Approaches and Applications.* Wallingford, UK: IAHS, 1995.

Morris, R. D., and others. "Chlorination, Chlorination By-Products, and Cancer: A Meta-Analysis." *American Journal of Public Health,* 1992, *82,* 955–963.

National Water Quality Assessment Program. Homepage. [http://water.usgs.gov/nawqa]. 2005.

New York City. "New York City's 2001 Watershed Protection Program Summary, Assessment and Long-term Plan." [http://www.nyc.gov/html/dep/html/fadplan.html]. 2002.

New York City Department of Environmental Protection. *Final Rules and Regulations for the Protection from Contamination, Degradation and Pollution of the New York City Water Supply and Its Sources.* [http://www.ci.nyc.ny.us/html/dep/html/ruleregs/finalrandr.html]. 1997.

New York City Department of Environmental Protection. *New York City's Water Supply System: History.* [http://www.nyc.gov/html/dep/html/history.html]. 2002.

O'Connor, D. R. *Report of the Walkerton Inquiry.* [http://www.attorneygeneral.jus.gov.on.ca/english/about/pubs/walkerton]. 2002.

Pacific Institute. *The World's Water.* [http://www.worldwater.org/default.htm]. 2003.

Pan American Health Organization. "Cholera in the Americas." *Epidemiological Bulletin,* 1995, *16,* 11–13.

Payment, P., Sartory, D. P., and Reasoner, D. J. "The History and Use of HPC in Drinking-Water Quality Management." In J. Bartram and others (eds.), *Heterotrophic Plate Counts and Drinking-Water Safety: The Significance of HPCs for Water Quality and the Human Health.* [http://www.who.int/water_sanitation_health/dwq/hpc/en]. 2003.

Pedley, S., and others (eds.). *Pathogenic Mycobacteria in Water: A Guide to Public Health Consequences, Monitoring and Management.* London: IWA, 2004.

Postel, S. *Last Oasis: Facing Water Scarcity.* (2nd ed.) New York: Norton, 1997.

Postel, S. *Pillar of Sand: Can the Irrigation Miracle Last?* New York: Norton, 1999.

Rose, J. B., and Grimes, D. J. *Reevaluation of Microbial Water Quality: Powerful New Tools for Detection and Risk Assessment.* [http://www.asm.org/academy/index.asp?bid=2156]. 2001.

Samrakandi, M. M., Ridenour, D. A., Yan, L., and Cirillo, J. D. "Entry into Host Cells by *Legionella.*" *Frontiers in Bioscience,* 2002, *7,* 1–11.

Schwarzenbach, R. P., Gschwend, P. M., and Imboden, D. M. *Environmental Organic Chemistry.* Hoboken, N.J.: Wiley-Interscience, 1993.

Shea, K. M. "Antibiotic Resistance: What Is the Impact of Agricultural Uses of Aantibiotics on Children's Health?" *Pediatrics,* 2003, *112,* 253–258.

Singh, A., and McFeters, G. A. "Injury of Enteropathogenic Bacteria in Drinking Water." In G. A. McFeters (ed.), *Drinking Water Microbiology.* New York: Springer, 1990.

Spearman, P. "Imported Dracunculiasis—United States, 1995 and 1997." *Morbidity and Mortality Weekly Report,* 1998, *47*(11), 209–211.

Stumm, W., and Morgan, J. J. *Aquatic Chemistry.* (3rd ed.) Hoboken, N.J.: Wiley, 1996.

Sulaiman, I. M., and others. "Differentiating Human from Animal Isolates of *Cryptosporidium Parvum.*" *Emerging Infectious Diseases,* 1998, *4,* 681–685.

Taylor, P. "Global Perspectives on Drinking Water: Water Supplies in Africa." In G. F. Craun (ed.), *Safety of Water Disinfection: Balancing Chemical and Microbial Risks.* Washington: ILSI Press, 1993.

United Nations Educational, Cultural and Scientific Organization, World Water Assessment Program. *Water for People, Water for Life: The UN World Water Development Report.* [http://unesdoc.unesco.org/images/0012/001295/129556e.pdf]. 2003.

U.S. Environmental Protection Agency. "Ground Water & Drinking Water." [www.epa.gov/safewater/ccr/ccrfact.html]. 1998.

U.S. Environmental Protection Agency. *Guidance Manual for Conducting Sanitary Surveys of Public Water Systems: Surface Water and Ground Water Under the Direct Influence* (GWUDI). EPA 815-R-99-016. [http://www.epa.gov/safewater/mdbp/pdf/sansurv/sansurv.pdf]. 1999.

U.S. Environmental Protection Agency. *Estimated per Capita Water Ingestion in the United States.* EPA-822-R00-008. [http://www.epa.gov/waterscience/drinking/percapita/Text.pdf]. 2000.

U.S. Environmental Protection Agency. *Bacterial Water Quality Standards for Recreational Waters (Freshwater and Marine Waters): Status Report.* EPA-823-R-03-008. [http://www.epa.gov/waterscience/beaches/local/statrept.pdf]. 2003.

U.S. Environmental Protection Agency. "Terms of the Environment." [http://www.epa.gov/OCEPAterms]. 2004.

U.S. Environmental Protection Agency. "Safe Drinking Water Act." [www.epa.gov/safewater/sdwa/sdwa.html]. 2005.

U.S. Geological Survey. *Pesticides Used on and Detected in Ground Water Beneath Golf Courses.* [http://ca.water.usgs.gov/pnsp/golf.html]. 1998.

U.S. Geological Survey. *Pesticides in Stream Sediment and Aquatic Biota: Current Understanding of Distribution and Major Influences.* [http://ca.water.usgs.gov/pnsp/rep/fs09200]. 2000.

U.S. Geological Survey. *High Plains Regional Ground Water (HPGW) Study.* [http://webserver.cr.usgs.gov/nawqa/hpgw]. 2004.

Van Donsel, D. J., and Geldreich, E. E. "Relationships of Salmonellae to Fecal Coliforms in Bottom Sediments." *Water Research,* 1971, *5,* 1079–1087.

Wing, S., Freedman, S., and Band, L. "The Potential Impact of Flooding on Confined Animal Feeding Operations in Eastern North Carolina." *Environmental Health Perspectives,* 2002, *110,* 387–391.

Winter, T. C., Harvey, J. W. Franke, O. L., and Alley, W. M. *Ground Water and Surface Water a Single Resource.* U.S. Geological Survey Circular 1139. [http://water.usgs.gov/pubs/circ/circ1139/index.html#pdf]. 2001.

Woods Hole Oceanographic Institution. "Red Tide." [http://www.whoi.edu/redtide]. 2005.

World Health Organization. *Guidelines for Drinking Water Quality,* Vol. 1: *Recommendations.* (2nd ed.) Geneva: World Health Organization, 1993.

World Health Organization. *World Health Report 1996: Fighting Disease, Fostering Development.* Geneva: World Health Organization, 1996.

World Health Organization. *Guidelines for Safe Recreational Waters,* Vol. 1: *Coastal and Fresh Waters.* [http://www.who.int/water_sanitation_health/bathing/en]. 2003a.

World Health Organization. *The Right to Water.* [http://www.who.int/water_sanitation_health/en/rtwintro.pdf]. 2003b.

World Health Organization. *The World Health Report 2003: Shaping the Future.* Geneva: World Health Organization, 2003c.

World Health Organization. *Dracunculiasis, Policy, Strategy and Objectives.* [http://www.who.int/ctd/dracun/strategies.htm]. 2004.

Yang, C. Y., Chiu, H. F., Cheng, M. F., and Tsai, S. S. "Chlorination of Drinking Water and Cancer Mortality in Taiwan." *Environmental Research,* 1998, *78,* 1–6.

Zwingle, E. "Ogallala Aquifer: Wellspring of the High Plains." *National Geographic,* Mar. 1993, pp. 80–109.

For Further Information

The American Water Works Association (AWWA) provides consumer information on drinking water and many other water-related topics. It also provides useful links to a number of sites, including a link to a unique site for physicians to help them improve "recognition of waterborne disease and health effects of water pollution":

American Water Works Association. Homepage. [http://www.awwa.org]. 2005.
Meinhardt, P. "Recognizing Waterborne Disease and The Health Effects of Water Pollution." [http://www.waterhealthconnection.org/index.asp]. 2005.

The Web site of the British Geological Survey provides information on the greatest mass poisoning from contaminated water ever recorded, the arsenic crisis in Bangladesh:

British Geological Survey. "Arsenic Contamination of Groundwater." [http://www.bgs.ac.uk/arsenic]. 2004.

The *Morbidity and Mortality Weekly Report* (MMWR) of the Centers for Disease Control and Prevention is the authoritative source on outbreaks of infectious disease in the United States. However, at least for waterborne disease, reports likely underestimate by orders of magnitude the actual incidence. Another useful CDC site provides information on drinking water, diarrheal disease, and recreational water quality.

Centers for Disease Control and Prevention. *Morbidity and Mortality Weekly Report.* [http://www.cdc.gov/mmwr]. (Weekly.)
Centers for Disease Control and Prevention, Division of Parasitic Diseases. "Parasitic Disease Information: Waterborne Illnesses." [http://www.cdc.gov/ncidod/dpd/parasites/waterborne/default.htm]. 2000.

The U.S. Environmental Protection Agency Web offers numerous useful resources related to water and health; see, for example:

U.S. Environmental Protection Agency. "Ground Water and Drinking Water." [http://www.epa.gov/safewater]. 2005.
U.S. Environmental Protection Agency. Homepage. [http://www.epa.gov]. 2005.
U.S. Environmental Protection Agency. "List of Contaminants and Their MCLs." [http://www.epa.gov/safewater/mcl.html#mcls]. 2005.
U.S. Environmental Protection Agency. "Safe Drinking Water Act." [http://www.epa.gov/safewater/sdwa/sdwa.html.] 2005.
U.S. Environmental Protection Agency. "Superfund Program." [http://www.epa.gov/superfund]. 2005.
U.S. Environmental Protection Agency. "Terms of the Environment." [http://www.epa.gov/OCEPAterms]. 2004.
U.S. Environmental Protection Agency, National Risk Management Research Laboratory (NRMRL). "Index of /ORD/NRMRL/Pub[lication]s." [http://www.epa.gov/ORD/NRMRL/Pubs]. 2005.

The Pacific Institute is "an independent, nonpartisan think tank studying issues at the intersection of development, environment, and security." Its Web site has links to a selection of publications on water that form a considerable database on, for example, global water availability and water use, as well as many other critical water issues:

Pacific Institute. Homepage. [http://www.pacinst.org]. 2005.

The United Nations offers a number of water-related Web sites; see, for example:

United Nations Children's Fund. "Water, Environment and Sanitation." [http://www.unicef.org/wes/index.html]. 2005.
United Nations Development Programme. "Water." [http://www.undp.org/water]. 2005.
United Nations Educational, Scientific and Cultural Organization. "Water." [http://www.unesco.org/water]. 2005.
United Nations Environment Programme. "Freshwater." [http://freshwater.unep.net]. 2005.
United Nations. Homepage. [http://www.un.org]. 2005.

The U.S. Geological Survey maintains an extremely useful resource with current assessments of ground and surface water quality in many U.S. river basins and aquifers:

U.S. Geological Survey. "National Water Quality Assessment Program." [http://water.usgs.gov/nawqa]. 2005.

The Water and Sanitation Program describes itself as "an integrated partnership to help the poor gain sustained access to improved water and sanitation":

Water and Sanitation Program. Homepage. [http://www.wsp.org]. 2005.

The Water Environment Federation (WEF) describes itself as a "technical and educational organization with members from varied disciplines who work toward the WEF vision of preservation and enhancement of the global water environment":

Water Environment Federation. Homepage. [http://www.wef.org]. 2005.

The Water Environment Research Foundation funds research to "address water quality issues as they impact water resources, the atmosphere, the lands, and quality of life." For examples of research projects on water and health, see

Water Environment Research Foundation. "News Highlights." [http://www.werf.org/index.cfm]. 2005.

The World Bank Web site provides links to major World Bank-funded projects; see, for example:

World Bank. Homepage. [http://www.worldbank.org]. 2005.
World Bank. "Water Resources Management." [http://lnweb18.worldbank.org/ESSD/ardext.nsf/18ParentDoc/WaterResourcesManagement?Opendocument]. 2004.
World Bank. "Water Supply and Sanitation." [http://www.worldbank.org/watsan]. 2005.

The Woods Hole Oceanographic Research Institution offers probably the best maintained source of on-line information on toxic algal blooms:

Woods Hole Oceanographic Research Institution. "Harmful Algae." [http://www.whoi.edu/redtide]. 2005.

The World Health Organization is arguably the leading source of information for internationally accepted statistics on human health, including water and health; see, for example:

World Health Organization. Homepage. [http://www.who.int/en]. 2005.
World Health Organization. "WHO Guidelines for Drinking Water Quality." [http://www.who.int/water_sanitation_health/dwq/guidelines/en]. 2005.
World Health Organization. "WHO Infectious Disease Index" (providing links to pages on diarrheal disease, cholera, dracunculiasis, malaria, and so forth). [http://www.who.int/health-topics/idindex.htm]. 2005.
World Health Organization. "Water, Sanitation and Health." [http://www.who.int/water_sanitation_health/en]. 2005.
World Health Organization. "WHO Weekly Epidemiological Record." [http://www.who.int/wer/en]. (Weekly.)
World Health Organization. "WHO World Health Report" (links to annual reports with data on the global burden of disease). [http://www.who.int/whr/en]. 2005.

The World Water Council, an "international water policy think tank," offers many articles on water policies and the barriers to and solutions for effective management of the world's water resources:

World Water Council. Homepage. [http://www.worldwatercouncil.org]. 2005.

PART FOUR

ENVIRONMENTAL HEALTH ON THE LOCAL SCALE

CHAPTER NINETEEN

SOLID AND HAZARDOUS WASTE

Sven Rodenbeck
Kenneth Orloff
Harvey Rogers
Henry Falk

Like all animal species, humans are producers of wastes. It is significant, however, that as humankind has evolved, the character of the wastes produced has changed markedly. No other species in the animal kingdom shares this trait. Like animal wastes, the wastes of early humans were highly organic and consisted of such materials as excreta, bedding materials, crude clothing, and implements. As humans evolved, however, refined and inorganic materials such as paper, cloth, ceramics, and metals were added to their wastes.

For many centuries, human waste products reflected a fundamentally agrarian lifestyle. As mankind's endeavors evolved to include more technology and industry, the mix of wastes produced by society changed radically and irrevocably. Mining spoils, ashes and slag from metal processing, and other industrial wastes became commonplace. As industry grew in complexity throughout the nineteenth and twentieth centuries, the waste mix became more varied and complex to manage. Waste management has emerged as a significant challenge because of the growing variety of wastes and the trend throughout the twentieth century toward more packaging and disposal features.

Finally, along with the industrialization and modernization of society, the steady trend toward urbanization of much of the population has affected waste management. As cities became more crowded, a shortage of space to accommodate all the waste developed. Open dumping and backyard burn barrels were no longer acceptable means of waste disposal. The rest of this chapter describes the types of wastes produced by modern society, the significance of those wastes with respect to human health and the environment, and some of the ways that wastes are managed.

What Is Solid Waste?

Determining whether something is solid waste is not a trivial matter. People have debated for years what solid waste is and how it should be managed. In fact, some material that is managed as solid waste is not a solid at room temperature but is rather a liquid or a gas (for example, gasses in cylinders). A fundamental premise is that a material is waste if it no longer has value or usable purpose. This requires a judgment that may be influenced by the eye of the beholder. Some materials once designated as wastes were later found to have value. For example, using new technology former mining wastes have been reextracted to recover residual metals. Cultural norms also influence the value judgment. Western industrial societies often throw away material with little thought of reuse or repair alternatives. However, as a starting point, the fundamental premise just described is probably adequate to characterize solid waste.

In the United States and generally in most modern industrial countries, waste material is typically divided into three broad categories:

1. Municipal solid waste
2. Special waste
3. Hazardous waste

Complex laws and regulations govern how these materials are identified, stored, collected, transported, treated, and finally disposed of.

Municipal Solid Waste

Municipal solid waste consists of everyday items that are commonly generated from homes. Over half of the U.S. municipal solid waste generated in 2001 consisted of containers, packaging, and nondurable goods such as newspapers and magazines (Figure 19.1). Other major components of municipal solid waste include yard trimmings, food wastes, and durable goods such as appliances, tires, and batteries. Local laws and regulations may prohibit the disposal of some of these materials (for example, tires) as municipal solid waste. More and more frequently, municipal and county governments are also prohibiting the disposal of yard clippings with municipal solid waste, requiring that the clippings be composted or disposed of in some other, more environmentally friendly manner.

FIGURE 19.1. COMPOSITION OF THE 229 MILLION TONS OF MUNICIPAL SOLID WASTE PRODUCED IN THE UNITED STATES (BEFORE RECYCLING), 2001.

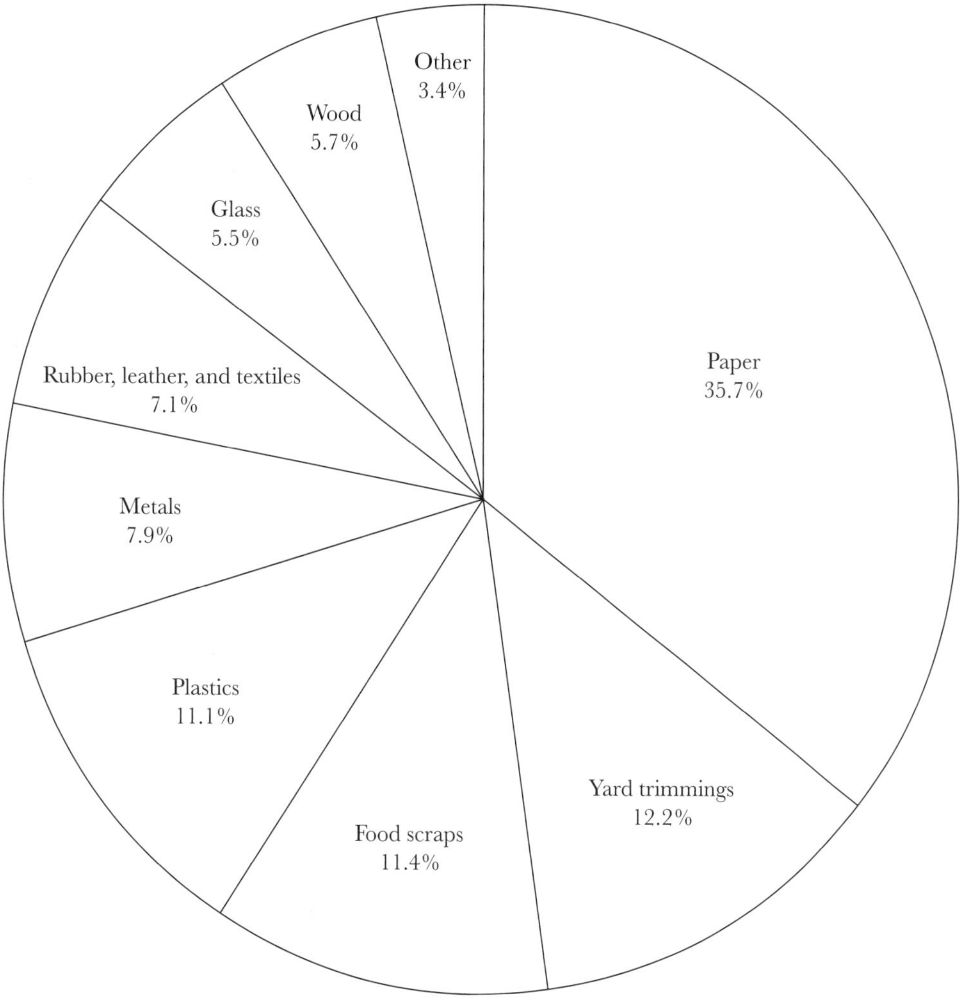

Source: Adapted from U.S. Environmental Protection Agency [EPA], 2003.

In the United States the per capita generation of municipal solid waste has increased steadily over the last forty years. In 2001, each person in the United States generated approximately 4.4 pounds of waste per day (Figure 19.2). This is an increase over the 1960 average of 2.7 pounds per person per day.

FIGURE 19.2. TOTAL AND PER CAPITA AMOUNTS OF MUNICIPAL SOLID WASTE PRODUCED IN THE UNITED STATES (BEFORE RECYCLING), 1960–2001.

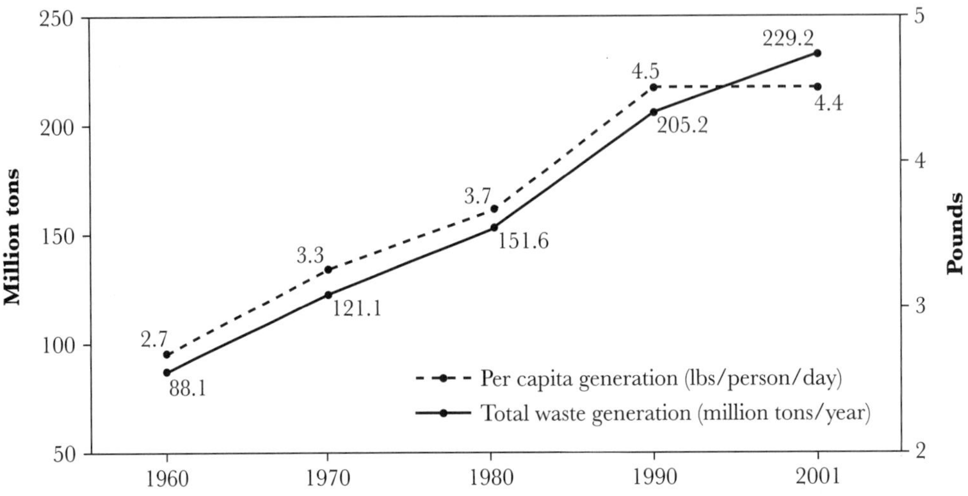

Source: Adapted from EPA, 2003.

Municipal solid waste from nonresidential sources such as office buildings is usually handled along with residential waste unless specifically regulated. For example, companies that discard large quantities of spent dry cell batteries may be required to manage them as hazardous waste.

Special Waste

This grouping is a catchall category of wastes. If a waste is neither municipal solid waste nor a designated hazardous waste, it will likely have a special designation with associated laws or regulations. Some commonly identified special wastes are

- Medical waste
- Construction debris
- Asbestos
- Mining waste
- Agricultural waste
- Radioactive waste
- Sewage sludge

Radioactive waste and sewage sludge are discussed in Chapters Twenty-Four and Eighteen, respectively.

Medical Waste. Medical waste includes items that are generated from health care treatment or research facilities (human and nonhuman) and that have come in contact with body fluids (for example, blood) or other material that may contain infectious or disease-causing agents, for example:

- Soiled or blood-soaked bandages
- Culture dishes and other associated glassware
- Gloves, gowns, scalpels, and other items used during surgery
- Needles used to give injections or draw blood
- Body fluids and tissues

One of the reasons medical waste is handled separately from municipal solid waste is to protect sanitation workers from infectious agents in the waste materials (Box 19.1).

Box 19.1. Health Risks of Medical Wastes

The proper management and disposal of waste material generated during health care activities has been a topic of discussion for several years. The U.S. public's concerns about medical waste heightened after medical materials washed up on East Coast beaches during the summers of 1987 and 1988. In addition to aesthetic concerns, fear of AIDS (acquired immunodeficiency syndrome) contributed heavily to the public's anxiety regarding medical waste.

The predominant health risk associated with medical waste is the presence of infectious pathological organisms (microorganisms—parasites, bacteria, and viruses—capable of causing infection and disease). It is important to remember that disease can occur only when all of the following occur together: the presence of an infectious agent, a sufficient number of infectious agents to cause infection, the availability of a susceptible host, and an appropriate portal of entry into that susceptible host. If any one of these factors does not exist, then disease will not occur. Because many infectious agents do not remain viable for an extended period of time outside a host, the potential for transmitting disease is greatest at the point where the waste is generated, usually in a hospital, clinic, or medical office. People who provide medical care at home may also be exposed to infectious wastes. In fact the greatest risk of disease transmission from medical waste is associated with accidental skin punctures from hypodermic needles and other *sharps.* This is particularly true for sharps contaminated with blood-borne pathogens (specifically, the Hepatitis B or C viruses and, to a much lesser extent, HIV).

FIGURE 19.3. LABELING ON MEDICAL WASTE CONTAINER.

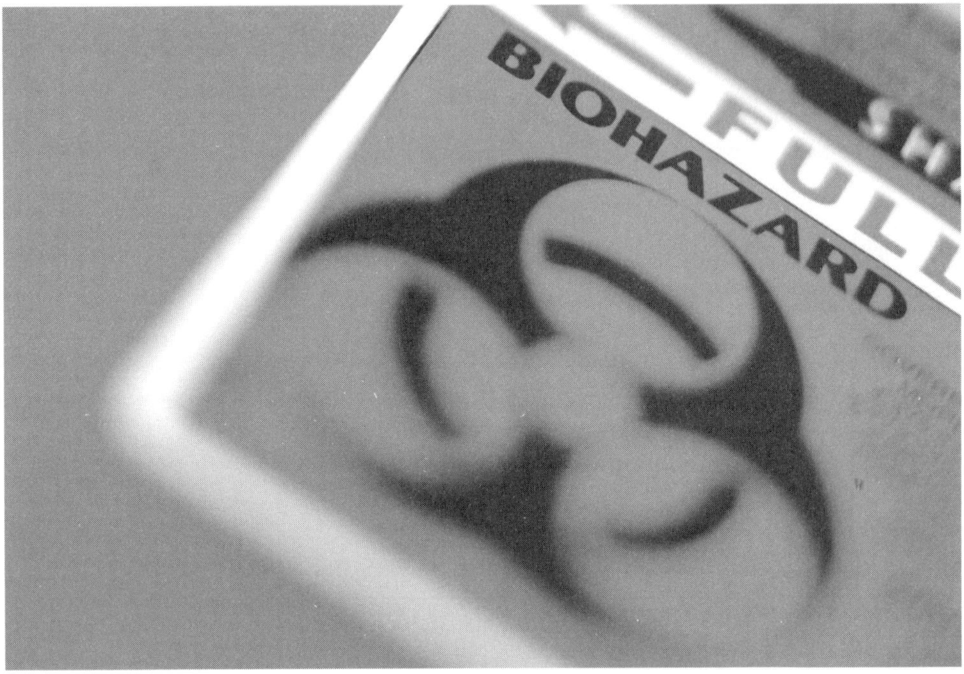

Owing to aesthetic concerns and studies that demonstrate that health care workers are at highest risk of being infected with Hepatitis B, Hepatitis C, or HIV by medical waste, medical waste is separated at the source from municipal solid waste. Separate containers are located in or near medical treatment areas in the health care facility (Figure 19.3). In particular, sharps are placed in penetration-resistant containers. Medical waste material is sealed in these containers and then usually shipped to specifically designed and managed medical waste incinerators. In some situations the waste material is treated in large autoclaves and then shipped to a secure landfill.

Construction Debris. Unless a construction material is regulated separately (as asbestos is, for example) the construction debris waste stream consists of material generated from the construction and demolition of buildings and other facilities. Typically, this *rubble* is disposed of in landfills specifically for construction debris or in municipal solid waste landfills.

Asbestos. In the United States, asbestos is designated a special waste, with its own rules and regulations. This class of fibrous minerals has, in the past, been used extensively in consumer products such as car brake linings and construction materials. Most uses of asbestos have been banned in the United States because of its demonstrated capacity to cause disease in workers and other people who have frequent contact with the minerals. To prevent the airborne release of asbestos fibers, federal regulations provide detailed guidance on the removal, packaging, and disposal of asbestos-containing material.

Mining Waste. The extraction of metals, coal, and oil from the earth's crust generates huge quantities of waste materials. The volume of wastes from mining operations exceeds the volume of wastes from all other categories combined. The disposal of leftover rubble and liquid material is regulated by solid waste laws and regulations and also by water pollution controls and land-use or land-reuse laws and regulations.

Agricultural Waste. In technologically advanced countries, the production of food has become highly industrialized. This has resulted in an increased concentration of animals and thus increased localized production of wastes. The clean water protection program regulates the liquid waste and sludge, or manure, from operations such as animal feedlots (see Chapter Eighteen). Those waste materials not regulated by federal laws are managed either by local authorities or through best practices developed by the industry.

Hazardous Waste

Hazardous waste can be simply defined as waste with properties that make it capable of harming human health or the environment. However, for regulatory purposes this simplistic definition is not sufficient. In the United States the Environmental Protection Agency's Resource Conservation and Recovery Act (RCRA) program has developed specific criteria for defining hazardous waste. RCRA regulations define hazardous waste by means of two different mechanisms. First, the materials from approximately 500 specific industrial waste streams are defined as hazardous. These listed wastes include materials such as spent solvents, electroplating wastes, and wood-preserving wastes. Second, wastes with specific characteristics are also defined as hazardous. The Environmental Protection Agency (EPA) has developed standardized test criteria to determine a waste's ignitability, corrosiveness, reactivity, and toxicity. If a waste possesses any of the criteria characteristics, it is classified as hazardous. However, many waste materials are specifically excluded from the hazardous waste definitions and regulations (for example, petroleum-related material is excluded).

In 2001, approximately 45 million tons of hazardous waste were generated in the United States. The states that generated the most hazardous waste tended to be those with large petrochemical industries. In general, other industrialized countries designate hazardous waste in much the same way the United States does, although they may use different coding or terminology.

Another issue in hazardous waste disposal is the information provided to nearby communities, which is discussed in Box 19.2.

Box 19.2. Community Right-to-Know

In the United States today, information is available to local communities regarding the release of hazardous materials into the environment. In 1986, Congress passed the Emergency Planning and Community Right-to-Know Act (EPCRA). That Act establishes planning and reporting requirements for federal, state, and local governments, Indian tribes, and industry, and it requires the involvement of the local community.

One of the centerpieces of the Act concerns advance planning for the accidental release of hazardous materials. Community emergency response plans, developed with the public, should

- Identify facilities and transportation routes of extremely hazardous substances
- Describe emergency response procedures, on site and off site
- Designate a community coordinator and facility coordinator(s) to implement the plan
- Outline emergency notification procedures
- Describe how to determine the probable area and population affected by releases
- Describe local emergency equipment and facilities and the persons responsible for them
- Outline evacuation plans
- Provide a training program for emergency responders (including schedules)
- Provide methods and schedules for exercising emergency response plans

Another centerpiece of EPCRA is the requirement that certain industrial facilities and operations annually report estimates of the quantities and types of hazardous materials stored on site, treated on site, and released to the environment. The EPA (2005) uses this information to maintain the national Toxics Release Inventory, or TRI.

The EPCRA requirements and information available from additional sources (for example, discharge permits for waste water and air releases) provide the public with a substantial amount of information to use in planing for growth and environmental protection. With this information the public can also better understand the potential for contact with and exposure to hazardous materials.

Solid Waste Management Strategies

Because solid and hazardous waste may affect human health, *waste management* is a fundamental part of environmental public health. Waste management is best accomplished through a multitiered approach. The first tier is primary waste stream reduction. Materials recycling, substitution of materials, and changes in consumer habits, among other methods, can help communities achieve waste stream reduction. All sectors of a modern society, when approached with effective informational campaigns and incentives, can practice waste reduction.

The second tier of solid waste management involves proper handling and disposal of waste in a manner that provides for protection of the public health and the environment. Although complete avoidance of solid waste generation is the ideal, it is likely that there will always be some residual of mankind's activities requiring disposal.

In the United States, landfilling is the means of disposal for 69 percent of hazardous waste and 55 percent of municipal waste. Other waste disposal options for hazardous waste include underground injection and storage in surface impoundments, underground mines, and salt dome formations. Each of these approaches has public health implications.

The next two sections of this chapter explore each of the two tiers of solid waste management in greater detail.

Primary Prevention of Waste

The ideal waste management strategy is to produce no waste in the first place. This goal can be approached in several ways; they can be summed up as *reduce, reuse,* and *recycle.* In an industrial setting this goal might be achieved by altering production processes to avoid or reduce the use of a hazardous chemical. For example, in some electroplating operations, less toxic alternatives can replace highly toxic cyanide salts. In office settings, converting to electronic commerce and records management can reduce waste paper production.

Waste reduction also applies to municipal wastes. The quantity of raw materials in food and beverage containers has been reduced because of economic pressures. In the past few decades manufacturers have reduced the amount of steel and aluminum in cans and the amount of plastic in milk jugs and plastic bags. These efforts have reduced the cost of these containers and decreased the amount of wastes needing disposal. Further reductions in packaging could be achieved if consumers carried reusable canvas shopping bags instead of expecting plastic or paper bags with each purchase.

If the generation of waste cannot be abated or reduced, then the next best alternative is to recycle the waste. Recycling can refer to using waste material to produce more of the original product or to using waste material in something else. Examples of the first kind of recycling are making glass or paper from used glass or paper and making new lead batteries from old lead batteries. An example of the second kind of recycling is using mining wastes as aggregate for asphalt and concrete production. In recent years, increased efforts to reduce the amount of trash dumped into landfills have led municipalities to encourage recycling of paper, plastic, aluminum, and glass. In some communities homeowners are also encouraged to compost yard waste, recycling it into a useful soil amendment. Recycling of municipal solid waste has steadily increased in the United States; today about 30 percent of this waste is recycled (Figure 19.4). Among municipal wastes, aluminum is the most valuable recyclable commodity. Approximately 49 percent of aluminum beer and soft drink cans in the United States are recycled. This results in large energy savings, because recycling aluminum uses 95 percent less energy than does extracting it from ore.

FIGURE 19.4. TOTAL AMOUNTS AND PERCENTAGES OF MUNICIPAL SOLID WASTE RECYCLED IN THE UNITED STATES, 1960–2001.

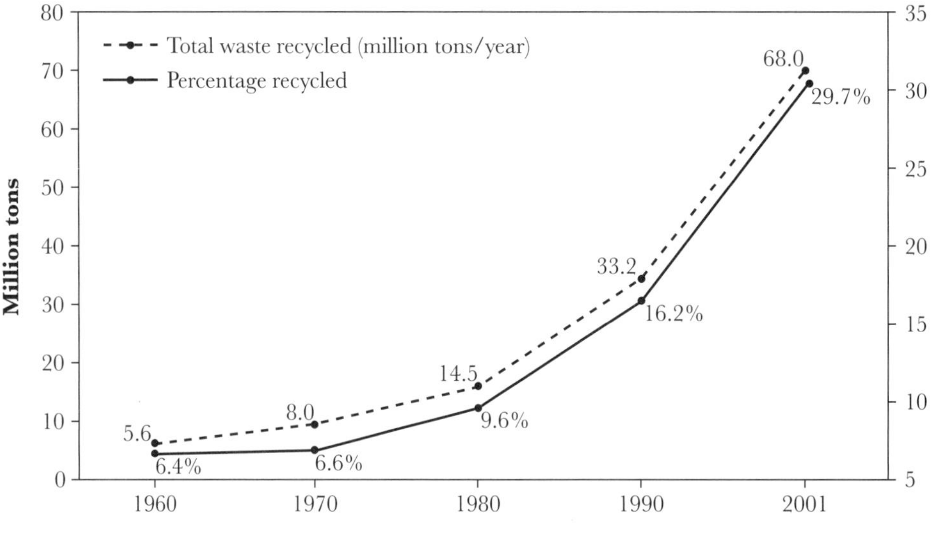

Source: Adapted from EPA, 2003.

Box 19.3. Tire Reuse and Recycling

Some types of wastes have evolved to pose unique challenges and opportunities. Just a little more than 100 years ago, solid waste from transportation operations consisted mainly of horse manure or ash and clinker produced from burning coal in steam engines. One century later these transportation wastes have been replaced with an estimated yearly production of a quarter of a billion waste rubber tires in the United States alone.

Waste tires are problematic for storage or disposal (Figure 19.5). They are hard to bury in landfills. Landfill operators report that tires tend to work their way up to the surface of the fill and disrupt the integrity of the landfill cover. Tires also serve as mosquito breeding sites when stored outdoors. And when stored in large piles, tires are vulnerable to fire. Tire fires are very difficult to extinguish and can cause substantial pollution of both the air and the underlying soil and water environment.

Approximately 20 percent of all used tires are recycled directly through the retreading process, leading to an interest in identifying additional ways of reusing or recycling waste tires. Tire material, in the form of chunks of rubber, can be used in the manufacture of truck bed liners, antifatigue mats, soaker hoses, shoe soles, and swings and can also be used as a civil engineering material, for example, as material for leachate drainage or for the daily cover at solid waste landfills. Ground, or crumb, rubber has been added to asphalt for paving, and research has been done on adding

FIGURE 19.5. WASTE TIRES.

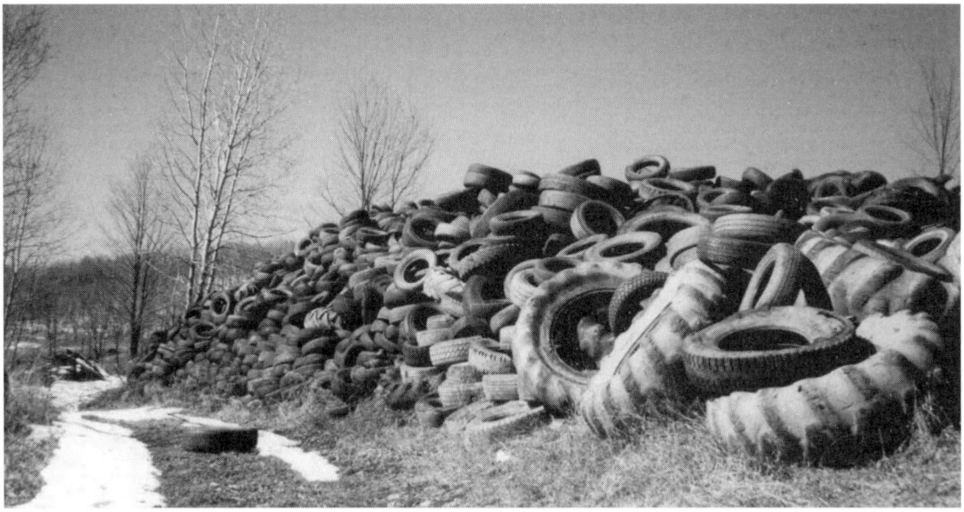

crumb rubber to concrete. When crumb rubber is blended with plastic, the resultant material can be processed like plastic but retains some of the elasticity of rubber. Pallets and railroad ties have been made from plastic-rubber blends.

As with any material recycling, economic factors enter into the ultimate fate of a particular waste stream, including that of used tires. For example, one potential use of waste tires is as tire derived fuel (TDF), a fuel supplement that can be blended with coal. Cement kilns have been considered good candidates for such fuel blends because the resultant ash can be incorporated directly into the final product and the air pollution impacts from the blended fuel are less than those from burning coal alone. As energy costs continue to escalate, the prospects for using more TDF seem favorable.

Waste Treatment and Disposal

It would be ideal if all solid, hazardous, and special waste could be recycled, reused, or avoided. Unfortunately, this ideal goal may not be attained, so society should strive to dispose of all such wastes in a manner that minimizes harm to human health and the environment. Both budgetary limitations and the need to comply with applicable regulations influence selection of the most practical option.

In years past it was common to burn wastes in backyard barrels, open dumps, and crude incinerators. All these methods had undesirable environmental and health impacts. During the second half of the twentieth century, public demand and government regulations led to improved waste treatment and disposal methods. Controlled, or sanitary, landfills replaced dumps. More sophisticated and controlled combustion systems replaced crude incinerators. Newer incinerators were specifically designed to burn a particular type of waste, such as medical waste, industrial waste, or municipal solid waste. Some industrial wastes, such as liquid brines, were discharged far beneath the earth's surface through deep well injection. Potentially harmful industrial wastes that had been previously discarded haphazardly in dumps or burial pits were also treated with remedial technologies designed to reduce or limit harmful impacts.

Sanitary Landfills

Open-burning municipal waste dumps, which were once prevalent throughout the United States, were the source of many environmental and public health problems. These problems included air pollution and groundwater pollution; increased populations of rats, flies, and other disease-carrying vectors; and nuisance odors and unsightly conditions. The creation of the EPA in 1970 prompted a major move in the United States to eliminate open dumps and replace them with the improved *sanitary landfill.* Careful site selection and preparation, the application of an earth cover for each day's accumulation of waste, and other procedural provisions eliminated most of the problems with open dumping. By 1996, approximately 3,500 municipal sanitary landfills operated in the United States.

Sanitary landfills vary in design, depending on local site considerations. However, by definition, all sanitary landfills share certain design features and operating principles. These are discussed in the following sections.

Site Selection and Preparation. Many technical and social factors go into selecting a site for a municipal sanitary landfill. Technical considerations include

- Adequate area to provide waste capacity for a reasonable time period
- Adequate elevation or separation to protect regional groundwater
- Available or appropriate soil for daily soil cover requirements
- Adequate buffer from surrounding populations
- Cost of the land

Normally, several candidate sites are identified and evaluated according to these considerations. In addition to these technical requirements, the selected site must also meet with community acceptance. Solid waste treatment or disposal sites of any kind are generally perceived as bad neighbors; consequently, community concerns (and sometimes outrage) and political pressures often influence actual site selection.

Once a landfill site has been selected, site preparation can begin. In addition to grading and installing sediment and erosion controls to protect local surface waters, provisions must also be made to protect groundwater from leachate. Leachate, a liquid organic waste decomposition product sometimes contaminated with chemicals, can migrate down and into the local aquifer. Installing an underlying natural or manmade impervious barrier can provide protection. Where significant amounts of leachate are anticipated, some landfills have systems to collect and treat it. Similarly, provisions are often made for collecting and controlling gaseous products of waste decomposition, consisting mainly of methane. In some cases the methane is cleaned and used as fuel for local energy production (Figure 19.6). Site preparation features may also include aesthetic screening of the landfill, scales for weighing incoming trash trucks, maintenance facilities, flares or gas vents, security arrangements, and monitoring wells to sample leachate.

Site Operations. Sanitary landfills are operated in a manner intended to contain and control waste. Each day's accumulation of waste is compacted and covered with earth in a cell. Usually waste is spread and compacted by heavy equipment

FIGURE 19.6. GENERALIZED DEPICTION OF A STATE-OF-THE-ART LANDFILL.

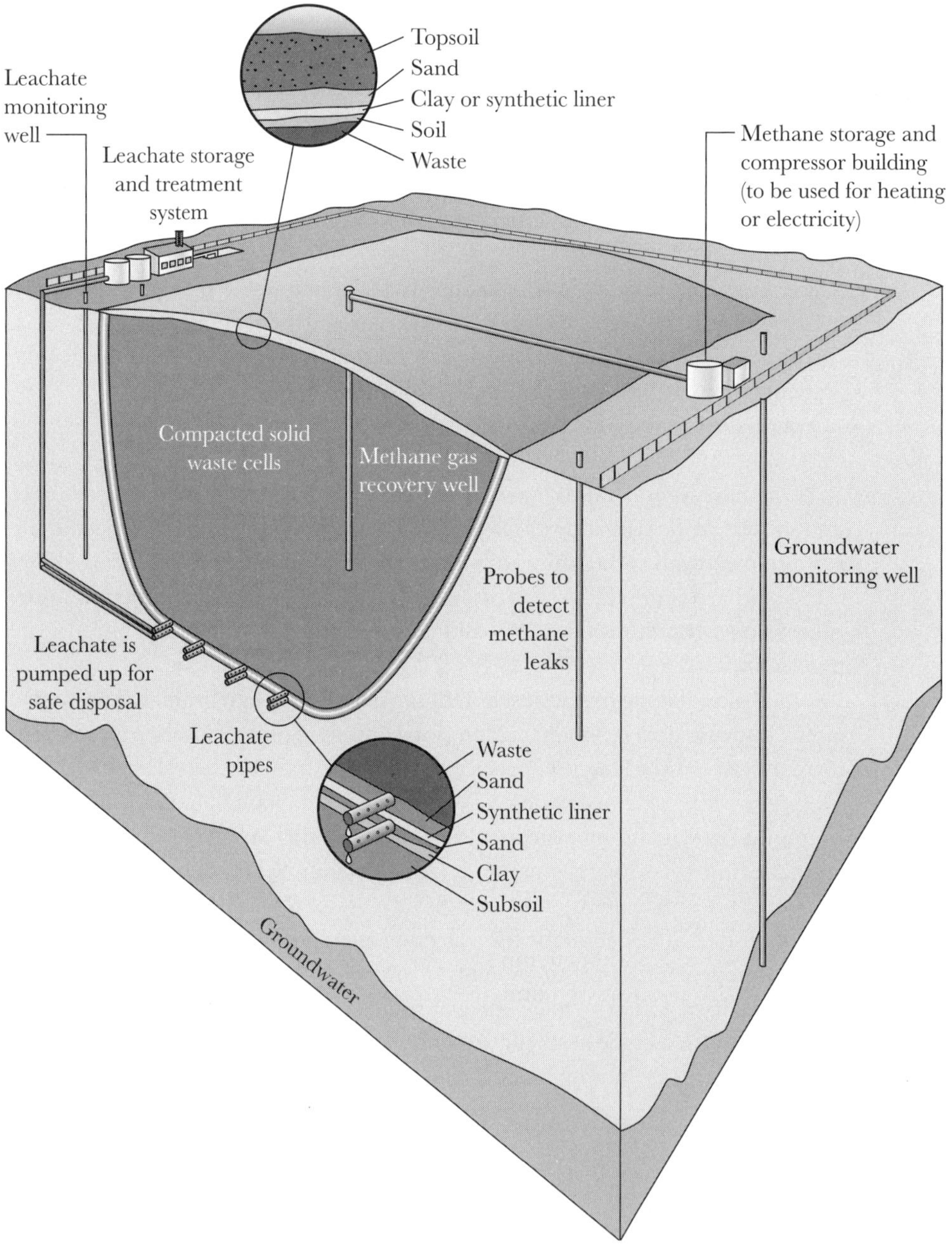

on a sloped working face within the cell. This compaction extends the life of the landfill and reduces the potential for fires. At the end of the day the working face and entire cell are covered with approximately 6 inches of compacted soil. This minimizes litter problems, helps control odors, and largely eliminates problems from animal and insect vectors. Some municipalities place solid waste in landfills in the form of precompacted bales, stacking these bales like building blocks each day and thereby maximizing site life.

Additional operating features help to minimize nuisance and health threats associated with landfills. For example, movable fence sections can be used to control blowing litter during particularly windy conditions. A supply of appropriate cover material may be stockpiled for use in cold or wet weather, when daily excavation for cover soil would not be practical. Odor and bird control techniques are sometimes used. Portions of the landfill may be dedicated to the disposal of hard-to-handle wastes, such as bulky demolition debris or large appliances. Lastly, the sanitary landfill may be designed so that after it is closed the land can be converted to a community asset such as a golf course or park.

Industrial and hazardous waste landfills share many of the containment and control features of sanitary landfills, but they are much more heavily regulated. The type of waste allowed in a given landfill is strictly defined in the operating permit. In some cases certain hazardous wastes must be specially treated, packaged, or stabilized before being placed in the landfill. Periodic analysis of the wastes may be required to ensure that adequate characterization of the fill is maintained.

Incineration

Broadly defined, *incineration* is the controlled combustion of a waste. Incineration has been used for all types of waste, including municipal solid waste, sewage sludge, industrial and hazardous waste, and medical waste. Some large municipal and industrial incinerators are designed to capture energy for reuse. The goals of incineration are to reduce the volume of the waste being processed, to reduce the hazardous characteristics of a particular waste stream, or to perform both these functions. All incineration attempts to control several variables in order to maximize the completeness of combustion. The *three T's* for ensuring complete combustion are

1. Time: the length of time that solids and combustion gases are in the ignition and burn zones of the incinerator
2. Temperature: an indication of the amount of heat energy in the combustion chambers available to break molecular bonds and facilitate oxidation toward the desired end products of combustion (carbon dioxide, water vapor, and inorganic ash)

3. Turbulence: the agitation of both solids and combustible by-products, providing the opportunity for complete oxidation to take place

The other major fundamental factor in combustion control is the provision of adequate oxygen, usually in the form of combustion air, to complete all oxidation reactions. The amount of air needed for complete combustion of a given waste stream is determined by chemical oxidation equations and is known as the stoichiometric air requirement. In actual incineration systems more than stoichiometric air is provided in order to force the reaction toward complete oxidation of the organic wastes. This excess air is usually reported as a percentage of the stoichiometric air.

Specific incineration designs vary widely in the ways that wastes are introduced into the units and in the ways that air control and mixing is achieved. Some incinerators have multiple chambers for combustion. Ignition and preliminary combustion take place in a *primary* chamber. The volatile products from the primary chamber are oxidized to completion in a *secondary* chamber, or *afterburner.* Some incinerators, sometimes known as starved air or pyrolytic combustors, seek to minimize entrainment of particulate matter in the primary chamber by keeping combustion air below the stoichiometric amount. Another way to reduce gas volume flow in the primary chamber is to use pure oxygen, rather than ambient air, for combustion.

Early incinerators were noted for smoke, odors, and sometimes even live embers coming out of the exhaust stacks. Because of these unacceptable conditions, regulations now require strict air pollution control technology. Now, devices such as wet or caustic scrubbers control acid gas. Electrostatic precipitators, venturi scrubbers, and baghouses capture fine particulates. Some of the newest hazardous waste incinerators have a final activated-carbon filtration system. This polishing device minimizes low-level products of incomplete combustion (PICs), such as dioxins and polycyclic aromatic hydrocarbons (PAHs). Inorganic waste contaminants, such as heavy metals (for example, mercury, lead, and chromium), can be difficult to control and can require special pollution control systems or their elimination from the waste being fed to the incinerator (Figure 19.7). Communities rarely, if ever, welcome incinerators or waste landfills.

Deep Well Injection

Deep well injection is a liquid waste disposal technology that uses deep injection wells to force treated or untreated liquid waste into geological formations that do not allow migration of contaminants into potential potable water aquifers. These wells, typically several thousand feet deep, extend into a permeable injection

FIGURE 19.7. GENERALIZED DIAGRAM OF INCINERATION MATERIAL AND PROCESS FLOW.

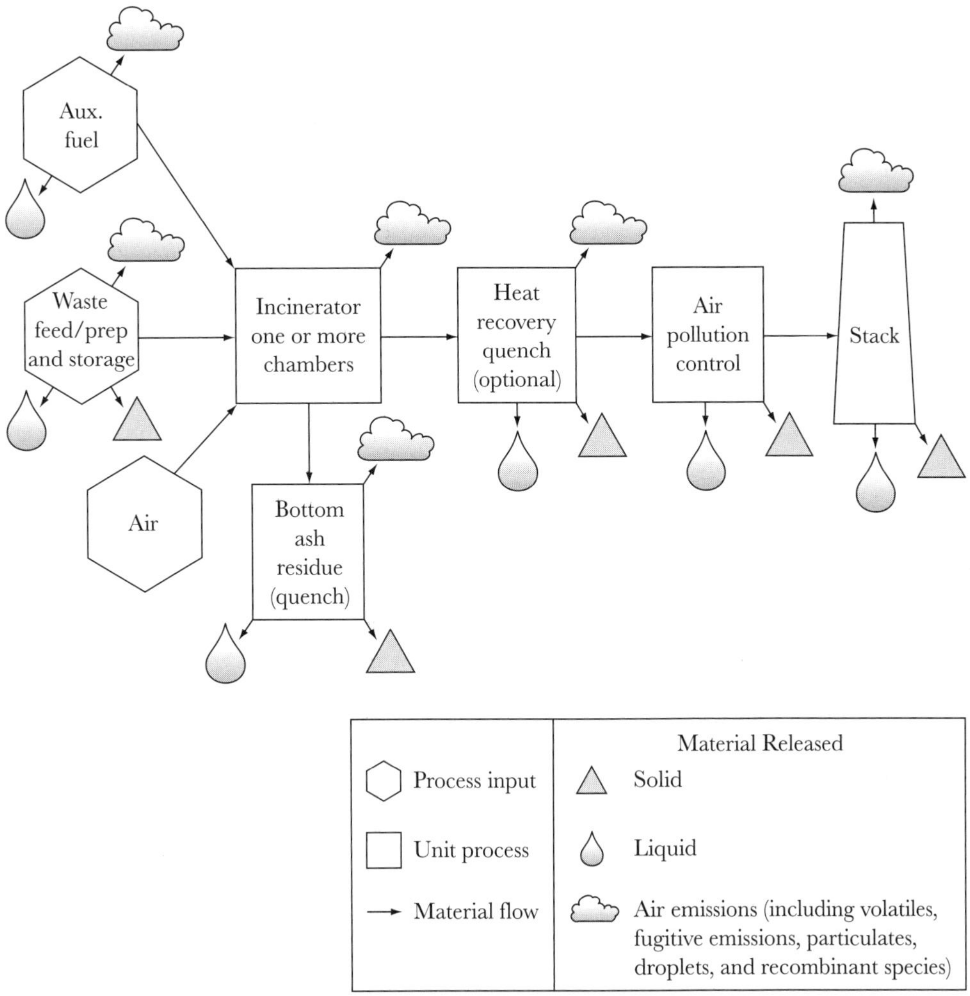

zone already containing highly saline brines. Impermeable rock or soil layers confine the injection zone vertically. The wastes injected can be radioactive wastes, hydrocarbon wastes, oil and gas drilling brines, hazardous wastes, and other wastes not suitable for landfill. In the United States, injection wells are regulated and classified under an EPA definition that addresses their uses and characteristics.

Injection wells can be located only in areas free of faults and other geological features that could allow wastes to migrate into potable water aquifers. Liquid wastes high in suspended solids, iron content, or organic substrates that could serve as food for microbial growth should not be disposed of in such wells because of their potential to foul or clog the well. Injection wells are double-sleeved; this allows monitoring for system integrity and places a dual boundary between intervening geological layers and the waste.

Other Technologies

This chapter has touched on some of the most prevalent methods for treating and disposing of wastes, but many other waste treatment techniques are in practice or evolving. Treatment methods such as supercritical water oxidation, molten metals and molten salt oxidation, glass melt and vitrification processes, and waste-specific biological treatment systems and composting are a few of these additional technologies. Dedicated treatment technologies, such as thermal desorption, have been developed for in situ and extractive remediation of old industrial waste disposal sites. Waste disposal technology has undergone tremendous technological evolution to keep pace with the changing character of society's waste products.

Health Concerns

Exposure to solid and hazardous wastes can adversely affect human health in several ways. The aesthetic impact of poor waste management—trash piling up in streets and vacant lots—can undermine the livability and even the safety of a community. At least five kinds of health hazards are well recognized:

1. Risks of infectious disease from poorly managed solid waste
2. Contamination of drinking water by biological and chemical wastes
3. Formation of air pollutants in landfills
4. Emission of air pollutants from incinerators
5. Contamination of food by waste chemicals that escape into the environment

Poorly operated landfills can be havens for flies, mosquitoes, rats, and mice. Uncovered garbage and trash provide them with food, shelter, and a breeding ground. These insects and animals can be vectors for disease, carrying pathogenic microbes into the surrounding community. Rats and mice can spread thirty-five diseases, including leptospirosis, salmonellosis, and rickettsialpox, to humans. Furthermore, rats can carry eighteen different kinds of mites, lice, fleas, and ticks.

Modern landfills, which require wastes to be covered daily with clean soil, have greatly reduced the spread of disease by these vectors.

Improper disposal of solid and hazardous wastes can contaminate drinking water. Both groundwater and surface water can be affected. Most old landfills or dumps lack liners; this absence allows chemicals buried in the landfill to leach down into the underlying aquifer. Volatile organic compounds (VOCs), such as trichloroethylene and tetrachloroethylene, and petroleum distillates, are common contaminants in municipal and industrial landfills. These organic solvents are widely used as degreasers, dry-cleaning fluids, and components of paints, varnishes, and adhesives. Because these chemicals are highly mobile, they readily migrate through unlined landfills into the underlying groundwater. Heavy metals in landfills, such as lead, cadmium, mercury, and chromium, can also be a source of groundwater contamination. Moreover, microbial degradation of garbage and vegetative wastes in a landfill can produce organic acids, which lower the pH of the milieu, making buried metals more soluble. Old industrial sites have also contaminated nearby groundwater, because waste chemicals were sometimes dumped into open pits or on the ground around the site. If the contaminated groundwater migrates off site, it can affect people who drink from down-gradient, private and public water wells.

In Hardeman County, Tennessee, leachate from a hazardous waste landfill contaminated private drinking water wells with carbon tetrachloride and other VOCs. People who drank from these wells experienced headaches, nausea, and visual disturbances. Physicians who examined the victims reported that several of them had enlarged livers (hepatomegaly). In addition, clinical laboratory tests documented the presence of elevated levels of liver enzymes and altered serum chemistries, evidence of liver toxicity. Fortunately, these abnormalities receded several months after the people stopped drinking the contaminated water.

Most old landfills also lack adequate leachate collection systems for aboveground discharges. As a result, leachate from these landfills can be carried by surface water runoff into nearby lakes and streams, introducing chemical contaminants. People who use these bodies of water for recreation or fishing can be exposed to this contamination.

The Kin-Buc landfill in Edison, New Jersey, is an example of this scenario (Figure 19.8). Municipal, industrial, and hazardous wastes, including liquids and oily wastes, were buried at the landfill during its thirty years of operation. Large quantities of oily liquids containing polychlorinated biphenyls (PCBs) leached out of the landfill into the adjacent wetlands. The PCBs contaminated a creek, which discharged into the Raritan river. Because PCBs resist biological metabolism and are lipophilic, they bioaccumulated in fish and shellfish in the river. State environmental officials tested striped bass, white perch, and blue crabs from the river

FIGURE 19.8. LEACHATE COLLECTION PONDS AT THE KIN-BUC LANDFILL IN EDISON, NEW JERSEY.

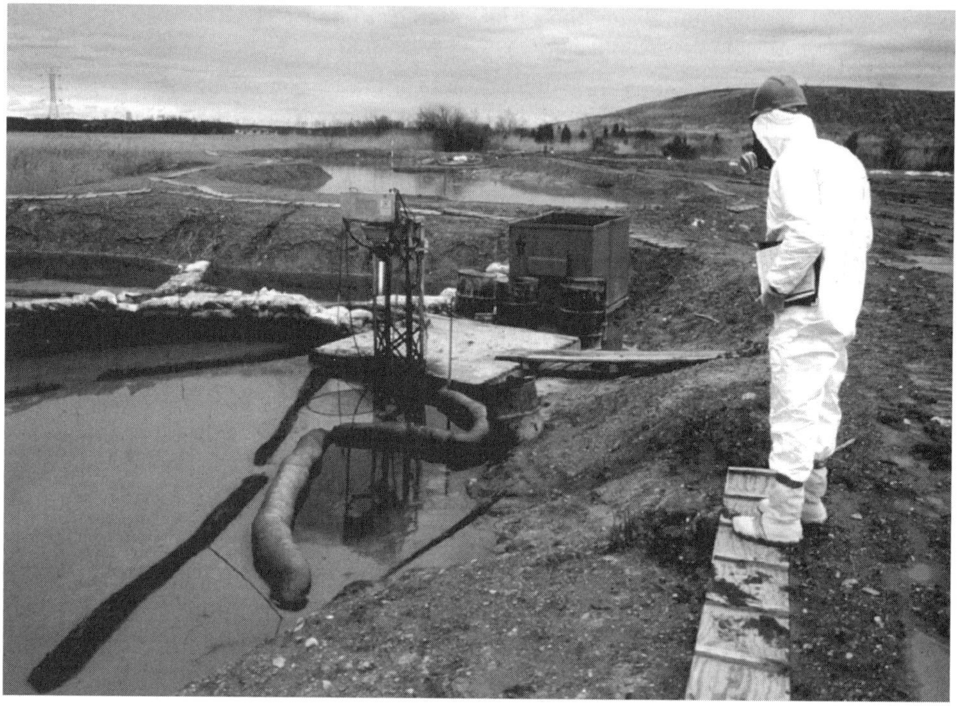

and detected elevated concentrations of PCBs. This finding prompted local health officials to issue a health advisory against eating fish and shellfish from the river, depriving people of recreation and a valuable food source.

Municipal landfills can also be a source of air pollutants such as methane, hydrogen sulfide, and VOCs. Anaerobic microbial digestion of organic matter buried in landfills generates large quantities of methane gas. In 1969, in Winston-Salem, North Carolina, methane gas from a landfill migrated underground through the soil into the basement of an armory building adjacent to the landfill. The methane built up to an explosive level in the basement, and a lit cigarette triggered an explosion that killed three men and injured five others. Methane and carbon dioxide released to the atmosphere from landfills can also have ecological effects because these gases may contribute to global climate change (see Chapter Eleven). It has been variously estimated that landfills account for 5 to 20 percent of methane emissions to the atmosphere.

Landfills can also be a source of odiferous gases such as hydrogen sulphide, mercaptans, and ammonia. The decay of organic material and some construction materials, such as gypsum wallboard, produces these gases. The concentrations of these gases in ambient air in neighborhoods near a landfill are usually not high enough to cause adverse health effects. However, their objectionable odor can adversely affect quality of life, and they may provoke respiratory irritation in sensitive individuals.

Wastes from mining and petroleum production form the largest category of solid wastes produced in the United States. Huge piles of mine tailings, left behind after the extraction of metals (Figure 19.9), are a potential source of environmental contamination. Residual metals can leach out of the tailings and contaminate groundwater and surface water resources. In China's Hu Nan Province, mining wastes containing arsenic were placed in an open-air dump. During the rainy season, leachate from the waste piles infiltrated groundwater being used as a

FIGURE 19.9. THIS MINE TAILINGS PILE IS THE LEGACY OF SIXTY YEARS OF LEAD AND ZINC MINING IN OTTAWA COUNTY, OKLAHOMA.

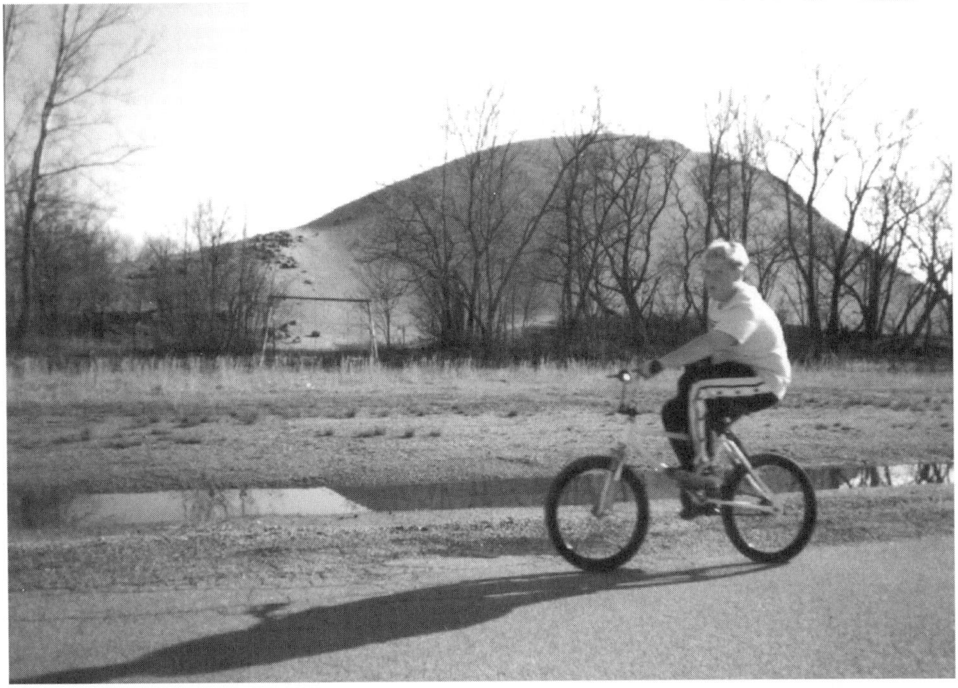

drinking-water source. Use of this contaminated groundwater caused acute arsenic poisoning in hundreds of people, and six people died.

Municipal and hazardous waste incinerators that release particulates, vapors, and gases to the ambient air are also of potential health concern. Burning even nontoxic materials, such as wood and paper, produces particulate matter, carbon monoxide, aldehydes, and polyaromatic hydrocarbons. Burning such commonplace materials as paints, solvents, insecticides, and plastics can form chlorinated dibenzodioxins and chlorinated dibenzofurans, collectively known as dioxins. Small amounts of dioxins are released from hazardous waste incinerators, which operate under strict environmental regulations. Backyard burning of household trash in open barrels can also be a significant source of atmospheric dioxin emissions. It has been estimated that backyard trash burning by only two to forty households can generate as much dioxin as a municipal waste incinerator.

Although inhalation of dioxins in ambient air is a potential source of exposure, the major source of exposure to dioxins is food consumption. Once dioxins are released to the environment, they resist chemical, physical, and biological degradation, and they can accumulate in aquatic and terrestrial animals. More than 90 percent of the dioxin exposure in the general population is derived from background, low-level dioxin contamination in dairy products, meats, fish, eggs, and other foods.

The improper disposal or treatment of waste materials can lead to releases of other environmentally stable chemicals, such as PCBs, polybrominated diphenyl ethers (flame retardants), and plasticizers, as well as heavy metals, such as mercury, cadmium, and lead. Migration of these chemicals into waterways and agricultural fields can result in contamination of food sources.

A classic example of such food contamination occurred in Minamata Bay in Japan in the 1950s. Inorganic mercury, used as a catalyst by a chemical company, was discharged into the bay. Bacteria in the sediment converted the inorganic mercury into methylmercury, which accumulated in fish. Residents who ate the local fish developed classic neurological symptoms of methylmercury toxicity, including paresthesia, ataxia, loss of hearing and vision, and tremors. Children born to methylmercury-exposed mothers developed a cerebral palsy-like syndrome that was sometimes fatal.

Some metals found in waste streams, such as cadmium, can accumulate in edible plants. In Japan, zinc mining in the Jinzu River basin contaminated the river with cadmium and other metals. Farmers used cadmium-contaminated water from the river to irrigate their rice fields, resulting in cadmium contamination of their rice crops. After years of exposure to high doses of cadmium from the rice they ate, many farmers developed kidney disease, which led to a loss of calcium from their bones. Postmenopausal women who had borne several children became especially prone to developing fragile, painful bones that spontaneously fractured, which gave the condition its name, *itai-itai byo,* or "ouch-ouch disease."

In spite of this historical experience, improper handling or disposal of chemical wastes continues to contaminate food and pose a risk to human health. In 1999, in Belgium, waste transformer oil containing PCBs was mixed into recycled animal fat that was added to animal feed. The contaminated feed was distributed to poultry farms in Belgium and resulted in widespread contamination of chickens and eggs with PCBs and dioxins. This contamination prompted the Belgian government to remove all poultry products, eggs, and derived products from the market and led to the destruction of 2 million chickens.

Another practice that poses a risk to human health is the disposal of wastes by shipping them to another country, typically a less developed nation, as discussed in Box 19.4.

Box 19.4. International Trafficking in Hazardous Wastes

As environmental laws for disposing of hazardous wastes in industrialized countries became more stringent and compliance became expensive, some waste generators began shipping wastes to other countries for disposal. The United Nations Environmental Programme estimates that about 10 percent of hazardous waste produced worldwide is shipped across international borders. In some cases the recipient country is ill prepared to handle the hazardous wastes safely. Hazardous waste workers often lack adequate personal protective equipment and training, which puts their health and safety at risk. Furthermore, when these wastes are not adequately treated and disposed of, they can create a potentially dangerous environmental legacy for the recipient country.

Concern over the international shipping of hazardous wastes led to a 1989 treaty known as the Basel Convention. The convention's goal is to regulate the international movement of hazardous materials and to ensure that these wastes are managed and disposed of in an environmentally sound manner. One of the key provisions is that hazardous wastes can cross national boundaries only upon prior written notification by the exporting state to competent authorities of the importing state.

As of May 2005, 165 countries and the European Union had ratified the Basel Convention. The United States signed the convention in 1992 but has not ratified it, which would require congressional action. The United States has not ratified the convention because its acceptance would likely necessitate changes in Resource Conservation and Recovery Act (RCRA) regulations that specify how hazardous wastes are defined and how those wastes are managed.

One of the challenges facing the convention is how to deal with trafficking in recyclable materials, such as spent lead-acid batteries and other nonferrous scrap metal. These wastes are valuable commodities on the world market, and recycling these materials provides jobs and generates income in countries with struggling economies. Under a proposed amendment to the convention, the transfer of such materials from industrialized to developing countries would be banned.

In recent years the practice of ship breaking has attracted the attention of the environmental community. Some environmental groups have characterized this practice as being a covert form of international trafficking in hazardous wastes. *Ship breaking* is the dismantling of decommissioned ships to recover steel and other recyclables, and ships are often sent to less developed countries for this process. Concerns have been raised because workers may not be protected from exposure to lead, asbestos, PCBs, mercury, and other hazardous materials during ship dismantling operations. India is the world's leader in ship breaking (38 percent), followed by China (25 percent), Bangladesh (19 percent), Pakistan (7 percent), and other countries (11 percent).

Public health practice emphasizes prevention over treatment. This principle is especially relevant in the field of environmental health because preventing environmental contamination is easier and less costly than cleaning it up after it has occurred. Therefore both industrialized and developing countries should learn from the mistakes of the past and strive to manage and treat wastes in a manner that protects public health.

Thought Questions

1. Discuss the different approaches to solid waste management and their advantages and disadvantages.
2. Discuss the different types of solid waste and how they are identified.
3. Name and discuss ways in which you can reduce the amount of waste you produce.
4. Select one of the waste treatment or disposal technologies discussed in this chapter, and explain how it could be used effectively in a solid waste management program. Discuss the type of solid waste that would be involved and how using the technology would protect the health of people and the environment.
5. Discuss how people can be exposed to the toxic substances found in solid and hazardous wastes.

References

U.S. Environmental Protection Agency. *Municipal Solid Waste in the United States: 2001 Facts and Figures.* Washington, D.C.: U.S. Environmental Protection Agency, 2003.

U.S. Environmental Protection Agency. "National Toxics Release Inventory" (TRI). [www.epa.gov/tri]. 2005.

For Further Information

Publications

Chang, H. O. *Hazardous and Radioactive Waste Treatment Technologies Handbook.* Boca Raton, Fla.: CRC Press, 2000.

Gorner, I. K. "Waste Incineration: European State of the Art and New Developments." Article no. 200303. *IFRF Combustion Journal.* [http://www.journal.ifrf.net]. July 2003.

Hickman, H. L. *Principles of Integrated Solid Waste Management.* Annapolis, Md.: American Academy of Environmental Engineers, 1999.

Johnson, B. L. *Impact of Hazardous Waste on Human Health: Hazard, Health Effects, Equity, and Communications Issues.* Boca Raton, Fla.: Lewis, 1999.

Manuel, J. S. "Unbuilding for the Environment." *Environmental Health Perspectives,* 2003, *111,* A881–A887.

National Research Council. *Environmental Epidemiology: Public Health and Hazardous Wastes.* Washington, D.C.: National Academies Press, 1991.

Orloff, K., and Falk, H. "An International Perspective on Hazardous Waste Practices." *International Journal of Hygiene and Environmental Health,* 2003, *206,* 291–302.

Rathje, W. L., and Murphy, C. *Rubbish! The Archaeology of Garbage.* Tucson: University of Arizona Press, 2001.

Schneider, A., and McCumber, D. *An Air That Kills.* New York: Putnum, 2004.

Taylor, D. "Talking Trash: The Economic and Environmental Issues of Landfills." *Environmental Health Perspectives,* 1999, *107,* A404–A409.

Tchobanoglous, G., and Kreith, F. *Handbook of Solid Waste Management.* (2nd ed.) New York: McGraw-Hill, 2002.

Federal Government Web Sites

Because federal government agencies frequently revise and update information and data posted on their Web sites, specific Web pages are not provided here. However, each of the following Web sites has a search engine for locating information on waste management and disposal and effects on health.

Agency for Toxic Substances and Disease Registry [http://www.atsdr.cdc.gov].
Centers for Disease Control and Prevention [http://www.cdc.gov].
U.S. Environmental Protection Agency [http://www.epa.gov].

CHAPTER TWENTY

PEST CONTROL AND PESTICIDES

Mark G. Robson
George C. Hamilton

Pests have plagued humankind since the beginning of time, as recorded in the ancient writings of the Chinese, Egyptian, and Hebrew peoples. For example, there is a vivid description of a serious pest invasion in the book of Exodus (10:14–15): ". . . and the locusts came up over all the land of Egypt and settled on the whole country of Egypt. They covered the face of the whole land so that the land was darkened and they ate all the plants in the land and all the fruit of the trees. Not a green thing remained, neither tree nor plant of the field, through all the land of Egypt." Diseases such as plague and malaria—both propagated by pests—have changed the course of human history (Zinsser, 1963; McNeill, 1976; Sullivan, 2004).

Efforts to control pests are also as old as history. Early control measures used chalk, plant extracts, mercury, arsenic, lead, and other compounds. Over time, people also have attempted to control pests through sacrifices, prayers, rituals, dancing, and other approaches. Some appear quite humorous to us today; during an outbreak of cutworms in Switzerland in 1476, "Several of the offending insects were hauled into court, proclaimed guilty, excommunicated by the archbishop, and banished from the land" (Nadakavukaren, 1995).

Over the last century or two, chemicals have come to dominate human efforts at pest control. As with medications, the ideal pesticide is both safe and effective—safe in terms of both human and ecosystem health and effective at controlling the target species. Historically, although many compounds were recommended to control pests, almost none were empirically tested and most turned out to be ineffective (Keifer, Wesseling, and McConnell, 2005). Paris green (copper acetoarsenate) was among the first compounds to be used on a large scale in agricultural production. In the 1860s, it was shown to have insecticidal properties and was used to control the Colorado potato beetle, *Leptinotarsa decemlineata.* Paris green was also an effective fungicide. Later in the nineteenth century lead arsenate became a popular pesticide and was widely used in agriculture. Chemical pest control changed dramatically in 1939. Paul Muller, a chemist with the Geigy Corporation in Switzerland, found that a synthetic compound synthesized more than half a century earlier was an effective insecticide while boasting low mammalian toxicity. This compound was dichlorodiphenyltrichloroethane, or DDT. DDT was widely used during World War II to control a number of insect problems that plagued the war effort, including body lice, the carriers of typhus, and mosquitoes, the carriers of yellow fever, malaria, and dengue. DDT is still used in many parts of the world for vector control, particularly for malaria and other mosquito-borne diseases. Muller received the Nobel Prize in Physiology or Medicine in 1948 for his work on DDT.

After the war DDT and similar chlorinated pesticides made their way into the agricultural marketplace. The introduction of these compounds into agriculture changed pest control and food production worldwide. However, public health and ecological research has increasingly revealed problems with pesticides, ranging from human toxicity to wildlife toxicity to ecosystem disruption. (Figures 20.1 and 20.2 display modes of applying agricultural pesticides.) Rachel Carson's *Silent Spring,* published in 1962, was a powerful wakeup call, alerting the public and policymakers to the downsides of widespread pesticide use. Modern pest control has therefore sought to move beyond exclusive reliance on pesticides, using combinations of chemical and nonchemical methods (Ware and Whitacre, 2004).

A *pest* can be any species of plant, animal, or microorganism that threatens human health and well-being. However, most pests fill specific ecological niches and have functions that are important to ecosystem integrity (even if not directly useful to humans). Bees sting but pollinate plants and make honey; ants interrupt picnics and may sting but play an essential role in nutrient cycles; termites destroy homes but are essential in processing fallen trees in forests. It is a rare pest that is *only* a pest (Figure 20.3).

The U.S. Environmental Protection Agency (EPA) defines seven categories of public health pests:

1. *Cockroaches.* Cockroaches are controlled to halt the spread of asthma, allergy, and food contamination.

FIGURE 20.1. APPLICATION OF LEAD ARSENATE IN THE EARLY 1900S.

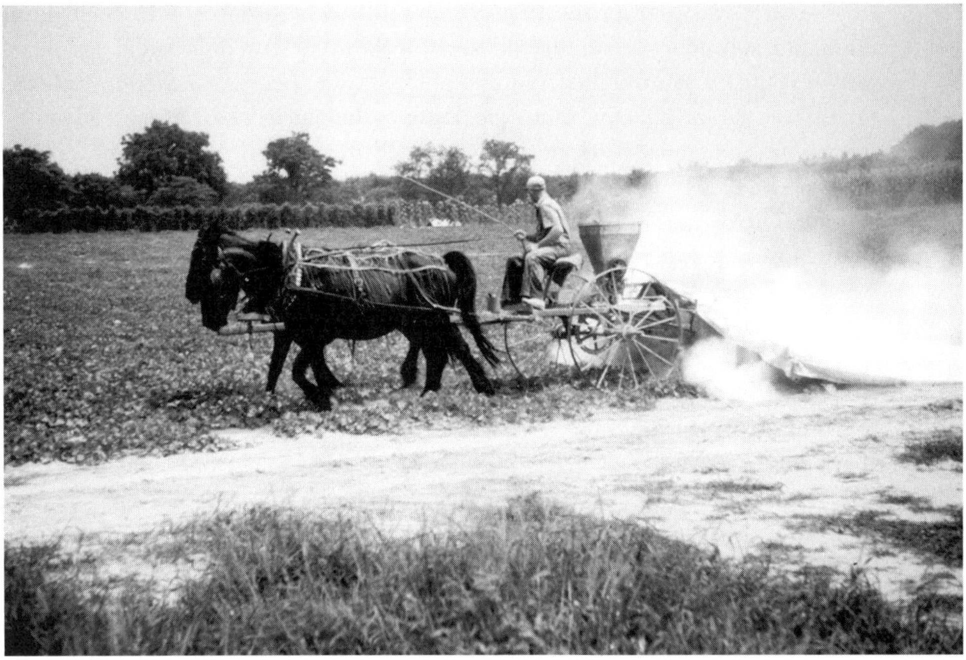

2. *Body, head, and crab lice.* These lice are controlled to prevent the spread of skin irritations and rashes and to prevent the occurrence of louse-borne diseases, such as epidemic typhus, trench fever, and epidemic relapsing fever.
3. *Mosquitoes.* Mosquitoes are controlled to prevent the spread of mosquito-borne diseases such as malaria; St. Louis, Eastern, Western, West Nile, and LaCrosse encephalitides; yellow fever; and dengue fever.
4. *Various rats and mice.* Rats and mice are controlled to prevent the spread of rodent-borne diseases and the contamination of food for human consumption.
5. *Various microorganisms, including bacteria, viruses, and protozoans.* Microorganisms listed as public health pests are controlled by public health agencies and hospitals for the purpose of preventing the spread of numerous diseases.
6. *Reptiles and birds.* Certain reptiles and birds are controlled to prevent the spread of disease and to prevent direct injury.
7. *Various mammals.* Certain mammals have the potential to inflict direct human injury and can act as disease reservoirs (for rabies, for example).

FIGURE 20.2. MODERN PESTICIDE APPLICATION EQUIPMENT.

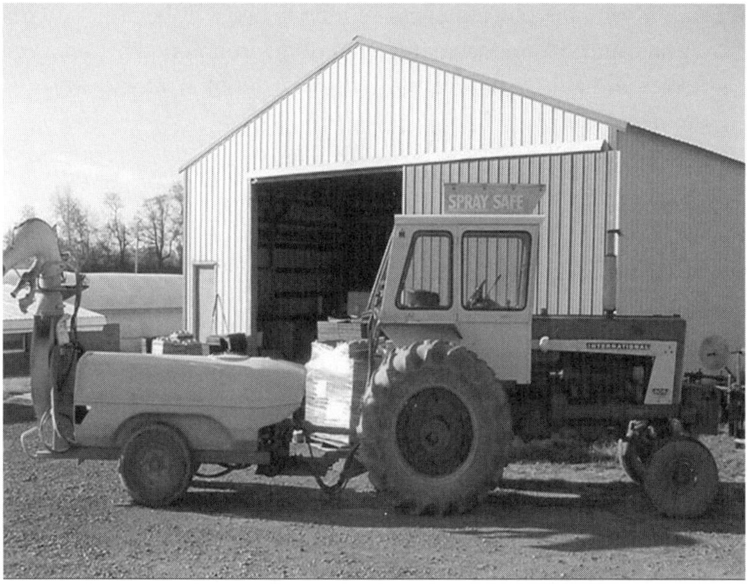

FIGURE 20.3. A CORN BORER, AN EXAMPLE OF AN INSECT PEST, CAUSING DAMAGE IN THE STALK OF A CORN PLANT.

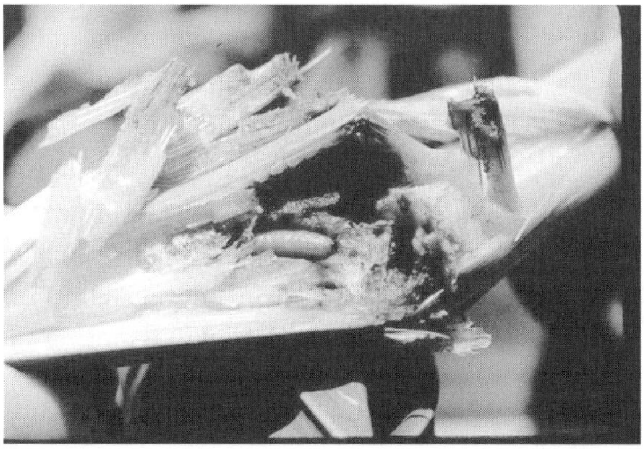

Note: The borers cause the stalks to lodge (fall over), making the corn difficult to harvest. One-fourth to one-third of the global corn harvest is lost to pests.

This chapter describes various categories of pests in some detail, including their physical characteristics, habitats, and impacts on human health. It begins with insects and moves next to vertebrate pests. It then turns to pest control, a traditional and still important function of environmental health, beginning with pesticides and concluding with the broader set of strategies known as *integrated pest management* (IPM).

Insect Pests

Insects belong to the class Insecta or Hexapoda and have three body regions (head, thorax, and abdomen), six legs that are connected to the thorax, and in the adults of most species, thoracic wings (Triplehorn and Johnson, 2005). Insects can have either chewing or sucking mouthparts. Those with chewing mouthparts, such as grasshoppers, termites and fleas, tear and crush plant material, insects, or other materials. Insects with sucking mouthparts, such as aphids, butterflies, and mosquitoes, pierce their food and then extract fluids in order to feed.

All insects go through one of two types of development, or metamorphosis: *gradual* (egg, nymph, and adult) or *complete* (egg, larva, pupa, and adult). Among insects that undergo incomplete metamorphosis, juveniles look identical to adults; as they mature they expand in size through a series of molts. Each time they molt, they develop external wing pads; during their final molt, to the adult form, fully functional wings and reproductive structures appear. Among insects that undergo complete metamorphosis, juveniles look dramatically different from the adults. They go through a series of larvae molts, culminating in a resting stage called the pupa. During this stage, the body tissues of the insect reorient themselves to produce the adult. When the final molt occurs, the insect breaks its way out of the pupal skin as a fully functional adult.

Bedbugs

Bedbugs are human *ectoparasites* (that is, they live on external surfaces) that are universal pests. They belong to the order Hemiptera and are flightless as adults (Triplehorn and Johnson, 2005). They undergo incomplete metamorphosis and must feed on blood in order to survive. Common names for the bedbug include mahogany flat, chinch, and red coat (Truman, Bennet, and Butts, 1982). The adult common bedbug, *Cimex lectularius,* is about 0.2 inches long, 0.1 inch wide, and oval. Its extremely flat body allows it get in cracks and crevices, making it more difficult to detect. Bedbugs have piercing-sucking mouthparts that are used to penetrate the host skin in order to feed on blood. Eggs are laid away from hosts and attached to surfaces and can hatch in six to seventeen days under normal room temperatures. Once the eggs hatch the small, colorless nymphs undergo gradual metamorphosis, taking blood meals as they develop. Humans are the preferred host of bedbugs, but bedbugs feed on canaries, cats, dogs, mice, poultry, and rats when humans are not available. Normally, they feed at night and hide in areas such as cracks and crevices, the folds of mattresses, the upholstery of chairs and sofas, or on bedsprings. Bedbugs give off a distinctive odor from thoracic glands; the odor can be quite strong during heavy infestations. In the laboratory, bedbugs are capable of transmitting anthrax, plague, tularemia, yellow fever, relapsing fever, and typhus, but there is little evidence that they transmit these diseases under normal conditions. Accordingly, they are not considered an important vector species. (Insect repellents, one line of defense against insect bites and insect-borne diseases, are discussed in Box 20.1.)

Box 20.1. Insect Repellants

Insect repellants are designed not to kill insects but to deter them from settling on skin and clothes. These are popular products, both to avoid the discomfort of bites by mosquitoes and other insects and to prevent disease transmission. The public health benefit of reducing insect bites is considerable. For instance, mosquitoes alone transmit disease to more than 700 million persons annually. Malaria remains a common disease in poor and middle-income countries (see Box 20.5), and in the United States, mosquitoes transmit eastern equine encephalitis, western equine encephalitis, St. Louis encephalitis, and La Crosse encephalitis, and since 1999, West Nile virus, serving as a reminder that no part of the world is immune from mosquito-borne diseases (Fradin and Day, 2002).

A variety of insect repellants are commercially available, some derived from plants and others consisting of synthetic chemicals. Many factors determine the effectiveness of a repellant, including the species of biting organism; the user's age, sex, level of activity, and biochemical attractiveness to biting arthropods; and the ambient temperature, humidity, and wind speed (Fradin and Day, 2002). As a result, any given repellent is not equally protective for all users.

The major component of nearly all consumer insect repellants is N,N-diethyl-m-toluamide, now called N,N-diethyl-3-methylbenzamide, or DEET (Bell, Veltri, and Page, 2002). Discovered by scientists at the U.S. Department of Agriculture and patented by the U.S. Army in 1946, DEET has been used in commercial repellants since the late 1950s ("DEET Is Hard to Beat," 2003). It is a broad-spectrum repellent, effective against many species of mosquitoes, biting flies, chiggers, fleas, and ticks (Fradin and Day, 2002). When compared to alternatives, including such synthetic chemicals as IR3535 and such "natural" repellants as citronella, soybean oil, peppermint oil, eucalyptus oil, and prickly pear cactus, DEET has generally been shown to be far superior in repelling insects.

Is DEET safe? Once applied to the skin it is absorbed, in quantities that have ranged between 5 percent and 15 percent in different studies (Sudakin and Trevathan, 2003). It is metabolized and excreted in the urine in twelve to twenty-four hours. Acute toxicity is extremely rare. Fewer than fifty cases of serious toxic effects have been documented in the medical literature since 1960; most of these followed extremely large exposures and resolved without lasting effects (Fradin and Day, 2002). However, some animal testing has suggested that DEET may cause neurological effects (Sudakin and Trevathan, 2003; Abdel-Rahman and others, 2004). It is therefore prudent to use DEET in moderation. Guidelines for use include the following:

- Do not use concentrations above 50 percent, as efficacy plateaus at that level (Buescher, Rutledge, Wirtz, and Nelson, 1983). Concentrations of 20 to 30 percent are generally sufficient.
- Apply DEET on or near all exposed skin surfaces; it is not effective more than about two inches from the point of application. To minimize skin absorption, DEET may be applied to clothing, but it is a plasticizer, capable of dissolving some synthetic fabrics.
- DEET is efficacious for a matter of hours (approximately five hours in one careful study; Fradin and Day, 2002) so periodic reapplication may be necessary.
- The efficacy of DEET decreases at higher temperatures.
- DEET is readily washed off by perspiration, rain, or other water sources, so reapplication is necessary after wetting.

It is important to remember that DEET is only one aspect of protection from arthropod bites. People should also avoid infested habitats, avoid outdoor exposure at times of the day when biting is most active, and wear protective clothing. (For further information see Fradin, 1998; Pollack, Kiszewski, and Spielman, 2002; Roberts and Reigart, 2004.)

Cockroaches

Cockroaches belong to the order Blattodea (Triplehorn and Johnson, 2005). Most cockroaches are tropical, and they are very common in the southern areas of the United States. In northern areas, those most commonly encountered are the ones that live indoors, in houses, restaurants, and other buildings. Cockroaches are not known to transmit any serious diseases. However, they contaminate food, produce an unpleasant odor, and can become a serious nuisance, and exposure to cockroach antigen is an important risk factor for developing asthma. The four most common problem species in the United States are the German, brown-banded, Oriental, and American cockroaches.

Cockroaches undergo gradual metamorphosis (Truman, Bennet, and Butts, 1982) and have egg, nymph, and adult stages. Adult females produce egg cases, called *ootheca.* These protect the eggs from desiccation and, depending on species, may be carried around by the female until hatching or deposition in protected areas. The wings of adult cockroaches may be long and fully functional or short and almost nonexistent. In some species only the males have functional wings and may or may not fly. Most cockroaches are nocturnal but may be seen during the day when population numbers are high.

The German cockroach, *Blatella germanica,* is the most common cockroach in homes in the United States. Adults are about 1.3 cm in length, pale brown, and have two dark stripes on the pronotum, or back, of the insect. Females carry their ootheca until the eggs are ready to hatch and are the only common house-infesting cockroach to do so. German cockroaches are generalist feeders but prefer fermented food, and if water is present, adults can live for about a month.

The American cockroach, *Periplaneta americana,* or water bug, Bombay canary, or flying water bug, is the largest of the house-dwelling cockroaches (4 cm or more). It is reddish-brown, and males and females are fully winged but seldom fly. Females drop or secure ootheca in areas where food may be present, along baseboards or outdoors in damp, decaying wood (southern United States). They prefer dark, moist areas and are common in basements. American cockroaches feed on a variety of food sources, including book bindings, manuscripts, and other starchy substances and syrup and other types of sweets.

The Oriental cockroach, *Blatella orientalis,* or water bug, black beetle, or shad roach, is a cosmopolitan pest, found throughout the world. These roaches are black in color and about 3 cm in length. Females have rudimentary wings; male wings cover about three-quarters of the abdomen. Females drop their eggs or attach them to protected surface near a food supply. Oriental cockroaches feed on filth and rubbish and are especially fond of garbage. They also like high-moisture areas and must have water to survive.

The brown-banded cockroach, *Supella longipalpa,* is a small cockroach (less than 1.5 cm), with two lighter transverse bands across the base of the wings and abdomen. Females carry ootheca for one or two days and then attach them to a protected surface. This species is found high on ceilings, hiding behind picture frames, and near motors and electrical devices that generate heat. They require less water than other cockroaches and are rarely found in kitchens and bathrooms. Brown-banded cockroaches feed on starchy substances but can be found feeding on just about anything.

Fleas

Fleas are small ectoparasites (2 to 4 mm long) belonging to the order Siphonaptera (Triplehorn and Johnson, 2005). They have chewing mouthparts as juveniles and piercing-sucking mouthparts as adults, which are used to feed on blood (Truman, Bennet, and Butts, 1982), Fleas go through complete metamorphosis. Eggs are laid on the host animal but fall off into carpets, upholstery, and pet bedding material. The eggs hatch into legless, wormlike larvae. Larvae feed on debris and other organic material, including the feces of adult fleas and bits of dried blood. Larvae go through three stages (*instars*) until they spin cocoons and enter the pupal stage. When the adults emerge (in seven to fourteen days) they are ready to feed and mate. Fleas are of great importance because they are carriers of diseases such as plague and murine typhus.

There are several species of fleas, including those that feed on humans and pets. The cat flea, *Ctenocephalides felis,* and the dog flea, *C. canis,* are common throughout the United States and prefer to feed on dogs, cats, and humans and sometimes rats. They prefer areas with high amounts of organic material and are common in houses, under buildings, and in yards. Both species are intermediate hosts for dog tapeworm *Dipylidium caninum,* which can be transmitted to children who accidentally ingest infested fleas while playing with pets. The human flea, *Pulex irritans,* is common through the United States, especially in the Pacific coast region. It feeds almost exclusively on humans but can be found on swine and occasionally dogs. It can carry plague under laboratory conditions but is not normally a carrier of this disease. The oriental rat flea, *Xenopsylla cheopis,* is commonly found on Norway and roof rats and has become distributed throughout the United States. It is the chief carrier of bubonic plague in rats. Rats are its preferred host, but it will occasionally feed on humans. The northern rat flea, *Nosopsyllus fasciatus,* is also found throughout the United States, feeding on rats and mice. Although it is a known carrier of the plague organism it rarely bites humans. The sticktight flea, *Echidnophage gallinacea,* is primarily a pest of poultry in the southern and southwestern United States; however, it will attack other animals including man. This flea can be infected with plague and murine typhus; however, because females tend to feed on only one host, its importance as a vector is reduced. The mouse flea, *Leptopsylla segnis,* is commonly found on rats in the Gulf states and California, and to a lesser extent on house mice, and is not known to transmit disease.

Lice

Lice are flightless, ectoparasitic insects that belong to either the order Anoplura (sucking lice) or Mallophaga (chewing lice) (Triplehorn and Johnson, 2005). They are small insects (2 to 3 mm long) that exhibit gradual metamorphosis. Sucking lice insert their mouthparts into their host in order to feed on blood (Truman, Bennet, and Butts, 1982). Chewing lice feed on host skin scales and secretions. Sucking lice can be differentiated from chewing lice by the relationship between head and thorax; sucking lice have heads that are conical and narrower than their thoraxes, whereas chewing lice have heads that are shield shaped and wider than the thorax. Both groups spend their entire life on their host.

There are approximately 500 species of sucking lice that feed on mammals. Only two species attack humans: *Pediculus humanus,* which includes the body louse (*P. humanus humanus*) and the head louse (*P. humanus capitus*), and the crab or pubic louse (*Phthirus pubis*). Eggs are laid on the host, connected to body hair. They hatch into nymphs that immediately begin feeding on the host. Body lice are known to spread typhus and relapsing fever. Head lice and pubic lice do not transmit disease but are rapidly transmitted in settings such as schools and day-care centers and can be a serious nuisance. There are roughly 2,600 species of chewing lice. All are parasitic on either birds or mammals but do not attack humans.

Mosquitoes

Mosquitoes and other biting flies belong to the order Diptera (Triplehorn and Johnson, 2005). Mosquitoes are a large (169 species in North America), well-known, and important group of biting flies that spend their larval life living in water and their adult life above the water's surface. Mosquitoes are the vector for numerous human diseases, including malaria, dengue fever, yellow fever, and several encephalitis viruses.

Mosquitoes undergo complete metamorphosis (Hamilton and Racz, 1998). Female mosquitoes lay their eggs either as rafts on the surface of water or singly in or near water. In the latter situation the eggs remain dormant until the presence of water stimulates their development. Upon hatching, larvae, or wrigglers, feed on algae and other organic debris. All mosquitoes need air to breathe and must periodically stop feeding to do so. How this occurs depends on the species. Larval culicine mosquitoes, except *Anopheles* spp., insert an air tube or siphon on the tip of the abdomen through the water's surface like a snorkel in order to breathe. Anopheline mosquitoes do not have an air tube and must position themselves horizontal to the water surface to breathe. Other mosquito species can insert their breathing apparatus into the roots of aquatic plants in order to breathe. Under optimal conditions, larvae pupate within seven days. The small, comma-shaped pupae hang in the surface tension of the water surface so that their breathing tubes maintain contact with air. When the adults emerge, both females and males feed on plant juices, such as nectar, in order to survive. Females, however, must also feed on blood in order to develop their eggs. Depending on the species, they may obtain blood from birds, mammals, reptiles, or amphibians. Only the species that feed on humans are directly associated with the transmission of disease.

There are several species of mosquitoes that are responsible for transmitting the most serious diseases. For example, malaria is transmitted by *Anopheles* species. *Aedes aegypti* transmits both yellow fever and dengue fever (Triplehorn and Johnson, 2005). Filariasis, which is caused by a filarial worm, is transmitted by *Culex* species. West Nile virus is spread by a variety of species, primarily in the genus *Culex*, that have fed on birds. Eastern equine encephalitis is known to be circulated by *Culiseta melanura* in birds, but *Aedes sollicitans*, *Aedes vexans*, and *Coquillettidia perturbans* are suspected as major vectors of the disease in humans (Hamilton and Racz, 1998). *Culex pipiens*, the common house mosquito, transmits St. Louis encephalitis. Because *C. pipiens* is an urban mosquito, St. Louis encephalitis is prevalent in urban centers when it occurs.

Termites

Termites are insects that belong to the order Isoptera and are responsible for millions of dollars of damage to wood and wooden structures throughout the world (Triplehorn and Johnson, 2005). Worldwide there are about 1,900 species of termites. There are four families of termites: Kalotermitidae (seventeen U.S. species), Termopsidae (three U.S. species), Rhinotermitidae (nine U.S. species) and Termitidae (fifteen U.S. species). Termites have moniliform (beadlike) or filiform (filament-like) antennae, a broad connection between the thorax and abdomen, and front and hind wings that are equal in shape and size—characteristics that distinguish termites from ants. (Unlike termites, ants have elbowed antennae, a thin connection, called a *petiole*, between the thorax and abdomen, and front wings that are larger than the hind wings.)

Termites live in highly organized societies with three distinct castes: reproductive females and males, workers, and soldiers. Reproductive termites have four wings. Termites undergo simple metamorphosis and feed on cast skins, feces of other termites, dead individuals, and plant materials such as wood and wood products. The cellulose in the wood and wood products that termites eat is digested by a myriad of flagellate protists that live in the termite's digestive system. Without these organisms termites would starve to death. Termites are not born with these organisms but obtain them from feeding on the anal fluids of other termites.

Termites are important to humans for several reasons. First, because of their affinity for wood, they are very destructive to wooden portions of buildings, furniture, books, utility poles, fence posts, and other structures. Worldwide they also produce large amounts of atmospheric methane. Termites are also important because they help convert dead trees and other plant substances into decayed matter that can be used by other organisms.

Three main groups of destructive termites are of concern in the United States: subterranean termites, drywood termites, and dampwood termites. Subterranean termites live in wood that is either buried in the soil or is in contact with the soil. They may also enter wood not in contact with soil but must maintain contact in some way with soil. These termites are serious pests in the eastern United States. One introduced member of this group is the Formosan termite, *Coptotermes formosanus.* This termite is native to China and Taiwan and is one of the most destructive termites in the world. It has been introduced into several countries, including Japan, Guam, and the United States. It was first introduced into Texas in 1965 and has since spread to Alabama, Louisiana, Mississippi, Georgia, Florida, Tennessee, and North and South Carolina. It attacks living trees as well as dead stumps and wooden structures. Drywood termites live aboveground in wooden posts, tree stumps, trees, and buildings made of wood and do not need to be in contact with soil. Dampwood termites live in moist, dead wood, tree roots, and similar structures. They occur in Florida and southern, western, and Pacific coast areas of the United States.

Ticks

Ticks belong to the order Acarina and are relatives of insects. Ticks have piercing-sucking mouthparts and undergo a development cycle similar to that of insects with gradual metamorphosis. Mating occurs while the females and males are on the host. Females then drop to the ground to lay eggs (Truman, Bennet, and Butts, 1982). When they hatch, the resultant larvae, or seed ticks, have six legs. They then seek out a host on which to feed. After receiving a blood meal, they drop to the ground and molt to the next stage, called the *nymph.* The larvae of some ticks that feed on only one host will remain on the host to molt. Nymphs have eight legs and resemble adults but have no genital pore. Like larvae, nymphs must find a host in order to receive a blood meal to survive. When they do, they molt to the adult stage. Adult male and female ticks may feed for several days before being able to reproduce. Most ticks can feed on a wide variety of hosts, including birds, reptiles, and mammals. In some species, such as the black-legged or deer tick, *Ixodes scapularis,* immature ticks and adult ticks feed on different hosts. Ticks can be divided into two categories: hard ticks (for example, the brown dog tick, American dog tick, and black-legged tick) and soft ticks (for example, the common fowl tick and relapsing fever tick). Ticks are responsible for at least nine human diseases in the United States, including Lyme disease, Rocky Mountain spotted fever, relapsing fever, babesiosis, and more recently, ehrlichiosis (American Lyme Disease Foundation [ALDF], 2005).

The brown dog tick, *Rhipicephalus sanguineus*, feeds on a wide range of hosts (Truman, Bennet, and Butts, 1982). Its most common host is dogs. Brown dog ticks are generally associated with structures that house dogs, such as kennels, veterinary hospitals, and homes. In the United States, *R. sanguineus* is a vector of canine ehrlichiosis (*Ehrlichia canis*) and canine babesiosis (*Babesia canis*) (Lord, 2001). These rarely cause disease in humans; only a few cases are known. In dogs, symptoms of canine ehrlichiosis include lameness and fever; babesiosis causes fever, anorexia, and anemia. In parts of Europe, Asia, and Africa, *R. sanguineus* is a vector of *Rickettsia conorii*, known locally as Mediterranean spotted fever, boutonneuse fever, or tick typhus. *R. sanguineus* has not been shown to transmit the bacteria that cause Lyme disease. Adult American dog ticks, *Dermacentor variabilis*, also prefer to feed on dogs but will feed on other larger mammals (Truman, Bennet, and Butts, 1982). Larvae and nymphs feed on small wild rodents such as mice. They may be found both indoors and outdoors and are the most widely distributed tick in the United States. American dog ticks are vectors for Rocky Mountain spotted fever and tick paralysis. All stages of the lone star tick, *Amblyomma americanum*, attack humans and other animals, such as cattle, sheep, horses, hogs, dogs, deer, and birds (North Carolina Agricultural Extension Service, 2005). The lone star tick is also a vector for Rocky Mountain spotted fever and tick paralysis and is a secondary vector for Lyme disease. The black-legged tick is a known vector for Lyme disease (ALDF, 2005). The black-legged tick larvae feed on small mammals found in the leaf litter. Nymphs feed on small mammals and birds and, if not already infected, usually acquire Lyme disease during this stage. Adults feed on larger mammals, such as deer. Nymphs and adults also feed on humans and, if infected, can transmit Lyme disease to humans. Black-legged ticks can also transmit babesiosis. The western deer tick, *Ixodes pacificus*, which is common in the Midwestern and Western United States, is also a carrier of Lyme disease and babesiosis.

Vertebrate Pests

Vertebrate pests include rats, mice, and birds.

Rats

Rats are relatively large rodents that are important pests (Truman, Bennet, and Butts, 1982). They contaminate grain, destroy food in processing and storage plants, and can bite sleeping children and adults. Rats, over time, have caused more human death, misery, and economic hardship than any other vertebrate pest. Rats are known carriers of insects (lice, fleas, and mites) that transit plague and murine typhus, and as such they helped cause the outbreaks of plague in the fourteenth century that killed an estimated 25 million people (Cantor, 2001). Rats can also transmit Weil's disease, or leptospirosis; trichinosis and acute food poisoning can occur from food contaminated with rat feces. Rats also harbor organisms that cause typhoid, dysentery, and rabies.

Rats are very adaptable and can change their habits to match different environments. The roof rat, *Rattus tattus,* is an excellent climber and is commonly found in higher levels of buildings but can also be found in sewers. The Norway rat, *Rattus norvegicus,* lives in burrows but can be found in conditions favoring roof rats.

Rats live in well-protected areas and make nests out of soft material that is chewed or separated into small pieces. Outdoors, nests may be in the ground or tangled in tree limbs, trash dumps, or piles of rubbish. Indoors, nests can be found in wall voids, underneath floors next to the ground, and in undisturbed rubbish or stored materials. Rats have poor vision but excellent hearing and senses of smell and touch. Rats need a supply of water in order to survive and can squeeze through holes as small as a quarter.

The Norway rat (house rat, brown rat, wharf rat, sewer rat, or water rat) weighs between 10 and 17 ounces and is 31.2 to 49 cm in length (tip of nose to tip of tail). These rats have a blunt muzzle and a thick, heavy body. The tail is shorter than the head and body together, and is light colored underneath. Their ears are small, close set, and appear half buried in fur. Norway rat fur is coarse and generally red-brown to gray-brown. Norway rats are well distributed and are adept at displacing other species. They prefer traveling over flat surfaces to climbing but will climb pipes, wires, and rough walls when necessary. They prefer food with a high carbohydrate and protein content but will eat almost anything, including their own young.

The roof rat (black rat, ship rat, or gray-bellied rat) weighs between 8 and 12 ounces and is 34.9 to 45.1 cm in length (tip of nose to tip of tail). These rats have a pointed muzzle and a slender body. The tail is longer than the head and body together and uniformly colored. Their ears are large, prominent, and stand out from their fur. Roof rat fur is black to slate-gray or tawny above and gray-white below, or tawny above with a white to lemon belly. These rats are common at seaports. They are excellent climbers and frequently build nests in tree holes, in underground burrows, inside buildings, and under rubbish piles. Roof rats prefer to eat seeds, fresh vegetables or fruits, potatoes, wheat, corn, and other related foods. Like Norway rats, however, they will eat just about anything to survive.

Mice

Several species of mice, including field mice and house mice, can invade homes and other structures. The house mouse, *Mus musculus,* is the species most often encountered (Truman, Bennet, and Butts, 1982). House mice are considerably smaller than rats, generally weighing between 0.5 and 0.75 ounces and being 15.2 to 19.1 cm in length (tip of nose to tip of tail). House mice have small heads and bodies. Their tails are equal in length to their heads and bodies together. Their ears are prominent and appear large for the size of the body. Their fur is silky and dusky gray in color. House mice can enter structures using holes the size of dimes.

House mice have a keen sense of smell, touch, and hearing and can run, jump, and swim very well. Their nests can be made up of any soft material. House mice can occasionally be found in large colonies in which several females communally raise their young. They prefer human foods and will eat cereals, seeds, fruit, vegetables, and especially sweet liquids. House mice do not need a source of free water to survive, as rats do, and can get all the water they need directly from their food.

Mice can transmit diseases to humans and can be a vector for rat-bite fever and Weil's disease. In addition, their droppings can carry organisms that cause food poisoning. House mice can also carry fleas that transmit murine typhus, and they harbor mites that transmit rickettsialpox.

Hantavirus pulmonary syndrome (HPS) is another disease transmitted by infected rodents, through urine, droppings, or saliva (Centers for Disease Control and Prevention, 2005). Humans can contract the disease when they inhale aerosolized virus. HPS was first recognized in 1993 and has since been identified throughout the United States. Although rare, HPS is potentially deadly. Rodent control in and around the home remains the primary strategy for preventing hantavirus infection. The deer mouse, *Peromyscus maniculatus,* is the primary reservoir of the hantavirus that causes HPS in the United States.

Birds

Many birds are common inhabitants of urban areas (Truman, Bennet, and Butts, 1982). Species such as pigeons (*Columba livia*), European starlings (*Sturnus vulgaris*), and English house sparrows (*Passer domesticus*) are common sights in parks, along sidewalks, and at feeders in our own yards. Most of the general public, however, is unaware that birds are associated with several diseases of humans and that a number of parasites they carry may irritate or bite humans and play a role in food contamination. The close association between birds and humans presents potential epidemiological problems, because birds harbor several serious diseases.

One of the best-recognized diseases is pigeon ornithosis (psittacosis in parrotlike birds). This disease is similar to viral pneumonia and is transmitted to man though infected droppings or respiratory droplets and may infect 30 to 75 percent of the pigeons in a given area without being noticed. Several species of birds, including pigeons, have been shown to be reservoirs for encephalitides. These diseases of the nervous system include West Nile virus, equine encephalitis, and St. Louis encephalitis, and are transmitted to man by bird-biting mosquitoes. More recently, outbreaks of avian flu in Asia have called attention to the potential of both free-living birds and domestic poultry to spread diseases. Systemic fungus diseases such as histoplamosis (*Histoplasma capsulatum*) and cryptococcosis (*Cryptococcus neoformans*) have been traced to pigeon and European starling manure. Pigeons have also been shown to harbor *Salmonella typhimurium,* which causes food poisoning, and the protozoan *Toxoplasma gondii,* which is responsible for toxoplasmosis and can appear in humans. Diseases carried by birds that are of lesser importance to man include Newcastle disease, aspergillosis, pseudotuberculosis, pigeon coccidiosis, swine erysipelas, and trichomoniasis.

Pesticides

Pesticides are a mainstay of pest control. They are sprayed on crops and alongside residential streets, poured in gardens, squirted along baseboards and in basements, and impregnated into bed nets. Over 900 active ingredients are in commercial use, and these are formulated into more than 35,000 commercial products. The EPA (2005a) estimates that in 1999 over 1 billion pounds of pesticides were applied in the United States and over 5.6 billion pounds were applied worldwide. It is common for an active pesticide to have several different formulations—a spray, a wettable powder, and a liquid concentrate, for example—each of which can be formulated at several different concentrations.

Pesticides are often classified according to the type of pest they control. For examples, insecticides control insects, herbicides control vegetation, fungicides control fungi, and so forth. Box 20.2 displays various categories of pesticides.

Box 20.2. Pesticides Classified by Target

Algicides	Substances that control algae in lakes, canals, swimming pools, water tanks, and other sites.
Antifouling agents	Substances that kill or repel organisms that attach to underwater surfaces, such as boat bottoms.
Antimicrobials	Substances that kill microorganisms (such as bacteria and viruses).

Attractants	Substances that attract pests (for example, to lure an insect or rodent to a trap; food, however, is not considered a pesticide when used as an attractant).
Biopesticides	Certain types of pesticides derived from such natural materials as animals, plants, bacteria, and certain minerals.
Biocides	Substances that kill microorganisms.
Disinfectants and sanitizers	Substances that kill or inactivate disease-producing microorganisms on inanimate objects.
Fungicides	Substances that kill fungi (including blights, mildews, molds, and rusts).
Fumigants	Substances that produce gas or vapor intended to destroy pests in buildings or soil.
Herbicides	Substances that kill weeds and other plants that grow where they are not wanted.
Insecticides	Substances that kill insects and other arthropods.
Miticides (also called acaricides)	Substances that kill mites that feed on plants and animals.
Microbial pesticides	Microorganisms that kill, inhibit, or outcompete pests, including insects and also other microorganisms.
Molluscicides	Substances that kill snails and slugs.
Nematicides	Substances that kill nematodes (microscopic, wormlike organisms that feed on plant roots).
Ovicides	Substances that kill the eggs of insects and mites.
Pheromones	Biochemicals that disrupt the mating behaviors of insects.
Repellents	Substances that repel pests, including insects (such as mosquitoes) and birds.
Rodenticides	Substances that control mice and other rodents.

The term *pesticide* also includes these substances:

Defoliants	Substances that cause leaves or other foliage to drop from a plant, usually to facilitate harvest.
Desiccants	Substances that promote drying of living tissues, such as unwanted plant tops.
Insect growth regulators	Substances that disrupt the molting, maturing from pupal to adult stage, or other life processes of insects.
Plant growth regulators	Substances (excluding fertilizers and other plant nutrients) that alter the expected growth, flowering, or reproduction rate of plants.

Pesticides may also be classified according to chemical structure. Although many categories of chemicals have some action against insects or other pests, four categories account for most pesticides in use: organophosphates, carbamates, organochlorines, and pyrethroids. A fifth important category, defined not so much by chemical structure as by origin, consists of the biopesticides.

Organophosphates were developed during the early nineteenth century, but their effects on insects, which are similar to their effects on humans, were not discovered until 1932. These pesticides are nervous system toxins. They function by phosphorylating, and therefore inactivating, molecules of acetylcholinesterase, the enzyme that regulates the neurotransmitter acetylcholine. Many species, from insects to humans, use this neurotransmitter, so many species are potentially susceptible to the effects of the organophosphates. In fact some of the more toxic organophosphates have been used as nerve gases, and one, Sarin, was used in the infamous Tokyo subway attacks in 1995 (Ohbu and others, 1997). Some examples of organophosphates in common use are chlorpyrifos, diazinon, malathion, parathion, and mevinphos. The organophosphates vary in toxicity and are usually are not persistent in the environment.

Carbamates function through a mechanism similar to that of the organophosphates—binding to and inactivating acetylcholinesterase. However, carbamates have lower affinity for acetylcholinesterase than do organophosphates, which reduces their toxicity to humans. Carbamate insecticides are widely used in homes, gardens, and agriculture. Examples include aldicarb, carbaryl, and methomyl. Carbamates are also nonpersistent in the environment.

Organochlorine insecticides were commonly used in the past. However, with growing recognition of their role as persistent organic pollutants (POPs)—chemicals that persist for many years, bioaccumulate, and may harm ecosystems and human health—many of them have been removed from use, including DDT, aldrin, dieldrin, chlordane, and heptachlor.

Pyrethroid pesticides were developed as a synthetic version of the naturally occurring pesticide pyrethrin, which is found in chrysanthemums. They have been modified to increase their stability in the environment. Examples include allethrin, cismethrin, fenvalerate, and remethrin. Some synthetic pyrethroids are toxic to the nervous system.

Biopesticides are pesticides of biological origin, derived from such natural materials as animals, plants, bacteria, and certain minerals. For example, canola oil and baking soda have pesticidal applications and are considered biopesticides. At the end of 2001, there were approximately 195 registered biopesticide active ingredients and 780 products. Biopesticides fall into three major classes:

- *Microbial pesticides* have a microorganism (for example, a bacterium, fungus, virus, or protozoan) as the active ingredient. Microbial pesticides can control many different kinds of pests, although each separate active ingredient is relatively specific for its target pest(s). For example, there are fungi that control certain weeds and other fungi that kill specific insects. The most widely used microbial pesticides are subspecies and strains of *Bacillus thuringiensis*, or Bt. Each strain of this bacterium produces a different mix of proteins, many of which are toxic to one or a few related species of insect larvae.

- *Plant-incorporated-protectants* (PIPs) are pesticidal substances that plants produce from genetic material that has been added to the plant. For example, scientists can introduce the gene for the Bt pesticidal protein into a plant's own genetic material, enabling the plant to manufacture the substance that destroys the pest. The protein and its genetic material, but not the plant itself, are regulated by EPA.
- *Biochemical pesticides* are naturally occurring substances that control pests by nontoxic mechanisms. Conventional pesticides, in contrast, are generally synthetic materials that directly kill or inactivate the pest. Biochemical pesticides include substances, such as insect sex pheromones, that interfere with mating and also include various scented plant extracts that attract insect pests to traps.

Patterns of Pesticide Use and Human Exposure

People encounter pesticides in many ways: inhalation of sprayed pesticides near farms or in offices, ingestion of pesticides on foods, or skin contact with recently applied pesticides (also see Box 20.3).

Box 20.3. Who Is Responsible for Applying Pesticides?

Humans and insects prefer many of the same ecosystems, so they encounter each other in many settings—on agricultural fields, in gardens, in homes, and elsewhere. As a result, efforts at pest control, including pesticide use, take many forms. Who actually applies pesticides?

Pesticides are divided into two categories: *general use* and *restricted use.* The difference between them is analogous to the difference between over-the-counter medications and prescription medications.

Homeowners can buy a variety of general use pesticides at garden centers, hardware stores, and grocery stores to combat day-to-day pests. These pesticides are usually less toxic and less concentrated than restricted use pesticides. Many are in ready-to-use formulations, such as fly sprays and garden sprays. Some substances defined as pesticides may seem surprising. For instance, common household bleach, because it claims germicidal properties, must be registered as a pesticide, and it has an EPA registration number under the Federal Insecticide, Fungicide, and Rodenticide Act.

Commercial pesticide use is more tightly regulated. It is generally carried out by private firms, which may be small local businesses or large national franchises. These firms must be registered as pest control businesses with the appropriate state agency, typically the state department of agriculture or the state department of environmental protection. They must have certified applicators on staff, and they must show proof of liability insurance, in case a misapplication should occur. Most specialize in a particular type of pest control, such as structural or turf and ornamental.

The people who apply pesticides for pest control firms are known as *commercial applicators.* State laws define their work in something like the following terms: the application of pesticides (including restricted use pesticides) to land, plants, seeds, animals, water, structures, or vehicles, using aerial, ground, or hand equipment, on a contractual or for-hire basis. Commercial applicators must pass a series of EPA-approved tests, which are administered by the state agency. They must demonstrate general knowledge about pesticides plus specific knowledge and training in their area of specialty. Any commercial application of a pesticide, even a general use pesticide, requires that the applicator be licensed and certified. To maintain a commercial license the applicator must undergo a recertification program every five years. This usually entails participating in educational programs and earning the required number of continuing education units.

Despite the requirement that commercial pesticide application be carried out by licensed and trained professionals, pesticides are sometimes applied by untrained individuals. For example, building superintendents and school custodians commonly apply "structural and household pest control" compounds without the necessary training and background. This can result in serious health and environmental problems.

Farmers are one of the largest users of pesticide products. Although some hire commercial applicators, some qualify as *private applicators* in order to apply pesticides to their own land. They must be trained and certified to perform this task, as commercial applicators are, and they must apply specified pesticides to specified crops in accordance with the notations on the pesticide labels. Pesticides registered for agricultural use may not be used for residential or interior needs.

Most mosquito and public health pest control is handled by county and state agencies. In many states it is the local mosquito control commission that sprays for a variety of mosquito pests.

Aquatic weed control is usually carried out by the application of herbicides. This too is a specialty task that should only be performed by individuals with special training, either working for private firms or for government agencies. This is a sensitive job because misapplication can have serious effects on humans, on fish and other marine animals, and on beneficial plants.

Other uses of pesticides are frequent as well. Veterinarians apply flea and tick dips to control these pests on cats and dogs. Physicians apply pesticides to patients suffering from body lice and head lice. Federal agencies apply pesticides to cargo ships and airplanes importing or exporting food and fiber products.

Overall, pesticides are applied by a wide variety of people and organizations in a wide variety of situations. Although federal and state regulations have gone a long way toward ensuring safety, unapproved or sloppy procedures can still result in potential hazards to people and the environment.

Residential exposure is common. Eighty percent of U.S. households use pesticides more than once a year in and around their homes (Davis, Brownson, and Garcia, 1992; Whitmore and others, 1994). Many of the pesticides applied indoors are semivolatile (Dalaker and Naifeh, 1997). Once applied, semivolatile pesticides can vaporize from treated surfaces and can distribute in and on targeted and nontargeted surfaces and objects (Gurunathan and others, 1998; Lewis, Fortune, Blanchard, and Camann, 2001; Hore and others, 2005). This raises concern about exposures because U.S. householders, including children, may spend up to 90 percent of their time indoors, within or around treated areas (Savage and others, 1981). Children in pesticide-treated homes may be exposed to pesticides via multiple routes and from multiple media. Given their inherent biological vulnerabilities and characteristic behaviors, which are different from those of adults, children can be particularly susceptible to the effects of pesticides (Freeman, Ettinger, Barry, and Rhoads, 1997; see Chapter Twenty-Eight).

Work by many researchers has indicated that pesticides can persist in the home for long periods of time. They can also accumulate on surfaces that pose a particular risk to children. The plush toys that small children often carry and sleep with, for example, can act as sinks for pesticides applied in the home.

Occupational exposure is also common among farmworkers and other high-risk occupations. Workers who directly handle pesticides, including mixers and loaders, are at highest risk (Figure 20.4), followed by those who apply the pesticides in agricultural or commercial settings. Finally, farmworkers who enter treated fields where pesticides have been applied to perform allowed tasks, such as weeding, irrigating, or picking crops, are also at risk.

Pesticide Toxicity

Pesticides are toxic. This is a desired property, responsible for the ability of pesticides to kill unwanted species. However, pesticide toxicity may also affect humans, making this a public health issue. Pesticide damage to unintended species, and therefore to entire ecosystems, is also a serious concern in some circumstances.

FIGURE 20.4. WORKERS IN GHANA MIXING AND LOADING AN ORGANOPHOSPHATE INSECTICIDE WITHOUT ADEQUATE PERSONAL PROTECTIVE EQUIPMENT.

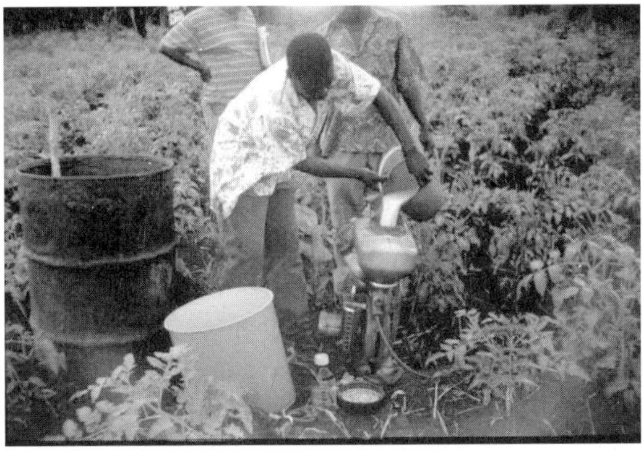

The EPA estimates that between 10,000 and 20,000 medically treated pesticide poisonings occur each year in the United States (Blondell, 1997), including suicides, attempted suicides, and unintentional poisonings. In the United States in 1983, the mortality rate from unintentional acute pesticide poisoning was estimated to be 2.7 per 10 million among men (and 0.5 among women) (Keifer, Wesseling, and McConnell, 2005).

Acute toxicity is most associated with the organophosphates and the carbamates. These compounds block the action of acetylcholinesterase at peripheral nerves and in the central nervous system. The early symptoms of poisoning include headache, hypersecretion, muscle twitching, nausea, and diarrhea. (Health care providers remember this syndrome with the mnemonic SLUDGE, for Salivation, Lacrimation, Urination, Diarrhea, GI upset, and pulmonary Edema, or DUMBELS, for Diarrhea, Urination, Miosis, Bronchospasm, Emesis, Lacrimation, and Salivation.) More severe poisoning can feature respiratory depression, loss of consciousness, and death. Victims who survive may develop weakness or paralysis of the arms and legs, known as organophosphate-induced delayed neuropathy (OPIDN), or they may exhibit an *intermediate syndrome* characterized by respiratory depression and muscular weakness.

Pesticides are required to carry warning statements on their labels, which are mostly based on acute toxicity. The label statements are based on oral LD_{50} (lethal dose for 50 percent; see Chapter Two), inhalation LD_{50}, dermal LD_{50}, eye effects, and skin effects. The toxicity warning categories are shown in Box 20.4.

Box 20.4. Pesticide Toxicity Categories and Labeling Requirements

Toxicity Category I—All pesticide products meeting the criteria of Toxicity Category I shall bear on the front panel the signal word "Danger." In addition if the product was assigned to Toxicity Category I on the basis of its oral, inhalation or dermal toxicity (as distinct from skin and eye local effects) the word "Poison" shall appear in red on a background of distinctly contrasting color and the skull and crossbones shall appear in immediate proximity to the word "Poison."

Toxicity Category II—All pesticide products meeting the criteria of Toxicity Category II shall bear on the front panel the signal word "Warning."

Toxicity Category III—All pesticide products meeting the criteria of Toxicity Category III shall bear on the front panel the signal word "Caution."

Toxicity Category IV—All pesticide products meeting the criteria of Toxicity Category IV shall bear on the front panel the signal word "Caution."

Child hazard warning—Every pesticide product label shall bear on the front panel the statement "keep out of reach of children." Only in cases where the likelihood of contact with children during distribution, marketing, storage, or use is demonstrated by the applicant to be extremely remote, or if the nature of the pesticide is such that it is approved for use on infants or small children, may the Administrator waive this requirement.

Further information on these criteria and labeling requirements is published in the Code of Federal Regulations (40 CFR 156.10).

Source: EPA, 2005b.

Chronic toxicity is also a growing concern as epidemiological and toxicological evidence accumulates. A review of epidemiological evidence reveals that pesticide exposure is associated with increases in the risk of several cancers, including non-Hodgkin's lymphoma (relative risk <2), leukemia (relative risk <1.5), multiple myeloma (an excess risk exists, although the specific exposure link is weak), soft-tissue sarcoma (inconsistent patterns have been observed), prostate cancer (relative risk <1.5), pancreatic cancer (increased risk found in some studies), lung cancer (causally associated with arsenical compounds), ovarian cancer (an association with triazine use has been found), breast cancer (possible estrogenic activity of chlorinated compounds), testicular cancer (antiandrogenic activity of chlorinated compounds), and Hodgkin's disease (small but significant excess risk found) (Alavanja, Hoppin, and Kamel, 2004).

In addition to acute neurotoxicity, pesticide exposure may have chronic effects on the nervous system, manifested by a range of symptoms, deficits in neurobehavioral performance, and abnormalities in nerve function. Neurotoxicity can result from high-level exposure to most types of pesticides, including organophosphates, carbamates, organochlorines, fungicides, and fumigants (Alavanja, Hoppin, and Kamel, 2004). There is also evidence linking pesticide exposure with chronic neurodegenerative diseases, especially Parkinson's disease (Priyadarshi, Khuder, Schaub, and Priyadarshi, 2001).

Pesticides may also have developmental, endocrine, and reproductive effects. This has been recognized for several decades; in fact Rachel Carson's landmark book, *Silent Spring,* took its title from the loss of songbirds that followed DDT-induced thinning of eggshells. Recent work has shown similar endocrine effects in other animals. Research at Lake Apopka, Florida, following contamination of the lake by organochlorine pesticides, dibromochloropropane, and ethylene dibromide, has shown marked changes in the alligator population, including decreased testosterone levels, smaller genitalia, and altered gender ratios in newborns, findings attributed to the effects of pesticides (Guillette and others, 1996; Semenza and others, 1997). Similarly, recent observations of demasculinization of atrazine-exposed frogs suggest that triazine compounds may have endocrine-disrupting effects (Hayes and others, 2002).

Pesticides also have direct and indirect effects on animal habitats. In the 1960s, the development of so-called no-till agriculture—a technique that involves heavy applications of chemicals, rather than tilling the soil, to control pests and weeds—caused widespread habitat destruction for many animals.

Pesticide Regulation

The EPA is the agency responsible for pesticide regulation, under the authority of two federal statutes: the Federal Insecticide, Fungicide, and Rodenticide Act (FIFRA) and the Federal Food, Drug, and Cosmetic Act (FFDCA).

According to the EPA (2005c):

> The Federal Insecticide, Fungicide, and Rodenticide Act (FIFRA) provides the basis for regulation, sale, distribution and use of pesticides in the U.S. This law authorizes EPA to review and register pesticides for specified uses. EPA also has the authority to suspend or cancel the registration of a pesticide if subsequent information shows that continued use would pose unreasonable risks. Some key elements of FIFRA include:
>
> - is a product licensing statute; pesticide products must obtain an EPA registration before manufacture, transport, and sale
> - registration based on a risk/benefit standard strong authority to require data—authority to issue data call-ins
> - ability to regulate pesticide use through labeling, packaging, composition, and disposal

- emergency exemption authority—permits approval of unregistered uses of registered products on a time limited basis
- ability to suspend or cancel a product's registration: appeals process, adjudicatory functions, etc.

The Federal Food, Drug, and Cosmetic Act (FFDCA) authorizes EPA to set maximum residue levels, or tolerances, for pesticides used in or on foods or animal feed. Features of FFDCA include:

- mandates strong provisions to protect infants and children
- provides the authority to set tolerances in foods and feeds (maximum pesticide residue levels)
- also provides authority to exempt a pesticide from the requirement of a tolerance
- rule-making process required to set tolerances or exemptions
- before a registration can be granted for a food use pesticide, a tolerance or tolerance exemption must be in place
- mandates primarily a health-based standard for setting the tolerance—"reasonable certainty of no harm"
- benefits may be considered only in limited extreme circumstances
- pesticide residues in foods are monitored and the tolerances enforced by FDA (fruits and vegetables, seafood) and USDA (meat, milk, poultry, eggs, and aquacultural foods)

The Food Quality Protection Act of 1996 (FQPA) amended FIFRA and FFDCA setting tougher safety standards for new and old pesticides and calling for uniform requirements regarding processed and unprocessed foods. Major provisions of this law include:

- amended both FIFRA and FFDCA, significantly changing the way EPA regulates pesticides:
- establishes a single safety standard for setting tolerances under FFDCA—*not* a risk/benefit standard (with some exceptions)
- assessment must include aggregate exposures including all dietary exposures, drinking water, and non-occupational (e.g., residential) exposures
- when assessing a tolerance, EPA must also consider cumulative effects and common mode of toxicity among related pesticides, the potential for endocrine disruption effects, and appropriate safety factor to incorporate
- requires a special finding for the protection of infants and children
- must incorporate a 10-fold safety factor to protect infants and children further unless reliable information in the database indicates that it can be reduced or removed

- establishes a tolerance reassessment program and lays out a schedule whereby EPA must reevaluate all tolerances that were in place as of August 1996 within 10 years
- requires a minor use program and provides that special considerations be afforded minor use actions
- requires review of antimicrobial actions within prescribed time frames
- EPA must now periodically review every pesticide registration every 15 years
- now required to set tolerances for use of pesticides under emergency exemptions (FIFRA Section 18)

Two other pieces of legislation are also relevant. The Pesticide Registration Improvement Act (PRIA) of 2003 "establishes pesticide registration service fees for registration actions in three pesticide program divisions: Antimicrobials, Biopesticides and Pollution Prevention, and Registration" (EPA, 2005c). The Endangered Species Act (ESA) of 1973 "prohibits any action that can adversely affect an endangered or threatened species or its habitat. In compliance with this law, EPA must ensure that use of the pesticides it registers will not harm these species" (EPA, 2005c).

Pesticide labeling was discussed in Box 20.4. Another important aspect of pesticide regulation is restrictions on use. In the United States and in many other countries, pesticides are sold either for *general use* or for *restricted use.* As mentioned earlier, the best analogy for the difference between these uses is the difference between over-the-counter medications and those requiring a prescription from a physician. General use pesticides are lower in toxicity, require few special precautions other than the standard safety measures, and are sold in lower concentrations. Restricted use pesticides are limited to sale to and use by a licensed pesticide applicator. Some compounds are general use at a low concentration or formulation and restricted use at a higher concentration. The licensed pesticide applicator will have received proper training for the use of these compounds and will have demonstrated to the state regulatory agency adequate knowledge for the safe and efficacious use of the product. Most states require examination and certification of the applicator, followed by continuing education and recertification. In most states commercial pest control can be carried out only by a licensed applicator.

Pesticide regulations have focused specifically on two high-risk groups: children and workers. *Children* are especially vulnerable to pesticide exposure. In 1996, the Food Quality Protection Act (FQPA) mandated that contributions from all routes of exposure and from all possible sources be considered when setting food tolerance levels for pesticides, paying particular attention to address the potential risks to infants and small children. The EPA subsequently undertook several actions to protect children:

- It set tougher standards to protect infants and children from pesticide risks, including an additional safety factor to account for developmental risks, incomplete data, and any special sensitivity and exposure to pesticide chemicals that infants and children may have.
- It restricted some uses of pesticides; for example, in 1999, the EPA disallowed major uses of the organophosphate methyl parathion in children's food and placed significant restrictions on the use of another organophosphate, azinphos methyl.
- It required additional studies on pesticides to clarify specific effects (such as developmental neurotoxicity and acute and subchronic neurotoxicity) in children.
- It developed new tests and risk assessment methods to target risk factors unique to infants and children.
- It increased consumer education; for example, a consumer information brochure was distributed to grocery stores nationwide and an interactive Web site (http://www.epa.gov/pesticides/food) was targeted to consumers.

Agricultural workers' risks of pesticide exposure are addressed by the EPA's Worker Protection Standard (WPS) that specifically protects agricultural workers. The WPS applies to over 3.5 million people who work with pesticides at over 560,000 workplaces. The WPS contains requirements for

- Pesticide safety training
- Notification of pesticide applications
- Use of personal protective equipment
- Restricted entry intervals following pesticide application
- Decontamination supplies
- Emergency medical assistance

Integrated Pest Management

Integrated pest management, or IPM, is an approach that uses multiple control techniques to maintain, or *manage,* pest populations below economically damaging levels while maintaining environmental quality. The IPM concept was first developed for use in agriculture in the 1960s, in response to environmental and developing pest-resistance issues caused by the use of various pesticides (Carson, 1962; Pedigo, 2002). In agriculture, IPM is defined as "a comprehensive approach to pest control that uses combined means to reduce the status of pests to tolerant levels while maintaining a quality environment" (Pedigo, 2002).

Since the 1960s, the IPM concept has been applied in numerous other settings, including turf and ornamental landscapes, homes, workplaces, and facilities such as schools, malls, restaurants, and hospitals. IPM is defined slightly differently for each of these applications. For turf and ornamental landscapes, for example, IPM definitions address maintaining "aesthetic quality." For buildings, homes, and schools, IPM definitions usually address sanitation, the preference for "low-impact" or "reduced-risk" chemicals, and the use of chemicals as a last resort. Finally, some states have also developed their own definitions of IPM and require the use of IPM in various situations (see, for example, New Jersey Department of Environmental Protection, 2005; "Pesticide Control Regulations," 2005). This complexity makes IPM difficult for the lay public to understand.

Common to all IPM definitions, however, are the goals of using more than one tool to control pests, keeping pest populations below damaging levels, maintaining environmental quality, and protecting human health. A useful overall definition of IPM is the following: A sustainable approach to managing pests by using all appropriate technology and management practices in a way that minimizes health, environmental and economic risks. In addition, IPM employs pest monitoring, consumer education, and cultural management techniques; sanitation and solid waste management; structural maintenance; and physical, mechanical, biological, and chemical controls.

Monitoring

Monitoring is the key to any good IPM program. Monitoring provides information on pest populations so that targeted, data-based control decisions can be made. The alternative to monitoring is to spray for pests whether they are present or not, which in today's society is unacceptable. Monitoring can also reveal how well a program is working and can identify problem areas that need more attention. A wide variety of species-specific monitoring methods are available, including the use of traps baited with various attractants.

Cultural Management Techniques

Cultural management techniques modify the environment to make it unattractive to pests. Practices such as covering garbage bins can eliminate a food source that rodents need to survive. Keeping dry food goods such as flour and sugar in sealed containers can keep storage pests from contaminating these products. Avoiding the placement of plants close to buildings can reduce the likelihood that carpenter ants will enter the structure. Removing or modifying areas that can hold water (gutters, empty cans, tires, low areas in the landscape) can remove potential breeding areas for mosquitoes. In the landscape, the use of cultural management techniques can make plants better able to withstand pest attack. Proper site selection and proper fertilization and watering, for example, reduce stress on plants, making them more vigorous and able to withstand attack. Another tactic is proper pruning. Pruning can remove diseased or insect-infested plant parts and can keep the pests from spreading to healthy tissue or further damaging the plant, providing control without the use of a pesticide.

Sanitation and Solid Waste Management

Sanitation and solid waste management can be a very important step toward controlling certain pests. This is especially important in food service and storage areas. Not leaving food out over night, cleaning under and behind kitchen appliances, and having regular refuse pickups are examples of practices that can keep pests such as cockroaches from gaining a foothold.

Structural Maintenance

Structural maintenance can keep pests from entering structures. Removing or repairing openings on a structure's facade can eliminate entry points for rodents. Placing screens over attic vents can keep insects from entering. Structural maintenance can also remove places were pests might obtain vital resources. Simple actions like fixing leaky facets can remove water sources that are vital to rats and several cockroach species. Fixing water leaks and reducing the subsequent decay of water-soaked wood also reduces the potential for carpenter ant infestations.

Control Measures

When pest-monitoring procedures indicate a pest problem and when measures such as sanitation and cultural management are either not available or not completely effective, use of a control measure may be warranted. Depending on the pest and the situation, several measures may be available: physical and mechanical interventions, biological control agents, or chemical pesticide applications. The optimal control measure is the one that is least harmful to the environment and human health while still providing effective control. Box 20.5 presents the pros and cons of using DDT as a control measure against malaria, and the subsequent discussion offers general considerations in selecting among various control tactics.

Box 20.5. DDT in Antimalarial Campaigns: An Example of Public Health Trade-Offs

Up through the first part of the twentieth century, malaria control relied on environmental approaches such as drainage and landfills to eliminate the larval mosquito habitat and on biological controls such as larvivorous fish in ponds and larvicidal applications of oil and Paris green (Mabaso, Sharp, and Lengeler, 2004; Najera, 2001). These methods were effective, especially in Europe and North America, but malaria continued to be a problem in many poor nations.

DDT, or dichlorodiphenyltrichloroethane, was introduced as an agricultural pesticide during the 1930s, and during World War II military forces used it for typhus control (Gahan, Travis, Morton, and Lindquist, 1945). During the 1950s and 1960s, as part of malaria control campaigns worldwide, DDT played an important role in reducing mosquito populations and reducing the burden of disease.

However, DDT belongs to a category of chemicals known as *persistent organic pollutants* (POPs); it persists for years in the environment, it is bioconcentrated as it moves up the food chain, and it may harm wildlife and even humans. Rachel Carson's *Silent Spring* alerted the public that chemicals such as DDT could have catastrophic ecosystem effects, killing not only insects but birds and other species. In addition, although DDT has low acute toxicity in humans, there is some evidence that it may disrupt reproductive and endocrine functions. Because of these concerns, Sweden banned the use of DDT in 1970, the United States did so in 1972, and many other countries have followed suit. The Stockholm Convention on Persistent Organic Pollutants, an international treaty that requires the elimination of DDT and other POPs, was signed in 2001 and took effect in 2004, when the fiftieth nation ratified it (Kapp, 2004b; Stockholm Convention on Persistent Organic Pollutants, 2001).

Malaria remains a common and deadly disease in much of the developing world. It kills 3 million people each year, including one child every thirty seconds, despite decades of research on vaccines, new drugs, and alternative control strategies. If DDT is effective in controlling malaria, should it continue to be used? This is a classic example of a trade-off in public health, a dilemma in which one public health goal—the elimination of a persistent chemical pollutant—collides with another public health goal—the control of a killer disease. Strong arguments have been advanced on both sides of the debate.

Arguments against continued DDT use:

- DDT accumulates in ecosystems, persists for years or even decades, bioconcentrates, and has been shown to cause reproductive failure and other adverse outcomes in fish, birds, and other species beyond target insect species (Turusov, Rakitsky, and Tomatis, 2002).
- DDT accumulates in the adipose tissue of humans and other organisms (World Health Organization [WHO], 1989).

- Although the acute toxicity of DDT is low, there is some evidence that DDT may disrupt reproductive and endocrine functions and neurological development (Longnecker, Klebanoff, Zhou, and Brock, 2001; Longnecker, Rogan, and Lucier, 1997). There is also laboratory evidence of carcinogenicity, leading the National Toxicology Program (2005) to classify DDT as "reasonably anticipated to be a human carcinogen," and the International Agency for Research on Cancer (1991) to classify it as "possibly carcinogenic to humans." A precautionary approach would dictate avoiding the use of such a chemical.
- Continued use of DDT will result in increasing insect resistance, so in the long run this will not be a useful strategy.
- Alternatives to DDT, including nonchemical approaches and synthetic pyrethroids, are readily available.

Arguments in favor of continued DDT use:

- DDT has very low acute toxicity for humans (Smith, 2000), and the evidence for human carcinogenicity and other adverse effects is weak (Smith, 2000; Curtis and Lines, 2000). In contrast the burden of mortality and morbidity from malaria is enormous. Therefore a cost-benefit analysis clearly favors the use of DDT.
- DDT is relatively inexpensive compared to alternatives and therefore more accessible for many poor countries. The cost of alternatives such as malathion and pyrethroid insecticides can be two times to twenty times that of DDT, and bed nets (at several dollars each) are also prohibitively expensive (Tren, 1999).
- DDT is easy to mix and apply, thereby eliminating the need for training and supervision (Tren, 1999). This makes it practical for widespread use in developing nations.
- Malaria (and other arthropod-borne diseases such as dengue fever and urban yellow fever) have surged in many areas following the phaseout of DDT, underlining the importance of DDT in malaria control (Roberts, Loughlin, Hshieh, and Legters, 1997; Roberts, Manguin, and Mouchet, 2000).
- DDT is now used for house spraying, a selective approach that requires much less volume than the previous agricultural and area spraying. This results in a much lower environmental load than resulted from applications in the past.

What do you think? Should the continued use of DDT be permitted for malaria control? (For further information see Kapp, 2004a; Roberts and others, 2004; Stolberg, 1999.)

Physical and mechanical controls include the use of techniques or materials that will keep pests from becoming a problem. These can include such simple measures as painting building foundations white and creating light-colored borders around foundations to help prevent rats and mice from entering buildings, or raising dumpsters and other outdoor refuse containers up off the ground to reduce hiding places for rats. Other possibilities include installing bug zappers at doors leading to the outside to help prevent flying insects from entering a building, caulking doors and windows to remove access points for insects and rodents, and using door sweeps or sealing voids around pipes to prevent the entry of pests. What can or should be used depends on the pest involved and the situation at hand. What is appropriate for one pest may not be appropriate for another. For example, window screens keep flying insects such as mosquitoes from entering a structure but have little impact on mice. Bug zappers used at the entrances to food preparation areas and warehouses help prevent flying insects from entering the structure but do not prevent termites from entering. Termite guards help prevent termite infestations but have little or no impact on other pest species. Bug zappers used outdoors do little more than attract insects into the areas, and sonic devices to repel pests have little or no effect. One should be careful to choose an appropriate, effective control measure.

Biological control involves the use, manipulation, and conservation of living organisms that feed on insects and weeds for the purpose of controlling a pest. By definition, biological control agents (natural enemies) are beneficial organisms that create or recreate a natural balance to control pests. Although biological control is used primarily in agriculture, this method, when feasible, can provide effective control in an environmentally friendly manner in many other situations. For example, nematodes, living organisms that attack certain insects, can be used in place of chemicals to control fungus gnats in house plant pots or white grubs in turf. Given the right conditions, gambusia (mosquito fish) released into ponds can control mosquito larvae. Using biological control also means avoiding management tactics that might be detrimental to beneficial organisms. Using environmentally friendly chemicals or alternative control measures can avoid reductions in natural enemy populations. Outdoors, certain measures can encourage natural enemies in an area and keep them there once they are present. Using plant species that are attractive to beneficial organisms and that provide alternative or supplemental food sources, such as nectar and pollen, will help control ornamental and garden pests and reduce the need to use pesticides.

The use of chemical pesticides to control pests should be seen as a last resort; they should be used only when other tactics are not available, practical, or effective. Many state universities and extension services provide information on pesticides. These recommendations can be used in deciding which chemicals are available to control specific pests and under what circumstances. Chemicals that are less harmful to the environment or the user should be used whenever possible. The pesticide chosen should be effective, so that repeated applications and the use of more chemicals are not necessary. Finally, all labeling directions should be followed, and quantities applied should never exceed the amount prescribed by the label.

Consumer Education

Education of potential users of IPM is also very important. The general public and potential users of IPM must not only be made aware of what IPM is but must also understand its different components and how these components fit into a complete management program, one that reduces hazards to themselves and the environment.

Thought Questions

1. Pesticides are economic poisons; unlike other toxins or contaminants with which people come into contact, pesticides are intentionally applied to food, living spaces, and people. What are some of the risk-benefit issues in the application of pesticides? Is it worth the risk to apply pesticides?
2. Integrated pest management is a logical approach for many pest problems, but it is not widely used. What are some of the societal trade-offs when using IPM?
3. Pesticide use continues to be a major part of agricultural production; nevertheless, after fifty years of intense chemical use, a quarter to a third of the global harvest is lost to pests. Is this progress? What else can we do to improve the world food supply?
4. Are current pesticide regulations protective of public health, especially for susceptible populations?
5. WHO and other agencies still apply DDT and similar compounds to control many vector-borne diseases, such as malaria. The risks associated with DDT have been known for many decades. Is it appropriate that these compounds are still used for vector control?

References

Abdel-Rahman, A. A., and others. "Neurological Deficits Induced by Malathion, DEET, and Permethrin, Alone or in Combination in Adult Rats." *Journal of Toxicology & Environmental Health Part A,* 2004, *67*(4), 331–356.

Alavanja, M.C.R., Hoppin, J. A., and Kamel, F. "Health Effects of Chronic Pesticide Exposure: Cancer and Neurotoxicity." *Annual Review of Public Health,* 2004, *24,* 155–197.

American Lyme Disease Foundation. "Deer Tick Ecology." [http://www.aldf.com/DeerTickEcology.asp]. 2005.

Bell, J. W., Veltri, J. C., and Page, B. C. "Human Exposure to N,N-Diethyl-m-Toluamide Insect Repellant Reported to the American Association of Poison Control Centers, 1993–1997." *International Journal of Toxicology,* 2002, *21,* 341–352.

Blondell, J. "Epidemiology of Pesticide Poisonings in the United States, with Special Reference to Occupational Cases." *Occupational Medicine,* 1997, *12,* 209–220.

Buescher, M. D., Rutledge, L. C., Wirtz, R. A., and Nelson, J. H. "The Dose-Persistence Relationship of DEET Against *Aedes Aegypti.*" *Mosquito News,* 1983, *43,* 364–366.

Cantor, N. *In the Wake of the Plague: The Black Death and the World It Made.* New York: Free Press, 2001.

Carson, R. *Silent Spring.* Boston: Houghton Mifflin, 1962.

Centers for Disease Control and Prevention. "Hantavirus Pulmonary Syndrome (HPS)." [http://www.cdc.gov/ncidod/diseases/hanta/hps]. 2005.

Curtis, C. F., and Lines, J. D. "Should DDT Be Banned by International Treaty?" *Parasitology Today,* 2000, *16*(3), 119–121.

Dalaker, J., and Naifeh, M. *Poverty in the United States.* U.S. Bureau of the Census, Current Population Reports, Series P60-201. Washington, D.C.: U.S. Government Printing Office, 1997.

Davis, J. R., Brownson, R. C., and Garcia, R. "Family Pesticide Use in the Home, Garden, Orchard, and Yard." *Archives of Environmental Contamination and Toxicology,* 1992, *22,* 260–266.

"DEET Is Hard to Beat." *Harvard Health Letter,* 2003, *28,* 1–3.

Fradin, M. S. "Mosquitoes and Mosquito Repellents: A Clinician's Guide." *Annals of Internal Medicine,* 1998, *128,* 931–940.

Fradin, M. S., and Day, J. F. "Comparative Efficacy of Insect Repellants Against Mosquito Bites." *New England Journal of Medicine,* 2002, *347,* 13–18.

Freeman, N.C.G., Ettinger, A., Barry, M., and Rhoads, G. "Hygiene- and Food-Related Behaviors Associated with Blood Lead Levels of Young Children from Lead-Contaminated Homes." *Journal of Exposure Analysis and Environmental Epidemiology,* 1997, *7,* 1–15.

Gahan, J. B., Travis, B. V., Morton, F. A., and Lindquist, A. W. "DDT as a Residual-Type Treatment to Control *Anopheles Quadrimaculatus:* Practical Tests." *Journal of Economic Entomology,* 1945, *38,* 223–235.

Guillette, L. J., and others. "Reduction in Penis Size and Plasma Testosterone Concentrations in Juvenile Alligators Living in a Contaminated Environment." *General and Comparative Endocrinology,* 1996, *101,* 32–42.

Gurunathan, S., and others. "Accumulation of Chlorpyrifos on Residential Surfaces and Toys Accessible to Children." *Environmental Health Perspectives,* 1998, *106,* 9–16.

Hamilton, G. C., and Racz, A. (eds.). *Pesticide Applicator Training Manual: Mosquito Pest Control, Category 8B.* New Brunswick, N.J.: Rutgers Cooperative Extension, 1998.

Hayes, T. B., and others. "Hermaphroditic, Demasculinized Frogs After Exposure to the Herbicide Atrazine at Low Ecologically Relevant Doses." *Proceedings of the National Academy of Sciences of the United States of America,* 2002, *99*(8), 5476–5480.

Hore, P., and others. "Chlorpyrifos Accumulation Patterns for Child-Accessible Surfaces and Objects and Urinary Metabolite Excretion by Children for Two Weeks After Crack-and-Crevice Application." *Environmental Health Perspectives,* 2005, *113,* 211–219.

International Agency for Research on Cancer. *Occupational Exposures in Insecticide Application, and Some Pesticides.* IARC Monographs on the Evaluation of Carcinogenic Risks to Humans, vol. 53. Lyon: IARC, 1991.

Kapp C. "Help or Hazard." *Lancet,* 2004a, *364,* 1113–1114.

Kapp, C. "New International Convention Allows Use of DDT for Malaria Control." *Bulletin of the World Health Organization,* 2004b, *82,* 472–473.

Keifer, M. C., Wesseling, C., and McConnell, R. "Pesticides and Related Compounds." In L. Rosenstock, M. Cullen, C. Brodkin, and C. Redlich (eds.), *Textbook of Clinical Occupational and Environmental Medicine.* New York: Elsevier, 2005.

Lewis, R. G., Fortune, C. R., Blanchard, F. T., and Camann, D. E. "Movement and Deposition of Two Organophosphorus Pesticides Within a Residence After Interior and Exterior Applications." *Journal of the Air and Waste Management Association,* 2001, *51,* 339–351.

Longnecker, M. P., Klebanoff, M. A., Zhou, H., and Brock, J. W. "Association Between Maternal Serum Concentration of the DDT Metabolite DDE and Preterm and Small-For-Gestational-Age Babies at Birth." *Lancet,* 2001, *358,* 110–114.

Longnecker, M. P., Rogan, W. J., and Lucier, G. "The Human Health Effects of DDT (Dichlorodiphenyltrichloroethane) and PCBs (Polychlorinated Biphenyls) and an Overview of Organochlorines in Public Health." *Annual Review of Public Health,* 1997, *18,* 211–244.

Lord, C. C. "Brown Dog Tick." [http://creatures.ifas.ufl.edu/urban/medical/brown_dog_tick.htm#medical]. 2001.

Mabaso, M. L., Sharp, B., and Lengeler, C. "Historical Review of Malarial Control in Southern Africa with Emphasis on the Use of Indoor Residual House-Spraying." *Tropical Medicine and International Health,* 2004, *9,* 846–856.

McNeill, W. *Plagues and Peoples.* New York: Anchor Books, 1976.

Nadakavukaren, A. *Our Global Environment: A Health Perspective.* (4th ed.) Prospect Heights, Ill.: Waveland Press, 1995.

Najera, J. A. "Malaria Control: Achievements, Problems and Strategies." *Parassitologia,* 2001, *43,* 1–89.

National Toxicology Program. *Report on Carcinogens.* (11th ed.) Washington, D.C.: U.S. Department of Health and Human Services, Public Health Service, National Toxicology Program, 2005.

New Jersey Department of Environmental Protection, Pesticide Control Program. "Integrated Pest Management." [http://www.nj.gov/dep/enforcement/pcp/pcp-pubs.htm]. 2005.

North Carolina Agricultural Extension Service. "Ticks." [http://ipm.ncsu.edu/AG369/notes/ticks.html]. 2005.

Ohbu S., and others. "Sarin Poisoning on Tokyo Subway." *Southern Medical Journal,* 1997, *90*(6), 587–593.

Pedigo, L. P. *Agricultural Entomology and Pest Management.* (4th ed.) Upper Saddle River, N.J.: Prentice Hall, 2002.

"Pesticide Control Regulations." *New Jersey Administrative Code (NJAC)* 7:30, Subchapter 1: Scope and Definitions. [http://www.nj.gov/dep/enforcement/pcp/regulations/sub01new.pdf]. 2005.

Pollack, R. J., Kiszewski, A. E., and Spielman A. "Repelling Mosquitoes." *New England Journal of Medicine,* 2002, *347,* 2–3.

Priyadarshi, A., Khuder, S. A., Schaub, E. A., and Priyadarshi, S. S. "Environmental Risk Factors and Parkinson's Disease: A Meta-Analysis." *Environmental Research,* 2001, *86,* 122–127.

Roberts, D. R., Loughlin, L. L., Hshieh, P., and Legters, L. J. "DDT, Global Strategies, and a Malaria Control Crisis in South America." *Emerging Infectious Diseases,* 1997, *3,* 295–302.

Roberts, D. R., Manguin, S., and Mouchet, J. "DDT House Spraying and Re-Emerging Malaria." *Lancet,* 2000, *356,* 330–332.

Roberts, D., and others. "Malaria Control and Public Health." *Emerging Infectious Diseases,* 2004, *10,* 1170–1171.

Roberts, J. R., and Reigart, J. R. "Does Anything Beat DEET?" *Pediatric Annals,* 2004, *33*(7), 443–453.

Savage, E. P., and others. "Household Pesticide Usage in the United States." *Archives of Environmental Health,* 1981, *36,* 304–309.

Semenza, J. C., and others. "Reproductive Toxins and Alligator Abnormalities at Lake Apopka, Florida." *Environmental Health Perspectives,* 1997, *105,* 1030–1032.

Smith, A. G. "How Toxic Is DDT?" *Lancet,* 2000, *356,* 267–268.

Stockholm Convention on Persistent Organic Pollutants. Convention text. [http://www.pops.int/documents/convtext/convtext_en.pdf]. 2001.

Stolberg, S. G. "DDT, Target of Global Ban, Finds Defenders in Experts on Malaria." *New York Times,* July 29, 1999, p. 1A.

Sudakin, D. L., and Trevathan, W. R. "DEET: Review and Update of Safety and Risk in the General Population." *Journal of Toxicology: Clinical Toxicology,* 2003, *41*(6), 831–839.

Sullivan, R. *Rats: Observations on the History and Habitat of the City's Most Unwanted Inhabitants.* New York: Bloomsbury, 2004.

Tren, R. *The Economic Cost of Malaria in South Africa: Malaria Control and the DDT Issue.* Johannesburg: Africa Fighting Malaria, 1999.

Triplehorn, C. A., and Johnson, N. F. *Borror and Delong's Introduction to the Study of Insects.* (7th ed.) Pacific Grove, Calif.: Brooks/Cole, 2005.

Truman, L. C., Bennet, G. W., and Butts, W. L. *Scientific Guide to Pest Control Operations.* Orlando: Harcourt Brace, 1982.

Turusov, V., Rakitsky, V., and Tomatis, L. "Dichlorodiphenyltrichloroethane (DDT): Ubiquity, Persistence, and Risks." *Environmental Health Perspectives,* 2002, *110,* 125–128.

U.S. Environmental Protection Agency. "About Pesticides: Annual Reports." [http://www.epa.gov/oppfead1/annual]. 2005a.

U.S. Environmental Protection Agency. "Pesticides: Health and Safety: Toxicity Categories and Pesticide Label Statements." [http://www.epa.gov/pesticides/health/tox_categories.htm]. 2005b.

U.S. Environmental Protection Agency. "Pesticides: Regulating Pesticides: Laws." {http://www.epa.gov/pesticides/regulating/laws.htm]. 2005c.

Ware, G. W., and Whitacre, D. M. *The Pesticide Book.* (6th ed.) Willoughby, Ohio: MeisterPro, 2004.

Whitmore, R. W., and others. "Non-Occupational Exposures to Pesticides for Residents of Two U.S. Cities." *Archives of Environmental Contamination and Toxicology,* 1994, *26,* 47–59.

World Health Organization. *DDT and Its Derivatives: Environmental Aspects.* Environmental Health Criteria 83. Albany, N.Y.: WHO Publication Center, 1989.

Zinsser, H. *Rats, Lice, and History.* Boston: Little, Brown, 1963.

For Further Information

More information can be found at U.S. Environmental Protection Agency Web sites:

U.S. Environmental Protection Agency. "Pesticides." [http://www.epa.gov/pesticides]. 2005.
U.S. Environmental Protection Agency. "Pesticides: Health & Safety." [http://www.epa.gov/pesticides/safety/healthcare/handbook/handbook.htm]. 2005.
U.S. Environmental Protection Agency. "About Pesticides." [http://www.epa.gov/pesticides/about/types.htm]. 2005.

In addition, the United States has a national network of poison control centers. The national hotline number for the American Association of Poison Control Centers is 1-800-222-1222.

The EPA's Office of Pesticide Programs publishes R. Reigart and J. Roberts (eds.), *Recognition and Management of Pesticide Poisonings*, in both English and Spanish. The fifth edition (1999) covers about 1,500 pesticide products, in an easy-to-use format. Toxicology, signs and symptoms of poisoning, and treatment are covered in nineteen chapters on major types of pesticides. The fifth edition adds pesticide products that have come on the market since 1989, includes a new chapter on disinfectants, reviews clinical experiences with pesticide poisonings, and contains detailed references.

CHAPTER TWENTY-ONE

FOOD SAFETY

David McSwane

The United States has one of the safest food supplies in the world. Yet each year millions of Americans become ill, some with potentially fatal diseases, from eating contaminated food. Foodborne illness poses a significant public health challenge, and prevention of foodborne disease is an essential function of public health, environmental health, and agricultural agencies throughout the nation.

Food safety is the component of environmental health that protects our food supply from farm to table. Food safety programs typically involve a cooperative effort between the food industry and regulatory agencies at the federal, state, and local levels. The collective goal of these programs is to enhance the safety of America's food supply and reduce the incidence of foodborne illness.

Foodborne Illness: Magnitude of the Problem

Foodborne illness is the sickness people experience after consuming food and beverages that are contaminated with pathogenic (disease-causing) microorganisms, chemicals, or physical agents. Victims of foodborne illness commonly experience one or more symptoms such as nausea, vomiting, diarrhea, abdominal pain, headache, fever, and dehydration. The type and the severity of a person's symptoms are influenced by the type of pathogen in the food, the amount of contaminated food consumed, and the individual's health status at the time the contaminated food was eaten.

Foodborne illnesses often occur in outbreaks, with two or more people experiencing the same illness as a result of eating contaminated food. The victims of a foodborne disease outbreak may have eaten contaminated food together during a meal or they may have eaten tainted food separately but from a common source, such as a restaurant, supermarket, or manufacturer.

Cases of foodborne illness are the individuals who become ill as a result of eating contaminated food. Cases that occur in outbreaks, together with sporadic cases, make up the incidence of foodborne illness—the number of cases per population per unit of time. Foodborne illness is substantially underreported for several reasons: victims frequently experience mild symptoms and do not seek medical care; those who do seek medical care frequently have nonspecific symptoms that are not recognized as foodborne; definitive laboratory diagnoses of vomit, feces, or blood are often not carried out; and even when a diagnosis is made, physicians may not report cases to public health agencies.

Estimates of the number of cases of foodborne illness that occur each year vary greatly, not only because of underreporting but also because many pathogens that cause foodborne illness can also be spread from person to person or through water, thus obscuring the role of foodborne transmission. According to the Centers for Disease Control and Prevention (CDC), the exact cause of a foodborne illness is known in less than 20 percent of cases. In 1993, the U.S. Food and Drug Administration (FDA) estimated an annual burden of between 24 and 81 million cases of foodborne illness, resulting in an estimated 10,000 deaths (FDA, 1993). In 1994, the Council for Agricultural Science and Technology (CAST) estimated the annual number of foodborne illnesses at between 6.5 and 33 million cases, with about 9,000 deaths (Foegeding and Roberts, 1994). In 1996, the CDC implemented the Foodborne Disease Active Surveillance Network (FoodNet), as part of its Emerging Infections Program, to monitor and quantify the incidence of foodborne illness more precisely. FoodNet collects data on ten foodborne diseases in nine states and follows trends in foodborne infections for diagnosed illnesses caused by pathogens transmitted through food. From the data collected through FoodNet and other sources, the CDC estimated in 1999 that there are 76 million cases of foodborne illness in the United States annually, resulting in approximately 325,000 hospitalizations and 5,000 deaths (Mead and others, 1999).

FoodNet data released in 2004 suggest some shifts in the pathogens recognized as causing foodborne illness. Although cases involving *Cryptosporidium, E. coli* O157:H7, *Salmonella* Typhi, *Campylobacter,* and *Yersinia* declined significantly between 1996 and 2003, cases involving *Listeria, Shigella,* and *Vibrio* did not decline (Shallow and others, 2004). Regional and year-to-year variation in the incidence of foodborne illness has occurred since active surveillance began in 1996. Despite the annual and regional fluctuations, reductions in the overall incidence of foodborne illness indicate progress is being made toward preventing foodborne illness and protecting public health. Although less well documented, the burden of foodborne illness in developing countries, where levels of hygiene and sanitation are often substandard, is likely far greater.

Behind all these statistics are real people who have suffered debilitating, even fatal, diseases from what most of us consider one of life's less risky activities—eating. In addition to pain and suffering, foodborne illness costs society billions of dollars each year in the form of medical expenses, lost productivity, punitive damages and lost business for food companies, and increased surveillance by regulatory agencies.

Foodborne illness remains a significant public health problem for the United States and the rest of the world for at least three major reasons. First, known pathogens are being found in a growing number of foods. *Salmonella* bacteria are commonly found in raw poultry and eggs and have caused foodborne illness for many years. Recently, however, these organisms have also been linked to outbreaks associated with alfalfa sprouts. *E. coli* O157:H7 bacteria have long been associated with raw or improperly cooked ground beef and pork, but these organisms have recently also been found in unpasteurized apple juice and radish sprouts.

Second, new pathogens are being discovered. *Listeria monocytogenes* and *Cyclospora cayetanensis* are two examples of emerging pathogens that have been recently identified as causes of foodborne illness. *Listeria* bacteria have been identified as the cause of recent foodborne outbreaks linked to soft cheeses made with improperly pasteurized milk and to contaminated hot dogs and luncheon meats. *Cyclospora* is a parasite that has been associated with fresh fruits and vegetables that were contaminated on the farm.

Third, there are more people in susceptible populations. Anyone can become ill from eating contaminated food. However, most healthy adults remain asymptomatic or have very mild flulike symptoms that resolve in a few days. The same is not true for people in susceptible populations: infants and young children, the elderly, pregnant women and nursing mothers, and people with impaired immune function due to HIV infection, cancer, diabetes, and certain medications. The risks associated with foodborne illness are much more serious for individuals in susceptible populations than they are for healthy adults. Susceptible individuals typically become ill from smaller doses of pathogens, and the symptoms and durations of their illnesses can be much more severe, even life threatening.

Sources of Food Contamination

Whether food is prepared "from scratch" or arrives ready to eat, it can become contaminated at many points as it flows from harvest through processing and distribution to the consumer. Some common sources of food contamination are presented in Figure 21.1.

FIGURE 21.1. COMMON SOURCES OF FOOD CONTAMINATION.

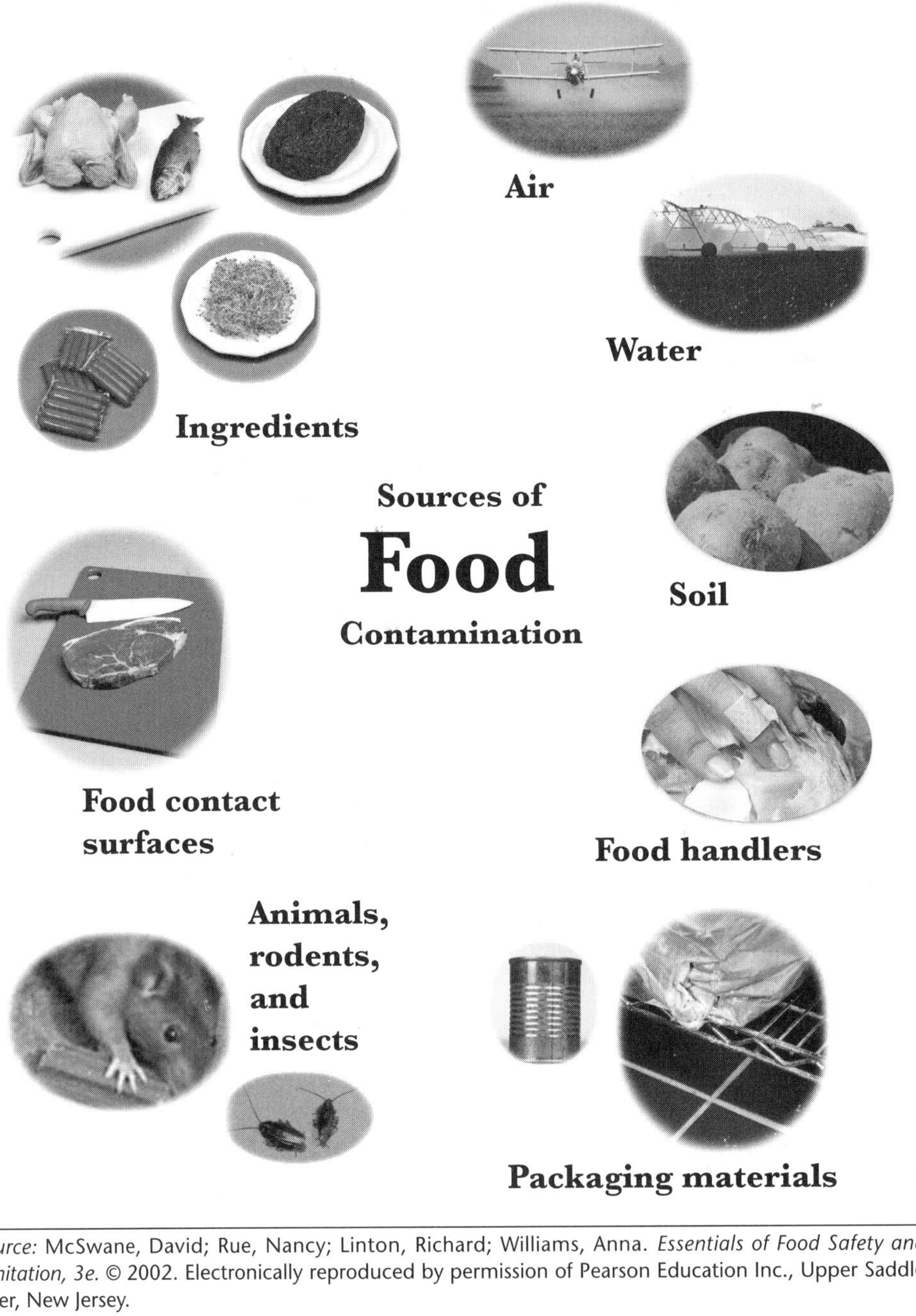
Air
Water
Ingredients
Sources of
Food
Contamination
Soil
Food contact surfaces
Food handlers
Animals, rodents, and insects
Packaging materials

Source: McSwane, David; Rue, Nancy; Linton, Richard; Williams, Anna. *Essentials of Food Safety and Sanitation, 3e.* © 2002. Electronically reproduced by permission of Pearson Education Inc., Upper Saddle River, New Jersey.

Raw foods can become contaminated at the farm, at the ranch, or on board a ship, among other places. Pathogens are present in the intestines of healthy animals raised for food. Similarly, fresh fruits and vegetables can be contaminated if they are washed or irrigated with water that is contaminated with animal manure or human sewage or if pesticides are applied close to the time they are harvested. Contamination can also occur as foods are handled during processing and distribution. Meat and poultry carcasses can become contaminated during slaughter by contact with small amounts of fecal material from the intestines of the animal. Biological hazards can also be introduced by infected food handlers or by cross-contamination, where pathogens from raw animal foods (beef, poultry, fish, and so forth) are transferred to ready-to-eat foods by contaminated hands, equipment, and utensils. Chemical contaminants, such as metals and organic chemicals, may be introduced accidentally during processing, causing outbreaks of toxic foodborne illness.

Foods used every day in the United States come from remote locations around the world. Eating food grown elsewhere in the world means depending on the soil, water, and sanitation conditions in those places and on the way workers in the various parts of the world produce, harvest, process, and transport the products. Because of the globalization of our food supply, the health hazards of one nation easily become those of another. Therefore measures to prevent and control contamination must begin when food is harvested and continue until the food is consumed.

Foodborne illness may be caused by biological, chemical, or physical hazards in food. *Biological hazards* are microscopic organisms, such as bacteria, viruses, and parasites, that pose an invisible challenge to food safety. Bacteria and viruses are the most common causes of foodborne illness, and controlling these biological hazards is a primary goal of every food safety program. *Chemical hazards* are toxic substances that can cause illness if ingested with food. These may be naturally occurring, such as the toxins associated with molds, plants (for example, mushrooms), and certain species of fish (for example, puffer fish) and shellfish, or of human origin, such as pesticides, cleaning agents, metals, and polychlorinated biphenyls (PCBs). *Physical hazards* are foreign objects such as stones, bone fragments from animals, pieces of glass, staples, and jewelry, which can get into food as a result of poor food-handling practices on the farm or ranch, in food-processing plants, and in retail food establishments.

In light of these three causes, acute foodborne illness may be classified as infection, intoxication, or toxin-mediated infection. Foodborne *infections* are caused when biological hazards are consumed along with food. After ingestion the pathogens multiply in the victim's stomach or intestines and produce such common symptoms of infection as nausea, abdominal pain, fever, and diarrhea.

Intoxications are poisonings caused by eating food that contains a toxic chemical. Some bacteria produce wastes that are toxic to humans. These toxins can produce illness when ingested with food even when the microbes that produced them are no longer present. Foodborne intoxication may also follow the consumption of poisonous plants or fish or the consumption of food that contains chemicals such as cleaning agents or pesticides. A *toxin-mediated infection* is caused by eating food that contains harmful microorganisms that produce a toxin once inside the human body. A toxin-mediated infection differs from an intoxication because the toxin is produced inside the human body.

Each foodborne illness has a characteristic onset time, the amount of time between the consumption of a contaminated food and the appearance of the first symptoms of illness. The onset time varies depending on such factors as the victim's age, health status, body weight, and the amount of contaminant ingested with the food, but usually ranges from a few hours to a few days. However, the onset time for hepatitis A and trichinosis can be several weeks.

It is not possible to cover all the foodborne illnesses of public health significance in this chapter; instead, a few examples are provided in each category. Readers wanting more detailed information or information about other foodborne illnesses are encouraged to consult the *Bad Bug Book* (FDA, 2003) or the CDC's food-related disease Web page (CDC, 2003).

Foodborne Illness Caused by Bacteria

Pathogenic bacteria can make people sick when they or their toxins are consumed with food. Unlike spoilage organisms, pathogenic bacteria do not typically change how a food looks, tastes, or smells. Therefore people eat the tainted food not suspecting they are exposing themselves to agents that can make them sick.

Bacterial contamination may occur in raw food, in cooked food that has not been properly handled, and on the surfaces of equipment and utensils that have been contaminated by raw animal foods, humans, and pests such as insects and rodents. However, certain food products support the rapid growth of infectious or toxin-producing microorganisms and thus account for most outbreaks. These items are called *potentially hazardous foods.* The FDA Food Code (2001) identifies the following groups of products as potentially hazardous foods:

- foods of animal origin that are raw or heat-treated (i.e., meat, poultry, eggs, fish, shellfish, and dairy products);
- foods of plant origin that are heat-treated or consist of raw seed sprouts, (i.e., cooked rice, steamed or baked potatoes, refried beans, cooked vegetables and sprouts); cut melons (i.e., cantaloupe); and

- garlic and oil mixtures that are not modified in a way to inhibit the growth of pathogenic microorganisms.

Because potentially hazardous foods have been frequently associated with foodborne disease outbreaks, they are a focal point of most food safety programs. Potentially hazardous foods must be handled and stored properly to prevent the bacterial growth and toxin production that can result in foodborne illness.

Bacterial causes of foodborne illness can be divided into two categories, the spore formers and the non-spore formers. This distinction is important because it has implications for prevention.

Foodborne Illness Caused by Spore-Forming Bacteria. All bacteria exist as vegetative cells that grow, reproduce, and produce wastes. However, some rod-shaped bacteria have the ability to form structures called *spores.* Spores are inactive or dormant forms of bacterial cells that enable the organism to survive when its environment is too hot, cold, dry, or acidic or when there is not enough food. Bacterial spores are commonly found in soil and in the general environment of farms, ranches, and other places where foods are produced. Bacteria can survive for many months as spores. When conditions become more favorable, the spores germinate, much like seeds, and the bacteria start to grow.

Spores are a common contaminant of foods that are grown in soil, such as vegetables and spices. They may also be found in raw animal foods if the animals have consumed grass and other foodstuffs that are contaminated with spores. Spores pose a special challenge for food safety because they are much harder to destroy than are vegetative forms of bacteria.

Clostridium perfringens is a species of anaerobic (unable to grow in the presence of oxygen) bacterium that is widely distributed in the environment and is found in the intestines of humans and many domestic and wild animals. Spores of this organism persist in soil, sediments, and areas subject to pollution by human or animal feces. Perfringens food poisoning is a toxin-mediated infection caused by *C. perfringens.* When *C. perfringens* bacteria cells are ingested with food, they colonize in the human intestinal tract and produce an enterotoxin that causes intense abdominal cramps and diarrhea. Symptoms usually begin between eight and twenty-two hours after consumption of foods containing *C. perfringens* bacteria, and the illness usually lasts a day or less. Perfringens is most often associated with potentially hazardous foods such as meat and poultry that have been subjected to temperature abuse. *Temperature abuse* refers to situations in which foods are held in the temperature danger zone [between 41° and 135°F (5° and 57°C)] for enough time to allow growth of harmful organisms or in which foods are not cooked or reheated sufficiently to destroy pathogens. In the case of *C. perfringens,* the bacterial spores can survive high temperatures during the initial cooking process. The spores that survive can germinate into vegetative forms of the bacteria and multiply in food that is not properly cooled. If served without adequate reheating, live vegetative forms of *C. perfringens* may be ingested with the food. The bacteria then produce the enterotoxin once they are inside the victim's body.

Clostridium botulinum bacteria are anaerobic organisms that have caused botulism outbreaks associated with improperly home-canned green beans, meats, fish, and garlic stored in oil. In many of the outbreaks these low-acid foods (pH above 4.6) were inadequately heat processed and then were placed in reduced oxygen food containers, such as cans, jars, and pouches. When held at room temperature the spores convert to vegetative cells and start to grow. The botulism bacteria then produce a neurotoxin that affects the victim's central nervous system. This toxin is one of the most deadly substances known. Symptoms of botulism usually start within eighteen to thirty-six hours of ingesting contaminated food, and include fatigue, headache, dizziness, double vision, and difficulty breathing and swallowing. If untreated, these symptoms may progress to paralysis of the arms, legs, trunk, and respiratory muscles, which may require ventilator support. After several weeks the paralysis slowly improves. If diagnosed early, foodborne botulism can be treated with an antitoxin that blocks the action of the toxin circulating in the blood.

Botulism toxin is not heat stable and can be destroyed if food is boiled for about twenty minutes. However, botulism cases occur because people do not make a practice of boiling their food sufficiently before eating it.

Foodborne Illness Caused by Non-Spore-Forming Bacteria. Many types of bacteria exist only as vegetative cells and do not form spores. Vegetative bacterial cells are easily destroyed by heat and can be effectively controlled by such processes as cooking and pasteurization. Examples of bacteria in this category that are significant causes of foodborne illness are *E. coli, Listeria, Salmonella,* and *Staphylococcus.*

Shiga Toxin–Producing E. Coli. The *Escherichia coli* group includes *E. coli* O157:H7 and other *E. coli* bacteria that produce shiga toxins. These are facultative anaerobic bacteria (that is, they can live with or without oxygen) that can cause an infection or a toxin-mediated infection. Shiga toxin–producing *E. coli* are commonly found in the intestines of warm-blooded animals, especially cows. These bacteria are frequently transferred to foods, such as beef, through contact with feces from the animal's intestines during slaughter. Shiga toxin–producing *E. coli* bacteria have also been found in juice and cider made from apples that have dropped to the ground in the orchard and have been contaminated with fecal waste from grazing animals. These organisms can also be spread by food handlers who are carriers of the bacteria and do not wash their hands properly after going to the toilet and by contaminated equipment and utensils.

The illness begins with flu-like symptoms including severe abdominal pain, nausea, vomiting, and watery or bloody diarrhea. The onset time for the Shiga toxin–producing *E. coli* group is twelve to seventy-two hours and the illness usually lasts from one to three days. In some people, particularly children under five years of age and the elderly, the infection can also cause a complication called hemolytic uremic syndrome (HUS), in which the red blood cells are destroyed and the kidneys fail. In the United States, HUS is a leading cause of acute kidney failure in children, and most cases of HUS are caused by E. coli O157:H7. Box 21.1 describes an outbreak of E. coli O157:H7 poisoning.

Box 21.1. Outbreak of *Escherichia Coli* O157:H7 Infections Associated with Drinking Unpasteurized Apple Juice

Widespread concern about *Escherichia coli* O157:H7 began in January 1993, during a multistate outbreak traced to eating undercooked ground beef from a Jack in the Box quick-service restaurant. Once a disease largely associated with contaminated raw or undercooked ground beef, this foodborne illness has since been linked with roast beef, dry salami, raw milk, lettuce, and unpasteurized apple juice.

On October 30, 1996, the Seattle-King County Department of Public Health and the Washington State Department of Health reported an outbreak of *E. coli* O157:H7 epidemiologically linked with drinking Odwalla brand unpasteurized apple juice or juice mixtures containing apple juice. The juice and juice mixtures were being sold by a coffee shop chain, grocery stores, and other retail outlets. The outbreak caused sixty-six people to become ill in Washington, Colorado, California, and British Columbia. Most of the victims of the illness were children, and a sixteen-month-old child in Colorado died as a result of hemolytic uremic syndrome caused by the *E. coli* infection.

Investigators could not pinpoint the exact source of the *E. coli* bacteria, but three of the most plausible theories were that (1) the apples used to make the juice were contaminated with animal feces, (2) the wooden crates used to ship the apples were contaminated, or (3) Odwalla employees did not wash their hands after using the toilet and before returning to work in the production areas of the plant.

Odwalla voluntarily recalled all its Odwalla brand apple juice and blended juice products containing apple juice after being notified by the Food and Drug Administration of the potential link to the outbreak. In a plea bargain with the government, Odwalla pleaded guilty to criminal charges of selling adulterated food products and agreed to pay a $1.5 million fine. A spokesperson for Odwalla said the company did not know unpasteurized apple juice could harbor *E. coli.* Since the outbreak, Odwalla has pasteurized the apple juice to reduce the number of bacteria in the product to safe levels.

Listeria Monocytogenes. Listeriosis is an infection caused by eating food contaminated with the bacterium *Listeria monocytogenes.* This disease affects primarily pregnant women, newborns, and adults with weakened immune systems. A person with listeriosis has fever, muscle aches, and sometimes gastrointestinal symptoms such as nausea or diarrhea. If the infection spreads to the nervous system, symptoms such as headache, stiff neck, confusion, loss of balance, or convulsions can occur. Pregnant women who contract listeriosis may experience only a mild, flulike illness. However, infections during pregnancy can lead to miscarriage or stillbirth, premature delivery, or infection of the newborn. Onset time is one day to three weeks, and the duration of the illness can be of indefinite duration, depending on when treatment is administered.

Listeria monocytogenes is found in soil and water. Vegetables can become contaminated from the soil or from manure used as fertilizer. Animals can carry this bacterium without appearing ill, and thus it can contaminate foods of animal origin such as meats and dairy products. The bacterium has been found in a variety of raw foods, such as uncooked meats and vegetables, as well as in processed foods that become contaminated after processing, such as soft cheeses and cold cuts at the deli counter. Unpasteurized (raw) milk or foods made from unpasteurized milk may contain the bacterium. Listeria is killed by pasteurization and cooking; however, in certain ready-to-eat foods such as hot dogs and deli luncheon meats, contamination may occur after cooking but before packaging, as illustrated in the case study in Box 21.2. *Listeria monocytogenes* is especially important to food safety because, unlike most other foodborne pathogens, this organism can grow at cold refrigeration temperatures, below 41°F (5°C).

Box 21.2. *Listeria* in Turkey Meat Causes Foodborne Disease Outbreak

Officials at the Centers for Disease Control and Prevention reported 120 cases of listeriosis during the summer and early fall of 2002. Cases appeared in eight states: Connecticut, Delaware, Maryland, Massachusetts, Michigan, New Jersey, New York, and Pennsylvania. Most of the victims were hospitalized, seven died, and three pregnant women had miscarriages or stillbirths.

The Food Safety Inspection Service of the U.S. Department of Agriculture conducted an inspection and found *Listeria* in turkey deli meats from two plants that manufacture fresh and frozen ready-to-eat turkey and chicken products. As a result of the outbreak the plants voluntarily recalled more than 200,000 pounds of fresh and frozen poultry products.

This outbreak reaffirms that people in highly susceptible populations (very young children, pregnant women, the elderly, and people with weakened immune systems are especially vulnerable to infections caused by foodborne bacteria such as *Listeria.* Individuals in high-risk groups should avoid eating

- Hot dogs and luncheon meats unless they are reheated until steaming hot
- Soft cheeses and foods made with raw, unpasteurized milk
- Refrigerated pâtés or meat spreads
- Smoked seafood unless it is contained in a cooked dish

Salmonella. *Salmonella* bacteria live in the intestinal tracts of humans and animals, especially birds. *Salmonella* is usually transmitted to humans through consumption of contaminated foods of animal origin such as beef, poultry, milk, or eggs. However, most foods, including vegetables, may become contaminated with fecal material from the unwashed hands of infected food handlers. Most persons infected with *Salmonella* develop diarrhea, fever, and abdominal cramps within twelve to seventy-two hours after infection. The illness usually lasts four to seven days, and most persons recover without treatment. However, elderly people, infants, and individuals with impaired immune systems are more likely to experience severe illness and may need to be hospitalized.

Staphylococcus Aureus. Some strains of *Staphylococcus aureus* bacteria produce enterotoxins that cause a condition called staphylococcal food poisoning. The most common symptoms of staphylococcal food poisoning are nausea, vomiting, abdominal cramping, and prostration. The onset of symptoms is usually within two to six hours of exposure, and a person can experience symptoms by consuming a small amount of toxin in food. Victims experience acute symptoms in many cases, but recovery generally occurs in a few days.

Humans and animals are the primary reservoirs of *Staphylococcus aureus.* Staphylococci are found in the nasal passages and throats and on the hair and skin of 30 to 50 percent of the population, including those who are otherwise healthy. These organisms are also found in infected burns, cuts, pimples, and boils. The bacteria are spread by droplets of saliva from talking, coughing, and sneezing. However, contamination from a worker's hands is the most common way the organism is introduced into foods. Some of the foods that have been incriminated in staphylococcal food-poisoning outbreaks are meat and meat products; poultry and egg products; salads such as egg, tuna, chicken, potato, and macaroni; and cream-filled bakery products. In most outbreaks these foods had been improperly handled by employees during preparation and were temperature abused during preparation, storage, and display.

Foodborne Illness Caused by Viruses

Viruses are assuming much greater importance as agents of foodborne illness. Food safety experts now believe the number of cases of foodborne illness caused by viruses is equal to or greater than the number of cases caused by bacteria. The viruses that cause foodborne disease differ from pathogenic bacteria in several ways. Viruses are much smaller in size and cannot grow outside a living host (human or animal). In addition, viruses are not affected by treatment with antibiotics, and a susceptible person needs to consume only a few viral particles in order to develop a foodborne infection. The two viruses of primary importance as food hazards are Hepatitis A virus and noroviruses.

Hepatitis A Virus. Hepatitis A virus causes a liver disease called *infectious hepatitis.* The hepatitis virus is a particular challenge for food establishments because employees can harbor the virus for up to six weeks and not show symptoms of illness. Food workers are generally contagious for one week before onset of symptoms and for two weeks after the symptoms of the disease appear. During that time infected workers may contaminate foods and expose other workers to the virus. The Hepatitis A virus is very hardy and can live for several hours in a suitable environment. Infectious hepatitis is usually mild and characterized by jaundice (yellow discoloration of the skin), fatigue, abdominal pain, loss of appetite, nausea, diarrhea, and fever. It can occasionally be severe, especially in people with liver disease.

The virus is most commonly transmitted by the fecal-oral route, when infected workers spread fecal material from unwashed hands and fingernails. Infectious hepatitis can also be spread by the ingestion of food and water that contain the Hepatitis A virus. Raw and lightly cooked shellfish harvested from polluted waters, vegetables exposed to polluted water during irrigation, and ready-to-eat foods handled by infected humans offer the largest threats of transmission and disease from Hepatitis A.

A large outbreak of infectious hepatitis occurred at a Pennsylvania restaurant in 2003 (Dato and others, 2003). The source was determined to be contaminated green onions. Investigators believe the green onions may have been contaminated with the Hepatitis A virus by infected farmworkers during harvesting and preparation and by contaminated water used during the irrigation, rinsing, processing, cooling, and icing of the onions.

Noroviruses. Noroviruses are a group of viruses that cause the "stomach flu," or gastroenteritis, in people. Several other names have been used for noroviruses, including Norwalk-like viruses, caliciviruses, and small round structured viruses. The symptoms of Norovirus illness usually include nausea, vomiting, diarrhea, and stomach cramping. Sometimes people additionally have a low-grade fever, chills, a headache, muscle aches, and a general sense of tiredness. The illness often begins suddenly, and the infected person may feel very sick. The illness is usually brief, with symptoms lasting only about one or two days. Sometimes people are unable to drink enough liquids to replace the fluids they have lost through vomiting and diarrhea. This problem with dehydration is usually seen only among the very young, the elderly, and persons with weakened immune systems.

People can become infected by eating food or drinking liquids that are contaminated with a norovirus, by touching surfaces or objects contaminated with a norovirus and then placing their hands in their mouth, and by having direct contact with another person who is infected and showing symptoms.

Noroviruses are very contagious and can spread easily from person to person, as illustrated in the case study in Box 21.3. People infected with a norovirus are contagious from the moment they begin feeling ill to at least three days after recovery. Some people may be contagious for as long as two weeks after recovery.

Box 21.3. Noroviruses Wreak Havoc on a Cruise Ships

During 2002, the CDC's Vessel Sanitation Program received reports of twenty-one outbreaks of acute gastroenteritis (AGE) on seventeen cruise ships sailing into U.S. ports. Of the twenty-one outbreaks, nine were confirmed by laboratory analysis of stool specimens from ill passengers and crew members to be caused by noroviruses (for example, Norwalk-like viruses). Noroviruses are among the most common causes of viral gastrointestinal outbreaks on cruise vessels. The symptoms of illness caused by Norovirus infection include nausea, vomiting, watery diarrhea, and abdominal pain. The illness usually develops within twelve to forty-eight hours of exposure and lasts from one to three days. Common modes of transmission for these viruses include person-to-person contact and consuming contaminated food or water.

Cruise ships dock in countries where levels of sanitation might be inadequate, thus increasing the risk of contamination in the water and food taken aboard and of having a passenger board with an active infection. After a passenger or crew member brings the virus on board, the close living quarters on ships amplify opportunities for person-to-person transmission. Furthermore, the arrival of new and susceptible passengers every one or two weeks on affected cruise ships provides an opportunity for sustained transmission during successive cruises. The continuation of these outbreaks on consecutive cruises with new passengers and the resurgence of outbreaks caused by the same virus strains that had appeared during previous cruises on the same ship, or even on different ships belonging to the same company, suggest that environmental contamination and infected crew members can serve as reservoirs of infection for passengers.

Because of noroviruses' high infectivity and persistence in the environment, transmission is difficult to control through routine sanitary measures. In addition to emphasizing basic food and water sanitation measures, control efforts should include thorough and prompt disinfection of ships during cruises and isolation of ill crew members and, if possible, passengers for seventy-two hours after clinical recovery. Cruise ships should promote frequent, vigorous hand washing with soap and water by passengers and crew. In addition, passengers and crew should avoid contact with other people on the ship when they are ill.

The increase in reported Norovirus outbreaks on cruise ships in 2002 might reflect an actual increase in these outbreaks or it might be attributable to improved surveillance, with an electronic reporting format implemented in January 2001, and increased application of sensitive molecular assays. The surveillance system captures cases of illness reported to the ship's infirmary or to designated staff on board the ship.

Foodborne Illness Caused by Parasites

Parasites are small creatures that live in or on a living host. Parasitic infections are far less common than either bacterial or viral foodborne illness. Nonetheless, parasites can become biological hazards if they are not properly controlled in retail food establishments. Two examples of foodborne parasites are *Anisakis* spp. and *Cyclospora cayetanensis.*

Anisakis spp. are roundworms found in some species of fish. The worms are about one inch long and the diameter of a human hair. They are beige, ivory, white, gray, brown, or pink. Humans are exposed to this parasite when they eat parasite-infested fish. Symptoms include coughing if worms attach in the throat, vomiting and abdominal pain if worms attach in the stomach, or sharp pain and fever if worms attach in the large intestine. Onset can occur anytime from one hour to two weeks after exposure.

Cyclospora cayetanensis is a parasite that has been associated with fresh fruits and vegetables contaminated at the farm. The parasite is passed from person to person by fecal-oral transmission. *Cyclospora* frequently finds its way into water and can then be transferred to foods or foods can be contaminated during handling. Symptoms of cyclosporiasis include watery and explosive diarrhea, loss of appetite, and bloating. The illness usually lasts one week or less. (Box 21.4 reviews the process of investigating the kinds of diseases discussed in these sections.)

Box 21.4. Investigating Foodborne Disease Outbreaks

Protecting the public from foodborne illness depends on rapid detection of outbreaks and a thorough knowledge of the agents and factors responsible for foodborne illness. Various state and local health departments and federal agencies are involved in disease surveillance to detect foodborne disease outbreaks. Surveillance attempts to link individual cases of illness to clusters of illness or outbreaks. The purposes of a foodborne illness investigation are to

- Determine the *cause* of the outbreak, including the etiologic agent, and verify that the agent is foodborne.
- Detect all cases, the food(s) or beverages involved in the transmission, and the environmental conditions and food-handling practices that may have contributed to the transmission of the agent.
- Control the outbreak, and prevent additional cases from occurring.
- Document foodborne disease occurrence to improve the knowledge of foodborne disease causation.
- Correct poor food-handling practices and provide training to prevent similar occurrences.
- Revise the HACCP plan (discussed on pp. 607–609) to prevent similar incidents in the future.
- Foster public confidence in the safety of the food supply and the integrity of the industry.

Local health departments play a key role in foodborne illness surveillance, as these agencies are often the first ones notified of cases of illness by family physicians, emergency department doctors, or complaints filed by victims or their families.

During the complaint investigation, a health department representative will gather information about the victims and the circumstances surrounding their illness. Individuals filing complainants will be asked to fully describe the situation in their own words and provide basic information such as their name, address, and home and work telephone numbers.

Many complainants attribute their illness to the last place at which they ate and may have already decided what food made them ill. The investigator must consider all possibilities, as the illness may not even be food related but may derive from another source or from person-to-person contact.

Although every outbreak is unique, the investigative process generally follows these nine steps (International Association for Food Protection [IAFP], 1999):

1. *Obtain a description of food items and secure any leftover food items.* If the outbreak is associated with a particular event, acquire a list of all food and beverages consumed at the event. If the outbreak is linked with a particular food establishment, obtain a copy of the menu or product list. Determine if leftovers are available from the event. If so, make sure they are collected, labeled, and stored at the proper temperature and where they will not be discarded.
2. *Gather basic data.* Obtain clinical and three-day food histories for the ill people through personal interviews or from medical personnel. This involves collecting information about the food consumed by the victim within the seventy-two hours prior to the onset of symptoms. This time frame is used because the onset time for many foodborne agents is seventy-two hours or less and because recall

becomes unreliable for foods consumed earlier than three days prior to onset. The seventy-two-hour food history should include all meals, snacks, and beverages, including water and ice, eaten either at home or commercial establishments. Determine where the foods were prepared, on site, at a caterer's kitchen, or elsewhere. If the foods were prepared at home, find out what ingredients were used, including herbs and spices, and where they were purchased. Ask if anything unusual was noticed about the foods, such as an off taste, odor, color, or texture. Find out if the foods appeared to be fully cooked and if they were served hot or cold prior to being eaten. The earlier this food history is obtained, the more reliable it is. Clinical information should include signs and symptoms, dates of onset, and common exposures categorized by person, place, and time.

3. *Formulate an initial hypothesis and case definition.* The initial case definition is based on facts about time, place, person, clinical signs, and mode of transmission. This tentative hypothesis is used to direct the investigation; however, it should not be too restrictive. Focusing too closely on one hypothesis can exclude potentially important cases or events. Case definitions can change as the investigations progresses.
4. *Collect clinical specimens for testing.* Determine if any clinical specimens have been collected by health care providers and obtain the results of any tests. If specimens were collected, contact the reference laboratories and have them save the specimens, if possible, for further testing. When specimens have not yet been collected, investigators should attempt to collect clinical specimens, first, from the people who are currently ill and, second, from those who were recently ill. Specimens should also be collected from food handlers who were ill before the outbreak as well as from those who were asymptomatic.
5. *Develop a questionnaire.* A standardized questionnaire is developed, using the initial case definition, food item description, and clinical data. This tool is used to collect

- Exposure data (time and place of exposure, approximate number exposed)
- Patient information (name, address, telephone number)
- Patient demographics (age, gender, and so forth)
- Illness history (whether subject is ill or well, any underlying conditions, medications)
- Clinical data (signs and symptoms, onset date and time, recovery date and time)
- Medical attention sought (provider, sample collection, test results, treatment)
- Contact with other ill individuals
- Menu from suspect meal(s)

It is extremely important to interview people who are well in addition to those who are ill. The cause of illness can be identified only by comparing the exposures (foods eaten) of those who are ill (cases) and of those who are not (controls).

6. *Analyze the questionnaires.* This is generally accomplished using a cohort or case-control study format. Analyze the data to identify differences in exposure frequencies between cases and controls to confirm or refute the hypothesis. As data from questionnaires are analyzed, it may be necessary to modify the course of the investigation by formulating a new hypothesis or case definition.
7. *Conduct an environmental investigation.* A health agency representative will audit HACCP processes (make observations and interview employees) and evaluate HACCP records.
8. *Implement control measures.* Control measures may include

   - Providing postexposure prophylaxis to control the spread of the disease
   - Recalling or destroying food
   - Making a public announcement of the outbreak
   - Providing educational information
   - Closing a food establishment to stop the ongoing spread of disease
   - Recommending antibiotic treatment or exclusion from work or child care or other measures

9. *Summarize the investigation.* It is important to prepare a document that summarizes the conditions and causes of the outbreak in order to prevent future occurrences. This summary also serves as the public record of the outbreak.

The publication *Procedures to Investigate Foodborne Illness* is available from the International Association for Food Protection (1999). The information in this manual is based on epidemiological principles and investigative techniques that have been found effective in determining causal factors of disease incidence. It can be a valuable guide for public health personnel or teams that are investigating reports of alleged foodborne illnesses.

Foodborne Illness Caused by Chemicals

Chemicals may occur naturally in food or may be added intentionally or unintentionally during food production and preparation. Naturally occurring chemicals include food allergens and toxins produced by biological organisms. Chemical contaminants of human origin include agricultural chemicals (for example, pesticides, fertilizers, and antibiotics), food additives (for example, preservatives and coloring agents), metals, and industrial by-products. Sometimes such chemicals are added intentionally but have unexpected adverse effects; for example, flavor enhancers such as monosodium glutamate (MSG) can cause headaches in some people. At other times chemicals are added improperly or unintentionally, and the results can be tragic. For example, during the winter of 1971–1972, Iraqi authorities distributed free wheat seeds to people in rural areas. These seeds had been treated with methylmercury as a fungicide and were intended for planting. However, some recipients ground the seeds into flour and made bread with it. An estimated 50,000 people were exposed to the contaminated bread, over 6,000 were hospitalized with acute mercury poisoning, and 459 died (Bakir and others, 1973; Al-Mufti and others, 1976). Ten years later, in 1981, malefactors in Spain denatured large amounts of rapeseed oil with aniline and illicitly sold it as pure olive oil. The contaminant triggered a previously unknown illness that included lung infiltrates, muscle pain, and a high blood count of eosinophils. Nearly 20,000 people became ill, and more than 300 died (Posada de la Paz, Philen, and Borda, 2001). Other chemical contaminants, such as lead and PCBs, have been introduced unintentionally into foods and linked to chronic conditions that developed over years.

Biomagnification occurs when the toxic burden of a large number of organisms at a lower trophic level is accumulated and concentrated by predators at a higher trophic level. For example, phytoplankton and bacteria in aquatic ecosystems take up heavy metals or toxic organic molecules from water or sediments. Their predators—zooplankton and small fish—collect and retain the toxins from many prey organisms, building up higher toxin concentrations. The top carnivores in the food chain—game fish and humans—can accumulate such high toxin levels that they suffer adverse health effects.

Vomiting is the most common symptom of acute chemical intoxication. It usually occurs within fifteen to thirty minutes after ingestion of the chemical, and in most instances victims feel better after expelling the chemical. In other cases more serious results can occur. Examples of chemicals that cause illness include food allergens; naturally occurring toxins, such as ciguatoxin and scombrotoxin; and mercury, PCBs, and pesticides.

Food Allergens. Food allergens can pose a serious health risk to children and adults who are sensitive to these substances. Five to 8 percent of children and 1 to 2 percent of adults are allergic to certain chemicals found in foods and food ingredients. Food allergens cause a person's immune system to overreact and may result in such symptoms as hives, swelling of the lips and tongue, difficulty breathing, vomiting, cramps, and diarrhea. These symptoms can occur within minutes of consuming the allergen. In severe situations a life-threatening allergic reaction called *anaphylaxis* can occur. Symptoms of anaphylaxis include itching and hives, swelling of the throat and difficulty breathing, dropping blood pressure, and unconsciousness.

Approximately 90 percent of all allergic reactions are caused by eight types of food: milk, eggs, wheat proteins, peanuts, soy, tree nuts, fish, and shellfish. In many instances a person who is allergic to a food does not have to eat much of that food in order to experience a severe reaction. As little as half a peanut can cause a severe reaction in a highly sensitive person. The only way people with food allergies can avoid allergic reactions is to avoid eating foods that contain allergens. Proper ingredient labeling and prevention of cross-contamination are important food safety measures for protecting people from food allergens. Cross-contamination is discussed on pp. 606–607.

Ciguatoxin. Ciguatoxin is produced by marine algae that live among certain coral reefs. When the algae are eaten by small reef fish, the toxin is stored in the flesh, skin, and organs. When the small reef fish are eaten by larger fish, such as barracuda, mackerel, and snapper, the toxin accumulates in the larger fish. Humans who eat these fish can then suffer ciguatoxin poisoning. Symptoms include vertigo, joint and muscle pain, numbness and tingling in the lips and mouth, temperature reversal sensation (hot things feel cold and vice versa), diarrhea, and vomiting. The onset time ranges from fifteen minutes to twenty-four hours. The toxin is not destroyed by cooking, and there is no commercially known method to determine whether ciguatoxin is present in fish. Purchasing seafood from a reputable supplier is considered the best preventative measure.

Scombrotoxin. The presence of large amounts of scombrotoxin in food can result in scombroid poisoning, also known as histamine poisoning. Histamine is produced by certain bacteria when they decompose foods containing the protein histidine. Tuna, mahi-mahi, sardines, mackerel, anchovies, and amberjack are examples of fish that have high levels of histidine that can be converted to histamine. Cooking does not inactivate the chemical once it has been formed. Symptoms of scombroid poisoning include dizziness, a burning feeling in the mouth, facial rash or hives, a peppery taste in the mouth, headache, itching, teary eyes, and runny nose. The onset time is thirty minutes or less.

Mercury. Mercury contamination of fish has attracted considerable public health attention in recent years. Mercury occurs naturally in the environment. Metallic and inorganic mercury can also be released into the air as industrial emissions, especially from coal-burning power plants (because coal often contains mercury) and from incinerators that burn mercury-containing refuse such as medical waste. Mercury then falls from the air and can enter surface water, accumulating in streams, rivers, and oceans. Mercury may also be a contaminant in wastes that drain directly into waterways from facilities such as paper and chloralkali chemical plants. Bacteria in the water organify the mercury to form methylmercury, which then enters the food chain. Fish absorb methylmercury from water as they feed on aquatic organisms. Long-lived, large predator fish such as sharks, swordfish, tilefish, and tuna may accumulate high levels of methylmercury and pose a risk to people who eat them regularly. Methylmercury is a nervous system toxin, and the developing fetus is especially susceptible to its effects. Women of childbearing age have long been warned to limit their fish intake to reduce the risk of exposing their unborn babies to mercury (see Box 21.5).

Box 21.5. FDA Recommendations for Avoiding Mercury in Fish

1. Do not eat shark, swordfish, king mackerel, or tilefish because they contain high levels of mercury.
2. Eat up to 12 ounces (two average meals) a week of a variety of fish and shellfish that are lower in mercury.

    Five of the most commonly eaten fish that are low in mercury are shrimp, canned light tuna, salmon, pollock, and catfish.

    Another commonly eaten fish, albacore ("white") tuna has more mercury than canned light tuna. So, when choosing your two meals of fish and shellfish, you may eat up to six ounces (one average meal) of albacore tuna per week.

3. Check local advisories about the safety of fish caught by family and friends in your local lakes, rivers, and coastal areas. If no advice is available, eat up to six ounces (one average meal) per week of fish you catch from local waters, but don't consume any other fish during that week.

Source: FDA, 2004.

Polychlorinated Biphenyls. Polychlorinated biphenyls (PCBs) are persistent chlorinated compounds that were manufactured from the 1920s to the 1970s for use in capacitors, transformers, and other applications. These compounds have entered the global ecosystem and have become widely distributed. They are fat soluble, so they concentrate in fatty tissues and are found at high levels in fish that are high on the marine food chain. Results of a recent study (Hites and others, 2004) showed that farmed salmon contain higher levels of PCBs and other persistent organic compounds than wild salmon. Part of the explanation for this is that farmed fish are fed fish meal, a concentrated preparation of smaller fish that represents a source of concentrated fat-soluble chemicals. The extent of the risk to humans is unclear, but based on evidence linking PCBs with cancer, nervous system toxicity, immune dysfunction, and other adverse outcomes, recommendations have also been issued to limit consumption of the most contaminated fish.

Chemical contaminants in fish pose an interesting example of the trade-offs inherent in food safety. Although fish may pose a risk if it is contaminated by mercury or PCBs, fish is an excellent dietary source of protein and omega-3 fatty acids (especially eicosapentaenoic acid, or EPA, and docosahexaenoic acid, or DHA), which are thought to promote cardiovascular health. Food safety involves a careful balance, minimizing the risks of contaminated fish and maximizing benefits by choosing the safest fish.

Pesticides. Pesticides are used widely in agriculture in the United States and worldwide, and many agricultural products such as fruits and vegetables contain trace quantities of pesticides, called *residues.* Foods are not systematically monitored for their content of pesticides, but available data suggest that some foods, in at least some instances, can carry nontrivial levels of pesticides. This has encouraged an interest in organic and so-called natural foods (Box 21.6). It is also a special issue for children, because their diets include large proportions of fruits and vegetables (or products derived from these foods, such as baby food and juices), resulting in large relative exposures to dietary pesticides. Children may also be more susceptible than adults to these contaminants (for reasons discussed in Chapter Twenty-Eight). This issue was studied by the National Academy of Sciences in 1993, and a groundbreaking report, *Pesticides in the Diets of Infants and Children,* recommended renewed attention to the dietary exposures that children sustain (National Research Council, 1993).

Box 21.6. Pros and Cons of Natural and Organic Foods

More and more consumers are buying natural and organic foods as they become aware of the connections between the foods they eat and their health and the health of their environment. Natural and organic foods have become a multibillion dollar industry, and sales of organic foods are likely to increase now that U.S. Department of Agriculture (USDA) national organic standards are in place to further boost consumer confidence.

The terms *natural* and *organic* are not synonymous when applied to foods. Natural foods are generally minimally processed and free of artificial ingredients but not necessarily organically grown. Natural foods may be organic, but it is not required that they be organic. In fact, there is no legal definition or system in place that governs what constitutes a *natural* food.

In contrast, a food that is sold as *organic* must meet certain standards. When food or feed is produced organically, it means that the crop is grown according to guidelines that prohibit the use of synthetic pesticides, synthetic growth regulators, and conventional, soluble fertilizers. Organic meat, poultry, eggs, and dairy products come from animals that are given no antibiotics or growth hormones. Organic produce is grown without using most conventional man-made insecticides and herbicides, fertilizers made with synthetic ingredients or sewage sludge, bioengineering, or ionizing radiation. Before a product can be labeled *organic,* a government-approved certifier must inspect the farm where the food is grown to make sure the farmer is following all the rules necessary to meet the USDA's national organic standards.

The Food Quality Protection Act (FQPA) directed the U.S. Environmental Protection Agency to conduct a reassessment of all food uses of pesticides, taking into account the heightened susceptibility of infants and children, the elderly, and other highly susceptible population groups. To improve the accuracy of FQPA pesticide dietary risk assessments, Congress funded the Pesticide Data Program (PDP) which focuses on the foods consumed most heavily by children, and food is tested, to the extent possible, as eaten.

Several years of PDP testing has greatly enhanced our understanding of pesticide residues in the U.S. food supply. The pattern of residues found in organic foods tested by the PDP differs markedly from the pattern in conventional samples in two important ways. First, produce grown organically is less likely to contain detectable levels of pesticide residues than is produce grown using conventional techniques. Second, produce grown using conventional techniques tends to contain multiple pesticide residues more often. Imported foods have consistently contained more residues than domestic samples.

Organic food differs from conventionally produced food in the way it is grown, handled, and processed. Yet USDA makes no claims that organically produced food is safer or more nutritious than conventionally produced food. One must not lose sight of the fact that bacteria and other pathogens are commonly found in the soil, barns, and general environment on all kinds of farms, including those where organic foods are grown. In addition, foods grown organically can still contain allergens that can trigger an adverse response if eaten by people who have sensitivities to these substances. Finally, organically grown foods are handled by people at various steps from harvest to retail, just as foods grown using conventional methods are. Organic foods are equally vulnerable to contamination from infected workers who do not practice good personal hygiene. For all these reasons, consumers should handle organic foods carefully to protect themselves and their families.

Prevention of Foodborne Illness Outbreaks

The CDC has identified several risk factors as primary contributors to foodborne disease outbreaks; these factors are therefore important focus areas for food safety programs. They include (Olsen and others, 2000)

- Improper holding temperatures
- Poor personal hygiene
- Improper cooking temperatures
- Foods from unsafe sources
- Contaminated equipment and cross-contamination

Improper Holding Temperatures

Keeping foods at improper holding temperatures permits the rapid growth of infectious and toxin-producing microorganisms. This rapid growth typically occurs when food is held at temperatures between 41°F and 135°F (5°C and 57°C). This temperature range is referred to as the *food temperature danger zone.* The relationship between temperature and microbial growth is illustrated in Figure 21.2. An

FIGURE 21.2. FOOD TEMPERATURE DANGER ZONE.

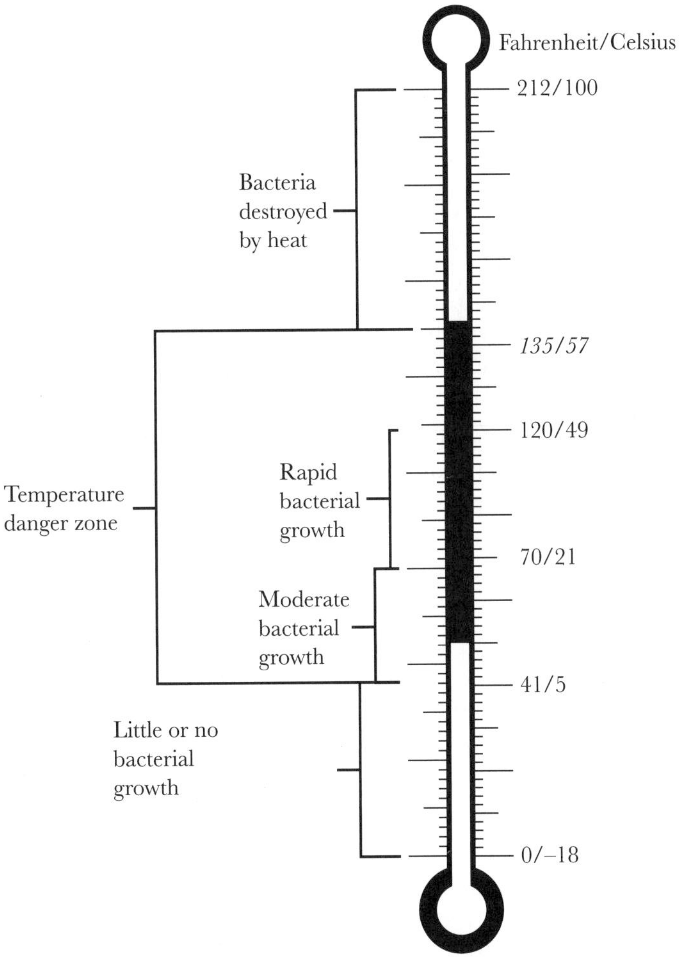

Source: McSwane, David; Rue, Nancy; Linton, Richard; Williams, Anna. *Essentials of Food Safety and Sanitation, 3e.* © 2002. Electronically reproduced by permission of Pearson Education Inc., Upper Saddle River, New Jersey.

important rule in food safety is "Keep it hot, keep it cold, or don't keep it." This requires keeping hot foods above 135°F (57°C) and cold foods below 41°F (5°C) whenever possible.

There are times during the cooking, cooling, reheating, and food preparation processes when a food must pass through the temperature danger zone. In order to control the growth of pathogens, it is necessary to minimize the amount of time the food remains in the temperature danger zone during these processes. The objective should be to pass food through the temperature danger zone as quickly as possible (through proper heating and cooling) and as infrequently as possible (by limiting the number of times a food is cooked, cooled, and reheated).

Poor Personal Hygiene

Even healthy people can be a source of the harmful microbes that cause foodborne illness. Therefore good personal hygiene is extremely important when handling foods. Soiled hands and clothing, infected food workers, and workers who do not practice good personal hygiene are major threats to food safety.

A food handler's hands and fingers can become contaminated when he or she eats, smokes, uses the toilet, handles raw foods, touches soiled items, or wipes up spills. Saliva, perspiration, feces, juices from raw animal food products, and various types of soil can be significant sources of contamination if they are allowed to get into food. Therefore food workers must wash their hands whenever they have been exposed to these contaminants. Workers should vigorously rub all surfaces of their fingers, fingertips, hands, wrists, and forearms for at ten to fifteen seconds, using soap or another approved cleaning compound. After washing, the hands and forearms must be rinsed under clean, warm running water and dried with a disposable paper towel or mechanical dryer, as illustrated in Figure 21.3.

Hand-sanitizing lotions may be used by food handlers to reduce the microbial load on clean hands. However, hand sanitizers should never be used as a substitute for proper hand washing.

Food workers may also use disposable gloves to help prevent contamination when handling foods. Gloves are especially useful when working with deli sandwiches, tacos, and other foods that require extensive manual contact during preparation. Workers must treat disposable gloves as a second skin. Whatever can contaminate human hands can also contaminate gloves. Therefore, whenever gloves become soiled, they should be discarded, the worker's hands should be washed thoroughly, and a new pair of disposable gloves put on.

FIGURE 21.3. THE PROPER HAND WASHING PROCEDURE.

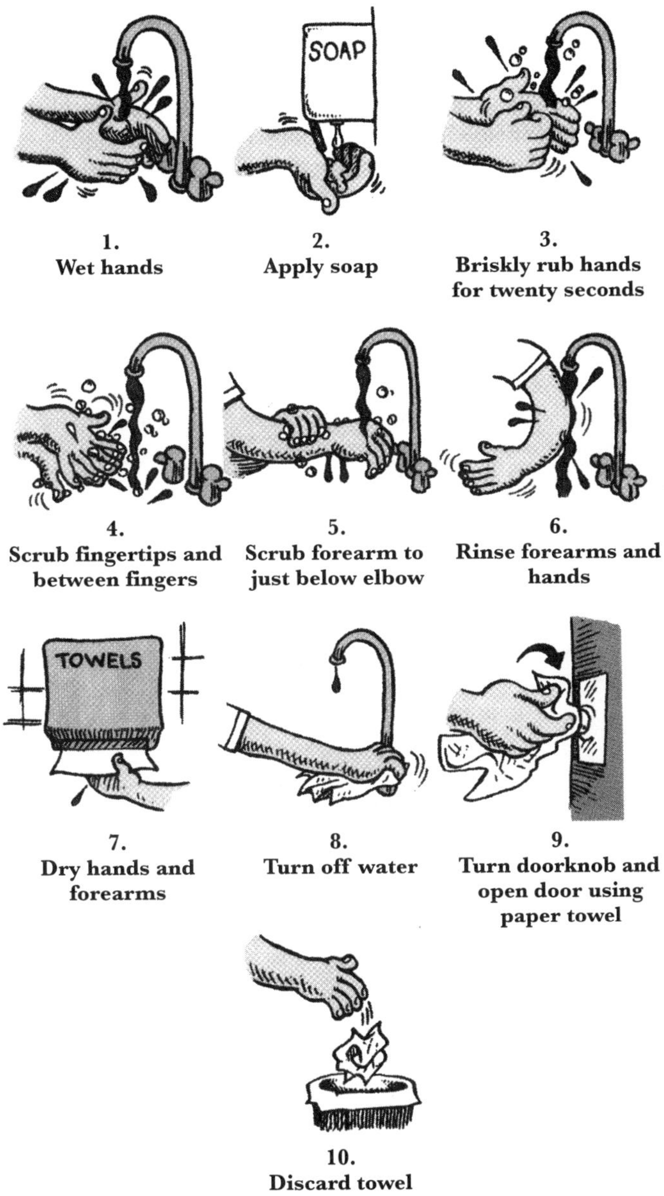

SOAP
1. Wet hands
2. Apply soap
3. Briskly rub hands for twenty seconds
4. Scrub fingertips and between fingers
5. Scrub forearm to just below elbow
6. Rinse forearms and hands
TOWELS
7. Dry hands and forearms
8. Turn off water
9. Turn doorknob and open door using paper towel
10. Discard towel

Source: McSwane, David; Rue, Nancy; Linton, Richard; Williams, Anna. *Essentials of Food Safety and Sanitation, 3e.* © 2002. Electronically reproduced by permission of Pearson Education Inc., Upper Saddle River, New Jersey.

Improper Cooking Temperatures

Raw foods of animal origin, such as red meats, poultry, eggs, fish, and shellfish, are frequently contaminated with microbial pathogens. Practices such as using raw eggs to make a Caesar salad, lightly cooking ground beef and ground pork, and consuming raw oysters on the half shell greatly increase a person's risk of contracting a foodborne illness.

Proper cooking makes food more palatable and safe to eat. When potentially hazardous foods such as meat, poultry, and fish are cooked to proper temperatures, pathogenic bacteria and other harmful organisms found in and on the products are destroyed. Destruction of pathogens depends on the internal temperature of the food product and the amount of time the food is held at that temperature. For instance, to ensure a safe Thanksgiving turkey, it should be cooked to an internal temperature of 165°F (74°C) and held at that temperature for at least fifteen seconds. The internal temperature of foods must be measured periodically throughout the cooking process. For most foods, the internal temperature is measured by inserting the sensing portion of a properly calibrated thermometer or thermocouple into the center or thickest part of the food. This will give an accurate measure of the internal temperature and ensure the food is heated sufficiently to destroy harmful organisms.

Foods from Unsafe Sources

Food from unsafe sources may be contaminated with biological, chemical, and physical hazards. This is the primary reason why foods prepared in a private home may not be used or sold in retail food establishments. These homemade foods are prohibited because of the increased risk of contamination from biological hazards such as *Clostridium botulinum* and *Staphylococcus aureus*. Shellfish harvested from polluted waters can be contaminated with Hepatitis A virus, and milk and milk products that are not pasteurized properly can be contaminated with a number of pathogens including *Listeria monocytogenes*. The safety and wholesomeness of foods can be enhanced by purchasing foods from sources that are routinely inspected by regulatory agencies and that are in compliance with applicable food safety laws.

Contamination and Cross-Contamination

Pathogens can be transferred to food by contaminated food-contact surfaces. Food-contact surfaces are the parts of equipment, utensils, and work surfaces that normally come into contact with food during storage, preparation, and service.

Proper cleaning and sanitizing of these surfaces enhances food safety and quality and increases the life expectancy of equipment and facilities.

Cross-contamination is the transfer of pathogens from one food to another via contaminated hands, equipment, or utensils. Cross-contamination commonly occurs when ready-to-eat foods come into contact with raw animal foods or surfaces that have had contact with these types of foods. For instance, if the knife and cutting board used when cutting raw chicken into pieces are then used when cutting up lettuce and tomatoes for a salad, the bacteria from the chicken can be transferred to the salad ingredients by the contaminated knife blade and cutting board. Cross-contamination can also occur when raw foods are stored above ready-to-eat foods, and juices from the raw product spill or splash onto the ready-to-eat food. Some measures that can be used to prevent cross-contamination between products are shown in Box 21.7.

Box 21.7. Preventing Cross-Contamination Between Products

- Use separate equipment, such as cutting boards, when preparing raw foods and ready-to-eat foods (color coding may be helpful for this task).
- Clean and sanitize food-contact surfaces of equipment and utensils in between working with raw animal foods and ready-to-eat foods.
- Avoid touching ready-to-eat foods with bare hands.
- Prepare ready-to-eat foods first, then the raw foods.
- Keep raw and ready-to-eat foods separate during storage or store ready-to-eat foods above raw products.

Controlling the risk factors that contribute to foodborne illness is not rocket science. However, it does require a concerted effort by both the food industry and consumers to ensure that foods are not temperature abused, proper personal hygiene is practiced, and necessary steps are taken to control contamination and cross-contamination.

Hazard Analysis Critical Control Point (HACCP) Food Safety System

The Hazard Analysis Critical Control Point (HACCP) approach is a central paradigm of food safety. It is designed to identify and control problems that may cause foodborne illness *before* they happen. The HACCP concept was developed in 1971 by the Pillsbury Company, in cooperation with the National Aeronautics and Space Administration (NASA) and the U.S. Army, when preparing to produce safe foods for the astronauts in the U.S. space program. By employing the HACCP food safety system, suppliers were able to produce food products for America's space travelers that were nearly 100 percent free of microbial hazards.

HACCP systems are currently used by food processors and retail food establishments to identify food safety hazards and prevent them from contaminating food. HACCP is not a stand-alone program. Rather it is part of a larger system of control procedures that must be in place to ensure food safety. The HACCP system must be supported by standard operating procedures (SOPs) such as good personal hygiene, pest control, and proper cleaning and sanitizing to prevent food from becoming contaminated at points throughout the production process. When SOPs are in place, the HACCP system enables managers to concentrate on food and how it is handled during storage, preparation, display, and service. A brief summary of the HACCP system is presented in Box 21.8.

Box 21.8. HACCP Food Safety System

The HACCP food safety system employs seven steps to identify, evaluate, and control food safety hazards.

Step 1: Conduct a Hazard Analysis

Hazard analysis is the process used to identify biological, chemical, or physical hazards of public health significance. The hazards might be found in food due to natural contamination (for example, from raw meat, poultry, or fish) or they may be introduced into the food by workers who practice poor personal hygiene, by improper food-handling practices, or by contaminated equipment. By conducting a hazard analysis, the HACCP team can decide which hazards and conditions are significant for food safety and therefore should be addressed by the HACCP system.

Step 2: Determine Critical Control Points

A *critical control point* (CCP) is a stage in the flow of food where control is essential if one is to prevent or eliminate a hazard or reduce it to an acceptable level. Receiving, storage, cooking, and chilling are a few examples of process stages where CCPs can be employed to control hazards. Loss of control at a CCP can result in an unacceptable health risk and can jeopardize the safety of the finished product and of the consumers who eat it.

Step 3: Establish Critical Limit(s)

Critical limits are the upper and lower boundaries of food safety. When these boundaries are exceeded, a hazard may exist or could develop. A critical limit must be set for each CCP to ensure that the CCP remains under control. When critical limits are not met, it could mean that the food is not safe.

Step 4: Establish a System to Monitor the CCPs

Once CCPs have been identified and critical limits set, someone must monitor food and food processes to ensure that critical limits are being met. Monitoring involves making observations and measurements of critical limits to determine if a CCP is under control. By routinely monitoring critical control points it is possible to determine when a critical limit has been exceeded before a food safety problem occurs.

Step 5: Establish the Corrective Action to Be Taken When a CCP Is Not Under Control

Corrective action must be taken immediately when monitoring reveals that a critical limit has not been met and it is suspected that a CCP is not under control. For example, if monitoring reveals that a food has not reached the required final cooking temperature, the cooking process must be continued until the required internal product temperature is reached.

Step 6: Verify That the HACCP System Is Working Effectively

The two components of the verification process are (a) verifying that the critical limits established for CCPs will effectively prevent, eliminate, or reduce hazards to acceptable levels, and (b) verifying that the overall HACCP plan is working properly. Verification involves making observations, reviewing monitoring records, and discussing corrective action procedures with employees.

Step 7: Establish Effective Record Keeping

Proper documentation is needed to verify that the HACCP system is working properly. Record keeping will normally involve written records produced during the monitoring and corrective action steps in the program. Record-keeping requirements must be as simple as possible, and employees must be trained to measure and record data accurately.

Food Safety Agencies and Initiatives

There are many opportunities for food products to become contaminated as they flow from the point of production to the point of consumption. Contamination can occur at the farm or ranch, in processing plants, at retail food establishments, and in a consumer's own kitchen. Making food safe is a responsibility that must be shared by producers, processors, transporters, retailers, government agencies, and consumers.

Protecting food safety is a function of regulatory agencies at all levels of government. Federal agencies are primarily responsible for regulating foods sold through interstate commerce, and state and local agencies enforce food safety rules and regulations in restaurants, supermarkets, institutional feeding operations, and other types of retail food establishments in their jurisdictions. State and local regulatory agencies provide a variety of essential services including facility and HACCP plan review, issuance of permits to operate, and routine inspections to assess compliance with food safety regulations. During food establishment inspections, inspectors examine food production, preparation, and service operations to look for evidence of time and temperature abuse, cross-contamination, and poor personal hygiene. In food establishments employing a HACCP system a major part of the inspection involves reviewing records kept as part of that system.

The federal agencies primarily responsible for food safety in America are the U.S. Department of Agriculture (USDA), the Food and Drug Administration (FDA), the Centers for Disease Control and Prevention (CDC), and the Environmental Protection Agency (EPA). A brief overview of each agency's role in food safety is presented in the following sections.

U.S. Department of Agriculture

The USDA regulates the production, processing, and interstate sale of domestic and imported meat (for example, cattle, sheep, and swine), poultry (for example, chicken, turkey, and duck), and egg products.

The Food Safety and Inspection Service (FSIS) is the agency within USDA that is responsible for ensuring the safety, wholesomeness, and correct labeling and packaging of meat, poultry, and egg products sold in interstate commerce, including imported products. In 2000, FSIS completed implementation of the Pathogen Reduction/Hazard Analysis and Critical Control Point (HACCP) rule. This rule addresses foodborne illness associated with meat and poultry products by focusing more attention on the prevention and reduction of illness-causing microbial pathogens on raw products. It also clarifies the respective roles of government and industry in food safety. Industry is accountable for producing safe food. Government is responsible for setting appropriate food safety standards, maintaining vigorous oversight to ensure that standards are met, and operating a strong enforcement program to deal with plants that do not comply with regulatory standards.

Meat and poultry slaughter and processing plants must implement HACCP programs to control factors affecting the ingredients, products, and processes in their manufacturing plants. The HACCP teams in the meat and poultry plants identify the processing steps they use to produce food commodities and determine what hazards, if any, are likely to occur at each step. After the hazards have been identified, the manufacturers identify critical control points (CCPs) that can be used to prevent, eliminate, or reduce hazards to acceptable levels. Critical limits are then set for each CCP and workers monitor the processes to assure that CCPs are kept under control and within critical limits. The objective of HACCP programs is to make products safe to consume and to make it possible to prove to agencies and consumers that products are safe.

FSIS inspectors examine animals before and after slaughter at slaughterhouses and processing plants. Inspections are performed on live animals to identify diseased animals and prevent them from entering the food supply. Carcasses are examined after slaughter to identify visible defects that can affect safety and quality. Products are also tested for the presence of harmful pathogens and drug and chemical residues. The traditional *organoleptic* method, in which inspectors used their senses (principally vision, smell, and touch) to identify high-risk animals is limited in its ability to identify contaminated foods, except in the most severe cases. This limitation was the driving force that prompted USDA officials to make a significant shift toward using HACCP for primary prevention of microbial hazards.

Progress is being made toward reducing pathogenic bacteria in meat, poultry, and eggs as the meat and poultry industries comply with the pathogen reduction and HACCP requirements. This success has prompted the FSIS to strengthen HACCP systems.

Food and Drug Administration

The FDA regulates the production, processing, manufacturing, and interstate sale of all food items except red meats, poultry, and eggs. The FDA's responsibility is to ensure that food is safe, wholesome, sanitary, and honestly packaged and labeled. Specialists at the FDA conduct inspections of food-processing plants, food storage facilities, and imported foods to ensure safety standards are maintained. The agency also promotes public health by protecting food from adulteration and misbranding. Food is considered *adulterated* when it contains filth or harmful substances, is decomposed, or is produced in unsanitary conditions. Food is *misbranded* when it is packaged or labeled in a false or misleading manner.

The FDA has created a variety of programs to protect food safety as products flow from farm to table. The agency has developed *good agricultural practices* (GAPs) to help farmers protect fruits and vegetables from contamination at the source. Contamination of produce can be reduced by employing GAPs that ensure proper manure management, water use, farmworker health and hygiene, sanitation of food production facilities, and transport of commodities to market.

The FDA has also created *good manufacturing practices* (GMPs), which are the minimum sanitary and processing requirements employed in food-processing plants. When implemented properly, GMPs help processing plants control the possibility of contamination from poor personal hygiene, pests, and contaminated facilities and equipment to ensure the production of safe and wholesome food. GMPs are an integral part of the nation's control over food safety problems.

In 1997, the FDA initiated a landmark seafood HACCP program to increase the safety of fish and shellfish and reduce seafood-related illnesses to the lowest possible levels. The seafood HACCP program requires seafood processors, repackers, and warehouses, both domestic firms and foreign exporters to this country, to follow HACCP principles and practices. Under the provisions of the seafood HACCP program, companies are required to identify hazards that in the absence of preventive controls are reasonably likely to affect the safety of seafood products. If even one hazard is identified, the seafood firm is required to adopt and implement an appropriate HACCP plan.

Outbreaks of foodborne illness have been traced to fresh juices that were not pasteurized or otherwise processed to eliminate harmful bacteria such as *E. coli* O157:H7 and *Salmonella* (Box 21.1). This led FDA to implement a new safety rule for juices in 2001. Under the rule, juice processors must implement a HACCP plan that addresses all points of production to prevent, reduce, or eliminate hazards in juices. Processors are required to evaluate their manufacturing process to determine whether there are any microbiological, chemical, or physical hazards that could contaminate their products. If a potential hazard is identified, processors are required to implement control measures to prevent, reduce, or eliminate those hazards. Processors are also required to use processes such as pasteurization or UV irradiation or a combination of techniques to achieve a 5-log (99.999 percent) reduction in the numbers of the most resistant pathogens in their finished products, compared to the levels present in the untreated juice.

HACCP systems are federally required for seafood, juice, meat, and poultry processors. These systems enable food processors to determine where hazards can occur in processing and implement control measures to prevent problems before

FIGURE 21.4. THE 2001 FDA FOOD CODE.

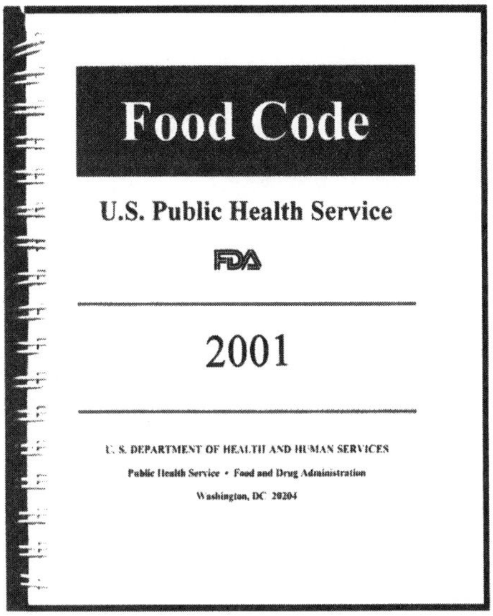

foodborne illness can occur. The HACCP approach offers a much more comprehensive and effective alternative to spot checks of manufacturing establishments and random sampling of final products to ensure safe foods.

The FDA promotes food safety in retail food establishments by publishing the Food Code, which serves as a model for retail food safety programs (Figure 21.4). The Food Code is not a federal law or regulation. Rather it is a set of recommendations put forth to promote food safety and sanitation nationwide.

Another function of the FDA is product recalls. The FDA can request a recall of a food product if it believes a potential hazard exists. Food recalls are typically voluntary, except when infant formula is involved. In the vast majority of cases, food processors willingly remove suspect products from the marketplace to keep consumers safe and avoid liability. However, if a company does not agree to a voluntary product recall, the FDA can issue public press releases and proceed to seize or embargo the product to remove it from commerce.

Centers for Disease Control and Prevention

The CDC contributes to food safety by helping state and local agencies conduct foodborne disease investigations and compiling statistics on foodborne and waterborne disease outbreaks. These activities support the CDC's goals of preventing and controlling diseases and supporting public health decision making by providing credible information on foodborne diseases.

Environmental Protection Agency (EPA)

The EPA contributes to food safety by regulating the use of toxic substances such as pesticides, sanitizers, and other chemicals. As described in Chapter Twenty, EPA regulates pesticides under the authority of the Federal Insecticide, Fungicide, and Rodenticide Act (FIFRA) and the Food Quality Protection Act (FQPA). Under FIFRA the EPA registers pesticides for use in the United States and prescribes labeling and other regulatory requirements to prevent unreasonable adverse effects on health or the environment. The Food Quality Protection Act mandates a single, health-based standard for all pesticides in all foods. It provides special protection for infants and children and expedites approval of safer pesticides. The FQPA requires periodic reevaluation of pesticide registrations and tolerances to ensure that the scientific data supporting pesticide registrations remain up to date.

Recent Initiatives in Food Safety

Government agencies and the food industry have joined forces to implement other food safety initiatives to lower the incidence of foodborne illness. A brief overview of selected programs is presented here.

PulseNet

PulseNet is a national network of public health laboratories, created by the CDC, that performs DNA "fingerprinting" of bacteria that cause foodborne illness. When cases of disease show similar fingerprint patterns, this finding suggests a common source, such as a contaminated food product. The fingerprints of strains of bacteria isolated from food products by regulatory agencies can also be compared with those isolated from ill persons. Identifying these connections can help investigators to detect outbreaks and can expedite the recall of foods suspected of being contaminated, removing them from the marketplace.

Fight BAC! Campaign

Consumers are the last line of defense in food safety. The Fight Bac!™ Campaign is an educational program designed to teach consumers about safe food handling. The

FIGURE 21.5. FIGHT BAC! CAMPAIGN LOGO.

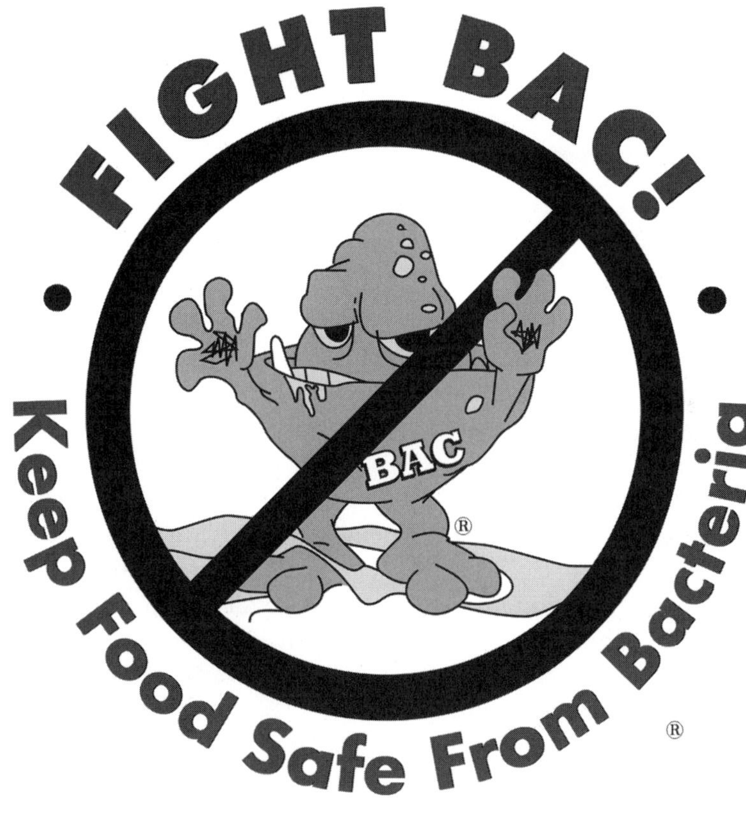

focal point of the campaign is BAC (short for *bacteria*), a character used to make consumers aware of the microbes that cause foodborne illness (Figure 21.5). More specifically, consumers are taught that even though they cannot see, smell, or taste BAC, it and millions more germs like it, may be in and on food and food-contact surfaces. The Fight Bac! Campaign uses a variety of media and community outreach programs to teach consumers how to keep food safe from pathogenic bacteria by washing their hands, cleaning and sanitizing surfaces that touch food, preventing cross-contamination, cooking foods to proper temperature, and cooling foods quickly.

Consumer Advisories

Food establishments are required to provide consumer advisories to inform their customers about the dangers of eating raw or undercooked animal foods or ingredients. The advisories must be provided at the point where customers order or purchase food to inform them of the fact that eating foods such as rare hamburgers, raw oysters, or Caesar salads made with raw eggs may increase their risk of foodborne illness, especially if they have certain medical conditions. Food establishments may use a variety of written communications (for example, brochures, deli case or menu advisories, or statements on labels or table tents) to satisfy the consumer advisory requirement.

Food Irradiation

Food irradiation is a promising new food safety technology that can be used to reduce or eliminate pathogenic bacteria, insects, and parasites. It reduces spoilage, and in certain fruits and vegetables, it inhibits sprouting and delays the ripening process.

Food irradiation uses high-energy radiation in any one of three approved forms: gamma ray, electron beam, or X-ray. Gamma rays may be generated by two approved sources, either cobalt-60 or cesium-137. These substances give off high-energy photons, called gamma rays, which can penetrate foods to a depth of several feet. An electron beam, or e-beam, is a stream of high-energy electrons propelled out of an electron gun. The electrons can penetrate food to a depth of a little over one inch, so the food to be treated must not be thicker than that if it is to be treated all the way through. X-ray irradiation is the newest technology. The X-ray machine employed is a more powerful version of the machines used in many hospitals and dental offices. X-rays can pass through thick foods. Use of this method does require heavy shielding for safety; however, as with e-beams, no radioactive sources are involved.

The FDA has concluded that food irradiation is safe and effective for many foods, a conclusion shared by the World Health Organization (WHO) and the USDA. To date, irradiation has been approved for red meat, poultry, spices, fruits, vegetables, fresh shell eggs, juices, and shellfish.

The FDA requires that irradiated foods be labeled with the statement "treated with radiation" (or "treated by irradiation") and the *radura*, the international symbol for irradiation. Irradiation labeling requirements apply only to foods sold in stores. For example, containers of irradiated spices must be labeled. However, the same spices do not need to be labeled when used as an ingredient in other foods. Irradiation labeling rules also do not apply to restaurant foods.

Irradiation is not a shortcut that means food hygiene efforts can be relaxed. Irradiated foods need to be stored, handled, and cooked in the same ways as unirradiated foods. They can still become contaminated with germs during processing after irradiation if the rules of basic hygiene are not followed.

Many consumers still question whether irradiation is safe. They wonder if the process transfers radiation to the product or if it causes chemical changes in the food that might be hazardous. Greater public acceptance of food irradiation awaits more understanding that irradiation does not make food radioactive, compromise nutritional quality, or noticeably change food taste, texture, or appearance when it is applied properly to a suitable product.

Safe Food as Healthy Food

Other recent initiatives address the public health aspects of food from a somewhat different perspective, focusing on food's nutritional value and the choices that shape what people in different environments eat. Box 21.9 offers three examples of this emerging concern.

Box 21.9. The Healthy Food Environment

Food safety, as a component of environmental public health, has traditionally focused on keeping hazardous microbes and chemical contaminants out of food. But in recent years a new environmental approach to food has emerged: an emphasis on the environmental context of nutrition and food choices. Three examples are illustrative: the availability of fresh food in poor neighborhoods, the density of liquor stores in poor neighborhoods, and the availability of "junk food" in schools.

Poor neighborhoods, such as those in central cities, have a relative scarcity of supermarkets and other sources of fresh fruits and vegetables. When these products are available, they are often sold in independent grocery stores rather than in national chain supermarkets, at prices out of reach for most neighborhood residents. At the same time, these poor neighborhoods typically have a high density of fast-food stores (Sooman, Macintyre, and Anderson, 1993; Mooney, 1990; Bolen and Hecht, 2003). For example, a study in Kansas City showed seventeen fast-food restaurants per 1,000 population in low-income neighborhoods, and only one per 1,000 in high-income neighborhoods (Poston and others, 2002). Evidence suggests that these environmental patterns—and the constrained nutritional choices they imply—predict lower than desirable fruit and vegetable consumption, at least in some ethnic and racial groups (Morland, Wing, and Diez Roux, 2002).

Similarly, poor neighborhoods feature a high density of liquor stores (LaVeist and Wallace, 2000), posing a different sort of environmental cue. Although this density has not been linked directly to drinking in poor neighborhoods, a study of college students showed that the density of liquor stores predicted the students' drinking habits (Weitzman, Folkman, Folkman, and Wechsler, 2002).

Finally, a lively debate has arisen about the increasingly common placement of soft drink and junk food vending machines in schools; this is part of a larger debate about what USDA (2000) has called the *school nutrition environment.* The CDC reported in 2001 that 43 percent of elementary schools, 74 percent of middle schools, and 98 percent of high schools have vending machines or snack bars for student food purchases. Of the schools surveyed, 76 percent sold soft drinks, sports drinks, and fruit drinks, and 63 percent sold salty snacks and baked goods not low in fat. In contrast, only 15 percent sold low-fat or nonfat yogurt, only 18 percent sold fruits or vegetables, and only 24 percent sold low-fat or skim milk (Wechsler, Brener, Kuester, and Miller, 2001). A 2003 survey in twenty-four states (Center for Science in the Public Interest, 2004), showed similar results. In 1,420 vending machines in 251 middle and high schools, 75 percent of the beverage options and 85 percent of the snacks were of poor nutritional quality; the choices included soda, imitation fruit juice, candy, chips, cookies, and snack cakes. Although available data do not conclusively link these aspects of the school nutrition environment with students' eating habits, critics point out that environmental interventions have been successful at increasing fruit consumption in schools (French and Stables, 2003), and charge that selling nonnutritious foods may discourage and even preclude healthy nutritional choices.

A broad view of food safety might well include attention to the nutritional opportunities and choices that play a role in shaping what people in different environments eat.

Emerging Threats to Food Safety

Over time, new threats to food safety can emerge. Two issues with which regulatory agencies, food producers, and the public are currently concerned are mad cow disease and bioterrorism.

Mad Cow Disease

Bovine spongiform encephalopathy (BSE), widely referred to as *mad cow disease,* is a chronic degenerative disease affecting the central nervous system in cattle. Affected animals may display agitated or aggressive behavior, abnormal posture, and lack of coordination. There is neither any treatment nor a vaccine to prevent the disease.

BSE was first diagnosed in 1986 in Great Britain. The first case discovered in the United States was diagnosed in Washington State in December of 2003. Even though the heifer affected with the disease appears to have been an anomaly, the episode created great concern in the United States and abroad. BSE belongs to the family of diseases known as the transmissible spongiform encephalopathies (TSEs). These diseases include scrapie, which affects sheep and goats, chronic wasting disease in deer and elk, and Creutzfeldt-Jakob disease in humans. TSEs create holes in the brain. As the disease progresses, more and more brain and central nervous system tissue is affected. Initial symptoms involve tremors and twitching. Later symptoms include blindness and loss of memory. Death follows.

The USDA's BSE surveillance program has historically focused on the cattle populations in which BSE is most likely to be found. These include cattle condemned at slaughter because of signs of central nervous system disorders; nonambulatory cattle; and cattle that die on farms.

In March 2004, Secretary of Agriculture Ann M. Veneman announced an expanded surveillance effort for BSE in the United States. The primary focus of USDA's enhanced surveillance effort will continue to be on the highest-risk populations for the disease, but the USDA will greatly increase the number of target animals surveyed and will include a random sampling of apparently normal, aged animals. According to statements released by the USDA, the enhanced program, when fully implemented, will be able to detect BSE at the rate of 1 positive in 10 million adult cattle with a 99 percent confidence level.

Bioterrorism

Since September 11, 2001, terrorism in the United States has become a national concern. Security experts believe the food supply is vulnerable to attacks by international terrorist groups, and this has prompted government agencies and the food industry to join forces to develop plans and guidelines for responding to threats to food security. Food security is different from food safety. *Food security* involves protecting food against deliberate contamination, whereas *food safety* is protecting food against accidental or unplanned contamination.

The CDC has identified and ranked several foodborne pathogens as agents for possible terrorist attacks. *Bacillus anthracis* (anthrax) and *Clostridium botulinum* (botulism) have been rated by the CDC as high-priority biological agents (Category A), because they are easy to disseminate and cause severe morbidity and moderate to high mortality. Most of the foodborne biological agents identified by CDC have been classified as Category B agents. because they are moderately easy to disseminate and cause moderate morbidity and low mortality. The Category B biological agents include *Salmonella* spp., *Shigella dysenteriae, E. coli* O157:H7, and ricin, a toxin. Several of the pathogens identified by CDC as critical biological agents are also known to pose a significant threat as unintentional food contaminants, as discussed earlier in this chapter. In addition, the CDC identified certain chemicals as possible agents for a terrorist attack. These include heavy metals, such as arsenic, lead, and mercury, and pesticides, dioxins, furans, and PCBs, all of which can be used to contaminate food. These toxins too have been introduced inadvertently into foods at times and linked to human health effects.

Terrorists frequently rely on readily available, low-technology approaches to induce fear and produce death and mass destruction. The ideal agent for a terrorist is one that is easily spread, produces high morbidity and mortality, and can be spread from person to person after the initial exposure. Security experts believe terrorists might use a combination of the biological and chemical agents noted here, attack in more than one location simultaneously, use new agents, or use organisms that are not on the critical list (for example, common, drug-resistant, or genetically engineered pathogens).

Some actions that have been recommended to producers, processors, and retailers for responding to the threat of sabotage in a rational manner include the following:

- Allow only employees who have proper identification into production areas.
- Use sign-in and sign-out records to track visitors and keep areas secure.
- Prohibit personal items, such as lunch containers, briefcases, purses, and similar items, from processing areas.
- Report any unusual or suspicious activity to supervisors or managers, and contact the Federal Bureau of Investigation (FBI) and the FDA's Office of Crime Investigation when a problem is identified.
- Designate a spokesperson to deal with media or other inquiries.

Managers and employees of the food industry are advised to be alert and to report any unusual activity promptly.

Food Safety Careers

Preventing foodborne illness and deaths remains a major public health challenge, and there are as many variations in food safety careers as there are challenges to solve. There has never been a case of foodborne illness that could not have been prevented, and prevention is a theme that is common to all food safety careers.

Food safety professionals protect and promote public health by investigating foodborne disease outbreaks to learn about their causes and by implementing food safety strategies to prevent future outbreaks from occurring. They also inspect production facilities, food-processing plants, and retail food establishments to ensure that products are safe, wholesome, and suitable for human consumption. Food safety professionals work in a variety of settings including private industries, government agencies, health care facilities, and academic institutions.

College and graduate areas of study for those who work in the food safety field range from veterinary medicine and microbiology to food science and environmental health. Those who choose a career in food safety use the principles of biology, chemistry, physics, and other sciences to solve problems. Food safety professionals routinely prepare reports, so good written and oral communication skills are essential.

Conclusion

Even though the United States has one of the safest food supplies in the world, foodborne illness poses a significant challenge to public health. Foodborne illness threatens the health and well-being of millions of Americans each year and costs billions of dollars in lost productivity, medical expenses, legal fees, lost business, and increased surveillance by regulatory agencies. Outbreaks of foodborne illness receive widespread media attention, and consumer confidence falls whenever a foodborne disease outbreak is reported. The bad publicity associated with such outbreaks can cause financial problems for the company whose product caused the outbreak and for the food industry. The entire food industry is affected when consumers begin to doubt the safety of food products.

Foodborne illness can be prevented, and the responsibility for making food safe must be shared by producers, processors, retailers, government officials, and consumers. A comprehensive and coordinated effort by all these entities is required to ensure the safety of our food supply from the farm to the table.

Data recently released by the CDC indicate measurable reductions in the incidence of some foodborne diseases. These data, although inconclusive for all foods, show that current approaches to combating pathogens in meat, poultry, egg products, seafood, and juices have been effective. Progress is being made toward the goal of preventing foodborne illness and protecting public health, but efforts to control foodborne pathogens are far from complete. The food industry, government agencies, and consumers must continue their vigilance over the nation's food supply to achieve even higher levels of safety and confidence.

Thought Questions

1. Explain how infections, intoxications, and toxin-mediated infections cause foodborne illness.
2. What four groups of people tend to be most highly susceptible to foodborne illness?
3. Identify the three classes of foodborne hazards, and give an example of each.
4. What is the temperature danger zone, and why is it important to food safety?

5. What is meant by poor personal hygiene, and how can it lead to foodborne illness?
6. What is cross-contamination, and what are some ways to prevent it?
7. What are the advantages of using HACCP rather than traditional food safety programs in retail food establishments?
8. What are critical control points and critical limits as they are used in HACCP programs?
9. Why is monitoring an important step in an HACCP system?
10. How do food recalls contribute to the safety of our nation's food supply?

References

Al-Mufti, A. W., and others. "Epidemiology of Organomercury Poisoning in Iraq, I: Incidence in a Defined Area and Relationship to the Eating of Contaminated Bread." *Bulletin of the World Health Organization,* 1976, *53*(suppl.), 23–36.

Bakir, F., and others. "Methylmercury Poisoning in Iraq." *Science,* 1973, *181*(96), 230–241.

Bolen, E., and Hecht, K. *Neighborhood Groceries: New Access to Healthy Food in Low-Income Communities.* [http://www.cfpa.net/Grocery.pdf]. 2003.

Center for Science in the Public Interest. *Dispensing Junk: How School Vending Undermines Efforts to Feed Children Well.* [http://cspinet.org/new/pdf/dispensing_junk.pdf]. 2004.

Centers for Disease Control and Prevention. "Infectious Disease Information: Food-Related Diseases." [http://www.cdc.gov/ncidod/diseases/food/index.htm]. 2003.

Dato, V., and others. "Hepatitis A Outbreak Associated with Green Onions at a Restaurant—Monaca, Pennsylvania, 2003." *Morbidity and Mortality Weekly Report,* 2003, *52*(47), 1155–1157.

Foegeding, P. M., and Roberts, T. *Foodborne Pathogens: Risks and Consequences.* Report R122. Ames, Iowa: Council for Agricultural Science and Technology, 1994.

French, S. A., and Stables, G. "Environmental Interventions to Promote Vegetable and Fruit Consumption Among Youth in School Settings." *Preventive Medicine,* 2003, *37,* 593–610.

Hites, R. A., and others. "Global Assessment of Organic Contaminants in Farmed Salmon." *Science,* 2004, *303,* 226–229.

International Association for Food Protection. *Procedures to Investigate Foodborne Illness.* (5th ed.) Des Moines, Iowa: International Association for Food Protection, 1999.

LaVeist, T. A., and Wallace, J. M., Jr. "Health Risk and Inequitable Distribution of Liquor Stores in African American Neighborhoods." *Social Science & Medicine,* 2000, *51*(4), 613–617.

McSwane, D., Rue, N., Linton, R., and Williams, A. *Essentials of Food Safety and Sanitation.* (3rd ed.) Upper Saddle River. N.J.: Pearson Education, 2002.

Mead, P. S., and others. "Food-Related Illness and Death in the United States." *Emerging Infectious Diseases,* 1999, *5*(5), 607–625.

Mooney, C. "Cost and Availability of Healthy Food Choices in a London Health District." *Journal of Human Nutrition and Dietetics,* 1990, *3,* 111–120.

Morland, K., Wing, S., and Diez Roux, A. "The Contextual Effect of the Local Food Environment on Residents' Diets: The Atherosclerosis Risk in Communities Study." *American Journal of Public Health,* 2002, *92,* 1761–1767.

National Research Council, Committee on Pesticides in the Diets of Infants and Children. *Pesticides in the Diets of Infants and Children.* Washington, D.C.: National Academies Press, 1993.

Olsen, S. J., and others. "Surveillance for Foodborne Disease Outbreaks—United States, 1993–1997." *Morbidity and Mortality Weekly Report: CDC Surveillance Summaries,* 2000, *49*(1), 1–51.

Posada de la Paz, M., Philen, R. M., and Borda, A. I. "Toxic Oil Syndrome: The Perspective After 20 Years." *Epidemiologic Reviews,* 2001, *23*(2), 231–247.

Poston, W.S.C., and others. "Obesity and the Environment: A Tale of Two Kansas Cities." Poster presented at the 23rd annual Scientific Sessions of the Society of Behavioral Medicine, San Diego, Apr. 2002.

Shallow, S., and others. "Preliminary FoodNet Data on the Incidence of Foodborne Illnesses—Selected Sites, United States, 2002. *Morbidity and Mortality Weekly Report,* 2004, *53*(16), 338–343.

Sooman, A., Macintyre, S., and Anderson, A. "Scotland's Health: A More Difficult Challenge for Some? The Price and Availability of Healthy Foods in Socially Contrasting Localities in the West of Scotland." *Health Bulletin,* 1993, *51*(5), 276–284.

U.S. Department of Agriculture. *Changing the Scene: Improving the School Nutrition Environment.* Alexandria, Va.: U.S. Department of Agriculture, 2000.

U.S. Food and Drug Administration. *1993 Food Code.* National Technical Information Services Publication PB94-113941. Washington, D.C.: U.S. Food and Drug Administration, 1993.

U.S. Food and Drug Administration. *2001 Food Code.* [http://www.cfsan.fda.gov/~dms/fc01-toc.html]. 2001.

U.S. Food and Drug Administration. *Foodborne Pathogenic Microorganisms and Natural Toxins Handbook: The "Bad Bug Book."* [http://vm.cfsan.fda.gov/~mow/intro.html]. 2003.

U.S. Food and Drug Administration. "What You Need to Know About Mercury in Fish and Shellfish." [http://www.cfsan.fda.gov/~dms/admehg3.html]. 2004.

Wechsler, H., Brener, N. D., Kuester, S., and Miller, C. "Food Service and Foods and Beverages Available at School: Results from the School Health Policies and Programs Study 2000." *Journal of School Health,* 2001, *71,* 313–324.

Weitzman, E. R., Folkman, A., Folkman, K. L., and Wechsler, H. "The Relationship of Alcohol Outlet Density to Heavy and Frequent Drinking and Drinking-Related Problems Among College Students at Eight Universities." *Health & Place,* 2002, *9*(1), 1–6.

For Further Information

Publications

Bryan, F. L., and others. *Procedures to Implement the Hazard Analysis Critical Control Point System.* Ames, Iowa: International Association for Food Protection, 1991.

Chin, J. (ed.). *Control of Communicable Diseases in Man.* (17th ed.) Washington, D.C.: American Public Health Association, 2000.

Jay, J. M. *Modern Food Microbiology.* (6th ed.) Gaithersburg, Md.: Aspen, 2000.

McSwane, D., Linton, R., and Rue, N. R. *Retail Best Practices and Guide to Food Safety and Sanitation.* Upper Saddle River, N.J.: Pearson Education, 2003.

McSwane, D., Rue, N. R., and Linton, R. *Essentials of Food Safety and Sanitation.* (4th ed.) Upper Saddle River, N.J.: Pearson Education, 2005.

Potter, N., and Hotchkiss, J. *Food Science.* (5th ed.) Gaithersburg, Md.: Aspen, 1998.

Organization Web Sites

Centers for Disease Control and Prevention [http://www.cdc.gov].

Food Allergy Network [http://www.foodallergy.org].

Food and Agriculture Organization of the United Nations [http://www.fao.org].

Food Marketing Institute [http://www.fmi.org].

Gateway to Government Food Safety Information [http://www.foodsafety.gov].

International Association for Food Protection [http://www.foodprotection.org]. (Use this site to order copies of *Procedures to Investigate Foodborne Illness.*)

International Food Information Council [http://www.ific.org].

National Restaurant Association [http://www.restaurant.org].

Partnerships for Food Safety Education [http://www.fightbac.org].

Prentice Hall [http://www.prenhall.com]. (Use this site to locate a range of textbooks, videos, and other training materials about retail food safety.)

U.S. Department of Agriculture [http://www.usda.gov].

U.S. Environmental Protection Agency [http://www.epa.gov].

U.S. Food and Drug Administration [http://www.fda.gov].

CHAPTER TWENTY-TWO

INDOOR AIR

Michael J. Hodgson

Since time immemorial humans have relied on sheltered places to protect them from the elements and to maintain comfort and safety. Caves, huts, igloos, yurts, plank or log cabins, and more sophisticated structures have provided shelter but have also posed health challenges from individuals' close proximity to pollutant sources in indoor spaces. Burning fuel in close, unventilated quarters is an ancient hazard; there is evidence of smoke damage in the sinuses of fossilized hunter-gatherers (Brimblecombe, 1987), and people in developing countries are still at risk of respiratory disease and lung cancer from indoor combustion. Over the last century, two striking changes of particular importance have occurred. First, we spend more and more of our time indoors (currently over 90 percent in developed countries). Second, building design has changed, especially since the oil shocks of the 1970s. This has resulted in substantially less exchange between indoor and outdoor air, in many cases by more than an order of magnitude. In addition, moisture retention, inoperable windows, and new materials have changed indoor pollutant characteristics over the last twenty-five years.

Since the turn of the nineteenth century, control of indoor environments has served two separate but overlapping purposes: to provide comfort and to protect

The views in this chapter represent only those of the author and not those of the Department of Veterans Affairs or the Veterans Health Administration.

health. The standards and guidelines pertinent to the indoor environment reflect these two goals, but they have changed dramatically since the mid-nineteenth century attempts at "indoor hygiene" (Jansen, 1994). In developed countries, indoor environments are generally no longer regulated by health but by housing departments, suggesting a very different set of institutional considerations and priorities. Indoor environment quality often presents a challenge to occupational and environmental health professionals. First, it involves exposures that cross the divide between occupational and nonoccupational settings. Second, little formal regulation exists. Although recommended exposure levels have been established by several organizations, these are nonenforceable guidelines, often lack a scientific basis, and do not address a substantial number of important pollutants. Third, at least in the built environment, exposures usually are better characterized by assessment of processes, potential sources, and exposure drivers than by quantitative measurements of specific pollutants, the traditional "gold standard" for industrial hygiene. Buildings and indoor environments in general must be examined to determine whether they were built and function as designed.

Major confusion can arise during investigations of complaints in the built environment, as at least three disciplines may be involved. Occupant complaints are best addressed by health professionals such as physicians, nurses, or others with an understanding of physiology and psychology and the ability to categorize and distinguish symptoms of disease from complaints. Building systems, such as envelopes or mechanical systems, require engineering knowledge. Finally, thinking about specific pollutants often requires detailed industrial hygiene and environmental science assessment skills. Each of these three disciplines may be useful at different stages of a building investigation, but each may also be misleading if it results in pursuing answers to the "wrong" questions. The case described in Box 22.1 presents an example.

Box 22.1. A Case of Building-Related Symptoms

Complaints of eye irritation, nasal stuffiness, headaches, and fatigue emerged over a period of six months after a major office reorganization. These complaints appeared centered around the members of one working unit that had suffered some loss of productivity.

The occupied space was the bottom three floors of a six-story, flat-roofed building. The building had been constructed thirty years before, but the air-handling system had been upgraded within the past five years. The flat roof membrane was intact, and no evidence of water leaks was seen on the roof or underneath in the ceilings. Each floor was served by a single air handler and divided into two zones.

The unit that was complaining had not been moved during the renovation because of workload issues. Painting had occurred during the unit's ongoing occupancy. Comparison of the "as built" drawings with the existing space suggested that a prior renovation had left that area underventilated, with too little outside air.

The unit members were moved temporarily while the supply ducts were upgraded. When they moved back in, two individuals on the first floor continued to complain of chest tightness and coughing. Their particular work area was in a corner of the building built into the earth berm. Examination of the cinder-block walls demonstrated some spalling (surface cracks and bulges), suggesting moisture damage. Peak flow tracings (breathing tests) were measured on the two occupants. One demonstrated a drop in air flow at work, with resolution of the problem away from work and resolution with the use of bronchodilators. The other individual showed no such changes at work. Examination of the wall and ground outside identified water drainage into that corner. A French drain was placed behind the building but led to no improvement in the second individual's presumed asthma. Finally, this individual was moved to the third floor and the symptoms resolved.

Three basic approaches are available when investigating building complaints or problems, arising from the three disciplines mentioned previously. The first approach focuses on *health problems* among building occupants, classifying syndromes, identifying diseases, and characterizing complaints. Although this approach is useful, it is unlikely to identify specific sources of problems within buildings because a specific pollutant may result from several different building components. For example, Legionnaires' disease may originate from either cooling tower aerosols or potable water systems, pulmonary disease from any one of a number of moisture sources, and mucosal irritation from entrained motor vehicle exhaust or inadequate ventilation. Therefore, although this approach may narrow the likely sources of the problem, it generally does not implicate a specific source.

The second approach focuses on *environmental control*, identifying deviations from good design, operations, and maintenance procedures. Deficiencies may be present and recognizable even if not associated with the complaints or illness. This approach is therefore independent of medical evaluations and may not predict actual exposures or disease at any given time, although it is necessary for any remediation.

The third approach focuses on *specific pollutants and exposures*. This is useful at the regulatory and scientific level but generally does not lead to the identification of a problem. In fact it may actually delay identification and resolution of problems, which may lead to unnecessary turmoil, lost productivity, and progressive adverse health effects.

In the following sections these three approaches are summarized separately, with discussion of disease identification, analysis of inadequate design, and recognition and measurement of pollutant sources.

Disorders Associated with the Built Environment

Health effects attributable to indoor pollutants have been recognized for centuries, at least since wood smoke in closed rooms was implicated in health problems in the eighteenth century. Actual ventilation requirements were first established in English coal mines in the early nineteenth century. In the mid-nineteenth century Max von Pettenkofer measured indoor carbon dioxide (CO_2) levels in an attempt to refine health requirements and define needed indoor ventilation rates. In the late nineteenth century, decreased ventilation was recognized as a contributing factor in the transmission of tuberculosis, leading to the first North American ventilation recommendations, in New York City in 1892 (Jansen, 1994). In the course of the twentieth century, ventilation for comfort gained its own importance, with the establishment of a comfort laboratory at the Harvard School of Public Health in the 1920s and 1930s.

Public health practitioners should recognize that health problems in buildings are best addressed by multidisciplinary teams. Most public health practitioners are unable to maintain a comprehensive knowledge of diagnostic and linkage criteria, nor will they have the clinical tools at hand to make such diagnoses. From such a perspective it is important to distinguish between disease and discomfort, recognizing the list of diseases defined in Table 22.1 and ensuring access to a skilled environmental and occupational health clinician.

Building-Related Illness

During the last twenty years, complaints attributed to buildings have generally been classified as either building-related illnesses (BRIs) or sick building syndrome (SBS). Classical BRIs, listed in Table 22.1, are diseases that usually have multiple etiologies, one of which is a specific factor that may arise in or from the indoor environment. (Readers may refer to other chapters or to references such as Hodgson, 1989, for a more detailed discussion.) Some, such as eosinophilic fungal sinusitis, remain controversial. BRIs are frequently distinguished from the symptom categories that define SBS (Table 22.2). Although the distinction between specific BRIs and SBS is widely used, outbreaks of specific diseases have often been associated with excess rates of nonspecific symptoms in individuals who do not meet formal case definitions. This has led

TABLE 22.1. SPECIFIC BUILDING-RELATED ILLNESSES AND THEIR CAUSES.

- RHINITIS, SINUSITIS
  Allergens
  Molds
  Spores
  Irritants, such as chemicals, cleaning agents, volatile organic compounds (VOCs)
- ASTHMA
  Irritant exposures, such as cleaning agents, VOCs, allergens, molds, phthalates
- HYPERSENSITIVITY PNEUMONITIS
  Molds
  Wood dust
  Methylene diisocyanate (MDI)
  Chemicals
  Thermotolerant bacteria related to moisture
- ORGANIC DUST TOXIC SYNDROME (INHALATION FEVERS)
  Gram-negative bacteria
  Molds
- INFECTIOUS AGENTS AND DISEASES
  Legionella pneumophila, which may result in Legionnaires' disease
  Mycobacterium tuberculosis, which may result in tuberculosis
  Viruses, which may result in upper respiratory tract infection
- DERMATITIS
  Fiberglass
  VOCs
  Low humidity
  Office products
- LUNG CANCER
  Radon
  Environmental tobacco smoke
  Asbestos
  Combustion Products
- ALLERGIC CONTACT DERMATITIS
  Formaldehyde
  Fungal antigens
  Rare blueprint or medical graphics equipment emissions
- IRRITANT CONTACT DERMATITIS
  Fiberglass
  Low relative humidity

to the suggestion that SBS may be an early stage of a BRI and, if left unchecked, may progress to a specific disease. (Clinical guidance for diagnostic and management criteria and more detailed discussions of specific etiologies and building sources of illnesses are available in standard textbooks of occupational and environmental health and on the Web; see, for example, Storey and others, 2004.)

TABLE 22.2. TYPICAL SYMPTOMS IN SICK BUILDING SYNDROME.

- MUCOUS MEMBRANE IRRITATION
  Eye irritation
  Nasal irritation
  Throat irritation
  Cough
- NEUROLOGICAL SYMPTOMS
  Headaches
  Fatigue
  Lack of concentration
  Memory loss
- RESPIRATORY SYMPTOMS
  Shortness of breath
  Cough
  Wheeze
- SKIN SYMPTOMS
  Rash
  Pruritus
  Dryness
- CHEMOSENSORY SYMPTOMS
  Dysosmia, or distorted sense of smell

Sick Building Syndrome

Despite much use, the term *sick building syndrome* remains without an operational definition. It is unclear whether the term refers to an *individual* with symptoms, to *buildings* that should be considered sick, or more likely, to a *conceptual model* of a systems problem (Jaakkola, 1998). Symptom prevalence varies from building to building, often without a recognized problem or an identified cause; a substantial number of building systems do not meet professional design criteria or are operated in substandard ways; and specific pollutants have been identified through reasonable measurement methods, physiological markers of exposure, and predictable dose-response relationships. Much of SBS has a clear etiology even though diagnosis at the individual level is difficult. Table 22.3 presents the etiologic factors that evidence suggests contribute to SBS.

In the 1980s and early 1990s, the results of numerous cross-sectional questionnaire investigations, conducted in several countries, were published, showing associations between complaint frequencies and a series of environmental risk factors (Mendell and Smith, 1990). The most prominent risk factor was mechanical ventilation, which was consistently associated with a 50 percent increase in symptoms (Mendell and Smith, 1990). Panel evaluations of office buildings in Denmark suggested that approximately 40 percent of the complaints could be attributed to

TABLE 22.3. DETERMINANTS OF INDOOR AIR QUALITY AND PEOPLE'S SYMPTOMS.

- AIR CONTAMINANTS
  Indoor sources: building materials, moisture, office and cleaning supplies
  Outdoor sources: automobile exhaust, industrial plants, moisture
- HVAC SYSTEM
  Ventilation
  Heating and air conditioning
  Humidification
- OFFICE ENVIRONMENT
  Carpeting
  Photoduplication
- WORK ORGANIZATION
  Job satisfaction
  Stress
  Social structures
- INDIVIDUAL FACTORS
  Sex
  Atopy
  Eczema
  Airway hyperreactivity
  Preexisting disease

ventilation systems, although it could not be determined if the pollutants were generated elsewhere and recirculated or if they were generated directly within the system. Environmental tobacco smoke (ETS), office machines, and human off-gassing contributed 25 percent, 20 percent, and 15 percent, respectively, to the remaining 60 percent (Fanger and others, 1988). During the 1990s, two major hypotheses evolved, one arguing that most symptoms were related to volatile organic compound (VOC) exposures (Hodgson and others, 1991; Ten Brinke, 1995) and inadequate ventilation (Wargocki and others, 2002), and the other arguing that many of these symptoms were related to moisture (Sieber and others, 1996; Bornehag and others, 2001; Bornehag, Sundell, and Sigsgaard, 2004). Subsequently, evidence for both views has accumulated (Pommer, 2004). Most recently, a randomized controlled trial of buildings (Menzies and others, 2003) suggests that bacterial growth on cooling coils, related to moisture, is the cause of many symptoms and that cleaning, by means of ultraviolet germicidal irradiation directly on the coils, will reduce those symptoms.

Over the last fifteen years our understanding of the relationships between health issues and the indoor environment has increased substantially. Mucosal irritation, itching, tearing and redness of the eyes, and throat symptoms are now generally attributed to stimulation of the irritant receptor, or the *common chemical sense.* (The common chemical sense is neither taste nor smell; it is a third chemosensory system that detects the irritating properties of substances in the mouth and odors in the nose—the burn of chili pepper, the tingle of ammonia.) Physiological techniques to measure these reactions are well defined (Doty and others, 2004). In addition, it appears that personal characteristics modify the likelihood of symptoms. Atopic individuals describe higher symptom frequencies, have been shown to respond to irritants at lower levels, and have lower irritant thresholds than nonatopic individuals do (Kjaergaard, Pedersen, and Molhave, 1992). Individuals with decreased tear film breakup time and less protection for the ocular mucosa have higher rates of symptoms. Finally, some individuals appear to cough more than others at specific levels of irritant exposures (Ternesten-Hasseus, Bende, and Millqvist, 2002). Therefore some symptom variability may result from biologically defined differences among individuals.

It is more difficult to address fatigue, headaches, lethargy, and other nonspecific symptoms. Some data suggest that such symptoms may be related to endotoxin exposure and associated with moisture or humidity (Teeuw, Vandenbroucke-Grauls, and Verhoef, 1994) or with decreased ventilation rates, although without a clear mechanism. Headaches are widely recognized as a symptom of a poor indoor environment; however, there are no studies that examine them using standard diagnostic classifications (Schwartz, Stewart, and Lipton, 1997), although data exist on headache treatment intervention effectiveness in the office (Warshaw and Burton, 1998). Work stress is also associated with all these symptoms (Mendell, 1993).

Building Systems: Environmental Design and Control

The first use of mechanical ventilation indoors occurred in eighteenth-century England when the new House of Parliament was fitted with blowers to distribute warmth from the furnaces. In 1860, Max von Pettenkofer calculated that indoor air was likely to be acceptable as long as the levels of carbon dioxide did not exceed 1,000 parts per million (ppm). Since 1892, the recommended indoor ventilation rate has ranged between 4 and 60 cubic feet per minute of outdoor air (cfm OA) per occupant. The latter rate was recommended for tuberculosis prevention in the 1890s and to decrease tobacco irritation in the 1990s; the former to keep miners alive in the early nineteenth century and during the "energy crisis" in the 1970s.

At present, buildings in the United States must be ventilated according to the local building code. Required outdoor air rates differ substantially between local building codes and professional design recommendations. The most widely recognized standard, Ventilation for Acceptable Indoor Air Quality, promulgated by the American Society of Heating, Refrigerating and Air-Conditioning Engineers (ASHRAE), recommends approximately 20 cfm OA per occupant for most commercial buildings. Additional specific standards offer guidelines for thermal, acoustical, and lighting comfort. None were developed explicitly to eliminate discomfort: by design at least 20 percent of occupants will be dissatisfied with their thermal environment at any given time. Nor does the ventilation standard address the diseases listed in Table 22.1. Careful scrutiny of the scientific basis for each of these standards, therefore, suggests major gaps and assumptions. Accordingly, health practitioners must remain aware that even when buildings "meet all professional standards," a substantial proportion of occupants may be dissatisfied or even ill from exposures. Newer building designs focus more on local control of the microenvironment, including lighting, thermal parameters, and acoustics in specific work zones. In the long run, such systems may serve the occupants better, support higher productivity, and lead to greater occupant satisfaction.

Heating, Ventilating, and Air-Conditioning Systems

The first system usually examined closely in a problem building is the heating, ventilating, and air-conditioning (HVAC) system. HVAC systems serve four simultaneous purposes: to deliver adequate quantities of outside air to the individual occupant (20 cfm); to condition the air (heating or cooling to offset ambient temperature and the heat load from both occupants and other sources, such as computers); to control the humidity (through latent heat removal); and to remove pollutants. They are expected to do this with a single control (thermostat) and with less than 10 percent excess (wasted) capacity, despite regular office moving and remodeling, changes in heat load from computers and office automation, and varying local pollutant sources (cleaning, machine emissions, and so on). Figure 22.1 displays a schematic of the design of a generic HVAC system.

Return air (air recirculated from indoor space) and outside air are mixed in a plenum. The first basic assumption, then, is that the outside air is clean. However, ambient air may not meet air quality guidelines. Moreover, entrained pollutants (ozone, oxides of nitrogen, or particulates) may occur in predictable patterns. For example, placement of air intakes may lead to circadian changes in pollutant loads (an intake at freeway level may result in elevated carbon monoxide, ozone, and nitrogen oxides during rush hours, for instance).

Air then passes through a filter bank to filter out the dust. All filters are rated for two specific factors. *Arrestance* refers to the ability to remove coarse dust. *Dust spot efficiency* refers to the ability to remove fine particulates of specific sizes, defined

FIGURE 22.1. SCHEMATIC OF A GENERIC HVAC SYSTEM.

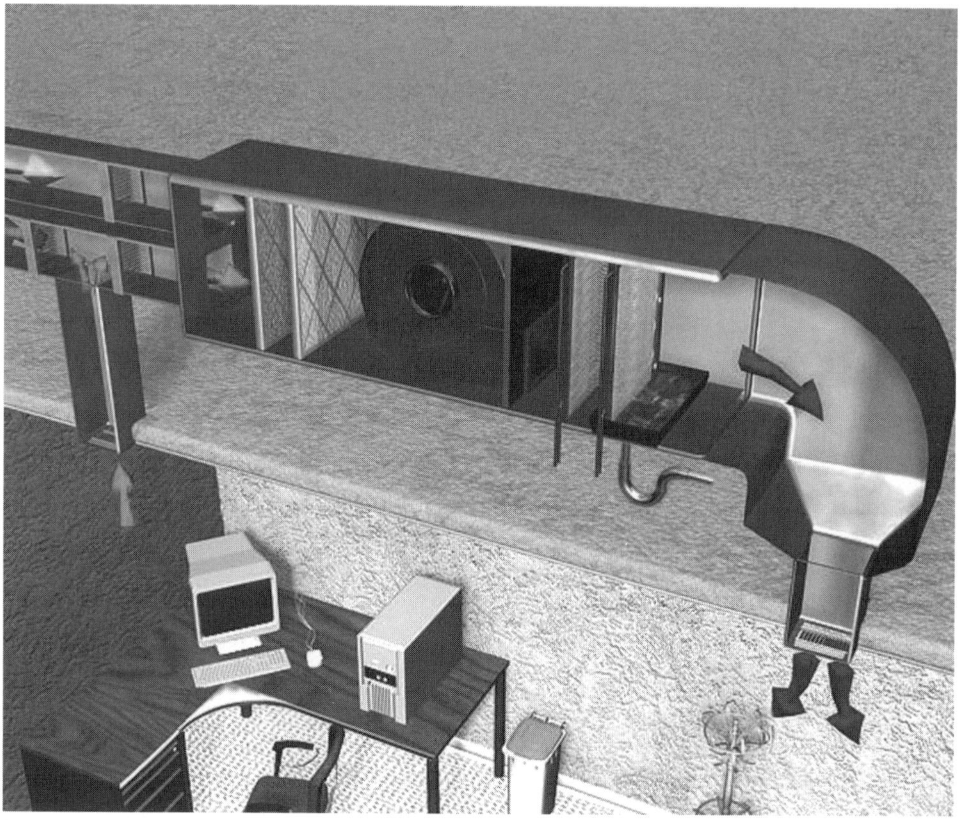

by mass median aerodynamic diameters. Serial filters of increasing efficiency are frequently used to decrease cost. In some settings, such as health care facilities, filtration is mandated. Most commercially available filters do not remove the particulate phase of ETS. Specific filters may remove gases and volatile organic compounds, but large banks of them are needed, with frequent replacement, for any useful filtration. The expense of such high-end filtration means it is rarely used. Where such filtration exists, it generally employs serial filters of increasing efficiency.

Next, air passes through a heat exchanger. Heating and cooling coils must dump their excess load elsewhere, either in cooling towers or some other outside process. As the air is cooled, water condenses on the cooling coils when the coil surface temperature is below the dew point of the air (based on the water content).

Deep (multiple rows of) coils remove proportionately more latent heat (water), and coils with a larger cross section remove more sensible heat (*dry-bulb temperature*). The latent heat ratio predicts, on average, how much moisture can be removed from the airstream. Operational strategies that rely on running less than the correct coolant temperature may then lead to less water removal, with more humid air delivered to occupied space. The condensed water collects in drain pans, and adequate drainage is important to prevent the growth of microbial agents and their dissemination in the airstream. Supply fans then disseminate air to louvers through ducts. These ducts may have internal or external insulation for sound control. Inadequate latent cooling may leave more water in the distributed air. Duct liners and plenums may become wet, attracting dust, and supporting growth of microorganisms.

Air is distributed to occupied spaces through supply air louvers, whose design (*throw*) ensures that air is brought to the occupants' breathing zone and thus to the microenvironment. If the throw is inadequate, short-circuiting will occur along the ceiling, without complete mixing of outside air. In the presence of mechanical obstacles such as partitions or thermal currents (such as may rise from copiers and computers), air may similarly bypass specific spaces, leading to increased pollution, decreased thermal comfort, and complaints.

Air is returned to the central system either through collecting ducts, open plenums, or open spaces.

Several basic forms of air conditioning are currently in use, either relying on variable air volume (VAV) or constant flow (CF) delivery. VAV systems mix air of different temperatures in mixing boxes to achieve a desired temperature in occupied spaces. That is, when the temperature in the occupied space has reached a preset level, no further air flow may occur until the temperature has exceeded the thermostat trigger. Dual duct systems convey cool air and warm air to such mixing boxes separately. CF systems, in contrast, regulate temperature by varying the amounts of initial conditioning and mixing, ensuring air flow at all times. Newer VAV systems often have provisions for minimal airflow even when temperatures are in a desired range, though many older systems do not. The balancing and maintenance of VAV systems requires substantially more expertise than the management of CF systems does.

Envelope Integrity

Envelope integrity refers to prevention of unwanted water incursion into a building. After adequate HVAC systems performance, this is the second most common problem. Water intrusion may result either from bulk moisture intrusion, as can occur through roof leaks, envelope penetration around windows or doors, or seepage up through concrete slabs. For years, such slabs were constructed without moisture barriers. Inadequate maintenance of windows and roofs is a major contributor to such problems. Also important are construction flaws, such as misaligned flashing and incomplete seals.

Space Design

Placement of ventilation air distribution louvers, furniture, and partitions may influence the distribution of air, the delivery of outside air to specific occupants, and the resulting adequacy of microenvironmental circulation. Retrofitting of walls in spaces without regard for the placement of louvers, and location of desks (people), partitions, and equipment (pollutant and heat sources) may lead to air quality complaints. The placement of thermostats and the sizes of the control zones represent major decisions that influence comfort, as heat loads may change with sun incursion, computer operations, and other variable activities.

Office Materials

A growing recognition that mucosal irritation is associated not only with inadequate ventilation but also with the accumulation of specific pollutant groups, such as VOCs, has led architects, designers, and building owners to scrutinize the emissions from newer office products. The screening of such products relies on information from existing databases and from manufacturers' data, although many of these sources report emissions in terms of *total volatile organic compounds,* an approach that ignores the striking differences in irritation potential between various agents (Wolkoff, 1999). Materials with large surface areas, such as carpets, drapes, and upholstery, may also serve as secondary sinks, adsorbing VOCs and dust. These sinks then contribute to local pollution later by re-releasing these agents and contributing to adverse health effects.

Design, Operations, and Maintenance

Several reports have examined whether buildings were designed according to professional standards in place at the time of design. More than 50 percent of buildings do not meet those standards (Woods, 1989). Also, many were constructed differently from their designs. For example, not infrequently there is inadequate space to run supply and return ducts after plumbing and electrical work has taken up space, leading to smaller-than-designed ducts and lower quantities of delivered air. In addition, many buildings are operated in a way that does not reflect system design intent. Finally, maintenance budgets are often inadequate, and the predictable deterioration of systems goes unchecked, with the predictable consequences.

An ASHRAE commissioning guide provides detailed procedures to ensure that buildings "work" at the beginning of their occupancy, but such guidelines are often not followed. Reviews of building systems suggest that the majority of buildings in the United States and elsewhere simply do not meet professional design standards and therefore contribute to health concerns and occupant discomfort (Woods, 1989; Sieber and others, 1996).

Specific Pollutants: Exposure Assessment

In general the pollutant-oriented literature on indoor environments addresses regulatory and scientific concerns. Still, approaches based on pollutant-by-pollutant analyses only rarely help identify specific sources of problems or problem control strategies. The relationship between criteria levels and systems performance (that is, between ventilation system efficiency and distribution effectiveness on the one hand and concentrations of particles, volatile organic compounds, and bioaerosols—fungi, bacteria, viruses—on the other) varies dramatically between buildings, so that specific measurements are only rarely useful. As discussed earlier, examination of systems and their performance is generally a far more effective solution strategy.

A fundamental recognition is that indoor environmental exposures represent complex mixtures of particulates and gases, with many potential interactions. The composition of the mixtures is not stable, so that the *indoor chemistry* leads to changing effects. Finally, additional exposures, involving such items as noise and vibration, lighting factors, and thermal parameters, affect people at least at the central nervous system level even if no interactions occur at the level of their peripheral receptors. Therefore use of environmental criteria alone, a common practice in applied occupational and environmental hygiene in the workplace, is unsuitable when evaluating the nonindustrial workplace. Although some attempts have defined such levels, they are not widely used and generally represent a distraction from more important approaches. In the regulatory and research communities, such pollutant-specific efforts do serve the purposes of defining hazards, examining dose-response relationships, changing building and housing codes, and developing prevention strategies based on rigorous scientific approaches.

Microbial Agents

There is evidence that microbial agents (fungi or bacteria or combinations of the two) can lead to allergic respiratory tract disease in public access buildings and residential environments and that viruses are transmitted as a function of ventilation rates. Symptoms appear more frequently in buildings with higher fungal and endotoxin levels or moisture problems and in atopic individuals. Microbial agents proliferate when growth nutrients, water, air, and heat coexist. Eradication requires interruption of at least one of these factors and is best done through moisture control and cleaning. The active agent components causing symptoms and disease remain unknown for most complaints, even for asthma associated with specific fungi.

Although quantitative sampling (for viable agents or spores) is commonly performed, most professional recommendations suggest doing this only to test a specific, well-designed scientific hypothesis (Macher, 1999). At times, sampling also serves the purpose of risk communication. Measurement of airborne levels is therefore primarily of scientific interest, useful for developing dose-response relationships and identifying specific active agent components but typically of little practical use in individual cases. When sampling is performed, speciation of the organisms is essential. Comparison of the indoor and outdoor levels of specific species, to determine whether the building is concentrating particular organisms, is essential. Finally, sampling may demonstrate the presence of certain species with the potential to form mycotoxins. However, this finding is of limited utility; there is widespread agreement that immunological testing, that is, documentation of antibodies, documents only exposure and has little predictive ability for disease (Trout and others, 2004). Usually, in practice, sources can be identified by visual inspection or smell and remediated without such testing.

There are no regulatory or voluntary standards for bioaerosols (as there are permissible exposure levels for chemicals), and most experts believe that no such standards are likely to develop in the next decade. More important, there is widespread agreement that the real problem—symptoms in the setting of bioaerosol exposure—is better addressed by focusing on moisture sources, pathways, consequences, and remediation.

Volatile Organic Compounds

Field epidemiology and controlled human exposure studies of volatile organic compounds (VOCs) have suggested that many of the complaints associated with indoor environments may result from exposure to low levels of VOCs (Hodgson, Levin, and Wolkoff, 1994; Wolkoff, 1999). Systematic assessment over the last ten years has identified irritant and odor thresholds for several homologous series of agents (aliphatic aldehydes, ketones, and alcohols). There are many sources of

VOCs in the indoor environment, including but not limited to paints, adhesives, cleaners, plastics, and fabric protectors. Modeling of these agents has identified a quantitative structure-activity relationship (Abraham, 1996) based on physicochemical properties of the molecules. On the one hand, in the presence of adequate ventilation and the absence of strong specific sources, these agents are generally below what are considered to be irritant thresholds, even for their combinations. On the other hand, in the presence of poor ventilation performance, these agents can clearly provide an adequate explanation for symptoms.

VOCs can be skin and mucous membrane irritants. These health symptoms appear to be related to the differences in VOC concentrations encountered on entering or leaving a room, to screening measures of VOC quantities, and to pollutants grouped by exposure sources (carpets, paints, and so forth). VOCs may trigger migraines, but most indoor headaches are not labeled as such. Central nervous system toxicity resulting from exposure to solvents has been described only after substantially higher exposures than are likely to occur in office buildings. The obvious exception is renovation during ongoing occupancy, but even here the exposure duration is substantially shorter than that encountered by such occupational groups as painters.

Environmental Tobacco Smoke

There is a well-established link between environmental tobacco smoke (ETS) and adverse health effects. Excess symptoms occur in buildings where smoking is permitted. Controversy exists within the engineering literature over whether smoking areas can really be separated from nonsmoking areas. Although this appears theoretically possible, field studies have consistently demonstrated ETS contamination in areas designated as nonsmoking. The engineering community is therefore deeply split on the topic.

A broader issue is raised by epidemiological literature that suggests a variety of chronic diseases are attributable to ETS, including lung cancer, heart disease, asthma, and chronic obstructive pulmonary disease. Much of this evidence is based on ETS as a risk factor among intense household contacts (spouses or parents), although some evidence has also accrued in the workplace. However, the proportion of chronic disease attributable to levels typically found in the office or other workplaces appears small.

Asbestos

Asbestos products were used in a broad range of applications in buildings. With inadequate maintenance these materials decay, leading to some degree of asbestos exposure. The intensity of this exposure varies considerably, depending on the activities of the individuals under scrutiny. Office workers, in general, are considered at very low risk for asbestos-related disease. Air sampling has rarely revealed fiber exposures above background levels. The risk from asbestos exposure in public access buildings can reasonably be considered negligible in most environments, despite clusters of mesothelioma, a cancer that has been linked to asbestos, among some nonexposed occupational groups.

Radon

Radon in indoor environments has come under considerable scrutiny as a cause of lung cancer. In the United States the risk from radon is primarily in residences and not the workplace. The U.S. Environmental Protection Agency has recommended remediation when levels in living space exceed 4 picocuries per liter (pCi/L), as measured over a three-month period. The risk of lung cancer at these low doses remains a focus of study. A substantial portion of the risk arises from radon's potentiation of smoking risk, so smoking cessation efforts may have substantially greater beneficial effects than radon intervention.

Biomass, Fossil Fuels, and Indoor Chemistry

In public access buildings the entrainment of vehicle exhaust sometimes leads to carbon monoxide and irritant (nitrogen oxide [NO_x] or sulfur dioxide [SO_2]) exposures. Usually, these exposures result from air intakes that are poorly designed and located, most often at street level or over loading docks. The irritants, as reactive agents, may form reaction products with unsaturated hydrocarbons indoors, and through the formation of Criegee radicals, may generate products more reactive and irritating than the original agents. This has been called *indoor chemistry*, and it represents a strong potentiation of the irritant effects of VOCs (Weschler, 2001).

Carbon Dioxide

CO_2 has been a subject of great interest in considerations of indoor air and is frequently (mis)named a pollutant. It is widely employed as an indicator of adequate ventilation, a use based on ASHRAE Standard 62, which uses CO_2 as a mass balance measure for adequate ventilation (pollutant removal) and generation (human sources). Because humans are the primary source of CO_2 in buildings, many consider it a reasonable indicator of ventilation adequacy. However, CO_2 levels do not always accurately reflect the ventilation. First, in spaces with relatively low occupant density (less than seven persons per 1,000 ft^2) or that have not reached steady state, due to an unstable number of occupants or insufficient elapsed time to reach equilibrium, measured CO_2 levels may be a poor indicator of overall ventilation and ventilation efficiency. Second, if there are unexpected, strong sources that far exceed the usually expected pollutant load, specific exposures may remain uncontrolled. Nevertheless, reviewing CO_2 levels is appropriate in many situations. Levels above 1,000 ppm (0.1 percent) indicate that a specific environment does not meet basic ventilation requirements.

Specific Building Environments

Common design principles are applied to the structures and mechanical systems of a wide range of buildings, but the populations that use these buildings often differ in important ways, with implications for health. This section considers indoor air quality in three specific building environments: homes, schools, and health care facilities.

Homes

Homes remain a major source of exposures, with no organized lobby to support public health efforts. Like commercial construction, home construction is regulated through the building code, which does not address ventilation rates, moisture control, or physical safety hazards.

Moisture and Disease. Since the late 1980s, data have suggested an association between childhood airways disease and moisture in the home. Moisture is associated with dust mite and cockroach exposures, and careful intervention has been shown to reduce dust mite antigen levels. More controversial is the relationship between fungi, bacteria, moisture, and asthma in adults and children. Although rare, case reports identify fungi as a possible cause of asthma. Recent studies link asthma with both fungi and endotoxin, which may serve as a reasonable marker of biomass or direct pulmonary effects. A recent Institute of Medicine report (IOM, 2004) outlines clearly the hazard of unwanted moisture.

A controversial issue is whether idiopathic pulmonary hemorrhage may be associated with the mold *Stachybotrys chartarum* in the home. After an initial report study of ten such cases in Cleveland, additional cases have been reported. An animal model was developed in rat pups, identifying capillary fragility as a consequence of controlled exposure to *Stachybotrys.* Toxins likely to cause protein synthesis inhibition can be measured with assays standardized to other well-known carcinogenic toxins, such as fumonisin. As for adult interstitial pneumonitis, the combination of an animal model with a suggested mechanism, an exposure pathway, a formal case-control study, and case reports suggests the possibility of a causal association (Hodgson and Dearborn, 2002).

The question of moisture sources in the home remains of great interest and concern. These sources may be any moisture incursion, including leaks through roofs, walls, windows, and doors, most of which represent straightforward construction defects. Additional moisture sources differ by geographic area. In the northern United States, below-grade moisture seepage remains a very common problem. In humid areas, inadequate enthalpy control (resulting in high indoor moisture content), caused by improper air-conditioning system sizing, represents a more common problem. Often it is a combination of below-grade moisture incursion, enthalpy design problems, and bulk moisture incursion that is associated with negative health effects (Bornehag and others, 2001; Bornehag, Sundell, and Sigsgaard, 2004; IOM, 2004).

Fossil Fuel Combustion. Also of concern is domestic exposure to the indoor combustion of wood, grass, dung (biomass fuels), coal, or petroleum derivatives, such as kerosene (fossil fuels), for cooking and heating. Combustion products include gaseous irritants (NO_x and SO_2), asphyxiants (carbon monoxide [CO]), and complex hydrocarbons in particulate matter (for example, polycyclic aromatic hydrocarbons). Exposure to these pollutants in unvented houses may reach industrial levels, especially in less developed countries (see Chapter Thirteen). Evidence suggests that stove exposures enhance the risk of this potentially fatal hazard, increasing the risk of low birthweight, lung cancer, and possibly obstructive airways disease. Low-technology solutions include the construction of flues and exhausts from local materials.

In developed countries, stove and heater exposures are considered a possible contributor to childhood respiratory infection and diminished lung function and to indoor moisture. These exposures may be a risk factor for the development of asthma or for more severe asthma in established cases. Long-term sequelae remain inadequately investigated. In addition, an association between indoor CO exposures and adverse cardiovascular and central nervous system effects has been suggested. Unusual point sources, entrainment of exhaust from portable grills, entrainment of exhaust from garages, and furnace air supply interruption are associated with mortality and morbidity.

Schools

Symptoms of nasal disease, asthma, and hypersensitivity pneumonitis are all well described in schools. Still, schools represent a building class with three particular sets of problems, relating to their function in society, their overlap of occupational and environmental exposures, and their governance.

First, schools are typically placed in less desirable building sites. Developers generally assign the most desirable land to residential or commercial use because of the obvious economic benefits. School land must generally be set aside as a condition of development. More often than not, the set-aside land has flaws, most often poor moisture drainage. For that reason, many schools are set in swampy land, with poor moisture drainage and moisture seepage into the slab.

Second, schools represent both a workplace for teachers and an environmental exposure setting for students. High occupant densities generate a particle load with cleaning needs that are far more dramatic than those found in most other settings. Control strategies are poorly developed. Lighting and acoustical performance also affect learning effectiveness.

Finally, school budget constraints often lead to deferred renovation, capital improvement, and maintenance. Mechanical systems are underdesigned. Retrofits are not adequately planned. A typical scenario takes the following pattern. A roof has a statistical life expectancy of twenty years. At twenty years, leaks begin. By the twenty-fifth year, parents and teachers are unhappy and propose a budget initiative. After some years of arguments, with increasing health complaints, expert investigations, and workers' compensation claims, a budget item is finally passed that will require two years for implementation.

Health Care Facilities

Tuberculosis transmission is a well-established concern in health care facilities and is closely related to indoor air handling (Nardell, 2003; Cookson and Jarvis, 1997). This suggests that low ventilation rates (Menzies, Fanning, Yuan, and FitzGerald, 2000) may well be related to transmission of viral illnesses to health care workers and patients, as has been documented for viral disease in offices (Myatt and others 2004). In addition, the presence of moisture and fungi (Streifel, 2002), particularly during renovation, represents a substantial risk for immunosuppressed patients. Accordingly, the Joint Commission on Accreditation of Healthcare Organizations has promulgated standards for risk assessment during construction. Finally, hospitals represent one of the few building types where humidification must occur in specific areas, with implications for fungal and bacterial growth. It is interesting in this regard that health care workers have the highest rates of asthma of any occupational group in the United States (Rosa and others, 2000).

Diagnostic Strategies and Prevention

Separate diagnostic strategies should be pursued for *people* and *buildings*. If a person's complaints fit a specific pattern (that is, indicate a specific BRI), the likely source should be identified and remediated. Where no prior reports of an exposure-effect relationship exist, a clinical diagnostic trial may be useful, that is, a trial removal of the person from work or the home. Identification of a specific physiological outcome allows the investigator to focus on a specific target organ under conditions that are measurable and reproducible. If an effect is identified, this may provide adequate evidence for intervention. If no change is identified, the patient can at least be reassured that no disease severe enough to lead to pathophysiological changes is present.

At the same time, the building should be evaluated, preferably by someone with ventilation expertise. Walk-throughs generally involve a review of the building's plans, inspection of various components of the HVAC system, and a review of other building systems and sources, such as may be present in mixed-use buildings (see Chapter Four). Occupant interviews or a questionnaire survey may be useful to characterize complaints, although these techniques are generally not helpful unless some specific disease is under investigation. Likely causes may be identified during the initial review, and a hypothesis should be formulated. Additional evidence may then be collected. Buildings must frequently be examined under various environmental conditions (for example, different temperatures and seasons), because many problems become evident only when the conditions and the associated systems change. If necessary, targeted sampling to document the presence of specific exposures may be useful to persuade the responsible parties of the appropriateness of or need for intervention. In general, extensive sampling is not helpful early in building investigations.

There is growing recognition of the importance of preventive maintenance and careful planning in renovation work. The former includes regular servicing of induction units, cleaning systems, and the like. None of these has been subjected to scientific scrutiny as new industries have arisen. Renovation requires careful planning as renovation during continued occupancy without isolation of the renovated space or isolation of the HVAC system serving the construction sites represents one of the two most common causes of building complaints. Premature occupancy, before commissioning, represents the other.

A widely discussed approach to ensuring indoor air quality is the healthy building movement, which focuses on prevention of sick buildings. This focus has led to several changes in design and construction practices, including closer coordination between architects and engineers, the use of outside peer reviewers for overall project evaluation, the rigorous evaluation and commissioning of newly constructed buildings, the selection of low-emitting materials, and the contractual hiring of designers and builders for a period after the completion to oversee building maintenance.

Finally, careful scrutiny of organizational functioning in the workplace may prevent the development of problems. Several studies have suggested that in addition to specific environmental contaminants, workplace stress may predict building-related complaints. The development of *crisis buildings* often reflects poor labor-management communication. The failure to act appropriately early in the course of building complaints and to take occupant concerns seriously may contribute to many of the health complaints that are clearly preventable.

Since the U.S. Occupational Safety and Health Administration withdrew its proposed standard on indoor air some years ago, no regulatory approach has appeared imminent. Some occupational environments, such as health care, have developed effective self-regulation managed by independent organizations. Office buildings and schools represent large enough classes of buildings, with enough hazards, to warrant some similar approach.

Thought Questions

1. A local developer constructed a set of low-rise (one-story), single-family, slab-on-grade housing units with attached garages. Several episodes of carbon monoxide poisoning, diagnosed in the local emergency room, have been reported to the poison control center. What questions do you ask? What sources do you look for? What solutions could you implement?
2. As a public health official, you are aware of an asthma problem in your local school. A review shows that the roof is leaking. How do you initiate a community process to get the roof replaced?
3. Your state is considering passing an indoor air quality act and asks you for help. What elements would you include?

References

Abraham, M. H. "The Potency of Gases and Vapors: QSARs—Anesthesia, Sensory Irritation, and Odor." In R. B. Gammage and B. A. Berven (eds.), *Indoor Air and Human Health.* (2nd ed.) Boca Raton, Fla.: Lewis, 1996.

Bornehag, C. G., Sundell, J., and Sigsgaard, T. "Dampness in Buildings and Health (DBH): Report from an Ongoing Epidemiological Investigation on the Association Between Indoor Environmental Factors and Health Effects Among Children in Sweden." *Indoor Air,* 2004, *14*(suppl. 7), 59–66.

Bornehag, C. G., and others. "Dampness in Buildings and Health: Nordic Interdisciplinary Review of the Scientific Evidence on Associations Between Exposure to 'Dampness' in Buildings and Health Effects (NORDDAMP)." *Indoor Air,* 2001, *11,* 72–86.

Brimblecombe, P. *The Big Smoke: A History of Air Pollution.* London: Methuen, 1987.

Cookson, S. T., and Jarvis, W. R. "Prevention of Nosocomial Transmission of Mycobacterium Tuberculosis." *Infectious Disease Clinics of North America,* 1997, *11*(2), 385–409.

Doty, R. L., and others. "Assessment of Upper Respiratory Tract and Ocular Irritative Effects of Volatile Chemicals in Humans." *Critical Reviews in Toxicology,* 2004, *34,* 1–58.

Fanger, P. O., and others. "Air Pollution Sources in Office and Assembly Halls, Quantified by the Olf-Unit." *Energy and Buildings,* 1988, *12,* 7–19.

Hodgson, M. J. "Clinical Diagnosis and Management of Building-Related Illness and the Sick-Building Syndrome." *Occupational Medicine,* 1989, *4,* 593–606.

Hodgson, M., and Dearborn, D. "Human Pulmonary Disease and Exposure to *Stachybotrys Chartarum* and other Toxigenic Fungi." *Journal of Occupational and Environmental Medicine,* 2002, *44,* 705–707.

Hodgson, M., Levin, H., and Wolkoff, P. "Volatile Organic Compounds and Indoor Air." *Journal of Allergy and Clinical Immunology,* 1994, *94,* 296–303.

Hodgson, M. J., and others. "Symptoms and Microenvironmental Measures in Nonproblem Buildings." *Journal of Occupational Medicine,* 1991, *33,* 527–533.

Institute of Medicine. *Damp Indoor Spaces and Health.* Washington, D.C.: National Academies Press, 2004.

Jaakkola, J. J. "The Office Environment Model: A Conceptual Analysis of the Sick Building Syndrome." *Indoor Air,* 1998, *8*(suppl. 4), 7–16.

Jansen J. "The 'V' in AHSVE: A Historical Perspective." *ASHRAE Journal* (American Society of Heating, Refrigerating and Air-Conditioning Engineers), 1994, pp. 126–132.

Kjaergaard, S. K., Pedersen, O. F., and Molhave, L. "Sensitivity of the Eyes to Airborne Irritant Stimuli: Influence of Individual Characteristics." *Archives of Environmental Health,* 1992, *47,* 45–51.

Macher J. (ed.). *Bioaerosols: Assessment and Control.* Cincinnati: American Conference of Governmental Industrial Hygienists, 1999.

Mendell, M. "Nonspecific Symptoms in Office Workers: A Review and Summary of the Epidemiologic Literature." *Indoor Air,* 1993, *3,* 227–236.

Mendell, M. J., and Smith, A. H. "Consistent Pattern of Elevated Symptoms in Air-Conditioned Office Buildings: A Reanalysis of Epidemiologic Studies." *American Journal of Public Health,* 1990, *80,* 1193–1199.

Menzies, D., Fanning, A., Yuan, L., and FitzGerald, J. M. "Hospital Ventilation and Risk for Tuberculous Infection in Canadian Health Care Workers." *Annals of Internal Medicine,* 2000, *133,* 779–789.

Menzies, D., and others. "Effect of Ultraviolet Germicidal Lights Installed in Office Ventilation Systems on Workers' Health and Well-Being: Double-Blind Multiple Crossover Trial." *Lancet,* 2003, *362,* 1785–1791.

Myatt, T. A., and others. "Detection of Airborne Rhinovirus and Its Relation to Outdoor Air Supply in Office Environments." *American Journal of Respiratory and Critical Care Medicine,* 2004, *169,* 1187–1190.

Nardell, E. A. "Environmental Infection Control of Tuberculosis." *Seminars in Respiratory Infections,* 2003, *18*(4), 307–319.

Pommer, L., and others. "Class Separation of Buildings with High and Low Prevalence of SBS by Principal Component Analysis." *Indoor Air,* 2004, *14,* 16–23.

Rosa, R. R., and others (eds.). *Worker Health Chartbook 2000.* DHHS (NIOSH) Publication no. 2000-127. [http://www.cdc.gov/niosh/00-127pd.html]. 2000.

Schwartz, B. S., Stewart, W. F., and Lipton, R. B. "Lost Workdays and Decreased Work Effectiveness Associated with Headache in the Workplace." *Journal of Occupational and Environmental Medicine,* 1997, *39,* 320–327.

Sieber, W. K., and others. "The NIOSH Indoor Evaluation Experience: Associations Between Environmental Factors and Self-Reported Health Conditions." *Applied Occupational and Environmental Hygiene,* 1996, *11,* 1387–1392.

Storey, E., and others. *Guidance for Clinicians on the Recognition and Management of Health Effects Related to Mold Exposure and Moisture Indoors.* University of Connecticut HealthCenter. [http://www.oehc.uchc.edu/clinser/MOLD%20GUIDE.pdf]. 2004.

Streifel, A. J. "In with the Good Air." *Infection Control and Hospital Epidemiology,* 2002, *23,* 488–490.

Teeuw, K., Vandenbroucke-Grauls, C. M., and Verhoef, J. "Airborne Gram Negative Bacteria and Endotoxin in SBS: A Study in Dutch Office Buildings." *Archives of Internal Medicine,* 1994, *154,* 2339–2345.

Ten Brinke, J. *Development of New VOC Exposure Metrics Related to "Sick Building Syndrome" Symptoms in Office Workers.* Lawrence Berkeley Laboratory Report LBL-37652. Berkeley, Calif.: Lawrence Berkeley Laboratory, 1995.

Ternesten-Hasseus, E., Bende, M., and Millqvist, E. "Increased Capsaicin Cough Sensitivity in Patients with Multiple Chemical Sensitivity." *Journal of Occupational and Environmental Medicine,* 2002, *44,* 1012–1017.

Trout, D. B., and others. "Clinical Use of Immunoassays in Assessing Exposure to Fungi and Potential Health Effects Related to Fungal Exposure." *Annals of Allergy, Asthma & Immunology,* 2004, *92,* 483–491.

Wargocki, P., and others. "Ventilation and Health in Non-Industrial Indoor Environments: Report from a European Multidisciplinary Scientific Consensus Meeting (EUROVEN)." *Indoor Air,* 2002, *12,* 113–128.

Warshaw, L. J., and Burton, W. N. "Cutting the Costs of Migraine: Role of the Employee Health Unit." *Journal of Occupational and Environmental Medicine,* 1998, *40,* 943–953.

Weschler, C. E. "Reactions Among Indoor Pollutants." *ScientificWorldJournal,* 2001, *1,* 443–457.

Wolkoff, P. "How to Measure and Evaluate Volatile Organic Compound Emissions from Building Products: A Perspective." *Science of the Total Environment,* 1999, *227,* 197–213.

Woods, J. E. "Cost Avoidance and Productivity in Owning and Operating Buildings." *Occupational Medicine,* 1989, *4,* 753–770.

For Further Information

Spengler, J., McCarthy, J., and Samet, J. (eds.). *Indoor Air Quality Handbook.* New York: McGraw Hill, 2000.

CHAPTER TWENTY-THREE

WORKPLACE HEALTH AND SAFETY

Melissa Perry
Howard Hu

The workplace can be thought of as a localized subset of the larger environment, a place where people confront environmental exposures each day as they earn their living. But occupational health is more than small-scale environmental health; it is a complex and fascinating topic that deserves special consideration. Why? First, work remains the central activity in which the world spends most its time outside of the home. In the work environment, people have enormous potential for exposures (both healthy and hazardous) over many years. Second, many hazardous exposures are experienced at their highest level in the workplace. In fact, this is reflected in longstanding policy; regulations typically allow higher exposures in the workplace than in the general environment. Third, the workplace presents an extraordinarily broad range of exposures, from acute chemical poisoning to catastrophic injuries, from long-term chemical effects to psychological stress. This variety is only partially captured in the term *occupational safety and health,* in which *safety* refers to protection from injuries and *health* refers to protection from illnesses. These long-term, high-level, and diverse exposures account for a fourth special feature of the workplace: it has been a "laboratory" for many exposures, with workers the inadvertent guinea pigs. Many environmental hazards were first recognized in the workplace, through observations of highly exposed workers. Fifth, occupational health is not only a subset of public health; it is also a subset of labor relations, a sociopolitical context that embodies unique issues of power, history, justice, and law. Finally, the workplace as a social construct offers many opportunities for health interventions, from health education to medical screening to drug screening. Occupational health is a unique and important part of environmental health.

History of Occupational Health

Since antiquity scholars have written about the specific exposures and diseases associated with occupations. Hippocrates recognized and recorded lead toxicity in the mining industry in the fourth century BCE. Pliny the Elder, a Roman scholar of the first century CE, described hazards associated with handling zinc and sulfur as well as perhaps the first recorded industrial hygiene protective device, a mask constructed from an animal bladder that was used by miners and smelter workers exposed to dust or fumes. Working conditions remained abysmal in the Middle Ages, but feudal guilds were established that assisted ill workers and their families. Formal study of occupational disease was undertaken by Ulrich Ellenbog in 1473, when he published a pamphlet on occupational diseases and injuries among gold miners, wrote about the toxic effects of carbon monoxide, mercury, lead, and nitric acid, and offered specific recommendations on hygiene and other preventive measures. In *De Re Metallica,* a book published in 1556, the Saxon physician and geologist Georgius Agricola described injuries and illnesses among miners, including silicosis—a deadly lung disease brought on by inhaling granite dust—and proposed methods for mine ventilation and other forms of worker protection.

In 1700, Bernardino Ramazzini (1633–1714), widely regarded as the "father of industrial medicine," published in Italy the first comprehensive book on industrial medicine, *De Morbis Artificum Diatriba* (The Diseases of Workmen). The book contained accurate descriptions of the occupational diseases of many of the trades of his time as well as his famous admonition that "when a doctor visits a working-class home he should be content to sit on a three-legged stool, if there isn't a gilded chair, and he should take time for examination; and to the questions recommended by Hippocrates, he should add one more: What is your occupation?" Ramazzini's writing also influenced the development of the field of industrial hygiene through the assertion that occupational diseases should be studied in the work environment rather than in hospital wards.

Later, in eighteenth-century England, Percival Pott (1715–1788) recognized soot as one of the causes of scrotal cancer among chimney sweeps, one of the first recorded connections between occupational exposures and cancer. Moreover, he used his reputation as a prominent London surgeon to advocate for passage of the Chimney-Sweepers Act of 1788, which formally recognized the disease connection and offered protections.

During the industrial revolution of the late eighteenth and nineteenth centuries, technology advanced rapidly, new and often dangerous machines were deployed in industry after industry, and mass production became common. Textile mills and factories sprung up, employing workers who worked for hourly wages and no longer owned the means of production and who had to depend on employers for their working conditions. These mills and factories also generated a huge increase in the use of—and worker exposure to—chemicals, such as the acids, alkalis, soaps, and mordants needed for processing textiles. The conditions in the mills and factories were often abominable.

Charles Turner Thackrah (1795–1833), a Yorkshire physician, developed an interest in the diseases he observed among the poorer classes of people living in the city of Leeds. He became a major figure in occupational health with the publication of his 200-page book titled *The Effects of the Principal Arts, Trades and Professions, and of Civic States and Habits of Living, on Health and Longevity, with Suggestions for the Removal of many of the Agents which produce Disease and Shorten the Duration of Life.* In it he proposed guidelines for the prevention of certain diseases, such as the elimination of lead as a glaze in the pottery industry and the use of ventilation and respiratory protection to protect knife grinders. Public outcry and the efforts of early Victorian reformers such as Thackrah led to passage of the Factory Act in 1833 and the Mines Act in 1842.

The first article on occupational disease in the United States appeared in 1837 and relied on Thackrah as an authority. But it was not until the turn of the twentieth century that the first major champion of occupational health in the United States, the remarkable Alice Hamilton (1869–1970), emerged (Figure 23.1). A keen firsthand observer of industrial conditions, she startled mine owners, factory managers, and state officials in Chicago with evidence of links between illness and exposure to toxins. Hamilton was appointed by the governor of Illinois to direct that state's Occupational Disease Commission from 1910 to 1919, and she became a key proponent of legislation establishing early forms of occupational health regulation and workers' compensation. In 1919, she moved to Boston and became the first female professor at Harvard Medical School, and later, in 1925, the Harvard School of Public Health. At Harvard, Hamilton conducted industrial research and, between 1924 and 1930, served on the League of Nations Health Committee, which allowed her to investigate industrial health conditions in other countries as well. She published *Industrial Poisons in the United States* in 1925, *Industrial Toxicology* in 1934, and perhaps the most inspiring of her works, the autobiography *Exploring the Dangerous Trades,* in 1943. In 1947, she was the first woman to receive the Albert Lasker Public Service Award.

The efforts of Hamilton and others to increase awareness of occupational health issues in the 1920s and 1930s were reinforced by a series of occupational health disasters. A prime example was the Gauley Bridge disaster (also

FIGURE 23.1. ALICE HAMILTON, PIONEER IN OCCUPATIONAL HEALTH IN THE UNITED STATES.

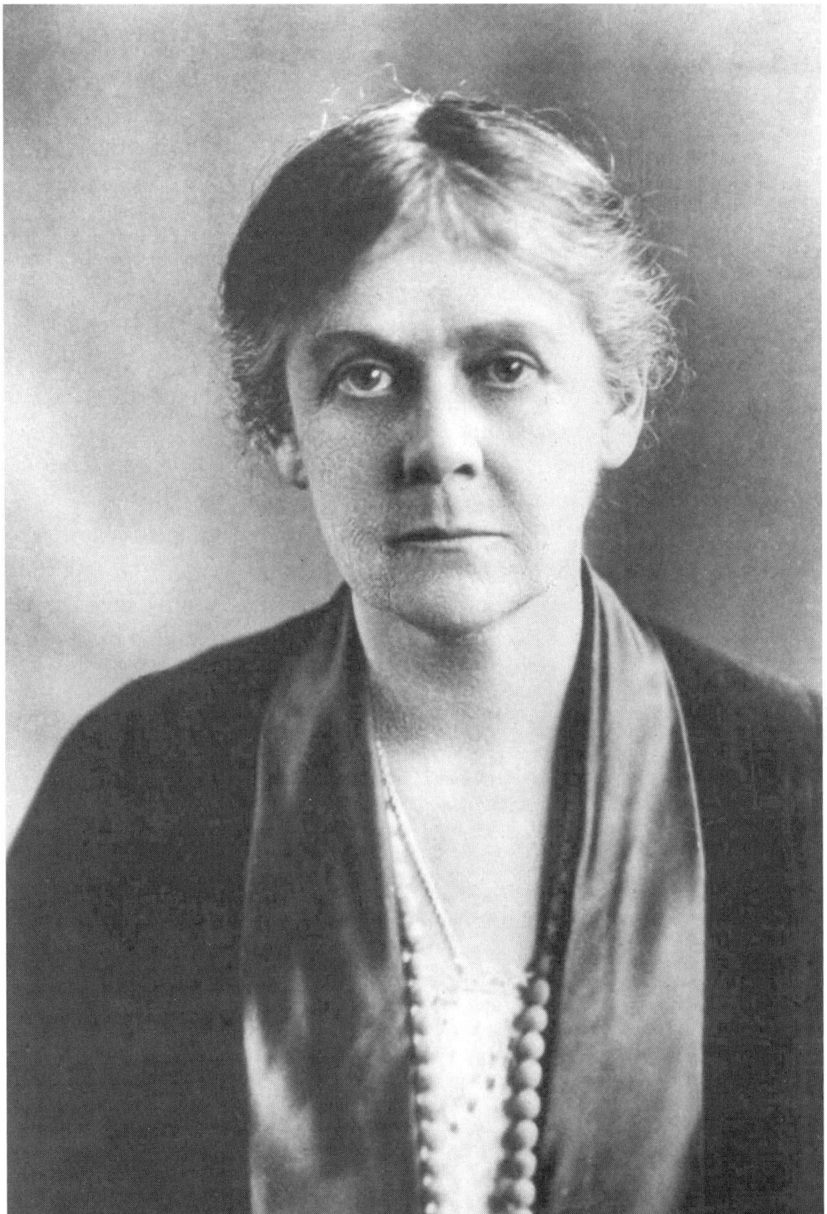

Source: AP/Wide World Photos.

known as the Hawk's Nest incident), in which several thousand workers, mostly African Americans, were employed to drill tunnels through rock as part of a new hydroelectric plant in West Virginia. Controls to reduce exposure to rock dust containing silica were nonexistent, and an estimated 700 workers died of acute silicosis—an inability to breath from lung damage brought on by silica fibers. By 1935, the West Virginia House of Delegates had promulgated a compensation program for silicosis victims.

The latter half of the twentieth century saw the development of modern academic departments of occupational health. One of the most prominent was led by Irving Selikoff (1915–1992) at the Mount Sinai School of Medicine. Selikoff was a physician who conducted some of the first studies linking asbestos exposure to the development of cancer and went on to lead the international effort to control asbestos exposure. Another winner of the Lasker Public Service Award (1952) and a tireless advocate who later lobbied for better recognition and control of other occupational carcinogens, Selikoff wrote: "By the time an agent is discovered and under control, millions of workers may have been exposed. Stopping cancer by stopping exposure may be too late. Tens of thousands will die of cancer because of seeds planted decades ago, unless those seeds can be destroyed. Their families may share the same risk because of contamination brought home, because of reproductive changes made by the same agents, and because of hazardous wastes in the air, water and on the land of their communities" (Ramazzini Institute for Occupational and Environmental Health Research, 2004).

Varieties of Workplace Environments

The nature of work has changed and continues to change for millions of workers, in parallel with profound changes in the world's economies. These changes include a rapid rise in the size of the service and information technology sectors, a relative contraction of manufacturing employment, and a marked transfer of some industries, particularly labor-intensive manufacturing and service work, from developed to developing countries. Such changes have radically changed the profile of workplace risks. Nevertheless, hazards remain, even in the advanced economies of the most developed countries.

The International Labour Organization (ILO) estimates that about half the world's population—about 2.95 billion people worldwide—are engaged in some form of economic activity. The amount of time workers spend at work varies, from 1,467 hours per year in Germany to 2,447 in Korea according to 2001 data (ILO, 2004). The U.S. figure was intermediate, at 1,821 hours per year.

Employment patterns vary in part by the level of a country's economic development. In most nations the largest share of employment is in the services sector, followed by industry, with a small proportion, usually less than 10 percent, in agriculture. In other nations, predominantly transitional economies, agriculture accounts for the largest proportion of employment, followed by services and then industry (ILO, 2003). China has a unique pattern: the largest share of employment is in agriculture, followed by industry and then the services sector. Manufacturing has been steadily declining as a proportion of employment; between 1990 and 2001, it declined in all nations except Honduras and Italy. By 2001, only seven nations still reported manufacturing employment at or above the 20 percent mark: Estonia, Finland, Italy, Japan, Poland, Portugal, and the Republic of Korea.

These trends might seem to signal progress toward safer and healthier workplaces. Indeed, improving occupational safety and health data have emerged in some places and in some industries. However, the reality is that all work—including work that at first glance would seem to be benign—may carry risks of injury or illness. Whereas some industries, such as mining and construction, present obvious dangers to life and limb, others pose more subtle threats—infectious diseases for health care workers, stress for office workers, chemical exposures for dry cleaners.

In many countries a *secondary,* or *informal,* economy accounts for a substantial proportion of employment. Window washers and vendors on the streets of Mexico City or Bangkok, undocumented farmworkers in the fields of California or North Carolina, Turkish construction workers in Germany, and African dishwashers in Spain, all labor in this setting. Such workers usually enjoy few labor rights and tend to be excluded from official statistics and workplace protection programs. Little is known about their health and safety status. However, it is likely that they work longer hours, face more uncontrolled hazards, suffer higher rates of injury and illness, and have fewer protections than workers in more mainstream employment do.

Workplace Health and Safety Problems

A wide range of health and safety problems can arise in the workplace:

- Occupational lung diseases
- Musculoskeletal disorders
- Occupational cancer
- Acute injuries
- Cardiovascular disease

- Disorders of reproduction
- Neurotoxic disorders
- Psychological disorders, including stress
- Noise-induced hearing loss
- Dermatologic conditions
- Infectious diseases
- Symptom-defined disorders, such as multiple-chemical sensitivity

Some of these, such as silicosis, have been recognized since ancient times, and others, such as reproductive toxicity from solvent exposure, have been more recently characterized. Some, such as asbestosis, are unique to the workplace (or nearly so), and others, such as lung cancer, may arise both from occupational and from nonoccupational exposures. Some are minor nuisances, and others are fatal. Each category is briefly described in the following sections.

Occupational Lung Diseases

Lung diseases among workers who breathe high concentrations of contaminated air have been recognized for centuries. One group of occupational lung diseases, the pneumoconioses, results when workers breathe dust that penetrates into the lungs, accumulates, and causes pathological reactions. Examples include asbestosis from breathing asbestos (for example, asbestos miners, insulators and other construction workers, and manufacturers of asbestos products such as brake linings and textiles are at risk), silicosis from breathing silica (miners, quarry workers, and sandblasters are at risk), coal workers' pneumoconiosis (or *black lung*) from breathing coal dust (miners are at risk), and berylliosis from breathing beryllium (hard metal workers are at risk). Victims of these diseases typically suffer from shortness of breath, cough, and weakness and have characteristic findings on chest X-ray. These diseases are largely irreversible and often progress even after exposure has ended.

A second group of occupational lung diseases affects the airways more than the lung parenchyma. Occupational asthma is one example. Hundreds of exposures have been reported to cause occupational asthma. These include chemicals such as toluene diisocyanate (for example, workers who make polyurethane foam products are at risk), trimellitic anhydride (workers exposed to epoxy resins are at risk), and polyvinyl chloride (meat wrappers are at risk). Other causes are naturally occurring molecules that are found in biological matter, such as wheat and other grains (for example, bakers and millers are at risk), certain wood dusts (timber cutters, carpenters, and cabinetmakers are at risk), colophony (solderers are at risk), and latex (health care workers are at risk). Occupational asthma was traditionally thought to result from long-term exposures, but in recent years immediate onset of asthma following acute, high-dose exposures such as chemical spills has been recognized. This unfortunate turn of events has been termed *reactive airways dysfunction syndrome.*

Some diseases affect both the lung parenchyma and the airways. An example is byssinosis (also called *brown lung* or *Monday morning asthma*). This disease, caused by inhaling the dust of cotton or other vegetable fibers (such as hemp, flax, or sisal), causes an asthmalike syndrome that improves after a few days away from work and flares upon returning.

A final category of occupational lung disease is lung cancer. Many workplace exposures have been linked to lung cancer. Examples include asbestos, diesel exhaust, chromium, nickel, and arsenic. A classic example of an occupational lung carcinogen is a chemical called bis-chloromethyl ether (BCME), which caused an outbreak of lung cancer affecting dozens of workers in a chemical factory in Philadelphia in the 1960s.

Musculoskeletal Disorders

Work-related musculoskeletal disorders (MSDs) affect primarily the tendons, muscles, and ligaments of the upper extremities and back. Physical factors, especially repetition, force, and vibration, play an important role in the onset of upper-extremity disorders, whereas heavy lifting, frequent bending and twisting, and whole body vibration are risk factors for low-back disorders (Bernard, 1997). Musculoskeletal disorders associated with office work have increased since the early 1990s and can range in severity from mild symptoms to functional impairment. These problems are quite prevalent in keyboard operators who type for prolonged periods, with more than 50 percent of newly hired computer users experiencing MSDs within the first year on a job (Gerr and others, 2002). Carpal tunnel syndrome of the wrist is a common example of a peripheral nerve entrapment syndrome that can occur in both wrists and be completely disabling. Tendonitis and nerve entrapments, as well as many back injuries, often result from cumulative trauma over time, rather than a single acute injury, accounting for terms such as *repetitive strain injuries* or *cumulative trauma disorders.* Although it is usually easy to identify the cause of such acute work injuries as fractures and lacerations, MSDs, by their nature, usually have a slow and insidious onset, which makes identifying causal factors especially difficult. Problems with recognition are complicated further by the fact that non-work-related activities can also cause MSDs.

Occupational Cancer

Workplace exposures can contribute to the causation of cancers. In general the cancers associated with workplace exposures occur at sites with extensive contact with chemicals—the lungs and skin when they are directly exposed or the liver and urinary tract when they are pathways for the metabolism and excretion of carcinogens—or at sites with unusually susceptible cells, such as bone marrow. In addition to the lung cancers, noted previously, examples include cancers of the skin (from sun exposure in outdoor workers and from arsenic, coal tar, and soot); the pleura and peritoneum, the linings of the lung and abdomen, respectively (almost exclusively from asbestos); the nasal cavity and sinuses (from chromium, nickel, wood, and leather dusts); the liver (from arsenic and vinyl chloride); the bone marrow (from benzene and ionizing radiation); and the bladder (from aromatic amines). In assessing individual cases of cancer, it is often difficult to quantify the relative roles of workplace carcinogens and other potential contributors such as cigarette smoking.

Acute Injuries

According to the National Institute for Occupational Safety and Health (NIOSH) about 10 million traumatic injuries occur in U.S. workplaces each year, of which 3 million are severe and between 5,000 and 10,000 are fatal. The full range of traumatic injuries occurs at work, including amputations, fractures, eye loss, and lacerations.

Fatal injury rates are highest in mining, agriculture, and construction (see Figure 23.2 and also the case example in Box 23.1), resulting from such incidents as mine collapses, tractor rollovers, and trench cave-ins. The transportation sector also features high fatality rates; in fact about half of work-related fatalities are motor vehicle related. Violence in the workplace is also an important cause of fatalities, accounting for the largest share of workplace deaths among women. The highest numbers of occupational homicides occur in retail stores (including liquor stores, gas stations, grocery stores, and jewelry stores), restaurants, hotels, and justice and public order facilities such as courts and prisons. Taxi drivers have the highest rate of occupational fatalities.

Box 23.1. Occupational Injuries Resulting from Falls

Falls have surpassed overall workplace homicides to become the second leading cause of work-related death across all industries. Between 1980 and 1994, deaths due to falls accounted for 10 percent of all occupational fatalities, with an average of 540 deaths per year—10 each week, 2 each working day. In 2000 alone, 717 workers died of injuries caused by falls from an elevation. In many of these fatalities, investigation reveals that noncompliance with regulations contributed to the falls and that the deaths were potentially preventable. Injury and fatality rates are high in

FIGURE 23.2. INCIDENCE RATE OF NONFATAL OCCUPATION INJURY CASES BY PRIVATE SECTOR, 2001.

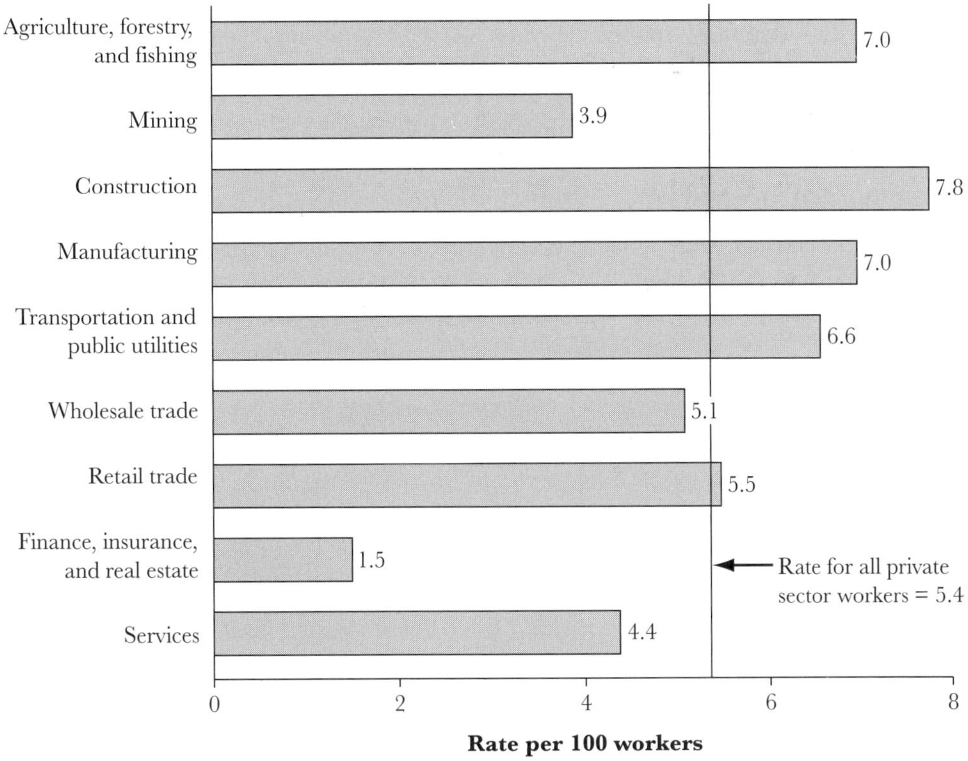

Source: NIOSH, 2004.

the construction industry, and falls are the leading cause of workplace fatalities among construction workers.

Case Presentation

On August 29, 2002, a twenty-three-year-old Hispanic roofer died from injuries he sustained when he fell over the unprotected edge of an elementary school gymnasium roof to an asphalt walkway approximately fifteen feet below. The victim was part of a seven-man roofing crew. He was last seen standing near the edge of the roof pulling on a power cord. No fall protection system was in place. A coworker standing nearby saw the victim fall over the edge. The foreman was working at ground level at the time of the incident and heard coworkers' calls for help. He called 911 from his cell phone while coworkers and school personnel ran to help the victim. Emergency responders arrived within a few minutes and, on observing the severity of the victim's head injury, called for a medical helicopter for transport. The medical helicopter was delayed by weather problems. A military helicopter responded approximately thirty minutes after the incident and transported the victim to a regional trauma center, where he was pronounced dead on arrival. The roofing company had operated for thirty-eight years and had thirty employees. Employees were trained and required to use fall protection, but none was used on the day of the incident (NIOSH, 2003).

Recommendations and Requirements

NIOSH recommends that employers should, at a minimum, (1) incorporate safety in work plans, (2) identify all fall hazards at a worksite, (3) conduct safety inspections regularly, (4) train employees in recognizing and avoiding unsafe conditions, and (5) provide employees with appropriate protective equipment and train them in its use. Passive fall prevention systems, such as guardrails and safety nets, are preferred over active systems, such as personal fall arrest systems (PFASs), because passive systems do not require workers actively to patrol their own safety. A PFAS involves a full-body harness that distributes the fall arrest forces over the body upon impact, self-retracting lifelines that limit the distance a worker can fall, and possibly also rope grabs, lanyards, and anchorage points. The Occupational Safety and Health Administration (OSHA) defines *low-slope* roofing as roofing with a slope less than or equal to a four-foot rise over twelve feet. For low-slope roofs six feet or more aboveground (as in this case), a warning line system is required; this involves a barrier erected on the roof to warn employees that they are approaching an unprotected roof edge. Within the warning line, employees are not required to use a guardrail, body belt, or safety net system. Employees working beyond the warning line require at least a safety monitor, a person responsible for recognizing fall hazards and warning employees about them. Safety monitors are the least protective of all fall protection systems permitted by OSHA, however, and combining the warning line system with other acceptable methods of fall protection is recommended. In this case no warning line system was in place nor was anyone assigned to be the safety monitor, despite the fact that both were required by the company's fall protection plan. In addition, instead of using battery-powered tools, the construction workers had plugged their tools into outlets at ground level. The worker is believed to have fallen while tugging on the entangled power cord of the electric screw gun he was using. Power cords should not be used in areas where they can become entangled (fall risk), near roof edges (fall risk), or where they could be damaged (electrocution risk).

Cardiovascular Disease

Several occupational exposures can contribute to cardiovascular disease. Some are chemicals, such as carbon monoxide, found in motor vehicle exhaust;

methylene chloride, a solvent used by furniture refinishers and others in paint stripping; and carbon disulfide, a chemical that is used in factories to produce rayon and that accelerates atherosclerotic plaque formation. An interesting example of work-related cardiovascular disease occurs among workers involved in nitroglycerin manufacturing; this chemical is used medically to dilate the coronary arteries, but when workers who have become habituated to it through workplace exposure leave the workplace for a few days, they may experience coronary vasoconstriction. Chronic lead exposure among, for example, workers who manufacture lead batteries or who remove lead paint, increases the risk of hypertension as well as abnormalities of cardiac conduction. Physical exposures such as noise and psychosocial stress may also contribute to cardiovascular disease.

Disorders of Reproduction

A number of workplace exposures can threaten reproduction. Examples include insecticides and herbicides, PCBs and polybrominated biphenyls (PBBs), ethylene oxide (a gas used in hospitals to sterilize equipment), metals (lead, arsenic, cadmium, mercury), and solvents. Dibromochloropropane, a nematicide, caused a well-known epidemic of sterility among production workers and farmers using the product. There is concern that exposures to some pesticides and other chlorinated organic chemicals may disrupt the function of the endocrine system, leading to disorders of development in children of exposed workers and contributing to the risk of such diseases as testicular cancer and breast cancer.

Neurotoxic Disorders

The central nervous system is a complex and delicate system that is a common target of toxic exposures. Most people are familiar with the neurotoxic effects of ethanol, a common chemical that is the active ingredient in alcoholic beverages. Many chemicals encountered in the workplace have similar effects. Painters, metal degreasers, plastics workers, cleaners, and other workers who are exposed to solvents such as toluene and perchloroethylene are at risk of central nervous system symptoms such as fatigue, memory loss, difficulty concentrating, and emotional lability. These effects may occur acutely and typically improve after hours or a day away from work. However, long-term exposures may lead to chronic effects and even to a syndrome termed *chronic solvent encephalopathy.* Abnormalities can often be detected on neurobehavioral testing. Some workers improve after discontinuation of exposure, but in some cases the effects appear to be irreversible. Other substances associated with neurobehavioral dysfunction include metals, particularly lead, mercury, arsenic, and manganese; pesticides, such as organophosphates and organochlorines; polychlorinated biphenyls (PCBs); and gases such as carbon monoxide. There is growing evidence that some nervous system toxicants may interact with genetic susceptibility factors to contribute to neurodegenerative diseases such as Alzheimer's, Parkinson's, and amyotrophic lateral sclerosis (Lou Gehrig's disease).

The peripheral nervous system may also be a target of workplace exposures. Organic solvents such as n-hexane, heavy metals such as lead and arsenic, and some organophosphate compounds can damage peripheral nerves, leading to weakness or even paralysis of the hands and feet. Some neurotoxins have unique and specific effects. For example, dimethylaminopropionitrile (DMAPN), an industrial catalyst, can cause paralysis of the bladder.

Psychological Disorders, Including Stress

Stress has emerged as a major occupational health concern. Not only does stress undermine quality of life, but it is a risk factor for hypertension, cardiovascular disease, immune dysfunction, asthma, and possibly other conditions (van der Doef and Maes, 1998). The leading model for understanding workplace stress was laid out by Karasek (1979, 1990) (Figure 23.3). This model emphasizes two dimensions of the workplace experience: job demand and decision control. People with high job demands perceive excessive task requirements or workload, time pressure, and conflicting demands. They describe themselves as "working very hard," "working very fast," and "not having enough time to get the job done." People with low workplace control say that they lack influence at work and are unable or unauthorized to make decisions or influence their jobs. Jobs with high demands and low control are those that are most stressful, as indicated by the downward arrow in Figure 23.3. However, high job demands are not necessarily bad; when combined with high control, demanding jobs can be highly stimulating and motivating. A third dimension of the workplace, social support, can mitigate some of the effects of stress.

Noise-Induced Hearing Loss

Loud noises are a feature of many workplaces. Exposure to noise can be acute, as with the sudden burst of an explosion, or chronic, as with the routine daily use of tools in construction trades, machines in manufacturing, or equipment in numerous other jobs. Noise causes hearing loss by damaging the delicate hair cells in the inner ear. According to NIOSH, 30 million Americans are exposed to hazardous noise at work, and 10 million have suffered permanent hearing loss as a result. Sound is measured in decibels. The decibel scale is logarithmic, so a noise

FIGURE 23.3. THE KARASEK JOB STRAIN MODEL.

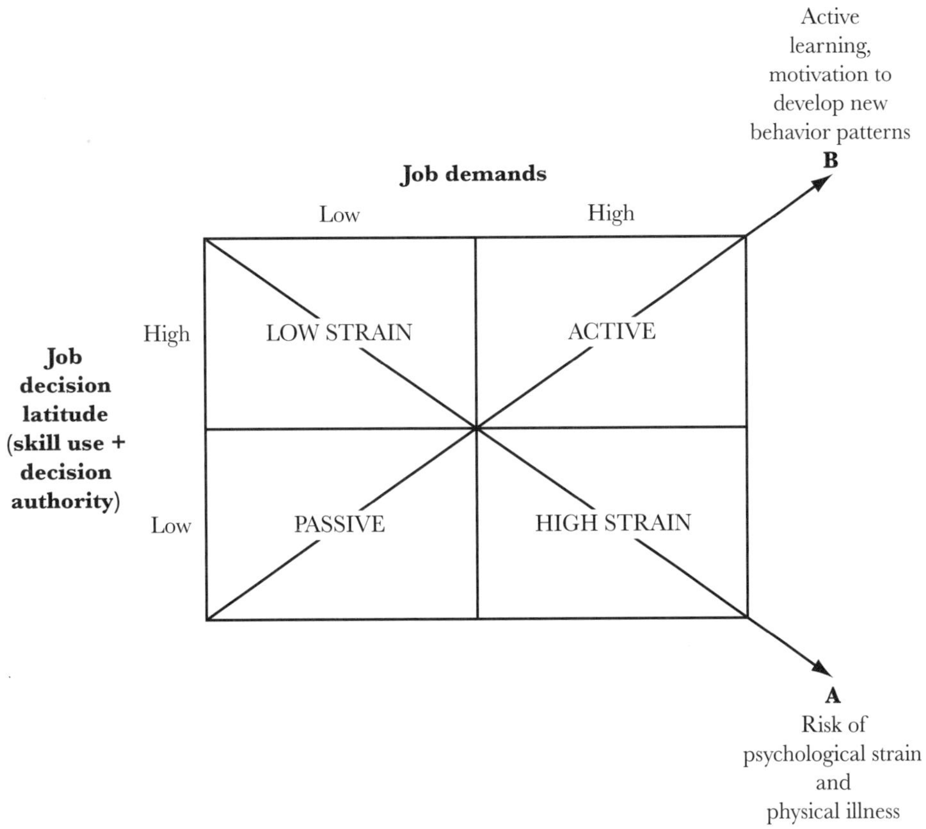

Source: Schnall, Landsbergis, and Baker, 1994.

at 110 decibels is 10 times louder than a noise at 100 decibels. A humming refrigerator reaches about 40 decibels, a normal conversation takes place at about 60 decibels, and traffic noise in a city may reach 80 decibels. In a woodshop the noise level is about 100 decibels, chainsaw noise measures about 110 decibels, and the loud noises produced by motorcycles, firecrackers, and firearms can reach 120 to 140 decibels. The noise levels of tools used in carpentry work can range well above 100 decibels, and prolonged exposure to noise above 85 decibels can cause hearing loss.

Like many occupational exposures, noise can be addressed through primary prevention—reducing the noise at the source, if possible, or enclosing it so it does not reach the work zone. If these measures are impossible, then personal protective equipment such as earplugs may be used. However, earplugs exemplify some of the limits of personal protective equipment. Many workers do not like them, they offer inadequate protection if selected or used improperly, and they may introduce problems of their own, such as inhibiting social interaction and blocking workers' ability to hear shouted warnings or alarms.

Dermatologic Conditions

Skin disorders account for about one in eight reported occupational diseases. Although several patterns may occur—such as burns, abrasions, and lacerations—the most common workplace skin disease is contact dermatitis. This condition is a reaction to substances that come into contact with the skin. It may represent an allergic reaction, or it may result simply from irritation. Not surprisingly, the most common site of contact dermatitis is the hands and arms. Rates of contact dermatitis are highest in agriculture, forestry, and fishing, followed by manufacturing. A wide range of chemicals and other materials can cause contact dermatitis, including cutting oils in the machine tool trades, grease and lubricating oils among mechanics, formaldehyde and dyes among textile workers, and latex (in gloves) among health care workers. With chronic contact dermatitis, a worker's skin may become thickened, hyperpigmented, dry, fissured, and itchy. Skin in this condition not only causes troubling symptoms for the worker but may also function poorly as a barrier, permitting chemicals to cross the skin and enter the person's general circulation. In fact, even intact skin may be a pathway by which chemicals enter the body, as described in Chapter Two. Chemicals that undergo percutaneous absorption include organophosphates, carbon disulfide, and methyl butyl ketone.

Infectious Diseases

Many categories of workers are at risk of occupational infections. Health care workers confront blood-borne pathogens such as Hepatitis B virus and HIV/AIDS; prevention requires scrupulous attention to avoiding contact with body fluids, handling needles and other sharps properly, and using protective equipment. Health care workers are also at risk of airborne infections, with tuberculosis being the most feared because of the associated bacterium's ability to be transported over relatively long distances in infectious droplet form. Other occupations at risk for infectious disease include farmworkers, slaughterhouse workers, and other workers who come into contact with animals and who may contract illnesses (the *zoonoses*) usually affecting animals; outdoor workers who may be bitten and infected by insects; and teachers and child-care workers who are exposed to diseases of children. Infections in workers may be a problem in broader public health terms as well. For examples, a restaurant worker with active hepatitis A may transmit the disease to large numbers of customers.

Symptom-Defined Disorders

The range of occupational illnesses also includes *syndromes* for which the biology and exact causal relationships remain obscure. One example is sick building syndrome (SBS), a constellation of symptoms including headache, fatigue, nasal irritation, and confusion. As explained in Chapter Twenty-Two, SBS typically presents as a cluster of symptoms among occupants of an office building with limited fresh air intake and point sources of indoor air pollution (such as copy machine emissions). Another symptom-based syndrome is multiple-chemical sensitivity (MCS), which is characterized by symptoms similar to those of sick building syndrome (headache, fatigue, respiratory irritation, confusion, muscle aches, abdominal distress). MCS sufferers, after an initial workplace (or nonoccupational) exposure event, begin to report exacerbations whenever exposed to relatively low levels of irritants such as fragrances, motor vehicle exhaust, and marker pen odors. Some cases of MCS begin as SBS.

Epidemiology of Occupational Injuries and Illnesses

Are workplace injuries and illnesses a large public health problem? To answer this question we need to assess data on the magnitude of the problem. And to do this we need to understand the data and where they come from.

There are two main sources of primary occupational injury and illness data: employer reports and insurance system reports. In the United States, employers are required to maintain records of injuries and illnesses in their workplaces. Each year the Department of Labor's Bureau of Labor Statistics collects these reports from a national sample of employers, compiles the data, extrapolates them to the entire workforce, and issues its annual *Survey of Occupational Injuries and Illnesses.* Insurance data in the United States come primarily from workers' compensation systems, but useful information may also come from private health insurance systems such as health maintenance organizations (HMOs). Both employer reports and workers' compensation data are likely to underreport; those who collect data have incentives not to report, and although most occupational injuries are readily recognized and attributed to work, many cases of illness go unrecognized or unacknowledged.

A third source of data is the health care system. For example, the Census of Fatal Occupational Injury (CFOI) compiles multiple data sources on workplace deaths, the National Electronic Injury Surveillance System uses hospital emergency department information, and the National Health Interview Survey annually surveys U.S. household members on health issues including injuries. These sources are informative only when information on occupation is collected at the time health care services are delivered. For example, emergency departments must seek and record information on the work-relatedness of injuries if this source is to yield useful occupational data.

Finally, a variety of secondary data sources—sources not specifically intended to collect occupation-related health data—can yield statistics on specific populations or types of illness or injury. These sources may offer an indirect way of accessing statistics that are normally hard to collect. Examples of secondary data sources on work-related injury and illness include vital records (death certificates), labor union pension records, police and justice system reports (data on transportation crashes and interpersonal violence events), government regulatory agency records (for example, national transportation agency records), emergency medical service (EMS) records, coroner's reports, employment records, and trauma registries (that collect work-related injury information).

With this general understanding of where occupational health statistics come from, we can consider the data available on occupational mortality (deaths) and morbidity (injuries and illnesses). In the United States, occupational fatalities have slowly declined over recent decades. Currently, between 5,000 and 6,000 workers are killed on the job each year, or about 100 every week. About half of these acute fatalities are motor vehicle related, and about 1 in 10 is a workplace homicide. The remaining fatalities represent a broad range of mishaps: the construction worker buried when a trench collapses, the farmworker entangled in a power take-off, the warehouse worker struck by a forklift, the petrochemical worker suffocated while cleaning out a chemical tank. The *numbers* of fatalities are highest in, in descending order, the construction, transportation, agriculture, and service sectors; however, the *rates* are highest in, in descending order, agriculture, mining, construction, and transportation (see Figure 23.2).

This fatality picture changes drastically once fatal illnesses are taken into account. In the United States, estimates of the annual number of fatalities from work-related disease range from 49,000 (Steenland and others, 2003) to 65,000 (Leigh and others, 1997), approximately ten times higher than the acute fatality count. The causes of these deaths include occupational cancer, respiratory and cardiovascular disease, chronic renal failure, and hepatitis. Many of these work-related deaths are not ordinarily attributed to occupational exposures and go uncounted in official data.

Globally, workplace injuries and illnesses are an even larger problem, due to the transfer of hazards from developed to developing nations and inadequate safeguards in many poor nations (see Chapter Thirteen). The International Labour Organization (ILO, 2004) recently estimated that occupational injuries and illnesses kill between 1.9 and 2.2 million workers each year, a number that exceeds the toll from traffic crashes and war combined. The occupational fatality rate varies greatly, from 5.3 per 100,000 workers per year in established market economies such as the United States, Europe, and Japan, to 21.0 in sub-Saharan Africa, 22.5 in the Middle East, and 23.1 in parts of Asia (Takala, 1999, 2000). Again, official statistics probably underestimate the true burden of occupational fatalities, due to underreporting, misdiagnosis, and in many poor countries, the existence of a substantial informal economy in which no reporting occurs at all. (Box 23.2, for example, describes fatal and nonfatal injuries in India.)

Box 23.2. Occupational Health in India

India is the world's second most populous nation, encompassing a diverse range of cultures and languages and spanning a broad range of climates and ecologies. It is also arguably the world's largest democracy, one that is undergoing huge and rapid changes related to rural-urban demographic shifts, industrialization and development, a globalizing economy, and associated alterations in people's lifestyles. India has grown a huge middle class, fueled by a productive education system and growth in the manufacturing, information technology, and biotechnology sectors—all while substantial segments of the population remain afflicted by poverty, unemployment, malnutrition, infectious diseases (such as malaria and tuberculosis), and disability.

One of the most prominent and universal symbols of the hazards of industrialization and globalization remains the 1984 disaster in Bhopal, India, in which a pesticide plant owned by the U.S.-based Union Carbide corporation experienced a chemical leak resulting in the release of massive clouds of methyl isocyanate over the city of Bhopal. By 1994, the death toll was estimated at 6,000. Independent agencies now estimate that the number of deaths related to this disaster has reached between 15,000 and 20,000, and several hundred thousand residents have experienced subsequent chronic health effects such as respiratory impairments, adverse reproductive outcomes, and cognitive deficits (Dhara and Dhara, 2002). Efforts to provide support for victims and settle claims resulting from the disaster became enmeshed in politics and a tug-of-war between the government's interests in justice and in continued foreign investment. Nevertheless Bhopal—and the rest of the country—have continued to develop, with the city now a thriving industrial hub of textile manufacturing, food processing, and electrical manufacturing.

Occupational health in India currently poses the same huge challenges that confront many rapidly developing countries. These challenges include enforcing lax health and safety standards, training a workforce with uneven levels of education, promoting health and safety concerns to the many thousands of small businesses and families that are engaged in home-based industries, and dealing with foreign industries that offer the promise of jobs but that also carry substantial occupational health risks. At the same time, some of India's occupational health issues are somewhat specific to India. For example, many of the estimated 100 million women in India who work outside the home are employed by industries engaged in such hazardous activities as the manufacturing of fireworks and matches (high exposures to potassium chloride, tetraphosphorous trisulfide, and lead tetraoxide and high risks of fire and explosions), the manufacturing of *bidi,* or cigarettes (nicotine exposures several times higher than those of smokers), agriculture (exposures to pesticides), and electronics manufacturing (exposures to solvents, arsine, phosphine, lead, and cadmium). Child labor is also a major problem in India (Venkateswarlu and others, 2003), with an estimated 70 to 115 million children between the ages of five and fourteen in the workforce, primarily in the agricultural sector (Figure 23.4). Many work twelve hours a day, are frequently exposed to pesticides, and are not provided with safety equipment or even shoes to protect their feet or water to wash their hands and clothes. Some materials banned for industrial use in other countries, such as asbestos, continue to be used in India, with an estimated 10 million industrial and mine workers in India exposed to asbestos or other dusts at concentrations of health concern.

When we turn from fatalities to nonfatal injuries and illnesses, the workplace is also an important contributor. According to the Bureau of Labor Statistics (BLS), a total of 4.4 million injuries and illnesses were reported in private industry workplaces during 2003, an annual incidence of 5.0 cases per 100 full-time worker equivalents. The highest incidence was in the construction and manufacturing sectors (each with 6.8 cases per 100,000 workers per year) and the lowest was in the financial services sector (BLS, 2004b). Although the most recent BLS data do not report the types of cases, data from the late 1990s suggest that nearly two-thirds of cases were accounted for by musculoskeletal diseases, such as carpal tunnel syndrome and tendonitis, and noise-induced hearing loss. Skin diseases such as dermatitis accounted for about one case in eight. Other diseases, such as asbestosis, cancers, and lead-induced hypertension, account for a small proportion of cases. However, diseases that develop over a long period (such as asbestosis) or that have workplace associations that are not immediately obvious (such as cancers or lead-induced hypertension) are known to be greatly underrecorded in databases such as the BLS survey.

These injuries and illnesses not only cause suffering for workers and inconvenience for both workers and employers but are also costly. The Liberty Mutual 2002 Workplace Safety Index estimated that direct costs for occupational injuries in 2002 rose to $49.6 billion (Liberty Mutual, 2004).

FIGURE 23.4. OCCUPATIONAL HEALTH IN INDIA: A CHILD WORKER IN A MARKETPLACE.

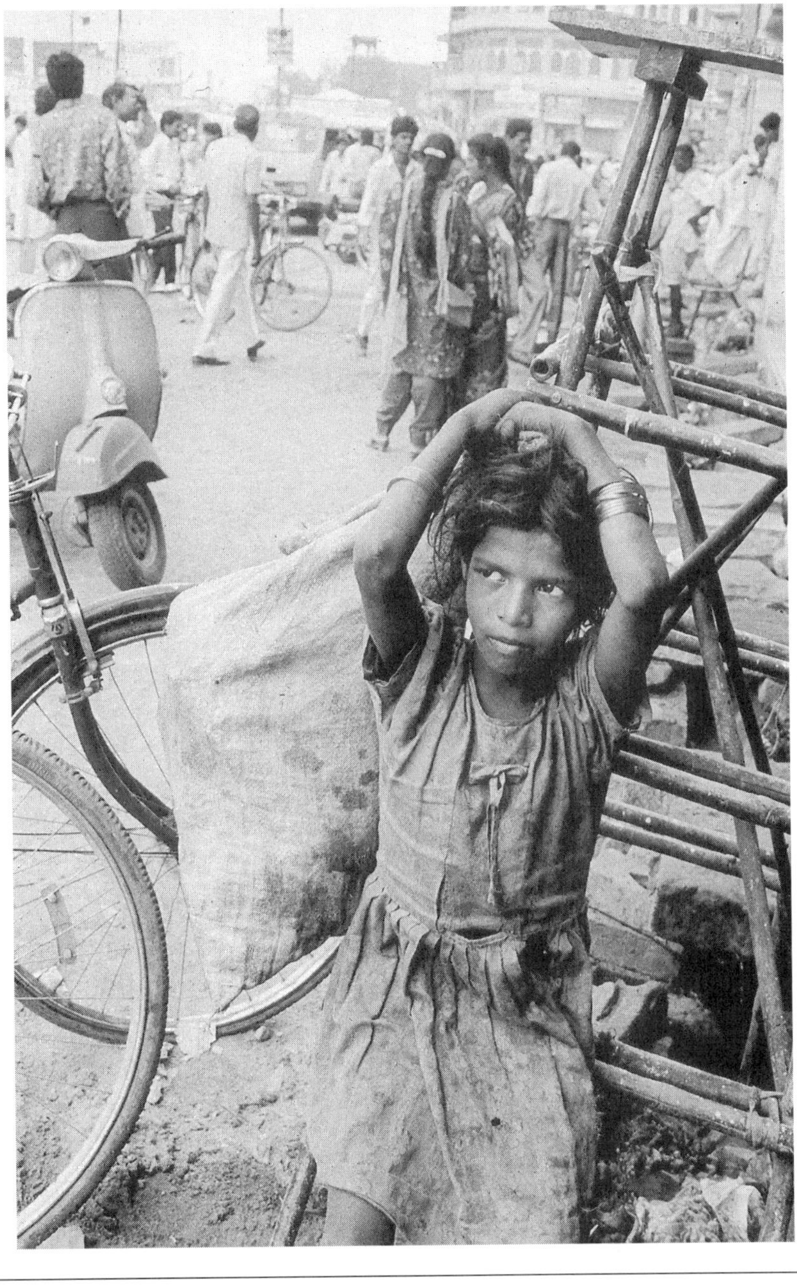

The risks of occupational injury and disease vary by age, occupation, industry, geographic location, and even the size of the workplace. An ironworker clearly faces a higher risk than an insurance underwriter (Figure 23.5). Similarly, two occupations accounted for more than 63 percent of work-related anxiety, stress, and neurotic disorder cases in the United States in 2001: technical, sales, and administrative support workers (2,250 cases) and managerial and professional specialty occupations (1,331 cases) (NIOSH, 2004). Workplace size is also an important variable; smaller workplaces generally experience higher rates of injury and illness, partly because fewer resources are available to control health and safety risks. In mining, for example, the highest fatal injury rates occur in mines employing fewer than ten workers. Internationally, the availability and adequacy of health and safety protections vary greatly, with workers in some countries facing a substantially higher risk than workers in other countries (even after accounting for differences in reporting).

Three industries deserve special mention, because they have unusually high work-related morbidity and mortality: mining, agriculture, and construction.

Mining

There are 500,000 miners in the United States, and at least 13 million miners working worldwide. Miners face risks of injuries from mine collapses, explosions, and power equipment and risks of illnesses from inhaling dusts and diesel fumes and from chemical exposures. In the United States, fatalities in mining have decreased over time due to the passage of mine health and safety legislation and due to improvements in mining technology, such as roof bolting to prevent roof cave-ins, dust suppression and ventilation techniques, and use of noncombustible materials to prevent fires and explosions. Despite these improvements, mining remains one of the most hazardous U.S. occupations.

Agriculture

Farming is also one of the most hazardous occupations. In the United States the leading agents of fatal and nonfatal injuries to farmers and farmworkers are tractors, farm machinery, livestock, building structures, falls, and bodies of water. Environmental exposures include pesticides, volatile organic compounds (fuel), noxious gases, airborne irritants, noise, vibration, zoonoses, and stress. Farm family members may also be exposed to these hazards, making agriculture a unique example of the intersection of occupational and environmental exposures. On the approximately 2.2 million farms in the United States in 1999, there were 1.3 million farmworkers and 4.6 million farm residents (U.S. Department of Agriculture, 2000). Farming is

FIGURE 23.5. FOUNDRY WORKER POURS MOLTEN METAL.

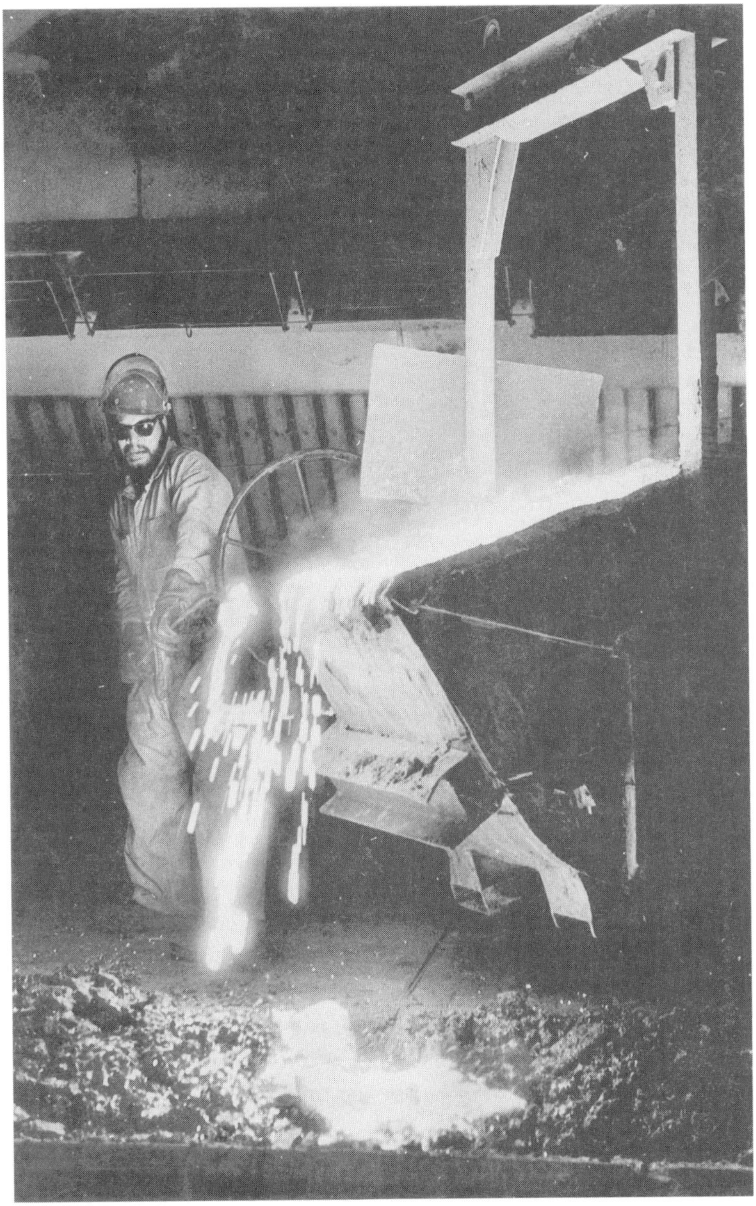

Note: Among the risks of foundry work are heat effects, burns, and silicosis (from shaking out the molds).

also unique in that child labor is common. As of 1991, the most recent year for which data are available, 27 percent of farm residents were youths less than twenty years old and at least 300,000 youths between the ages of fifteen and seventeen worked alongside their parents as farmworkers (Dacquel and Dahmann, 1993). Children account for about 20 percent of all farm fatalities and a higher proportion of the total number of nonfatal farm injuries. An estimated 38,000 children under the age of twenty years who lived on, worked on, or visited farms and ranches were injured in 1998, and approximately 100 unintentional injury deaths occur annually among children and adolescents on U.S. farms (Myers and Hendricks, 2001). Although the exact number of youths exposed to farm hazards annually is unknown, it has been estimated at more than 2 million.

Construction

The construction trades also rank high on the list of most hazardous occupations, in terms of both fatal and nonfatal occupational injuries. These injury rates vary by specific construction occupation, a common pattern in many industries. For example, the rate of lost-worktime injuries and illnesses in 2001 ranged from 131.2 per 10,000 workers for painters to 751.8 for ironworkers, nearly a sixfold difference. Falls to a lower level accounted for the highest number of fatal injuries among construction workers (4.3 per 100,000 full-time workers), and highway crashes accounted for the next highest number (1.7 per 100,000 full-time workers) (NIOSH, 2004).

Special Working Populations

Occupational health professionals are concerned with the safety of all workers, but certain populations of workers are especially vulnerable to workplace risks. This may occur for one or more of several reasons: they may confront excessive risks on the job, they may be susceptible to certain risks due to social or biological factors, or they may enjoy fewer protections than other workers. Four categories of workers deserve mention: women, socially and economically disadvantaged groups, children, and elders.

Women Workers

Women in the United States and internationally are more likely than men to work in low-skill, low-paying jobs. These jobs may feature exposures to chemicals that can threaten reproductive health, repetitive movements that can lead to musculoskeletal injuries, and other hazards. The reasons women are at higher risk than men are for work-related health problems have more to do with the social and economic influences affecting women's work than with biological sex differences. Less attention is paid to health risks specific to female-dominated occupations such as health care worker, cleaner, or keyboard operator; there is a (mis)perception that women's work is harmless and does not require major occupational health consideration; and the dual roles that women usually face as wage earners and family caregivers are not accommodated in the workplace.

Although over 47 million women worked full time at wage and salary jobs in the United States in 2002 (BLS, 2004a), women remain at a salary disadvantage when compared to men. Full-time working women as a group earned only about 78 percent of what men earned in 2002 (BLS, 2003). A 1998 Department of Labor study of employment and wage patterns attributed this disparity, in part, to the overrepresentation of women in traditionally lower-paying jobs. A much higher proportion of working women than working men were employed in technical, sales, and administrative support occupations (41 percent of women versus 19 percent of men). A higher proportion of working men, conversely, were employed in production jobs (20 percent of men versus 2 percent of women) where median weekly earnings were 20 percent higher than those for technical, sales, and administrative support jobs (Bowler, 1999).

Lower-paying positions can mean more mentally and physically demanding work. Many female-dominated jobs, such as cleaning and child care, are also socially isolating. Women's work is erroneously perceived as not being overtly dangerous compared to male-dominated work such as mining or construction. However, injury statistics demonstrate that injury rates in female-dominated industries are excessive. Health care workers experience high rates of overexertion from physically handling patients and are at risk of blood-borne pathogen exposures due to needlestick injuries, and precision industry assemblers and food service workers experience high rates of repetitive strain and cumulative trauma injuries due to repetitive manual work and static postures. Underestimating the health risks in such gender-segregated jobs results in insufficient health and safety protections for women.

Socially and Economically Disadvantaged Workers

In the United States and internationally, ethnic minorities who are socially marginalized are also more likely to be employed in physically demanding jobs with inherent hazards, such as construction, farmwork, mining, or meat packing (Frumkin, Walker, and Friedman-Jiménez, 1999). In the United States, problems related to this marginalization are compounded for undocumented immigrant workers, who are frequently employed in farm or service work but who are hidden from occupational safety regulatory authority. Undocumented immigrants often have no alternative to enduring unsafe working conditions and have no recourse if they are injured or become ill as a result of their work. The vulnerability of undocumented immigrant workers in the United States is now starting to receive increased attention among workplace safety advocates, and addressing their circumstances is becoming a major thrust of occupational health advocacy campaigns. This issue, like many other social and economic injustice problems, will likely be solved only if the requisite political will is in place to realize broad-reaching legislative protections for immigrant workers. The next decade will undoubtedly witness active debate around this issue, and occupational health professionals from clinicians to safety professionals to labor union representatives will contribute to that debate, with their ultimate goal being the protection of immigrant workers.

Child Workers

Another example of an especially vulnerable group in terms of workplace health and safety protections is young workers. In the United States, child labor laws are in place that are intended to recognize the inherent vulnerabilities that youths face, including the increased risk that they will be exploited in the workplace. However, the lack of comprehensive regulatory enforcement and the wide-scale lack of information among child workers, parents, and employers about child worker rights and protections contribute to the thousands of preventable work-related injuries and illnesses among youths each year. The conditions of child farmworkers are illustrative (also see Box 23.3). Child labor laws include exceptions for youths working in agriculture, and enforcement programs are weak. These two realities result in excessively hazardous conditions for teenage and younger farmworkers.

Box 23.3. Recollections of a Child Farmworker

When I was fourteen I worked in the fields for two weeks, chopping the weeds around the cotton plants. . . . I woke up one night, I couldn't breathe; I was allergic to something they were spraying in the fields. I stopped breathing . . . I tried to drink water but I couldn't so I ran into my mom's room 'cause I didn't have no air in me and I was like [wheezing gasps] trying to get air in there but I couldn't . . .

At the hospital they said I was allergic to something out there . . . something they were spraying. . . . They sprayed the fields in the morning. We'd be out there when they were doing it, or when they were leaving, or we could see them doing other fields. They'd spray by plane.

Source: Richard M., seventeen years old, in an interview conducted in Casa Grande, Arizona, Oct. 27, 1998; quoted in Human Rights Watch, 2000.

Older Workers

Another special workplace population consists of older workers. With average life expectancy now over seventy-five years in developed countries and sixty-four years in developing countries, people are staying in the workplace at older ages than they used to in the twentieth century. Productivity might be expected to decline with age, but occupational capacity studies to date do not consistently support this relationship (Wegman, 2000). In many contexts both life experience and years of experience on the job better predict job performance. It is perhaps most useful to think about age and work performance in terms of specific tasks. Performance in jobs requiring making knowledge-based judgments without time pressure is enhanced by age; skilled manual work is not necessarily affected by age if it requires average exertion; however, fast-paced data-processing performance can be impaired by age.

Special health concerns of older workers pertain most to injury. In general the frequency of injury decreases with age, although injury severity, including the likelihood of death, increases with age. However, as with the relationship between age and job performance, the relationship between injury severity and age varies by job type. Older construction workers are at higher risk than younger workers for nonfatal falls from ladders, whereas younger farmers are at higher risk for fatal machinery accidents. Older workers are at risk for unfair treatment when they are selectively used as part-time or occasional workers without the same pay and benefits as full-time coworkers. Hiring and employment practices must be equitable regardless of age to ensure that older workers are not forced into marginalized positions.

Prevention of Occupational Injuries and Illnesses

Prevention is the overwhelmingly most important element of the approach to any occupational health problem. It is critical to appreciate that prevention is most effective when it is considered and practiced on multiple levels.

Approaches to Prevention

In a workplace with an assortment of hazards, what is the best approach to preventing injuries and disease? A useful way of thinking about prevention is to adopt an integrated strategy that draws on key aspects from public health, industrial hygiene, and environmental stewardship models. Occupational disease and injury are caused by exposure to hazards on the job, and prevention requires controlling exposures. Anticipation of hazardous exposures, surveillance of hazards and health effects, analysis of health effects, and ultimately hazard control are all critical parts of an integrated approach to prevention. (Prevention strategies are discussed further in Chapter Twenty-Nine.)

A wide variety of tactics and technologies is available for controlling hazards. Four basic choices are production process reengineering, work environment controls, administrative controls, and worker behavior controls including personal protective devices. As explained in more detail in Chapter Twenty-Nine, a hierarchy of strategies exists, with a clear preference for workplace design that eliminates or minimizes exposures.

An example of healthy workplace design, and one of the best strategies, is *product* or *process substitution,* that is, replacing a toxic hazard or risky process with a safer alternative. For example, polyvinyl chloride (PVC) manufacturing might be replaced by production of another plastic. This would definitively eliminate hazardous workplace exposures to vinyl chloride monomer, and it would also offer upstream and downstream benefits: a reduced need for chlorine production (which often occurs at hazardous chloralkali plants), a reduced need for phthalate plasticizers (which can enter the human food chain), and a reduced need for incineration of chlorine-containing plastic products (which form dioxins when burned). Such changes require consideration of occupational hygiene at the earliest stage of planning a new industry or industrial plant. This consideration remains underemphasized in the training of most engineering and business executives, but it comprises a strategic goal that should be a part of the movement to make industry *green* (protective of the environment) in the twenty-first century.

Examples of possible work environment controls, continuing with the case of PVC manufacturing, are setting up automatic unloading of vinyl chloride monomer (instead of having workers manually open and pour from the bags), installing ventilation to reduce dust exposure, and enclosing the polymerization process to reduce worker exposures. Least preferable are protocols that call for workers to wear personal protective equipment, such as protective clothing and respirators, because this equipment relies for its effectiveness on human behavior and compliance (which is never infallible), is often uncomfortable to wear (especially for an eight-hour work shift), and sometimes poses safety hazards of its own (for example, a respirator reduces the worker's ability to communicate during an emergency). Occupational health specialists prefer using worker-focused interventions only when no other control alternatives exist.

Finally, administrative controls involve changes in how tasks are organized and performed. For example, in a workplace with a record of back injuries from lifting, the employer might provide training in proper lifting techniques and require that all lifts above a certain weight be performed by teams of two workers rather than by individuals. Another administrative control strategy is to restrict hazardous jobs to workers considered less susceptible to their effects, but such an approach can discriminate against certain classes of workers. For example, one firm that used lead in its production process restricted women of childbearing age from lead-exposed jobs (unless they could show that they were unable to bear children). This practice was challenged as discriminatory, and a landmark Supreme Court decision, *UAW* v. *Johnson Controls,* found for the plaintiff, limiting the scope of administrative controls (see the case example in Box 23.4).

Box 23.4. Occupational Lead Exposure and Reproductive Health

General population exposures to lead in the United States have declined over 70 percent in the past twenty years, largely due to the phaseout of leaded gasoline and the elimination of lead solder in food cans. However high exposures to lead can still occur in many different ways, including occupational exposure.

Case Presentation

A twenty-eight-year-old woman works as a torch burner, cutting steel coated with lead paint. She is now considering having a child. During the past eight years, her blood lead level has twice exceeded 40 μg/dL, the OSHA occupational standard, but currently it is 22 μg/dL. She is concerned that if she has a child it may face risks stemming from her current and past lead exposures.

Toxicity of Lead

High exposure to lead can occur through eating food contaminated by lead (from cooking in lead-based ceramic ware, for example), drinking water contaminated by lead-soldered plumbing, taking part in hobbies that use lead (such as making stained glass), using personal products that contain lead (such as *kohl,* an eyeliner cosmetic sometimes contaminated with lead), living in a home where lead paint was used and is now peeling, and working in an environment where lead is used or handled (such as automobile battery plants [see Figure 23.6], smelters, or construction projects that involve disturbing existing lead paint). NIOSH recently estimated that occupational exposures alone mean that every year more than 25,000 workers experience blood lead levels exceeding 40 μg/dL, the maximum allowable level under current regulations.

The routes of lead absorption are inhalation and ingestion. After lead is absorbed it reaches the blood and is rapidly distributed across membranes into organs such as the brain, testes, and bone. High exposures in both children and adults (producing

FIGURE 23.6. WORKERS IN AN AUTOMOBILE BATTERY PLANT, A SOURCE OF OCCUPATIONAL LEAD EXPOSURE.

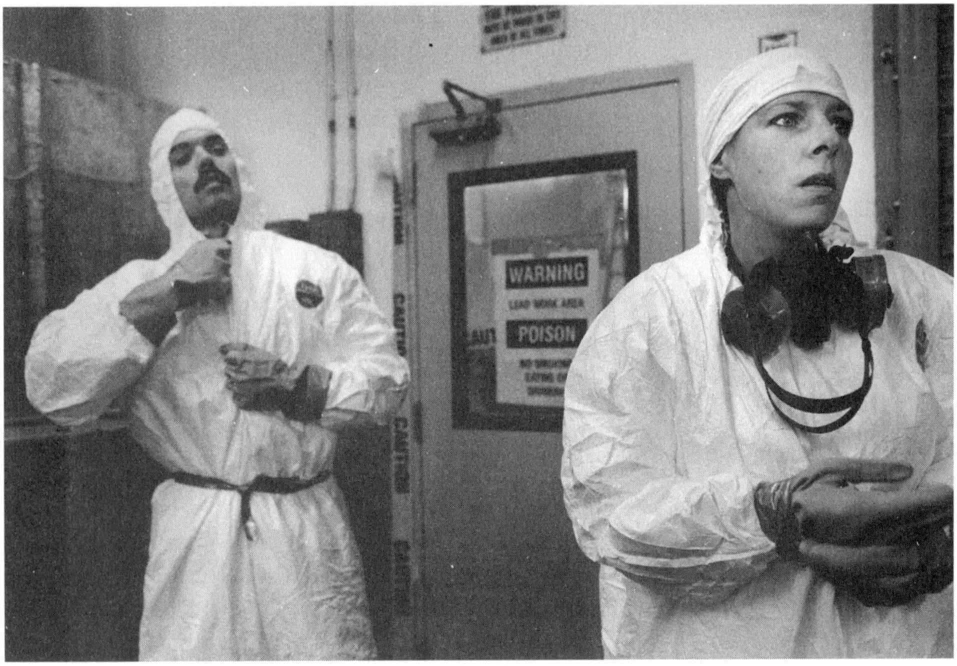

www.earldotter.com

blood lead levels greater than 40 to 80 μg/dL) can result in a wide spectrum of nonspecific symptoms of poisoning, including abdominal pain, lethargy and confusion, and joint pain. In children, recent studies indicate that even relatively modest levels of exposure (for example, a crawling toddler who lives for several weeks in a house with peeling lead paint and whose blood lead level reaches 10 or 15 μg/dL) can be enough to impair mental development. Screening for blood lead levels in children six months to five years of age is mandatory in many states, with current federal guidelines recommending interventions when blood lead levels exceed 10 μg/dL. Excretion occurs primarily through the kidneys into urine; treatment with chelating agents (drugs that bind with metal and hasten their excretion) is sometimes warranted.

In addition to creating a threat of acute toxicity, lead accumulates in bone, where it can reside for many years after exposure ends and from which it can reenter the blood stream. This internal source, operating over long periods of time, can increase the risk of central nervous system toxicity, kidney damage, hypertension, and reproductive effects. The rate of reentry is greatly accelerated during times of high bone resorption, such as pregnancy. Recent studies suggest that during pregnancy maternal bone lead stores are transferred into blood, cross the placenta, and affect fetal development, resulting in reduced birthweight, reduced skeletal growth, and lower performance on cognitive testing at two years of age (Hu and Hernández-Avila, 2002). Calcium supplementation has been suggested as a potential therapeutic intervention during pregnancy and lactation because it may decrease bone resorption during high-demand periods and in turn reduce lead mobilization from bone; studies to test this hypothesis are ongoing.

Legal Issues

A famous class action suit occurred in 1984 after Johnson Controls, a large manufacturing company, passed a policy excluding women of childbearing age from lead-exposed jobs in that company (unless they could provide medical evidence that they were unable to bear a child). After a long court battle that saw the policy upheld in federal district and appeals courts, the U.S. Supreme Court overturned the lower court decisions, saying that "the bias in the policy was obvious and that fertile men but not fertile women are given a choice as to whether they wish to risk their reproductive health for a particular job" (Annas, 1991). This case set a landmark precedent that has essentially restricted OSHA from promulgating regulations that protect female workers in ways different from protections for male workers.

OSHA's lead standard sets forth lengthy and detailed regulations for different kinds of potential occupational lead exposures. These regulations specify under what conditions an employee may be exposed to lead, what levels of exposure are permissible, and in what ways an employer is responsible for monitoring these exposures. The regulations also outline the steps that must be taken for an employee who has had an unacceptable exposure (over the limits), including access to medical care and wage protection during time off from work. However, pursuant to the Johnson Controls decision, there is no provision for gender differences in exposure, and should a woman become pregnant the fetus is not protected from lead exposure. The regulations do state that an employee can seek out medical advice "with respect to reproductive health . . . and may request pregnancy testing or lab evaluation of male fertility" (OSHA, 2005).

Occupational Safety and Health Regulation

Regulatory approaches should be considered central to any discussion of occupational hazard prevention. Workplace regulations—what they are, which government agency creates and enforces them, their effectiveness, and so on—vary widely from region to region and from country to country. In most countries, government has intervened in the private market, with standard setting, enforcement, and health and safety training, in response to a range of factors: the inability of voluntary efforts in the free market to protect workers adequately, the regular occurrence of widely publicized occupational health disasters, pressure by labor unions, and the existence of international guidelines from the International Labour Organization. Some countries subscribe to regional policies (such as those set by the European Union), but most have developed their own approaches to safety and health regulation.

In the United States (the focus of most of the ensuing discussion), the primary law regulating health in the workplace is the Occupational Safety and Health Act (OSH Act) of 1970. This legislation established the federal Occupational Safety and Health Administration (OSHA) to set and enforce standards and the National Institute for Occupational Safety and Health to conduct research and carry out site-specific health hazard evaluations. Other important laws include the Mine Safety and Health Act (MSHA) of 1969 and the Toxic Substances Control Act (TSCA) of 1976.

There are limits to OSHA's regulatory authority. In 1979, Congress exempted businesses with ten or fewer employees from routine OSHA inspections (although specific complaints can still trigger inspections). States may opt to maintain their own occupational safety and health regulatory programs; in theory these must be at least as protective as OSHA regulations, although some states have been notably lax in their enforcement. OSHA's jurisdiction also does not extend to federal or state workers; such workers must be covered by safety and health programs maintained by their own agencies.

What is OSHA's obligation in terms of setting standards? Section 6(b)(5) of the OSH Act requires the U.S. secretary of labor to set a standard that "most adequately assures, to the extent feasible, on the basis of the best available evidence, that no employee will suffer material impairment of health or functional capacity, even if such employee has a regular exposure to the hazard dealt with by such standard for the period of his working life." With regard to toxics, the burden of proving that a substance is hazardous is placed on OSHA. OSHA is also required to prove that any controls that it proposes are technically feasible.

Not surprisingly, many of the regulations proposed by OSHA are heavily contested, usually by the affected industries or labor unions, or by both, and several challenges have had to be addressed in federal court. Among precedents that have been set in such rulings are that OSHA must conduct quantitative risk assessment as part of the standard-setting process (the benzene standard), that OSHA may require medical monitoring and, based on that monitoring, may require removal of an employee from work while maintaining full pay and benefits (the lead standard), and that an OSHA standard is legally acceptable even if some employers are forced out of business, as long as the entire affected industry is not disrupted (the asbestos standard).

Perhaps the most far-reaching of all OSHA standards was established under the Hazards Communication Act (also known as the *right-to-know* standard), which requires manufacturers and employers to disclose information regarding chemical exposures to their employees (and to select others, such as their health providers). Under this Act, employers need to make available *material safety data sheets* (MSDSs) that list chemical ingredients and associated health risks for all potentially toxic substances used in the workplace. The Act also gives employees legal access to their workplace medical and exposure records.

Of course the effectiveness of regulations is dependent on enforcement. Enforcement is carried out in large part by a national network of regional and area offices that perform workplace inspections to check for violations of health and safety standards. OSHA makes random inspections of workplaces (sometimes without advance notice), with an emphasis on workplaces entailing a higher than average level of risks. In addition, certain events, such as workplace fatalities, trigger automatic inspections, and any employee can request an OSHA inspection while also requesting that his or her name be kept confidential. Violations of standards that are uncovered in such inspections are punishable by fines. However, OSHA's capacity to perform inspections is limited by the small number of OSHA inspectors (around 1,000) relative to the millions of U.S. workplaces and by antiregulatory political pressure. Instead of conducting inspections, OSHA often simply relays a complaint to an employer by mail, requiring as a response only a reply that discusses how a complaint will be addressed. Industries with high risks of toxic chemical exposures—as opposed to high risks of injuries—are often given less attention. Finally, OSHA's ability to conduct its work is heavily dependent on a budget that has historically been vulnerable to political interventions.

Conclusion

The workplace is a keenly important environment in terms of human health and safety. For many people, it rivals the home as the environment in which the most time is passed. It is also the environment in which the risks of hazardous exposures are highest. In fact much of what we know about the toxic effects of environmental chemicals derives from workplace studies, underlining the role of the workplace as an unintentional laboratory of human exposures. Workplace exposures also occur in settings that are socially complex, politically complex, and shaped by labor-management relations. Efforts to control workplace hazards have been highly contested, with labor unions claiming safe, healthy work as a human right, and employers insisting on their right to control workplace conditions and their need to control production costs.

In the United States, workplace injuries and illnesses have declined in recent years, as a result of numerous factors. One factor may be progressive underreporting.

Other factors reflect real improvements: technical improvements in many industrial processes and the shift in the economy from manufacturing to services and information, which entails a reduction in risk. Still others involve the export of hazards to poorer countries, as part of the globalization of production. In the coming century, occupational health and safety will increasingly need to focus on vulnerable working populations—those in the United States that are marginalized, such as migrant and undocumented workers, and those in poor nations that lack effective regulatory protection. For all these working populations, public health protection will grow out of traditional workplace protection strategies: workplace redesign, workplace exposure controls, personal protection, and administrative controls.

Thought Questions

1. Other than the fact that the workplace is where many people spend much of their lives, what environmental health characteristics distinguish the workplace from other settings?
2. What role did the textile industry play in the history of occupational health?
3. Discuss the various health effects that can be caused by the inhalation of asbestos.
4. Identify at least two workplace exposures that can increase the risk of heart disease.
5. Why are earplugs a less than ideal solution for protecting workers from noise-induced hearing loss?
6. What factors play a role in the underreporting of workplace illnesses and deaths?
7. Why are children particularly vulnerable to occupational health risks, and in what industries do children make up a major segment of the workforce?
8. What are *administrative controls* in the context of occupational health prevention strategies?
9. In the United States, occupational health regulations are set by the Occupational Safety and Health Administration (OSHA). What are some of the major factors that limit their effectiveness?

References

Annas, G. J. "Fetal Protection and Employment Discrimination: The Johnson Controls Case." *New England Journal of Medicine,* 1991, *325,* 740–743.

Bernard, B. P. *Musculoskeletal Disorders (MSDs) and Workplace Factors.* National Institute for Occupational Safety and Health. [http://www.cdc.gov/niosh/ergosci1.html]. 1997.

Bowler, M. "Women's Earnings: An Overview." *Monthly Labor Review.* [http://www.bls.gov/opub/mlr/1999/12/art2full.pdf]. 1999.

Bureau of Labor Statistics. "Women at Work: A Visual Essay." *Monthly Labor Review,* 2003, *126,* 45–50.

Bureau of Labor Statistics. "Current Population Survey 2002: Employed Persons by Full- and Part-Time Status and Sex, 1970–2002 Annual Averages." U.S. Department of Labor. [http://www.bls.gov/cps/wlf-tables16.pdf]. 2004a.

Bureau of Labor Statistics. "Workplace Injuries and Illnesses in 2003." [http://www.bls.gov/iif/oshwc/osh/os/osnr0021.txt]. 2004b.

Dacquel, L. T., and Dahmann, D. C. *Residents of Farms and Rural Areas: 1991.* Current Population Reports, Series P-20, no. 472. Washington, D.C.: U.S. Government Printing Office, 1993.

Dhara, V. R., and Dhara, R. "The Union Carbide Disaster in Bhopal: A Review of Health Effects." *Archives of Environmental Health,* 2002, *57,* 391–404.

Frumkin, H., Walker, E. D., and Friedman-Jiménez, G. "Minority Workers and Communities." *Occupational Medicine State of the Art Reviews,* 1999, *14,* 495–518.

Gerr, F., and others. "A Prospective Study of Computer Users, I: Study Design and Incidence of Musculoskeletal Symptoms and Disorders." *American Journal of Industrial Medicine,* 2002, *41,* 221–235.

Hu, H., and Hernández-Avila, M. "Lead, Bones, Women, and Pregnancy: The Poison Within?" *American Journal of Epidemiology,* 2002, *156,* 1088–1091.

Human Rights Watch. *Fingers to the Bone: United States Failure to Protect Child Farmworkers.* [http://www.hrw.org/reports/2000/frmwrkr]. 2000.

International Labour Organization. "Key Indicators of the Labor Market." [http://www.ilo.org/public/english/employment/strat/kilm/trends.htm#figure%204b]. 2003.

International Labour Organization. "Global Estimates of Fatalities Caused by Work-Related Diseases and Occupational Accidents, 2002." [http://www.ilo.org/public/english/protection/safework/accidis/globest_2002/dis_world.htm]. 2004.

Karasek, R. "Job Demands, Job Decision Latitude, and Mental Strain: Implications for Job Redesign." *Administrative Science Quarterly,* 1979, *24,* 285–308.

Karasek, R. "Health Risk with Increased Job Control Among White-Collar Workers." *Journal of Organizational Behavior,* 1990, *11*(3), 171–185.

Karasek, R., and Theorell, T. *Healthy Work: Stress, Productivity, and the Reconstruction of Working Life.* New York: Basic Books, 1990.

Leigh, J. P., and others. "Occupational Injury and Illness in the United States: Estimates of Costs, Morbidity, and Mortality." *Archives of Internal Medicine,* 1997, *157,* 1557–1568.

Liberty Mutual. "Liberty Mutual Workplace Safety Index." [http://www.libertymutual.com/omapps/ContentServer?cid=1078439448036&pagename=ResearchCenter%2FDocument%2FShowDoc&c=Document]. 2004.

Myers, J., and Hendricks, K. J. *Injuries Among Youth on Farms in the United States, 1998.* DHHS (NIOSH) Publication no. 2001-154. Cincinnati: National Institute for Occupational Safety and Health, 2001.

National Institute for Occupational Safety and Health. "Hispanic Roofer Dies After 15-Foot Fall from a Roof—North Carolina." Fatality Assessment Control Evaluation Program. [http://www.cdc.gov/niosh/face/In-house/full200303.html]. 2003.

National Institute for Occupational Safety and Health. *Worker Health Chartbook, 2004.* NIOSH Publication no. 2004—146. [http://www2a.cdc.gov/niosh-chartbook/ch2/ch2-1.asp] and [http://www2a.cdc.gov/niosh-chartbook/imagedetail.asp?imgid=116]. 2004.

Occupational Safety and Health Administration. Regulations (Preambles to Final Rules): Section 4-IV: Summary and Explanation of the Standard: Occupational Exposure to Lead. [http://www.osha.gov/pls/oshaweb/owadisp.show_document?p_table=PREAMBLES&p_id=950]. 2005.

Ramazzini Institute for Occupational and Environmental Health Research. "The Selikoff Fund for Environmental and Occupational Cancer Research." [http://www.ramazziniusa.org/oct00/selikoff_fund.htm]. 2004.

Schnall, P. L., Landsbergis, P. A., and Baker, D. "Job Strain and Cardiovascular Disease." *Annual Review of Public Health,* 1994, *15,* 381–411.

Steenland, K., and others. "Dying for Work: The Magnitude of U.S. Mortality from Selected Causes of Death Associated with Occupation." *American Journal of Industrial Medicine,* 2003, *43*(5), 461–482.

Takala, J. "Global Estimates of Fatal Occupational Accidents." *Epidemiology,* 1999, *10,* 640–646.

Takala, J. "Indicators of Death, Disability and Disease at Work." *Asian-Pacific Newsletter on Occupational Health and Safety,* 2000, *7*(1), 4–8.

U.S. Department of Agriculture, National Agricultural Statistics Service. *Agricultural Statistics 2000.* [http://www.usda.gov/nass/pubs/agr00/acro00.htm]. 2000.

Van der Doef, M., and Maes, S. "The Job Demand-Control(-Support) Model and Physical Health Outcomes: A Review of the Strain and Buffer Hypotheses." *Psychology and Health,* 1998, *13,* 909–936.

Venkateswarlu, D., and others. "Child Labour in India: A Health and Human Rights Perspective." *Lancet,* 2003, *362* (suppl.), S32–S33.

Wegman, D. H. "Older Workers." In B. S. Levy and D. H. Wegman (eds.), *Occupational Health: Recognizing and Preventing Work-Related Disease and Injury.* (4th ed.) Philadelphia: Lippincott, 2000.

For Further Information

LaDou, J. (ed.). *Current Occupational & Environmental Medicine.* (3rd ed.) New York: Lange Medical Books/McGraw–Hill, 2004.

Levenstein, C., and Wooding, J. (eds.). *Work, Health and Environment: Old Problems, New Solutions.* New York: Guilford Press, 1997.

Levy, B. S., and Wegman, D. H. (eds.). *Occupational Health: Recognizing and Preventing Work-Related Disease and Injury.* (4th ed.) Philadelphia: Lippincott, 2000.

Rosenstock, L., Cullen, M. R., Brodkin, C. A., and Redlich, C. A. (eds.). *Textbook of Clinical Occupational and Environmental Medicine.* (2nd ed.) Philadelphia: Elsevier Saunders, 2005.

Weeks, J. L., Levy, B. S., and Wagner, G. R. (eds.). *Preventing Occupational Disease and Injury.* Washington D.C.: American Public Health Association, 1991.

CHAPTER TWENTY-FOUR

RADIATION

Arthur C. Upton

Radiant energy exists in two forms: (1) electromagnetic waves of widely differing energies and wavelengths and (2) accelerated atomic particles varying in energy, mass, and charge. The diverse forms of radiation are shown in Figure 24.1. They differ in their physical characteristics and, accordingly, in the ways in which they transfer energy to an absorbing medium. Some types of radiation can deposit enough sharply localized energy to disrupt atoms and molecules in their paths, whereas others can deposit only enough energy to excite atoms and molecules. Radiations of different types thus vary markedly in their biological effects. For this reason the health effects of each form of radiation are considered separately in this chapter. This chapter also considers the health effects of ultrasound, a form of energy that is often classified with radiation for public health purposes but that actually consists of high-frequency mechanical vibrations and is not a component of the electromagnetic spectrum.

Historical Background

Since time immemorial the sun and fire flames have both been known to be sources of light and heat that could injure individuals overexposed to them. Other sources of potentially hazardous radiation were not generally recognized, however, until after Roentgen's discovery of the X-ray, in 1895. The X-ray was

FIGURE 24.1. THE ELECTROMAGNETIC SPECTRUM.

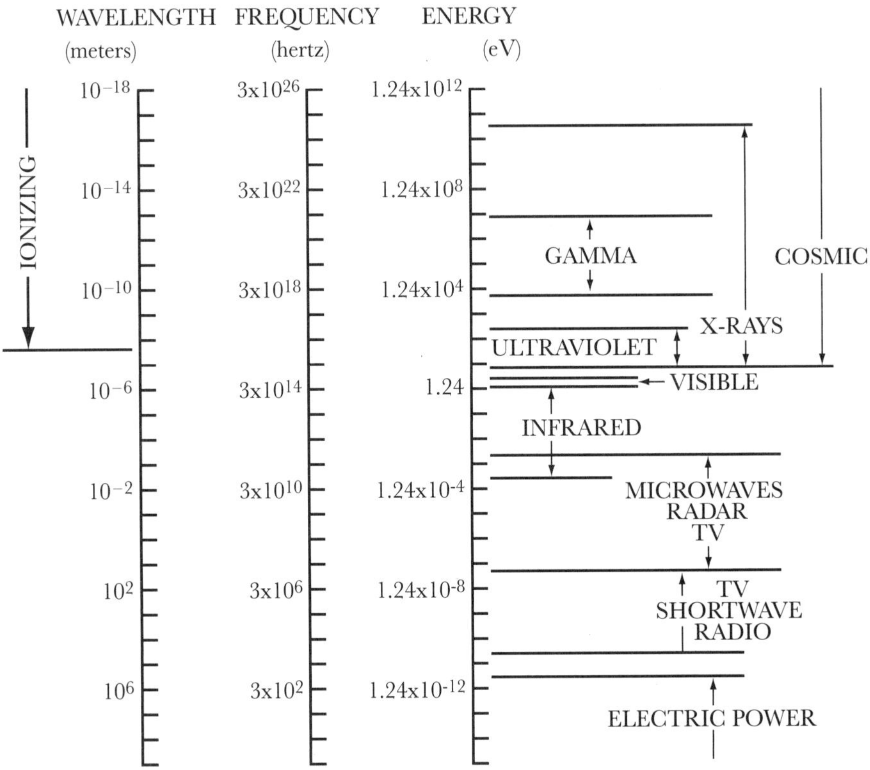

Source: Reprinted from *Medical Effects of Ionizing Radiation, 2nd Edition,* Fred A. Mettler, © Copyright 1995, with permission from Elsevier.

then introduced into medical practice so rapidly that within barely a year ninety-six cases of radiation injury were reported (Stone-Scott, 1897). Most of the injuries initially seen were acute skin reactions on the hands of those working with the early radiation equipment, but in a short time many other types of injury were also being reported, including the first cancers attributed to ionizing radiation (see Table 24.1 and Figure 24.2).

In the century that has elapsed since Roentgen's discovery, our knowledge of radiation injuries has been greatly advanced by extensive studies of the effects of radiation in humans, laboratory animals, and other model systems (Upton, 1986, 1987). Historical findings of particular public health significance include, first, the occurrence of rapidly fatal reactions to irradiation in heavily exposed radiation accident victims and atomic bomb victims; second, the delayed

TABLE 24.1. RADIATION INJURIES FOLLOWING ROENTGEN'S 1895 DISCOVERY OF THE X-RAY, 1896–1912.

Date	Type of Injury	Reported By
1896	Dermatitis of hands	Grubbe
1896	Smarting of eyes	Edison
1897	Epilation	Daniel
1897	Constitutional symptoms	Walsh
1899	Degeneration of blood vessels	Gassman
1902	Cancer in X-ray ulcer	Frieben
1903	Inhibition of bone growth	Perthes
1903	Sterilization	Albers-Schonberg
1904	Blood changes	Milchner and Mosse
1906	Bone marrow changes	Warthin
1911	Leukemia in five radiation workers	Jagic
1912	Anemia in two X-ray workers	Belere

Source: Stone, 1959.

FIGURE 24.2. A PIONEER RADIOLOGIST TESTING HIS FLUOROSCOPE BY EXAMINING HIS OWN HAND, FULLY EXPOSING HIMSELF AND HIS PATIENT IN THE PROCESS.

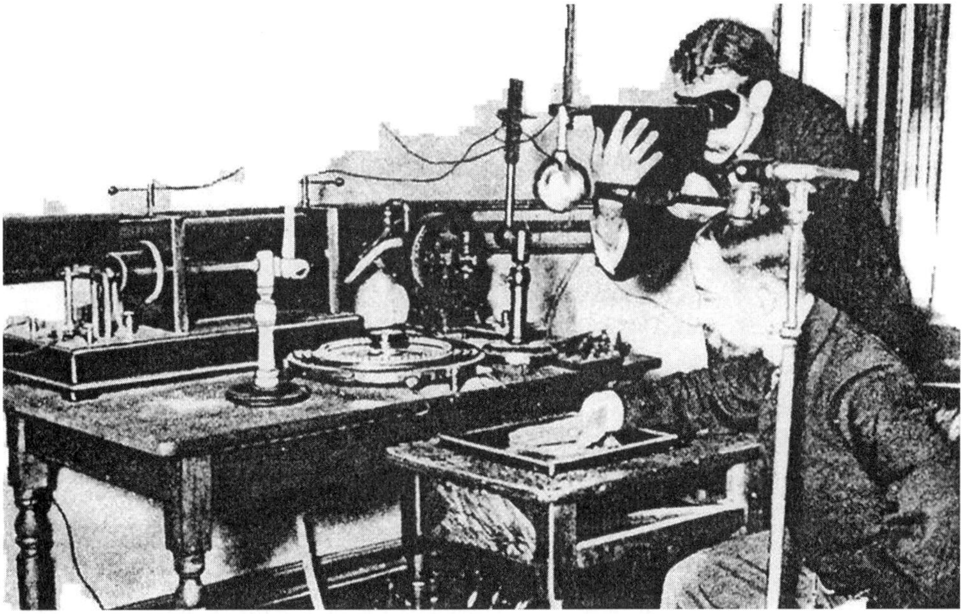

Source: From Percy Brown, *American Martyrs to Science Through the Roentgen Rays,* 1936. Courtesy of Charles C. Thomas Publisher, Ltd., Springfield, Illinois. 1936.

occurrence of dose-dependent increases in the frequency of lung cancers in underground hardrock miners, skeletal cancers in radium dial painters, skin cancers and leukemias in early radiologists, and cancers of the many types that developed in atomic bomb survivors and other irradiated populations; and third, the occurrence of dose-dependent increases in the frequency of severe mental retardation and other developmental disturbances in children irradiated prenatally (Upton, 1986, 1987; Mettler and Upton, 1995). Over the years, research into the health effects of various forms of radiation has received continuing impetus from radiation's expanding uses in medicine, science, and industry. The resulting knowledge of radiation effects has contributed importantly to the development of measures for protecting human health against other environmental hazards as well.

In the following sections, the discussion of each radiation type begins with an introduction to its nature, sources, and levels in the environment and then moves on to address such further issues as the types and mechanisms of injury and means of prevention and protection.

Ionizing Radiation

Ionizing radiations are those forms of radiation that can deposit enough localized energy in living cells to break chemical bonds and give rise to ions and free radicals. Such radiations feature electromagnetic waves of extremely short wavelengths (Figure 24.1) and accelerated atomic particles (for example, electrons, protons, neutrons, and alpha particles). Doses of ionizing radiation are customarily measured in terms of the corresponding amounts of energy that are deposited in the absorbing tissues (Table 24.2).

Natural sources of ionizing radiation include cosmic rays; radium and other radioactive elements in the earth's crust; internally deposited potassium-40, carbon-14, and other radionuclides normally present in living cells; and inhaled radon and its daughter elements (Table 24.3). The dose received from cosmic rays varies with elevation, being twice as high in mountainous regions as at sea level and up to two orders of magnitude higher at jet aircraft altitudes (National Council on Radiation Protection and Measurements [NCRP], 1987; United Nations Scientific Committee on the Effects of Atomic Radiation [UNSCEAR], 2000). Likewise, the dose received from radium may be increased by a factor of two or more in regions where the earth is rich in this element (NCRP, 1987). The largest dose from natural sources is typically the dose to the bronchial epithelium from inhaled radon (Table 24.3), which can vary by an order of magnitude or more, depending on the concentration of radon in indoor air (NCRP, 1984; UNSCEAR,

TABLE 24.2. QUANTITIES AND DOSE UNITS OF IONIZING RADIATION.

Quantity	Dose Unit	Definition
Absorbed dose	Gray (Gy)[a]	Energy deposited in tissue (1 joule/kg)
Equivalent dose	Sievert (Sv)[b]	Absorbed dose weighted for the ion density (potency) of the radiation
Effective dose	Sievert (Sv)	Equivalent dose weighted for the sensitivity of the exposed organ(s)
Collective effective dose	Person-Sv	Effective dose applied to a population
Committed effective dose	Sievert (Sv)	Cumulative effective dose to be received from a given intake of radioactivity
Radioactivity	Becquerel (Bq)[c]	One disintegration per second

[a]Another unit used for the same purpose is the rad: 1 rad = 100 ergs per gm = 0.01 Gy.

[b]Another unit used for the same purpose is the rem: 1 rem = 0.01 Sv.

[c]Another unit used for the same purpose is the curie (Ci): 1 Ci = 3.7×10^{10} disintegrations per second = 3.7×10^{10} Bq.

2000). In cigarette smokers, even larger doses—up to 0.2 Sv (20 rem) per year—may be received by the bronchial epithelium from polonium, another alpha emitter that is normally present in tobacco smoke (NCRP, 1984).

In addition to radiation received from natural sources, people are also exposed to radiation from artificial sources, the largest being the use of X-rays in medical diagnosis (Table 24.3). The effective doses received in various types of diagnostic examinations vary widely, ranging from less than 0.01 mSv (millisieverts) for examination of the arm or leg to more than 4 mSv for a barium enema. Lesser sources of exposure to man-made radiation include radioactive minerals (for example, uranium-238, thorium-232, potassium-40, and radium-226) in building materials, phosphate fertilizers, crushed rock, and combustible fuels; radiation-emitting components of TV sets, video display terminals, smoke detectors, and other consumer products; radioactive fallout from atomic weapons (for example, cesium-137, strontium-90, strontium-89, carbon-14, hydrogen-3, zirconium-95); nuclear power (for example, hydrogen-3, carbon-14, krypton-85, iodine-129, and cesium-137), and nuclear waste (Table 24.3). Contrary to popular misconception, the irradiation of food to rid it of microbial contaminants does not render the

TABLE 24.3. AVERAGE AMOUNTS OF IONIZING RADIATION RECEIVED ANNUALLY BY A RESIDENT OF THE UNITED STATES.

	Dose[a]	
Source	**mSv**	**%**
Natural		
Radon[b]	2.0	55
Cosmic	0.27	8
Terrestrial	0.28	8
Internal	0.39	11
Total natural	2.94	82
Artificial		
X-ray diagnosis	0.39	11
Nuclear medicine	0.14	4
Consumer products	0.10	3
Occupational	<0.01	<0.3
Nuclear fuel cycle	<0.01	<0.03
Nuclear fallout	<0.01	<0.03
Miscellaneous[c]	<0.01	<0.03
Total artificial	0.63	18
Total natural and artificial	3.57	100

Note: The values tabulated represent averages for the entire population; doses to specific individuals and subgroups may be substantially lower or higher.

[a]Average effective dose to soft tissues.

[b]Average effective dose to bronchial epithelium alone.

[c]Department of Energy facilities, smelters, transportation, and so forth.

Source: Adapted from National Research Council, 1990.

food radioactive or cause subsequent consumers of the food to be exposed to radiation.

Workers in certain occupations receive additional doses, depending on their job assignments and working conditions. Such occupations include, among others, medical and industrial radiography, nuclear reactor construction and operation, well logging, uranium mining and enrichment, and working on an airline crew. The average dose received occupationally by monitored radiation workers in the United States each year is less than that received from natural sources, and less than 1 percent of such workers receive a dose approaching the maximum permissible limit (50 mSv, or 5 rem) in any given year (NCRP, 1989). In less developed countries, however, where adequate facilities, equipment, and safety measures are often lacking, occupational doses tend to be larger (UNSCEAR, 1988, 2000).

Types and Mechanisms of Injury

Ionizing radiation, impinging on a living cell, collides randomly with atoms and molecules in its path, giving rise to ions and free radicals, which break chemical bonds and cause other molecular alterations that may injure the cell and its immediate neighbors. The spatial distribution of such events along the path of the radiation, known as the *linear energy transfer* (LET) of the radiation, depends on the energy, mass, and charge of the radiation. X-rays and gamma rays are sparsely ionizing in comparison with charged particles; for example, an alpha particle typically gives up all its energy in traversing only a few cells (Goodhead, 1988). The initial physicochemical changes that are produced occur almost instantaneously, but the evolution and expression of any resulting biological effects may take minutes, days, or years, depending on the types of effects in question.

Any molecule in the cell may be altered by radiation, but DNA is the most critical biological target because of the limited redundancy of the genetic information it contains. A dose of radiation that is large enough to kill the average dividing cell (2 Sv, or 200 rem) suffices to cause hundreds of lesions in that cell's DNA (Ward, 1988). Most such lesions are reparable, but those produced by a densely ionizing radiation (such as a proton or an alpha particle) are generally less reparable than those produced by a sparsely ionizing radiation (such as an X-ray or a gamma ray) (Goodhead, 1988; Ward, 1988). For this reason the relative biological effectiveness (RBE) of densely ionizing radiations exceeds that of sparsely ionizing radiations for most forms of injury (International Commission on Radiological Protection [ICRP], 1991).

Genetic Effects

Damage to DNA that remains unrepaired or that is misrepaired may be expressed in the form of mutations, the frequency of which approximates 10^{-5} to 10^{-6} per locus per Sv (National Research Council [NCR], 1990). The mutation rate appears to increase as a linear-nonthreshold function of the dose, implying that a single ionizing particle traversing the DNA may suffice to cause a mutation (NRC, 1990; UNSCEAR, 2000; NCRP, 2001). With low-LET (sparsely ionizing) radiation, however, the yield of mutations per unit dose typically decreases with decreasing dose rate, passing through a minimum in the range of 0.1 to 1.0 cGy (centigray) per minute, below which it rises again with further reduction of the dose rate (Vilenchik and Knudson, 2000). This variation in the mutagenic effectiveness of low-LET radiation is interpreted to signify that dose rates in the range of 0.1 to 1.0 cGy per minute are optimal for the error-free repair of DNA damage and that the adaptive response required for such repair is elicited progressively less effectively as the dose rate is reduced below about 0.1 cGy per minute (Vilenchik and Knudson, 2000). In this connection it is noteworthy that a similar, DNA repair-enhancing adaptive response can be elicited by prior exposure to an appropriate *conditioning* dose of radiation in some cells (UNSCEAR, 1994, 2000; NCRP, 2001); however, it is not clear whether the repair of all types of DNA lesions is enhanced by the response or how widely such a response is shared among different types of cells (Wojcik, 2000). Furthermore, it is noteworthy that the mechanisms that normally act to facilitate DNA repair or to eliminate cells in which the damage remains unrepaired may not operate effectively in cells in which one or more of the responsible homeostatic genes (for example, p53) has been mutated or lost (Nicholson and Thornberry, 1997).

In addition to its mutagenic effects, radiation may also cause changes in chromosome number and chromosome structure, the types and frequencies of which vary, depending on the stage of the cell cycle in which they are produced. The dose-response relationships for such chromosome aberrations are typically linear-quadratic at high doses and dose rates, and more nearly linear, with shallower slopes, at lower doses and dose rates of low-LET radiation (NCRP, 2001). Such aberrations in blood lymphocytes are elevated to a similar extent in radiation workers and in human populations residing in areas of high natural background radiation levels; and they serve as a useful biological dosimeter in radiation workers, radiation accident victims, and other exposed persons (Bender and others, 1988; Wang and others, 1990). Irradiation can also cause chromosome aberrations to arise in the progeny of exposed cells many cell generations later, owing to the induction of a transmissable genomic instability in the exposed cells (Morgan and others, 1996). In some types of cells, moreover, preexposure to a conditioning dose can reduce the frequency of chromosome aberrations produced by a subsequent test dose delivered in vitro (UNSCEAR, 1994). However, it is questionable whether such an adaptive response can be assumed to afford significant protection against the effects of chronic low-level irradiation, because a dose of at least 5 mGy (milligrays) delivered at a rate of at least 50 mGy per minute appears to be required to elicit the response; the protective effect of the response lasts but a few hours, and the response varies markedly from person to person, some individuals appearing to be entirely nonresponsive (Wojcik, 2000).

Heritable genetic effects of irradiation have been well documented in other organisms but have yet to be demonstrated conclusively in humans. Extensive studies in the more than 76,000 children of Japanese atomic bomb survivors have not detected any elevations in untoward pregnancy outcomes, neonatal deaths, malignancies, balanced chromosomal rearrangements, sex-chromosome aneuploids, alterations of serum or erythrocyte protein phenotypes, changes in sex ratio, or disturbances in growth and development (NRC, 1990). Likewise, although a case-control study has suggested that an excess of leukemia and non-Hodgkin's lymphoma in young people residing in the village of Seascale, England, might have resulted from the inheritance of genetic changes caused by the occupational irradiation of their fathers (Gardner and others, 1990), there are strong reasons for rejecting this hypothesis (Doll, Evans, and Darby, 1994; Wakeford and others, 1994a, 1994b).

In the absence of definitive evidence of heritable effects of radiation in humans, estimates of the risks of such effects must rely heavily on extrapolation from findings in laboratory animals. From the available data it is inferred that human germ cells are probably no more radiosensitive than those of the mouse and that a dose of at least 1.0 Sv would be required to double the rate of heritable mutations in the human species (NRC, 1990; Neel and others, 1990). On this basis, it is estimated that less than 1 percent of inherited disease in the human population is attributable to natural background irradiation (NRC, 1990; UNSCEAR, 1993).

Somatic Effects

The early, acute effects of radiation damage to genes, chromosomes, and other vital organelles can cause the deaths of affected cells, especially dividing cells, which are highly radiosensitive as a class (ICRP, 1984). Measured in terms of proliferative capacity, the survival of dividing cells tends to decrease exponentially with increasing dose, 1 to 2 Sv (100 to 200 rem) generally sufficing to reduce the surviving population by about 50 percent (Hall, 1988). Although a dose below 0.5 Sv (50 rem) kills too few cells to cause clinically detectable injury in most organs other than those of the embryo, a larger dose may kill enough of the progenitor cells in a tissue to interfere with the orderly replacement of its senescent cells, thereby causing the tissue to undergo atrophy. The rapidity with which the atrophy ensues will depend in part on the cell population dynamics within the affected tissue; in organs characterized by slow cell turnover, such as the liver and vascular endothelium, the process is typically much slower than in organs characterized by rapid cell turnover, such as the bone marrow, epidermis, and intestinal mucosa (ICRP, 1984). Also, if only a small volume of tissue is irradiated or if the dose is accumulated gradually over an extended period of time, the severity of the injury tends to be reduced by the compensatory proliferation of cells in the tissue that survive.

The acute effects of radiation include diverse types of reactions, which vary markedly in their dose-response relationships, clinical manifestations, timing, and prognosis (Mettler and Upton, 1995). Such reactions generally result from the severe depletion of progenitor cells in the exposed tissues and can be elicited only by doses above the thresholds that are high enough to kill many such cells. The reactions are therefore classified as *nonstochastic* (or *deterministic*) (ICRP, 1984), in contrast to the mutagenic and carcinogenic effects of radiation, which are classified as *stochastic* effects because they are thought to result from random molecular alterations in individual cells that increase in frequency as linear-nonthreshold functions of the dose (ICRP, 1991; NCRP, 2001).

Although some degree of radiation injury is inevitable in radiotherapy patients, few treated with modern methods experience severe or disabling radiation injuries. By the same token, modern safety practices have all but eliminated injuries from excessive occupational exposure such as were prevalent among pioneer radiation workers. Radiation accidents, however, remain a significant cause of injury. Some 285 nuclear reactor accidents (excluding the Chernobyl accident) were reported in various countries between 1945 and 1987, resulting in the irradiation of more than 1,350 persons, 33 of whom were injured fatally (Lushbaugh, Fry, and Ricks, 1987). The most serious such accident to date was the Chernobyl accident, which occurred in April 1986 in Ukraine and which released enough radiation and radioactive materials to cause radiation sickness and burns in more than 200 emergency personnel and firefighters, injuring 31 of them fatally. The heaviest contamination occurred in the vicinity of the reactor itself, necessitating evacuation of tens of thousands of inhabitants from the area, but doses to the thyroid gland averaging more than 20 mSv (2 rem) were sustained by infants in some areas of neighboring countries, largely through the ingestion of radioiodine via cow's milk, and the prevalence of thyroid cancer in such children has since risen dramatically (Astakhova and others, 1998; Tronko and others, 1999). Organs other than the thyroid typically receive such a small fraction of the dose normally accumulated each year from natural background radiation that the long-term health effects of such exposure cannot be predicted with certainty. The collective dose commitment to the population of the Northern Hemisphere as a whole, however, is estimated to approximate 600,000 person-Sv (60 million person-rem) (UNSCEAR, 1988), which could be predicted (on the basis of the non-threshold risk models discussed later) to cause up to 30,000 extra cancer deaths within the next seventy years (U.S. Department of Energy [DOE], 1987).

Radiation accidents have become less frequent but continue to occur from time to time. One of the latest occurred in a processing plant near Tokyo in 1999, when a critical mass of enriched uranium, produced accidentally, released large amounts of radiation, injuring three workers seriously and exposing more than sixty others, including golfers on a neighboring golf course (Normile, 1999). Also, accidents involving medical and industrial gamma ray sources, although less catastrophic than reactor accidents, have been far more numerous and have sometimes also caused severe injury and loss of life. The improper disposal of a cesium-137 source in Goiania, Brazil, in 1987, for example, resulted in the irradiation of dozens of unsuspecting victims, four of whom were injured fatally (UNSCEAR, 1993).

Prominent features of the acute effects of ionizing radiation on the more radiosensitive tissues of the body are described briefly in the following paragraphs:

Skin. Brief exposure of the skin to a dose of 6 Sv or more suffices to produce a sunburn-like rash and loss of hair in the exposed area. If the dose exceeds 10 to 20 Sv, blistering and ulceration may ensue, followed by scarring of the underlying tissue, and a second wave of atrophy and ulceration months or years later (ICRP, 1984; Mettler and Upton, 1995).

Bone marrow and lymphoid tissue. A dose of 2 to 3 Sv delivered rapidly to the whole body leads to a marked depression of the lymphocyte count and immune response within hours and a comparable depression of the leukocyte and platelet counts within three to five weeks. After a larger dose the latter changes may be severe enough to result in fatal infection or hemorrhage (see Table 24.4).

Intestine. An acute dose of 10 Sv causes the lining of the small intestine to become denuded within days (ICRP, 1984; UNSCEAR, 1988; Mettler and Upton, 1995), and if a large enough area of the lining is affected, a fulminating, rapidly fatal, dysentery-like syndrome results (Table 24.4).

Gonads. A dose of 0.15 Sv delivered rapidly to both testes can kill enough immature sperm-forming cells to lower the sperm count, and a dose of 2 to 4 Sv is likely to cause permanent sterility. Likewise, a dose of 1.5 to 2.0 Sv delivered rapidly to both ovaries kills enough oocytes to cause temporary sterility, and a larger dose may cause permanent sterility, depending on the age of the woman at the time of exposure (ICRP, 1984; Mettler and Upton, 1995).

Respiratory tract. The lung is not highly radiosensitive, but a dose of 6 to 10 Sv can cause the exposed area to become severely inflamed within the following one to three months. If a large enough volume of the lung is affected, the process may terminate in respiratory failure within the ensuing weeks or in other complications months or years later (ICRP, 1984; UNSCEAR, 1988; Upton and Mettler, 1995).

Lens of the eye. Acute exposure of the lens to more than 1 Sv may be followed within months by the formation of a microscopic lens opacity, and 2 to 3 Sv received in a single brief exposure (or 5.5 to 14 Sv accumulated over a period of months) may cause a vision-impairing cataract (ICRP, 1984; Mettler and Upton, 1995).

Other tissues. The other tissues of the body have thresholds for acute injury that are substantially higher than those for the reactions described above (Mettler and Upton, 1995). All tissues, however, tend to be more radiosensitive when in a rapidly growing state (ICRP, 1984; Mettler and Upton, 1995).

TABLE 24.4. MAJOR FORMS AND FEATURES OF ACUTE RADIATION SYNDROME.

Time After Irradiation	Cerebral Form (>50 Sv)	Gastrointestinal Form (10–20 Sv)	Hemopoietic Form (2–10 Sv)	Pulmonary Form (>6 Sv to lungs)
First day	Nausea Vomiting Diarrhea Headache Disorientation Ataxia Coma Convulsions Death	Nausea Vomiting Diarrhea	Nausea Vomiting Diarrhea	Nausea Vomiting
Second week		Nausea Vomiting Diarrhea Fever Erythema Prostration Death		
Third to sixth weeks			Weakness Fatigue Anorexia Fever Hemorrhage Epilation Recovery (?) Death (?)	
Second to eighth months				Cough Dyspnea Fever Chest pain Respiratory failure (?)

Whole-body radiation injury. Rapid exposure of a major part of the body to more than 1 Sv may cause *acute radiation syndrome,* or *radiation sickness.* This syndrome is characterized by a prodromal stage with malaise, anorexia, nausea, and vomiting; an ensuing asymptomatic, latent period; a second (main) phase of illness; and finally, either recovery or death (Table 24.4). The main phase of the illness typically takes one of the following four forms, depending on the predominant locus of radiation injury: hematological, gastrointestinal, cerebral, or pulmonary. Another syndrome, termed *chronic radiation sickness,* has been reported in chronically exposed workers of the Mayak nuclear facility and in persons residing downriver from that facility who were exposed to its radioactive effluents. The clinical findings in such persons, yet to be reported in other irradiated populations, include varying and persistent leukopenia, thrombocytopenia, arthralgia, asthenia, and various other ill-defined neurological complaints (Kossenko and others, 1994).

Localized radiation injury. In contrast to the clinical manifestations of acute whole-body radiation injury, which are often dramatic and prompt, the reaction to sharply localized irradiation, whether from an external radiation source or from an internally deposited radionuclide, tends to evolve more slowly and to produce few symptoms, unless the volume of tissue irradiated or the dose is relatively large. In this connection it is noteworthy that some radionuclides (such as tritium, carbon-14, and cesium-137) tend to be distributed systemically and to irradiate the whole body to varying degrees, whereas others are characteristically concentrated in specific organs. Radium and strontium-90, for example, are deposited predominantly in bone, causing skeletal injuries primarily, whereas radioactive iodine concentrates in the thyroid gland, which is the chief site of any resulting injury (Stannard, 1988; Mettler and Upton, 1995).

Carcinogenic Effects

The carcinogenic effects of ionizing radiation, first manifested early in this century by skin cancers and leukemia in pioneer radiation workers, have since been documented extensively by the occurrence of dose-dependent excesses of osteosarcomas and cranial sinus carcinomas in radium dial painters, carcinomas of the respiratory tract in underground hardrock miners, and cancers of many organs in atomic bomb survivors, radiotherapy patients, and experimentally irradiated laboratory animals (Upton, 1986; Mettler and Upton, 1995). The tumors caused by irradiation characteristically take years or decades to appear and exhibit no features distinguishing them from other growths. With few exceptions, moreover, they have been detectable only after relatively large doses (>0.5 Sv, or 50 rem) and have varied in frequency with the type of neoplasm as well as the age and sex of the exposed individuals. The neoplasms typically evolve through a succession of stages, and in experimental animals the carcinogenic effects of radiation have been observed to include initiating effects, promoting effects, and effects on the progression of neoplasia, depending on the experimental conditions in question (NRC, 1990). The molecular mechanisms of these effects remain to be fully elucidated, but the activation of oncogenes or the inactivation or loss of tumor-suppressor genes appear to be involved in many if not all instances (NRC, 1990). Furthermore, the carcinogenic effects of radiation resemble those of chemical carcinogens in being subject to modification, in varying degrees, by hormones, nutritional variables, and other modifying factors; and in combination with chemical carcinogens, the effects of radiation may be additive, synergistic, or mutually antagonistic, depending on the specific chemicals and exposure conditions in question (UNSCEAR, 2000).

Effects on the Developing Embryo

Radiosensitivity is relatively high throughout prenatal life. The effects of a given dose can vary markedly, however, depending on the developmental stage of the embryo or fetus at the time of exposure (Mettler and Upton, 1995). During the preimplantation period, the embryo is maximally susceptible to killing by irradiation. Subsequently, during critical stages in organogenesis, it is susceptible to the induction of malformations and other disturbances of development. The latter are dramatically exemplified in the dose-dependent increase in the frequency of mental retardation and the dose-dependent decrease in IQ test scores observed in atomic bomb survivors who were irradiated between the eighth and fifteenth weeks (and to a lesser extent, between the sixteenth and twenty-fifth weeks) after conception (UNSCEAR, 1986; NRC, 1990). Susceptibility to the carcinogenic effects of radiation also appears to be comparatively high throughout the prenatal period; the available data suggest that irradiation in utero may increase a child's risk of leukemia and other cancers by as much as 40 percent per Sv (Doll and Wakeford, 1997).

Risk Assessment

Although nonstochastic effects of radiation are produced only by relatively large doses, genetic and carcinogenic effects appear to increase in frequency as non-threshold functions of the dose (NCRP, 1993, 2001). The existing data, however, do not suffice to describe the dose-incidence relationship unambiguously for any type of neoplasm in the low-dose domain or to define how long after irradiation the risk of the growth may remain elevated in an exposed population. Therefore any risks attributable to low-level irradiation can be estimated only by extrapolation, based on models (NCRP, 1997, 2001), a process described in detail in Chapter Thirty-Two. Various dose-effect models have been used to estimate the risks of low-level irradiation, most of which involve the assumption that the overall risk of cancer increases in proportion with the dose at low-dose levels; however, because the carcinogenic potency of X-rays and gamma rays in laboratory animals has been found to be reduced by as much as an order of magnitude when the exposure is prolonged, the risk to humans is generally estimated to increase less steeply with the dose at low doses and dose rates than at high doses and dose rates. Furthermore, as has been emphasized elsewhere (NCRP, 2001), the available data do not exclude the possibility that there may be a threshold in the mSv dose range, below which the carcinogenicity of radiation is lacking altogether. For this reason the existing estimates must be used with caution when attempting to predict the risks of cancer that may be attributable to small doses or doses accumulated over weeks, months, or years.

These uncertainties notwithstanding, models have been applied to epidemiological data from the atomic bomb survivors and other irradiated populations, and these models have yielded estimates of the lifetime risks of different forms of cancer that may be attributable to ionizing irradiation (see, for example, Table 24.5). In interpreting the estimates, however, it must be recognized that they are based on population averages and hence cannot be assumed to apply equally to all individuals. Susceptibility to certain types of cancer (notably cancers of the thyroid and breast) is substantially higher in children than in adults, and susceptibility is also increased in association with certain hereditary disorders, such as retinoblastoma and nevoid basal cell carcinoma syndrome (Sankaranarayanan and Chakraborty, 1995; ICRP, 1998; Little, 2000). Although quantitative estimates are therefore limited by various sources of uncertainty, they are nevertheless judged in some quarters to provide the only rational basis for assessing the extent to which a cancer arising in a previously irradiated person can be attributed to the dose of radiation in question (National Institutes of Health, 1985).

TABLE 24.5. ESTIMATED LIFETIME RISKS OF FATAL CANCERS FROM ACUTE EXPOSURE TO IONIZING RADIATION.

	Excess Cancer Deaths per 10^6 per Sv	
Type or Site of Cancer	**Number**	**%[a]**
Stomach	110	18
Lung	85	3
Colon	85	5
Bone marrow (leukemia)	50	10
Urinary bladder	30	5
Esophagus	30	10
Breast	20	1
Liver	15	8
Gonads	10	2
Thyroid	8	8
Bone	5	5
Skin	2	2
Remainder	50	1
Total	500	2

[a]Percentage increase over background expectation for a nonirradiated population.

Source: Adapted from ICRP, 1991; Puskin and Nelson, 1995.

Studies to ascertain whether the rates of cancer and other diseases do, in fact, vary detectably with natural background radiation levels have been inconclusive thus far. A few studies have even suggested an inverse relationship, which has been interpreted by some observers as evidence for the existence of beneficial (or hormetic) effects of low-level irradiation (Luckey, 1991); however, such a relationship has not usually persisted after controlling for the effects of confounding variables (UNSCEAR, 2000; NCRP, 2001; Upton, 2001). The fact that populations residing in areas of elevated natural background radiation have not exhibited significant increases in cancer rates (UNSCEAR, 2000) is not unexpected in view of the low levels of exposure in question; that is, the estimates in Table 24.5 imply that although up to 10 percent of lung cancers in the U.S. population may conceivably result from residential exposure to radon (NRC, 1998), no more than 3 percent of all cancers in the population are attributable to natural background radiation (NRC, 1990).

By the same token, although some cohorts of underground hardrock miners continue to exhibit elevated mortality from lung cancer (NRC, 1998), carcinogenic effects of occupational irradiation are no longer readily demonstrable in most U.S. radiation workers, thanks to modern radiation protection practices. The data for several large cohorts of nuclear workers, however, suggest a dose-dependent excess of leukemia in this population (Cardis and others, 1995) that is comparable in magnitude with the estimate shown in Table 24.5. Excesses of multiple myeloma and other forms of cancer have also been reported in some cohorts of occupationally exposed workers, but such excesses have been observed only inconsistently and are of equivocal significance (Mettler and Upton, 1995; NCRP, 1997; UNSCEAR, 2000).

Among populations exposed to radioactive fallout, carcinogenic effects on the thyroid gland have been well documented in Marshall Islanders who received large doses to the thyroid in childhood and infancy (possibly up to 20 Gy, or 2,000 rad) from radioactive iodine, tellurium, and external gamma ray emitters in fallout released by a thermonuclear weapons test at Bikini atoll in 1954 (Robbins and Adams, 1989). The incidence of thyroid cancer has also been observed to be increased in U.S. children who resided downwind from the Nevada nuclear weapons test site (Kerber and others, 1993) and in children living in areas of Belarus and Ukraine that were contaminated by radionuclides released in the Chernobyl accident (Astakhova and others, 1998; Heidenreich and others, 1999).

Radiation Protection and Prevention

To minimize any associated risks of radiation injury, it is recommended that (1) no activity involving exposure to ionizing radiation should be considered justifiable unless it produces a sufficient benefit to those who are exposed, or to society at large, to offset any harm it may cause; (2) in any such activity the dose or likelihood of exposure should be kept *as low as reasonably achievable* (ALARA), taking all relevant economic and social factors into account; and (3) the radiation exposure of individuals resulting from any combination of such activities should be subject to dose limits that are low enough to prevent nonstochastic effects altogether and also low enough to prevent the risks of any stochastic effects (which may have no thresholds) from exceeding socially acceptable levels. For members of the public, therefore, the effective dose is conventionally recommended not exceed 5 mSv in any given year, or 1 mSv per year on average (NCRP, 1993).

To comply with the above precautionary guidelines, any facility dealing with ionizing radiation must be properly designed, must carefully plan and oversee its operating procedures, must have in place a well-conceived radiation protection program, must ensure that its workers are adequately trained and supervised, and must maintain a well-developed and well-rehearsed emergency preparedness plan, in order to be able to respond promptly and effectively in the event of a malfunction, spill, or other type of radiation accident (Shapiro, 1990).

Because medical radiographic examinations and indoor radon constitute the most important controllable sources of exposure to ionizing radiation for members of the general public (Table 24.2), prudent measures to limit irradiation from these sources also are warranted (Upton, Shore, and Harley, 1990). Other potential risks to human health and the environment that call for increased attention are the millions of cubic feet of radioactive and mixed wastes (mine and mill tailings, spent nuclear fuel, waste from the decommissioning of nuclear power plants, dismantled industrial and medical radiation sources, radioactive pharmaceuticals and reagents, heavy metals, polyaromatic hydrocarbons, and other contaminants) that are present in ever-growing quantities and that severely tax existing storage capacities at numerous sites (see, for example, NRC, 1989; DOE, 1993). Also needed in less developed countries are more adequate safeguards to protect occupationally exposed workers and members of the public against excessive exposure to radiation (UNSCEAR, 1988).

Ultraviolet Radiation

Ultraviolet radiations (UVRs) consist of electromagnetic waves, subdivided for convenience into three bands of the spectrum (Figure 24.1): UVA, 315–440 nm (nanometers) (sometimes called *black light*); UVB, 280–315 nm; and UVC, 100–280 nm (which is germicidal). The chief source of UVR for members of the public is sunlight, which varies in intensity with latitude, elevation, and season (AMA Council on Scientific Affairs, 1989). Important man-made sources of high-intensity exposure include sunlamps and tanning lamps, welding arcs, plasma torches, germicidal and blacklight lamps, electric arc furnaces, hot-metal operations, mercury-vapor lamps, and lasers. Common low-intensity sources include fluorescent lamps and certain laboratory equipment (Driscoll and Cridland, 2000).

Types and Mechanisms of Injury

UVR does not penetrate deeply into human tissues, so the injuries it causes are confined chiefly to the skin and eyes. Reactions of the skin to UVR, common among fair-skinned people, include sunburn, pigmentation, skin cancers (basal cell and squamous cell carcinomas and, to a lesser extent, melanomas), aging of the skin, telangiectasia, solar elastoses, and solar keratoses (Figure 24.3) (English, Armstrong, Kricker, and Fleming, 1997; Driscoll and Cridland, 2000; Yashar and

FIGURE 24.3. A BASAL CELL CARCINOMA OF THE SKIN OF TWENTY YEARS DURATION IN A FIFTY-EIGHT-YEAR-OLD MAN.

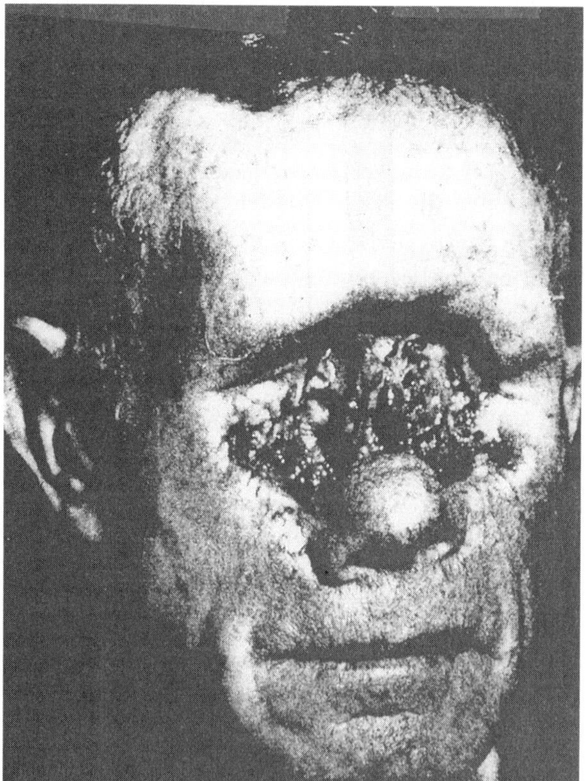

Note: Such tumors are the commonest of cancers and occur primarily in sun-exposed areas of the skin.

Source: Reprinted from *Anderson's Pathology,* Warren Shields, Copyright 1953, with permission from Elsevier.

Lim, 2003). Injuries of the eye include photokeratitis and photoconjunctivitis, which may result from brief exposure to a high-intensity UVR source (*welder's flash,* for example) or from more prolonged exposure to intense sunlight (*snow blindness,* for example); prolonged exposure may also cause pterygium, climatic droplet keratopathy, cortical lens cataract, solar retinitis, and macular degeneration (Driscoll and Cridland, 2000; McCarty and Taylor, 2002; Sliney, 2002).

The effects of UVR result chiefly from its absorption in DNA, leading to the production of pyrimidine dimers and mutational changes in exposed cells (Ehrhart, Gosselet, Culerrier, and Sarasin, 2003). Sensitivity to UVR may therefore be increased by DNA repair defects (for example, xeroderma pigmentosum), by agents (such as caffeine) that inhibit the repair enzymes, and by photosensitizing agents (such as psoralens, sulfonamides, tetracyclines, nalidixic acid, sulfonylureas, thiazides, phenothiazines, furocoumarins, and coal tar) that produce UVR-absorbing DNA photoproducts (Harper and Bickers, 1989; Yashar and Lim, 2003). The carcinogenic action of UVR is mediated primarily through direct effects on the exposed cells but may involve depression of local immunity as well (Kripke, 1993; Ichihashi and others, 2003). UVB, although far less intense than UVA in sunlight, plays a more important role in sunburn and skin carcinogenesis (English, Armstrong, Kricker, and Fleming, 1997), but UVA also contributes to the latter, as well as to tanning, some photosensitivity reactions, aging of the skin, photokeratitis, and cortical lens opacities (AMA Council on Scientific Affairs, 1989; Driscoll and Cridland, 2000).

Radiation Protection and Prevention

Excessive exposure to sunlight or other sources of UVR should be avoided, especially by fair-skinned individuals. In addition to engineering and administrative controls for limiting exposure (enclosures, interlocks, restriction of access, training, supervision, and so forth), protective clothing, UVR-screening lotions or creams, and UVR-blocking sunglasses should be used for the purpose when necessary. To protect occupationally exposed workers under conditions where the duration of exposure is not less than 0.1 μs, it is recommended that exposures of the skin and eye to UVR be kept below 30 J/m^2 effective irradiance and that exposure of the eye to UVA be kept below 10^4 J/m^2 (Driscoll and Cridland, 2000).

From a global perspective it is significant that the protective layer of ozone in the stratosphere has been gradually depleted by chlorofluorocarbons and other air pollutants (Rex and others, 1997; McKenzie, Bjorn, Bais, and Ilyasd, 2003; Diffey, 2004), and that every 1 percent decrease in ozone is estimated to increase the UVR reaching the earth by 1 to 2 percent and thereby to increase the rate of nonmelanotic skin cancer by 2 to 6 percent (Henriksen, Dahlback, Larsen, and

Moan, 1990). Also, of course, the rise in cancer rates is only one of the adverse outcomes to be expected from the increased levels of UVR, the most serious, perhaps, being the far-reaching impacts on vegetation and crop production that may result (Worrest and Grant, 1989; Caldwell and others, 2003).

Visible Light

Visible light consists of electromagnetic waves ranging in wavelength from 380 nm (violet) to 760 nm (red) (Figure 24.1). Sources of visible light in the environment vary widely in the intensity of their emissions. Common high-intensity sources other than the sun include lasers, electric welding or carbon arcs, and tungsten filament lamps.

Types and Mechanisms of Injury

A light that is too bright can injure the eye through photochemical reactions in the retina. Sustained exposure to intensities exceeding 0.1 mW/cm^2, such as can result from gazing at a bright source of light, may produce photochemical blue-light injury, and brief exposure of the retina to intensities exceeding 10 W/cm^2, depending on image size, may cause a retinal burn, resulting in a scotoma (blind spot) which may be permanent (Sliney and Wolbarsht, 1980; Frank and Slesin, 1998). The lens, iris, cornea, and skin also are vulnerable to injury from the thermal effects of laser radiation (Sliney and Wolbarsht, 1980). Too little illumination, conversely, can also be harmful, causing eyestrain (Huer, 1983) or seasonal affective disorder (SAD) (Rosenthal and others, 1988).

Radiation Protection and Prevention

Bright, continuously visible light normally elicits an aversion response that acts to protect the eye against injury so that few sources of light are sufficiently large and bright to cause a retinal burn under normal viewing conditions. A solar eclipse must never be viewed directly, however, and in situations involving potential exposure to carbon arcs, lasers, or other high-intensity sources, appropriate training, equipment, and protective eye shields are indicated (American National Standards Institute, 1986; American Conference of Governmental Industrial Hygienists [ACGIH], 1999).

Infrared Radiation

Infrared radiation (IR) consists of electromagnetic waves ranging in wavelength from 7×10^{-5} m to 3×10^{-2} m (Figure 24.1). Such radiation is emitted by all objects with temperatures above absolute zero, but potentially hazardous sources of IR include furnaces, ovens, welding arcs, molten glass, molten metal, and heating lamps.

Types and Mechanisms of Injury

The injuries caused by IR are mainly burns of the skin and cataracts of the lens of the eye. The warning sensation of heat usually prompts aversion in time to prevent the skin from being burned by IR, but the lens of the eye is vulnerable in lacking heat-sensing and heat-dissipating ability. Consequently, glassblowers, blacksmiths, oven operators, and those working around heating and drying lamps are at risk of IR-induced cataracts (Lydahl, 1984).

Radiation Protection and Prevention

Control of IR hazards requires appropriate shielding of sources, proper training and supervision of potentially exposed persons, and use of protective clothing and goggles. As a further precaution, it is recommended that exposures to IR not exceed 10 mW/cm^2 (ACGIH, 1999).

Microwave Radiation

Microwave and radiofrequency radiation (MW/RFR) consists of electromagnetic waves ranging in frequency from about 3 kHz to 300 GHz (Figure 24.1). Sources of MW/RFR occur in radar, television, radio, cellular phones, cell phone towers, and other telecommunications systems and are also used in various industrial operations (for example, heating, welding, and melting of metals; processing of wood and plastic; high-temperature plasma), household appliances (such as microwave ovens), and medical applications (for example, diathermy and hyperthermia) (International Labour Organization, 1986).

Types and Mechanisms of Injury

The biological effects of MW/RFR appear to be primarily thermal in nature. MW/RFR can penetrate deeply enough, however, so that the cutaneous burns it causes tend to involve dermal and subcutaneous tissues and to heal slowly. Cataracts of the lens of the eye also can result from high-intensity exposures (>1.5 kW/m^2) (Lipman, Tripathi, and Tripathi, 1988), and even death from hyperthermia has been encountered in the industrial use of MW/RFR sources (Roberts and Michaelson, 1985). MW/RFR can also interfere with cardiac pacemakers and other medical devices. Although the biological effects of

MW/RFR are attributed primarily to thermal mechanisms, there is growing evidence suggesting that MW/RFR may elicit some types of effects through nonthermal mechanisms as well. It has been suggested that such effects, yet to be demonstrated conclusively, include damage to DNA, impairment of fertility, developmental disturbances, neurobehavioral abnormalities, depression of immunity, stimulation of cell proliferation, and carcinogenic effects (Tenforde, 1998); to date, however, the relevant epidemiological and experimental data provide no firm evidence of the carcinogenicity or genotoxicity of such radiations (Moulder and others, 1999; Elwood, 2003; Anane and others, 2003; Zeni and others, 2003). As cellular phone use becomes more common, it will become a leading source of RFR exposure, and epidemiological data will help clarify whether there are any adverse health effects (see Box 24.1 and Figure 24.4).

FIGURE 24.4. CELL PHONES, NOW VIRTUALLY UBIQUITOUS, INCREASE THE LEVEL OF RADIOFREQUENCY RADIATION THROUGHOUT THE ENVIRONMENT.

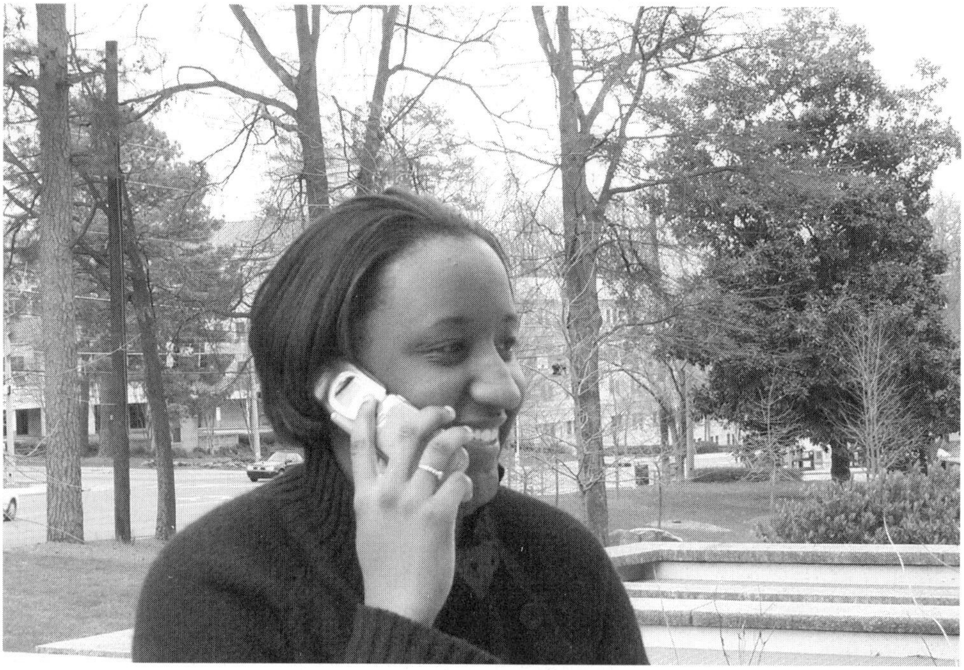

Box 24.1. Cell Phones and Cancer

Suggestions that the radiofrequency radiation from cell phones and cell phone towers may increase the risk of cancer have caused growing concern in recent years, prompting public objections to the siting of TV, radio, and cell phone transmission towers. As yet, however, the available epidemiological and experimental data are inconclusive (Frumkin, Jacobson, Gansler, and Thun, 2001; Kundi, Mild, Hardell, and Mattsson, 2004), providing no firm evidence that the low levels of radiofrequency radiation emitted by such sources pose cancer risks.

Radiation Protection and Prevention

Prevention of injury from MW/RFR requires proper design and shielding of MW/RFR sources, along with appropriate training and supervision of potentially exposed persons (especially those wearing cardiac pacemakers or other sensitive devices). To prevent detectable heating of tissue, exposures to MW/RFR of different frequencies should be kept below the relevant threshold limit values (ACGIH, 1999; International Commission on Non-Ionizing Radiation Protection, 1998; Sliney and Colville, 2000).

Extremely Low Frequency Electromagnetic Fields

Extremely low frequency (ELF) electromagnetic fields (EMFs) consist of time-varying magnetic fields with frequencies below 300 Hz. They are widely present throughout the environment, the largest arising intermittently from solar activity and thunderstorms, and reaching intensities on the order of 0.5 T (Teslas) (Grandolfo and Vecchia, 1985). Stronger EMFs, however, are the localized 50 to 60 Hz fields generated by electric power lines, transformers, motors, household appliances, video display terminals (VDTs), and various medical devices, notably magnetic resonance imaging (MRI) systems (Office of Technology Assessment [OTA], 1989; Tenforde, 1992). For example, the field strength on the ground beneath a 765 kV, 60 Hz power line carrying 1 kA (kiloampere) per phase is on the order of 15 T, and the field strength in close proximity to common household appliances may range up to 2.5 mT (milliteslas) (Tenforde, 1992). The strength of such fields decreases rapidly with distance, however, so that the average ambient value in the home environment is less than 0.3 T (3 mG [milligauss]) (Silva, Hummon, Rutter, and Hooper, 1989). By the same token, although field strengths at video display terminals typically range up to 5 T, those at the location of the operator are generally less than 1 T (Tenforde, 1992).

Types and Mechanisms of Injury

Extremely low frequency EMFs may have biological effects. The electrical currents they induce can alter electrical activity in the body—in cell membranes, in electrically active tissues such as nerves, muscles, and the retina, and in cardiac pacemakers. Low exposures (current density under 10 mA/m^2) produce few if any effects, because this level of electrical activity occurs naturally in many tissues. However, higher exposures (current densities above 10 mA/m^2) can change the biochemistry and physiology of some cells. These changes may include alterations in growth rate, melatonin secretion, endocrine activity, and immune response, although probably not genotoxicity. And even higher exposures (current densities above 1 A) can excite nerves and cause potentially irreversible effects, such as cardiac fibrillation (Tenforde, 1992, 1998).

There is some evidence that long-continued exposure to weaker EMFs may cause other, severe effects. Epidemiological observations suggest that the risks of leukemia in children may be increased by residential exposure to household EMFs, the risks of brain cancer and leukemia may be increased in utility workers by occupational exposure to EMFs, and the risks of reproductive disorders may be increased in pregnant women by chronic exposure to EMFs through the operation of VDTs (Tenforde, 1992, 1996; NRC, 1996). Although the weight of evidence argues against the latter possibility, the relevant epidemiological data are inconclusive as yet, and their interpretation is complicated by uncertainties in exposure assessment and by the lack of established biological mechanisms for the effects in question (NRC, 1996; Tenforde, 1998). Nevertheless, the fact that such fields have been reported to influence ion transport, melatonin secretion, and tumor promotion in some model systems (Tenforde, 1992, 1998) has reinforced public health concern (OTA, 1989; NRC, 1996).

Radiation Protection and Prevention

Areas containing EMFs stronger than 0.5 mT (such as exist around transformers, accelerators, MRI systems, and other electric devices) should be posted with warning signs and should be avoided by persons wearing pacemakers. In addition, it is recommended that the strength of any 60 Hz time-varying magnetic field, such as typically exists around an MRI system, should be limited to 1 mT for occupational exposures, and to 0.1 mT for exposure of those wearing cardiac pacemakers or for continuous exposures involving members of the general public (ACGIH, 1999). Also, as a precautionary measure to minimize any risks that might be associated with the use of electric blankets or VDTs, most manufacturers have introduced design changes to eliminate or reduce the EMFs to which the users of such devices could otherwise be exposed (Tenforde, 1992, 1996; Sliney and Colville, 2000).

Ultrasound

Ultrasound is often classified for public health purposes with nonionizing radiation, but it is not a component of the electromagnetic spectrum and actually consists of mechanical vibrations at frequencies above the audible range (that is, >16 kHz). Sources of high-power, low-frequency ultrasound are used widely in science and industry for cleaning, degreasing, plastic welding, liquid extracting, atomizing, homogenizing, and emulsifying operations and are also used in medicine for lithotripsy and other applications. Low-power, high-frequency ultrasound is used widely in analytical work and in medical diagnosis, such as in ultrasonography (NCRP, 1983, 1992, 2002).

Types and Mechanisms of Injury

The biological effects of ultrasound are produced through mechanisms similar in many respects to those of mechanical vibration, involving thermal (NCRP, 1992) as well as nonthermal (NCRP, 2002) changes. High-power, low-frequency ultrasound, transmitted through the air or through bodily contact with the generating source, has been observed to cause a variety of effects in occupationally exposed workers, including headache, earache, tinnitus, vertigo, malaise, photophobia, hypercusia, peripheral neuritis, and autonomic polyneuritis. The possibility that it may cause adverse effects on the embryo has also been suggested (NCRP, 1983, 1992, 2002).

Excessive exposure to high-frequency ultrasound through bodily contact with its source may be expected, in principle, to cause complaints similar to those just noted; however, no adverse effects have been shown to result from exposure to high-frequency ultrasound at the low power levels used in medical ultrasonography (NCRP, 2002). Nevertheless, the existing epidemiological data do not suffice to exclude the possibility that ultrasonography as it is currently employed in clinical practice may carry a small risk of adverse effects (NCRP, 2002).

Ultrasound Protection and Prevention

Protection against potential injury by ultrasound requires appropriate isolation and insulation of generating sources, as well as proper training and use of ear protective devices by those working around such sources. In addition, yearly audiometric and neurological examinations of occupationally exposed workers are recommended (World Health Organization, 1982).

Conclusion

The adverse health effects of different forms of radiant energy are highly diverse, ranging from rapidly fatal reactions to cancers, birth defects, and hereditary disorders that do not appear until months, years, or decades later. The nature, frequency, and severity of the effects depend on the type of radiant energy in question and the particular conditions of exposure. Most such effects are produced only by moderate to high levels of exposure and can therefore be prevented by keeping any exposures below the relevant thresholds. However, the genotoxic and carcinogenic effects of ionizing and ultraviolet radiations appear to increase in frequency as linear-nonthreshold functions of the dose and may therefore not be entirely preventable without avoiding exposure to these forms of radiation altogether. Because complete avoidance is not feasible, the exposure should be limited sufficiently to prevent any resulting risks of mutagenic and carcinogenic effects from exceeding acceptable levels.

To achieve the desired level of protection against each of the different forms of radiation requires appropriate design, control, and operation of all radiation sources; proper training and supervision of operating and potentially exposed personnel; and education of the public in prudent protective health measures. These requirements can be met satisfactorily in most situations involving radiation hazards if the necessary effort and resources are provided. Public health problems that remain to be adequately addressed at this time include (1) the risks associated with residential exposure to indoor radon, (2) the hazards posed by the large and growing quantities of radioactive and mixed wastes, (3) assessment of the potential risks that may be associated with exposure to radiofrequency radiation and 60 Hz electromagnetic fields, and (4) the ultraviolet radiation–induced impacts on human health and the environment that can be expected to result from further depletion of stratospheric ozone levels.

Thought Questions

1. What types of injury of public health concern are associated with exposure to each of the different forms of radiation, and how do the risks of such injuries vary with the radiation dose?
2. Dental X-rays are performed on a routine basis in many dental offices and clinics. How would you evaluate the risks and benefits of routine dental X-rays?

3. A cell phone company proposes to erect a cell tower on the roof of your university building. Would you approve this installation? Why or why not?

References

AMA Council on Scientific Affairs. "Harmful Effects of Ultraviolet Radiation." *Journal of the American Medical Association,* 1989, *262,* 380–384.

American Conference of Governmental Industrial Hygienists. *Threshold Limit Values and Biological Exposure Indices for 1999.* Cincinnati: American Conference of Governmental Industrial Hygienists, 1999.

American National Standards Institute. *Safe Use of Lasers.* New York: American National Standards Institute, 1986.

Anane, R., and others. "Effects of GSM-900 Microwaves on DMBA-Induced Mammary Tumors in Female Sprague-Dawley Rats." *Radiation Research,* 2003, *160,* 492–497.

Astakhova, L. N., and others. "Chernobyl-Related Thyroid Cancer in Children of Belarus: A Case-Control Study." *Radiation Research,* 1998, *150,* 340–356.

Bender, M. A., and others. "Current Status of Cytogenetic Procedures to Detect and Quantify Previous Exposures to Radiation." *Mutation Research,* 1988, *196,* 103–159.

Brown, P. *American Martyrs to Science Through the Roentgen Rays.* Springfield, Ill.: Thomas, 1936.

Caldwell, M. M., and others. "Terrestrial Ecosystems, Increased Solar Ultraviolet Radiation and Interactions with Other Climatic Change Factors." P*hotochemical & Photobiological Sciences,* 2003, *2,* 29–38.

Cardis, E., and others. "Effects of Low Doses and Low Dose Rates of External Ionizing Radiation: Cancer Mortality Among Nuclear Industry Workers in Three Countries." *Radiation Research,* 1995, *142,* 117–132.

Diffey, B. "Climate Change, Ozone Depletion and the Impact on Ultraviolet Exposure of Human Skin." *Physics in Medicine and Biology,* 2004, *49*(1), R1–R11.

Doll, R., Evans, N. J., and Darby, S. C. "Paternal Exposure Not to Blame." *Nature,* 1994, *367,* 678–680.

Doll, R., and Wakeford, R. "Risk of Childhood Cancer from Fetal Irradiation." *British Journal of Radiology,* 1997, *70,* 130–139.

Driscoll, C.M.H., and Cridland, N. A. "Ultraviolet Radiation." In M. Lippmann (ed.), *Environmental Toxicants.* (2nd ed.) New York: Wiley-Interscience, 2000.

Ehrhart, J. C., Gosselet, F. P., Culerrier, R. M., and Sarasin, A. "UVB-Induced Mutations in Human Key Gatekeeper Genes Governing Signaling Pathways and Consequences for Skin Tumourigenesis." P*hotochemical & Photobiological Sciences,* 2003, *2,* 825–834.

Elwood, J. M. "Epidemiologic Studies of Radiofrequency Exposures and Human Cancer." *Bioelectromagnetics,* 2003, (suppl. 6), S63–S73.

English, D. R., Armstrong, B. K., Kricker, A., and Fleming, C. "Sunlight and Cancer." *Cancer Causes & Control,* 1997, *8,* 271–283.

Frank, A. L., and Slesin, L. "Nonionizing Radiation." In R. B. Wallace (ed.), *Maxcy-Rosenau-Last Public Health and Preventive Medicine.* (14th ed.) Stamford, Conn.: Appleton & Lang, 1998.

Frumkin, H., Jacobson, A., Gansler, T., and Thun, M. J. "Cellular Phones and Risk of Brain Tumors." *Ca: A Cancer Journal for Clinicians,* 2001, *51*(2), 137–141.

Gardner, M. J., and others. Results of Case-Control Study of Leukaemia and Lymphoma Among Young People Near Sellafield Nuclear Plant in West Cumbria." *British Medical Journal,* 1990, *300,* 423–429.

Goodhead, D. J. "Spatial and Temporal Distribution of Energy." *Health Physics,* 1988, *55,* 231–240.

Grandolfo, M., and Vecchia, P. "Natural and Man-Made Exposures to Static and ELF Magnetic Fields." In M. Grandolfo, S. M. Michaelson, and A. Rindi (eds.), *Biological Effects and Dosimetry of Static and ELF Electromagnetic Fields.* New York: Plenum, 1985.

Hall, E. J. *Radiobiology for the Radiologist.* (3rd ed.) Philadelphia: Lippincott, 1988.

Harper, L. C., and Bickers, D. R. *Photosensitivity Diseases: Principles of Diagnosis and Treatment.* (2nd ed.) Toronto: Decker, 1989.

Heidenreich, W. F., and others. "Time Trends of Thyroid Cancer Incidence in Belarus After the Chernobyl Accident." *Radiation Research,* 1999, *181,* 617–625.

Henriksen, T., Dahlback, A., Larsen, S., and Moan, J. "Ultraviolet Radiation and Skin Cancer: Effect of an Ozone Layer Depletion." *Photochemistry and Photobiology,* 1990, *51,* 579–582.

Huer, H. H. "Lighting." In L. Parmeggiana (ed.), *Encyclopedia of Occupational Health and Safety.* Geneva: International Labour Organization, 1983.

Ichihashi, M., and others. "UV-Induced Skin Damage." *Toxicology,* 2003, *189,* 21–39.

International Commission on Non-Ionizing Radiation Protection. "Guidelines for Limiting Exposure to Time-Varying Electric, Magnetic, and Electromagnetic Fields (up to 300GHz)." *Health Physics,* 1998, *74,* 494–522.

International Commission on Radiological Protection. "Nonstochastic Effects of Ionizing Radiation." ICRP Publication 41. *Annals of the ICRP,* 1984, *14*(entire issue 3).

International Commission on Radiological Protection. "1990 Recommendations of the International Commission on Radiological Protection." ICRP Publication 60. *Annals of the ICRP,* 1991, *21*(entire issue 1–3).

International Commission on Radiological Protection. "Genetic Susceptibility to Cancer." ICRP Publication 79. *Annals of the ICRP,* 1998, *28*(1–2), 1–157.

International Labour Organization. *Protection of Workers against Radiofrequency and Microwave Radiation: A Technical Review.* Occupational Safety and Health Series Report no. 57. Geneva: International Labour Organization, 1986.

Kerber, R. A., and others. "A Cohort Study of Thyroid Disease in Relation to Fallout from Nuclear Weapons Testing." *Journal of the American Medical Association,* 1993, *270,* 2076–2082.

Kossenko, M. M., and others. *Analysis of Chronic Radiation Sickness in the Population of the Southern Urals.* AFFRI Contract Report 94-1. Springfield, Va.: Armed Forces Radiobiological Research Institute, 1994.

Kripke, M. L. "Immunosuppressive Action of UV Radiation." In F. R. deGruijl (ed.), *The Dark Side of Sunlight.* Utrecht: University of Utrecht, 1993.

Kundi, M., Mild, K., Hardell, L., and Mattsson, M. O. "Mobile Telephones and Cancer: A Review of Epidemiological Evidence." *Journal of Toxicology & Environmental Health Part B: Critical Reviews,* 2004, *7*(5), 351–384.

Lipman, R. M., Tripathi, B. J., and Tripathi, R. C. "Cataracts Induced by Microwave and Ionizing Radiation." *Survey of Ophthalmology,* 1988, *33,* 200–210.

Little, J. B. "Radiation Carcinogenesis." *Carcinogenesis,* 2000, *21,* 397–404.

Luckey, T. D. *Radiation Hormesis.* Boca Raton, Fla.: CRC Press, 1991.

Lushbaugh, C. C., Fry, S. A., and Ricks, R. C. "Nuclear Reactor Accidents: Preparedness and Consequences." *British Journal of Radiology,* 1987, *60,* 1159–1183.

Lydahl, E. "Infrared Radiation and Cataract." *Acta Ophthalmologica Supplement,* 1984, *166,* 1–63.

McCarty, C. A., and Taylor, H. R. "A Review of the Epidemiological Evidence Linking Ultraviolet Radiation and Cataracts." *Developments in Ophthalmology,* 2002, *35,* 21–31.

McKenzie, R. L., Bjorn, L. O., Bais, A., and Ilyasd, M. "Changes in Biologically Active Ultraviolet Radiation Reaching the Earth's Surface." *Photochemical & Photobiological Sciences,* 2003, *2,* 5–15.

Mettler, F. A., and Upton, A. C. *Medical Effects of Ionizing Radiation.* New York: Grune & Stratton, 1995.

Morgan, W. F., and others. "Genomic Instability Induced by Ionizing Radiation." *Radiation Research,* 1996, *146,* 247–258.

Moulder, J. E., and others. "Cell Phones and Cancer: What Is the Evidence for a Connection?" *Radiation Research,* 1999, *151,* 513–531.

National Council on Radiation Protection and Measurements. *Biological Effects of Ultrasound: Mechanisms and Clinical Implications.* NCRP Report no. 74. Bethesda, Md.: National Council on Radiation Protection and Measurements, 1983.

National Council on Radiation Protection and Measurements. *Evaluation of Occupational and Environmental Exposures to Radon and Radon Daughters in the United States.* NCRP Report no. 78. Bethesda, Md.: National Council on Radiation Protection and Measurements, 1984.

National Council on Radiation Protection and Measurements. *Ionizing Radiation Exposure of the Population of the United States.* NCRP Report no. 93. Bethesda, Md.: National Council on Radiation Protection and Measurements, 1987.

National Council on Radiation Protection and Measurements. *Exposure of the U.S. Population from Occupational Radiation.* NCRP Report no. 101. Bethesda, Md.: National Council on Radiation Protection and Measurements, 1989.

National Council on Radiation Protection and Measurements. *Exposure Criteria for Medical Diagnostic Ultrasound, I: Criteria Based on Thermal Mechanisms.* NCRP Report no. 113. Bethesda, Md.: National Council on Radiation Protection and Measurements, 1992.

National Council on Radiation Protection and Measurements. *Limitation of Exposure to Ionizing Radiation.* NCRP Report no. 116. Bethesda, Md.: National Council on Radiation Protection and Measurements, 1993.

National Council on Radiation Protection and Measurements. *Uncertainties in Fatal Risk Estimates Used in Radiation Protection.* NCRP Report no. 126. Bethesda, Md.: National Council on Radiation Protection and Measurements, 1997.

National Council on Radiation Protection and Measurements. *Evaluation of the Linear-Nonthreshold Dose-Response Model For Ionizing Radiation.* NCRP Report no. 136. Bethesda, Md.: National Council on Radiation Protection and Measurements, 2001.

National Council on Radiation Protection and Measurements. *Exposure Criteria for Medical Diagnostic Ultrasound, II: Criteria Based on All Known Mechanisms.* NCRP Report no. 140. Bethesda, Md.: National Council on Radiation Protection and Measurements, 2002.

National Institutes of Health. *Report of the National Institutes of Health Working Group to Develop Radioepidemiological Tables.* NIH Publication no. 85-2748. Washington, D.C.: U.S. Government Printing Office, 1985.

National Research Council. *The Nuclear Weapons Complex.* Washington, D.C.: National Academies Press, 1989.

National Research Council. *Health Effects of Exposure to Low Levels of Ionizing Radiation: BEIR V.* Washington, D.C.: National Academies Press, 1990.

National Research Council. *Possible Health Effects of Exposure to Residential Electric and Magnetic Fields.* Washington, D.C.: National Academies Press, 1996.

National Research Council. *Health Effects of Exposure to Radon.* Washington, D.C.: National Academies Press, 1998.

Neel, J. V., and others. "The Children of Parents Exposed to Atomic Bombs: Estimates of the Genetic Doubling Dose of Radiation for Humans." *American Journal of Human Genetics,* 1990, *46,* 1053–1072.

Nicholson, D. W., and Thornberry, N. A. "Caspas Killer Proteases." *Trends in Biochemical Sciences,* 1997, *22,* 299–306.

Normile, D. "Nuclear Accident: Special Treatment Set for Radiation Victim." *Science,* 1999, *286,* 207–208.

Office of Technology Assessment. *Biological Effects of Power Frequency Electric & Magnetic Fields.* Background Paper OTA-BP-E-53. Washington, D.C.: U.S. Government Printing Office, 1989.

Puskin, J. S., and Nelson, C. B. "Estimates of Radiogenic Cancer Risks." *Health Physics,* 1995, *69,* 93–101.

Rex, M., and others. "Prolonged Stratospheric Ozone Loss in the 1995–96 Arctic Winter." *Nature,* 1997, *389,* 835–838.

Robbins, J., and Adams, W. "Radiation Effects in the Marshall Islands." In S. Nagataki (ed.), *Radiation and the Thyroid.* Amsterdam: Excerpta Medica, 1989.

Roberts, N. J., Jr., and Michaelson, S. M. "Epidemiological Studies of Human Exposures to Microwave Radiation: A Critical Review." *International Archives of Occupational and Environmental Health,* 1985, *56,* 169–178.

Rosenthal, N. E., and others. "Phototherapy for Seasonal Affective Disorder." *Journal of Biological Rhythms,* 1988, *3,* 101–120.

Sankaranarayanan, K., and Chakraborty, R. "Cancer Predisposition, Radiosensitivity and the Risk of Radiation-Induced Cancers, I: Background." *Radiation Research,* 1995, *143,* 121–143.

Shapiro, J. *Radiation Protection: A Guide for Scientists and Physicians.* (3rd ed.) Cambridge, Mass.: Harvard University Press, 1990.

Silva, M., Hummon, N., Rutter, D., and Hooper, C. "Power Frequency Magnetic Fields in the Home." *IEEE Transactions on Power Delivery,* 1989, *4,* 465–477.

Sliney, D. H. "How Light Reaches the Eye and Its Components." *International Journal of Toxicology,* 2002, *21,* 501–509.

Sliney, D. H., and Colville, F. "Microwaves and Electromagnetic Fields." In M. Lippmann (ed.), *Environmental Toxicants.* (2nd ed.) New York: Wiley-Interscience, 2000.

Sliney, D. H., and Wolbarsht, M. *Safety with Lasers.* New York: Plenum, 1980.

Stannard, J. N. *Radioactivity and Health: A History.* U.S. Department of Energy Report DOE/RL/01830-T5. Washington, D.C.: National Technical Information Services, 1988.

Stone, R. S. "Maximum Permissible Standards." In B. P. Sonnenblick (ed.), *Protection in Diagnostic Radiology.* New Brunswick, N.J.: Rutgers University Press, 1959.

Stone-Scott, N. "X-Ray Injuries." *American X-Ray Journal,* 1897, *1,* 57–67.

Tenforde, T. S. "Biological Interactions and Potential Health Effects of Extremely-Low-Frequency Magnetic Fields from Power Lines and Other Common Sources." *Annual Review of Public Health,* 1992, *13,* 173–196.

Tenforde, T. S. "Interaction of ELF Magnetic Fields with Living Systems." In C. Polk and E. Postow (eds.), *Handbook of Biological Effects of Electromagnetic Fields.* (2nd ed.) Boca Raton, Fla.: CRC Press, 1996.

Tenforde, T. S. "Electromagnetic Fields and Carcinogenesis: An Analysis of Biological Mechanisms." In G. L. Carlo (ed.), *Wireless Phones and Health: Scientific Progress.* Norwell, Mass.: Kluwer Academic, 1998.

Tronko, M. D., and others. "Thyroid Carcinoma in Children and Adolescents in Ukraine After the Chernobyl Nuclear Accident: Statistical Data and Clinicomorphologic Characteristics." *Cancer,* 1999, *86,* 149–156.

United Nations Scientific Committee on the Effects of Atomic Radiation. *Genetic and Somatic Effects of Ionizing Radiation.* Report to the General Assembly, with Annexes. New York: United Nations, 1986.

United Nations Scientific Committee on the Effects of Atomic Radiation. *Sources, Effects, and Risks of Ionizing Radiation.* Report to the General Assembly, with Annexes. New York: United Nations, 1988.

United Nations Scientific Committee on the Effects of Atomic Radiation. *Sources and Effects of Ionizing Radiation.* Report to the General Assembly, with Annexes. New York: United Nations, 1993.

United Nations Scientific Committee on the Effects of Atomic Radiation. *Sources and Effects of Ionizing Radiation.* Report to the General Assembly, with Annexes. New York: United Nations, 1994.

United Nations Scientific Committee on the Effects of Atomic Radiation. *Sources and Effects of Ionizing Radiation.* Report to the General Assembly, with Annexes. New York: United Nations, 2000.

U.S. Department of Energy. *Health and Environmental Consequences of the Chernobyl Nuclear Power Plant Accident.* DOE/ER-0332. Washington, D.C.: U.S. Department of Energy, 1987.

U.S. Department of Energy. *U.S. Department of Energy Interim Mixed Waste Inventory Report: Waste Streams, Treatment Capacities and Technologies.* DOE/NBM-1100. Springfield, Va.: National Technical Information Services, 1993.

Upton, A. C. "Historical Perspectives on Radiation Carcinogenesis." In A. C. Upton, R. E. Albert, F. J. Burns, and R. E. Shore (eds.), *Radiation Carcinogenesis.* New York: Elsevier, 1986.

Upton, A. C. "Prevention of Work-Related Injuries and Diseases: Lessons from Our Experience with Ionizing Radiation." *American Journal of Industrial Medicine,* 1987, *12,* 291–309.

Upton, A. C. "Radiation Hormesis: Data and Interpretations." *Critical Reviews in Toxicology,* 2001, *31,* 681–695.

Upton, A. C., Shore, R. E., and Harley, N. H. "The Health Effects of Low-Level Ionizing Radiation." *Annual Review of Public Health,* 1990, *13,* 127–150.

Vilenchik, M. M., and Knudson, A. G., Jr. "Inverse Radiation Dose-Rate Effects on Somatic and Germ-Line Mutations and DNA Damage Rates." *Proceedings of the National Academy of Sciences of the United States of America,* 2000, *97,* 5381–5386.

Wakeford, R., and others. "The Descriptive Statistics and Health Implications of Occupational Radiation Doses Received by Men at the Sellafield Nuclear Installation Before the Conception of Their Children." *Journal of Radiological Protection,* 1994a, *14,* 3–16.

Wakeford, R., and others. "The Seascale Childhood Leukaemia Cases: The Mutation Rates Implied by Paternal Preconceptional Radiation Doses." *Journal of Radiological Protection,* 1994b, *14,* 17–24.

Wang, J. X., and others. "Thyroid Nodularity and Chromosome Aberrations Among Women in Areas of High Background Radiation in China." *Journal of the National Cancer Institute,* 1990, *82,* 478–485.

Ward, J. F. "DNA Damage Produced by Ionizing Radiation in Mammalian Cells: Identities, Mechanisms of Formation, and Repairability." *Progress in Nucleic Acid Research and Molecular Biology,* 1988, *35,* 96–128.

Warren, S. "Neoplasms." In W.A.D. Anderson (ed.), *Anderson's Pathology.* St. Louis: Mosby, 1953.

Wojcik, A. "The Current Status of the Adaptive Response to Ionizing Radiation in Mammalian Cells." *Human Ecology and Risk Assessment,* 2000, *6,* 281–300.

World Health Organization. *Ultrasound: Environmental Health Criteria 22.* Geneva: World Health Organization, 1982.

Worrest, R. C., and Grant, L. D. "Effects of Ultraviolet-B Radiation on Terrestrial Plants and Marine Organisms." In R. R. Jones and T. Wigley (eds.), *Ozone Depletion: Health and Environmental Consequences.* New York: Wiley, 1989.

Yashar, S. S., and Lim, H. W. "Classification and Evaluation of Photodermatoses." *Dermatologic Therapy,* 2003, *16,* 1–7.

Zeni, O., and others. "Lack of Genotoxic Effects (Micronucleus Induction) in Human Lymphocytes Exposed in Vitro to 900 MHz Electromagnetic Fields." *Radiation Research,* 2003, *160,* 152–158.

For Further Information

Shapiro, J. *Radiation Protection: A Guide for Scientists, Regulators and Physicians.* (4th ed.) Cambridge, Mass.: Harvard University Press, 2002.

Wakeford, R. "The Cancer Epidemiology of Radiation." *Oncogene,* 2004, *23,* 6404–6428.

CHAPTER TWENTY-FIVE

INJURIES

Junaid A. Razzak
Jeremy J. Hess
Arthur L. Kellermann

The word *injury* originates from the Latin *in* + *jur* (from *jus*), which literally means "not right." In cellular terms, injury is physical damage caused by the excessive transfer of energy (whether mechanical, electrical, chemical, thermal, or radiation) or by the lack of essential factors for energy production, such as oxygen (resulting in suffocation or drowning, for example), or for maintenance of homeostasis (resulting in frostbite, for example).

Traditionally, public health officials ignored injuries because they were assumed to be random, unavoidable "accidents," without a clear causal pathway. We now know, however, that many injuries, like diseases, affect identifiable high-risk groups, follow a predictable chain of events, and are therefore preventable. When prevention fails, the severity of an injury may be reduced. The likelihood of death or long-term disability can be reduced by prompt provision of acute care and subsequently, of rehabilitation. The combination of these three strategies—prevention, acute care, and rehabilitation—is termed *injury control.*

This chapter provides a general outline of injuries, following a public health approach and focusing on environmental factors. It begins with definitions, provides some epidemiological data to frame the scope of the injury problem, and proceeds to a general analysis of injury outcomes as well as risk and preventive factors. It then discusses general principles of prevention and control, and examines certain injuries and environments in greater detail, to illustrate key points about injury causes and prevention. This last section illustrates ways to conceptualize injuries and creative strategies to reduce the significant burdens that injuries impose.

The Public Health Approach to Injury Prevention and Control

Injury control draws on the expertise of many disciplines, including epidemiology, disease prevention, health promotion, biomechanics, acute care, rehabilitation, law, and public administration. It follows the traditional public health approach, which involves four generic steps (Centers for Disease Control and Prevention, 2002):

1. Define the health problem;
2. Identify causes, risk factors, and protective factors associated with the problem;
3. Develop and test interventions to reduce the problem's impact; and
4. Implement successful interventions, evaluate their impact, and ensure widespread acceptance and implementation of prevention principles and strategies of control.

Defining the Problem

Injuries, as we noted in our introduction, are any of a number of events that result in physical damage and, typically, in impaired or lost function. The World Health Organization (WHO) defines injury as "the physical damage when a human body is suddenly or briefly subjected to intolerable levels of energy. It can be a bodily lesion resulting from acute exposure to energy in amounts that exceed the threshold of physiological tolerance, or it can be an impairment of function resulting from the lack of one or more vital elements (i.e., air, water, warmth), as in drowning, strangulation, or freezing. The time between exposure to the energy and the appearance of an injury is short" (Holder and others, 2001, p. 5).

It is important to characterize the distribution of injuries in given populations, to quantify the scope of an injury problem, to monitor patterns and trends, and to evaluate the impact of countermeasures. Several sources of information may be used for this purpose. Vital records or death certificates can be used to document overall rates of mortality, but they do not provide information about nonfatal injuries. Hospital records as well as trauma registries, emergency department (ED) data, emergency medical services (EMS) reports, and police reports, or a combination of these sources, may be used to provide essential information about cases of major trauma, depending on local resources and the nature of the information being sought. In the United States the National Hospital Discharge Survey and the National Hospital Ambulatory Medical Care Survey: Emergency Department Summary are important sources of injury data. Other high-income countries (HICs) have similar systems for monitoring morbidity and mortality data associated with injuries. Although middle-income and low-income countries (MICs and LICs, respectively) often do not have similar extensive surveillance systems in place, data on injuries can be gathered from death certificates, hospital discharge summaries, emergency department records, and other sources (Razzak and Luby, 1998; Razzak, Marsh, and Stansfield, 2002).

Types of Injuries. Relying on these sources of data, investigators have identified a wide range of injuries and classified them according to several schemes. The most widely used approach divides injuries by intent. Purposefully inflicted injuries, known as *intentional,* are subdivided into those caused by self-directed harm, such as suicide, attempted suicide, or a suicidal gesture (sometimes called *parasuicide*), and those due to interpersonal violence. Violence-related injuries are further subdivided into individual violence (for example, assault or homicide), group violence (for example, gang violence), and collective violence (for example, religious or ethnic violence or state-sanctioned warfare). *Unintentional* injuries are often subdivided by mechanism—road traffic injuries, falls, burns, poisonings, drownings, and so on. Injuries may also be classified in other ways: according to the environment or circumstances in which they occur (for example, home, workplace, or roadways), by the body parts or systems most affected (for example, spinal cord injury), or by a particular pattern or context that results in injuries, (for example, intimate partner violence).

Global Burden of Injury. Injuries are a significant cause of both morbidity and mortality throughout the world, ranking among the ten leading causes of death worldwide (Krug, 1999). According to WHO, injury ranks as a leading cause of death and disability among all age groups up to the age of sixty (Peden, McGee, and Krug, 2002). An estimated 5 million people worldwide died from injuries in 2000, accounting for 9 percent of global deaths and 12 percent of the global burden of disease. As injuries commonly target young men during their most productive years, the burden of injuries is often distributed far beyond the injured individual.

Injuries place a disproportionate burden on the world's poor; more than 90 percent of injuries in 2000 occurred in LICs and MICs (Peden, McGee, and Krug, 2002). The LICs and MICs of Europe have the highest injury mortality rates, but the Southeast Asia and Western Pacific regions account for the highest number of injury deaths worldwide. Even in HICs such as the United States, injuries account for about one in four ED visits (McCaig and Burt, 2003). In the United States, injuries are the number one cause of death between the ages of one and forty-four and account for more years of potential life lost before age sixty-five than all causes of cancer and all causes of heart disease combined.

Injury mortality has a multimodal age distribution, most heavily affecting children, adolescents, young adults, and parents of young children. Young people between the ages of fifteen and forty-four years account for nearly half of the world's fatal injuries. Because of their vulnerability and often close proximity to water and fire, children under five years of age account for approximately 25 percent of drowning deaths and just over 15 percent of fire-related deaths worldwide.

Injury rates are higher in males than in females. For example, global injury mortality is twice as high among males as among females, and for some types of injuries—road traffic injuries and interpersonal violence—the disparity approaches threefold. However, this pattern varies by injury type; in some regions female mortality rates from suicide and burns are as high as or even higher than male rates.

In contrast to the progress that has been made in the control of many infectious diseases, little has been done to stem the tide of injuries around the world. In fact the World Bank predicts that the global burden of injuries, especially those caused by interpersonal violence, war, self-inflicted injuries, and road traffic, will increase dramatically by the year 2020 (Murray and Lopez, 1996). Road traffic injuries alone are expected to rise from the ninth leading cause of lost disability-adjusted life years (DALYs) worldwide to third by 2020 (Table 25.1).

The Injury Pyramid. Injury mortality data represent only a small fraction of the total injury burden. For every injured victim who dies, there are typically

TABLE 25.1. RANKING OF INJURY-RELATED MORTALITY AND BURDEN OF DISEASE (DALYS LOST), 1990 AND 2020.

	Rank (number of deaths)		*Rank (DALYs lost)*	
	1990	**2020**	**1990**	**2020**
Road traffic injuries	9	6	9	3
Self-inflicted injuries	12	10	17	14
Interpersonal violence	16	14	19	12
War	20	15	16	8

Source: Murray and Lopez, 1996.

FIGURE 25.1. THE INJURY PYRAMID.

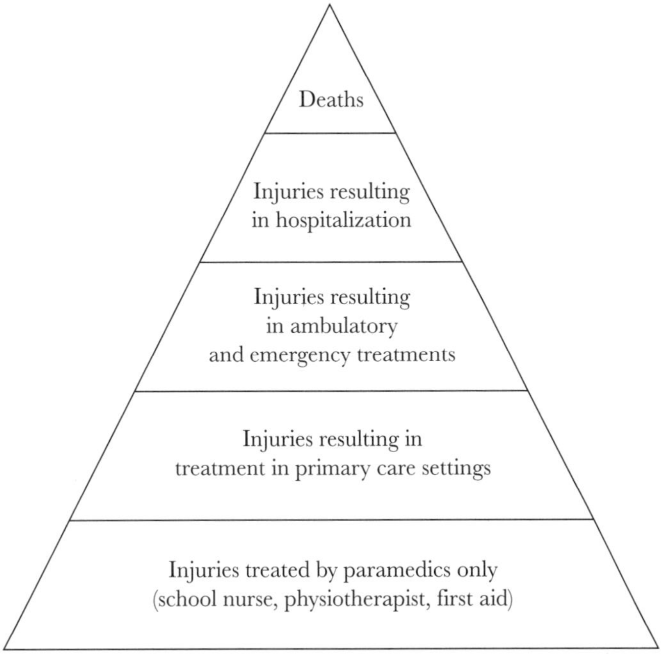

many more who sustain serious but nonfatal injuries. Many of these victims suffer long-lasting or even permanent disabilities. Because, in general, nonfatal events greatly outnumber fatalities, the relationship among injury deaths, hospitalizations, and ED or office visits can be viewed as an *injury pyramid* (Figure 25.1). For example, a recent study of injuries in Missouri and Nebraska during the three-year period from 1996 through 1998 identified 13,052 fatal injuries, 131,210 hospital admissions for injuries, and 1.9 million injury visits to emergency departments. Road traffic injuries and firearm-related injuries were the leading causes of fatal injury in both states, but falls were a far more common cause of hospital admissions and ED visits than firearms were, ranking second only to road traffic injuries (Wadman, Muelleman, Coto, and Kellermann, 2003).

It is likely that similar ratios of fatal to nonfatal injuries by cause prevail in LICs and MICs. However, many countries lack the data systems necessary to tabulate these counts routinely and reliably. As a result, mortality data are often the only information available to quantify the public health impact of injuries. This means that conclusions are based on only the tip of a very large pyramid.

Identifying Risk and Protective Factors

The second step of the public health approach calls for characterizing risk and protective factors associated with injuries. In practice this is done through descriptive epidemiological studies. These studies characterize *who* is injured, *what* injuries are involved, and *where, when,* and, *why* particular injuries occur. These data can also generate hypotheses for further investigation with analytical studies. In some cases the link between a risk factor and injury is so strong that no additional research is needed. For example, early studies of road traffic injuries in the United States revealed that half of all fatal crashes and 60 percent of fatal single-vehicle crashes involved alcohol (Polen and Friedman, 1988). In other cases, in order to quantify the impact of particular risk factors, it is necessary to compare the rate of injury among those *with* the risk factors of interest to the rate among similar individuals *without* these risk factors. Conversely, protective factors, essentially negative risk factors, can diminish the effect of an injury or prevent it from occurring at all. The protective effect of bicycle helmets against closed head injuries is an excellent example of a strong protective factor that mitigates the effect of a potentially devastating injury.

Developing and Testing Interventions

Once risk and protective factors have been investigated, interventions can be conceived, developed, and tested. Careful attention must be given to the characteristics of the target population, the feasibility of the candidate countermeasure(s), the acceptability of the countermeasures among the target population, and the countermeasure cost. Pilot programs are often helpful to test various strategies. The most promising can then be selected for widespread implementation. The Haddon matrix is particularly useful for managing this process of injury prevention and control.

William Haddon, a physician, established the field of injury control by applying the core principles of public health to the prevention and mitigation of injuries. Using the time-tested concept of the *epidemiological triangle*—the idea that many diseases result from harmful interactions among the *host,* the disease *vector,* and the *environment*—Haddon showed how these same three factors interact to cause many injuries. To facilitate the identification of opportunities for prevention and control, Haddon divided injury-causing events into three temporal phases: the pre-event phase, the event itself, and the post-event phase. This yielded a phase-factor matrix of nine cells, as shown in Table 25.2 (Haddon, 1972). Examining each cell can suggest various strategies to prevent or control injuries. Since its introduction in 1972, the Haddon matrix has proven to be an invaluable tool for injury prevention and control.

TABLE 25.2. THE HADDON MATRIX APPLIED TO MOTOR VEHICLE CRASHES.

	Factors		
Phases	**Host**	**Agent**	**Environment**
Pre-event	Alcohol; speed	Tires; brakes	Signs; signals; surface
Event	Belt use; helmet use	Seat belt; air bags	Side slope; guardrails
Post-event	Health; age	Fuel system; materials	EMS response; road shoulders

Source: Haddon, 1972.

TABLE 25.3. OPTIONS ANALYSIS IN INJURY CONTROL.

Options	**Examples**
1. Prevent creation of hazard.	Ban production and civilian sale of assault weapons.
2. Reduce the amount of hazard.	Limit water heater temperature to 125°F (47.25°C).
3. Prevent the release of a hazard that already exists.	Put dangerous medications in "childproof" containers.
4. Modify the rate of distribution of release of the hazard from its source.	Require fire-safe cigarettes that cannot easily ignite furniture or bedding.
5. Separate, by time or space, the hazard from the host.	Construct overpasses or underpasses to eliminate crossing streams of traffic.
6. Physically separate, by barriers, the hazard from the host.	Equip taxicabs with bulletproof and knifeproof partitions.
7. Modify surfaces and basic structures to minimize injury.	Equip all new cars with driver-side and passenger-side air bags.
8. Make that which is to be protected more resistant to damage.	Issue bulletproof vests to law enforcement officers and security guards.
9. Mitigate damage already done.	Promote citizen training in first aid and cardiopulmonary resuscitation (CPR).
10. Stabilize, repair, and rehabilitate the injured person.	Implement trauma care.

Source: Haddon, 1973.

Haddon (1973) later outlined ten generic injury-control strategies that can be used to break the chain of injury causation (Table 25.3). Examining this list to identify the most promising approaches is known as *options analysis.* The best strategy is not always the most obvious one or the one most proximate to the injury itself. Often a combination of strategies is superior to any single one.

Haddon's ideas were first applied to the prevention and control of motor vehicle crashes, an application that is illustrated in Box 25.1. They yielded dramatic results. According to the Centers for Disease Control and Prevention (CDC), between 1925 and 1999 the number of drivers increased sixfold, the number of motor vehicles increased elevenfold, and the number of vehicle miles traveled (VMTs) increased tenfold. Despite this dramatic increase in automobile use, the death rate per 100 million VMTs plummeted from 18 in 1925 to only 1.7 in 1997, a 90 percent decrease (CDC, 1999). On the strength of this accomplishment the CDC acclaimed the reduction in road and traffic fatalities as one of the top ten public health achievements of the twentieth century. Other developed countries, such as Sweden and United Kingdom, have achieved equal if not more impressive improvements in road traffic safety (Evans, 2004). Assuredly, this reduction in mortality began before Haddon applied his theories to injury control, and there were significant advances in road safety and automobile engineering that resulted in substantial safety gains. Nevertheless, Haddon's approach to traffic safety was revolutionary and facilitated a great public health accomplishment.

Box 25.1. The Car Crash in Which Princess Diana Died

On August 31, 1997, Diana Princess of Wales and her companion, Dodi al Fayed, were involved in a high-speed car crash in a roadway underpass in Paris, France. The Princess, her companion, and the car's chauffeur, Henri Paul, were all killed; Trevor Rees-Jones, a restrained front-seat passenger, survived with facial trauma. The crash—the details of which are well known and have been broadcast around the world—the crash response, and the ultimately fatal outcomes lend themselves to Haddon Matrix analysis. This analysis illustrates several principles of injury prevention and control.

Using the terms of Haddon's matrix, the hosts of the injury were the princess, al Fayed, Rees-Jones, and Paul; only Rees-Jones was restrained. The princess and al Fayed were in the backseat. The vector was deceleration precipitated by the impact of the car against a supporting column in the underpass, and in turn the deceleration injuries sustained by the vehicle's passengers. The hosts' environment included the interior of the car and the backseat in particular; the car's environment included an underpass with central support columns, rather than a smooth wall or a guardrail to separate the columns from the road way.

Dividing the event further, important pre-event phase factors included the chauffeur's intoxication and the car's high speed. Important factors affecting the event itself included the lack of restraints (seat belts) in use and the lack of supplemental passive measures (airbags) that deployed during the fatal impact. A key post-event factor affecting the outcome was the emergency medical service (EMS) response, which was focused on on-scene extraction and treatment rather than expedited transport to a trauma care facility. Rees-Jones was extricated and treated for facial injuries; the chauffeur and al Fayed were pronounced dead on EMS arrival; the princess was still alive when EMS arrived. The delay in transporting the extricated princess to a hospital was approximately forty-five minutes to an hour. Despite her significant injuries, had the post-event phase of her injury been managed more expeditiously, the ultimate outcome might have been less tragic, illustrating another key component of injury control: mitigation of an injury's effect.

This brief analysis illustrates a host of injury prevention and control principles and suggests multiple ways in which injuries can be prevented and their effects mitigated and controlled.

Implementing Interventions and Ensuring Widespread Acceptance of Control Strategies

The fourth component of the public health approach, implementing interventions and pursuing widespread adoption of the most effective strategies, is best considered jointly with the third component, developing and testing interventions. So in this section we outline some of the basic concepts of injury prevention strategies and illustrate that developing such strategies and ensuring their widespread adoption form something of a continuum. (Another part of the fourth component is evaluation, and we discuss that separately later.)

Active Versus Passive Interventions. Most injury prevention strategies can be classified as either active or passive. *Active* countermeasures require the conscious cooperation of the individual to be effective. Examples include the use of manual safety belts, motorcycle helmets, child safety seats, and protective eyewear in the workplace. *Passive* countermeasures require little or no cooperation by the person being protected. Examples include air bags in cars, sprinkler systems in public buildings, flotation hulls on watercraft, and shields that prevent workers from becoming ensnared in hazardous equipment.

The Three E's of Injury Control. Most injury control countermeasures, whether active or passive, employ one of three generic strategies: *education, enforcement* of regulations, or *engineering* of physical structures (including *environmental* changes). Each approach offers advantages and disadvantages.

Education is often the first approach taken to promote safe behavior. Educational interventions encourage the public to adopt safe behaviors and practices voluntarily. Implicit in this approach is the belief that once people know what to do to reduce their risk of injury, they will change their behavior. Examples of such interventions are driver's education, child pedestrian training (Burke and others, 1996), education of parents and caregivers to reduce playground injuries among children (Withaneachi and Meehan, 1998), posters and videos that promote safe behavior in the workplace (Smith, 2001), and various training materials that promote burn prevention (Herd, Widdowson, and Tanner, 1986; Keswani, 1986).

Public education campaigns are popular because they are voluntary. Although educational programs do lead to an increase in *knowledge,* they may have little impact on *behavior* and on injury rates, especially if they are carried out in isolation. For example, a systematic review of randomized, controlled trials on improving pedestrian safety showed improvements in some road safety behaviors among trained pedestrians but no consistent, overall behavioral change (Duperrex, Bunn, and Roberts, 2002).

The impact of public education is often blunted by *attenuation of effect.* No matter how powerful, pervasive, and repetitive a safety message may be, some people never encounter it. Among those who do, some will actively reject the message. Some who accept the message will be insufficiently motivated to change their behavior. Among those who change their behavior, some will relapse over time. Others will fail to follow the message consistently. Finally, not everyone who adopts a protective strategy escapes injury.

Enforcement of laws and regulations may increase compliance when voluntary acceptance of an effective countermeasure is poor. Motorcycle helmets provide a telling example. Wearing a motorcycle helmet reduces the risk of death or severe traumatic brain injury in a crash by approximately 55 percent. In states where helmet use is voluntary, only about half of motorcyclists wear one, whereas in states where helmet use is mandated and the law is aggressively enforced, helmet usage exceeds 98 percent (National Highway Traffic Safety Administration, 2003). Evaluations have conclusively shown that states with mandatory helmet laws have lower motorcycle crash fatality rates than do states that lack these laws (Ulmer and Preusser, 2003). Bicycle helmet use can be increased with legislation as well (Graitcer, Kellermann, and Christoffel, 1995). In Montgomery County, Maryland, educational efforts to encourage bicycle helmet use increased self-reported use from 8 to 13 percent. In nearby Howard County, where educational efforts were supplemented by a mandatory bicycle helmet law, helmet use increased from 11 to 37 percent (Dannenberg and others, 1993).

Combining education and enforcement usually works better than relying on either strategy alone. In Elmira, New York, a publicity campaign combined with high-visibility enforcement of the state's safety belt law boosted rates of use from 49 to 77 percent. Four months after the effort ceased, safety belt use declined to 66 percent, but it rebounded to 80 percent during a reminder campaign (Williams, Preusser, Blomberg, and Lund, 1987). In Houston, Texas, the use of safety belts increased from 39 to 54 percent after a multifaceted program that included education, a media campaign, and high-profile law enforcement (Hanfling,

Mangus, Gill, and Bailey, 2000). In Brazil a 20 percent reduction in traffic fatalities followed the implementation of speed limits (Poli de Figueiredo and others, 2001). In the cities of Bogotá and Cali, Colombia, a widely publicized and visibly enforced ban on the carrying of firearms during elections and high-risk holidays was associated with a significant decrease in the rate of homicides compared to the rate when the ban was not in effect (Villaveces and others, 2000).

Although mandatory use laws are often effective, they may be difficult to enact. Opponents of such laws argue that they infringe on personal freedom and that individuals have the right to choose hazardous behavior if the risk is acceptable to them. Moreover, enforcement of regulations can be difficult in many LICs due to limited resources. In Ghana, for example, a nation of 18 million, the entire 16,000-member police force has only 145 vehicles available for enforcement and other purposes (Forjuoh, 2003).

In workplace settings, rules to promote safe behavior by employees may be easily introduced, but they are unlikely to be effective unless they are visibly and consistently enforced. Examples include requiring the use of hard hats in construction zones, safety goggles near ocular hazards, and safety straps when working in high places and enforcing a strict no-smoking policy around flammable materials.

Engineering solutions are the injury control strategy that draws most directly on the preventive paradigm of environmental health (see Chapter Twenty-Nine). Many injuries can be prevented by designing and building safety into products or environments. The up-front cost of engineering may exceed the cost of education or enforcement campaigns, but the downstream effects are often greater as well. Engineering is usually more effective than behavioral change because it does not require the cooperation of users to exert its protective effects.

Consider the following examples. In contrast to unsuccessful efforts to "fix the nut behind the wheel," adoption of federal standards for passenger restraint systems (seat belts), safety glass, fuel system integrity, and nonflammable interior fabric saved an estimated 37,000 lives between 1975 and 1978 alone. The subsequent introduction of air bags cut the annual toll of crash-related deaths and injuries still further (Kahane, 1998).

Seat belts in cars are a good example of successful engineering for injury prevention. When properly used, they reduce motor vehicle fatalities by about 50 percent and serious injury by about 55 percent. They are affordable and feasible in countries where automobile use is prevalent or rapidly increasing, but it is difficult to encourage widespread use of safety belts without high-visibility enforcement (Forjuoh, 2003).

LICs differ from HICs in their patterns of road traffic deaths. Whereas in HICs motor vehicle occupants make up the majority of fatal road traffic injury victims, in LICs the majority of victims are "vulnerable road users"—pedestrians, passengers riding in large vehicles such as trucks and buses, and riders of two-wheelers (bicycles and motorcycles) (Razzak, Laflamme, Luby, and Chotani, 2004; Peden and others, 2004). Because it is very difficult if not impossible to get pedestrians to change their behavior consistently, engineering interventions are often the most effective strategy for protecting them. Options include installation of sidewalks, imposition of roadway barriers between pedestrians and traffic, placement of flexible "pedestrian crossing" signs in the center of a roadway, creation of one-way-street networks in urban areas, school zone signage and other measures, and installation of adequate lighting so that pedestrians crossing roadways are visible at night (Retting, Ferguson, and McCartt, 2003). Many of these interventions can be adopted by LICs, particularly in locations where pedestrian injuries occur with great frequency (Forjuoh, 2003).

In South Asia, high burn death rates among females result from using portable stoves on uneven surfaces (where they can overturn and explode) or on the floor (where long skirts can catch fire and where refueling and maintenance are difficult) (Fauveau and Blancet, 1989; Marsh and others, 1996). Simple changes in stove design to keep heat and flames away from clothing and out of reach of children could prevent many burns. Loose, flammable clothing is another important risk factor for burns among children and women in some LICs. Proven interventions from HICs (Baker, O'Neill, Ginsburg, and Li, 1992), such as use of fabrics that are less flammable, fire-resistance standards for children's sleepwear, and a change from loose, frilly dresses to more close-fitting clothes, can be applied in LIC settings with significant advantage.

Engineering strategies can be applied to equipment and devices, or they can be applied on a larger scale, to environments. Seat belts are an example of an engineering change within an automobile; banked curves, guardrails, and separation of opposing lanes of traffic are examples of larger-scale environmental changes. Both kinds of change are usually considered engineering strategies, but in the examples later in this chapter, we distinguish engineering and environmental change, in part to emphasize the role of environmental health approaches in injury control.

Because engineering solutions can increase the cost of a product, they are often unpopular with manufacturers. For this reason many advocates of injury prevention support consumer product safety laws to compel manufacturers to act. Manufacturers often oppose product safety legislation because they fear it will raise the prices of their products, discourage sales, and reduce their ability to compete with nonregulated manufacturers in other countries. When efforts to regulate a hazardous product fail, product liability lawsuits may be the only way to force a needed change in product design. That can elicit another form of legislative backlash, as manufacturers seek protection from product liability lawsuits under the guise of "tort reform" (Vernick, Mair, Teret, and Sapsin, 2003).

Evaluating and Refining Interventions

Program evaluation is an important part of the public health approach. Without continuing surveillance and other well-designed modes of program evaluation, it is difficult to assess which interventions have the greatest impact and, therefore, which should be reinforced and which curtailed. Program evaluation uses established methods to reach valid conclusions about the effects of a given intervention; this large field is beyond the scope of this chapter. In general, however, many prevention programs are evaluated by determining their impact on morbidity or mortality in the target population. When good surveillance systems are in place, this approach is worthwhile and can produce valid results. However, large-scale surveillance is not always possible or might fail to detect the effects of small-scale demonstration projects. In some instances surrogate measures may be used to assess program impact. For example, rates of smoke detector use in a target neighborhood before and after a promotional program might be used in evaluating that program because quantifying fire-related injuries—which are rare events—might take too long. Also, as surveillance is time consuming and expensive, sampling techniques can establish patterns in subsets of a given population; these patterns can then be extrapolated to the population as a whole. This technique can be useful for MICs and LICs, where resource constraints can limit sample size. Regardless of the form the evaluation takes, it must be tailored to the intervention and the outcome of interest, and the methodology should yield valid results. Once a good program evaluation has been performed, intervention priorities can be reorganized, the Haddon matrix can be revisited, and new prevention goals can be pursued.

Injury Prevention in Practice

Now that we have outlined the public health approach and explored several of its key components with regard to injury control, we turn to several specific types of injuries to illustrate how that approach is applied.

Intentional Injuries (Violence)

The World Health Organization defines violence as "the intentional use of physical force or power, threatened or actual, against oneself, another person, or against a group or community that either results in or has a high likelihood of resulting in injury, death, psychological harm, mal-development or deprivation" (Krug and others, 2002, p. 5).

The *World Report on Violence and Health,* published by the WHO Department of Violence and Injury Prevention in 2002, divides violence into three broad categories: self-directed violence; interpersonal violence, and collective violence (Krug and others, 2002). These terms describe, respectively, attempted and completed suicides (as well as parasuicides); violence inflicted by another individual or by small groups of individuals; and violence inflicted by larger groups such as states, organized political groups, militia groups, and terrorist organizations. These three broad categories may each be divided further to reflect specific subsets of violence, including physical, sexual, and psychological violence and violence involving deprivation or neglect. This typology is graphically presented in Figure 25.2.

Epidemiology and Risk Factors. Violence caused 51,326 deaths and 2,058,547 injuries in 2001 in the United States (National Center for Injury Prevention and Control [NCIPC], 2004). The economic impact of gunshot wounds in the United States alone is estimated at $126 billion (Cook and Ludwig, 2000). Cutting or stab wounds cost an additional $51 billion (Miller and Cohen, 1997). In 2000, an estimated 1.6 million people worldwide died as a result of violence. Violence is a leading cause of death for people aged fifteen to forty-four worldwide, accounting for about 14 percent of deaths among males and 7 percent of deaths among females. Most of these deaths occur in low- and middle-income countries. Nearly half of violence-related deaths in any given year are suicides, almost one-third are homicides, and about one-fifth are war related. Mortality figures represent the tip of the iceberg. For every person who dies as a result of violence, many more sustain nonfatal injuries. Many survivors of violence suffer a range of physical, sexual, reproductive, and mental health problems.

Countermeasures. Countermeasures for intentional injuries include a range of strategies. Many countries attempt to reduce the degree of harm caused by violence by controlling access to or use of firearms, the most common means of interpersonal violence (Krug and others, 2002; Kellermann, Lee, Mercy, and Banton, 1991). Although some of the best-known violence countermeasures rely on education and enforcement, a surprising number relate to environmental change. These measures are sometimes known as *crime prevention through environmental design,* or CPTED (Sherman and others, 1998), and some examples are shown in Table 25.4.

Burns

A burn occurs when some or all of the layers of the skin are destroyed by a hot liquid (scald), a hot solid (contact burn), or a flame (flame burn). Burns can also be produced by exposure to ultraviolet radiation, radioactivity, electricity, or certain chemicals.

FIGURE 25.2. TYPOLOGY OF VIOLENCE.

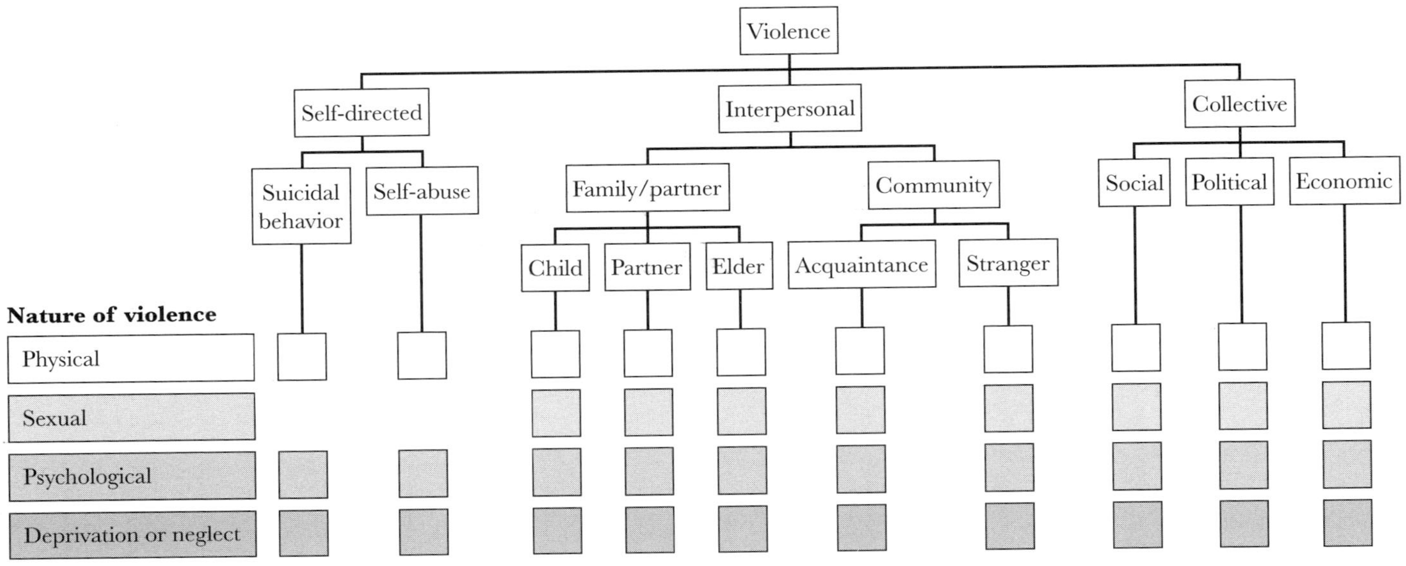

Source: Krug and others, 2002, © World Health Organization.

TABLE 25.4. COUNTERMEASURES FOR INTENTIONAL INJURIES.

Education	Anger management interventions
Enforcement	Community policing Targeted patrols, to discourage the carrying of concealed weapons Earlier closing hours for bars
Engineering	Safety locks on guns
Environmental change	Improved street lighting Safe pedestrian routes Bulletproof booths at all-night gas stations and selected retail outlets Drop safes, to limit cash on hand Protective shields between the front and back seats in taxicabs

TABLE 25.5. COUNTERMEASURES FOR BURNS.

Education	Burn prevention campaigns
Enforcement	Building codes Smoking rules around flammable material
Engineering	Tap water temperature reduction Temperature regulating valves Modified handles Smoke detectors Automatic sprinklers Control of ignition sources (cigarettes, matches, and lighters) Reduction of clothing flammability
Environmental change	Elevated hearth for the fire

Epidemiology and Risk Factors. In the United States there are 2,600 deaths and 14,000 injuries due to fire each year. Residential fires alone result in more than $6 billion in property damage annually (Karter, 2003). Globally, fire-related burns accounted for 238,000 deaths in 2000. At least 80 percent of these deaths occurred in homes. More than 95 percent of fatal fire-related burns worldwide occur in LICs and MICs. Females in Southeast Asia have the highest fire-related burn mortality rates worldwide, followed by males in Africa and females in the Eastern Mediterranean. Children under five years of age and the elderly (those over seventy years old) have the highest burn mortality rates. In India alone there are approximately 100,000 deaths due to burns each year; 600,000 burn victims require hospital admission and treatment in a burn unit.

Countermeasures. Countermeasures for burns include a wide range of strategies, as shown in Table 25.5.

Poisoning

A poison exposure is the ingestion of or contact with a substance that can produce toxic effects. Poisonings can be acute or chronic, as discussed in Chapter Two. Acute poisonings are classified as injuries.

Epidemiology and Risk Factors. In 2000, poison centers in the United States reported approximately 2.2 million poison exposures, an average of one exposure every fifteen seconds. More than 90 percent of poison exposures occur at home, and just over half of exposures involve children younger than age six. The most common poison exposures for children are ingestion of household products such as cosmetics and personal care products, cleaning substances, pain relievers, foreign bodies, and plants. For adults, the most common poison exposures are pain relievers, sedatives, cleaning substances, antidepressants, and bites or stings. Carbon monoxide (CO) results in more fatal unintentional poisonings in the United States than any other agent, with the highest number occurring during the winter months. Medical spending for poisoning treatment totaled $3 billion in 1992. Spending would be considerably higher in the United States without the established network of poison control centers that aid in the triage and treatment of acute poisonings (Darwin, 2003; Miller and Lestina, 1997).

Worldwide, poisonings rank sixth as a cause of injury. However, data on poisonings in developing countries are scarce. The spectrum of poisoning in LICs is probably different from that in developed countries. Pesticides, kerosene, and other chemicals are common causes of poisoning in LIC settings.

Countermeasures. Countermeasures for poisoning rely more heavily on education, enforcement, and engineering than on environmental changes, as shown in Table 25.6.

TABLE 25.6. COUNTERMEASURES FOR POISONING.

Education	Warning labels Physician-based education programs Community-based education programs Poison control centers
Enforcement	Carbon monoxide alarms
Engineering	Child-resistant packaging Carbon monoxide alarms Shape and size of tablets of medicine
Environmental change	Locked storage for pesticide stocks on farms

Falls

A fall is an event that results in a person coming to rest inadvertently on the ground or floor or other lower level.

Epidemiology and Risk Factors. More than one in three U.S. adults aged sixty-five and older falls each year, making falls a leading cause of fatal injuries and the most common cause of nonfatal injuries and hospital admissions for trauma among that age group in the United States. Globally, an estimated 283,000 people died due to falls in 2000. A quarter of all fatal falls occurred in the HICs. Europe and the Western Pacific region combined account for nearly 60 percent of the total number of fall-related deaths worldwide. Males in the LICs and MICs of Europe have by far the highest fall-related mortality rates worldwide.

There are two distinct at-risk populations for falls, children and the elderly. In all regions of the world, adults over the age of seventy years, particularly females, have significantly higher fall-related mortality rates than younger people do. However, children account for the most morbidity, with almost 50 percent of the total number of DALYs lost. In lowland areas of tropical countries where tree agriculture is widespread, occupational falls from trees and other tree-related injuries are a leading cause of death, hospitalization, or permanent disability from spinal cord injury. In some countries, building-related falls from unprotected rooftops, windows, and stairs are a common source of injury for children. The home environment has been identified as a potential contributor to as many as 50 percent of falls occurring to the elderly. Falls among children, in contrast, are related to their age. Young children most frequently fall in and around the home, for example, from chairs, from beds, and down stairs. Older children fall from playground equipment, during play and recreational activities, and during sports.

Countermeasures. Countermeasures for falls rely heavily on environmental interventions, as shown in Table 25.7.

TABLE 25.7. COUNTERMEASURES FOR FALLS.

Education	Physical activity and balancing exercises
Enforcement	Legislation for barriers in high-rise buildings
Engineering	Barriers in high-rise buildings
Environmental change	Removal of obstructed pathways and loose throw rugs Well-maintained stairways Improved lighting and visibility Modification of hard surfaces on which people might fall Safety devices, such as grab bars Barriers in high-rise buildings

TABLE 25.8. COUNTERMEASURES FOR DROWNING.

Education	Swimming instruction Training in resuscitation techniques
Enforcement	Supervision; lifeguards
Engineering	Pool alarms; pool covers Personal flotation devices
Environmental change	Four-sided fencing around pools

Drowning

Drowning is fatal respiratory impairment from submersion or immersion in liquid.

Epidemiology and Risk Factors. In the United States more than 3,000 people die in unintentional drownings each year, averaging 9 people per day. About three times that number receive care in emergency departments for near drownings. In 2000, an estimated 450,000 people drowned worldwide, making drowning the second leading cause of unintentional injury death after road traffic injuries. These global burden of disease figures underestimate drowning deaths, because they exclude drowning due to floods, boating, and water transport. Ninety-seven percent of all drowning deaths occur in LICs and MICs. The Western Pacific and Southeast Asia regions account for 60 percent of the mortality and DALYs. Males in Africa and in the Western Pacific have the highest drowning mortality rates worldwide. Among the various age groups, children under five years of age have the highest drowning mortality rates. Over half the global mortality due to drowning and 60 percent of the total number of DALYs lost due to drowning occur among children younger than fifteen years old.

Countermeasures. Drowning countermeasures are summarized in Table 25.8.

Injury Control in Special Settings

Certain settings have special importance for injury control, either because they pose a particular risk or because specific control strategies are available. This section discusses four such settings: the workplace, playgrounds, roadways, and the home.

The Workplace

Occupational injuries represent a considerable part of the injury burden on society, affecting people in the most productive years of their lives.

Epidemiology. Globally, almost 1,000 workers are killed by injuries every day, and about 6 of every 1,000 workers will be fatally injured at work during a forty-year worklife. Nonfatal injuries are an even more pervasive problem. In the United States alone, almost 16,000 workers are hurt on the job each day, producing 6 million occupational injury cases annually. Nevertheless, this represents a significant improvement over historical levels of injury. In the past sixty years, the annual rate of workplace injury fatalities in the United States has declined from 37 per 100,000 full-time workers in 1933 to 4 per 100,000 in 1997.

Occupational injuries cover a wide spectrum. They range from skin cuts to piercing wounds, burns, amputations, crush injuries, eye injuries, and chemical exposures. In certain occupational groups, such as law enforcement personnel and commercial truck drivers, violence or road traffic injuries are leading causes of occupational injuries and deaths.

Countermeasures. Countermeasures for workplace injuries are shown in Table 25.9 (and are discussed in more detail in Chapter Twenty-Three).

Playgrounds

In terms of Haddon's approach, children are the host of playground injuries; the vector is often potential energy, in the form of gravity, as many playground injuries result from falls (from swings, slides, or other equipment, for example). As children may not be supervised and cannot be relied on to generate active injury control themselves, the playground environment must be engineered with passive injury control in mind.

Epidemiology. More than 200,000 children are treated for playground equipment–related injuries in U.S. hospital emergency rooms each year. Two-thirds of these injuries occur on public playgrounds. Four out of five injuries involve falls, primarily to the surface below the equipment (Tinsworth and McDonald, 2001).

TABLE 25.9. COUNTERMEASURES FOR WORKPLACE INJURIES.

Education	Job safety training
Enforcement	Occupational safety and health standards that require use of protective gear, such as eyewear, hard hats, and safety belts
Engineering	Machine guards; automated sensors to interrupt hazardous equipment
Environmental change	Conversion to automated production lines; barriers that divide workers from vehicles

TABLE 25.10. COUNTERMEASURES FOR PLAYGROUND INJURIES.

Education	Education of children, parents, and teachers
Enforcement	Adult playground supervision to prevent bullying and hazardous behavior
Engineering	Limiting the average incline of a slide to <30 degrees Handrails on stairways and stepladders Cover playground surfaces with wood chips, double-shredded bark mulch, or pea gravel.
Environmental change	Organization of equipment to prevent injuries from conflicting activities and from children running between activities Separation of equipment by user age

Countermeasures. Countermeasures for playground injuries rely heavily on engineering and environmental changes, as shown in Table 25.10.

Roadways

Transportation injuries, especially those that occur on and near roadways, represent one of the leading categories of injuries worldwide. (These injuries are also discussed in Chapter Seventeen.) A *road traffic injury* is defined as any injury due to a crash involving one or more vehicles and originating or terminating on a public roadway.

Epidemiology. The worldwide epidemic of road traffic injuries is only just beginning. At present over a million people die each year and some 10 million people sustain permanent disabilities in road traffic crashes. For people under forty-four years of age, road traffic crashes are a leading cause of death and disability, second only to HIV and AIDS. Many developing countries are still at comparatively low levels of motorization, and the incidence of road traffic injuries in these countries is likely to increase. It is estimated that by 2020, road traffic crashes will have moved from ninth to third in the world disease burden ranking, as measured in DALYs.

Several categories of risk factors for road injuries can be identified. These relate to road users, the road itself, and vehicles. These factors, in turn, suggest a variety of injury control strategies (Peden and others, 2004). All road users are at risk of being injured or killed in a road traffic crash, although *vulnerable road users,* such as pedestrians and two-wheelers, usually bear the greatest burden. In a review of road traffic collisions in thirty-eight developing countries, it was found that pedestrian fatalities outnumbered other road-user deaths in 75 percent of the studies (Odero, Garner, and Zwi, 1997). Young male drivers and their passengers were at higher risk. Multicountry studies have shown that individuals from less privileged socioeconomic groups or living in poorer areas are at greatest risk of being killed or injured. Seat belt use among drivers and vehicle occupants has been found to decrease death and nonfatal injuries by 50 percent. Similarly, a child who is properly restrained in a safety seat is 71 percent less likely to die in a crash than is a child who is not properly restrained. Another major risk factor for road traffic injuries is use of alcohol. Alcohol consumption increases the probability both that a crash will occur and that death or serious injury will follow. A survey of studies in LICs and MICs found that a positive blood alcohol level was noted in 8 to 29 percent of drivers involved in crashes who were not fatally injured and in 33 to 69 percent of fatally injured drivers.

Roadway factors are also extremely important. Roads built to facilitate transport without consideration of safety can dramatically increase the incidence of serious and fatal traffic injuries. In many countries roads have multiple users, ranging from pedestrians to two-wheelers to automobiles and large vehicles. From the perspective of pedestrians and cyclists, proximity to motor vehicles capable of traveling at high speeds is the most important road safety problem. A road network planned for safety includes a hierarchy of roads, each intended to serve a certain function. It should also include infrastructure that protects pedestrians and bicyclists from automobiles and large transport vehicles. Each road should be designed according to its particular function in the network. A key characteristic of a well-designed road is that it protects vulnerable road users from large vehicles and makes compliance with the intended speed limit a natural choice for drivers. Such design can not only prevent injuries but also achieve other public health goals, such as promoting walking and bicycling (see Chapter Seventeen).

Vehicle design can have considerable influence on crash injuries. Many factors can increase the risk of injury, such as poor design of the crush zone so it fails to absorb energy, failure of the structural cage around the passenger compartment to provide a protective shell, absence of features that protect occupants from side impacts or stop them from being ejected from the vehicle, and lack of high-mounted brake lights in the rear. Similarly, vehicles that are not clearly visible are at high risk of involvement in crashes, especially at night, and slow-moving vehicles on fast-moving roadways are at risk for rear-end crashes. Daytime running lights for cars, though not required in many countries, reduce the incidence of daytime crashes by 10 to 15 percent (Elvik, 1996). Bus and truck fronts designed to reduce injuries to pedestrians and cyclists could also lower the injury burden, as could minimizing differences in vehicle design in ways that

TABLE 25.11. COUNTERMEASURES FOR ROAD INJURIES.

Education	Pedestrian safety education Bicyclist training schemes Motorist education Helmet and safety belt promotion
Enforcement	Speed limits Graduated driver's licenses Strategies for reducing alcohol-impaired driving Helmet and safety belt use laws
Engineering	Puncture-resistant gas tanks Energy-absorbing interiors Crush zones and reinforced cages around occupants Air bags
Environmental change	Areawide traffic calming Bicycle paths and lanes Energy-absorbing materials in front of bridge columns and other fixed objects Breakaway light poles Roadway lighting at high-frequency pedestrian crossings

would reduce injuries when a higher-riding vehicle and a lower-riding vehicle collide.

Countermeasures. Countermeasures to reduce road injuries draw on a broad spectrum of strategies from driver and pedestrian education to environmental modifications. Examples appear in Table 25.11 and Box 25.2.

Box 25.2. Highway-Railroad Crossings

The United States has over 200,000 miles of railroad tracks, and railroads carry approximately 40 percent of the country's freight traffic. In 2003, according to the Federal Railway Administration (FRA), there were over 750 million train miles traveled, and there were 368 fatalities involving highway-rail crossings. According to FRA surveillance data, the rate of fatalities at highway-rail crossings has steadily declined since the 1990s while total rail traffic has significantly increased. Safety officials attribute the drop in fatality rates to several factors. These measures include education, engineering, and enforcement activities and provide an interesting example of injury prevention and control.

Railroad crossings are engineered environments. Crash injuries at crossings involve kinetic energy transferred from a moving train, with limited capacity to brake, to a moving or stationary highway vehicle and its passengers. Engineering solutions to crossing injuries have been aimed at limiting the ability of motor vehicles to enter the crossing—and thus the zone where injury is likely to occur—at the same time a train enters the crossing. Passive measures are the most reliable as they do not require active motorist compliance. Crossing arms are a longstanding example of a passive measure, though motorists may circumvent simple arms and enter the crossing. Innovations have included medians that tightly direct traffic flow at crossings, cable netting at crossing sites, and automated regional traffic redirection systems to redirect automobile traffic based on rail traffic flow. Driver education about crossings and safety measures, as well as increased enforcement of laws specific to highway-rail crossings (whistle laws and moving violations, for example), have also contributed to mortality reduction in recent years.

Although no studies have been done to show a clear causal relationship between any particular interventions and changes in mortality rates, highway-rail intersections offer an excellent model of a unique environment in which engineering, education, and enforcement have all been profitably used to control injury. (See Federal Railroad Administration, 2005, for surveillance data and additional information.)

Home Injuries

Injuries that occur in the home are conceptually grouped according to the environment in which they occur, rather than by the particular mechanism of injury or by intent. The most common home injuries are burns, scalds, smoke inhalation, animal bites, choking, strangulation, and poisoning; other injuries that often occur in the home are falls and certain intentional injuries such as those that result from intimate partner violence, child abuse, and suicides and parasuicides. Injuries from fires and falls are the primary injuries that occur at home.

Epidemiology. Given their wide range, it is difficult to present a unifying epidemiological picture of injuries in the home. Epidemiological data on some of the most common home injuries have been presented in other sections of this chapter. Generally, home injuries are responsible for more than 10 million ED visits annually in the United States, and account for approximately 20 percent of ED visits for injuries as a whole (NCIPC, 2002).

Countermeasures. A wide range of interventions have been shown to be effective at reducing home injuries. Some of the more notable interventions that have not been presented in other parts of this chapter are displayed in Table 25.12.

TABLE 25.12. COUNTERMEASURES FOR HOME INJURIES.

Education	Educating children and families about fire hazards and escape routes Educating children about poison control Babysitter training Choking response training Store guns safely or no guns at home
Enforcement	Building code enforcement Sprinkler and fire alarm system code enforcement
Engineering	Hot water heater temperature controls Gun trigger locks; trigger fingerprint recognition Childproof cigarette lighters Fire-resistant fabrics for sleepwear and furnishings Fire escapes and escape routes Child safety caps on medications
Environmental change	Cupboard locks Electrical outlet covers Fire hazard reduction Fire alarms Stair gates

Conclusion

Injury, whether caused by unintentional or intentional events, is a significant public health problem. The burden of injury is greatest in LICs and MICs and among individuals of low socioeconomic status in HICs. Most of these injuries are preventable. Public health professionals can play an important role in reducing the global burden of injuries by identifying, implementing, and evaluating population-based countermeasures to prevent and control injuries. Which strategy is employed in a particular country will depend in large part on the nature of the local problem, the concerns of the population, the availability of resources, and competing demands. Nonetheless, there is ample reason to believe that even simple countermeasures may make a big impact on reducing the global burden of death and disability due to injury.

Thought Questions

1. What is the difference between an injury and an accident? Why is it important to make the distinction? Discuss some strategies for highlighting the difference between accidents and injuries.

2. Consider an injury sustained by you or a member of your family: (a) describe the injury and how it meets the injury definition laid out in this chapter, (b) create a Haddon matrix for the injury, and (c) generate several solutions that could minimize the incidence or impact of the injury among others. Make sure you have at least one educational, one environmental, and one engineering solution.
3. Scan the headlines of the last week, and identify a type of injury mentioned there. Outline a possible public health approach toward reducing morbidity and mortality from that injury. Your response should (a) create a precise definition of the injury; (b) outline strategies for clarifying its distribution, risk factors, and protective factors; (c) suggest intervention strategies for reducing the injury's morbidity and mortality; and (d) describe how you would evaluate the effectiveness of your proposed interventions.
4. Gun violence poses a significant burden on citizens of the United States. Create a Haddon matrix for interpersonal violence involving firearms in the United States (identify a subset of gun violence, such as shootings in the home or hunting injuries, if you wish); generate at least three interventions not listed in this chapter for reducing morbidity and mortality from gun-related injuries; and conduct an options analysis of the various possible interventions and identify those that you believe would have the highest yield.
5. Discuss the overlap between injury control and environmental health.
6. For one hour of your day, catalogue all the injury prevention mechanisms that you encounter (directly or indirectly). For instance, when you get in your car, list the major injury prevention and control measures there, including seat belts, air bags and supplemental restraint systems, and so forth. Attempt to include educational, environmental, and engineering solutions in your list.

References

Baker, S. P., O'Neill, B., Ginsburg, M. J., and Li, G. *The Injury Fact Book.* (2nd ed.) New York: Oxford University Press, 1992.

Burke, G., and others. "Evaluation of the Effectiveness of a Pavement Stencil in Promoting Safe Behavior Among Elementary School Children at School Bus Stops." *Pediatrics,* 1996, *97,* 520–530.

Centers for Disease Control and Prevention. "Achievements in Public Health, 1900–1999 Motor-Vehicle Safety: A 20th Century Public Health Achievement." *Morbidity and Mortality Weekly Report,* 1999, *48*(18), 369–374.

Centers for Disease Control and Prevention. *Injury Fact Book 2001–2002.* Atlanta, Ga.: Centers for Disease Control and Prevention, National Center for Injury Prevention and Control, 2002.

Cook, P. J., and Ludwig, J. *Gun Violence: The Real Costs.* New York: Oxford University Press, 2000.

Dannenberg, A. L., and others. "Bicycle Helmet Laws and Educational Campaigns: An Evaluation of Strategies to Increase Children's Helmet Use." *American Journal of Public Health,* 1993, *83,* 667–674.

Darwin, J. "Reaffirmed Cost-Effectiveness of Poison Centers." *Annals of Emergency Medicine,* 2003, *41,* 159–160.

Duperrex, O., Bunn, F., and Roberts, I. "Safety Education of Pedestrians for Injury Prevention: A Systematic Review of Randomised Controlled Trials." *British Medical Journal,* 2002, *324,* 1129.

Elvik, R. "A Meta-Analysis of Studies Concerning the Safety Effects of Daytime Running Lights on Cars." *Accident Analysis and Prevention,* 1996, *28,* 685–694.

Evans, L. "Evans Responds to Letters on Roles of Litigation and Safety Belts." *American Journal of Public Health,* 2004, *94,* 171–172.

Fauveau, U., and Blancet, T. "Deaths from Injuries and Induced Abortion Among Rural Bangladesh Women." *Social Science & Medicine,* 1989, *29,* 1121–1127.

Federal Railroad Administration, Office of Safety Analysis. "Query." [http://safetydata.fra.dot.gov/OfficeofSafety/Query]. 2005.

Forjuoh, S. N. "Traffic-Related Injury Prevention Interventions for Low-Income Countries." *Injury Control and Safety Promotion,* 2003, *10,* 109–118.

Graitcer, P. L., Kellermann, A. L., and Christoffel, T. "A Review of Educational and Legislative Strategies to Promote Bicycle Helmets." *Injury Prevention,* 1995, *1,* 122–129.

Haddon, W. "A Logical Framework for Categorizing Highway Safety Phenomena and Activity." *Journal of Trauma: Injury, Infection, and Critical Care,* 1972, *12,* 193–207.

Haddon, W. "Energy Damage and the Ten Countermeasure Strategies." *Journal of Trauma: Injury, Infection, and Critical Care,* 1973, *13,* 321–331.

Hanfling, M. J., Mangus, L. G., Gill, A. C., and Bailey, R. "A Multifaceted Approach to Improving Motor Vehicle Restraint Compliance." *Injury Prevention,* 2000, *6,* 125–129.

Herd, A. N., Widdowson, P., and Tanner, N.S.B. "Scalds in the Very Young: Prevention or Cure?" *Burns,* 1986, *12,* 246–249.

Holder, Y., and others (eds.). *Injury Surveillance Guidelines.* Geneva: World Health Organization, in Conjunction with the Centers for Disease Control, 2001.

Kahane, C. J. *Fatality Reduction by Air Bags: Analysis of Accident Data Through Early 1996.* National Highway Traffic Safety Administration (NHTSA) Report no. DOT-HS-808-470. Washington, D.C.: National Highway Traffic Safety Administration, 1998.

Karter, M. J. *Fire Loss in the United States During 2002.* Quincy, Mass.: National Fire Protection Association, Fire Analysis and Research Division, 2003.

Kellermann, A. L., Lee, R. K., Mercy, J. A., and Banton, J. "The Epidemiological Basis for the Prevention of Firearm Injuries." *Annual Review of Public Health,* 1991, *12,* 17–40.

Keswani, M. H. "The Prevention of Burning Injury." *Burns,* 1986, *12,* 533–539.

Krug, E. (ed.). *Injury: A Leading Cause of the Global Burden of Disease.* Geneva: World Health Organization, 1999.

Krug, E., and others (eds.). *World Report on Violence and Health.* Geneva: World Health Organization, 2002.

Marsh, D., and others. "Epidemiology of Adults Hospitalized with Burns in Karachi, Pakistan." *Burns,* 1996, *22,* 225–229.

McCaig, F. L., and Burt, C. W. *National Hospital Ambulatory Medical Care Survey: 2001 Emergency Department Summary.* Advance data from Vital and Health Statistics, no. 335. Hyattsville, Md.: National Center for Health Statistics, 2003.

Miller, T. R., and Cohen, M. A. "Costs of Gunshot and Cut/Stab Wounds in the United States, with Some Canadian Comparisons." *Accident Analysis and Prevention,* 1997, *29,* 329–341.

Miller, T. R., and Lestina, D. C. "Costs of Poisoning in the United States and Savings from Poison Control Centers: A Benefit-Cost Analysis." *Annals of Emergency Medicine,* 1997, *49*(2), 239–245.

Murray, C. J., and Lopez, A. D. *The Global Burden of Disease: A Comprehensive Assessment of Mortality and Disability from Diseases, Injuries and Risk Factors in 1990 and Projected to 2020.* Global Burden of Disease and Injury Series, Vol. I. Cambridge, Mass.: Harvard School of Public Health, 1996.

National Center for Injury Prevention and Control. *Injury Research Agenda.* Atlanta, Ga.: National Center for Injury Prevention and Control, 2002.

National Center for Injury Prevention and Control. "Web-Based Injury Statistics Query and Reporting System (WISQARS)." [http://www.cdc.gov/ncipc/wisqars]. 2004.

National Highway Traffic Safety Administration. *Motorcycle Safety Program.* Washington, D.C.: U.S. Department of Transportation, 2003.

Odero, W., Garner, P., and Zwi, A. "Road Traffic Injuries in Developing Countries: A Comprehensive Review of Epidemiological Studies." *Tropical Medicine and International Health,* 1997, *2,* 445–460.

Peden, M., McGee, K., and Krug, E. (eds.). *Injury: A Leading Cause of the Global Burden of Disease, 2000.* Geneva: World Health Organization, 2002.

Peden, M., and others (eds.). *World Report on Road Traffic Injury Prevention.* Geneva: World Health Organization, 2004.

Polen, M. R., and Friedman, G. D. (U.S. Preventive Services Task Force). "Automobile Injury: Selected Risk Factors and Prevention in the Health Care Setting." *Journal of the American Medical Association,* 1988, *259,* 76–80.

Poli de Figueiredo, L. F., and others. "Increases in Fines and Driver License Withdrawal Have Effectively Reduced Immediate Deaths from Trauma on Brazilian Roads: First-Year Report on the New Traffic Code." *Injury,* 2001, *32*(2), 91–94.

Razzak, J. A., Laflamme, L., Luby, S. P., and Chotani, H. "Childhood Injuries in Pakistan: When, Where and How?" *Public Health,* 2004, *118*(2), 114–120.

Razzak, J. A., and Luby, S. P. "Estimating Deaths and Injuries Due to Road Traffic Accidents in Karachi, Pakistan, Through the Capture-Recapture Method." *International Journal of Epidemiology,* 1998, *27,* 866–870.

Razzak, J. A., Marsh, D. M., and Stansfield, S. "District Hospital-Based Injury Data: Is It an Option in a Developing Country?" *Injury Prevention,* 2002, *8,* 345–346.

Retting, R. A., Ferguson, S. A., and McCartt, A. T. "A Review of Evidence-Based Traffic Engineering Measures Designed to Reduce Pedestrian-Motor Vehicle Crashes." *American Journal of Public Health,* 2003, *93,* 1456–1462.

Sherman, L. W., and others. *Preventing Crime: What Works, What Doesn't, What's Promising.* Washington, D.C.: National Institute of Justice, 1998.

Smith, G. S. "Public Health Approaches to Occupational Injury Prevention: Do They Work?" *Injury Prevention,* 2001, *7,* 3–10.

Tinsworth, D. K., and McDonald, J. E. *Special Study: Injuries and Deaths Associated with Children's Playground Equipment.* Washington D.C.: U.S. Consumer Product Safety Commission, Apr. 2001.

Ulmer, R. G., and Preusser, D. F. *Evaluation of the Repeal of Motorcycle Helmet Laws in Kentucky and Louisiana*. NHTSA Report no. DOT-HS-809-530. Washington D.C.: National Highway Traffic Safety Administration, Oct. 2003.

Vernick, J. S., Mair, J. S., Teret, S. P., and Sapsin, J. W. "Role of Litigation in Preventing Product-Related Injuries." *Epidemiologic Reviews,* 2003, *25,* 90–98.

Villaveces, A., and others. "Effect of a Ban on Carrying Firearms on Homicide Rates in Two Colombian Cities." *Journal of the American Medical Association,* 2000, *283,* 1205–1209.

Wadman, M. C., Muelleman, R. L., Coto, J. A., and Kellermann, A. L. "The Pyramid of Injury: Using E-Codes to Accurately Describe the Burden of Injury." *Annals of Emergency Medicine,* 2003, *42,* 468–478.

Williams, A. F., Preusser, D. F., Blomberg, R. D., and Lund, A. D. "Seat Belt Use Law Enforcement and Publicity in Elmira, New York: A Reminder Campaign." *American Journal of Public Health,* 1987, *77,* 1450–1451.

Withaneachi, D., and Meehan, T. "Promoting Safer Play Equipment in Primary Schools: Evaluation of an Educational Campaign." *Health Promotion Journal of Australia,* 1998, *8,* 125–129.

For Further Information

Web Sites

The Web site of the American College of Emergency Physicians (ACEP) contains a primer for health care providers interested in injury control and provides links to various injury prevention organizations as well as a short bibliography of seminal injury control books and articles:

American College of Emergency Physicians. "General Injury Control Resources." [http://www.acep.org/webportal/MemberCenter/SectionsofMembership/TraumaandInjuryPrevention/InjuryPreventionResources]. 2005.

The Centers for Disease Control and Prevention's National Center for Injury Control and Prevention maintains information on injury control, including surveillance data and statistics, for the United States. The NCICP's Web site also offers program information and funding sources:

Centers for Disease Control and Prevention, National Center for Injury Control and Prevention. Homepage. [http://www.cdc.gov/ncipc]. 2005.

The Injury Prevention Web is a meta-site that hosts the Web pages of several injury prevention organizations and serves as an excellent source for injury prevention resources.

Injury Prevention Web. Homepage. [http://www.injuryprevention.org]. 2005.

SafetyLit is an online resource for recent injury prevention research:

SafetyLit. Homepage. [http://www.safetylit.org]. 2005.

The World Health Organization's Department of Injuries and Violence Prevention maintains a clearinghouse for information about injury control, including epidemiology and prevention, the world over, with a regularly updated list of campaigns, conferences, and other injury control activities:

World Health Organization. "Injuries and Violence Prevention." [http://www.who.int/violence_injury_prevention/en]. 2005.

Publications

Barss, P., Smith, G. S., Baker, S. P., and Mohan, D. *Injury Prevention: An International Perspective: Epidemiology, Surveillance and Policy.* New York: Oxford University Press, 1998.

Christoffel, T., and Gallagher, S. S. *Injury Prevention and Public Health Practical Knowledge, Skills, and Strategies.* Gaithersburg, Md.: Aspen, 1999.

Mohan, D., and Tiwari, G. (eds.). *Injury Prevention and Control.* Boca Raton, Fla.: CRC Press, 2000.

Rivara, F. P., and others. *Injury Control: Research and Program Evaluation.* New York: Cambridge University Press, 2000.

Robertson, L. S. *Injury Epidemiology.* New York: Oxford University Press, 1999.

Smith, G., and others. *Injury Prevention: An International Perspective: Epidemiology, Surveillance, and Policy.* New York: Oxford University Press, 1998.

Journals

Accident Analysis and Prevention. Elsevier. [http://authors.elsevier.com/JournalDetail.html?PubID=336&Precis=DESC].

Injury Control and Safety Promotion. Taylor & Francis. [http://www.tandf.co.uk/journals/titles/17457300.asp].

Injury Prevention. BMJ Publishing Group. [http://ip.bmjjournals.com].

Journal of Safety Research. Elsevier for the National Safety Council (NSC). [http://www.nsc.org/lrs/res/jsr.htm] and [http://authors.elsevier.com/JournalDetail.html?PubID=679&Precis=DESC].

Traffic Injury Prevention. Taylor & Francis for Association for the Advancement of Automotive Medicine (AAAM), International Traffic Medicine Association (ITMA), International Council on Alcohol, Drugs and Traffic Safety (ICADTS), and International Research Council on the Biomechanics of Impact (IRCOBI). [http://www.tandf.co.uk/journals/titles/15389588.asp].

CHAPTER TWENTY-SIX

DISASTER PREPAREDNESS

Eric K. Noji
Catherine Y. Lee

Throughout history natural disasters have exacted a heavy toll of death and suffering. During the past thirty years they have claimed about 4 million lives worldwide, adversely affected the lives of at least a billion more people, and resulted in property damage exceeding $75 billion. Why discuss disasters in a textbook of Environmental Health? First, many disasters result from environmental conditions, either natural occurrences, such as hurricanes, or events of human origin, such as factory explosions. Second, disasters can create environmental health challenges, such as disrupted water treatment systems after a hurricane or toxic airborne chemicals after a factory explosion. Finally, disaster management exemplifies many of the public health principles that are applied in other arenas of environmental health.

Recent natural catastrophes have included the Bam earthquake in Iran (2004), a series of devastating hurricanes in the Caribbean (1998) (including Hurricanes Mitch and Georges); severe flooding in Mozambique (2000), France (2003), and California (1998); tornadoes in Oklahoma and Texas (1999); tsunamis in Sri Lanka, Indonesia, Thailand, India, and neighboring countries following the Indian Ocean earthquake (2004); and global adverse weather conditions related to the El Niño phenomenon (1997 and 1998) (see Table 26.1). The future appears likely to be even more frightening. Global climate change is increasing the potential for severe weather events and flooding and introducing tropical vector-borne diseases into more temperate regions (see Chapter Eleven). Increasing

TABLE 26.1. SELECTED NATURAL DISASTERS, 1970–2004.

Year	Event	Location	Approximate Death Toll
1970	Earthquake and landslide	Peru	70,000
1970	Tropical cyclone	Bangladesh	300,000
1971	Tropical cyclone	India	25,000
1972	Earthquake	Nicaragua	6,000
1976	Earthquake	China	250,000
1976	Earthquake	Guatemala	24,000
1976	Earthquake	Italy	900
1977	Tropical cyclone	India	20,000
1978	Earthquake	Iran	25,000
1980	Earthquake	Italy	1,300
1982	Volcanic eruption	Mexico	1,700
1985	Tropical cyclone	Bangladesh	10,000
1985	Earthquake	Mexico	10,000
1985	Volcanic eruption	Columbia	22,000
1988	Hurricane Gilbert	Caribbean	343
1988	Earthquake	Armenia SSR	25,000
1989	Hurricane Hugo	Caribbean	56
1990	Earthquake	Iran	40,000
1990	Earthquake	Philippines	2,000
1991	Tropical cyclone	Bangladesh	140,000
1991	Volcanic eruption	Philippines	800
1991	Typhoon and flood	Philippines	6,000
1991	Flood	China	1,500
1992	Hurricane Andrew	USA	52
1993	Earthquake	India	10,000
1995	Earthquake	Japan	6,000
1998	Hurricane Mitch	Central America	10,000
1999	Earthquake	Turkey	18,000
1999	Earthquake	Taiwan	1,000
2001	Earthquake	India	20,000
2003	Earthquake	Algeria	3,000
2004	Earthquake	Iran	25,000
2004	Tsunami	Sri Lanka, Indonesia, Thailand	150,000

Source: Data from Office of U.S. Foreign Disaster Assistance, 2004; National Geographic Society, 1987.

population density in floodplains and in earthquake- and hurricane-prone areas points to the probability of future catastrophic natural disasters with millions of casualties. Many large-scale natural disasters occur in remote areas, far from towns and hospitals. Roads frequently become impassable, bridges collapse, and inclement weather adds to the difficulties. The more remote the area, the longer it takes for external assistance to arrive, and the more the community will have to rely on its own resources, at least for the first several hours, if not days. Friends, neighbors, and relatives conduct the initial search and rescue of victims, provide basic first aid, and transport the injured to the nearest health care facilities.

The Public Health Approach to Disasters

Good disaster management must link data collection and analysis to an immediate decision-making process. The overall objectives of disaster management from a public health perspective are to assess the needs of disaster-affected populations, match available resources to those needs, prevent further adverse health effects, implement disease control strategies for well-defined problems, evaluate the effectiveness of disaster relief programs, and improve contingency plans for various types of future disasters.

The effects of disasters on the health of populations are quantifiable. Common patterns of morbidity and mortality following certain disasters can be identified. Better epidemiological knowledge of the causes of death and the types of injuries and illnesses associated with natural disasters is essential for determining the relief supplies, equipment, and personnel needed to respond effectively. In addition, results of disaster research serve as the basis for providing informed advice about the probable health effects of future disasters, for establishing priorities for action by emergency medical services, and for emphasizing the importance of accurate information in making relief management decisions.

Proper planning and execution of disaster medical aid programs requires knowledge of the types of disasters that might occur, the morbidity and mortality that might result, and the consequent medical care needs. Emergency responders should be experts on ways of handling the type of disaster most prevalent in their own community, because each type of disaster is characterized by different morbidity and mortality patterns and has different health care requirements. For example, hospitals along the Gulf Coast of the United States should plan for hurricanes, and those in California should plan for earthquakes. In addition, specific types of medical and health problems tend to occur at different times following a natural disaster's impact. With earthquakes, for example, the problem of severe injuries that require immediate trauma care must be handled mainly at the time and place of impact. The problem of increased risk of disease transmission can be handled later, however, because it takes longer to develop and the greatest danger occurs with crowding and poor sanitation. Effective emergency medical response depends on anticipating the different medical and health problems before they arise and on delivering the appropriate interventions at the precise times and places where they are needed most.

What Is a Disaster?

There are many definitions of disaster, but most include three components. First, a disaster is a disruption of normal conditions. Second, a disaster features human suffering or property damage, or both, generally on a large scale. Third, a disaster exceeds the capacity of the affected community or area to respond and requires outside assistance. True disasters affect a community in numerous ways. Roads, telephone lines, and other transportation and communication links are often destroyed. Public utilities and energy supplies may be disrupted. Substantial numbers of victims may be rendered homeless (Figure 26.1). Portions of the community's industrial or economic base may be destroyed or damaged. Casualties may require medical care, and damage to food sources and utilities may create public health threats (Table 26.2).

Past Problems in Natural Disaster Management

In ancient times little mitigation of the effects of disaster was possible (Noji and Toole, 1997). Today, in contrast, communications inform us rapidly of disasters and allow us to initiate medical and other aid to victims quickly and efficiently. An effective response requires adequate planning and brisk execution.

FIGURE 26.1. KOSOVO WAR REFUGEE CAMP OUTSIDE THE VILLAGE OF CEGRANE, MACEDONIA, 1999: AN EXAMPLE OF THE SOCIAL DISPLACEMENT AND POOR ENVIRONMENTAL CONDITIONS THAT CAN FOLLOW DISASTERS OF NATURAL OR HUMAN ORIGIN.

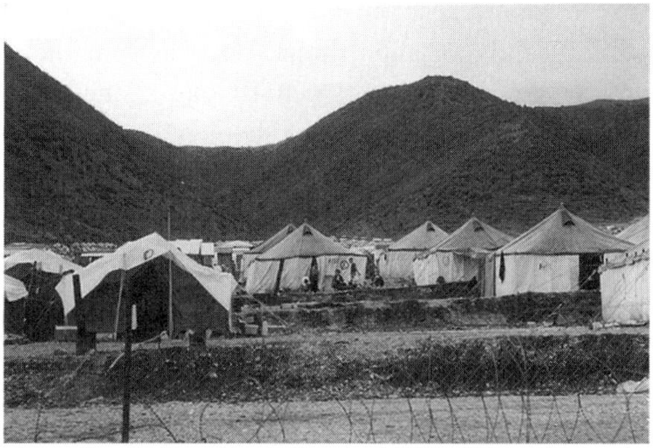

Source: Photo by D. Coop.

TABLE 26.2. SHORT-TERM EFFECTS OF MAJOR NATURAL DISASTERS.

	Earthquakes	High winds (without flooding)	Tsunamis	Floods (including flash floods)
Deaths	Many	Few	Many	Few
Severe injuries requiring extensive care	Overwhelming	Moderate	Few	Few
Increased risk of communicable diseases	Potential (but small) risk following all major disasters (probability rises as overcrowding increases and sanitation deteriorates)			
Food scarcity	Rare (may occur because of factors other than food shortage)		Common	Common
Major population movements	Rare	Rare	Common	Common

Source: Adapted from Pan American Health Organization, 2002.

Aid in many previous disasters has been well intentioned but poorly organized and thus has had limited benefits. Health decisions made during emergencies have often been based on insufficient, nonexistent, or even false information, which has resulted in inappropriate, insufficient, or unnecessary health aid, waste of health resources, and even counter-effective measures. For example, large amounts of useless drugs and other consumable supplies have frequently been sent to disaster sites. After the 1976 earthquake in Guatemala, 100 tons of unsorted medicines were airlifted to the country from foreign donors. Of these medicines, 90 percent were of no value because they had expired, had already been opened, or carried labels written in foreign languages (de Ville de Goyet and others, 1976). A similar situation occurred after the 1988 Armenian earthquake, when international relief operations sent at least 5,000 tons of drugs and consumable medical supplies. Because of the difficulties with identification and sorting, only 30 percent of the drugs were immediately usable by the health workers in Armenia; 11 percent were useless, and 8 percent had expired. Ultimately, 20 percent of all the drugs provided by international aid had to be destroyed (Autier and others, 1990). Other examples of inappropriate aid include sending mobile hospitals and teams of specialized trauma or emergency medicine specialists that arrive much too late and sending unprepared medical volunteers when nonmedical relief workers (such as sanitary engineers) would probably be more appropriate. The arrival of unprepared and inexperienced foreign personnel may damage the relief effort by tying up communications, transportation, and housing. These problems are all compounded in the resource vacuum typically created by a disaster—communications, transportation, local supplies and support, and a decision-making structure are usually lacking. These problems with relief operations are often closely covered and widely reported by the media; the conspicuous failure to deliver services effectively and efficiently is sometimes pejoratively termed "the second disaster."

Information Management Systems for Disaster Response

Over the past several years, efforts have been made to develop rapid and valid disaster damage assessment techniques. These techniques must be able to define the overall effects of the disaster, the nature and extent of the health problems, the population groups at particular risk for adverse health events, the survivors' specific health care needs, the local resources available to cope with the event, and the extent and effectiveness of the response to the disaster by local authorities, and this information must be assembled accurately and quickly. Guha-Sapir and Lechat (1986; see also Guha-Sapir, 1991) have proposed useful attributes for indicators used for needs assessment following earthquakes ("quick and dirty" surveys). These attributes include simplicity, speed of use, and operational feasibility. The techniques employed (sample and systematic surveys and simple reporting systems) are methodologically straightforward. Given suitable personnel and transport, reasonably accurate estimates of relief needs could be obtained quickly. Problems may arise, however, with the interpretation of data, particularly incomplete data, and in developing countries where predisaster health and nutritional levels are unknown.

The ultimate goal of such surveillance is to prevent or reduce the adverse health consequences of the disaster itself as well as to optimize the decision-making processes associated with relief effort management. These epidemiological objectives can be simply defined as the *surveillance cycle:* the collection of data, analysis of data, and response to data. The surveillance cycle must be repeated many times: immediately with "quick and dirty" assessments of problems, using the most rudimentary data collection techniques; then with short-term assessments involving the establishment of simple but reliable sources of data; and subsequently with ongoing surveillance to identify continuing problems and to monitor the response to the interventions chosen.

Field surveillance methods vary greatly by disaster setting and by the personnel and time available (Seaman, 1984, 1990; Lechat, 1990; 1993-94). Early field surveys must be simple and must address essential questions requiring immediate answers that will directly prevent loss of life or injury. Subsequently, surveys can address issues such as the availability of medical care, the need for specific interventions, and epidemic control (including a rumor clearinghouse), each of which demands more careful investigation. Surveillance must be sensitive to monitor the impact of relief on the health problems of the population and to determine whether the effort is having a tangible impact on the population or whether new strategies are needed. Surveillance becomes an iterative, cyclical process in which simple health outcomes are constantly monitored and interventions assessed for efficacy.

Finally, linking the information gathered to a management decision process is important. The information is clearly an essential requirement for determining the relief supplies, equipment, and personnel needed to respond appropriately and effectively to a catastrophic event. In the rapid evolution of a disaster relief program, major decisions regarding relief are made early, hastily, and often irreversibly, so reliable early data are vital. An organized approach to data collection in disaster situations can greatly improve decision making and can predict a variety of options that disaster managers need to face. The availability of questionnaires prepared before the disaster and able to be quickly adapted and modified assists in efficient data collection. Standardized procedures for collecting data during disasters need to be developed so that appropriate and timely information can be made available for operational decisions and action.

Operational decisions vary depending on the phase of the disaster. In the early phase of relief, basic needs for water, food, clothing, shelter, and medical care must be met, after which the longer-term process of rebuilding proceeds. Relief aid can often be squandered as relief workers overreact to minor problems when excitement is great, needs are extensive, and scrutiny by the media is intense. Everyone in the disaster area feels needs, experiences loss, and is moved to act; the challenge of the early assessment is to decide where early intervention will prevent the greatest loss of life or severe morbidity. The postimpact phase requires information on long-term rehabilitation and restoration of health services. Making an epidemiological assessment, prioritizing needs, and ordering an appropriate response can have a major impact on the community's ability to return to normalcy in both the short and the long term.

Health Care Needs in Specific Disasters

Natural hazards that can cause substantial property damage, economic dislocation, and medical problems include earthquakes and associated phenomena, volcanic eruptions, and extreme weather incidents such as heat waves and blizzards. Accounts of morbidity and mortality recorded after previous disasters can predict the medical care needs of future disasters and provide a foundation for disaster response planning. Disasters of human origin addressed in this section are industrial disasters and terrorist acts. Other disasters, such as fires and train wrecks, are not specifically discussed, but similar principles apply.

Floods

Floods are the most common natural disasters. They affect more people worldwide and cause greater mortality than any other type of natural disaster. They occur in almost every country, but 70 percent of all flood deaths occur in India and Bangladesh. In the United States, floods cause more deaths than any other natural disaster, with most fatalities resulting from flash floods.

Fast-flowing water carrying debris such as boulders and fallen trees accounts for the primary flood-related injuries and deaths. Not surprisingly, the main cause of death during floods is drowning, followed by various combinations of trauma, drowning, and hypothermia with or without submersion. Persons submerged in cold water for up to about forty minutes have been successfully resuscitated with 100 percent recovery of neurological function. Unfortunately, such resuscitations from clinical death require technologically advanced measures, which may not be available for days following a flood, even in a highly developed country such as the United States.

The proportion of flood survivors requiring emergency medical care is reported to vary between 0.2 and 2 percent. Most injuries requiring urgent medical attention are minor and include lacerations, skin rashes, and ulcers. Increased incidence of snakebites has been reported following floods in India and the Philippines. In India most snakebites have been inflicted by cobras, driven by rising floodwaters to seek higher ground near towns and villages. After some floods, substantial numbers of casualties caused by fire have been documented. Fast-flowing water can break oil or gasoline storage tanks. If the resulting film of oil is ignited, the fire may spread to buildings on dry land.

From a public health viewpoint, floods may disrupt water purification and sewage disposal systems, cause toxic waste sites to overflow, or dislodge chemicals stored above ground. In addition, makeshift evacuation centers with insufficient sanitary facilities may become substantially overcrowded. The combination of these events may contribute to increased exposures to highly toxic biological and chemical agents. For example, there may be a potential for waterborne disease transmission of such agents as enterotoxigenic *Escherichia coli, Shigella, Salmonella,* and Hepatitis A virus. The risk of transmission of malaria and yellow fever may be increased because of enhanced vector-breeding conditions. Ussher (1973) reported that the most serious problems encountered after a Philippine flood were viral upper respiratory tract infections, which were probably caused by crowded conditions in temporary shelters.

Despite the potential for communicable diseases to follow floods, large-scale outbreaks rarely occur (Aghababian and Teuscher, 1992; Toole, 1992), and mass vaccination programs are counterproductive. They not only divert limited personnel and resources from other critical relief tasks but may also create a false sense of security and cause persons who have been vaccinated to neglect basic hygiene. Although the public often demands typhoid vaccine and tetanus toxoid after floods, no epidemics of typhoid after floods have ever been documented in the United States. In addition, antibodies to typhoid take several weeks to develop following immunization, and even then vaccination protects only moderately. Likewise, mass tetanus vaccination programs are not indicated. Management of flood-associated wounds should include appropriate evaluation of the injured person's tetanus immunization history, and vaccination only if indicated.

The threat of communicable diseases should be addressed by establishing an epidemiological surveillance system, so that an increase in cases of communicable diseases in the flood-stricken area can be identified quickly. Particular attention should be given to diseases endemic to the area. For example, when floods occur in areas with endemic arthropod-borne encephalitides, arthropods known to transmit these diseases should be monitored and areas should be sprayed if the vector population increases significantly after the flood.

Tropical Cyclones (Hurricanes and Typhoons)

Tropical cyclones are low-pressure weather systems, such as hurricanes and typhoons, that usually form in the tropics (see Box 26.1). Worldwide, these storms have killed hundreds of thousands and injured millions of people during the last twenty years. In the United States from 1900 to 2003, more than 14,000 people lost their lives in hurricanes. The greatest natural disaster in U.S. history occurred on September 8, 1900, when a hurricane struck Galveston, Texas, and killed more than 6,000 people. In 1970, deaths resulting from a single tropical cyclone striking Bangladesh were estimated to exceed 250,000. As population growth continues along vulnerable coastal areas, deaths and injuries resulting from tropical cyclones will increase.

Box 26.1. Varieties of Tropical Typhoons

Tropical cyclone is a generic term for a low-pressure weather system that forms over water in tropical climates. Powerful thunderstorms typically accompany tropical cyclones, with winds that circle counterclockwise in the Northern Hemisphere and clockwise in the Southern Hemisphere. A tropical cyclone with relatively mild maximum sustained surface winds is called a *tropical depression,* and when wind speeds rise to intermediate levels, the term *tropical storm* is applied. When wind speeds reach a high level, then different names are applied, depending on the region of the world:

- *Hurricane*—in the North Atlantic, Caribbean, and Eastern Pacific Oceans
- *Typhoon*—in the Northwest Pacific Ocean
- *Severe tropical cyclone*—in the Southwest Pacific or the Southeast Indian Oceans
- *Severe cyclonic storm*—in the North Indian Ocean
- *Tropical cyclone*—in the Southwest Indian Ocean

Although hurricane (and typhoon) winds do great damage (Figure 26.2), wind is not the biggest killer in a hurricane. Hurricanes are classic examples of disasters that trigger secondary effects. They lead to tornadoes and flooding (Figure 26.3) that together with storm surges can cause extraordinarily high rates of morbidity and mortality. This was seen following the 1991 cyclone and sea surge in Bangladesh, in which 140,000 people drowned, and during Hurricane

FIGURE 26.2. DEBRIS AND DAMAGED BUILDINGS IN PENSACOLA, FLORIDA, RESULTING FROM HURRICANE IVAN, SEPTEMBER 2004.

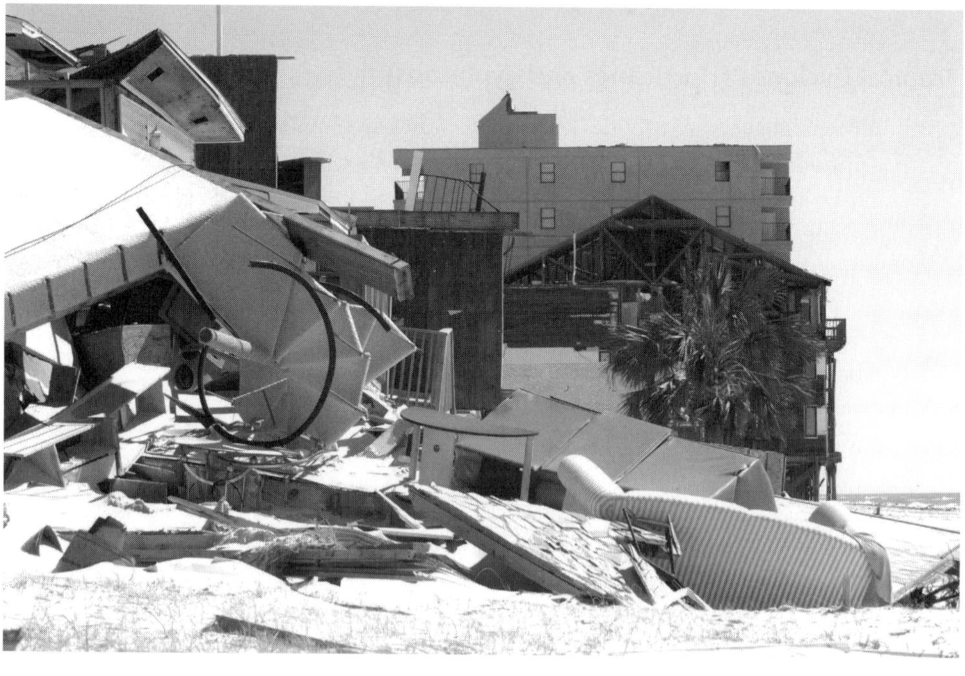

Source: FEMA (Federal Emergency Management Agency) photo, Jocelyn Augustino.

FIGURE 26.3. DESTRUCTION OF NORTH CAROLINA HWY 12 ALONG HATTERAS ISLAND, RESULTING FROM HURRICANE ISABEL, SEPTEMBER 2003.

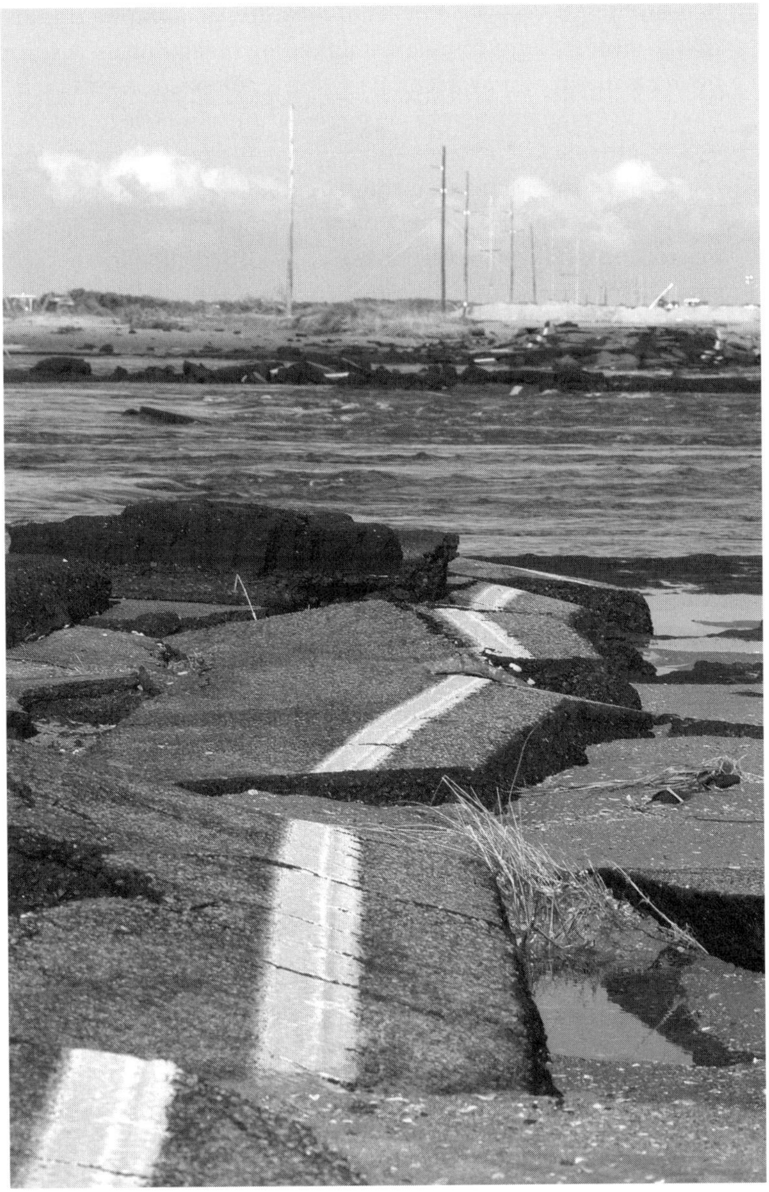

Source: FEMA news photo, Cynthia Hunter.

Mitch in Central America in 1998, which led to thousands of drowning deaths. Nine out of ten hurricane fatalities are drownings associated with storm surges. The major rescue problem is locating people stranded by rising waters and evacuating them to higher land. Other causes of deaths and injuries include burial beneath houses collapsed by wind or water, penetrating trauma from broken glass or wood, blunt trauma from floating objects or debris, and entrapment by mudslides that may accompany hurricane-associated floods. Many of the most severe injuries occur to persons who are in mobile homes during the storm or who are injured or electrocuted during the postdisaster cleanup.

Most persons who seek medical care after hurricanes do not require sophisticated surgical or intensive care services and can be treated as outpatients. The great majority have suffered lacerations caused by flying glass or other debris; a few have closed fractures and other, mostly penetrating injuries. Longmire and associates studied injuries associated with Hurricane Frederic and Hurricane Elena (Longmire and Ten Eyck, 1984; Longmire, Burch, and Broom, 1988). They found a statistically significant increase in lacerations, puncture wounds, chain saw injuries, burns, gasoline aspiration, gastrointestinal complaints, insect stings, and spouse abuse in the two weeks after the hurricane, signaling a need for primary care physicians and nurses skilled in managing minor surgical emergencies. However, trauma after a cyclone is not usually a major public health problem when compared with the need for water, food, clothing, sanitation, and other hygienic measures.

Infectious disease outbreaks are often a major concern following a hurricane. The probability of an outbreak is influenced by (Malilay, 1997)

- Preexisting levels of disease
- Ecological changes following the hurricane
- Population displacement
- Changes in population density (for example, crowding in storm shelters)
- Disruption of public utilities
- Interruption of basic public health services

Although infectious disease outbreaks are not common after tropical cyclones, there have been notable exceptions—a malaria outbreak after Hurricane Flora in Haiti in 1963; increases in typhoid, hepatitis, and other diseases after Hurricanes David and Frederick in the Dominican Republic in 1979; and possible increases in diarrheal diseases after a 1991 cyclone in Bangladesh (Malilay, 1997). The possibility of disease emphasizes the need for rapid assessments of public health in the aftermath of a disaster.

A public health approach to hurricanes involves a number of preventive strategies. Appropriate building design and construction materials can minimize building destruction and associated injuries; so can appropriate land-use planning that limits construction in vulnerable areas. Early warning systems allow people time to prepare and, if necessary, to evacuate areas in the path of a hurricane. Adequate shelter during hurricanes (brick or concrete shelters instead of, say, mobile homes) offers important protection. Public education is essential, so that people pay attention to and comply with advisories and are aware of impending hurricanes.

Tornadoes

Tornadoes are among the most violent of all natural atmospheric phenomena. They are windstorms that form over land when air masses collide, forming a vortex, often with a typical funnel-shaped appearance. Winds in tornadoes may reach 250 miles per hour. North America is the most tornado-prone continent; they are particularly common in a swath running from Texas north through Oklahoma, Kansas, and Nebraska. Over 700 tornadoes occur in the United States each year, and over the last fifty years tornadoes have been responsible for more than 9,000 deaths. However, most tornadoes are not catastrophic events; of the 14,600 tornadoes studied between 1952 and 1973, only 497 caused fatalities, and 26 of those accounted for almost half of the fatalities. The Centers for Disease Control and Prevention (CDC) has reviewed the public health impact of tornadoes in great detail (Brenner and Noji, 1993; Lillibridge, 1997).

The destruction caused by tornadoes results from the combined action of their strong rotary winds and the partial vacuum in the center of the vortex. For example, when a tornado passes over a building, the winds twist and rip at the outside. Simultaneously, the abrupt pressure reduction in the tornado's eye causes explosive pressures inside the building. Walls collapse or topple outward, windows explode, and debris from this destruction can be propelled through the air as high-velocity missiles. Buildings with unreinforced masonry, wood frames, or large window areas are likely to suffer the most extensive damage. Thus building practices may be largely responsible for the severity of injury resulting from tornadoes.

Victims of tornado disasters suffer characteristic patterns of injuries (Carter, Millson, and Allen, 1989; Bohonos and Hogan, 1999). The leading cause of death is craniocerebral trauma, followed by crushing wounds of the chest and trunk, both often occurring because a person has become airborne and then hits something or falls. Fractures are the most frequent nonfatal injury. Also frequent are lacerations, penetrating trauma with retained foreign bodies, and other soft tissue injuries. A high percentage of wounds among tornado casualties are heavily contaminated. In many instances foreign materials such as glass, wood splinters, tar, dirt, grass, and manure are deeply embedded in areas of soft tissue injury.

The public health approach to tornadoes parallels the approach to hurricanes. Early warning systems are key, and the severe storm warning system of the National Weather Service is credited with the downward trend in the annual number of tornado deaths during the twentieth century, despite a growing population and an increase in the number of reported tornadoes (Lillibridge, 1997). Adequate shelter during tornadoes, especially underground shelter, has demonstrated efficacy and offers particular advantages over fragile structures such as mobile homes. Effective means of communication, ranging from warning sirens in tornado-prone residential areas to radio warning systems, are essential, as is public education, so that people pay attention to and comply with advisories and are aware of impending tornadoes.

Volcanic Eruptions

Volcanic eruptions have claimed more than 266,000 lives in the past 400 years, with fatalities occurring in about 5 percent of all eruptions. One of history's most famous eruptions was that of Mount Vesuvius, near present-day Naples, in 79 CE, which buried the cities of Pompeii and Herculaneum. In 1631, after several centuries of quiescence, another eruption of Vesuvius killed an additional 4,000 people. Subsequently, catastrophic eruptions occurred at Krakatoa (Indonesia) in 1883, which caused the deaths of 36,000 people; Mount Pelee in 1902, which caused the destruction of St. Pierre in Martinique and the deaths of 28,000 people; Nevado del Ruiz, in Colombia, which claimed 25,000 lives in 1985; and Mount Pinatubo in the Philippines, with effects still ongoing since eruptions in the early 1990s because of persistent mudflows. The U.S. Geological Survey has identified about thirty-five volcanoes in the Western United States and Alaska that are likely to erupt in the future. Most are in remote rural areas and are not likely to result in disaster. A few, such as Mount Hood, Mount Shasta, Mount Rainier, and the volcano underlying Mammoth Lakes in California, are near population centers. Because of increasing population density in areas of volcanic activity, volcanic hazards are of growing concern.

Eruptions have immediate life-threatening health effects through suffocation from inhalation of massive quantities of airborne ash, scalding from blasts of superheated steam, and the effects of toxic gases. Pyroclastic flows and surges are particularly lethal. These are currents of extremely hot gases and particles that flow down the slopes of a volcano at tens to hundreds of meters per second and cover hundreds of square kilometers. Because of their suddenness and speed, pyroclastic flows and surges are difficult to escape. Mudflows, or lahars, account for at least 10 percent of volcano-related deaths. These are flowing masses of volcanic debris mixed with water. The mud is sometimes scalding hot, and entrapped persons may sustain severe burns. A relatively minor eruption of Nevado del Ruiz in 1985 triggered lahars from that Andean volcano's ice cap that buried more than 22,000 persons.

An indirect effect of volcanic activity is the accumulation of toxic volcanic gases in deep crater lakes. Sudden releases of these gases can be catastrophic; carbon dioxide released from Lake Monoun and Lake Nyos in Cameroon in 1984 and 1986, respectively, claimed 1,800 lives. Other toxic effects of these gas releases include pulmonary edema, irritant conjunctivitis, joint pain, muscle weakness, and cutaneous bullae. In the rare event of a ground-level release of toxic gases or aerosols (for example, from a vent in the side of a volcano opening to the atmosphere), equipment for monitoring atmospheric concentrations of sulfur dioxide, hydrogen sulfide, hydrofluoric acid, carbon dioxide, and other gases should be available.

A volcanic eruption may also generate tremendous quantities of ashfall. Buildings have been reported to collapse from the weight of ash accumulating on roofs, resulting in severe trauma to the occupants. The ash can also be irritating to the eyes (causing corneal abrasions), mucous membranes, and respiratory system. Upper airway irritation, cough, and bronchospasm, as well as exacerbation of chronic lung diseases, are common findings in symptomatic patients. In extremely high concentrations (for example, in the path of a pyroclastic flow or near the volcanic vent during an ashfall), volcanic ash may cause severe tracheal injury, pulmonary edema, and bronchial obstruction leading to death from acute pulmonary injury or from suffocation. After the eruption of Mount St. Helens in 1980, twenty-three immediate deaths were reported. Postmortem examinations revealed that eighteen of these resulted from asphyxia. In the majority of the asphyxiated victims the ash mixed with mucus and formed plugs that obstructed the principal airways (trachea and main bronchi). Finally, a delayed onset of ash-induced mucus hypersecretion or obstructive airways disease may occur.

Public health responses to volcanoes are limited by the difficulty of predicting the timing or magnitude of eruptions with any certainty. However, in instances where advance warnings were generated—at Mount Pinatubo in 1991 and at Rabaul, New Guinea—mass evacuations of 50,000 and 30,000 people, respectively, were carried out, and tens of thousands of lives were saved. Preparation for such an evacuation had been in place in Rabaul for a decade, which facilitated a successful intervention. These examples highlight the importance of identifying at-risk areas, planning evacuation procedures, and implementing notification measures. In addition, preparation in volcanic areas may involve having emergency air-monitoring equipment, masks, and emergency medical facilities available (Baxter, 1997).

Earthquakes

An earthquake is a series of shock waves in the earth's crust, representing a release of accumulated energy. Most earthquakes occur at the boundary zones between tectonic plates, sections of the earth's crust that are in motion relative to each other. About 75 percent of the world's seismic energy is released at the edge of the Pacific Ocean, where the thinner Pacific plate is forced beneath thicker continental crust along *subduction zones.* The affected areas extend up the west coasts of South and Central America to the California coast and also involve Alaska, the Aleutians, Japan, China, the Philippines, Indonesia, and Australasia. Another 15 percent of the world's seismic energy is released at the collision of the Eurasian and African plates, forming an earthquake-prone band stretching from Myanmar west to the Himalayas, the Caucasus, and the Mediterranean.

A powerful earthquake is one of the most destructive events in nature. During the past twenty years, earthquakes have caused more than a million deaths and injuries worldwide. In the United States, approximately 1,600 deaths attributed to earthquakes have been recorded since colonial times, of which more than 1,000 have occurred in California. Deaths resulting from major earthquakes can be instantaneous, rapid, or delayed. The major cause of *instantaneous* death is crush injuries from the collapse of buildings that are not adequately designed for earthquake resistance, are built with inadequate materials, or are poorly constructed. Factors determining the number of people killed when a building collapses include how badly they are trapped, how severely they are injured, how long they must wait for rescue, and how long they can survive without medical attention. Instantaneous death can also occur through drowning in earthquake-induced tidal waves (tsunamis). *Rapid* death occurs within minutes or hours as the result of asphyxia from dust inhalation (collapsing buildings generate heavy dust clouds that may contain toxic materials such as asbestos), delayed effects of injuries, or effects of exposure (for example, hypothermia). *Delayed* death occurs within days and can be caused by dehydration, hypothermia, hyperthermia, crush syndrome, or postoperative sepsis.

Burns and smoke inhalation from fires used to be major hazards after an earthquake. For example, following the 1923 earthquake in Tokyo, more than 140,000 people perished, principally because of fires that broke out in a city where most buildings were constructed from highly flammable paper (*shoji*) and wood materials. Since 1950, however, the incidence of burns following earthquakes has decreased considerably.

In addition to needing care for injuries related to building collapse, large numbers of earthquake victims may require medical care for acute myocardial infarction; exacerbation of chronic diseases such as diabetes or hypertension, anxiety and other mental health problems; respiratory disease from exposure to dust from rubble; and near drowning because of flooding from broken dams. An example of the medical consequences of an earthquake was observed after a magnitude 6.7 earthquake in Athens, Greece. Mortality from myocardial infarction rose by 50 percent during the first three days after the earthquake, peaking on the third day (Katsouyanni, Kogevinas, and Trichopoulos, 1986; Trichopoulos and others, 1983). Finally, an earthquake may precipitate a major technological disaster by damaging or destroying nuclear power stations, hospitals with dangerous biological products, hydrocarbon storage areas, and hazardous chemical plants.

Preventing earthquakes is obviously impossible, but preventive actions include avoiding building in highly seismic areas, and using earthquake-resistant building techniques, both for new construction and when retrofitting older buildings. Among these techniques are anchoring houses and bracing walls. Inside buildings, heavy furniture, appliances, and other large objects that could fall or be thrown about during an earthquake should be firmly anchored. Earthquake prediction is not well developed, so advance warnings are impractical. However, once an earthquake occurs, if people have been trained in protective behaviors they may be able to increase their safety. Some evidence suggests that people are safer outside buildings than inside them, on lower floors than on upper floors, and under structural supports such as furniture or door frames than exposed in rooms (although much of this evidence is equivocal) (Noji, 1997).

Medical disaster planning for earthquakes is a challenge. Hospitals and other health care facilities are particularly vulnerable to the damaging effects of an earthquake. Because of loss of power and water supplies, equipment such as X-ray machines, kidney dialysis machines, ventilators, and blood analyzers, and hospital facilities such as intensive care units and surgical theaters, cannot function normally when they are most needed. In the immediate aftermath of an earthquake, search and rescue operations and emergency medical care are crucial. To increase trapped victims' chances of survival, search and rescue teams must respond rapidly after a building collapses. Studies of the 1980 Campania-Irpinia, Italy, earthquake (de Bruycker and others, 1983) and the 1976 Tangshan, China, earthquake (Sheng, 1987) showed that the proportion of trapped people found alive declined as delay in extrication increased. In the Italian study a survey of 3,619 survivors showed that 93 percent of those who were trapped and survived were extricated within the first twenty-four hours and that 95 percent of the deaths recorded occurred while the victims were still trapped in rubble. Estimates of the survival times of victims buried under collapsed earthen buildings in Turkey and China indicate that within two to six hours less than 50 percent of those buried are still alive (de Bruycker, Greco, and Lechat, 1985). Although we cannot determine whether a trapped person dies immediately or survives for some time under the debris, it is safe to assume that more people would be saved if they were extricated sooner. Safar (1986), studying the 1980 earthquake in Italy, concluded that 25 to 50 percent of the victims who were injured and died slowly could have been saved if lifesaving first aid had been rendered immediately. As suggested by these data, if any significant reduction in earthquake mortality is to be achieved, appropriate search and rescue action must be provided within the first two days after the impact.

Paralleling the speed required for effective search and extrication is the speed with which emergency medical services must be provided. The greatest demand occurs within the first twenty-four hours, and emergency medical admissions return to normal after three to five days. Consequently, field hospitals that arrive a week after an earthquake may be too late to be of use (Noji, 1997).

This chapter does not address fires as a separate category of disaster, but many of the same issues of preparation and response that apply to floods, eruptions, and earthquakes apply to large fires (Figure 26.4).

Industrial Disasters

The 1984 chemical disaster in Bhopal, India, and the 1986 nuclear reactor fire and explosion at Chernobyl, Ukraine, may serve as case examples for almost any discipline taught in a school of public health. Such technological disasters have elements of acute and chronic epidemiology, industrial hygiene, toxicology, environmental pollution and planning, disaster preparedness and management, health economics, medical ethics, and environmental protection law, to name a few. The key to reducing the public health impact of industrial disasters is to prevent them. The location of industrial plants, their proximity to populated areas, and their methods of storing chemicals can all be controlled. Safe plant design is one of the most effective methods of interrupting the causal chain leading to industrial disasters. Design elements include the use of less hazardous materials, the storage of explosive or otherwise hazardous chemicals in small amounts, and the installation and proper maintenance of adequate backup and safety systems.

On the local level (for example, in a community surrounding a single plant) the planning effort may be directed primarily at the inventory and storage of chemicals. On the broader scale, surveillance activities need to be pursued to evaluate the distribution of chemical plant and transportation releases, the types of chemicals involved, the nature of any acute morbidity and mortality associated with the releases, the population groups most affected, and so forth. On the basis of studies of past industrial disasters, public health officials and others can

FIGURE 26.4. MALIBU, CALIFORNIA, WILDFIRE, 1996: STATE OFFICE OF EMERGENCY SERVICES FIREFIGHTERS MONITOR THE FIRE'S SPREAD ACROSS THE DRY BRUSH ON A HILLSIDE.

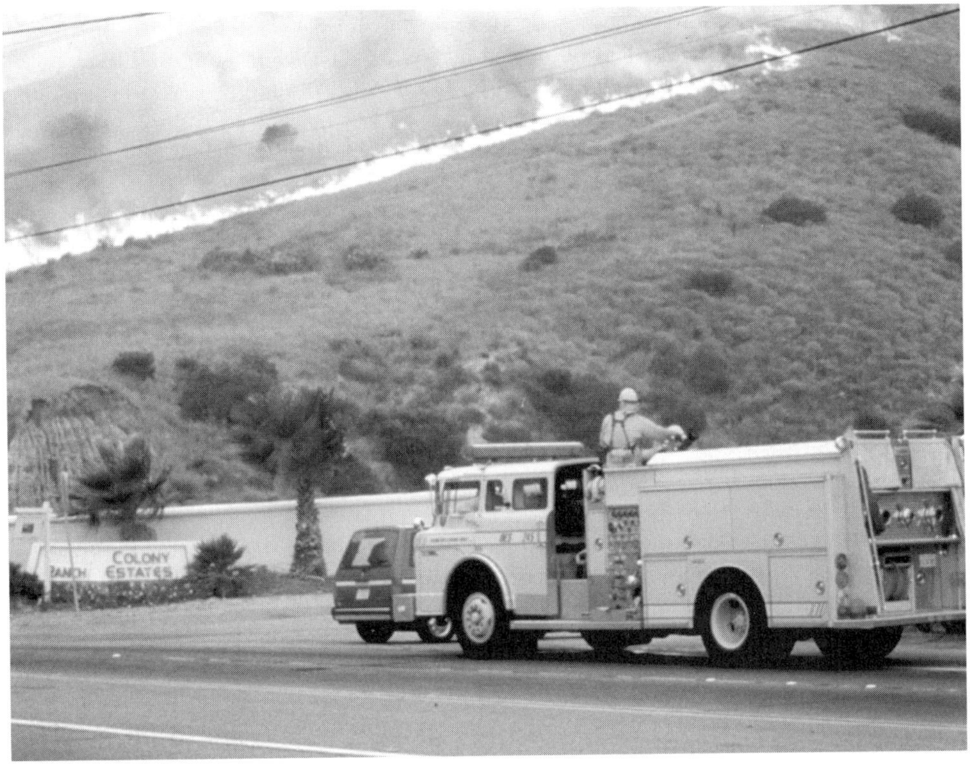

Source: FEMA news photo.

recommend preventive action in these settings and supply the information needed for developing remedial and regulatory measures to prevent industrial disasters.

Medical preparedness for an industrial disaster should include training medical personnel to care for patients in a contaminated environment and to treat chemically contaminated patients. A reasonable strategy for local public health officials would begin by training medical personnel at the industrial site and by training emergency medical personnel in the nearby community. Personal protective equipment (PPE) and respirators to protect the airways from the effects of harmful chemicals will be required to protect industrial workers and hazardous materials emergency responders who may be required to work in hazardous environments.

Other protective measures may be required to protect people's skin and eyes. Four levels of personal protective equipment (A, B, C, and D) have been defined. Although increasing the level used has been recommended by the U.S. Environmental Protection Agency (EPA), depending on the magnitude of the hazard, level B is generally recommended for entering an environment where the extent of the chemical hazard is not fully known. Level B protection consists of chemical-resistant clothing, boots, and hood; double-layered chemical-resistant gloves; and a positive-pressure, self-contained breathing apparatus. Clearly, having to wear this equipment imposes performance impediments that limit the effectiveness of emergency-response personnel in the field.

Generally, providing protective gear (such as gas masks) to the general population is impractical and potentially dangerous. The training needed by laypeople to use PPE effectively and the level of ongoing PPE maintenance and refresher courses required have generally been seen as prohibitive when balanced against the relatively low probability of hazardous materials disasters. Resources are often better spent on developing other industrial-disaster-mitigation strategies, such as evacuating people from the site of chemical exposure.

Planning for mass decontamination generally requires that the decontamination occur outdoors. Ensuring that chemically contaminated patients do not enter treatment facilities or emergency vehicles without first undergoing decontamination is vital if emergency medical operations are to be sustained during an industrial disaster. Specific equipment needs for decontamination include a water source, brushes, and mild soaps and detergents. Managing the effluent properly after patient decontamination is also part of hazardous materials medical preparedness. Effective patient decontamination requires training and should be part of routine industrial disaster drills. Medical planning for industrial disasters must include mechanisms to refer disaster victims from primary care sites to other medical facilities where critical specialty services such as burn care are available. Before an industrial disaster occurs, referral arrangements should be made with hospitals that have the capability of providing burn care services and hyperbaric oxygen and surgical subspecialty services such as plastic surgery to potential victims. Patients may sustain burns and inhalation damage from fires in addition to the full range of traumatic injuries associated with explosions. For instance, primary blast injuries resulting from the direct effects of blast shock waves may threaten the lives of patients who may not show external signs of life-threatening injury.

Terrorism

Terrorist incidents in the United States and elsewhere involving bacterial pathogens, nerve gas, and a lethal plant toxin (ricin), have demonstrated that the

United States is vulnerable to biological and chemical threats as well as to terrorist use of explosives. Recipes for preparing "homemade" agents are readily available, and reports of arsenals of military bioweapons raise the possibility that terrorists might have access to highly dangerous agents that have been engineered for mass dissemination in the form of small-particle aerosols. Such agents as the variola virus, the causative agent of smallpox, are highly contagious and often fatal. Responding to large-scale outbreaks caused by these agents will require the rapid mobilization of public health workers, emergency responders, and private health care providers. Large-scale outbreaks will also require rapid procurement and distribution of large quantities of drugs and vaccines, which must be available quickly.

In the past most planning for emergency response to terrorism has been concerned with overt attacks (for example, bombings like the attack on the Oklahoma City Federal Building in 1995 and on Madrid trains in 2004). Some terrorist attacks are almost impossible to foresee or prevent, like planes crashing into the double towers of the World Trade Center on September 11, 2001, the worst terrorist attack in history. Chemical terrorism acts, like the Sarin release in the Tokyo subway system in 1995, are likely to be overt because the acute effects of chemical agents are usually obvious. Such attacks elicit immediate response from police, fire, and EMS personnel.

In contrast, attacks with biological agents are more likely to be covert. They present different challenges and require an additional dimension of emergency planning that involves the public health infrastructure. Because the initial detection of and response to a covert biological or chemical attack will probably occur at the local level, disease surveillance systems at local hospitals and state and local health agencies must be capable of detecting unusual patterns of disease or injury, including those caused by unusual or unknown threat agents. Epidemiologists at state and local health agencies must have expertise and resources for responding to reports of clusters of rare, unusual, or unexplained illnesses.

Covert dissemination of a biological agent in a public place will not have an immediate impact because of the delay between exposure and onset of illness (the incubation period). Consequently, the first casualties of a covert attack will most likely be identified by physicians or other primary health care providers. For example, in the event of a covert release of the contagious variola virus, patients will appear in doctors' offices, clinics, and emergency rooms during the first or second week, complaining of fever, back pain, headache, nausea, and other symptoms of what initially might appear to be an ordinary viral infection. As the disease progresses, these patients will develop the papular rash characteristic of early-stage smallpox, a rash that physicians might not recognize immediately. By the time the rash becomes pustular and patients begin to die, the terrorists would be far away and the disease disseminated through the population by person-to-person contact.

Only a short window of opportunity will exist between the time the first cases are identified and the time a second wave of the population becomes ill. During that brief period public health officials will need to determine that an attack has occurred, identify the organism, and avoid further casualties through prevention strategies (for example, mass vaccination in the case of smallpox or prophylactic treatment in the case of anthrax). In the case of smallpox, as person-to-person contact continues, successive waves of transmission could carry infection to distant locations, as occurred during the 2003 SARS virus outbreak and the 2004 avian flu outbreak. These issues might also be relevant for other person-to-person transmissible etiologic agents (for example, plague or certain viral hemorrhagic fevers).

Certain chemical agents can also be delivered covertly through contaminated food or water. In 1999, the vulnerability of the food supply was illustrated when chickens in Belgium were unintentionally exposed to dioxin-contaminated fat through their feed. Dioxin, a cancer-causing chemical that does not cause immediate symptoms in humans, was probably present in chicken meat and eggs sold in Europe as early as 1999, because the contamination was not discovered for months. This incident underscores the need for prompt diagnoses of unusual or suspicious health problems in animals as well as humans, a lesson that was also demonstrated by the winter 1999 outbreak of mosquito-borne West Nile virus in the United States, first diagnosed in birds and humans in New York City. The dioxin episode also demonstrates how a covert act of foodborne biological or chemical terrorism could affect commerce and human or animal health.

Practical Issues in Disaster Response

A disaster may create numbers of casualties that exceed the capacity of the local health care system. The approach to patient evaluation and treatment under such conditions is quite different in style and quality from usual health care practice. Although some principles of medical care remain unchanged in a mass casualty incident, others must be altered to achieve the best overall result. The health care system must adapt to this situation with four measures: simplifying care (austerity); rationing care (adopting a triage ethic); calling for outside help; and in circumstances of catastrophe, instituting mass care measures typical of battlefield medicine. Many compromises in work methods eliminate attention to details that would be the norm in less urgent situations. Physicians and nurses often perform procedures beyond the scope of their usual practices. Professional functions and roles are widely shared among physicians, nurses, and paramedics. These adaptations allow available resources to serve more victims.

Austerity

To be effective, disaster medical care must be confined to basic measures adequate to preserve life and function. Examinations, techniques, appliances, and drugs that are not essential to patient survival or preservation of function are luxuries. It may be necessary to perform fracture reductions and other minor surgical procedures with oral narcotic analgesia only. Orthopedic devices are often improvised. Use of outdated drugs is sometimes acceptable when the alternative is no drugs. The level of austerity is determined by the health care personnel, supplies, and equipment available at the disaster treatment site.

Triage and Rationing

Initial management of mass casualties includes triage, basic field stabilization, and transportation. In general *triage* may be defined as the prioritization of patient care based on severity of injury or illness, prognosis, and availability of resources. The goal of triage therefore is to select those patients in greatest need of immediate medical attention and to arrange for that treatment. This concept originated on the world's battlefields, where victims are classified and treated based on the seriousness of their injuries. Military surgeons long ago recognized that the number of victims produced in battle could overwhelm medical resources. Some injuries would be fatal even under ideal circumstances where resources are unlimited. In mass casualty situations, one no longer can concentrate all resources on the management of a single critically ill patient. Attempts at salvaging mortally wounded individuals with heroic measures under conditions of limited personnel and supplies may deprive other victims of care for life-threatening but readily correctable, conditions. The walking wounded sustain injuries that are survivable even if the provision of definitive medical care is significantly delayed. Thus, in the humanitarian interest of providing the greatest good for the greatest number of persons, methods of classification have been developed that facilitate treatment prioritization. The first victims treated are those with life-threatening injuries that can be readily stabilized without the expenditure of massive amounts of limited resources. The next priority is persons who have sustained injuries likely to have significant morbidity that could be appreciably lessened by early intervention. Catastrophically injured patients (for example, those with burns involving 95 percent of the body surface area), who have a minimal chance for survival despite optimal medical care, are provided comfort measures and may need to be left to die. Spending time on patients who are not likely to live leaves other patients who might be saved awaiting care. If too much time passes, these patients also may become unsalvageable. In addition to attending to the nature and urgency of the patient's systemic condition, triage decisions must be sensitive to other factors affecting prognosis, such as the patient's age, general health, and physical condition; the responders' qualifications; and the availability of key supplies and equipment.

Triage procedures are routinely used in civilian multiple or mass casualty incidents and are essential in disaster incidents. Prioritization of victims may be needed with smaller numbers of casualties when environmental conditions, remote settings, or unusual circumstances limit availability of medical care or ease of evacuation. The decision to evacuate persons who stand a reasonable chance of survival before others who are mortally injured may be necessary in settings of high-angle technical mountain rescue, complicated cave rescue, or extended overland transport from isolated wilderness regions, particularly when air evacuation is unavailable or infeasible. Effective triage is critical to the success of any disaster care operation and should be performed by a senior and knowledgeable provider. The essential differentiation to be made is *now* versus *not now.* In disaster triage the moribund patient unlikely to survive is classified as *not now,* when in ordinary circumstances he or she would be *immediate.*

Numerous triage methods have been discussed in the medical literature (Garner, Lee, Harrison, and Schultz, 2001; Kilner, 2002; Benson, Koenig, and Schultz, 1996; Schultz, Koenig, and Noji, 1996; Wesson and Scorpio, 1992; American College of Surgeons, 1986). These methods fall into two classes: qualitative and quantitative. Qualitative methods classify patients into subjective categories (immediate, delayed, minor, expectant, and so on). Two-tier, three-tier, four-tier, and five-tier systems have been described. Any qualitative triage method can be used successfully in a disaster. Each ranks patients relative to others and to the available care, and each requires periodic reconsideration for treatment. Quantitative methods assign an objective score to each patient based on initial clinical status. Various schemes based on anatomic indicators of injury severity, physiological measurements, and mechanisms of injury have been developed to predict certain categories of outcomes, such as survival (Gabbe, Cameron, and Finch, 2003; Champion, 2002). The Trauma Score is one such system, used in trauma research as a predictor of outcome. Many emergency medical systems use the revised Trauma Score for field triage and as a guide for patient routing in tiered trauma treatment systems. Although experienced physicians frequently rely on their best medical judgment to triage patients, medically inexperienced personnel may benefit from this algorithmic approach to assessment and triage. Suppose that several residents of an isolated mountain village were injured during an earthquake, that the village had only one health care worker, and that evacuation and treatment resources were limited. Decisions would have to be made regarding who would be evacuated first and who would be treated first. A trauma assessment based on physiological variables could provide a relatively objective evaluation of each patient's condition and a rational basis for the allocation of scarce resources. The use of such standardized scoring systems for triage decisions, however, remains to be studied in the disaster setting. Triage methods founded on scoring systems require familiarity with the scoring systems. They cannot be used by disaster medical personnel unfamiliar with their application or modification.

Mechanics of the Triage Process. Triage should begin as soon as trained medical personnel arrive on the scene. A rapid survey is performed, noting the number of victims, hazards to victims and rescuers, and the need for additional help. This information should be relayed rapidly to the communication centers responsible for the dispatch of emergency services so that additional help can be mobilized as early as possible. The most qualified medical person present should be designated the provisional triage officer. The triage officer should not be assigned other duties and should not become extensively involved in patient care. During the initial survey each victim is rapidly assessed for immediately correctable life-threatening problems such as airway obstruction, vigorous hemorrhage, or nonfatal penetrating chest injuries. Initial care should be limited to correction of these problems. In other words, resuscitation and definitive care clearly have no role at this stage. Care should be limited to manually opening airways and controlling external hemorrhage. Physical hazards may influence the decision to provide further care on site or to delay additional therapy until victims are transported a safe distance away to a casualty collection point. As additional experienced emergency medical personnel arrive, the role of triage officer should be assumed by the most experienced and knowledgeable person(s) present. Advanced medical knowledge is an asset in minimizing triage errors. However, field-experienced physicians are relatively rare. Successful disaster triage can be performed by appropriately trained advanced emergency medical technicians or by experienced nurses. Triage is a dynamic process. Continued clinical deterioration or improvement may change the initial decision to evacuate or treat a victim. Triage should be performed each time the responsibility for the care of a victim is transferred.

Adjuncts to Triage. A *triage tag* is a paper tag intended to show a patient's triage category, usually by means of a color code. All such tags enforce the use of the particular scheme of categorization for which they were designed. For example, they might refer to categories such as immediate, delayed, minor, and expectant.

Most are deliberately simple (the METTAG is an example) and bear only minimal information to identify the patient and indicate triage class and site of injury. Others carry more information and serve as an abbreviated medical record. Vayer, Ten Eyck, and Cowan (1986) reviewed the use of triage tags in disasters and reported that the tags had been used effectively in only a few multiple casualty incidents. These authors recommend that triage tags be abandoned and replaced by a system of geographic triage that sorts casualties into areas reserved for patients of similar priority for treatment. Simultaneously, some disaster medical systems are recasting their triage tags as victim-tracking tags intended for use in an elaborate evacuation system.

On-Site Medical Care

Determining how much and what type of care to administer at the disaster site depends on several factors. If the number of patients is small and sufficient prehospital personnel and transportation resources are available, on-site medical care can proceed in a fairly normal manner, with rapid stabilization and transportation to nearby hospitals. When extrication is prolonged, potentially lifesaving interventions, such as intravenous fluids for hypovolemic shock, should be instituted. Nonetheless, early rapid transportation with a minimum of treatment should be practiced when further casualties are likely to occur from fire, explosion, falling buildings, hazardous materials, or extreme weather conditions if people remain on site.

With an overwhelming number of casualties that exceed transportation capacities, advanced field medical treatment may be beneficial because hours may pass before seriously injured patients can be evacuated. This may necessitate the establishment of field hospitals with operating theater capabilities. Such a field hospital may be set up in a large building such as a school or church. Casualties are brought to the field hospital from the disaster site for further assessment and initial treatment of injuries. After a period of observation and stabilization, they are either sent home or transported to a hospital. Also, evacuation of the ambulatory and those with minor injuries may rapidly overwhelm local hospitals before the arrival of the more severely injured. Under these conditions it may be better not to evacuate the severely injured, but to treat them locally.

Communication Between Disaster Site and Hospital

Local emergency communications or the disaster operations center should alert hospitals in the affected area of a possible mass or multiple casualty situation. This report should include the number of injured and more specifically the number of seriously injured and the number for whom ambulatory treatment is sufficient. Hospitals should report to the local emergency communications center the following information:

- Bed availability
- Number of casualties received thus far
- Number of additional casualties that the hospital is prepared to accept
- Specific items in short supply

Terrorism Preparedness and Emergency Response

Preparedness for terrorist-caused outbreaks and injuries is an essential component of the U.S. public health system, which is designed to protect the population against any unusual public health event (for example, influenza pandemics, contaminated municipal water supplies, or intentional dissemination of *Yersinia pestis,* the causative agent of plague). Early detection of and response to biological or chemical terrorism are just as crucial. Without special preparation at the local and state levels, a large-scale attack with variola virus, aerosolized anthrax spores, a nerve gas, or a foodborne biological or chemical agent could overwhelm the local and perhaps national public health infrastructure. Large numbers of patients, including both infected persons and the "worried well," would seek medical attention, with a corresponding need for medical supplies, diagnostic tests, and hospital beds. Emergency responders, health care workers, and public health officials could be at special risk.

The epidemiological skills, surveillance methods, diagnostic techniques, and physical resources required to detect and investigate unusual or unknown diseases, as well as syndromes or injuries caused by chemical accidents, are similar to those needed to identify and respond to an attack with a biological or chemical agent. However, public health agencies must prepare also for the special features a terrorist attack probably would have, for example, mass casualties or the use of rare agents. Terrorists might use combinations of chemical and biological agents, attack in two or more locations simultaneously, use new agents, or use organisms that are not on the critical list (for example, common, drug-resistant, or genetically engineered pathogens). Lists of critical biological and chemical agents will need to be modified as new information becomes available. In addition, each state and locality will need to adapt these lists to local conditions and preparedness needs. Chemical and other agents have been developed for use as weapons, and other potentially dangerous agents are readily found in U.S. society. All may cause severe public health risks and require multiagency planning and preparation for an appropriate response.

Potential biological and chemical agents are numerous, and the public health, hospital, and health care organization infrastructure must be equipped to quickly resolve crises that would arise from a biological or chemical attack. Because of the hundreds of new chemicals introduced internationally each month, treating exposed persons by clinical syndrome rather than by specific agent is more useful for public health planning and emergency medical response purposes. Public health agencies and first responders might render the most aggressive, timely, and clinically relevant treatment possible by using treatment modalities based on syndromic categories (for example, burns and trauma, cardiorespiratory failure, neurological damage, and shock). These activities must be linked with information coming from the authorities responsible for environmental sampling and decontamination.

To best protect the public, preparedness efforts must be focused on agents that might have the greatest impact on U.S. health and security, especially agents that are highly contagious or that can be engineered for widespread dissemination via small-particle aerosols (for example, one preparedness effort is focusing on mass smallpox vaccination of the U.S. population). Preparing the nation to address such dangers is a major challenge for U.S. public health systems and health care providers. Early detection requires increased biological and chemical terrorism awareness among frontline health care providers because they are in the best position to report suspicious illnesses and injuries. Also, early detection will require improved communication systems between those providers and public health officials. State and local health care agencies must have enhanced capacity to investigate unusual events and unexplained illnesses, and diagnostic laboratories must be equipped to identify biological and chemical agents that are rarely seen in the United States. Fundamental to these efforts is comprehensive, integrated training designed to ensure core competency in public health preparedness and the highest levels of scientific expertise among local, state, and federal partners.

Concept of Operations. In the event of a confirmed terrorist attack, the Office of the Assistant Secretary for Public Health Emergency Preparedness, U.S. Department of Health and Human Services (DHHS), is responsible for coordinating with other federal agencies, in accord with Presidential Decision Directive (PDD) 39. PDD 39 designates the Federal Bureau of Investigation (FBI) as the lead agency for the crisis plan and charges the Federal Emergency Management Agency (FEMA) with ensuring that the management of the federal response is adequate to address the consequences of terrorism. Presidential Decision Directive 62 states that "HHS and the PHS [Public Health Service] is the lead agency to plan and to prepare for a national response to medical emergencies arising from the terrorist use of weapons of mass destruction." If requested by a state health agency, the DHHS will deploy response teams to investigate unexplained or suspicious illnesses or unusual etiologic agents and provide on-site consultation regarding medical management and disease control. The DHHS, with the support of other federal agencies, will

- Provide enhanced local response capabilities through the development of Metropolitan Medical Strike Team systems (now known as Metropolitan Medical Response Systems, or MMRS).
- Develop and maintain the National Disaster Medical System (NDMS), including the National Medical Response Teams.
- Work with the Department of Defense (DOD) to ensure deployability of NDMS response teams, supplies, and equipment.
- Work with the Department of Veterans Affairs (VA) to ensure adequate stockpiles of antidotes and other necessary pharmaceuticals nationwide and the training of medical personnel in NDMS hospitals.

National Pharmaceutical Stockpile. To ensure the availability, procurement, and delivery of medical supplies, devices, and equipment that might be needed to respond to terrorist-caused illness or injury, the CDC maintains the National Pharmaceutical Stockpile (NPS) program to make available lifesaving pharmaceuticals, vaccines, antidotes, and other medical supplies and equipment necessary to counter the effects of nerve agents, biological pathogens, and chemical agents and to augment depleted state and local resources for responding to terrorist attacks and other emergencies. The NPS program is capable of immediate deployment to any U.S. location in the event of a terrorist attack using a biological, toxin, or chemical agent directed against a civilian population. Both *12-hour push packages* and *vendor managed inventory* (VMI) are stored in strategic locations around the United States to ensure rapid delivery anywhere in the country.

A comprehensive medical and public health response to a biological or chemical terrorist event involves epidemiological investigation, medical treatment, and prophylaxis for affected persons and the initiation of disease prevention or environmental decontamination measures. The CDC is responsible for assisting state and local health agencies in developing resources and expertise for investigating unusual events and unexplained illnesses.

National Disaster Medical System and Disaster Medical Assistance Teams. The National Disaster Medical System (NDMS) is a federally coordinated initiative designed to augment the nation's emergency medical response capability in the event of a catastrophic disaster. This system is a cooperative program of four federal agencies: the DOD, FEMA, the VA, and the Department of Homeland Security (DHS). NDMS provides an interstate medical mutual aid system linking the federal government, state and local agencies, and private sector institutions to address the medical care needs of victims of catastrophic disasters. The program was designed to supplement the activities of state and local governments in a massive civil disaster or to back up the military medical care system in the event of an overseas conventional conflict. NDMS contains a medical response element to bring organized aid to a disaster-affected area, an evacuation system, and a network of precommitted hospital beds throughout the United States. Its medical response element includes dozens of volunteer civilian *disaster medical assistance teams,* or DMATs, that operate supplemental casualty clearing facilities for triage, stabilization, and holding care for disaster victims, and evacuation facilities for patients in excess of local hospital capacity. Specialized National Medical Response Team—Weapons of Mass Destruction (NMRT-WMD) teams are designed to provide medical care following nuclear, biological, or chemical incidents. These teams are capable of providing mass casualty decontamination, medical triage, and primary and secondary medical care to stabilize victims for transportation to tertiary care facilities in a hazardous materials environment. Four NMRTs-WMD are geographically dispersed throughout the United States.

U.S. preparedness to mitigate the medical and public health consequences of biological and chemical terrorism depends on the coordinated activities of well-trained health care and public health personnel throughout the United States who have access to up-to-the-minute emergency information. Effective communication with the public through the news media will also be essential to limit terrorists' ability to induce public panic and disrupt daily life. During the first decade of the twenty-first century, DHHS is working with state and local health agencies to

- Develop a state-of-the-art communication system that will support disease surveillance.
- Initiate rapid notification and information exchange regarding disease outbreaks that are possibly related to bioterrorism.
- Disseminate diagnostic results and emergency health information.
- Coordinate emergency response activities.

Through this network and similar mechanisms, DHHS aims to provide terrorism-related training to epidemiologists and laboratorians, emergency responders, emergency department personnel and other frontline health care providers, and health and safety personnel.

Public Concerns Associated with Disasters

Two public concerns that arise, particularly in the most severe disasters, are the potential for epidemics and the disposition of dead bodies. In each case the public health response involves both minimizing hazards and providing information.

Epidemics

Natural disasters are often followed by rampant rumors about impending epidemics (such as typhoid, cholera, or rabies) or about unusual conditions such as increased snakebites and dog bites. Such unsubstantiated reports gain great public credibility when printed as facts in newspapers or reported on television or radio. For example, following disasters in developing countries, any disruption of the water supply or sewage treatment facilities has usually been accompanied by rumors of outbreaks of cholera or typhoid. Such rumors may reflect fears and anxieties about a disastrous event rather than the true perception of an imminent problem. Although natural disasters do not usually result in outbreaks of infectious disease, under certain circumstances disasters may increase disease transmission. In addition, information on disease incidence in most developing countries is poor, and some outbreaks may have been missed by public health authorities. The most frequently observed increases in communicable disease are caused by fecal contamination of water and by respiratory spread (for example, of measles in refugee camps).

During the past forty years, outbreaks of communicable disease following natural disasters have been unusual; however, disasters do have elements that can contribute to transmission of disease, and persons responsible for managing disaster relief operations should establish a surveillance system and institute appropriate sanitary and medical measures to prevent outbreaks. Mass vaccination programs, however, are rarely necessary. Finally, a clearinghouse for rumors should be established to investigate those that have merit in a timely fashion, dispel those that are obviously false, and inform the public of hazards where a response is required. This concept has been helpful not only in developing countries but also in urban settings in industrialized countries.

Disposition of Dead Bodies

The public and government authorities are usually greatly concerned about the danger of disease transmission from decaying corpses. Responsible health authorities should recognize, however, that the health hazards associated with unburied bodies are minimal, particularly when death has resulted from trauma (de Ville de Goyet, 2004). Such bodies are unlikely to cause outbreaks of diseases such as typhoid, cholera, or plague, although they may transmit agents of gastroenteritis or food poisoning to survivors if the bodies contaminate streams, wells, or other water sources. Despite the negligible health risk, dead bodies represent a delicate social problem. Demands for mass burial or cremation are certainly not justified on public health grounds, and mass cremations require tremendous quantities of fuel.

The Future of Public Health Preparedness

On January 10, 2002, President Bush signed appropriations legislation providing $2.9 billion for the Department of Health and Human Services, a tenfold increase in DHHS funding for bioterrorism preparedness. The funds have been used to develop comprehensive bioterrorism preparedness plans, upgrade infectious disease surveillance and investigation through the Health Alert Network (HAN), enhance the readiness of hospital systems to deal with large numbers of casualties, expand public health laboratory and communication capacities, and improve connectivity between hospitals and city, local, and state health departments to enhance disease reporting. As the lead federal agency in preparing for the threat of bioterrorism, DHHS works closely with the states, local government, and the private sector to build the needed new public health infrastructure and to accelerate research into likely bioterror diseases. In addition, staff from various DHHS agencies, including the CDC, Health Resources and Services Administration (HRSA), and Office of Public Health Emergency Preparedness, have participated in developing a strategic WMD plan, reflecting a general need for broad-based public health involvement in terrorism preparedness and planning. The CDC targets state and local programs supporting bioterrorism, infectious diseases, and public health emergency preparedness activities statewide. HRSA provides funding, to be used by states to create regional hospital plans for response in the event of a bioterrorism attack.

Future goals of federal public health preparedness efforts include

- Having at least one epidemiologist in each metropolitan area with a population greater than 500,000
- Developing an education and training plan that will reach health professionals, emergency room physicians and nurses, local public health officials, and the public with information relating to bioterrorism, new and emerging diseases, and other infectious agents

- Targeting bioterrorism research toward new vaccines, antiviral drugs, and new diagnostic tools to better protect against biologic agents

Implementation of the objectives outlined in the DHHS's strategic plan is coordinated through the DHHS Office of the Assistant Secretary for Emergency Preparedness and Response. DHHS program personnel are charged with

- Helping to build local and state preparedness
- Developing U.S. medical expertise regarding potential threat agents, and coordinating medical response activities during actual bioterrorist events

Implementation will require collaboration with state and local public health agencies and with other persons and groups, including

- Public health organizations
- Medical research centers
- Health care providers and their networks
- Professional societies
- Medical examiners
- Emergency response units and responder organizations
- Safety and medical equipment manufacturers
- Other federal agencies
- International organizations

Conclusion

This chapter discussed the health effects of some of the more important sudden-impact natural and technological disasters and of potential future threats (such as intentionally released biological agents) and outlined the requirements for effective emergency medical and public health response to these events. The overall objective of disaster management is to assess the needs of disaster-affected populations, to match resources to needs efficiently, to prevent further adverse health effects, to evaluate relief program effectiveness, and to plan for future disasters.

Thought Questions

1. List two major categories of natural disasters and provide an example of each.
2. Describe public health and medical preparedness for an industrial disaster.

3. State two reasons why disasters are a public health problem.
4. What is the disaster surveillance cycle?
5. Four common disaster myths are that (a) foreign medical volunteers with any kind of medical background are needed, (b) epidemics and plagues are inevitable after every disaster, (c) disasters are random killers, and (d) things get back to normal within a few weeks. Briefly describe the reality in each instance.

References

Aghababian, R. V., and Teuscher, J. "Infectious Diseases Following Major Disasters." *Annals of Emergency Medicine,* 1992, *21,* 362–367.

American College of Surgeons, Committee on Trauma. "Field Categorization of Trauma Victims." *Bulletin of the American College of Surgeons,* 1986, *71,* 17–21.

Autier, P., and others. "Drug Supply in the Aftermath of the 1988 Armenian Earthquake." *Lancet,* 1990, *335,* 1388–1390.

Baxter, P. J. "Volcanoes." In E. K. Noji (ed.), *The Public Health Consequences of Disasters.* New York: Oxford University Press, 1997.

Benson, M., Koenig, K. L., and Schultz, C. H. "Disaster Triage: START, Then SAVE: A New Method of Dynamic Triage for Victims of a Catastrophic Earthquake." *Prehospital and Disaster Medicine,* 1996, *11,* 117–124.

Bohonos, J. J., and Hogan, D. E. "The Medical Impact of Tornadoes in North America." *Journal of Emergency Medicine,* 1999, *17*(1), 67–73.

Brenner, S. A., and Noji, E. K. "Risk Factors for Death and Injury in Tornadoes: An Epidemiologic Approach." In C. Church, D. Burgess, C. Doswell, and R. Davies-Jones (eds.), *The Tornado: Its Structure, Dynamics, Prediction, and Hazards.* Washington, D.C.: American Geophysical Union, 1993.

Carter, A. O., Millson, M. E., and Allen, D. E. "Epidemiologic Study of Deaths and Injuries Due to Tornadoes." *American Journal of Epidemiology,* 1989, *130,* 1209–1218.

Champion, H. R. "Trauma Scoring." *Scandinavian Journal of Surgery,* 2002, *91*(1), 12–22.

de Bruycker, M., Greco, D., and Lechat, M. F. "The 1980 Earthquake in Southern Italy: Morbidity and Mortality." *International Journal of Epidemiology,* 1985, *14,* 113–117.

de Bruycker, M., and others. "The 1980 Earthquake in Southern Italy: Rescue of Trapped Victims and Mortality." *Bulletin of the World Health Organization,* 1983, *61,* 1021–1025.

de Ville de Goyet, C. "Epidemics Caused by Dead Bodies: A Disaster Myth That Does Not Want to Die." *Pan American Journal of Public Health,* 2004, *15*(5), 297–299.

de Ville de Goyet, C., and others. "Earthquake in Guatemala: Epidemiologic Evaluation of the Relief Effort." *Bulletin of the Pan American Health Organization,* 1976, *10*(2), 95–109.

Gabbe, B. J., Cameron, P. A., and Finch, C. F. "Is the Revised Trauma Score Still Useful?" *ANZ Journal of Surgery,* 2003, *73,* 944–948.

Garner, A., Lee, A., Harrison, K., and Schultz, C. H. "Comparative Analysis of Multiple-Casualty Incident Triage Algorithms." *Annals of Emergency Medicine,* 2001, *38,* 541–548.

Guha-Sapir, D. "Rapid Needs Assessment in Mass Emergencies: Review of Current Concepts and Methods." *World Health Statistics Quarterly,* 1991, *44,* 171–181.

Guha-Sapir, D., and Lechat, M. F. "Information Systems and Needs Assessment in Natural Disasters: An Approach for Better Disaster Relief Management." *Disasters,* 1986, *10,* 232–237.

Katsouyanni, K., Kogevinas, M., and Trichopoulos, D. "Earthquake-Related Stress and Cardiac Mortality." *International Journal of Epidemiology,* 1986, *15,* 326–330.

Kilner, T. "Triage Decisions of Prehospital Emergency Health Care Providers, Using a Multiple Casualty Scenario Paper Exercise." *Emergency Medicine Journal,* 2002, *19,* 348–353.

Lechat, M. F. "Updates: The Epidemiology of Health Effects of Disasters." *Epidemiologic Reviews,* 1990, *12,* 192–97.

Lechat, M. F. "Accident and Disaster Epidemiology." *Public Health Reviews,* 1993–1994, *21*(3–4), 243–253.

Lillibridge, D. R. "Tornadoes." In E. K. Noji (ed.), *The Public Health Consequences of Disasters.* New York: Oxford University Press, 1997.

Longmire, A. W., Burch, J., and Broom, L. A. "Morbidity of Hurricane Elena." *Southern Medical Journal,* 1988, *81,* 1343–1346.

Longmire, A. W., and Ten Eyck, R. P. "Morbidity of Hurricane Frederic." *Annals of Emergency Medicine,* 1984, *13,* 334–338.

Malilay, J. "Tropical Cyclones." In E. K. Noji (ed.), *The Public Health Consequences of Disasters.* New York: Oxford University Press, 1997.

National Geographic Society. *Nature on the Rampage: Our Violent Earth.* Washington, D.C.: National Geographic Society, 1987.

Noji, E. K. "Earthquakes." In E. K. Noji (ed.), *The Public Health Consequences of Disasters.* New York: Oxford University Press, 1997.

Noji, E. K., and Toole, M. J. "Public Health and Disasters: The Historical Development of Public Health Responses to Disasters." *Disasters,* 1997, *21,* 369–379.

Office of U.S. Foreign Disaster Assistance. *Disaster History: Significant Data on Major Disasters Worldwide, 1900-Present.* Washington, D.C.: U.S. Agency for International Development, 2004.

Pan American Health Organization. *Emergency Health Management After Natural Disaster.* Scientific Publication no. 407. Washington, D.C.: Pan American Health Organization, Office of Emergency Preparedness and Disaster Relief Coordination, 2002.

Safar, P. "Resuscitation Potentials in Earthquakes: An International Panel." *Prehospital and Disaster Medicine,* 1986, *3,* 77.

Schultz, C. H., Koenig, K. L., and Noji, E. K. "A Medical Disaster Response to Reduce Immediate Mortality After an Earthquake." *New England Journal of Medicine,* 1996, *334,* 438–444.

Seaman, J. *Epidemiology of Natural Disasters.* Basel: Karger, 1984.

Seaman, J. "Disaster Epidemiology: Or, Why Most International Disaster Relief Is Ineffective." *Injury,* 1990, *21,* 5–8.

Sheng, Z. Y. "Medical Support in the Tangshan Earthquake: A Review of the Management of Mass Casualties and Certain Major Injuries." *Journal of Trauma,* 1987, *27,* 1130–1135.

Toole, M. J. "Communicable Disease Epidemiology Following Disasters." *Annals of Emergency Medicine,* 1992, *21,* 418–420.

Trichopoulos, D., and others. "Psychological Stress and Fatal Heart Attack: The Athens (1981) Earthquake Natural Experiment." *Lancet,* 1983, *1,* 441–444.

Ussher, J. H. "Philippine Flood Disaster." *Journal of the Royal Naval Medical Service,* 1973, *59,* 81–83.

Vayer, J. S., Ten Eyck, R. P., and Cowan, M. L. "New Concepts in Triage." *Annals of Emergency Medicine,* 1986, *15,* 927–930.

Wesson, D. E., and Scorpio, R. "Field Triage: Help or Hindrance?" *Canadian Journal of Surgery,* 1992, *35,* 19–21.

For Further Information

Baskett, P., and Weller, R. (eds.). *Medicine for Disasters.* London: Wright, 1988.

Beinin, L. *Medical Consequences of Natural Disasters.* Berlin: Springer-Verlag, 1985.

Jenkins, A. L., and van de Leuv, J. H. *Disaster Planning in Emergency Department Organization and Management.* (2nd ed.) St. Louis: Mosby, 1978.

National Research Council. *Confronting Natural Disasters: An International Decade for Natural Hazard Reduction.* Washington, D.C.: National Academies Press, 1987.

National Research Council, U.S. National Committee for the Decade for Natural Disaster Reduction. *A Safer Future: Reducing the Impacts of Natural Disasters.* Washington, D.C.: National Academies Press, 1991.

Noji, E. K. (ed.). *The Public Health Consequences of Disasters.* New York: Oxford University Press, 1997.

Pan American Health Organization. *Assessing Needs in the Health Sector After Floods and Hurricanes.* Technical Paper no. 11. Washington, D.C.: Pan American Health Organization, 1987.

Tomasik, K. M. (ed.). *Emergency Preparedness: When Disaster Strikes.* Plant, Technology & Safety Management Series. Oakbrook Terrace, Ill.: Joint Commission on the Accreditation of Healthcare Organizations, 1994.

UCLA Center for Public Health and Disasters. Homepage. [http://www.cphd.ucla.edu]. 2005.

U.S. Department of Health and Human Services. "National Disaster Medical System." [http://ndms.dhhs.gov]. 2005.

CHAPTER TWENTY-SEVEN

NATURE CONTACT: A HEALTH BENEFIT?

Howard Frumkin

Much of this book is about hazards. We learn that contaminated food can cause diarrheal diseases (Chapter Twenty-One), that air pollution can cause respiratory disease (Chapter Fourteen), that poorly designed roadways can result in injuries (Chapters Seventeen and Twenty-Five), that degraded urban environments may encourage violence (Chapter Sixteen). Clearly, environmental exposures can threaten health—and this is a central focus of the environmental health field.

But the environment, broadly conceived, may also *enhance* health. One example is the many pharmaceuticals that derive from plants and animals, a compelling argument for preserving biodiversity (Wilson, 1992; Daily, 1997; Cassis, 1998). Another example is even more intuitive: contact with the natural world may directly benefit health. If so, then the field of environmental health needs to extend its interest beyond toxicity to consider possible health benefits. This chapter reviews the evidence for health benefits of the natural environment.

This chapter is adapted from H. Frumkin, "Beyond Toxicity: The Greening of Environmental Health," *American Journal of Preventive Medicine,* 2001, *20,* 234–240.

The Links Between Health and Environment

Many people appreciate a walk in the park or the sound of a bird's song or the sight of ocean waves lapping at the seashore. Even if these were only aesthetic preferences they would deserve our attention because they are so common as to seem nearly universal. In the words of University of Michigan psychologist Rachel Kaplan (1983): "Nature matters to people. Big trees and small trees, glistening water, chirping birds, budding bushes, colorful flowers—these are important ingredients in a good life" (p. 155). But perhaps these are more than aesthetic preferences. Perhaps we as a species find tranquility in certain natural environments, a soothing, restorative, even a healing sense. If so, contact with nature might be an important component of our well-being.

From an evolutionary perspective, a deep-seated connection with the natural world would be no surprise. Primate evolution began at least 65 million years ago, and the first hominids appeared as much as 5 million years ago. Two million years ago *australopithecines* were fashioning primitive stone tools and hunting in bands on the grassy savannas of Africa. *Homo habilis* probably appeared 2 or 3 million years ago, and our immediate predecessor, *homo erectus,* appeared about 1.5 million years ago. Human history as we now know it began during the Neolithic period, just 10,000 or 15,000 years ago, when the last great ice age ended and climate and ecology came to resemble those of our current world. Our ancestors—true *homo sapiens*—began to form settlements, cultivate crops, domesticate animals, dig mines, and even make art. If the last 2 million years of our species' history were scaled to a single human lifetime of seventy years, then the first humans would not have begun settling into villages until eight months after their sixty-ninth birthday. Some people—aboriginal groups in Australia, South America, the Pacific Islands, and elsewhere—would remain hunter-gatherers until a day or two before their seventieth birthday. We have broken with long-established patterns of living rather late in our life as a species.

For the great majority of human existence, human lives have been embedded in the natural environment. Those who could navigate it well—who could smell the water, find the plants, follow the animals, recognize the safe havens—must have enjoyed survival advantages. According to biologist E. O. Wilson (1993), "It would . . . be quite extraordinary to find that all learning rules related to that world have been erased in a few thousand years, even in the tiny minority of peoples who have existed for more than one or two generations in wholly urban environments" (p. 32). In a 1984 book, Wilson hypothesized the existence of *biophilia,* "the innately emotional affiliation of human beings to other living organisms" (Wilson, 1984, p. 31). Building on this theory, others have postulated an affinity for nature that goes beyond living things to include streams, ocean waves, and wind (Heerwagen and Orians, 1993).

The human connection to nature and the idea that this connection might be a component of good health have a long history in philosophy, art, and popular culture (see, for example, Nash, 1982; McLuhan, 1994). The New England transcendentalists, almost two centuries ago, argued that the human spirit was rooted in nature, and a leading exponent, Henry David Thoreau, wrote of the "tonic of wildness." A century later the conservationist John Muir observed, "Thousands of tired, nerve-shaken, over-civilized people are beginning to find out that going to the mountains is going home; that wilderness is a necessity; and that mountain parks and reservations are useful not only as fountains of timber and irrigating rivers, but as fountains of life" (Fox, 1981, p. 116).

But the history of human culture has also in many ways been the history of separation from nature. David Abram (1996) argues that this separation began with the very development of language, which replaced nature images with abstract symbols as central elements of human cognition and communication. Although our ancestors lived in close proximity to nature, their struggle to survive was in many ways a struggle to vanquish nature, or at least to shape it to their ends and to control its most extreme and unpredictable actions. The book of Genesis, which dates from about 3,000 years ago, included the often-repeated divine mandate, "Be fertile and multiply. Fill the land and conquer it. Dominate the fish of the sea, the birds of the sky, and every beast that walks the land." (As described in Chapter Nine, contemporary thinkers have imputed a gentler meaning to this passage, emphasizing stewardship rather than conquest.) The ancient Greeks abstracted human learning from nature. In the Platonic dialogue *Phaedrus,* Socrates finds himself outside the city walls, and grumbles to his companion, "I'm a lover of learning, and trees and open country won't teach me anything, whereas men in town do" (Hamilton and Cairns, 1961, p. 479). By now, wisdom and comfort were to be found in human society, apart from, and superior to, the world of nature. And subsequent developments have led most people, at least in developed nations, to live lives that are effectively insulated from the natural world. In the words of historian Roderick Nash (1982), "For thousands of years after our race opted for a civilized existence, we dreamed of and labored toward an escape from the anxieties of a wilderness condition only to find, when we reached the promised land of supermarkets and air conditioners, that we had forfeited something of great value" (p. 267).

Through what mechanisms might nature contact benefit health? Environmental psychology offers some possible answers to this question. Kaplan and Kaplan (1982) emphasized the importance of *directed attention,* the ability to block competing stimuli during purposeful activity. They proposed that people can develop *attentional fatigue* from overusing their attentional mechanisms, resulting in memory loss, diminished ability to focus, and greater impatience and frustration in interpersonal interactions. Moreover, they suggested that contact with nature could be restorative by renewing attention and improving cognitive abilities (Kaplan, 1995). Research has supported this view. For example, a study of college students (Tennessen and Cimprich, 1995) showed that those with more natural views from their dormitory windows had higher levels of attention and cognitive function. A study of apartment dwellers (Kaplan, 2001) showed that those with nature views from their windows scored higher on measures of effective functioning (including "focused," "effective," and "attentive") and lower on measures of being distracted (including "forgetful," "disorganized," and "difficult to finish things you have started"). Among the components of nature views, landscaping and gardens were most important in predicting effective functioning, and the presence of trees, farms, and fields was most important in predicting less distraction. And a study of children with attention deficit/hyperactivity disorder (Kuo and Taylor, 2004), using parents' ratings of their children's symptoms, found that playing in relatively *green*, or natural, settings reduced ADHD symptoms substantially more than playing in built outdoor and indoor settings. Nature contact may help, at least in part, through attention restoration.

Nature contact may also help by reducing stress. This is an intuitive notion; many people choose vacations in beautiful natural locations, probably expecting some stress reduction. Again, research supports this notion. For example, Ulrich and others (1991) exposed undergraduate students to a stressful film, followed by a variety of videotapes of natural and urban settings. The students' stress recovery, as measured by self-report and measures of cardiovascular variables, was significantly faster when they viewed the nature scenes. In another study (Parsons and others, 1998), students viewed a stressful film (showing workplace injuries), followed by a video of a roadside scene (either a forest, a golf course, a mixed development, or a commercial urban setting), followed by a second stressor (solving mathematical problems under time pressure). As measured by several (but not all) stress-related outcomes, such as blood pressure and skin conductance, students experienced higher levels of stress and recovered more slowly after viewing the artifact-dominated scenes relative to the nature-dominated scenes. And in a third study (Wells and Evans, 2003), 337 children in rural towns in upstate New York were classified according to the "naturalness" of their homes, including the views from the windows, the number of plants inside the home, and the composition of the yard. Children in the high-nature homes reacted to stressful life events with significantly less psychological distress compared to children in the low-nature homes. Results such as these suggest that nature contact may function, at least acutely, to mitigate stress.

Nature contact might be healthy in a third way, by playing a role in wholesome child development. Psychologists and others (Nabhan and Trimble, 1994; Kahn, 1999; Kahn and Kellert, 2002; Louv, 2005) have argued that children's ability to develop perceptual and expressive skills, imagination, moral judgments, and other attributes is greatly enhanced by contact with nature. Chapter Twenty-Eight introduces the concept that children have windows of vulnerability to toxic exposures; children may also have developmental windows during which nature contact fills important needs.

In considering the benefits of animal contact, Beck and Katcher (2003) suggest a fourth mechanism—social support. They point out that social contact is a strong predictor of good health and that pets provide companionship and intimacy for many people. This may be a beneficial aspect of nature contact more generally. For example, a family study in Zurich found that children who regularly played outside in natural areas had more than twice as many playmates as children restricted to indoor play because of heavy nearby traffic (Hüttenmoser, 1995). Interestingly, the same disparity in the quantity of friends was found among the corresponding groups of parents as well. Perhaps both biophilia-related mechanisms and social mechanisms function to yield health benefits.

Suppose, then, that humans have an affiliation with nature, an affiliation that conferred a survival advantage over evolutionary time, and that is now part of our genetic heritage. Suppose further that in modern life we more and more contain and suppress this affiliation—not only with our steam engines and Saran wrap but even with such basic means as our use of language. Is there any evidence that we can promote health by promoting this affiliation?

Domains of Nature Contact

Evidence that our contacts with nature can be beneficial to health is available from at least four aspects of the natural world—animals, plants, landscapes, and wilderness experiences.

Animals

Animals have always played a prominent part in human life (Clutton-Brock, 1981). Today more people go to zoos each year than to all professional sporting events (Wilson, 1993, p. 32). Fifty-six percent of U.S. households own pets (Beck and Meyers, 1996). More than 90 percent of the characters used in children's preschool books to help children with language acquisition and counting are animals (Kellert, 1993, p. 52). Numerous studies have established that household animals are considered family members; people talk to their pets as if they were human, carry their photographs, and share their bedrooms with them (Beck and Katcher, 1983). Fifty percent of adults and 70 percent of adolescents confide in their animals (Beck and Meyers, 1996).

A wide body of evidence links animals with human health. In a study in a Melbourne cardiovascular disease risk clinic, nearly 6,000 patients were divided into those who owned pets and those who did not. Among men the pet owners had statistically significantly lower systolic blood pressure, cholesterol, and triglycerides than the non-pet owners. Among women a similar trend was observed. These findings did not appear to be due to differences in exercise levels (say, from dog walking), in diet, in social class, or in other confounders (Anderson, Reid, and Jennings, 1992). In a 1995 study, 369 survivors of myocardial infarction were followed for one year. Of these, 112 owned pets and 257 did not. The dog owners had a one-year survival rate six times higher than that of the non-dog owners, and this benefit was not due to physiological differences (cat owners showed no such advantage) (Friedmann and Thomas, 1995).

Investigators in Cambridge, England, followed seventy-one adults who had just acquired pets and compared them with twenty-six petless controls over a ten-month period. Within a month of acquiring the pet the pet owners showed a statistically significant decrease in minor health problems. In the dog owners (but not the cat owners) this improvement was sustained for the entire ten months of observation (Serpell, 1991). In another study, this one in the United States, 938 Medicare enrollees were divided into pet owners and non-pet owners. The pet owners, especially the dog owners, had fewer physician visits than non-pet owners. Moreover, stressful life events were associated with more doctor visits among the non-pet owners but not among the pet owners, suggesting that owning a pet helped mediate stress (Siegel, 1990). (Not all studies have found decreased use of medical services among elderly pet owners; see Jorm and others, 1997.)

Animal-assisted therapy has been evaluated in the treatment of mental illness. For example, in a Virginia psychiatric hospital, 230 patients with mood disorders, schizophrenia, substance abuse disorders, and other diagnoses were treated with both a session of animal-assisted therapy (featuring interaction with a dog) and a session of conventional recreational therapy, using a crossover design. Both therapies reduced the patients' anxiety levels as measured by the State-Trait Anxiety Inventory, but in all diagnostic groups except mood disorders, the animal-assisted therapy achieved substantially greater reductions (Barker and Dawson, 1998).

The role of animals in helping people handle stress has been tested specifically. In one study patients about to undergo oral surgery were randomly assigned to one of five conditions: a half-hour of looking at an aquarium, with or without hypnosis, a half-hour of looking at a picture of a waterfall, with or without hypnosis, and a half-hour of sitting quietly (the control group). The patients' comfort and relaxation during surgery were graded independently by the oral surgeon, the investigator, and the patients themselves. The most relaxed patients were those who looked at the aquarium, irrespective of whether they had been hypnotized. The patients who looked at the waterfall picture and were also hypnotized were almost as relaxed. Those who looked at the waterfall picture without being hypnotized, however, had low relaxation scores, as low as those of the control patients (Katcher, Segal, and Beck, 1984). In another study, forty-five women were exposed to a stressful stimulus alone, in the presence of a human friend, and in the presence of their dog. Their autonomic nervous system responses to stress, such as heart rate, were measured. The stress response was marked when subjects were alone and even more marked when a friend was present. But having a dog present significantly reduced the stress response (Allen, 1997). *Animal-facilitated therapy* in the treatment of psychiatric conditions is widely used (Draper, Gerber, and Layng, 1990; Beck and Katcher, 2003).

Evidence such as this supports the conclusion of animal researchers Alan Beck and N. Marshall Meyers (1996): "Preserving the bond between people and their animals, like encouraging good nutrition and exercise, appears to be in the best interests of those concerned with public health" (p. 249).

Plants

People feel good around plants. In the 1989 National Gardening Survey of more than 2,000 randomly selected households, 50.1 percent of respondents agreed with the statement, "The flowers and plants at theme parks, historic sites, golf courses, and restaurants are important to my enjoyment of visiting there," and 40 percent agreed with the statement, "Being around plants makes me feel calmer and more relaxed" (Butterfield and Relf, 1992). Among residents of retirement communities, 99 percent indicate that "living within pleasant landscaped grounds" is either essential or important, and 95 percent indicate that windows facing green, landscaped grounds are either essential or important (Browne, 1992). Office employees report that plants make them feel calmer and more relaxed, and that an office with plants is a more desirable place to work (Randall, Shoemaker, Relf, and Geller, 1992; Larsen and others, 1998), although work performance does not necessarily improve (Larsen and others, 1998). In urban settings, gardens and gardening have been linked to a range of social benefits, ranging from improved property values to greater conviviality (for example, Patel, 1992). Psychologist Michael Perlman (1994) has written of the psychological power of trees, as evidenced by mythology, dreams, and self-reported emotional responses.

Indeed, the concept that plants have a role in mental health has been applied in *horticultural therapy,* a form of treatment based on the presumed therapeutic effects of gardening (Lewis, 1996). Horticultural therapy is also used in community-based programs, geriatrics programs, prisons, developmental disabilities programs, and special education (Mattson, 1992). In prisons, observers have noted that gardening has a "strangely soothing effect," making "pacifists of potential battlers" (Neese, 1959) and seeming to decrease the numbers of assaults among prisoners (Hunter, 1970, reported in Lewis, 1990).

Could contact with plants also contribute to healing from physical ailments (Lewis, 1990)? Oliver Sacks raised this possibility in a memorable passage in his 1984 account of recovery from a serious leg injury, *A Leg to Stand On.* After more than two weeks in a small hospital room with no outside view, and a third week on a dreary surgical ward, he was finally taken out to the hospital garden:

> This was a great joy—to be out in the air—for I had not been outside in almost a month. A pure and intense joy, a blessing, to feel the sun on my face and the wind in my hair, to hear birds, to see, touch, and fondle the living plants. Some essential connection and communion with nature was re-established after the horrible isolation and alienation I had known. Some part of me came alive, when I was taken to the garden, which had been starved, and died, perhaps without my knowing it [pp. 133–134].

Sacks credited his garden contact with an important role in his recovery and mused that perhaps more hospitals should have gardens or even be set in the countryside or near woods.

Another anecdotal account comes from Swee-Lian Yi, a twenty-nine-year-old severe stroke victim who was hospitalized in New York's Rusk Institute for Rehabilitation. Like Sacks, she found her first visit to the hospital greenhouse a turning point. "It was when I walked through that building, perfectly quiet, filled with green and growing plants and the sweet smell of healthy soil that my anxiety began to ebb away. In its place came a tranquility I had not experienced since the day of my stroke" (Yi, 1985). In fact hospitals have traditionally had gardens as an adjunct to recuperation and healing, and despite the depredations of managed care, notable examples survive in many parts of the country (Gerlach-Spriggs, Kaufman, and Warner, 1998). Although empirical evidence of efficacy is scarce (Frumkin, 2004), this time-honored practice reflects a perception that proximity to plants, like proximity to animals, may in some circumstances enhance health (also see Box 27.1).

Box 27.1. Nature Contact in the Inner City

An important line of research from the University of Illinois Human-Environment Research Laboratory has focused on nature contact in a rarely studied setting: inner-city housing projects. Investigators took advantage of a natural experiment at Chicago's Robert Taylor Homes. This complex consists of twenty-eight identical high-rise buildings arrayed along a three-mile stretch of land, bounded by busy roadways and railway lines. Some of the buildings are surrounded by pleasant stands of trees, whereas others open onto barren stretches of ground (Figure 27.1). Residents are essentially randomly assigned to a building with one landscape type or the other, because assignment depends on where a vacancy exists when their names come up on the Housing Authority list. The research compared residents of the buildings with and without trees, and was limited to those who lived on the lower floors (to ensure that participants in buildings surrounded by trees did have tree views from their windows).

This research has yielded surprising and important findings. Compared to living in buildings with barren surroundings, living in buildings with trees was associated with

- Higher levels of attention and greater effectiveness in managing major life issues (Kuo, 2001)
- Substantially lower levels of aggression and violence (both as victims and as perpetrators) among women (Kuo and Sullivan, 2001a)
- Lower levels of reported crime (Kuo and Sullivan, 2001b)
- Higher levels of self-discipline (as measured by tests of concentration, impulse inhibition, and delay of gratification) among girls (but not among boys) (Taylor, Kuo, and Sullivan, 2002)

These findings suggest that nature contact in otherwise deprived urban environments—even relatively simple forms of contact such as having trees outside an apartment building—can offer powerful benefits to the people who live there.

Landscapes

Natural landscapes may have a similar effect. Returning to an evolutionary perspective, human history probably began on the African savanna, a region of open grasslands punctuated by scattered copses of trees and denser woods near rivers and lakes. If this sounds like the choicest real estate in most cities and towns, that may not be a coincidence. As E. O. Wilson (1984) points out, "certain key features of the ancient physical habitat match the choices made by modern human beings when they have a say in the matter" (p. 109)—a pattern that repeats in

FIGURE 27.1. THREE VIEWS OF ROBERT TAYLOR HOMES: AERIAL VIEW (TOP), BARREN SURROUNDINGS (MIDDLE), AND SURROUNDINGS WITH TREES (BOTTOM).

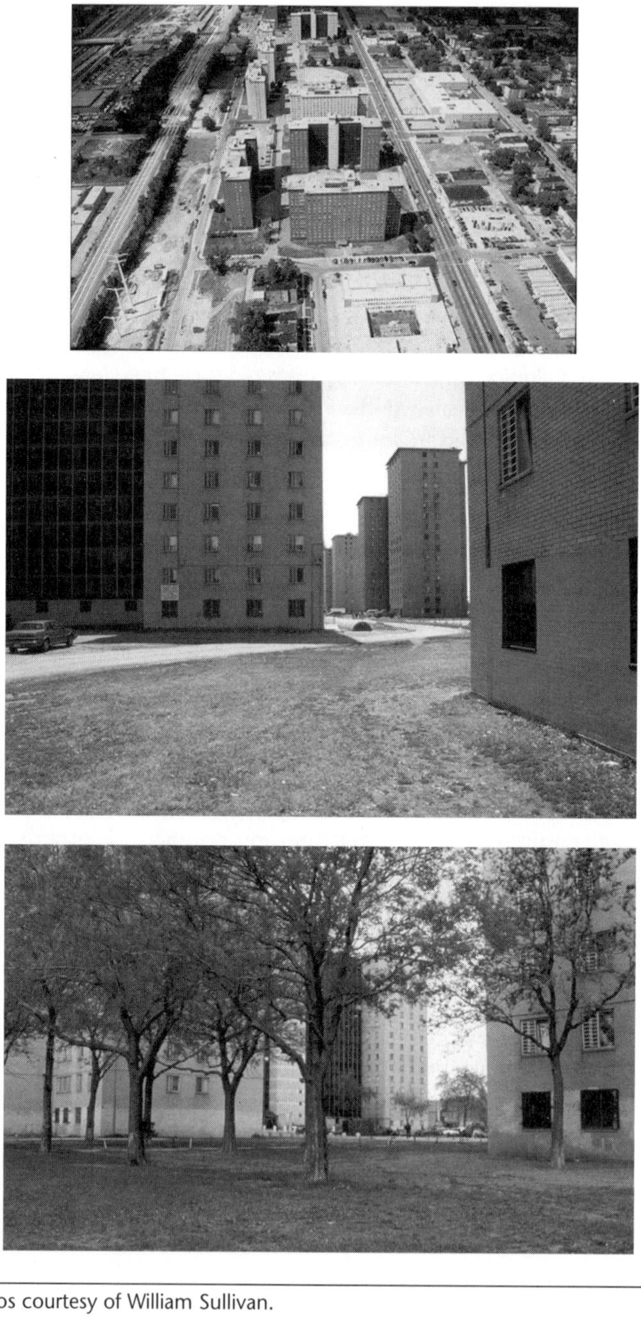

Source: Photos courtesy of William Sullivan.

parks, cemeteries, golf courses, and lawns. "It seems that whenever people are given a free choice, they move to open tree-studded land on prominences overlooking water" (p. 110).

Could evolution have selected for certain landscape preferences? Perhaps. "A crucial step in the lives of most organisms, including humans, is selection of a habitat. If a creature gets into the right place, everything else is likely to be easier. Habitat selection depends on the recognition of objects, sounds, and odors to which the organism responds as if it understood their significance for future behavior and success" (Heerwagen and Orians, 1993, p. 140). For example, many birds use patterns of tree density and vertical arrangement of branches as primary settling cues; presumably these cues correlate with crucial information about such benefits as food availability and concealment from predators. For early humans a place with an open view would have offered better opportunities than a spatially restricted setting to identify food and shelter and to avoid predators. But not too open a view: clumps of trees would offer hiding places in a pinch and, like streams and lakes, might also signal the presence of prey for the hunter (Ulrich, 1993). Going further, perhaps the ability to identify relaxing, restorative settings, and the capacity to recover from fatigue and stress, could also have been adaptive (Ulrich, 1993; Kaplan and Kaplan, 1989). If you can run away from a saber-toothed tiger, your survival is enhanced. But if, having run away, you can then get to a peaceful place, relax, and regather your strength, that may further enhance your survival. Perhaps individuals who chose such settings gained a survival advantage (Ulrich, 1993).

There is considerable evidence that people's aesthetic preferences conform to this prediction. When offered a variety of landscapes, people react most positively to savanna-like settings, with moderate to high depth or openness, relatively smooth or uniform-length grassy vegetation or ground surfaces, scattered trees or small groupings of trees, and water (Schroeder and Green, 1985; Kaplan, 1984). Notably, these findings emerge cross-culturally, in studies of North Americans, Europeans, Asians, and Africans (see, for example, Hull and Revell, 1989; Purcell, Lamb, Peron, and Falchero, 1994; Korpela and Hartig, 1996).

The effect of landscapes may extend beyond aesthetics to restoration or stress recovery. Research on recreational activities has shown that savanna-like settings are associated with self-reported feelings of "peacefulness," "tranquility," or "relaxation" (Ulrich, 1983). Viewing such settings leads to decreased fear and anger and enhanced positive affect on the Zuckerman Inventory of Personal Reactions (ZIPERS) (Honeyman, 1992). Moreover, viewing nature scenes is associated with enhanced mental alertness, attention, and cognitive performance, as measured by tasks such as proofreading and by formal psychological testing (Hartig, Mang, and Evans, 1991; Cimprich, 2003; Tennessen and Cimprich, 1995).

The same results emerge from studies that directly consider conventional health end points. In 1981, Ernest Moore, a University of Michigan architect, took advantage of a natural experiment at the State Prison of Southern Michigan, a massive depression-era structure. Half the prisoners occupied cells along the outside wall, with a window view of rolling farmland and trees, and the other half occupied cells that faced the prison courtyard. Assignment to one or the other kind of cell was random. Compared to the prisoners in the exterior cells, the prisoners in the inside cells had a 24 percent higher frequency of sick call visits. Moore could not identify any design feature to explain this difference and concluded that the outside view "may provide some stress reduction" (Moore, 1981–1982). Likewise, employees with views of nature at work report fewer headaches (as well as less job pressure and greater job satisfaction) than do those without such a view (Kaplan, Talbot, and Kaplan, 1988, reported in Kaplan, 1992).

Similar observations have come from health care settings. A short 1984 article in *Science* bore the provocative title "View Through a Window May Influence Recovery from Surgery." Like the Michigan prison study, this study also took advantage of an inadvertent architectural experiment. On the surgical floors of a 200-bed suburban Pennsylvania hospital, some rooms faced a stand of deciduous trees, and others faced a brown brick wall. Postoperative patients were assigned essentially randomly to one or the other kind of room. The records of all cholecystectomy patients over a ten-year interval, restricted to the summer months when the trees were in foliage, were reviewed. End points were the length of hospitalization, the need for pain and anxiety medications, the occurrence of minor medical complications, and nurses' notes. Compared to patients with brick views, patients with tree views had statistically significantly shorter hospitalizations (7.96 days compared to 8.70 days), less need for pain medications, and fewer negative comments in the nurses' notes (Ulrich, 1984).

Other evidence is available from therapeutic settings. In a study of dental patients, researchers placed a large mural of an open, natural scene on the wall of a dental waiting room on some days and removed it on others. Dental patients with appointments on the days when the mural was visible had lower blood pressure and less self-reported anxiety than the patients with appointments on the days when the mural was taken down (Heerwagen, 1990). In a study of psychiatric inpatients, patients were exposed to two kinds of wall art: nature scenes such as landscapes and abstract or symbolic art. Interviews suggested more positive responses to the nature scenes. And in fifteen years of records on patient attacks on the wall art, every attack was on abstract art, none was on a nature scene (Ulrich, 1986, reported in Ulrich, 1993). (No information was provided on how many of the psychiatric patients were artists or art critics.) And in a randomized clinical trial of patients undergoing bronchoscopy (insertion of a flexible fiber-optic tube through the trachea into the lungs), patients who viewed a nature scene (a mountain stream in a spring meadow) and heard recorded nature sounds (water in a stream or chirping birds) experienced better pain control than did patients who received only conventional sedation (although anxiety levels did not differ between the two groups) (Diette and others, 2003). Viewing landscapes and related nature scenes, whether in actuality or in pictures, seems to have a salutary effect.

Wilderness Experiences

Wilderness experiences—entering the landscape rather than only viewing it—may also be therapeutic. David Cumes (1998a, 1998b) has described *wilderness rapture,* involving self-awareness; feelings of awe, wonder, and humility; a sense of comfort in and connection to nature; increased appreciation of others; and a feeling of renewal and vigor. Others have described the spiritual inspiration that comes from wilderness experiences (Fredrickson and Anderson, 1999). These outcomes are often cited in favorable accounts of so-called wilderness therapy for psychiatric patients (Jerstad and Stelzer, 1973; Witman, 1987; Plakun, Tucker, and Harris, 1981; Berman and Anton, 1988), emotionally disturbed children and adolescents (Hobbs and Shelton, 1972; Marx, 1988; Davis-Berman and Berman, 1989), bereaved persons (Moyer, 1988; Birnbaum, 1991), and rape and incest survivors (Levine, 1994) and also for patients with cancer (Pearson, 1989), end-stage renal disease (Warady, 1994), posttraumatic stress disorder (PTSD) (Hyer and others, 1996), addiction disorders (Bennett, Cardone, and Jarczyk, 1998; Kennedy and Minami, 1993), and other ailments (Easley, Passineau, and Driver, 1990). *Green exercise* may represent a less intense version of this same phenomenon (Box 27.2).

Box 27.2. Green Exercise

Exercise is clearly good for health; the benefits include weight loss, blood pressure and cholesterol reduction, and decreased risk of heart attacks, stroke, diabetes, and some cancers. Exercise is also good for mental health; it improves attention, lifts mood, and relieves depression. Could it matter where you exercise?

In recent years research has suggested that exercise in natural settings may be more beneficial than exercise in barren or heavily built settings (Pretty, Griffin, Sellens, and Pretty, 2003). In a Swedish study twelve regular runners took two hour-long runs, one through a nature reserve featuring pine-birch forest, open fields, and a lakeshore and the other through an urban route featuring mid-rise apartment houses, commercial development, and heavy traffic. The runners preferred the park route and perceived it as more psychologically restorative than the urban route, scoring it substantially higher on a *perceived restorativeness scale* (with such dimensions as "being away" from daily routine, fascination, and compatibility with personal tastes). In addition, self-rated anxiety or depression and anger decreased more and self-rated revitalization and tranquility improved more with the park compared to the urban route (although these differences did not reach statistical significance) (Bodin and Hartig, 2003).

In another study volunteers exercised on a treadmill while viewing different scenes on a screen—some rural and other urban, some pleasant and others unpleasant. Exercising while viewing the pleasant rural scenes resulted in a greater decrease in blood pressure than any other condition, and when measured on several psychological measures—self-esteem, anger-hostility, fatigue-inertia, tension-anxiety, and vigor-activity—people viewing the rural pleasant scenes had more consistent improvements than they did in any other condition (although again, not always with statistical significance) (Pretty, Peacock, Sellens, and Griffin, forthcoming).

If these findings can be replicated, they suggest that the well-known health benefits of exercise may be further enhanced by exercising in pleasing natural settings—something that golfers, hikers, and resort owners (among others) may already believe.

Most documented examples of beneficial effects from wilderness experiences relate to mental health endpoints. A group of 5.5- to 11.5-year-old emotionally disturbed boys attending an outdoor day camp was compared to a group of similar boys not attending the camp. The campers' self-ratings of their emotional adjustment and also their teachers' ratings were significantly better than those of the controls, although neither parents' ratings nor scores on formal psychological testing showed an improvement (Shniderman, 1974). A group of adolescents being treated for depression, substance abuse, or adjustment reactions improved on measures of cooperation and trust following a wilderness experience, whereas controls did not (Witman, 1987). Psychiatric inpatients showed improvements in coping ability and locus of control following a wilderness adventure program (Plakun, Tucker, and Harris, 1981). Inpatients at the Oregon State Mental Hospital showed improved function and greater probability of discharge following wilderness adventure programs (Jerstad and Stelzer, 1973). In a convenience sample of more than 700 people who had participated in wilderness excursions lasting two to four weeks, 90 percent described "an increased sense of aliveness, well-being, and energy," and 90 percent reported that the experience had helped them break an addiction (defined broadly and ranging from nicotine to chocolate) (Greenway, 1995).

This literature is more extensive than the literature on plants and animals (Colan, 1986), but several limitations make it difficult to interpret (McNeil, 1957; Byers, 1979). Much of the published research comes from proponents such as adventure companies with a personal or commercial interest in wilderness experiences. Much of the research refers to structured trips or summer camp programs rather than to the more general phenomenon of contact with wilderness. Beneficial outcomes may be due to the vacation quality of the experience, to the psychological value of setting and achieving difficult goals, or to the group bonding that occurs on some such trips (or to some combination of these), rather than (or in addition to) the wilderness contact itself. Few studies have been randomized, and selection bias can rarely be excluded. Blinding of subjects has been impossible, and blinding of investigators has not been attempted.

Despite these limitations, many published accounts do suggest some benefit from wilderness experiences. Mental health has been more studied than somatic conditions, and short-term benefit has been demonstrated more than long-term benefit.

There is evidence, then, that contact with the natural world—with animals, plants, landscapes, and wilderness—may offer health benefits. Perhaps this reflects ancient learning habits, preferences, and tastes, echoes of our origins as creatures of the wild. Satisfying these preferences—taking seriously our affiliation with the natural world—may be an effective way to enhance health, not to mention cheaper and freer of side effects than medications. If so, this implies a broad vision of environmental health, one that stretches from urban planning to landscape architecture, from interior design to forestry, from botany to veterinary medicine.

Steps Toward the Greening of Environmental Health

A paradigm of environmental health that considers good places as well as bad ones, health as well as illness, has implications in at least three arenas: research, collaboration, and public health intervention.

Research

Clinical and epidemiological research in environmental health addresses many variants of the same question: Is there an association between exposure and outcome? A focus on nature contact suggests a research agenda directed not only at potentially *hazardous* exposures but also at potentially *healthy ones*, and at outcomes that reflect not only impaired health but also enhanced health (Frumkin, 2003). If people have regular contact with flowers or trees, do they report greater well-being, better sleep, fewer headaches, reduced joint pain? Do inner-city children who attend a rural summer camp have better health during the next semester of school than their friends who spent the summer in the city? Do patients with cancer or AIDS survive longer, or have fewer infections or less pain or higher T cell counts, if they have pets? Do gardens in hospitals speed postoperative recovery? Can psychotherapy that employs contact with nature—known as *ecopsychology* (Roszak, Gomes, and Kanner, 1995)—have an empirical basis? If any of these therapeutic approaches shows promise, which patients will benefit and what kinds of contact with nature have the greatest efficacy and cost effectiveness?

Answering these questions requires an orientation toward empirical research among professions that have traditionally not emphasized it, from landscape architecture to horticulture. It also requires an ability to define and operationalize variables currently unfamiliar to health researchers. What is *exposure* to nature, what does the concept of a *dose* mean in this context, and how do we measure it? Similarly, the outcome variables that reflect health instead of disease are less familiar and need to be developed and validated. These challenges offer broad opportunities for methods development and hypothesis testing.

Collaboration

Environmental health specialists, from researchers to clinicians, have long recognized the need to collaborate with other professionals. They work with mechanical engineers to build exposure chambers, with chemists to measure exposures, and with software engineers to apply geographic information systems to health data. A focus on natural environments requires collaborations with other kinds of professionals: landscape architects to help identify the salient features of outdoor exposures, interior designers to do the same for microenvironments, veterinarians to help understand more about human relationships with animals, and urban and regional planners to help link environmental health principles with large-scale environmental design.

Public Health Intervention

Finally, as we learn more about the health benefits of particular environments, we need to act on these findings. On the clinical level this may have implications for patient care. Perhaps physicians and nurses will advise patients to take a few days in the country, to spend time gardening, or to adopt a pet if clinical evidence offers support for such measures. Perhaps we will build hospitals in scenic locations or plant gardens in rehabilitation centers. Perhaps the employers and managed care organizations that pay for health care will come to fund such interventions, especially if they prove to rival pharmaceuticals in cost and efficacy.

On the public health level, environmental health has a long history of providing data, and advocating action based on these data, to achieve control of environmental hazards—more protective air pollution regulations, lower automobile emissions, safer pesticide practices, and cleaner rivers and streams. In the same way, public health will need to act on emerging evidence of environmental health benefits. We take it for granted that health experts play a prominent role at the Food and Drug Administration and the Environmental Protection Agency; how about a role at the National Park Service or the local zoo? As we learn more about the health benefits of contact with the natural world, we need to apply this knowledge in ways that directly enhance the health of the public.

Thought Questions

1. Describe your last contact with a natural setting—on a vacation, a weekend outing, or even a recent visit to a park. How did it make you feel? How would you design research to demonstrate the effects across a broad population?
2. Consider the availability of parks and green space in your city or town. Are they available near the places where people live and work? Do some sections have better access to them than others? What about poor and minority communities? Is this an environmental justice issue?
3. Suppose your community is considering a land conservation initiative that would set aside tracts of green space and prohibit future development on them. Environmental advocates are leading this effort, but they ask you to support it based on public health considerations. How would you make the case?

References

Abram, D. *The Spell of the Sensuous: Perception and Language in a More-Than-Human World.* New York: Vintage Books, 1996.

Allen, D. T. "Effects of Dogs on Human Health." *Journal of the American Veterinary Medicine Association,* 1997, *210,* 1136–1139.

Anderson, W. P., Reid, C., and Jennings, G. "Pet Ownership and Risk Factors for Cardiovascular Disease." *Medical Journal of Australia,* 1992, *157,* 298–301.

Barker, S. B., and Dawson, K. S. "The Effects of Animal-Assisted Therapy on Anxiety Ratings of Hospitalized Psychiatric Patients." *Psychiatric Services,* 1998, *49*(6), 797–801.

Beck, A. M., and Katcher, A. H. *Between Pets and People: The Importance of Animal Companionship.* New York: Perigree Books, 1983.

Beck, A., and Katcher, A. "Future Directions in Human-Animal Bond Research." *American Behavioral Scientist,* 2003, *47,* 79–93.

Beck, A. M., and Meyers, N. M. "Health Enhancement and Companion Animal Ownership." *Annual Review of Public Health,* 1996, *17,* 247–257.

Bennett, L. W., Cardone, S., and Jarczyk, J. "Effects of a Therapeutic Camping Program on Addiction Recovery: The Algonquin Relapse Prevention Program." *Journal of Substance Abuse Treatment,* 1998, *15,* 469–474.

Berman, D. S., and Anton, M. T. "A Wilderness Therapy Program as an Alternative to Adolescent Psychiatric Hospitalization." *Residential Treatment for Children and Youth,* 1988, *5,* 41–53.

Birnbaum, A. "Haven Hugs & Bugs." *American Journal of Hospice Palliative Care,* 1991, *8,* 23–29.

Bodin, M., and Hartig, T. "Does the Outdoor Environment Matter for Psychological Restoration Gained Through Running?" *Psychology of Sport and Exercise,* 2003, *4,* 141–153.

Browne, A. "The Role of Nature for the Promotion of Well-Being in the Elderly." In D. Relf (ed.), *The Role of Horticulture in Human Well-Being and Social Development.* Portland, Ore.: Timber Press, 1992.

Butterfield, B., and Relf, D. "National Survey of Attitudes Toward Plants and Gardening." In D. Relf (ed.), *The Role of Horticulture in Human Well-Being and Social Development.* Portland, Ore.: Timber Press, 1992.

Byers, E. S. "Wilderness Camping as a Therapy for Emotionally Disturbed Children: A Critical Review." *Exceptional Children,* 1979, *45,* 628–635.

Cassis, G. "Biodiversity Loss: A Human Health Issue." *Medical Journal of Australia,* 1998, *169,* 568–569.

Cimprich, B. "An Environmental Intervention to Restore Attention in Women with Newly Diagnosed Breast Cancer." *Cancer Nursing,* 2003, *26,* 284–292.

Clutton-Brock, J. *Domesticated Animals from Early Times.* Austin: University of Texas Press, 1981.

Colan, N. B. *Outward Bound: An Annotated Bibliography (1976–1985).* Greenwich, Conn.: Outward Bound USA, 1986.

Cumes, D. *Inner Passages Outer Journeys: Wilderness, Healing, and the Discovery of Self.* Minneapolis: Llewellyn, 1998a.

Cumes, D. "Nature as Medicine: The Healing Power of the Wilderness." *Alternative Therapies,* 1998b, *4,* 79–86.

Daily, G. C. (ed.). *Nature's Services: Societal Dependence on Natural Ecosystems.* Washington D.C.: Island Press, 1997.

Davis-Berman, J., and Berman, D. S. "The Wilderness Therapy Program: An Empirical Study of Its Effects with Adolescents in an Outpatient Setting." *Journal of Contemporary Psychotherapy,* 1989, *19,* 271–281.

Diette, G. B., and others. "Distraction Therapy with Nature Sights and Sounds Reduces Pain During Flexible Bronchoscopy." *Chest,* 2003, *123,* 141–148.

Draper, R. J., Gerber, G. J., and Layng, E. M. "Defining the Role of Pet Animals in Psychotherapy." *Psychiatric Journal of the University of Ottawa,* 1990, *15*(3), 169–172.

Easley, A. T., Passineau, J. F., and Driver, B. L. (comps.). *The Use of Wilderness for Personal Growth, Therapy, and Education.* Fort Collins, Colo.: U.S. Department of Agriculture, Forest Service, Rocky Mountain Forest and Range Experiment Station, 1990.

Fox, S. *John Muir and His Legacy.* Boston: Little, Brown, 1981.

Fredrickson, L. M., and Anderson, D. H. "A Qualitative Exploration of the Wilderness Experience as a Source of Spiritual Inspiration." *Journal of Environmental Psychology,* 1999, *19,* 21–39.

Friedmann, E., and Thomas, S. A. "Pet Ownership, Social Support, and One-Year Survival After Acute Myocardial Infarction in the Cardiac Arrhythmia Suppression Trial (CAST)." *American Journal of Cardiology,* 1995, *76,* 1213–1217.

Frumkin, H. "Healthy Places: Exploring the Evidence." *American Journal of Public Health,* 2003, *93,* 1451–1455.

Frumkin, H. "White Coats, Green Plants: Clinical Epidemiology Meets Horticulture." *Acta Horticulturae,* 2004, *639,* 15–26.

Gerlach-Spriggs, N., Kaufman, R. E., and Warner, S. B. *Restorative Gardens: The Healing Landscape.* New Haven, Conn.: Yale University Press, 1998.

Greenway, R. "The Wilderness Effect and Ecopsychology." In T. Roszak, M. E. Gomes, and A. D. Kanner (eds.), *Ecopsychology: Restoring the Earth, Healing the Mind.* San Francisco: Sierra Club Books, 1995.

Hamilton, E., and Cairns, H. (eds.). *Plato: The Collected Dialogues.* Princeton, N.J.: Princeton University Press, 1961.

Hartig, T., Mang, M., and Evans, G. "Restorative Effects of Natural Environmental Experiences." *Environment and Behavior,* 1991, *23,* 3–26.

Heerwagen, J. H. "The Psychological Aspects of Windows and Window Design." In K. H. Anthony, J. Choi, and B. Orland (eds.), *Proceedings of the 21st Annual Conference of the Environmental Design Research Association.* Oklahoma City, Okla.: EDRA, 1990.

Heerwagen, J. H., and Orians, G. H. "Humans, Habitats, and Aesthetics." In S. R. Kellert and E. O. Wilson (eds.), *The Biophilia Hypothesis.* Washington, D.C.: Island Press, 1993.

Hobbs, T. R., and Shelton, G. C. "Therapeutic Camping for Emotionally Disturbed Adolescents." *Hospital & Community Psychiatry,* 1972, *23,* 298–301.

Honeyman, M. K. "Vegetation and Stress: A Comparison Study of Varying Amounts of Vegetation in Countryside and Urban Scenes." In D. Relf (ed.), *The Role of Horticulture in Human Well-Being and Social Development.* Portland, Ore.: Timber Press, 1992.

Hull, R. B., and Revell, G.R.B. "Cross-Cultural Comparison on Landscape Scenic Beauty Evaluations: A Case Study in Bali." *Journal of Environmental Psychology,* 1989, *9,* 177–191.

Hunter, N. L. *Horticulture Programs in Prisons.* San Luis Obispo: Horticulture Department, California State Polytechnic College, 1970.

Hüttenmoser, M. "Children and Their Living Surroundings: Empirical Investigations into the Significance of Living Surroundings for the Everyday Life and Development of Children." *Children's Environments,* 1995, *12,* 403–413.

Hyer, L., and others. "Effects of Outward Bound Experience as an Adjunct to Inpatient PTSD Treatment of War Veterans." *Journal of Clinical Psychology,* 1996, *52,* 263–278.

Jerstad, L., and Stelzer, J. "Adventure Experiences as Treatment for Residential Mental Patients." *Therapeutic Recreation,* 1973, *7,* 8–11.

Jorm, A. F., and others. "Impact of Pet Ownership on Elderly Australians' Use of Medical Services: An Analysis Using Medicare Data." *Medical Journal of Australia,* 1997, *166,* 376–377.

Kahn, P. H., Jr. *The Human Relationship with Nature: Development and Culture.* Cambridge, Mass.: MIT Press, 1999.

Kahn, P. H., Jr., and Kellert, S. R. (eds.). *Children and Nature: Psychological, Sociocultural, and Evolutionary Investigations.* Cambridge, Mass.: MIT Press, 2002.

Kaplan, R. "The Role of Nature in the Urban Context." In I. Altman and J. F. Wohlwill (eds.), *Behavior and the Natural Environment.* New York: Plenum, 1983.

Kaplan, R. "Dominant and Variable Values in Environmental Preference." In A. S. Devlin and S. L. Taylor (eds.), *Environmental Preference and Landscape Preference.* New London: Connecticut College, 1984.

Kaplan, R. "The Psychological Benefits of Nearby Nature." In D. Relf (ed.), *The Role of Horticulture in Human Well-Being and Social Development.* Portland, Ore.: Timber Press, 1992.

Kaplan, R. "The Nature of the View from Home: Psychological Benefits." *Environment and Behavior,* 2001, *33,* 507–542.

Kaplan, R., and Kaplan, S. *The Experience of Nature: A Psychological Perspective.* New York: Cambridge University Press, 1989.

Kaplan, S. "The Restorative Benefits of Nature: Toward an Integrative Framework." *Journal of Environmental Psychology,* 1995, *15,* 169–182.

Kaplan, S., and Kaplan, R. *Cognition and Environment.* New York: Praeger, 1982.

Kaplan, S., Talbot, J. F., and Kaplan, R. "Coping with Daily Hassles: The Impact of Nearby Nature on the Work Environment." Washington, D.C.: USDA Forest Service, North Central Forest Experiment Station, 1988.

Katcher, A., Segal, H., and Beck, A. "Comparison of Contemplation and Hypnosis for the Reduction of Anxiety and Discomfort During Dental Surgery." *American Journal of Clinical Hypnosis,* 1984, *27,* 14–21.

Kellert, S. R. "The Biological Basis for Human Values of Nature." In S. R. Kellert and E. O. Wilson (eds.), *The Biophilia Hypothesis.* Washington, D.C.: Island Press, 1993.

Kennedy, B. P., and Minami, M. "The Beech Hill Hospital/Outward Bound Adolescent Chemical Dependency Treatment Program." *Journal of Substance Abuse Treatment,* 1993, *10,* 395–406.

Korpela, K., and Hartig, T. "Restorative Qualities of Favorite Places." *Journal of Environmental Psychology,* 1996, *16,* 221–233.

Kuo, F. E. "Coping with Poverty: Impacts of Environment and Attention in the Inner City." *Environment and Behavior,* 2001, *33*(1), 5–34.

Kuo, F. E., and Sullivan, W. C. "Aggression and Violence in the Inner City: Effects of Environment Via Mental Fatigue." *Environment and Behavior,* 2001a, *33*(4), 543–571.

Kuo, F. E., and Sullivan, W. C. "Environment and Crime in the Inner City: Does Vegetation Reduce Crime?" *Environment and Behavior,* 2001b, *33*(3), 343–367.

Kuo, F. E., and Taylor, A. F. "A Potential Natural Treatment for Attention-Deficit/Hyperactivity Disorder: Evidence from a National Study." *American Journal of Public Health,* 2004, *94,* 1580–1586.

Larsen, L., and others. "Plants in the Workplace: The Effects of Plant Density on Productivity, Attitudes, and Perceptions." *Environment and Behavior,* 1998, *30,* 261–282.

Levine, D. "Breaking Through Barriers: Wilderness Therapy for Sexual Assault Survivors." *Women and Therapy,* 1994, *15*(3–4), 175–184.

Lewis, C. A. "Gardening as Healing Process." In M. Francis and R. T. Hester (eds.), *The Meaning of Gardens.* Cambridge, Mass.: MIT Press, 1990.

Lewis, C. A. *Green Nature/Human Nature: The Meaning of Plants in Our Lives.* Urbana: University of Illinois Press, 1996.

Louv, R. *Last Child in the Woods: Saving our Children from Nature-Deficit Disorder.* Chapel Hill, N.C.: Algonquin Press, 2005.

Marx, J. D. "An Outdoor Adventure Counseling Program for Adolescents." *Social Work,* 1988, *33,* 517–520.

Mattson, R. H. "Prescribing Health Benefits Through Horticultural Activities." In D. Relf (ed.), *The Role of Horticulture in Human Well-Being and Social Development.* Portland, Ore.: Timber Press, 1992.

McLuhan, T. C. *The Way of the Earth: Encounters with Nature in Ancient and Contemporary Thought.* New York: Simon & Schuster, 1994.

McNeil, E. B. "The Background of Therapeutic Camping." *Journal of Social Issues,* 1957, *13,* 3–14.

Moore, E. O. "A Prison Environment's Effect on Health Care Service Demands." *Journal of Environmental Systems,* 1981–1982, *11,* 17–34.

Moyer, J. A. "Bannock Bereavement Retreat: A Camping Experience for Surviving Children." *American Journal of Hospice Care,* 1988, *5,* 26–30.

Nabhan, G. P., and Trimble, S. *The Geography of Childhood: Why Children Need Wild Places.* Boston: Beacon Press, 1994.

Nash, R. *Wilderness and the American Mind.* (3rd ed.) New Haven, Conn.: Yale University Press, 1982.

Neese, R. "Prisoner's Escape." *Flower Grower,* 1959, *46,* 39–40.

Parsons, R., and others. "The View from the Road: Implications for Stress Recovery and Immunization." *Journal of Environmental Psychology,* 1998, *18,* 113–140.

Patel, I. C. "Socio-Economic Impact of Community Gardening in an Urban Setting." In D. Relf (ed.), *The Role of Horticulture in Human Well-Being and Social Development.* Portland, Ore.: Timber Press, 1992.

Pearson, J. "A Wilderness Program for Adolescents with Cancer." *Journal of the Association of Pediatric Oncology Nurses,* 1989, *6,* 24–25.

Perlman, M. *The Power of Trees: The Reforesting of the Soul.* Dallas: Spring, 1994.

Plakun, E., Tucker, G. J., and Harris, P. Q. "Outward Bound: An Adjunctive Psychiatric Therapy." *Journal of Psychiatric Treatment and Evaluation,* 1981, *3,* 33–37.

Pretty, J., Griffin, M., Sellens, M., and Pretty, C. *Green Exercise: Complementary Roles of Nature, Exercise and Diet in Physical and Emotional Well-Being and Implications for Public Policy.* CES Occasional Paper 2003-1. Centre for Environment and Society, University of Essex. [http://www2.essex.ac.uk/ces/ResearchProgrammes/CESOccasionalPapers/GreenExercise.pdf]. Mar. 2003.

Pretty, J., Peacock, J., Sellens, M., and Griffin, M. "The Mental and Physical Health Outcomes of Green Exercise." *International Journal of Environmental Health Research,* forthcoming.

Purcell, A. T., Lamb, R. J., Peron, E. M., and Falchero, S. "Preference or Preferences for Landscape?" *Journal of Environmental Psychology,* 1994, *14,* 195–209.

Randall, K., Shoemaker, C. A., Relf, D., and Geller, E. S. "Effects of Plantscapes in an Office Environment on Worker Satisfaction." In D. Relf (ed.), *The Role of Horticulture in Human Well-Being and Social Development.* Portland, Ore.: Timber Press, 1992.

Roszak, T., Gomes, M. E., and Kanner, A. D. (eds.). *Ecopsychology: Restoring the Earth, Healing the Mind.* San Francisco: Sierra Club Books, 1995.

Sacks, O. *A Leg to Stand On.* New York: HarperCollins, 1984.

Schroeder, H. W., and Green, T. L. "Public Preferences for Tree Density in Municipal Parks." *Journal of Arboriculture,* 1985, *11,* 272–277.

Serpell, J. "Beneficial Effects of Pet Ownership on Some Aspects of Human Health and Behaviour." *Journal of the Royal Society of Medicine,* 1991, *84,* 717–720.

Shniderman, C. M. "Impact of Therapeutic Camping." *Social Work,* 1974, *19,* 354–357.

Siegel, J. "Stressful Life Events and Use of Physician Services Among the Elderly: The Moderating Role of Pet Ownership." *Journal of Personality and Social Psychology,* 1990, *58,* 1081–1086.

Taylor, A. F., Kuo, F. E., and Sullivan, W. C. "Views of Nature and Self-Discipline: Evidence from Inner City Children." *Journal of Environmental Psychology,* 2002, *22*(1–2), 49–63.
Tennessen, C. M., and Cimprich, B. "Views to Nature: Effects on Attention." *Journal of Environmental Psychology,* 1995, *15,* 77–85.
Ulrich, R. S. "Aesthetic and Affective Response to Natural Environment." In I. Altman and J. F. Wohlwill (eds.), *Human Behavior and Environment,* Vol. 6: *Behavior and the Natural Environment.* New York: Plenum, 1983.
Ulrich, R. S. "View Through a Window May Influence Recovery from Surgery." *Science,* 1984, *224,* 420–421.
Ulrich, R. S. *Effects of Hospital Environments on Patient Well-Being.* Research Report 9(55). Trondheim, Norway: Department of Psychiatry and Behavioral Medicine, University of Trondheim, 1986.
Ulrich, R. S. "Biophilia, Biophobia, and Natural Landscapes." In S. R. Kellert and E. O. Wilson (eds.), *The Biophilia Hypothesis.* Washington, D.C.: Island Press, 1993.
Ulrich, R. S., and others. "Stress Recovery During Exposure to Natural and Urban Environments." *Journal of Environmental Psychology,* 1991, *11,* 201–230.
Warady, B. A. "Therapeutic Camping for Children with End-Stage Renal Disease." *Pediatric Nephrology,* 1994, *8,* 387–390.
Wells, N. M., and Evans, G. W. "Nearby Nature: A Buffer of Life Stress Among Rural Children." *Environment and Behavior,* 2003, *35,* 311–330.
Wilson, E. O. *Biophilia: The Human Bond with Other Species.* Cambridge, Mass.: Harvard University Press, 1984.
Wilson, E. O. *The Diversity of Life.* Cambridge, Mass.: Harvard University Press, 1992.
Wilson, E. O. "Biophilia and the Conservation Ethic." In S. R. Kellert and E. O. Wilson (eds.), *The Biophilia Hypothesis.* Washington, D.C.: Island Press, 1993.
Witman, J. P. "The Efficacy of Adventure Programming in the Development of Cooperation and Trust with Adolescents in Treatment." *Therapeutic Recreation Journal,* 1987, *21,* 22–29.
Yi, S.-L. "A Life Renewed." *National Gardening,* 1985, *8,* 19–21.

For Further Information

University-Based Web Sites

The Human-Environment Research Laboratory at the University of Illinois is a leader in research on benefits of nature contact. Its Web site contains information in a variety of interesting categories, such as "Canopy & Crime," "Girls & Greenery," "Kids & Concentration," "Neighbors & Nature," "Plants & Poverty," and "Vegetation & Violence":

Human-Environment Research Laboratory. Homepage. [http://www.herl.uiuc.edu]. 2005.

An excellent, in-depth review of the health benefits of nature contact has been produced by researchers at Deakin University, in Melbourne, in collaboration with Parks Victoria, the state parks agency, as part of that agency's Healthy Parks,

Healthy People theme. For the full 2002 report, *Healthy Parks, Healthy People: The Health Benefits of Contact with Nature in a Park Context: A Review of Current Literature,* and an associated annotated bibliography, see

Parks Victoria. "Healthy Parks Healthy People." [http://www.parkweb.vic.gov.au/1process_content.cfm?section=99&page=16]. 2002.

The University of Essex Center for Environment and Society has a research focus on human health, including the benefits of nature contact. Its Web site offers research papers on topics such as green exercise and links to other useful sites:

University of Essex, Center for Environment and Society. "Collaborative Research Programs." [http://www2.essex.ac.uk/ces/ResearchProgrammes/NewPageCollaborativeResProg.htm]. 2005.

OPENspace is a "research center for inclusive access to outdoor environments" at the Edinburgh College of Art. Its Web site includes reviews on the health benefits of access to open space and nature (with titles like "Health, Well-Being, and Open Space" focusing on such groups as ethnic minorities and teenagers):

Edinburgh College of Art, OPENspace. Homepage. [http://openspace.eca.ac.uk/index.htm]. 2005.

Purdue University's Center for the Human-Animal Bond carries out research and education on the health effects of animal contact. Its Web site provides research results and links to a number of related sites:

Purdue University School of Veterinary Medicine, Center for the Human-Animal Bond. Homepage. [http://www.vet.purdue.edu/depts/vad/cae]. 2000.

Professional Organizations

People-Plant Council [http://www.hort.vt.edu/HUMAN/PPC.html].
American Horticultural Therapy Association [http://www.ahta.org].
Delta Society (the human-animal health connection) [http://www.deltasociety.org].

Publications

Altman, I., and Wohlwill, J. F. (eds.). *Behavior and the Natural Environment.* New York: Plenum, 1983.

Caras, R. A. *A Perfect Harmony: The Intertwining Lives of Animals and Humans Throughout History.* New York: Fireside, 1996.

Fine, A. (ed.) *Handbook on Animal-Assisted Therapy: Theoretical Foundations and Guidelines for Practice.* San Diego: Academic Press, 2000.

Flagler, J., and Poincelot, R. P. *People-Plant Relationships: Setting Research Priorities.* Binghamton, N.Y.: Food Products Press, 1994.

Francis, M., Lindsey, P., and Rice, J. S. (eds.). *The Healing Dimensions of People-Plant Relations: Proceedings of a Research Symposium.* Davis: Center for Design Research, University of California Davis, 1994.

Gerlach-Spriggs, N., Kaufman, R. E., and Warner, S. B., Jr. *Restorative Gardens: The Healing Landscape.* New Haven, Conn.: Yale University Press, 1998.

Kellert, S. R., and Wilson, E. O. (eds.). *The Biophilia Hypothesis.* Washington, D.C.: Island Press, 1993.

Lewis, C. A. *Green Nature, Human Nature: The Meaning of Plants in Our Lives.* Urbana: University of Illinois Press, 1996.

Marcus, C. C., and Barnes, M. *Healing Gardens: Therapeutic Benefits and Design Recommendations.* New York: Wiley, 1999.

Relf, D. (ed.). *The Role of Horticulture in Human Well-Being and Social Development: A National Symposium, 19–21 April 1990, Arlington, Virginia.* Portland, Ore.: Timber Press, 1992.

Tyson, M. M. *The Healing Landscape: Therapeutic Outdoor Environments.* New York: McGraw-Hill, 1998.

CHAPTER TWENTY-EIGHT

CHILDREN

Maida Galvez
Joel Forman
Philip J. Landrigan

The environment in which children live today is very different from that of fifty years ago. The chemical revolution has been one major engine of environmental change. As the result of advances in chemistry, there now exist more than 80,000 synthetic chemicals, nearly all of them invented since the 1950s (U.S. Environmental Protection Agency [EPA], 1998). They include plastics, pesticides, motor fuels, building materials, antibiotics, chemotherapeutic agents, flame retardants, and synthetic hormones. Children are especially at risk of exposure to the 2,800 synthetic chemicals that are produced in quantities of 1 million pounds or more per year (EPA, 1998). These high production volume (HPV) chemicals are distributed widely in the environment—in air, food, water, and consumer products. In recent national surveys HPV synthetic chemicals have been detected and quantified in the bodies of children (Centers for Disease Control and Prevention [CDC], 2003). Only 43 percent of HPV chemicals have been tested for their potential to cause toxicity, and fewer than 20 percent for their capacity to interfere with children's development (National Academy of Sciences [NAS], 1984). This dearth of toxicological data creates a setting in which new chemicals can cause and have caused adverse effects in children (and in adults) without warning.

Population growth, rapid urbanization, and development of the macroenvironment represent a second dimension of environmental change in the past fifty years. Especially rapid evolution has occurred in the built environment—housing, roads and walkways, transportation networks, shops and markets, and parks and public spaces (Weich and others, 2001). Urban, rural, suburban, agricultural, and developing areas each have their unique environmental features, and the impacts of chemical exposures on children's health are mediated by the contextual settings of these built environments.

It is now understood that the environment on both a micro (chemical) and macro (structural) level has a profound ability to affect children's growth and development, exerting positive as well as negative influences (Briggs, 2003). Health and disease are the products of complex interactions among multiple genetic, behavioral, cultural, familial, socioeconomic, and environmental factors. The study of environmental factors and their effects on children's health is critical to understanding the etiology of a vast array of common childhood conditions from asthma to obesity, and to developing evidence-based strategies for disease prevention and health promotion.

Children's environmental health issues are important not only to parents and pediatricians but to society at large. The U.S. government's failure to require premarket testing of synthetic chemicals compels pediatricians and the American public to learn about toxicities through recognition of the unanticipated consequences of human exposure, making all inhabitants of the earth "canaries in a coal mine." Children's unknowing exposure to hundreds of new chemicals makes them the experimental subjects in a lifelong uncontrolled experiment. Children unduly bear the burden of such permanent and irreversible effects of toxic environmental exposures as decreased intelligence, birth defects, and developmental delays. This chapter introduces the field of children's environmental health with a historical account of the recognition that children are a special population, discusses general considerations in examining environmental etiologies for children's health problems, and presents case studies of specific environmental exposures, including pesticides, lead, solvents, mold, and neighborhood design. It concludes with a discussion of risk assessment and risk communication as they apply to children.

Children as a Special Population

Our understanding that children's environmental health requires special attention involves the changing patterns of disease among children, the economic burden of children's diseases, and children's particular sensitivity to environmental exposures.

Changing Patterns of Disease

Patterns of illness among children in the United States and other industrially developed nations have changed substantially in the past century (Haggerty and

Rothmann, 1975). The major diseases confronting children in developed nations today are chronic illnesses of multifactorial origin, such as asthma, which has doubled in prevalence since 1980 (Harada, 1978; "Asthma Mortality and Hospitalization Among Children and Young Adults," 1996; Mannino and others, 1998); birth defects, which remain the leading cause of infant death (MacDorman and Atkinson, 1999); developmental disorders, such as attention deficit/hyperactivity disorder and autism; and childhood leukemia and brain cancer (Gurney and others, 1996; Legler and others, 1999), which have increased in incidence since the 1970s. Collectively, these diseases are termed the *new pediatric morbidity.* The classic infectious diseases are much reduced in incidence and in developed nations (in contrast to the situation in developing nations) they are no longer the leading causes of illness and death (DiLiberti and Jackson, 1999). Infant mortality has been lowered, although not equally across U.S. society, and life expectancy increased. Evidence is increasing that toxic chemicals in the environment are important causes of disease in children. It is now hypothesized that the majority of disease in childhood is the consequence of interactions between the environment—defined broadly to include diet and lifestyle factors as well as toxic chemical exposures—and individual, genetically determined susceptibility (Olden and Wilson, 2000).

Economic Burden of Pediatric Environmental Disease

The contribution of environmental pollutants to the incidence, prevalence, mortality, and costs of disease in U.S. children is substantial. Landrigan and others (2002) examined this burden for four categories of illness—lead poisoning, asthma, cancer, and neurobehavioral disorders. They found that the costs of these environmentally related diseases in children amount to $54.9 billion annually, approximately 2.8 percent of the total annual cost of illness in the United States. These costs may be compared to the annual health care costs attributable to motor vehicle crashes ($80.6 billion) and those due to stroke ($51.5 billion) (Duke University Center for Health Policy, Law & Management, 2000). The annual estimated costs of military weapons research are $35 billion and of veterans' benefits $39 billion (Center for Defense Information, 1996). The costs of pediatric disease of environmental origin are large compared with the relatively meager amount of money spent on research related to children (Office of Science and Technology Policy, 1997). Landrigan and others concluded that diseases of toxic environmental origin among children make an important and insufficiently recognized contribution to total health care costs in the United States.

The costs of pediatric disease of environmental origin will likely become yet greater in the years ahead if children's exposures to inadequately tested chemicals are permitted to continue. Increased investment is required in tracking and surveillance

(Pew Environmental Health Commission, 2000), in basic studies of disease mechanisms, and in prevention-oriented epidemiological research (Berkowitz and others, 2001). Most important, increased investment is needed to prevent pollution.

Historical Perspective

Environmental pediatrics originated in early studies of major outbreaks of acute disease of toxic origin in children. These analyses formed the basis for the current understanding that children are uniquely vulnerable to many toxins in the environment. Among these early reports were

- A 1904 report from Queensland, Australia, describing an epidemic of lead poisoning in young children (Gibson, 1904). Clinical and epidemiological investigation traced the source of the outbreak to the ingestion of lead-based paint by children playing on verandas. This study was the first report of lead paint poisoning in children, and it led to the banning of lead-based paint in many nations.
- A study of an epidemic of leukemia in the 1940s and 1950s among young children in Hiroshima and Nagasaki who were exposed to ionizing radiation in the 1945 atomic bombings (Miller, 1956). This study and subsequent studies of fetuses exposed in utero (see, for example, Gurney and others, 1996) established that infants and fetuses are more susceptible than adults to leukemia after radiation exposure. In addition, an increased risk of microcephaly was observed among infants who were exposed to radiation in the first trimester of pregnancy during the bombings (Miller and Blot, 1972).
- A report from Minamata, Japan, in the 1960s of an epidemic of cerebral palsy, mental retardation, and convulsions among children living in a fishing village on the Inland Sea (Harada, 1978). This epidemic was traced to ingestion of fish and shellfish contaminated with methylmercury. The source of the mercury was found to be a plastics factory that had discharged metallic mercury into the sediments on the floor of Minamata Bay. The mercury was transformed by microorganisms into methylmercury, and it then bioaccumulated as it moved up the marine food chain, eventually reaching people who ate fish and shellfish. The most devastating effects were seen among children exposed in utero. Similar epidemics occurred subsequently in Guatemala (Ordonez, Carrillo, Miranda, and Gale, 1966), Iraq (Bakir and others, 1973), and New Mexico (Pierce and others, 1972).
- Studies of the epidemic of phocomelia (congenital limb malformations) that followed the ingestion of thalidomide as an antiemetic agent in early pregnancy (McBride, 1961; Taussig, 1962). More than 15,000 cases were reported worldwide.

- A report on cases of adenocarcinoma of the vagina among young women who had been exposed in utero to the synthetic estrogen diethylstilbestrol, taken in pregnancy by their mothers to prevent premature labor (Herbst, Hubby, Azizi, and Makii, 1981).

Robert W. Miller, a pediatrician who served for many years as an epidemiologist with the U.S. National Cancer Institute, deserves great recognition as the first scientist to move beyond the study of specific outbreaks of acute environmental disease in children to the realization that children are unusually sensitive to a broad range of environmental toxins. Miller stressed the key role of the *alert clinician* in identifying associations between environmental exposures and pediatric disease. Early in his career Miller was assigned by the U.S. Public Health Service to the Atomic Bomb Casualty Commission (now the Radiation Effects Research Foundation) in Hiroshima, Japan. His research there elucidated the epidemiology of leukemia in children exposed to the atomic bombings (Miller, 1956). He returned to the United States, and in the late 1960s he established the Committee on Environmental Hazards (now the Committee on Environmental Health) of the American Academy of Pediatrics, a scholarly body that has been of seminal importance for development of the discipline of environmental pediatrics.

Herbert L. Needleman is a second pediatrician who has contributed enormously to the development of environmental pediatrics. Needleman's research has centered on the study of lead neurotoxicity in children (Needleman and others, 1979, 1990). His seminal contribution was the recognition that lead can cause toxic effects at levels of exposure too low to produce clinically overt symptoms. This recognition gave rise to the now widely applied concept of *subclinical toxicity,* the idea that toxic agents such as lead produce a spectrum of effects ranging from coma, convulsions, and death at high-end exposures to silent brain injury with loss of intelligence and disruption of behavior at low-end exposures. Needleman's other great contribution was in the realm of evidence-based advocacy. When he was charged falsely by the lead industry with having fabricated his results, he demonstrated great courage in standing his ground and in allowing his data to be examined objectively by the National Institutes of Health. For his scientific contributions to the health of children as well as for his courage, Needleman was subsequently awarded the Heinz Medal for the Environment.

Three key historical milestones, events that further advanced the development of environmental pediatrics, were the publication by the National Research Council in 1993 of *Pesticides in the Diets of Infants and Children,* passage of the Food Quality Protection Act in 1996, and promulgation of a presidential Executive Order on children's health and the environment in 1997.

Report on Pesticides in the Diets of Infants and Children, 1993. An event of catalytic importance in bringing environmental threats to children's health to the attention of policymakers was the formation in 1988 of the National Research Council (NRC) Committee on Pesticides in the Diets of Infants and Children. This committee, chaired by physician Philip Landrigan, was convened at the request of the Senate Committee on Agriculture. The congressional charge to the committee was threefold:

1. To explore differences in exposure to pesticides between children and adults and the implications of those differences for risk assessment
2. To explore differences in susceptibility to pesticides between children and adults and their implications for risk assessment
3. To analyze federal laws and regulations regarding food use pesticides to determine whether those rules adequately protected the health of infants and children

The committee issued its final report in 1993 (NRC, 1993). The major conclusion was that "children are not little adults." By that phrase the committee meant that children are qualitatively different from adults both in their patterns of exposure and in their vulnerability to pesticides and other toxic chemicals (see Box 28.1). Specifically, the committee noted four fundamental differences between children and adults:

1. Children have disproportionately heavy exposures to environmental toxicants.
2. Children's metabolic pathways, especially in the first months after birth, are immature. In many instances children are less able than adults are to deal with toxic compounds.
3. Children are undergoing rapid growth and development. These developmental processes create windows of unique vulnerability in which the course of development can be disrupted permanently by environmental toxins.
4. Because children have more future years of life than do most adults, they have more time to develop chronic diseases that may be triggered by early exposures with long latency periods.

Box 28.1. The Unique Susceptibility of Children

Children are uniquely vulnerable to environmental toxins. Their heightened susceptibility stems from several sources. Children have greater exposures to environmental toxins than adults do (NRC, 1993). Children drink more water, eat more food, and breathe more air per kilogram of body weight than adults do. For example, in the first six months of life infants consume seven times as much water (in total) per kilogram as do average adults. Children aged one through five years eat three to four times more food per kilogram than do adults. Furthermore, children have unique food preferences. For example, the average one-year-old drinks twenty-one times more apple juice and eleven times more grape juice and eats two to seven times more grapes, bananas, pears, carrots, and broccoli than does the average adult (Wiles and Campbell, 1993). The air intake of a resting infant is twice that of an adult. These patterns of increased consumption reflect the rapid metabolism of children as well as their need to fuel growth and development.

The implication for health is that children have substantially greater exposure per kilogram to any toxic materials that are present in water, food, or air. Two additional characteristics of children further magnify their exposures to toxins in the environment: they frequently put their hands in their mouths, which increases their ingestion of any toxins in dust or soil, and they play close to the ground, which increases their exposure to toxins in dust, soil, and carpets as well as to toxins that form low-lying layers in the air, as certain pesticide vapors do.

The metabolic pathways of children, especially in the first months after birth, are immature compared with those of adults (Spielberg, 1992). As a consequence of this biochemical immaturity, the ability of a child to detoxify and excrete certain toxins is different from that of an adult. In some instances children are actually better able than adults to deal with environmental toxins. More commonly, however, they are less able than adults to deal with toxic chemicals and thus are more vulnerable to them (NRC, 1993).

Children undergo rapid growth and development, and their delicate developmental processes are easily disrupted (NRC, 1993). Many organ systems in young children, such as the nervous, reproductive, and immune systems, undergo very rapid growth, development, and differentiation during the first months and years of life. During this period, structures are developed and vital connections are established. These developmental processes create windows of great vulnerability to environmental toxicants, in which even minute exposures can produce devastating results. The nervous system, for example, is not well able to repair any structural damage that is caused by environmental toxins. If cells in the developing brain are destroyed by chemicals such as lead, mercury, or solvents or if formation of vital connections between nerve cells is blocked, then there is a high risk that the resulting neurobehavioral dysfunction will be permanent and irreversible. The consequences can be loss of intelligence and alteration of normal behavior (Eriksson and others, 2001). Similar considerations pertain in the reproductive, immune, endocrine, and cardiovascular systems.

The NRC committee also concluded that the federal laws and regulations governing the use of agricultural pesticides were not sufficiently strict to protect the health of children. The committee found that these laws and regulations were targeted toward protecting the health of healthy adults and accounted for neither the unique exposures nor the special susceptibilities of children. The committee recommended that federal policies for regulating agricultural pesticides be revamped fundamentally. Specific recommendations included the following:

- Collect better data on children's exposure to pesticides.
- Improve toxicological testing of pesticides to include assessments of developmental toxicity.
- Perform toxicological studies that examine the long-term and delayed effects of early exposures to pesticides.
- Examine the possible interactive effects among multiple pesticides, especially those that act through similar mechanisms of action.
- Protect the health of children by imposing an extra margin of safety in setting standards for pesticides when data on children's unique exposures or special susceptibilities to a particular pesticide are lacking or when the data show that children are uniquely susceptible to that pesticide.

Food Quality Protection Act, 1996. In 1996, three years after release of the NRC report *Pesticides in the Diets of Infants and Children*, the U.S. Congress, by unanimous vote of both Houses, passed the Food Quality Protection Act (FQPA), the major federal legislation governing the use of pesticides in agriculture. The FQPA incorporates all the major recommendations of the NRC committee. It requires that pesticide standards be based primarily on health considerations and that standards be set at levels that protect the health of infants and children. It requires that an extra margin of safety be incorporated into pesticide risk assessment when data show that a particular pesticide is especially toxic to infants and children or when data on the toxicity to infants and children are lacking. It requires that interactive effects among pesticides be considered. Finally, the FQPA requires that pesticides be assessed systematically for possible endocrine-disrupting effects.

Passage of the FQPA was a watershed event for children's environmental health. As the first federal environmental statute to call explicitly for protecting children's health against environmental hazards, it marked a paradigm shift in federal policy. The consequences of the FQPA have extended far beyond the regulation of agricultural pesticides.

Executive Order on Children's Health and the Environment, 1997. In April 1997, President Clinton and Vice President Gore signed the Executive Order on Children's Environmental Health and Safety. This order declared that protection of children's environmental health would be a high priority of that administration.

It established a cabinet-level oversight committee on children's environmental health, cochaired by the administrator of the U.S. Environmental Protection Agency (EPA) and the secretary of the U.S. Department of Health and Human Services. This committee was given broad responsibility to review the programs of all cabinet agencies to ensure that they were protective of children's health. Never previously had children's environmental health enjoyed such a high profile within the federal government. Consequences of the work of this cabinet-level committee include the establishment of a national network of *children's environmental health and disease prevention research centers* and the launching of the National Children's Study; both of these developments are discussed later in this chapter.

As a consequence of these advances, environmental pediatrics has emerged as a new field of research and practice and has systematically begun to address questions about the role of environmental factors in the etiology of a diverse range of childhood illnesses. Since the late 1990s, children's environmental health has become an increasingly important and visible component of pediatric practice. The American Academy of Pediatrics (AAP) published the *Handbook of Pediatric Environmental Health* in 1999 (and a second edition five years later), a resource commonly referred to as the "green book." National conferences have been held on the impact of environmental toxins on the health of children, and journals have devoted entire issues to topics in children's environmental health (Weiss and Landrigan, 2000). The national network of children's environmental health research centers and a parallel network of clinically oriented *pediatric environmental health specialty units* have been established in the United States and abroad. As the field of environmental pediatrics grows as a specialty so does the body of research by leading scientists and clinicians who seek to further our understanding of the impact of environmental exposures on the growth and development of children.

Case Studies in Environmental Pediatrics

Clinicians who evaluate patients need to consider the possibility of environmental contributions to symptoms and disease (as described in Chapter Thirty-Five). This is as true for children as it is for adults. A high index of suspicion is critical to making a correct diagnosis. This suspicion will guide environmental screening questions when taking a history. Integral to an environmental history is obtaining information about current and past exposures, potential sources of toxic exposures, exposure settings, and potential routes of exposures (Figures 28.1 and 28.2). Particular attention must be paid to those factors unique to the age and developmental stage of the child. These principles are illustrated

FIGURE 28.1. A CHILDREN'S PLAYGROUND LOCATED NEAR A SOURCE OF TOXIC EMISSIONS.

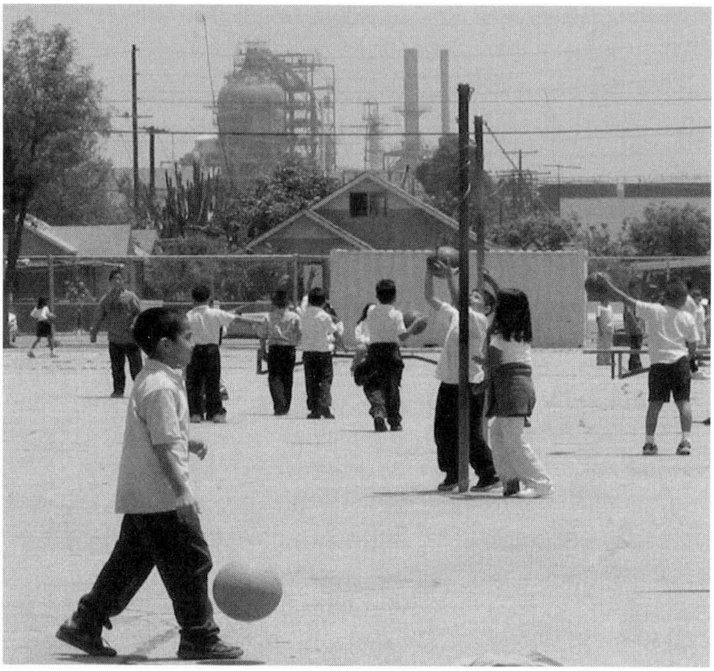

Source: Photo by Andrea Hricko; used with permission.

in the case studies that follow and that examine typical routes of exposure and exposure settings.

Routes of Exposure

When the possibility of environmental etiology is under diagnostic consideration, it is important to determine whether a plausible pathway of exposure exists. Exposure pathways vary by chemical and by stage of life. As described in Chapter Two, the major routes for adults are inhalation, ingestion, and skin absorption, with parenteral (intravenous and intramuscular) routes sometimes being important. For children, it is important also to consider transplacental transfer and breast milk (see Box 28.2). At times multiple pathways may be involved—for example, both skin absorption and inhalation, as in the case of metallic mercury, to which children may be exposed both by skin contact and by inhalation of vapors.

FIGURE 28.2. CHILDREN BATHING IN A DRUM THAT ONCE HELD A TOXIC CHEMICAL.

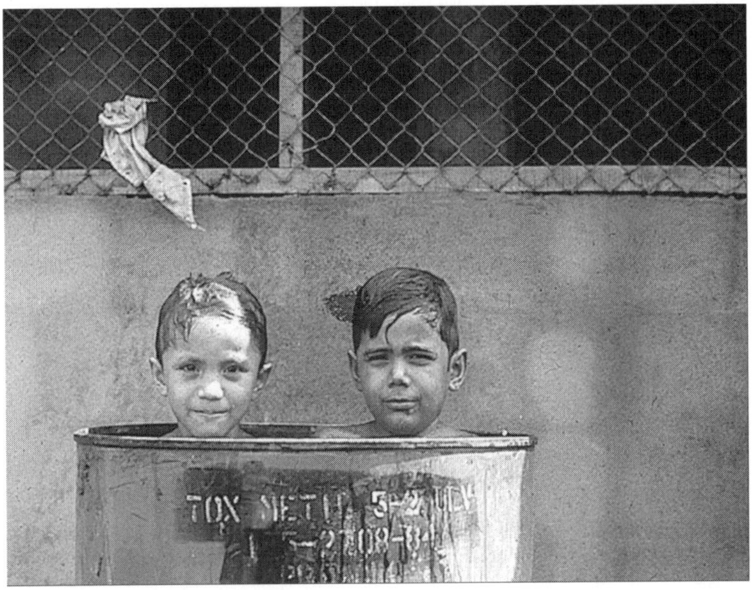

Source: Photo by Don Cole; used with permission.

Box 28.2. The Dilemma of Breast Feeding

Human milk is without question the best source of nutrition for human infants. Breast milk contains the optimal balance of fats, carbohydrates, and proteins for developing babies, and it provides a range of benefits for growth, immunity, and development (Institute of Medicine, 1991). Breast milk contains immune factors that help infants fight infections (Oddy, 2001), and it contains growth factors that appear to influence brain development and increase resistance to chronic diseases such as asthma, allergies, and diabetes. Breastfeeding builds a bond between a mother and her child, and this bond enhances health and well-being across the generations. For these reasons, breast feeding is recommended by the American Academy of Pediatrics for a minimum of six months.

Unfortunately, breast milk is not pristine. Contamination of human milk is widespread, the result of decades of inadequately controlled pollution of the environment by toxic chemicals. Polychlorinated biphenyls (PCBs), dichlorodiphenyltrichloroethane (DDT) and its metabolites, dioxins, dibenzofurans, polybrominated diphenyl ethers (PBDEs), and heavy metals are among the toxic chemicals most often found in breast milk (Sonawane, 1995; Hooper and McDonald, 2000). These compounds are encountered to varying extents among women in developed as well as developing nations. Some of the highest levels of contamination are seen among women in agricultural areas of the developing world that are extensively treated with pesticides (Hooper and others, 1999) and among women in remote areas. An example of the latter are the Canadian Inuit, who eat a diet rich in seal, whale, and other species high on the marine food chain that accumulate heavy burdens of persistent organic pollutants (POPs) (Dewailly and others, 1993).

The finding of toxic chemicals in breast milk raises a series of important issues for pediatric practice, for the practice of public health, and for the environmental health research community. It also illuminates gaps in current knowledge, including insufficient information on the nature and levels of contaminants in breast milk, lack of consistent protocols for collecting and analyzing breast milk samples, lack of toxicokinetic data, and lack of data on children's health outcomes following exposure to chemicals in breast milk. These gaps impede risk assessment and make it difficult to formulate evidence-based health guidance.

In the clinical setting mothers often pose the question of potential harms from breast feeding. Yet the longitudinal studies of babies who consumed breast milk that are needed to answer this question are lacking. Though there are tests available to measure the levels of chemical contaminants such as dioxins in breast milk, there are no standard reference values that define a "safe" level of exposure. In the absence of such standards the information that results from breast milk testing is, except in extreme cases, difficult to interpret and of little use clinically.

The American Academy of Pediatrics does not recommend that mothers routinely have their breast milk tested for environmental contaminants. The benefits of human milk far outweigh the risks, so women should not stop breast feeding because of concerns about environmental contamination, unless specifically advised to do so by a pediatrician or pediatric environmental specialist. The take-home message is that "breast is best" in terms of infant feedings, but large-scale, prospective studies are still needed to clarify the health effects of environmental contaminants commonly found in breast milk.

In keeping with the principles of developmental toxicology, the diagnostic evaluation should identify specific behaviors unique to a child's age that may place him or her at increased risk. The following cases illustrate routes of exposure and highlight the unique susceptibility of children to environmental exposures in the context of everyday experiences.

Exposure Through Inhalation: Case Study on Air Pollutants. In a New York inner-city neighborhood, community-based organizations, environmental justice coalitions, parents' associations, community board members, and schools came together to oppose the reopening of a depot for diesel-powered buses across the street from a public elementary school and adjacent to low-income housing projects (Northridge and others, 1999; West Harlem Environmental Action, 2005). The primary concern was the potential health effects, particularly asthma, related to diesel exhaust. This neighborhood has the highest rates of asthma citywide.

Diesel exhaust is recognized to be a serious health hazard (as discussed in Chapters Fourteen and Seventeen). It is a known respiratory irritant and has been shown to exacerbate asthma in susceptible individuals. It contains many toxic chemicals, and two pose especially critical risks to human health. The first, oxides of nitrogen (NO_x), is a major contributor to ground-level ozone. These oxides are corrosive to lung tissue and act as powerful respiratory irritants, worsening asthma and causing bronchitis. The second, particulate matter, can also be inhaled and can lodge deep in the lungs. The particulates contain abundant polycyclic aromatic hydrocarbons (PAHs), a class of chemicals recognized by the Environmental Protection Agency as human carcinogens.

Children are particularly sensitive to NO_x and airborne particulate matter in diesel exhaust for several reasons. First, children breathe more rapidly than adults, allowing for the inhalation of more pollutants per kilogram of body weight. Children also spend more time playing outdoors and close to the ground, increasing the likelihood of being exposed to outdoor air pollutants. Also, children have an entire lifetime over which to develop chronic illnesses related to environmental exposures incurred early on.

Grassroots activism has raised awareness of the disproportionate siting of bus depots in predominantly low-income, minority communities as an environmental justice issue (see Chapter Eight). Despite these efforts the groups were unable to defeat the opening of the bus depot in 2003. Still, concessions were made, including the addition of a roof on the depot building. Activists have not backed down, however, and continue to press for conversion of the city's bus fleet to ultra low sulfur diesel fuel or compressed natural gas. They are also advocating for enforcement of anti-idling laws, which prohibit buses from running their engines while standing in the city streets.

Exposure Through Ingestion: Case Study on Pesticides in Food and Water. A program in the Yakima and Columbia river valleys in Washington State is reaching out to adolescent and adult female migrant and seasonal farmworkers at risk for health effects from pesticide exposure. By definition, migrant workers move from one agricultural community to another, as dictated by the crops that are in season. For these workers and their children the risk of pesticide exposure is heightened by the indoor and outdoor contamination of their homes through spraying, take-home exposures, and soil and water contamination. This combination of exposures from many routes may result in widespread contamination of areas where children eat, sleep, and play. Both the water supply and food products, including locally grown produce, may also be affected.

Ingestion of contaminated food products is the predominant source of exposure to pesticides for the general population. In a study by Curl, Fenske, and Elgethun (2003), children who consumed foods that were at least 75 percent organic were likely to have significantly lower levels of pesticides detected in their urine than were children who ate a diet of nonorganic food products. The authors conclude that "consumption of organic fruits, vegetables and juices can reduce children's exposure levels from above to below the U.S. Environmental Protection Agency's current guidelines, thereby shifting exposures from a range of uncertain risk to a range of negligible risk. Consumption of organic produce appears to provide a relatively simple way for parents to reduce their children's exposure to organophosphate pesticides" (p. 382).

Even though there are known benefits to pesticide use, such as increased crop yield and prevention of insect- and rodent-borne diseases, the benefits must be tempered by consideration of potential risks (see Chapter Twenty). Depending on the pesticide of concern, a variety of health effects have been detected. Multiple organ systems may be involved, including the lungs, kidneys, digestive tract, immune system, and central nervous system. In addition, the EPA considers several organophosphate pesticides to be probable carcinogens. Epidemiological studies support a relationship between pesticide exposure and subsequent development of brain cancer, non-Hodgkin's lymphoma, and leukemia (Zahm and Ward, 1998). In examining the effects of exposures to pesticides during pregnancy, studies have suggested an association with limb reduction defects (Engel, O'Meara, and Schwartz, 2000); cryptorchidism, or undescended testes (Weidner, Moller, Jensen, and Skakkebaek, 1998); neural tube defects (Shaw and others, 1999); heart problems (Loffredo, Silbergeld, Ferencz, and Zhang, 2001); and impaired fetal growth (Longnecker, Klebanoff, Zhou, and Brock, 2001).

To remove pesticide residues from produce, parents are advised to rinse fresh produce thoroughly with water before it is cooked or eaten. Peeling reduces the levels of pesticides that may be on the surface, though some residues remain because they have been absorbed into the food. Eating a diet with many different fruits, vegetables, and grains is a healthy practice that may also prevent overexposure to a single pesticide residue found in a particular crop. The most effective method to reduce intake is consumption of certified organic produce grown with minimal or no synthetic chemicals.

For seasonal and migrant workers, pesticide exposures from the food supply are compounded by occupational exposures. Many farmworkers are not aware of the risks associated with pesticide exposure or have not been educated about preventive measures that can reduce negative health impacts of such exposure. Some workers choose not to practice behaviors that could minimize negative health effects. A cooperative effort of the National Catholic Rural Life Conference (NCRLC), organizations engaged in pesticide education or providing services to migrants, Radio Cadena and other Hispanic media, the Diocese of Yakima, and four Catholic parishes is helping adolescent and adult female migrant and seasonal farmworkers reduce the negative health impacts of agricultural pesticides. As part of this project the parishes involved have developed, implemented, and are now evaluating educational sessions to reduce the health impacts of agricultural pesticides and have created an educational series of radio minidramas, news pieces, and public service announcements. This is one example of how a religious group has identified a need in the community and mobilized resources to provide pesticide safety and sanitation education. Church-based initiatives such as this one provide a unique opportunity to reach many members of a community (see Chapter Nine).

Exposure Through the Skin: Case Study on DEET. The members of a family living in the United States are returning to their native country in sub-Saharan Africa for a four-week vacation and are discussing concerns about malaria with their family pediatrician. The parents are bringing along on the trip their three children: a fifteen-month-old infant son, a four-year-old son, and a nine-year-old daughter. They plan to use malaria prophylaxis in addition to insecticide-treated mosquito netting at night. However, they have also seen a number of insect repellants available in the local pharmacy. Today they are bringing in a specific repellant for the pediatrician's review; they want to know if it is approved for use in children. The active ingredient is DEET (N,N-diethyl-m-toluamide, also known as N,N-diethyl-3-methylbenzamide), at a concentration of 10 percent.

The pediatrician advises the family that DEET is a widely used product that repels a variety of insects including mosquitoes and ticks. Concentrations range from 10 to 100 percent, but only concentrations below 30 percent are recommended for children. The main route of DEET exposure is dermal, and very high exposures may occur with frequent reapplication, as has been reported with combination sunscreens and insect repellants. For this reason combination sunscreens and repellants are not recommended. The pediatrician also recommends that the children wear long-sleeved clothing that covers their extremities as a protective measure. DEET may then be applied to their clothing rather than directly on the skin. Otherwise, DEET should be applied only once daily, in sparse amounts, to exposed areas of the skin. Strict avoidance of the child's face and hands is necessary to prevent accidental ingestion through hand-to-mouth behaviors.

Acute DEET toxicity is rare but may include skin or eye irritation and, following high-dose exposures, central nervous system disorders such as seizures (Lipscomb, Kramer, and Leikin, 1992) and encephalopathy (Briassoulis, Narlioglou, and Hatzis, 2001). Animal studies of acute and chronic high-dose exposure suggest potential effects on the liver, kidney, and brain.

Exposure in Utero: Case Study on Polychlorinated Biphenyls. Polychlorinated biphenyls (PCBs) are a family of synthetic chlorinated hydrocarbon compounds that were used widely from the 1930s until the 1970s as coolants, lubricants, and insulators in transformers, electrical equipment, capacitors, insulation, the fluorescent lighting of the time, and air conditioners. They were also used as solvents in carbonless carbon paper, plastics, and paints. They resist burning and are difficult to break down, traits that made them ideal for these uses. In 1977, use of PCBs was banned because of concerns about their persistence in the environment and their effects on human health.

Much was learned about the devastating effects of high-dose PCB exposure in utero from a large-scale community outbreak that occurred in Kyushu province, Japan, in 1968 (Masuda, 1985). The source of the contamination was PCBs that had leaked from heat exchangers to contaminate rice oil. Rice oil is widely used for cooking in that area, and women who consumed food cooked with the contaminated oil accumulated PCBs in their fatty tissue. When these women subsequently became pregnant, the lipophilic PCBs were able to cross the placenta, thus exposing babies in utero. PCBs also concentrated in breast milk. Approximately 1,000 babies were affected. Infants born to the PCB-poisoned mothers had a constellation of symptoms, including mental retardation, developmental delays, eye and skin defects, darkening of the skin, and liver disease. These health effects came to be known as *Yusho disease* (Taylor, Lawrence, Hwang, and Paulson, 1984).

Lower-dose exposure to PCBs in the prenatal period, at levels too low to produce obvious symptoms, has also been shown to have adverse effects on central nervous function, including decreased intelligence, memory, and attention span (Tilson, Jacobson, and Rogan, 1990; Yu, Hsu, Gladen, and Rogan, 1991). These effects appear permanent and irreversible. Quite strikingly, similar effects have not been seen following exposure to PCBs during infancy and childhood. This difference in susceptibility suggests a special window of vulnerability for the developing brain in utero.

Though levels of PCBs can be measured accurately in blood and in breast milk, there are no standard reference values that define a "normal" level of exposure. All Americans have some level of PCBs in their bodies as a result of environmental contamination decades ago, but the link between low-level adult exposure to PCBs and health effects is not clear. For that reason, results of PCB testing are difficult to interpret and of little use clinically.

There is no known treatment to reduce the levels of PCBs in the body. The mainstay of therapy is to minimize exposure to PCBs; the most important action is to avoid eating fish caught from PCB-contaminated waters. Adherence to fish consumption advisories is particularly critical for pregnant women and women who hope to become pregnant in the future. State health departments issue advisories that list local areas considered unsafe for fishing due to PCB contamination.

Exposure Settings

Routes of exposure are often very much tied to a particular exposure setting. Exposure settings for children include the home, day-care centers, schools, public areas, and neighborhoods. The nature of the exposure setting may either enhance or mitigate the impact of the exposure, depending on the amount of time the child spends there, the condition of the area, and the degree of social control. Often all areas in which a child spends time must be explored in determining the exact source of an exposure. The following cases highlight the interactions between an exposure setting and a specific contaminant.

Home Exposure: Case Study on Lead. On routine blood testing a two-year-old girl was found to have a blood lead level of 22 micrograms per deciliter ($\mu g/dL$). A prior lead level obtained one year earlier was 8 $\mu g/dL$. She is currently healthy though she has also been diagnosed with a mild iron deficiency anemia. According to her parents she has never been diagnosed with developmental delays, and her behavior has not been out of the range of normal for a typical two-year-old. The child's seven-year-old sister was also tested and found to have a lead level of 2 $\mu g/dL$. The Centers for Disease Control and Prevention's current level of concern is 10 $\mu g/dL$. Blood lead levels greater than 10 $\mu g/dL$, but even as low as 5 $\mu g/dL$, have been associated with behavioral problems and decreased intelligence. Children with blood lead levels above 20$\mu g/dL$ may exhibit gastrointestinal symptoms such as poor appetite, nausea, vomiting, abdominal pain, and constipation. These children may have difficulty with learning and school performance and also behavioral problems such as hyperactivity. Severe lead poisoning, with blood lead levels above 60 $\mu g/dL$, may be associated with neurological symptoms such as changes in mental status, difficulty walking, seizures, and coma.

The two-year-old girl's pediatrician elicited an environmental history, adapted from the AAP green book, to determine whether there were any potential sources of exposure in the home (Etzel and Balk, 2003). Here are the key questions asked in that history; each question is followed by the parents' answer in italics:

- What is the age and condition of the home? U.S. homes built pre-1978 may contain leaded paint. *We live in a two-bedroom apartment in a building that was built in the early 1900s. We have lived there for about ten years.*
- Are the windowsills peeling? Do the window wells contain solid material? Friction areas such as windows and door jambs can produce lead-containing dust and paint chips, which young children may then ingest through hand-to-mouth behaviors. *The window wells are solid but the windowsills have been peeling for many years now. We have complained to our landlord, but he has never addressed the problem.*
- Are you renovating a room or planning to? Renovations in older homes, without proper precautions for lead-based paint hazards, can be a potential source of exposure to pregnant women and children. *The rooms have not been renovated while we have been living here.*
- Have there been any recent renovations in common areas of your building or in your neighborhood? Renovations in close proximity to the home, such as a neighbor's home, or in common areas of a building, such as the fire escape or basement, may also generate leaded dust and paint chips. *No renovations that we are aware of.*
- Does your neighborhood have any local industries that may be potential sources of lead exposure? *Our neighborhood is predominantly residential.*
- Do you use tap water? Some older homes have leaded pipes, which may then contaminate the water supply. *We drink city tap water, which is safe to drink according to the department of health.*
- Do you use imported herbal remedies? Some traditional and herbal remedies contain lead; this is especially important in communities with new immigrants. *We don't use any herbal remedies.*
- What do you and your spouse do for a living? Are there any potential occupational take-home exposures? *My husband works in a restaurant as a manager, and I am a full-time mom.*
- Do you work at home with substances that may be hazardous? *No hobbies or projects at home.*
- Do you use any imported spices or products that may contain lead? *None.*
- Do you use any traditional ceramic pottery or other imported dishware where lead may be found in the glaze? *No.*
- Have you recently traveled outside the country, as there are a variety of lead exposures to consider in foreign settings and in fact leaded gasoline is still used in many parts of the world? *No travel outside of the U.S.*

- Does your child exhibit frequent hand-to-mouth behaviors? Has she been observed directly ingesting paint chips? *She constantly has her hands in her mouth though we have never witnessed her ingesting paint chips.*

As part of the investigation, the local department of health (DOH) conducted an evaluation to identify any lead hazards in the home. This evaluation included an inventory of the child's daily activities, including time spent outside the home. X-ray fluorescence (XRF) identified the presence of leaded paint throughout the apartment and multiple areas of chipped peeling paint, particularly around the door frames and windows. This was a clear violation of the city's local lead laws. No other sources of lead were found. Local lead laws require landlords in this city to conduct annual visits to homes with children aged six years old and under. Lead hazards must be identified and appropriately abated by a certified lead abatement contractor within a specified time period. In this case the family was relocated while abatement was conducted. Lead dust swipe sampling was conducted after the renovations had been completed and prior to the family's return to the apartment. Blood lead levels were followed every three months for the two-year-old girl and her lead levels subsequently declined to below 10 μg/dL without the need for chelation therapy. The child was placed on supplemental iron for iron deficiency anemia, and her parents were advised to ensure that her diet was rich in iron and calcium.

Day-Care Exposure: Case Study on Solvents. Several families raised concerns to the Environmental Protection Agency and the local DOH about work going on in close proximity to a suburban day-care center, sited in a former industrial area. A hazardous material team had been seen conducting testing of outdoor areas within fifty yards of the center. The day-care center had been in operation for five years and served about 150 children aged six weeks to five years old. The building had fourteen rooms, and there was an outside play area.

Investigation by the EPA and local DOH revealed that a steel company had been in operation for thirty years on a site adjacent to the site where the day-care center was now located. The steel company site had been designated an EPA Superfund hazardous waste site. Degreasers had been used, including tetrachloroethylene (PERC), trichloroethylene, and trichloroethane. Sludge from the degreasing equipment was stored in drums. The steel company had been cited in the past for improper spill control, and ensuing investigations revealed elevated levels of the degreasers at depths down to forty feet below the ground surface. Levels of these chemicals were also found in groundwater samples collected from monitoring wells.

Due to concerns that exposures from the Superfund site might pose a problem to nearby facilities, including the day-care center, environmental testing was conducted for PERC, the chemical being found at the highest levels. Other volatile organic compounds (VOCs) were also measured. Air samples were collected by means of passive organic vapor sampling devices for twenty-four-hour periods on three separate occasions. The results for PERC in the day-care center ranged from 46 to 260 micrograms per cubic meter ($\mu g/m^3$). The New York State Department of Health recommends that the air level of PERC in a residential community not exceed 100 $\mu g/m^3$. These levels are set to protect the health of healthy adults and do not take into consideration vulnerable populations such as young children. Repeat testing conducted after improvements to the day-care center's ventilation system revealed levels of 7.0 to 20.7 $\mu g/m^3$. Families with children attending the day-care center were notified about the elevated levels of PERC found there. A series of community forums was convened, and representatives from the EPA, the local DOH, the regional pediatric environmental health specialty unit, and the department of pediatrics at a nearby community hospital were present in order to help explain the potential health impacts form these exposures.

According to the Agency for Toxic Substances and Disease Registry (ATSDR, 2004), tetrachloroethylene (also known as perchloroethylene [PCE, or PERC] and tetrachloroethene) is a synthetic chemical widely used for fabric dry cleaning and metal degreasing. At room temperature it is nonflammable and liquid in form. It evaporates easily into the air and has a sharp, sweet odor. Most people can smell tetrachloroethylene when it is present in air at a level of 30,000 $\mu g/m^3$ or more, although some people can detect it at even lower levels. High concentrations of tetrachloroethylene can cause dizziness, headache, sleepiness, confusion, nausea, difficulty in speaking and walking, unconsciousness, and death. Skin irritation may result from repeated or extended skin contact. These symptoms occur almost entirely in work environments when people have been accidentally exposed to high concentrations. The health effects of breathing air or drinking water with low levels of tetrachloroethylene are not known. Results of animal studies, conducted with amounts much higher than those that most people are exposed to, show that tetrachloroethylene can cause liver and kidney damage.

Given the levels found at the day-care center and information from prior studies assessing levels of exposure in children living adjacent to dry-cleaning stores, the consensus was that the children who had been at the center were not at significant risk for long-term health effects related to their exposures. However, given the fact that the levels were elevated above background levels and that children may in fact be particularly vulnerable to exposures incurred early in life, due to their rapid growth and ongoing development, in general it was felt to be prudent to minimize these exposures. The day-care center voluntarily closed upon receiving the results of the elevated PERC levels. The children remained asymptomatic. Although blood or urine testing is available for some of these exposures, it was not recommended for these families as there are no standardized reference values for "normal" levels of exposure, particularly for children. Further studies are needed to assess the health effects of chronic, low-level PERC exposures for children.

School Exposure: Case Study on Mold. One October a school nurse at a public elementary school noted an increased frequency of asthma exacerbations in fourth-grade students from one particular homeroom. In an effort to identify potential triggers the nurse surveyed the room. There were no carpets or pets present in the classroom, and it had not undergone any recent renovations. The classroom was used for history and English classes, and no arts and crafts or scientific experiments were conducted there. Upon entering the room the nurse noted a musty odor. The ceiling was found to have an area of water damage, with a small area of mold visible on the ceiling. The principal of the school was notified. In order to obtain further information about potential health effects related to mold, the local department of health was consulted, in addition to the regional pediatric environmental health specialty unit. The school also elected to have an industrial hygienist survey the school to make recommendations for mold abatement.

Health effects from mold range from irritant effects such as eye, ear, nose, and throat irritations to allergy or asthma symptoms such as sneezing, coughing, and wheezing. (See Chapter Twenty-Two for further information.) It is not known whether mold exposure causes asthma. For susceptible individuals it may exacerbate asthmatic conditions. The relationship between mold exposure and chronic symptoms such as fatigue is unclear. Some molds, such as *Stachybotrus,* produce toxins, but it is not known whether exposure to these toxins causes chronic health effects. If a family has a strong family history of atopy (allergy symptoms), it is possible that the children are predisposed to allergies and that the subsequent exposure to mold is exacerbating their symptoms. In general the best test to determine sensitivity is to observe whether the symptoms improve when the exposure is removed. Do the child's symptoms improve when the child is out of the school for a significant period of time, such as during vacations? If so, this is the best evidence that symptoms are being aggravated by mold exposure. Usually, mold-related symptoms resolve once exposure has been removed.

Determining the source of the moisture is of utmost importance in preventing any further mold growth. Ideally, humidity in schools should be kept between 30 and 50 percent, and any water leaks should be addressed immediately. It is recommended that a certified industrial hygienist evaluate the area of concern to make recommendations about further cleanup. Extensive areas of mold (more than 100 square feet) should be addressed by certified contractors, as outlined in the Environmental Protection Agency's "Mold in Schools" fact sheet (EPA, Indoor Environments Division, 2004).

In this case, the hygienist, after surveying the affected classroom and other classrooms, determined the etiology to be an isolated pipe leak affecting this classroom alone. Children were removed from the classroom for the duration of the abatement. Parents were informed of the proceedings from the start of the investigation, were provided with information about the health effects of mold, and were given the opportunity to discuss their concerns with health professionals through the local DOH and the regional pediatric environmental health specialty unit. Parents were also referred to the Healthy Schools Network (HSN) for further information. Founded in 1995, HSN is a national not-for-profit organization centered on children's environmental health and dedicated to assuring every child and school employee an environmentally safe and healthy school through research, information, referral, and advocacy.

For further assistance, the IAQ (Indoor Air Quality) Design Tools for Schools (EPA, 2005) provide guidance and links to other information resources for those involved in the design of new schools and the repair, renovation, and maintenance of existing school facilities. Though the primary focus is on indoor air quality, the IAQ tools Web site also promotes energy efficiency, day lighting, materials efficiency, and safety.

Play Area Exposure: Case Study on Arsenic. A news release alerted the public to the potential hazards of arsenic-treated wood, used commonly since the 1930s in decks, in playground equipment, and for other outdoor uses. Upon hearing the news, families in a suburban California community became concerned about the playground equipment in the nearby state park. The playground, refurbished two years previously, was widely used by the community year round. One family identified the manufacturer of the playground equipment and found that the lumber did in fact consist of wood treated with chromated copper arsenic (CCA). This preservative is used to protect wood against rot and fungus.

A child's hand-to-mouth behavior is the major source of exposure to arsenic from CCA-treated play sets. Children aged six and younger frequently exhibit hand-to-mouth behaviors, which allow the direct ingestion of arsenic. The risk of exposure to arsenic is greatest when the wood is in poor condition. As this playground set was only two years old, it was in fairly good condition, though there were a few areas of obvious wear. The playground surface was made from recycled rubber, which diminished potential exposures from arsenic leaching into soil and subsequent hand-to-mouth ingestion through this pathway.

Although the predominant sources of exposure to arsenic are food, soil, and water (especially the groundwater of certain areas, as described in Chapter Thirteen), arsenic exposure via playgrounds may contribute to a child's daily level of exposure. Concerns have been raised about arsenic due to its association with an increased risk of developing lung or bladder cancer over a child's lifetime (ATSDR, 2003). Epidemiological studies from Taiwan have shown an increased incidence of lung and bladder cancer from elevated levels of arsenic in the drinking water (Chiou and others, 1995, 2001). Due to these potential health effects, the manufacturers of CCA treated products reached a voluntary agreement with the EPA to end the manufacture of CCA-treated wood for most consumer applications as of December 2003. However, according to the EPA, some CCA-treated wood may still have been stocked on store shelves through mid-2004.

To minimize exposure to arsenic-treated wood, diligent maintenance of playground equipment is warranted to prevent wear and tear and the subsequent leaching of arsenic. One method of upkeep is routine annual staining of the wood with a polyurethane stain to prevent deterioration. Alternatively, one can choose wood alternatives that do not require pretreatment, such as cedar or redwood. Frequent hand washing is recommended, particularly after outdoor play, in order to decrease potential for direct ingestion.

In this case, local parents spearheaded an effort to replace the CCA-treated equipment with a cedar play set. In the meantime the local parks department performed regular upkeep and maintenance of the equipment.

Exposure Through Urban and Suburban Neighborhood Design: Childhood Obesity. Obesity is a global problem. The World Health Organization (2002) has declared overweight to be one of the top ten health risks in the world and one of the top five in developed nations. Studies designed to assess the impact of environmental determinants of overweight are now exploring how neighborhood design (urban, suburban, or rural) influences diet and physical activity levels and the subsequent prevalence of childhood obesity.

Many of the structural features of the urban built environment—its enormous size, its large and densely clustered population, its social institutions, its psychosocial stressors, its economy, its rapid pace, its violence, the configuration of its streets, parks, schools, and play spaces—affect children's health, growth, and development. The adverse effects of the urban environment are especially magnified in low-income, predominantly minority communities where crowded streets, lack of outdoor play spaces, limited access to fresh and healthy food, and substandard housing all contribute to substantial and well-documented disparities in child health (Jackson, 2003; also see Chapter Sixteen in this volume).

In suburban and rural communities, environmental factors contribute to childhood overweight and obesity in a unique way. As cities rapidly encroach upon neighboring areas, the phenomenon of *urban sprawl* is becoming common. Urban sprawl is characterized by low-density land use and poor integration of residential areas with public amenities. In the United States and other developed countries, people are relying more and more on cars to get from place to place instead of walking or taking public transportation. Too many suburban towns have no sidewalks and no safe bicycle paths (Frumkin, Frank, and Jackson, 2004). Neighborhood design is one factor promoting this method of transportation, as residential areas are segregated from stores, schools, and other resources.

The impression is widespread that obesity is solely a problem of the individual. Although it is true that individual choice is an important factor in the genesis of obesity, it is also true, especially in the case of childhood obesity, that environmental factors in the home, school, and neighborhood that promote poor dietary habits and sedentary lifestyles are important. Obesity is a problem not only of the individual but also of neighborhoods, schools, modes of transportation, local food availability, food advertising practices, and government policies. Further exploration of the impact of the environment on everyday behaviors is critical to understanding the current trend of rising obesity.

Environmental risk factors that may influence everyday behaviors and risk of obesity include a *food environment* that poses increased exposure to high-calorie fast foods, "junk" foods, and refined sugars (see Box 21.9). Low-income families must often depend on smaller stores that have a limited selection of fresh foods, often at relatively higher cost. The presence of a supermarket within a census tract is associated with a 32 percent increase in fruit and vegetable intake compared to the average intake in neighborhoods without supermarkets (Morland, Wing, and Diez Roux, 2002). Supermarkets have twice the amount of healthy foods that neighborhood grocery stores do and four times the amount carried by convenience stores (Sallis and others, 1986). Yet there are four times as many supermarkets located in white neighborhoods as there are in black neighborhoods (Morland, Wing, Diez Roux, and Poole, 2002). Public health workers and health care providers need to consider factors in the local food environment level when recommending dietary changes.

Patterns of physical activity may also be influenced by the built environment. Lack of access to playgrounds, a dearth of organized sports activities, and concerns for physical safety that lead parents to keep their children indoors may further increase the risk of childhood obesity. Increased television viewing, which may be a marker of an increasingly sedentary lifestyle, is now widely recognized as a risk factor for childhood obesity, and this is one potential area in which to target interventions (Dietz and Gortmaker, 1985). In fact, reducing television viewing has been shown in several studies to reduce childhood obesity (Robinson, 1999; Dennison, Russo, Burdick, and Jenkins, 2004).

Improved access to recreational facilities is associated with higher levels of participation in vigorous activity, regardless of individuals' socioeconomic status (Sallis and others, 1990). Disadvantaged areas tend to have fewer recreational facilities, raising concerns that lack of access is a barrier to physical activity, putting some communities at higher risk for inactivity and obesity (MacIntyre, MacIver, and Sooman, 1993). This reinforces the role of the built environment as a potentially modifiable risk factor for physical inactivity.

Recognizing the contribution of the environment to this growing epidemic is just the beginning. Further work is needed to develop and implement strategies to prevent and control obesity. Identifying and addressing environmental determinants of obesity through research studies provides a unique opportunity to institute change on a population-wide level through both structural changes in the environment and public policy changes in conjunction with individual behavioral changes (Srinivasan, O'Fallon, and Dearry, 2003).

Risk Assessment and Communication

Traditional risk assessment has generally failed to consider the special exposures and the unique susceptibilities of infants and children. Children represent a unique subgroup within the population, one that requires special consideration in risk assessment. In calling for a new paradigm for environmental research and risk assessment, Landrigan and Carlson (1995) wrote: "The essence of this paradigm is to place the child, not the chemical or hazard, at the center of the analysis. The analysis would then begin with the child, his or her biology, exposure patterns, and developmental stage. This paradigm calls for a new way of thinking, and a retooling of the risk assessment process so that it takes into account not only the increased vulnerability of children but also the effects of multiple and cumulative exposures over the course of a lifetime" (p. 50).

Adoption of a new child-centered agenda for research and risk assessment will be necessary if disease of toxic environmental origin in children is to be identified, understood, controlled, and prevented. This agenda needs to be multidisciplinary. Specific requirements of the new agenda are (1) exploration and quantification of unique patterns of exposure for children; (2) adoption of new, more sensitive approaches to testing chemicals that can recognize the consequences of exposure during early development; (3) identification, through clinical and epidemiological studies, of etiologic associations between environmental exposures and pediatric diseases; and (4) elucidation, at the cellular and molecular levels, of the pathogenetic mechanisms of pediatric environmental illness.

If high-risk groups such as children do not receive appropriate consideration, then risk assessment and the regulatory decisions that follow from it will in many cases fail to protect these most vulnerable members of society from environmentally induced disease and dysfunction. Several specific tasks need to be part of developing and implementing this new child-centered paradigm, including improved exposure assessment, enhanced toxicity testing, new toxicodynamic and toxicokinetic models, a mechanistic approach to hazard assessment, and application of uncertainty and safety factors that specifically consider children's risks. In addition, application of the precautionary principle can provide an overarching framework for considering children's risks.

Improved Exposure Assessment

Additional data are needed on children's patterns and levels of exposures to chemicals in the environment. Because exposures vary by age, this information will need to be collected for different age groups, from the developing baby in utero through adolescence. Accurate and frequently updated information is needed on children's diets at different ages and on the concentrations of xenobiotics (chemicals foreign to the human body) in those diets. Surveys also should be regularly conducted of levels of chemical contaminants in breast milk. Better data are needed on the extent of exposure that results from children's unique mouthing behaviors.

All sources of exposure need to be considered in evaluating the potential risks of environmental chemicals to infants and children (NRC, 1993). Models need to be developed that can account for children's simultaneous exposures to multiple chemicals of differing potency via multiple routes of exposure. These models need to be able to assess the cumulative effects of chemicals that may have either synergistic or antagonistic actions. The EPA's recent work in assessing exposures to multiple organophosphate pesticides is a useful first step in this direction.

Exposure estimates for acute effects and exposure estimates for chronic effects need to be constructed differently. The incorporation of biomarkers into data collection may be useful. Most important, it is essential to examine the full distribution of children's exposures to chemicals in the environment. Point estimates of average exposure are no longer sufficient. The actual distribution of the range of children's exposures across the population needs to be determined through field studies. Appropriate mathematical models, such as Monte Carlo models (see Chapter Thirty-Two), must be constructed in order to permit the combination of various data sets and thus an examination of full exposure distributions (National Academy of Sciences, 1992). Of special concern are children whose exposures fall into the top 10, 5, or 1 percent of the population.

Enhanced Toxicity Testing

New, more sensitive approaches to chemical toxicity testing are needed that can reliably detect the unanticipated developmental consequences of exposures during critical windows of prenatal and postnatal vulnerability (Selevan, Kimmel, and Mendola, 2000). These new models of developmental toxicity testing need to generate data on organ systems that have not been adequately addressed in the past, for example, the nervous, immune, respiratory, reproductive, cardiovascular, and endocrine systems.

A shortcoming of much current toxicity testing is that test chemicals are administered to experimental animals in adolescence, and the animals are subsequently sacrificed at a point in life that corresponds roughly to a human age of sixty to sixty-five years. Thus both the unique effects of early exposures and any late effects of early exposures are not captured (EPA, Risk Assessment Forum, 2002); these effects might include cancer, heart disease, neurological disorders, or diabetes. To improve current toxicity testing for certain classes of chemicals, investigators may need to undertake studies in which chemicals are administered to experimental animals either in utero or shortly after birth and the subjects then followed over their entire natural life spans. For other classes of compounds, it may be necessary to expose animals throughout the life span. The approach should attempt to replicate the human experience and may enhance detection of delayed effects (NAS, 1992).

Excessive reliance on observation of birth anomalies and insufficient testing of organ system function have been features of much traditional toxicity testing. To improve the situation, enhanced functional tests of neurobehavioral, immune, endocrine, and reproductive toxicity will be of great importance (EPA, 1986; EPA, Risk Assessment Forum, 1991, 2002). One particular area of growing concern is the potential for recently introduced chemicals such as phthalates to act as endocrine disrupters (EDs). Recent national surveys conducted by the Centers for Disease Control and Prevention found that biomarker residues of EDs are present almost universally in Americans but also that significant disparities in body burdens by age, sex, and race and ethnicity exist, with the highest levels found in children and minorities. Animal studies have shown a relationship between phthalates and fetal death, malformations, and reproductive toxicity (Shea, 2003). This calls for an exploration of the potential for endocrine disruption through phthalate exposure from commonplace items such as plastic toys. Yet, "no short- or long-term follow-up studies have evaluated possible phthalate toxicity in medically exposed infants" (Shea, 2003). These functional assessments need to be applied on a more routine basis, especially when data from other studies, for example, adult target organ toxicity or multigeneration studies, raise concerns about possible developmental effects.

New Toxicodynamic and Toxicokinetic Models

The physiological and biochemical characteristics of children that influence the metabolism and disposition of chemicals at different stages of development need to be considered in risk assessment. Physiological parameters, such as tissue growth rates, and biochemical parameters, such as enzyme induction, may differentially affect the responses of infants and children at different developmental stages to environmental chemicals (Cresteil, 1998; Ginsberg and others, 2002). Physiologically based pharmacokinetic models can be used to estimate the dose of toxic metabolites reaching target tissues at different developmental stages (O'Flaherty, 1997; Welsch, Blumenthal, and Conolly, 1995).

A Mechanistic Approach to Hazard Assessment

The pathogenic mechanisms of environmentally induced disease in children need to be elucidated at functional, organ, cellular, and molecular levels (Birnbaum, 1994; Campbell, Seidler, and Slotkin, 1997; Whitney and others, 1995). These assessments could be undertaken in conjunction with toxicity testing of chemicals and also in the context of epidemiological studies. Clinical and epidemiological studies are of proven value for studying etiologic associations between environmental exposures and pediatric disease (Bellinger and others, 1987; Jacobson and Jacobson, 1996; Needleman and others, 1990). A major multiyear, prospective, epidemiological study of children's health, the National Children's Study, has been proposed and will be an invaluable means of identifying and characterizing the consequences of multiple, early, low-level exposures, as called for in the Children's Health Act of 2000 (Berkowitz and others, 2001).

Application of Uncertainty and Safety Factors Specific to Children's Risks

In the absence of data to the contrary, children must be presumed to be more vulnerable than adults to environmental toxic agents, a presumption specifically recommended by the NRC Committee on Pesticides in the Diets of Infants and Children (1993). Traditional approaches to risk assessment are now being modified to account more carefully and explicitly for risks to children (EPA, Risk

Assessment Forum, 2002). However, a number of data gaps in exposure assessment and in developmental toxicity must be addressed through the development and implementation of additional testing guideline protocols (EPA, 1999; EPA, Risk Assessment Forum, 2002), the acquisition of better information on children's exposure patterns and sources, and basic research both on mechanisms of underlying development and on chemical interactions of environmental agents with developing organ systems (NRC, 2000).

The Precautionary Principle

The 1998 Wingspread "Statement on the Precautionary Principle" summarizes the precautionary principle as follows: "When an activity raises threats of harm to human health or the environment, precautionary measures should be taken even if some cause and effect relationships are not fully established scientifically." (This principle is described in detail in Chapter Twenty-Nine.) It has special relevance to children, because the notion of protecting children from harm is so widely accepted.

Risk Communication

Concern for one's children's health and well-being is a defining aspect of parenting. Indeed, even adults who minimize the risks of their own environmental exposures may have deep concerns about those their children confront. Clear communication on the part of health care providers and collaborative partnerships with agencies and academic centers can do much to provide parents with useful information and to help them respond appropriately to environmental exposures. Examples of this exchange of information appear in the case studies presented earlier and in Box 28.3.

Box 28.3. Risk Communication and the World Trade Center

A difficulty in risk assessment targeted toward children is that we have so little knowledge about normal background levels of exposure for the general population aged zero to eighteen years and babies in utero. Current acceptable thresholds of exposure for many environmental exposures are based on studies of healthy adults in the workplace setting and do not take into account vulnerable populations.

After the fall of the World Trade Center (WTC) towers in New York City, officials and investigators were faced with concerns about pediatric exposures to environmental toxins for which there are no good child health standards. The strategy they employed was to compare the WTC exposures to both the current and the historical background exposure levels. This method is useful for comparison of both dose and duration of exposure. Although this information has a limited ability to answer questions about health effects related to the exposure or about safety, it provides families with a frame of reference. When the magnitude of the exposure is in line with either current or historical background levels and is of brief duration, this sort of comparison can provide some reassurance even when a true risk assessment is not possible in the absence of evidence-based reference values or environmental thresholds specific to children.

This general approach proved very useful when dealing with such WTC exposures as releases of volatile organic compounds, dioxins, polychlorinated biphenyls, and even toxins with reference ranges for sensitive populations, such as particulate matter and lead. For example, the collapse of the World Trade Center led to the release of particulate matter ($PM_{2.5}$ and PM_{10}) from the breakdown of the building's structures and contents. This resulted in tons of dust, rubble, and debris at Ground Zero. The fact that gases, dust, soot, and smoke were also released, as a result of the fires at the site, was clearly evidenced by the smoke plumes seen in varying degrees for the duration of the fires through December 2001.

In the immediate aftermath of the WTC collapse, EPA data indicated large increases in hourly levels of $PM_{2.5}$ at and above the Air Quality Index level of 40 $\mu g/m^3$. In general these short-term elevations of particulate matter followed the path of the smoke plumes as determined by wind direction. Levels of particulate matter were higher at nighttime and lower on rainy days because moisture decreased the amounts of airborne particulate matter. Though some hourly levels were reported to be as high as 200 $\mu g/m^3$, twenty-four-hour averages for these same areas were significantly lower at 40 to 90 $\mu g/m^3$.

Although these twenty-four-hour levels were elevated, they were similar to background levels of air pollution seen previously in New York City. Routine EPA monitoring of particulate matter provides us with these historical levels. Data prior to September 2001 indicated outdoor particulate matter levels of 18.4 $\mu g/m^3$ for $PM_{2.5}$ (year 2000 average) and levels of 25 $\mu g/m^3$ for PM_{10} (1998 average). Twenty-four-hour levels for New York City as high as 40 to 89 $\mu g/m^3$ for $PM_{2.5}$ and 51 to 121 $\mu g/m^3$ for PM_{10} (1996 to 2001) had been previously reported. This indicated that even pre-9/11 levels of particulate matter exceeded the National Ambient Air Quality Standards (NAAQS), most likely reflecting background levels of air pollution in urban areas. This stresses that much work has yet to be done to improve the overall quality of outdoor air.

Guidance provided to families in the surrounding community explained that long-term health effects were unlikely to result from short-term exposures to particulate matter. However, acute reversible health effects, including asthma exacerbations and eye, ear, nose, and throat irritation, were possible. This was in contrast to the more substantial exposures experienced by the workers and volunteers at Ground Zero, for whom significant long-term health effects were possible. Studies are now underway to assess whether health effects are seen in the infants of pregnant women present at the WTC site the day of the collapse of the towers. A registry of Ground Zero workers and volunteers is also underway, enabling long-term follow-up of health conditions with long latency periods.

The Future of Children's Environmental Health: National Children's Study

In December 2000, the U.S. Congress appropriated funds to plan the National Children's Study, a national, longitudinal cohort study of children's health (National Children's Study, 2005). An important goal of this study is to examine systematically the impact on children's health and development of early exposure to environmental toxins. In addition, the study will examine interactions among environmental toxins, socioeconomic factors, behavioral factors, and genetic inheritance in their effects on the health of children. It is anticipated that the study will enroll as many as 100,000 children and families and that it will follow the children prospectively to at least age eighteen (Berkowitz and others, 2001)—a pediatric counterpart to the landmark Framingham Heart Study, one of the major sources of insight into adult health over the last half century (Futterman and Lemberg, 2000; Messerli and Mittler, 1998). Although other cohort studies have studied children prospectively (Broman, 1984; Rutter, 1989; Silva, 1990), no longitudinal study has examined the impact of environmental toxins on children's health or has studied the interactions between environmental toxins and other social, behavioral, and environmental risk factors.

The National Children's Study will have the statistical power to explore the simultaneous impact of many risk factors—environmental toxicants, health behaviors, socioeconomic factors, and genetics—on the long-term health of U.S. children. Prospective epidemiological research can quantify environmental exposures and evaluate factors that are not recorded routinely in medical charts or birth certificates. Such research can also assess the effects of early exposures to environmental toxicants on neurobehavioral development. The longitudinal design will permit direct examination of risk factors from earliest exposure through to the clinical appearance of dysfunction, thus permitting recognition of the sequence of causality. Recent advances in epidemiological technique, in computer technology, in the management of biological specimens, and in the evaluation of genetic markers increase the potential of this study to yield important etiologic insights (Berkowitz and others, 2001).

Establishing this national longitudinal study will be an enormously complex and costly task (Berkowitz and others, 2001). When focusing on relatively rare outcomes, such as some of those that may occur in children, a large sample size is required, and this study will enroll thousands of participants, resulting in enough new cases of disease and death to ensure statistically reliable findings. Retaining and tracking thousands of participants over many years is a challenge. The collection, processing, storage, and maintenance of biological specimens will need to be controlled carefully. Data will be obtained on environmental exposures and psychosocial aspects in the home environment. Standardized, age-appropriate, developmental assessments will be the main outcome measures. The successful establishment and maintenance of such a cohort will require teams drawn from a range of disciplines, including epidemiology, exposure assessment, toxicology, developmental psychology, neurobiology, biostatistics, and pediatrics. In return, however, the National Children's Study promises to yield unprecedented insights into the determinants of health and illness in children.

Conclusion

Environmental pediatrics is an area of pediatric medicine that has advanced remarkably in the past fifty years. It has risen to importance in parallel with two developments: first, the conquest in the industrialized nations of the major infectious diseases and the corresponding rise in chronic conditions such as asthma, cancer, developmental disabilities, and birth defects as the primary causes of illness and death in children and, second, the growing recognition that environment factors are responsible, at least in part, for these changes in patterns of disease.

The challenge now for children's environmental health is to understand better the impact of environmental exposures on the patterns of health and disease in children and to design evidence-based approaches to the prevention and treatment of childhood disease of environmental origin. "Children are not merely a special vulnerable group within our population but rather the current inhabitants of a developmental stage through which all future generations must pass. Protection of fetuses, infants and children is essential for the sustainability of the human species" (Landrigan, Kimmel, Correa, and Eskenazi, 2004, p. 263). We have a strong foundation of data, clinicians and researchers, concerned parents, policymakers, and training programs; we must continue the tradition of inquiry into the role of the environment in children's health and into action that can protect children from environmental hazards.

Thought Questions

1. Examine the statistics on childhood lead poisoning in your area to determine which populations are at risk. In particular, carefully examine demographics and geographic distributions of childhood lead poisoning cases. Explore the local lead laws and compare them to the lead laws of other areas to determine

whether they are adequately protective. If necessary, how might you advocate for stricter lead laws in your area?

2. Name potential pathways of exposure for a specific toxin (such as cigarette smoke, carbon monoxide, endocrine disruptors, or dioxins) and name the factors unique to a child's developmental stage that may place him or her at increased risk. Explore the current scientific literature on subsequent health effects related to this exposure at each critical window of vulnerability (pregnancy, infancy, early childhood, and adolescence).
3. What are the current recommendations for fish intake in pregnant women and children? Where can families in your area obtain information on local fish advisories? What are the potential health effects related to in utero or childhood exposures to mercury or PCBs in fish? Use the current scientific literature, including population-based studies of fish intake, to support your response. Explore current regulations on mercury and PCB pollution, and identify areas where your advocacy may be beneficial.
4. Neighborhood factors influence lifestyle habits. What are some of the neighborhood design factors that might improve a child's level of physical activity? Differentiate between urban and suburban design. In particular, address factors in the schools that might be addressed to improve both diet and physical activity. Which groups in your area could you convene to address making positive changes in these various factors?
5. What are the environmental justice (EJ) issues in your area that may disproportionately affect children's health? How might you reach out to communities at risk that are disproportionately affected by environmental toxins? Explore past EJ issues that have negatively affected children's health, and identify the groups or factors that were largely responsible for implementing change.
6. What can be done on the local, state, national, and international levels to secure the future of children's environmental health research, clinical services, advocacy, and policy? Use a current environmental concern as an example.

References

Agency for Toxic Substances and Disease Registry. "ToxFaqs for Arsenic." [http://www.atsdr.cdc.gov/tfacts2.html]. 2003.

Agency for Toxic Substances and Disease Registry. "ToxFaqs for Tetrachloroethylene (PERC)." [http://www.atsdr.cdc.gov/tfacts18.html]. 2004.

"Asthma Mortality and Hospitalization Among Children and Young Adults—United States, 1980–1993." *Morbidity and Mortality Weekly Report,* 1996, *45*(17), 350–353.

Bakir, F., and others. "Methylmercury Poisoning in Iraq." *Science,* 1973, *181*(96), 230–241.

Bellinger, D., and others. "Longitudinal Analyses of Prenatal and Postnatal Lead Exposure and Early Cognitive Development." *New England Journal of Medicine,* 1987, *316,* 1037–1043.

Berkowitz, G. S., and others. "The Rationale for a National Prospective Cohort Study of Environmental Exposure and Childhood Development." *Environmental Research,* 2001, *85*(2), 59–68.

Birnbaum, L. S. "The Mechanism of Dioxin Toxicity: Relationship to Risk Assessment." *Environmental Health Perspectives,* 1994, *102*(suppl. 9), 157–167.

Briassoulis, G., Narlioglou, M., and Hatzis, T. "Toxic Encephalopathy Associated with Use of DEET Insect Repellents: A Case Analysis of Its Toxicity in Children." *Human & Experimental Toxicology,* 2001, *20*(1), 8–14.

Briggs, D. *Making a Difference: Indicators to Improve Children's Environmental Health.* World Health Organization. [http://www.who.int/phe/children/en/cehindic.pdf]. 2003.

Broman, S. "The Collaborative Perinatal Project: An Overview." In S. A. Mednick, M. Harway, and K. M. Finello (eds.), *Handbook of Longitudinal Research.* New York: Praeger, 1984.

Campbell, C. G., Seidler, F. J., and Slotkin, T. A. "Chlorpyrifos Interferes with Cell Development in Rat Brain Regions." *Brain Research Bulletin,* 1997, *43*(2), 179–189.

Center for Defense Information. "Military Costs: The Real Total." [http://www.cdi.org/issues/realtota.html]. 1996.

Centers for Disease Control and Prevention. *Second National Report on Human Exposure to Environmental Chemicals.* NCEH Publication no. 02-0716. Atlanta, Ga.: Centers for Disease Control and Prevention, 2003.

Chiou, H. Y., and others. "Incidence of Internal Cancers and Ingested Inorganic Arsenic: A Seven-Year Follow-Up Study in Taiwan." *Cancer Research,* 1995, *55*(6), 1296–1300.

Chiou, H. Y., and others. "Incidence of Transitional Cell Carcinoma and Arsenic in Drinking Water: A Follow-Up Study of 8,102 Residents in an Arseniasis-Endemic Area in Northeastern Taiwan. *American Journal of Epidemiology,* 2001, *153,* 411–418.

Cresteil, T. "Onset of Xenobiotic Metabolism in Children: Toxicological Implications." *Food Additives and Contaminants,* 1998, *15*(suppl.), 45–51.

Curl, C. L., Fenske, R. A., and Elgethun, K. "Organophosphorus Pesticide Exposure of Urban and Suburban Preschool Children with Organic and Conventional Diets." *Environmental Health Perspectives,* 2003, *111,* 377–382.

Dennison, B. A., Russo, T. J., Burdick, P. A., and Jenkins, P. L. "An Intervention to Reduce Television Viewing by Preschool Children." *Archives of Pediatrics & Adolescent Medicine,* 2004, *158*(2), 170–176.

Dewailly, E., and others. "Inuit Exposure to Organochlorines Through the Aquatic Food Chain in Arctic Quebec." *Environmental Health Perspectives,* 1993, *101,* 618–620.

Dietz, W. H., Jr., and Gortmaker, S. L. "Do We Fatten Our Children at the Television Set? Obesity and Television Viewing in Children and Adolescents." *Pediatrics,* 1985, *75*(5), 807–812.

DiLiberti, J. H., and Jackson, C. R. "Long-Term Trends in Childhood Infectious Disease Mortality Rates." *American Journal of Public Health,* 1999, *89,* 1883–1885.

Duke University Center for Health Policy, Law & Management. "Cost of Illness by Disease: Rankings." [http://www.hpolicy.duke.edu/cyberexchange/coirank.htm]. 2000.

Engel, L. S., O'Meara, E. S., and Schwartz, S. M. "Maternal Occupation in Agriculture and Risk of Limb Defects in Washington State, 1980–1993." *Scandinavian Journal of Work, Environment & Health,* 2000, *26*(3), 193–198.

Eriksson, J. G., and others. "Early Growth and Coronary Heart Disease in Later Life: Longitudinal Study." *British Medical Journal,* 2001, *322,* 949–953.

Etzel, R. A., and Balk, S. J. (eds.). *Handbook of Pediatric Environmental Health.* (2nd ed.) Elk Grove, Ill.: American Academy of Pediatrics, 2003.

Frumkin, H., Frank, L., and Jackson, R. J. *Urban Sprawl and Public Health.* Washington, D.C.: Island Press, 2004.

Futterman, L. G., and Lemberg, L. "The Framingham Heart Study: A Pivotal Legacy of the Last Millennium." *American Journal of Critical Care,* 2000, *9*(2), 147–151.

Gibson, J. L. "A Plea for Painted Railing and Painted Walls of Rooms as the Source of Lead Poisoning Among Queensland Children." *Australian Medical Gazette,* 1904, *23,* 149–153.

Ginsberg, G., and others. "Evaluation of Child/Adult Pharmacokinetic Differences from a Database Derived from the Therapeutic Drug Literature." *Toxicological Sciences,* 2002, *66,* 185–200.

Gurney, J. G., and others. "Trends in Cancer Incidence Among Children in the U.S." *Cancer,* 1996, *78*(3), 532–541.

Haggerty, R., and Rothmann, J. *Child Health and the Community.* New York: Wiley, 1975.

Harada, H. "Congenital Minamata Disease: Intrauterine Methylmercury Poisoning." *Teratology,* 1978, *18,* 285–288.

Herbst, A. L., Hubby, M. M., Azizi, F., and Makii, M. M. "Reproductive and Gynecologic Surgical Experience in Diethylstilbestrol-Exposed Daughters." *American Journal of Obstetrics and Gynecology,* 1981, *141*(8), 1019–1028.

Hooper, K., and McDonald, T. A. "The PBDEs: An Emerging Environmental Challenge and Another Reason for Breast-Milk Monitoring Programs." *Environmental Health Perspectives,* 2000, *108,* 387–392.

Hooper, K., and others. "Analysis of Breast Milk to Assess Exposure to Chlorinated Contaminants in Kazakhstan: Sources of 2,3,7,8-Tetrachlorodibenzo-p-Dioxin (TCDD) Exposures in an Agricultural Region of Southern Kazakhstan." *Environmental Health Perspectives,* 1999, *107,* 447–457.

Institute of Medicine, Food and Nutrition Board. *Nutrition During Lactation.* Washington, D.C.: National Academies Press, 1991.

Jackson, R. J. "The Impact of the Built Environment on Health: An Emerging Field." *American Journal of Public Health,* 2003, *93,* 1382–1384.

Jacobson, J. L., and Jacobson, S. W. "Intellectual Impairment in Children Exposed to Polychlorinated Biphenyls in Utero." *New England Journal of Medicine,* 1996, *335,* 783–789.

Landrigan, P. J., and Carlson, J. E. "Environmental Policy and Children's Health." *Future Child,* 1995, *5*(2), 34–52.

Landrigan P. J., Kimmel, C. A., Correa, A., and Eskenazi, B. "Children's Health and the Environment: Public Health Issues and Challenges for Risk Assessment." *Environmental Health Perspectives,* 2004, *112,* 257–265.

Landrigan, P. J., and others. "Environmental Pollutants and Disease in American Children: Estimates of Morbidity, Mortality, and Costs for Lead Poisoning, Asthma, Cancer, and Developmental Disabilities." *Environmental Health Perspectives,* 2002, *110,* 721–728.

Legler, J. M., and others. "Cancer Surveillance Series [Corrected]: Brain and Other Central Nervous System Cancers: Recent Trends in Incidence and Mortality." *Journal of the National Cancer Institute,* 1999, *91*(16), 1382–1390.

Lipscomb, J. W., Kramer, J. E., and Leikin, J. B. "Seizure Following Brief Exposure to the Insect Repellent N,N-Diethyl-m-Toluamide." *Annals of Emergency Medicine,* 1992, *21,* 315–317.

Loffredo, C. A., Silbergeld, E. K., Ferencz, C., and Zhang, J. "Association of Transposition of the Great Arteries in Infants with Maternal Exposures to Herbicides and Rodenticides." *American Journal of Epidemiology,* 2001, *153,* 529–536.

Longnecker, M. P., Klebanoff, M. A., Zhou, H., and Brock, J. W. "Association Between Maternal Serum Concentration of the DDT Metabolite DDE and Preterm and Small-for-Gestational-Age Babies at Birth." *Lancet,* 2001, *358,* 110–114.

MacDorman, M. F., and Atkinson, J. O. "Infant Mortality Statistics from the 1997 Period Linked Birth/Infant Death Data Set." *National Vital Statistics Reports,* 1999, *47*(23), 1–23.

MacIntyre, S., MacIver, S., and Sooman, A. "Area, Class and Health: Should We Be Focusing on Places or People?" *Journal of Social Policy,* 1993, *22*(2), 213–243.

Mannino, D. M., and others. "Surveillance for Asthma—United States, 1960–1995." *Morbidity and Mortality Weekly Report: CDC Surveillance Summaries,* 1998, *47*(1), 1–27.

Masuda, Y. "Health Status of Japanese and Taiwanese After Exposure to Contaminated Rice Oil." *Environmental Health Perspectives,* 1985, *60,* 321–325.

McBride, W. G. "Thalidomide and Congenital Abnormalities." *Lancet,* 1961, *2,* 1358.

Messerli, F. H., and Mittler B. S. "Framingham at 50." *Lancet,* 1998, *352,* 1006.

Miller, R. W. "Delayed Effects Occurring Within the First Decade After Exposure of Young Individuals to the Hiroshima Atomic Bomb." *Pediatrics,* 1956, *18*(1), 1–18.

Miller, R. W., and Blot, W. J. "Small Head Size After in-Utero Exposure to Atomic Radiation." *Lancet,* 1972, *2,* 784–787.

Morland, K., Wing, S., and Diez Roux, A. "The Contextual Effect of the Local Food Environment on Residents' Diets: The Atherosclerosis Risk in Communities Study." *American Journal of Public Health,* 2002, *92,* 1761–1767.

Morland, K., Wing, S., Diez Roux, A., and Poole, C. "Neighborhood Characteristics Associated with the Location of Food Stores and Food Service Places." *American Journal of Preventive Medicine,* 2002, *22,* 23–29.

National Academy of Sciences. *Toxicity Testing: Needs and Priorities.* Washington, D.C.: National Academies Press, 1984.

National Academy of Sciences. *Environmental Neurotoxicology.* Washington, D.C.: National Academies Press, 1992.

National Children's Study. Homepage. [www.nationalchildrensstudy.gov]. 2005.

National Research Council, Committee on Pesticides in the Diets of Infants and Children. *Pesticides in the Diets of Infants and Children.* Washington, D.C.: National Academies Press, 1993.

National Research Council. *Scientific Frontiers in Developmental Toxicology and Risk Assessment.* Washington, D.C.: National Academies Press, 2000.

Needleman, H. L., and others. "Deficits in Psychologic and Classroom Performance of Children with Elevated Dentine Lead Levels." *New England Journal of Medicine,* 1979, *300,* 689–695.

Needleman, H. L., and others. "The Long-Term Effects of Exposure to Low Doses of Lead in Childhood: An 11-Year Follow-Up Report." *New England Journal of Medicine,* 1990, *322,* 83–88.

Northridge, M. E., and others. "Diesel Exhaust Exposure Among Adolescents in Harlem: A Community-Driven Study." *American Journal of Public Health,* 1999, *89,* 998–1002.

Oddy, W. H. "Breastfeeding Protects Against Illness and Infection in Infants and Children: A Review of the Evidence." *Breastfeeding Review,* 2001, *9*(2), 11–18.

Office of Science and Technology Policy, National Science and Technology Council. *Investing in Our Future: A National Research Initiative for America's Children for the 21st Century.* Washington, D.C.: Executive Office of the President, Office of Science and Technology Policy, 1997.

O'Flaherty, E. J. "Pharmacokinetics, Pharmacodynamics, and Prediction of Developmental Abnormalities." *Reproductive Toxicology,* 1997, *11*(2–3), 413–416.

Olden, K., and Wilson, S. "Environmental Health and Genomics: Visions and Implications." *Nature Reviews: Genetics,* 2000, *1*(2), 149–153.

Ordonez, J. V., Carrillo, J. A., Miranda, M., and Gale, J. L. [Epidemiologic study of a disease believed to be encephalitis in the region of the highlands of Guatemala.] [Article in Spanish.] *Boletin de la Oficina Sanitaria Panamericana,* 1966, *60*(6), 510–519.

Pew Environmental Health Commission. *Attack Asthma: Why America Needs a Public Health Defense System to Battle Environmental Threats.* [http://healthyamericans.org/reports/files/asthma.pdf]. Apr. 2000.

Pierce, P. E., and others. "Alkyl Mercury Poisoning in Humans: Report of an Outbreak." *Journal of the American Medical Association,* 1972, *220,* 1439–1442.

Robinson, T. N. "Reducing Children's Television Viewing to Prevent Obesity: A Randomized Controlled Trial." *Journal of the American Medical Association,* 1999, *282,* 1561–1567.

Rutter, M. "Isle of Wight Revisited: Twenty-Five Years of Child Psychiatric Epidemiology." *Journal of the American Academy of Child and Adolescent Psychiatry,* 1989, *28*(5), 633–653.

Sallis, J. F., and others. "San Diego Surveyed for Heart-Healthy Foods and Exercise Facilities." *Public Health Reports,* 1986, *101,* 216–219.

Sallis, J. F., and others. "Distance Between Homes and Exercise Facilities Related to Frequency of Exercise Among San Diego Residents." *Public Health Reports,* 1990, *105,* 179–185.

Selevan, S. G., Kimmel, C. A., and Mendola, P. "Identifying Critical Windows of Exposure for Children's Health." *Environmental Health Perspectives,* 2000, *108*(suppl. 3), 451–455.

Shaw, G. M., and others. "Maternal Pesticide Exposure from Multiple Sources and Selected Congenital Anomalies." *Epidemiology,* 1999, *10,* 60–66.

Shea, K. M. (American Academy of Pediatrics Committee on Environmental Health). "Pediatric Exposure and Potential Toxicity of Phthalate Plasticizers." *Pediatrics,* 2003, *111*(6, pt. 1), 1467–1474.

Silva, P. A. "The Dunedin Multidisciplinary Health and Development Study: A 15-Year Longitudinal Study." *Paediatric and Perinatal Epidemiology,* 1990, *4*(1), 76–107.

Sonawane, B. R. "Chemical Contaminants in Human Milk: An Overview." *Environmental Health Perspectives,* 1995, *103*(suppl. 6), 197–205.

Spielberg, S. P. "Anticonvulsant Adverse Drug Reactions: Age Dependent and Age Independent." In P. S. Guzelian, C. J. Henry, and S. S. Olin (eds.), *Similarities and Differences Between Children and Adults: Implications for Risk Assessment.* Washington, D.C.: International Life Sciences Institute Press, 1992.

Srinivasan, S., O'Fallon, L. R., and Dearry, A. "Creating Healthy Communities, Healthy Homes, Healthy People: Initiating a Research Agenda on the Built Environment and Public Health." *American Journal of Public Health,* 2003, *93,* 1446–1450.

Taussig, H. "A Study of the German Outbreak of Phocomelia." *Journal of the American Medical Association,* 1962, *180,* 1106–1114.

Taylor, P. R., Lawrence, C. E., Hwang, H. L., and Paulson, A. S. "Polychlorinated Biphenyls: Influence on Birthweight and Gestation." *American Journal of Public Health,* 1984, *74,* 1153–1154.

Tilson, H. A., Jacobson, J. L., and Rogan, W. J. "Polychlorinated Biphenyls and the Developing Nervous System: Cross-Species Comparisons." *Neurotoxicology and Teratology,* 1990, *12,* 239–248.

U.S. Environmental Protection Agency. "Guidelines for the Health Assessment of Suspect Developmental Toxicants." *Federal Register,* 51, 1986, 34028–34040.

U.S. Environmental Protection Agency. *Chemicals-in Commerce Information System: Chemical Update System Database.* Washington, D.C.: U.S. Environmental Protection Agency, 1998.

U.S. Environmental Protection Agency. *Toxicology Data Requirements for Assessing Risks of Pesticide Exposure to Children's Health.* Report of the Toxicology Working Group of the 10X Task Force. [http://www.epa.gov/scipoly/sap/1999/may/10xtx428.pdf]. 1999.

U.S. Environmental Protection Agency. "Indoor Air—IAQ Tools for Schools." [http://www.epa.gov/iaq/schools/index.html]. 2005.

U.S. Environmental Protection Agency, Indoor Environments Division. "Fact Sheet: Mold in Schools." EPA-402-F-03-029. [http://www.epa.gov/iaq/schools/images/moldfactsheet.pdf]. 2004.

U.S. Environmental Protection Agency, Office of Pesticide Programs. *Determination of the Appropriate FQPA Safety Factor(s) for Use in the Tolerance-Setting Process.* [http://www.epa.gov/pesticides/trac/science/determ.pdf]. 2002.

U.S. Environmental Protection Agency, Risk Assessment Forum. *Guidelines for Developmental Toxicity Risk Assessment.* EPA/600/FR-91/001. [http://cfpub1.epa.gov/ncea/cfm/recordisplay.cfm?deid=23162]. 1991.

U.S. Environmental Protection Agency, Risk Assessment Forum. *A Review of the Reference Dose and Reference Concentration Processes.* EPA/630/P-02/002F. [http://cfpub.epa.gov/ncea/cfm/recordisplay.cfm?deid=55365]. 2002.

Weich, S., and others. "Measuring the Built Environment: Validity of a Site Survey Instrument for Use in Urban Settings." *Health & Place,* 2001, *7*(4), 283–292.

Weidner, I. S., Moller, H., Jensen, T. K., and Skakkebaek, N. E. "Cryptorchidism and Hypospadias in Sons of Gardeners and Farmers." *Environmental Health Perspectives,* 1998, *106,* 793–796.

Weiss, B., and Landrigan, P. J. "The Developing Brain and the Environment: An Introduction." *Environmental Health Perspectives,* 2000, *108* (suppl. 3), 373–374.

Welsch, F., Blumenthal, G. M., and Conolly, R. B. "Physiologically Based Pharmacokinetic Models Applicable to Organogenesis: Extrapolation Between Species and Potential Use in Prenatal Toxicity Risk Assessments." *Toxicology Letters,* 1995, *82–83,* 539–547.

West Harlem Environmental Action. "We Act." [www.weact.org]. 2005.

Whitney, K. D., Seidler, F. J., and Slotkin, T. A. "Developmental Neurotoxicity of Chlorpyrifos: Cellular Mechanisms." *Toxicology and Applied Pharmacology,* 1995, *134,* 53–62.

Wiles, R., and Campbell, C. *Pesticides in Children's Food.* Washington, D.C.: Environmental Working Group, 1993.

World Health Organization. *The World Health Report 2002: Reducing Risks, Promoting Healthy Life.* Geneva: World Health Organization, 2002.

Yu, M. L., Hsu, C. C., Gladen, B. C., and Rogan, W. J. "In Utero PCB/PCDF Exposure: Relation of Developmental Delay to Dysmorphology and Dose." *Neurotoxicology and Teratology,* 1991, *13,* 195–202.

Zahm, S. H., and Ward, M. H. "Pesticides and Childhood Cancer." *Environmental Health Perspectives,* 1998, *106* (suppl. 3), 893–908.

For Further Information

Governmental Agencies

The U.S. Environmental Protection Agency's Office of Children's Health Protection coordinates children's environmental health activity within EPA and with other partners. Its Web site is an excellent source of information and links to other Web sites:

U.S. Environmental Protection Agency, Office of Children's Health Protection. Homepage. [http://yosemite.epa.gov/ochp/ochpweb.nsf/homepage]. 2005.

Environmental Health Perspectives, the journal of the National Institute of Environmental Health Sciences (NIEHS), has a monthly section dedicated to children's environmental health and is a valuable source of emerging research in this area.

Environmental Health Perspectives. Homepage. [http://ehp.niehs.nih.gov]. 2005.

Medical Organizations

The American Academy of Pediatrics Committee on Environmental Health has been active in promoting children's environmental health within the pediatrics profession and more broadly. It produces the *Handbook of Pediatric Environmental Health,* issues policy statements, and maintains an informative Web site:

American Academy of Pediatrics, Committee on Environmental Health. Homepage. [http://www.aap.org/visit/cmte16.htm]. 2005.

Clinical Services and Training Programs

In 1998, the Association of Occupational and Environmental Clinics (AOEC), in association with the EPA and the Agency for Toxic Substances and Disease Registry, established a new network of clinical centers in children's environmental health, the *pediatric environmental health specialty units* (PEHSUs). PEHSUs exist throughout the United States and in some foreign countries, providing clinical assessments, education, and consultation. For information about the PEHSUs, including links to each unit, see

Association of Occupational and Environmental Clinics. "Pediatric Environmental Health Specialty Units." [http://www.aoec.org/PEHSU.htm]. 2005.

In 2001, the Ambulatory Pediatric Association (APA) established the Pediatric Environmental Health Fellowship Program, a national training program in environmental pediatrics. The training is available at Boston Children's Hospital of Harvard Medical School, Mount Sinai School of Medicine, Cincinnati Children's Hospital, and Children's National Medical Center.

Research

In 1998, the EPA, the NIEHS, and the CDC jointly established the *centers for children's environment health and disease prevention research,* a national network of research centers at major medical centers. The creation of these centers marked the largest federal research investment to date in children's environmental health. For information on these centers see

National Institute of Environmental Health Sciences. "Centers for Children's Environmental Health and Disease Prevention Research." [http://www.niehs.nih.gov/translat/children/children.htm]. 2005.

The CDC periodically publishes the National Report on Human Exposure to Environmental Chemicals, an ongoing assessment, using biomonitoring, of the exposure of the U.S. population, including children, to environmental chemicals. For information on methods and results and existing reports, see

Centers for Disease Control and Prevention. National Report Homepage. [http://www.cdc.gov/exposurereport]. 2005.

Nongovernmental Organizations

Children's Environmental Health Network (CEHN) [http://www.cehn.org].
Children's Health Environment Coalition (CHEC) [http://www.checnet.org].
Healthy Schools Network, Inc (HSN) [http://www.healthyschools.org].
Learning Disabilities Association of America [http://www.ldanatl.org].

Publications

Etzel, R. A., and Balk, S. J. (eds.). *Handbook of Pediatric Environmental Health.* (2nd ed.) Elk Grove, Ill.: American Academy of Pediatrics, 2003.

Needleman, H. L., and Landrigan, P. J. *Raising Children Toxic Free: How to Keep Your Child Safe from Lead, Asbestos, Pesticides, and Other Environmental Hazards.* New York: HarperCollins, 1994.

Wigle, D. T. *Child Health and the Environment.* New York: Oxford University Press, 2003.

Possible Student Activities

- Identify local environmental health issues in your community, and partner with grassroots organizations in advocacy efforts.
- Take a "toxic" tour of your neighborhood to identify major sources of pollutants and to better understand the microenvironmental and macroenvironmental issues pertinent to your community.
- Volunteer with an organization such as Children's Health Environmental Coalition (CHEC) or Children's Environmental Health Network (CEHN), both to learn about children's environmental health issues in more detail and to share your own expertise.
- Promote the *greening* of day-care facilities, schools, and hospitals in your neighborhood.
- Advocate for the development of environmental health education curriculums for grade school, high school, and even college and graduate students in a diversity of fields.
- Be active in parents' associations in the schools and on community boards to ensure that children's environmental health issues are on their agendas.
- Join in educational and outreach efforts through community forums or health fairs to foster awareness of children's environmental health issues.
- Keep abreast of local, state, national, and international policies that may affect children's environmental health, such as the policies affecting the regulation of lead, industrial sources of hazardous pollutants, and zoning and development.
- Participate in children's environmental health research, either as a researcher or as an active member of a community advisory board.
- Contribute editorials and articles about children's environmental health issues to newsletters, newspapers, and journals.
- Advocate for increased federal funding for children's environmental health and especially for the National Children's Study, fellowship training programs, and the centers for children's environmental health and disease prevention research.

PART FIVE

THE PRACTICE OF ENVIRONMENTAL HEALTH

CHAPTER TWENTY-NINE

PREVENTION

Joel A. Tickner

Because environmental health risks are caused directly or indirectly by human activities, they are largely preventable. Indeed, it is the responsibility of the environmental health practitioner to understand this relationship and to act to minimize preventable impacts on human health. The opportunity to act will depend on the nature of the problem (uncertainty about it, its magnitude and scale) as well as available resources. Although seemingly commonsense, prevention is frequently not the focus of environmental health research, policy, or other interventions. It is important that students and environmental health practitioners understand the fundamental concepts of prevention and the options that exist if they are to address the underlying causes of effects on human health from environmental sources.

In this chapter we examine the concept of prevention and its application in environmental health. Because many environmental health risks are global, complex, and highly uncertain, this chapter introduces the concept of the precautionary principle, which can be a guide to health protective decision making in the absence of certain proof. Taken together, prevention and precaution offer a paradigm for environmental health that focuses on understanding the underlying

The author thanks Melissa Coffin and Cathy Crumbley for their assistance with chapter editing and the preparation of some of the boxes included in this chapter.

causes of environmentally induced illness and injury as well as the design and implementation of anticipatory interventions that are intended to avoid problems in the first place. In other words, a focus on prevention takes us from a reactive to a proactive and solutions-oriented approach to environmental health.

The Public Health Model of Prevention

Public health generally responds to health threats through cures and remediation, but it also aims to prevent illness by promoting healthy behaviors, addressing the causes of disease, and attempting to understand the complex web of determinants underlying disease. Although there are many examples of successful preventive environmental interventions in public health history, such as modern sanitation and the chlorination of drinking water, in general the historical focus on prevention and health promotion has not been extended to modern-day action on the impacts of environmental degradation on human health.

C.E.A. Winslow's now classic definition of *public health* outlines this preventive purpose:

> Public health is the Science and Art of preventing disease, prolonging life, and promoting physical and mental health and efficiency through organized community efforts for the sanitation of the environment, the control of community infections, the education of the individual in principles of personal hygiene, the organization of medical and nursing service for the early diagnosis and preventive treatment of disease, and the development of the social machinery which will ensure to every individual in the community a standard of living adequate for the maintenance of health [Winslow, 1920, p. 183].

In essence, prevention depends on taking appropriate measures to counteract or intercept the causes of disease or degradation. To intercept those causes requires developing an awareness and an understanding of the causes and of the populations or individuals that might be particularly susceptible, developing surveillance and monitoring systems to identify both potential causes before they cause damage and opportunities to intervene in those causes, and developing effective interventions to prevent impacts from occurring.

The impacts of environmental degradation on human health are the result of a complex set of factors—genetic, environmental, and social. In other words they are multicausal, the result of the confluence of humans (and their specific genetic or physiological susceptibilities), an agent or agents (a toxic substance,

FIGURE 29.1. AN ENVIRONMENTAL HEALTH INTERVENTION MODEL.

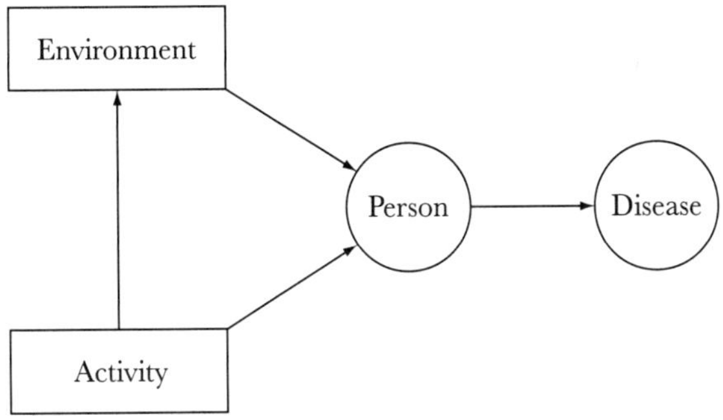

microbe, or other stressor), and the environment (environmental conditions, social factors, and so forth, that bring the agent and human together). Effective prevention requires understanding this complex set of determinants, which can in turn provide clues to the most effective prevention options.

Another way to think about options for prevention is to consider toward whom or what the prevention intervention is directed. Is it directed toward the individual, toward the environment, or toward the activity (overpopulation, socioeconomic disparities, deforestation, a production process that emits hazardous chemicals, and so forth)? This approach, depicted in Figure 29.1, might be referred to as the source-path-receptor (worker, community member) model. For example, West Nile virus may be prevented at the individual level through wearing protective clothing, using screens on windows, purchasing insect zappers, educating older people and those with compromised immune systems to avoid outside evening activities in summer, and applying repellents. It may be prevented at the environmental level by removing mosquito habitats, such as standing water; applying larvicides to kill mosquito larvae; and reducing global climate change, a possible contributor to the spread of this virus to northern regions (Epstein, 2000). At the disease or impact level, the consequences of West Nile virus may be mitigated through support therapy or immunization to prevent the virus or reduce its impacts.

Human risk is a function of both exposure to some potentially harmful agent or activity and the inherent hazard of that agent or activity. Exposures and hazards (and hence risk) can often vary greatly in a population due to genetic, physiological, or social susceptibility. In the environmental health intervention model it is possible to prevent risks by *reducing exposure* (applying controls to reduce or eliminate exposures) or by *reducing hazard* (replacing a toxic material with a less toxic material). Consideration of both hazard and exposure provides more options for preventive interventions.

Levels of Prevention

Prevention can take many forms, from stopping a potentially harmful activity before it causes damage to acting to prevent further degradation once impacts on health have been identified. Both are important in environmental health efforts, and the approach to prevention may differ by region (technical and economic capacity) or by particular environmental health risk. However, primary prevention—preventing risks at their source—is of course a first priority. (Specific examples of tools for prevention are outlined later in this chapter.) In 1958, Leavell and Clark identified primary, secondary, and tertiary levels of prevention, a model that is still well recognized.

Primary prevention involves intervening in systems to address risk factors for disease (and to reduce or eliminate exposure to harmful agents) before diagnosis and to develop measures designed to promote general optimum health. Primary prevention can be divided into two types:

- *Health promotion:* procedures not directed at any particular disease but that serve to further general health and well-being. An example of health promotion is education about the impacts of pesticides on health.
- *Specific protection:* measures taken to intercept the causes of disease before they adversely affect health. An example of specific protection is the use of gloves to prevent dermal exposure to pesticides, or the avoidance of pesticides.

Secondary prevention is early detection, often at the preclinical stage, before disease is evident. Early detection and prompt treatment reduce the lag time between diagnosis, treatment, and preventive action; this is necessary to prevent further illness from occurring. Secondary prevention ends further degradation of health by removing the precipitating behavior or activity. An example of secondary prevention is workplace surveillance that allows a worker to be removed from a potentially hazardous situation once some indicator of effects or level of personal exposure has occurred.

Tertiary prevention involves limiting health damage through treatment and rehabilitation once disease occurs. An example of tertiary prevention is rehabilitation therapy for a worker with lower back strain caused by work conditions. (Box 29.1 presents some further examples.)

Box 29.1. The Levels of Prevention Applied to Environmental Risks

Primary Prevention

- Identifying a hazardous material in a workplace and replacing it with a less toxic one
- Changing a production process to reduce emissions
- Developing hybrid gasoline-electric cars that achieve greater fuel efficiency while releasing fewer pollutants
- Avoiding grazing cattle near drinking-water sources
- Educating consumers about recycling and consuming fewer disposable products
- Encouraging women of childbearing age to avoid eating fish containing mercury

Secondary Prevention

- Establishing a biomonitoring system to identify levels of contaminants in human body fluids
- Using sewage treatment plants to treat industrial wastes
- Using postmarketing surveillance and testing to identify potential hazards associated with a chemical used in cleaning products

Tertiary Prevention

- Remediating soil at a contaminated site
- Treating farmworkers for early signs of pesticide poisoning
- Removing lead paint from inner-city housing of children with elevated blood lead levels

We can also consider a fourth type of prevention, which might be termed *primordial prevention*. This is action taken due to knowledge about what might happen in the future, for example, increases in smoking and subsequent cardiovascular disease in developing countries or increases in infectious disease caused by climate change. This type of prevention may involve taking strategic action to reach specified, future system goals. This is far-reaching, anticipatory prevention, corresponding to what has been called *backcasting* (discussed later, in Box 29.7).

In the practice of industrial hygiene in occupational health, an established hierarchy of prevention states that hazards should be controlled in the following order:

- *Substitution* that includes using safer chemicals or other products or activities in order to keep hazards from entering the workplace
- *Engineering controls* that include using equipment that mitigates exposure

- *Administrative controls* that include changing the way workers do their jobs to reduce their exposure to hazards
- *Personal protective equipment* (PPE) that includes respirators, hard hats, face and eye protection, hearing protection, gloves, and protective clothing and footwear

More recently in the fields of occupational health and environmental protection, hierarchies of prevention have been established. Under these hierarchies primary prevention refers to prevention of pollution or exposure at the source, and secondary prevention refers to both medical surveillance and what might be termed *end-of-pipe* controls that reduce, but do not fully prevent, exposure (these are discussed in further detail below). Tertiary prevention refers to early therapeutic interventions as well as to cleanup of contaminated sites and avoidance of further problems.

Substitution is the only way to eliminate a hazard completely and is the preferred approach. Engineering controls can be expensive and can shift hazards from the workers to the environment. Finally, the use of personal protective equipment can be burdensome (think of wearing a respirator for hours a day, for example, or wearing gloves and protective clothing in a hot, sunny setting such as a farm field) and as a result subject to noncompliance. PPE also can fail and is costly to maintain (Levy and Wegman, 2000; also see Chapter Four in this volume).

A fundamental change in environmental protection paradigms occurred with the passage of the Pollution Prevention Act of 1990. Prior to this Act most environmental protection efforts focused either on treating pollution once it entered the environment—in landfills or waste treatment facilities—or on controlling emissions through expensive technologies such as scrubbers and filters that tended to shift pollutants from one medium (air or water or workplace or community) to another. The Pollution Prevention Act states: "The Congress hereby declares it to be the national policy of the United States that pollution should be prevented or reduced at the source whenever feasible; pollution that cannot be prevented should be recycled in an environmentally safe manner whenever feasible; pollution that cannot be prevented or recycled should be treated in an environmentally safe manner whenever feasible; and disposal or other release into the environment should be employed only as a last resort and should be conducted in an environmentally safe manner."

Pollution prevention differs from control in several important ways: first, prevention is integrated into product and process development and operation whereas control is brought in after problems arise; second, prevention focuses on why pollution is created and the processes and activities that lead to it whereas control focuses on treatment and characterization of impacts after pollution is created; and third, prevention is achieved through technical and nontechnical approaches, including social and management change, whereas control is almost always purely technology based.

Moving Upstream: Proximate Cause and Root Cause Prevention

Clearly, all prevention is not the same. It is possible to prevent impacts of environmental degradation at their source or at some point in the causal chain before they cause disease. The ways we frame problems and the types of questions we ask about them are critical to the types of interventions and solutions we seek. For example, if we are concerned about preventing the impacts of dioxin (a by-product of combustion of chlorine-containing materials) being emitted from an incinerator, we could focus on more efficient combustion technology, we could focus on segregating wastes so that materials that contribute to forming dioxin are not incinerated, or we could focus on reducing the waste that needs to be incinerated in the first place. Or, if we are concerned about preventing the emission of a contaminant from a factory, we could ask what the cancer risk is to the local population that is consuming that contaminant in its drinking water (and then use controls to reduce exposure to just below the level of concern), or we could ask why that emission is occurring in the first place and try to redesign the production process to avoid it.

Many environmental health prevention activities represent what might be termed *proximate cause prevention* (or *proximal primary prevention*). Proximate cause prevention focuses intervention at the link in the causal chain that is closest to disease and impact: for example, advising women not to eat mercury-contaminated fish to avoid fetal exposure to methylmercury. Compared to other interventions, it tends to be short-term action oriented, cheaper, and involves less intensive societal intervention. Focusing only on proximate causes, however, may yield only a short-term solution and fail to fully address the problem, or it may address the wrong problem.

Root cause prevention (or *distal primary prevention*) focuses on the early links in the causal chain, often far removed from the ultimate impact or disease: for example, reducing mercury emissions from coal-fired power plants and other sources or redesigning power production and products to avoid mercury use (and emissions) in the first place. It focuses on how a myriad of environmental, social, and other factors come together to affect human health. It tends to be long-term action oriented, to require social and political change, to be costly in the short term to implement, and to yield benefits that are often uncertain and do not occur until far in the future. For example, consider the impacts of overpopulation in developing countries. One route to addressing concerns about overpopulation is family planning, educating men and women about birth control and encouraging reduced family size. Family planning has played an important role in reducing birthrates in developing nations. However, it tends not to address the root question of why so many babies are born in developing countries or why impacts are occurring. Root cause prevention would focus on education and job creation for women, addressing disproportionate land tenure, reducing poverty, improving maternal and child health (addressing factors in health impacts and access to health care), and changing policies that encourage people to destroy natural resources. (Box 29.2 gives an example of proximate and root cause prevention related to food safety.) In the end, environmental health practitioners need to examine problems broadly, identifying opportunities for proximate prevention and for root cause prevention.

Box 29.2. Proximate and Root Cause Prevention: The Case of Food Safety

Despite having one of the safest food supplies in the world, the United States still experiences widespread problems with microbial contamination (see Chapter Twenty-One). Every year there are as many as 76 million cases of foodborne illness, which are responsible for as many as 10,000 deaths and 325,000 hospitalizations. The economic costs of microbial contamination of food may be as high as $17 billion per year. Several approaches have been suggested to prevent this contamination, including increased meat and dairy inspections, irradiation of meats and fruits and vegetables to kill any microbes, and the use of the Hazard Analysis and Critical Point (HACCP) system. The HACCP system is a voluntary food safety system in which producers identify potential sources of contamination of food sources, the critical points of contaminant entry into the production process, and methods for monitoring and taking preventive action when a prescribed level of contamination has been surpassed. Hand washing and good personal hygiene are always an important final defense against microbial contamination in the home, restaurants, and schools.

Little attention, however, has been paid to the reasons why microbial contamination of the food supply occurs in the first place. Several potential root sources of microbial contamination can be identified: factory farming, where animals are in close proximity and can spread disease; consolidated factory production of meats, with very few processors accounting for most of the nation's production and a labor force with a high proportion of poor, immigrant meatpackers with few health benefits, who must come to work even when ill; the increased consumption of food that is imported, particularly from developing nations with lower health standards; the increased production of highly processed foods, with multiple opportunities for contamination in those processes; and quite possibly global climate change and globalization, which may introduce new contaminants into the food supply (Nestle, 2003).

The Complexity of Environmental Health Risks

Previous chapters of this book have introduced a wide variety of environmental health risks that vary in cause, complexity, and impact. Traditional risks (unsafe drinking water, inadequate sanitation, and indoor air pollution) are well established and arguably the most serious current threats to health. Particularly in developing countries and those in transition, it is important that public health interventions be strengthened to prevent these risks.

More modern, and often highly uncertain, risks occur when industrialization and rapid growth proceed with little concern for environmental and health protection. Exposures to dangerous chemicals, hazardous wastes, radiation and electromagnetic fields, and industrial pollutants through food, water, air, direct exposure from everyday products, and global climate change are increasingly important factors in environmentally related illness. These sources of exposure can result in health effects long after the initial exposure or contact, making discovery of causal links all the more difficult. They can also result in effects that are irreversible or that take many generations to remediate. For example, some persistent (long-lasting in the environment) and bioaccumulative (concentrating in fatty tissue) pollutants can remain in the environment for decades or even centuries, affect people far away (in space and time) from their actual use, and can cause impacts long after their use has been discontinued. In many indigenous Arctic communities, fish and other food sources have become contaminated with mercury, PCBs, and other pollutants (Suk and others, 2004). Traditional food sources are of vital nutritional, cultural, and social value to these communities, and they confront the dilemma of feeding their children contaminated foods or depriving them of these important benefits.

In addition to these uncertain yet direct impacts of environmental pollution on health, there are indirect effects that are often difficult to link back to their root causes. For example, global warming caused by industrial pollution may result in extreme weather events and drought, leading to the spread of new infectious disease or otherwise adversely affecting health (Chapter Eleven). Poor land-use patterns and lack of public transportation can lead to increased use of automobiles and air pollution and also safety risks, childhood obesity, and subsequent diabetes (Chapters Sixteen and Seventeen). The World Health Organization's *World Health Report 2002* (WHO, 2002) discusses concerns about *risk transition,* in which nations move from one set of environmental health risks (for example, risks such as diarrheal disease from poor water quality or inadequate sanitation) to another (risks such as respiratory disease or cancer from industrial pollution and increased consumption) (see Chapter Thirteen).

With our increasing knowledge about the complexities of ecosystems, the human body, and the impacts of various stressors, scientists are realizing that they understand much less about the links between environmental degradation and disease than they had thought. As zoologist and former president of the American Association for the Advancement of Science Jane Lubchenco (1998) has noted: "Humans have unwittingly embarked upon a grand experiment with our planet. The outcome of this experiment is unknown but has profound implications for all of life on Earth" (p. 492).

Limitations in Scientific Knowledge

Our capacity to identify adverse human health or environmental effects is limited by the present state of scientific knowledge. A lack of comprehensive knowledge about many environmental health risks makes knowing what to look for and where to look extremely difficult (Box 29.3 offers an example). Scientific knowledge is especially limited on the variability of ecological systems and the effects of pollution on health. The question for decision makers is, How can science establish an *assimilative capacity*—a predicable level of harm from which an ecosystem can recover—or a "safe" level of exposure when the exact effect and its magnitude, distribution, and interconnections are poorly characterized?

Box 29.3. Lack of Knowledge of Chemical Toxicity

Most people think that industrial chemicals on the market and in everyday products such as cleaners have been tested for their toxicity and have been "approved" for use. Unfortunately, this is not the case. Toxicity testing for industrial chemicals provides an important example of the uncertainties involved and the limitations of current approaches to environmental decision making. Under the Toxic Substances Control Act, chemical manufacturers and importers are required to submit available data related to the potential health effects of new chemicals. The U.S. Environmental Protection Agency (EPA) may then require additional testing before that chemical reaches the market. Companies are also required under Section 8(e) of the Act to submit evidence of substantial risk if that becomes available once the substance is on the market. They are also required to submit data when test rules are issued by the EPA. As early as 1984, the U.S. National Academy of Sciences noted the overwhelming lack of data on the health effects of industrial chemicals. The academy found that 78 percent of the chemicals in highest-volume commercial use had not undergone even "minimal" toxicity testing.

Studies in the late 1990s by the Environmental Defense Fund (now Environmental Defense) and the EPA found that the situation had not improved some fourteen years later. For the almost 3,000 high production volume (HPV) chemicals, those produced in or imported into the United States in quantities of over 1 million pounds per year, the studies noted the following: 93 percent lack some basic chemical-screening data; 43 percent have no basic toxicity data; 51 percent of chemicals on the EPA's Toxics Release Inventory lack basic toxicity information; and a large percentage of the available information deals only with acute toxicity. As a result of this lack of information, in 1998 Vice President Gore ordered screening-level testing for these HPV chemicals, to be conducted by industry. Although this initiative will provide important screening data on a good number of the HPV chemicals, it will not yield information on health effects not covered by the screening (such as developmental toxicity) or on exposure, interactions, or human risk. Further, the EPA, which will collect the data and place publicly available summaries on the Internet, has yet to determine which if any preventive actions it might take on the basis of the data received.

Source: Adapted from Environmental Defense, 2005; EPA, 1998.

Many substances once thought benign, such as chlorofluorocarbons (used in propellants and ultimately demonstrated to affect the ozone layer), have been shown to harm human health or the environment. Case studies and commonsense scientific observation often suggest causal links decades before those links are proven. For example, concerns about the health hazards of asbestos and benzene were identified as early as 1898, yet preventive actions for workplace exposures did not occur until the 1980s. The health effects of lead have been known for hundreds of years, yet a large percentage of children around the world are still exposed at levels above the 10 $\mu g/dl$ level of concern for cognitive effects (and the level of concern is dropping below 10 $\mu g/dl$ as our understanding of the effects of lead on the developing brain increases). Waiting for "convincing" human evidence is often costly in terms of human health, ecological damage, and the resources needed for remediation (see Box 29.4). Further, even when preventive action is taken, problems may persist for long periods of time after direct exposure is stopped. For example Dutch research indicates that children exposed to current background levels of PCBs are at risk of adverse cognitive effects, despite the restrictions placed on these chemicals some twenty-five years ago (Vreugdenhil and others, 2003; European Environment Agency, 2002).

Box 29.4. Late Lessons from Early Warnings

There are numerous examples of preventive actions that took place years or decades after early evidence suggested that environmental hazards existed. For example, in 2002 the European Environment Agency (EEA) published a report titled *Late Lessons from Early Warnings* that outlined fourteen case studies of precaution and prevention not taken. Not acting on early warnings can have very high costs for human health and the economy. Consider the examples of asbestos and lead.

Asbestos

Throughout Western Europe during the early 1900s, reports on lung diseases and cancers linked these diseases to exposure to asbestos dust. While European and American medical communities were documenting emerging associations between illness and exposure, however, governments were slow to implement restrictions. One example of government's unwillingness to act in the absence of hard proof of a link between asbestos exposure and lung disease occurred in The Netherlands.

By 1949, the Dutch government had recognized asbestosis as an occupational disease, but it did not act to prevent exposure until 1977, with a ban on the spraying of so-called blue asbestos. Despite mounting evidence that linked asbestos to mesothelioma, a cancer in the lining of the chest or abdomen, almost thirty years passed after asbestos was recognized as a threat to health before preventive measures were taken. Similarly, evidence that all types of asbestos were toxic, not just the blue type, continued to accumulate throughout the 1980s, yet it was not until 1993 that all asbestos was banned from manufacturing. Again the government delayed restriction, this time until 1998, when it extended the ban to the greater public, after almost a century of warnings.

Had the Dutch government acted in 1949 when it first suspected that asbestos posed a health risk, 3,000 consumer products containing asbestos would have been kept from the market. Instead, 1.4 million tons of asbestos were added to the environment, and it is estimated that tens of thousands of workers were exposed to airborne fibers before the 1993 ban. The ultimate cost in lives and dollars can not yet be totaled, because just under half of the asbestos manufactured in the Netherlands remains in products and buildings. Researchers estimate that the number of people sickened by asbestos will peak in 2018, with over 1,400 patients per year, when asbestos-containing products begin to enter the waste stream. It is estimated that had action been taken in the late 1960s, as many as 34,000 lives would have been saved.

Lead

In the United States lead has long been recognized as a poison. By 1912, the National Lead Company was already taking extensive safety measures to protect its workers. Experts advised that leadless paints be developed in reaction to the growing number of painters hospitalized for lead poisoning—indeed, in 1910 and the decade that followed, several European countries banned the use of lead in paint. Despite these early warnings, General Motors soon introduced leaded gasoline to American motorists. By 1924, reports of lead-related neurological disorders were becoming more common, and doctors cautioned that widespread damage could be done before the public or the government would be aware of it. Those warnings were ignored and leaded gasoline continued to be produced for another sixty years.

Years later, the consequences of this exposure have been seen mostly in children. A 1997 study found that the lead concentration in the blood of American five-year-olds (some twenty years after lead was banned in gasoline) was still sufficient to cause an average drop of .675 IQ points per child. Quite apart from the social implications of such widespread effects on a generation, researchers estimate that this effect over the years on IQs results in a national economic loss of $43.4 billion per year. More recent research indicates that previous estimates of safe levels of lead exposure may not be sufficient to protect children from neurological impacts.

Source: Asbestos example adapted from Heerings, 2000; lead example adapted from Markowitz and Rosner, 2002; Landrigan and others, 2002.

Cumulative and Interactive Effects

Traditional decision-making strategies have focused on single-agent, single-medium effects, when in reality humans and ecosystems are exposed to a wide variety of physical, biological, and chemical stressors. For example, in developing countries such as those in Africa or Central America, citizens are faced with such stressors as poverty, microbial contamination of water and food, severe air pollution in cities, and exposure to pesticides used in agriculture. How these stressors interact to result in health impacts is unknown. In general, complex systems pose greater uncertainty in defining and analyzing problems. Environmental science is only beginning to address the cumulative effects of the wide range of stressors to which humans and ecosystems are subjected.

Susceptible Subpopulations

Evidence and understanding of the disproportionate impacts of environmental degradation on specific populations are increasing. Certain groups may be at higher risk of adverse effects owing to genetic predisposition, disease status, developmental status, social status, and geographic location. For example, children have a unique susceptibility to the effects of toxic substances due to their immature metabolic processes, rapid development, and higher exposures (see Chapter Twenty-Eight). The responses of sensitive subpopulations and the highly variable responses to environmental insults among members of any exposed group are frequently overlooked in environmental decision-making.

Uncertainty: A Frequent Obstacle to Prevention

Uncertainty is an inevitable aspect of many environmental risks. It is inevitable because humans operate in open, dynamic environments that are difficult to control. For example, variability among individuals generally cannot be reduced.

Complex, unpredictable, and uncertain systems may produce consequences that are unpredictable and irreversible.

Unfortunately, uncertainty is often ignored or its impacts minimized in environmental health research and policy. This can work against preventive activities: for example, preventive actions may be stalled while researchers are reducing uncertainties. Several types of uncertainty are involved when hazards to health and the environment are characterized, but only the first two in the following list are typically addressed in environmental health research and policy:

- *Parameter uncertainty.* This uncertainty arises when information about specific components of an analysis is missing or ambiguous. Typically, parameter uncertainty can be reduced by acquiring more information.
- *Model uncertainty.* Models are theoretical constructs with the purpose of explaining or predicting events. Models of environmental systems, at best, show only a simplified and incomplete picture of reality. Model uncertainty arises when gaps in scientific theory or information result in imprecision in a model, such as a dose-response model.
- *Systemic or epistemic uncertainty.* This is uncertainty about the effects of cumulative or additive exposures and about interconnections that science cannot readily understand. This type of uncertainty increases as the scope of an analysis increases.

Two nonscientific forms of uncertainty also exist. *Smokescreen uncertainty* is what is created by critics of preventive public policy measures when they hide or fail to study potential impacts or when they set up studies to increase the appearance of uncertainty (Fagin and Lavelle, 1996). *Politically induced uncertainty* is what is created when governmental agencies decide not to study a hazard, purposely limit the list of alternatives considered or the scope of analysis, or hide uncertainty in quantitative models. A large determinant of ignorance and uncertainty may be the choice not to perform research in certain areas.

Uncertainty analysis tends to address only known uncertainties. Two more profound uncertainties—indeterminacy and ignorance—are rarely considered. *Indeterminacy* is a quality that results in the inability to know something. When indeterminacy is present it reflects not only a lack of observed association between cause and effect but also a lack of linear relationships between upstream actions and downstream effects in open-ended systems with multiple influences. For example, it is nearly impossible to predict a chemical plant explosion because such explosions result from many overlapping technical and social factors (Perrow, 1984). Similarly, in developing countries, political and economic insecurity combined with biological and chemical stressors may make characterizing a particular environmental risk nearly impossible. *Ignorance* is the state of not knowing what we do not know (for example, not knowing what we are uncertain about). It too is intrinsic to the complexity of environmental problems and the limitations of analytical tools.

From this discussion on uncertainty, one might conclude that if only we had more scientific knowledge, we might be better able to prevent the impacts of the environment on health. Although this is partly true, preventive actions for even well-established risks are often slow and inadequate and often address only proximate causal factors and not root causes of illness (as demonstrated in Box 29.2). Thus it is important to institute policies to address both known risks, such as water contamination, and the more uncertain and often indirect contemporary risks that could in the future become important factors in disease and illness in humans.

A New Environmental Health Paradigm: Precaution

What society should do in the face of uncertainty about cause-and-effect relationships is necessarily a question of public policy, not science. The policy may be to act in the face of uncertainty, or it may be not to act and instead to study the problem further; both can be considered actions. Decision makers are called upon to bridge the gap between uncertain science (and the need for more information) and the political need to take action to prevent harm.

The concept of the *precautionary principle* is increasingly being raised in debates about such threats to health and the environment as climate change, as these threats become more complex, uncertain, and global. The need for precaution arises because of uncertainty and the potential costs of inaction in the face of uncertainty. If all potential hazards could be quantitatively assessed with minimal error, then it would be relatively easy to base policy decisions on quantitative analyses and little else. But in a world in which global weather, aquifers, and growing children still hold many mysteries, the best environmental policies need to be informed by the best available science but also guided by a principle of erring on the side of caution.

The precautionary principle encourages policies that protect human health and the environment in the face of uncertain risks. In this broad sense it is not a new concept. Precaution, like prevention, is firmly rooted in centuries of medical and public health theory and practice, as noted earlier in this chapter. The Hippocratic injunction, "First do no harm," underscores a duty to prevent damage to health. Public health practitioners study the story of John Snow, who famously removed the handle from the Broad Street pump and stopped a cholera epidemic, basing his decision to do so solely on observation, informed judgment, and an incomplete understanding of the illness. Florence Nightingale, the mother of modern nursing, noted that pure air and pure water—"removing the offensive thing, not its smell"—were critical to a healthy home, even though the impacts of particular contaminants were not well known to her or others at the time (Tickner, 2002).

In 1998, the U.S. Institute of Medicine issued a report on the future of public health affirming the public health requirement "that [both] continuing and emerging threats to the health of the public be successfully countered. These threats include the immediate crises, such as the AIDS epidemic; enduring problems, such as injuries and chronic illness; and growing challenges, such as the aging of our population and the toxic by-products of a modern economy, transmitted through air, water, soil, or food" (IOM, 1988, p. 19). This definition suggests that a preventive approach to environmental health should also be precautionary, addressing known risk factors as well as complex and uncertain determinants and creating more sustainable policies, economic activities, and lifestyles.

Roots of the Precautionary Principle

As a principle of environmental and health decision making, the precautionary principle has its roots in the German *Vorsorgeprinzip.* An alternative translation of this word is "forecaring principle," or "foresight principle," which has the advantage of emphasizing anticipatory action, a proactive idea with a connotation slightly different from precautionary action, which to many sounds reactive and even negative. The *Vorsorgeprinzip* was established to deal with serious emerging, but not proven, risks to ecosystems and health. It is based on the concept that society should seek to avoid environmental damage by careful social planning that can stimulate innovation, job creation, and sustainable development. Although it has its roots in 1970s German environmental policy, over the past twenty-five years this principle has served as a guiding element in international treaties addressing marine pollution, ozone-depleting chemicals, genetically modified organisms, fisheries, climate change, and sustainable development (Raffensperger and Tickner, 1999; O'Riordan, Cameron, and Jordan, 2001).

The 1994 Maastricht Treaty, which formed the European Union, establishes precaution, the prevention of pollution at its source, and the "polluter pays" principle, as central elements of European environmental health policy. Though not explicitly mentioned, precaution also underscores many health and environmental policies enacted throughout the world and designed to protect health and the environment in the face of uncertain risks. These include food safety policies, clean water and clean air policies, and occupational health and chemical substitution policies. For example, drug regulation throughout much of the world is based on the precautionary notion that pharmaceuticals should be proven safe and effective before people are exposed to them and that manufacturers have a responsibility to act on knowledge of unintended impacts.

Definitions of the Precautionary Principle

There are two commonly cited definitions of the precautionary principle. One appears in the declaration of the 1992 United Nations Conference on Environment and Development (known as the Rio Declaration) and the other in the 1998 Wingspread Statement on the Precautionary Principle.

The Rio Declaration states: "In order to protect the environment, the precautionary approach shall be widely applied by States according to their capabilities. Where there are threats of serious or irreversible damage, lack of full scientific certainty shall not be used as a reason for postponing cost-effective measures to prevent environmental degradation." The Wingspread Statement on the Precautionary Principle states: "When an activity raises threats of harm to human health or the environment, precautionary measures should be taken even if some cause and effect relationships are not fully established scientifically" (Raffensperger and Tickner, 1999, pp. 353–354).

Even though definitions of the precautionary principle differ (as is often the case in international policy), they all have similar elements: if there is uncertainty, yet credible scientific evidence or concern about threats to health exists, precautionary measures should be taken. In other words, preventive action should be taken on early warnings even though the nature and magnitude of the risk are not fully understood.

Implementing the Precautionary Principle

Implementing the precautionary principle in order to protect health and ecosystems from risks requires new approaches to environmental science and policymaking to make them more effective at anticipating those risks and at promoting cost-effective alternatives to risky activities, products, and processes. Applying the precautionary principle in environmental health should involve the elements outlined in the following paragraphs.

Shifting the Questions Asked in Environmental and Health Policy. One fundamental change the precautionary principle encourages is that scientists and policymakers begin to ask a new set of questions about activities and potential hazards. Instead of asking, What level of risk is acceptable? or, How much contamination can a human or ecosystem assimilate? we ask, How much contamination can we avoid while still achieving our goals? What are the alternatives or opportunities for prevention? and, Is this activity needed in the first place?

This shift reorients the focus of environmental policies and regulations, moving it from analysis of problems to analysis of solutions and establishment of goals. It fosters examining a product or activity as a whole and asking whether its purpose can be served in a less harmful and possibly more effective way, rather than simply narrowly examining one aspect of that product or activity (the amount of harm it might cause). A focus on seeking safer alternatives may also allow decision makers to partially bypass contentious and costly debates over proof of harm and causality, dedicating scarce public health resources to solutions.

Shifting Presumptions. In addition to switching the questions decision makers ask about environmental risks, the precautionary principle shifts the presumptions used in decision making. Rather than presume that specific substances or economic activities are safe until proven dangerous, the precautionary principle establishes a presumption in favor of protecting the environment and public health in the face of uncertain risks. This places the responsibility for developing information, regular monitoring, demonstrating relative safety, analyzing alternatives, and preventing harm on those undertaking potentially harmful activities.

Conducting Transparent and Inclusive Decision-Making Processes. Environmental health decisions tend to be primarily policy decisions informed by science and values. A more participatory process for decision making would be appropriate to the precautionary principle and could improve the ability of decision makers to anticipate and prevent harm to ecosystems and human health. There are several important reasons for establishing more democratic environmental decision-making processes. Nonexperts, thinking broadly and not being bound by disciplinary constraints, see problems, issues, and solutions that experts miss; lay judgments reflect a sensitivity to social and political values and common sense that experts' models do not acknowledge; and the lay public may have a better capacity than experts alone for accommodating uncertainty and correcting errors. Finally, broader public participation may increase the quality, legitimacy, and accountability of complex decisions (Tickner, 2001).

Although the terms *precaution* and *prevention* are often used interchangeably, a preventive decision is not necessarily also precautionary: for example, the preventive decisions to phase out lead in gasoline and to take action to prevent smoking were not also precautionary. But precautionary decisions should necessarily be preventive as well. They should not simply transfer risks from humans to ecosystems, from workers to consumers, and so on. Ideally, implementing precaution involves shifting our attention upstream in the chain of health determinants.

Critiques of the Precautionary Approach

Although the precautionary principle may sound like common sense, it has engendered substantial criticism. In particular it has been criticized for being against the tenets of sound science, stifling innovation, causing unintended consequences potentially more serious than the problem that triggered the precautionary action in the first place, creating *false positives* (apparent risks that waste resources and distract from real problems), and providing insufficient guidance for decision making (Holm and Harris, 1999; Graham and Weiner, 1995; Tickner, Kriebel, and Wright, 2003). These critiques, and also complaints about the high costs of action, have often been applied to prevention measures as well. The following sections address each of these criticisms of the precautionary principle.

It Is Against the Norms of Sound Science. When the precautionary principle is discussed in the context of its relationship to science, it is often portrayed either as antiscience or as a risk-management principle that is implemented only after objective scientific enquiry takes place. In practice this is not the case. The current focus and methods of scientific inquiry may often implicitly work against action in the face of uncertainty, narrowly focusing inquiry on single disciplines and phenomena in spite of the fact that the environmental problems we face are much more complex than any single set of research methods can evaluate. Current scientific practice also focuses on those aspects of a problem that are quantifiable or researchable with limited resources and often misses the multiple stressors to which humans are exposed or overlooks vulnerable subpopulations. A narrowed research focus may mean that important aspects of the problem are missed. Worse, scientists and policymakers might mistakenly conclude that there is no evidence of harm when in fact the problem is a lack of evidence.

As environmental science faces the increasing challenges presented by more complex risks with greater uncertainty and ignorance, the nexus between science and preventive policy becomes ever more important. In this context, precaution is entirely consistent with good science; rather than demanding less science, it demands more rigorous and transparent science that provides insights into the ways health and ecosystems are disrupted by technologies, identifies and assesses opportunities for prevention and restoration, and makes clear where the gaps are in our current understanding of risks. A shift to more precautionary policies creates opportunities and challenges for scientists to think differently about the way they conduct studies and communicate results. The 2001 Lowell Statement on Science and the Precautionary Principle, drafted by eighty-five scientists from seventeen countries, outlines changes in science and science policy that would allow scientific inquiry to more effectively address uncertain, complex risks, including the following changes (Tickner, 2003):

- A more effective linkage between research on hazards and expanded research on primary prevention, safer technological options, and restoration;
- Increased use of interdisciplinary approaches to science and policy, including better integration of qualitative and quantitative data;
- Innovative research methods for analyzing the cumulative and interactive effects of various hazards to which ecosystems and people are exposed; for examining impacts on populations and systems; and for analyzing the impacts of hazards on vulnerable sub-populations and disproportionately affected communities;
- Systems for continuous monitoring and surveillance to avoid unintended consequences of actions, and to identify early warnings of risks; and
- More comprehensive techniques for analyzing and communicating potential hazards and uncertainties (what is known, not known, and can be known).

A more precautionary approach to science would ensure that research is informed by the most *appropriate science,* which can be understood as choosing methods and tools to fit the nature and complexity of the problem. This would include identifying ways to involve numerous data sources and constituencies in the scientific evaluation process, as well as examining the whole of the evidence rather than its separate parts.

It Stifles Innovation. Adopting the precautionary principle does not mean adopting rigid prohibitions against new technologies. Absolute proof of safety is impossible; the challenge for policymakers is to find the balance between potential risk and social benefit. For example, some proponents of genetically modified food claim that the precautionary principle blocks development and use of this technology on the basis of a hypothetical risk, with negative consequences for feeding the hungry in less developed countries. However, a precautionary approach to regulation of this technology would begin by clarifying its intended purposes. Is the purpose of genetic modification of food to increase food production, to support a more ecologically sustainable form of agriculture, or to create business opportunities? Once the purpose is identified, alternative methods of achieving this purpose should be identified and weighed against the genetic technology, both in terms of efficacy and potential risks (costs and benefits). This alternatives analysis should be very broad—examining a wide range of food production strategies and including the full range of interested parties. A thorough search for alternative ways to achieve the same social goals will often identify technologies that should be encouraged.

It Creates New Risks and Unintended Consequences. Avoiding unintended negative consequences of technologies or policies is an important aspect of the precautionary principle. Well-intended precautionary public health interventions can and often do result in serious adverse consequences (sometimes called risk trade-offs). Often, however, these adverse consequences are the result of incomplete analysis, lack of foresight, and inadequate consideration of uncertainties rather than a failure of precaution.

Critics have suggested, for example, that the precautionary principle might dictate a ban on the pesticide DDT because of that pesticide's long-term environmental effects, with serious negative consequences for the control of mosquitoes that spread malaria. DDT is cheap, effective, and readily available but also persistent in the environment, with significant ecological and possible human impacts. Application of the precautionary principle would not result in simply banning DDT and abandoning those at risk for malaria. Precaution would demand evaluation of a variety of potential mechanisms of harm, the assessment of alternatives, and the participation of those potentially affected by the choice of malaria prevention strategies. The nonprecautionary error is to begin from too small a set of options—either spray a pesticide with uncertain human impacts or let people die from malaria.

It Creates False Positives. Another concern raised against precaution is that it may lead to acting against false-positive risks, to overregulation that diverts important resources from real risks. A decision to act on limited knowledge about a hazard may ultimately turn out to have been due to a false positive, but if it spurs innovation, stimulates new economic forces, and raises awareness of ecological cycles and other lessons of sustainability, then it may still be judged to have been a worthwhile decision.

For example, arguments that organic food is safer than conventional food because of its lack of pesticide residues may in the end be considered a false positive because research has not demonstrated clear health benefits associated with organic food. A 2003 study found that compared to children fed conventional foods, children who consumed a primarily organic diet had one-sixth the levels of organophosphate pesticide metabolites in their urine (Curl, Fenske, and Elgethun, 2003). This study is important because it indicates that an organic diet may reduce exposure to certain pesticides. One might decide, on a precautionary basis, that this reduction in exposure is sufficient justification to buy organic foods, but this is very different from the risk-based approach in which one would wait for strong evidence that these levels of pesticides were harmful before trying to avoid them. Because of the limits of observational epidemiology, this strong evidence of risk may never be found. Thus, from the narrow perspective of traditional risk assessment, buying organic foods for health reasons may represent a false positive.

However, there are myriad other indirect benefits from promoting organic agriculture, including increased biodiversity, reduced use of synthetic fertilizer and pesticides (which can contaminate soil, air, and surface water and groundwater, and lead to human exposure), reduced energy use, and improved farmworker health.

It Does Not Provide Enough Guidance on How Decisions Should Be Made. By itself the precautionary principle (and, indeed, prevention too) provide little guidance on methods for evaluating problems and solutions and making decisions. There is no recipe for precaution (or for prevention); however, a heuristic—a process flow that guides sound decision making—can be useful. Such an approach (outlined in Box 29.5) allows learning based on accumulated knowledge; it also allows understanding and the flexibility to adapt decisions to the specific characteristics of an environmental health problem.

Box 29.5. A Preventive and Precautionary Decision-Making Process Flow

1. Problem Scoping (defining the problem broadly so as to examine proximate and root causes of impacts)

- What is the activity to be addressed, and why is it of concern as an environmental health risk?
- What is the full range of plausible impacts, and do indirect impacts need to be considered?
- Who or what are the affected populations, and will some be disproportionately affected?
- What are the research and information needs for characterizing the risk?
- Who is responsible for studying the risk, providing information, or taking appropriate preventive actions?
- Who should be involved in decision making, and at what points during the process?

2. Environmental and Health Impact Analysis (conducting a multidisciplinary examination of potential impacts)

- How severe are potential impacts from the activity?
- What is the nature and intensity of exposure, who is exposed, and are there disproportionate exposures?
- How strong is the evidence of existing or potential impacts from the activity?
- What are the types of uncertainties, and what is their significance?
- Can the uncertainties be reduced through further study?
- What are the magnitude and the severity of potential impacts, including spatial and temporal scales, susceptible subpopulations, reversibility, cumulative effects, and links to other hazards?

3. **Alternatives Assessment (examining a wide range of alternatives to the activity)**

- Are technology or policy options available that would reduce or eliminate the impacts of this activity?
- Is this activity necessary, or what is the purpose of the agent?
- Do alternative options present potential trade-off risks or unintended consequences that should be considered and addressed in implementation?
- What are the pros and cons of the various options?

4. **Implementation of Preventive and Precautionary Actions (determining the appropriate course of action)**

- What other considerations must be included in the decision—cost effectiveness, least burdensome option, technical feasibility, political and cultural feasibility, adaptability?
- What interventions, such as technical assistance, information, or technology support, are needed to ensure adoption of the precautionary changes?
- Can uncertainty be reduced in practical timescales and without excessive cost?
- Can the full cooperation of the activity proponent be ensured in monitoring, reviewing, and implementing the action?
- What types of monitoring, surveillance, and feedback should be instituted to ensure early warnings of unintended consequences and continuous reductions of environmental impacts?

Causality: When Do We Know Enough to Act or Not to Act?

As noted throughout this chapter, many environmental health risks are complex and the result of multiple interacting variables. Establishing causal relationships, linking a particular exposure with a particular adverse outcome, can be very difficult and often misleading. Traditionally, while additional information on the risks of an activity is sought, the default assumption—either implicitly or explicitly—is that the risk is not real.

In 1965, statistician Bradford Hill proposed a set of considerations to guide scientists and policymakers in assessing whether an observed association is likely to be causal. Now widely used (and often misinterpreted) by scientists and decision makers to make determinations of causality, these considerations are strength of association, consistency across studies, specificity of effects, dose-response, temporality of effects, plausibility of effects, coherence with other knowledge, evidence from experiments, and analogy based on experience. Hill advised broad interpretation of the evidence with respect to these considerations, to ensure that associations not be discounted simply because there is insufficient evidence or understanding about a hazard at a particular point in time. He noted: "What I do not believe—and this has been suggested—is that we can usefully lay down some hard and fast rules of evidence that must be obeyed before we accept cause and effect." According to Hill, causal judgments must not require perfect information, and causality must be considered in the context of available knowledge, informed judgment, and a responsibility to prevent impacts to health. Hill noted: "All scientific work is incomplete—whether it be observational or experimental. All scientific work is liable to be upset or modified by advancing knowledge. That does not confer upon us a freedom to ignore the knowledge we already have or to postpone the action that it appears to demand at a given time" (pp. 299–300).

The critical question for decision makers and public health practitioners under a precautionary and preventive approach is not causality but rather whether there is enough evidence to act to prevent a particular risk (Box 29.6 offers an example). In this respect environmental science, being an applied science, serves the purpose of informing policy, of helping decision makers understand when and if there is enough evidence to act. How one determines whether there is enough evidence to act should vary depending on the nature of the problem and be a function of the following:

- The available knowledge and accumulated understanding
- The complexity, magnitude, and uncertainty of the risk
- The presence of high-risk populations
- The availability of options to prevent the risk
- The potential implications of not acting to prevent the risk
- Social and public values
- A public health responsibility to protect health

Box 29.6. When Do We Know Enough to Act? The Case of Phthalates in Baby Toys

An environmental health example of redefining when we know enough to act is the approach taken by the Danish government over the use of phthalate plasticizers in children's toys. Phthalates are used to make polyvinyl chloride toys flexible and are also used as solvents in cosmetics (such as nail polish). They are among the most widely dispersed chemicals in the environment and are widely found in human blood and urine as well as household dust. The most widely used phthalate, diethylhexyl phthalate, is an animal carcinogen and adversely affects the kidneys and respiratory system. Of greatest concern is the fetal and neonatal reproductive toxicity of the phthalates, which can affect the testes and sperm production and development and can cause defects in the developing embryo.

When concerns were raised about the use of these chemicals (in particular, diisononyl phthalate) in children's teething toys, the Danish government weighed the clear evidence of exposure and the uncertain toxicity of the chemical, the unique vulnerability of children to environmental insults, the existing availability of alternatives, and the need for such toys and then determined that precaution should be applied to phase these chemicals out of toys used by small children. In the United States, in contrast, the Consumer Product Safety Commission (CPSC)—which must quantitatively demonstrate harm before acting—undertook expensive and somewhat unrealistic research that used adult volunteers to measure children's exposure. The CSPC came to the conclusion that the risk to children was likely low but also that there was a great deal of uncertainty about the risk and that companies should voluntarily remove phthalates from toys. The ultimate result in both the United States and Denmark was the same—the chemicals were removed from the toys—but the cost in time (resulting in additional exposures to children) and resources to achieve that result was much greater in the United States.

Source: Adapted from Kriebel and others, 2001.

Tools for Applying a Preventive and Precautionary Approach to Environmental Health

Precautionary and preventive actions may involve instituting surveillance of workers and communities, informing the public about risks and uncertainties while further study is undertaken to characterize the risks, setting workplace exposure limits and restrictions on potentially harmful activities, and phasing out activities that have been found particularly problematic. Multiple preventive actions should be taken and should be case specific, depending on the nature of the risk, who is exposed (for example, disproportionately affected or highly vulnerable communities), technological and economic feasibility, and preventability of the risk. Taking preventive action should be considered a continuous, iterative process. Such interventions should designed to be cost effective (meaning least costly for achieving a particular goal) and when possible should have effects that are synergistic (addressing several risks at once) and win-win (good for health and the economy). (See the example in Box 29.7.)

Box 29.7. The Natural Step: Systems Thinking for Environmental Health and Sustainability

Karl-Henrik Robèrt

In the 1980s, Swedish physician and cancer researcher Karl-Henrik Robèrt had some important insights. Studying the growth of normal and malignant cells, he observed that human cells, animal cells, and plant cells shared many structures and functions; we are very much a part of nature. He also found that the parents of his pediatric cancer patients were wonderfully dedicated; there seemed to be no limit to the sacrifices they were prepared to make for their children. Meanwhile, casting his gaze outside the hospital, he saw a global decline in per capita productivity of renewable resources. He felt that mankind was running into the open end of a funnel, squeezed by both declining life-sustaining resources and increasing demands. Each unit of production from forests, farmland, and waterways was requiring progressively more inputs—more pesticides and fertilizers for the same harvest, larger fishing boats to catch the same fish. The main problem, he thought, was not that we were running out of nonrenewable resources such as petroleum. Rather, the life-sustaining resources that provide clean water, fresh air, and food, and also spiritual inspiration, were being progressively sullied by waste. Heavy metals were accumulating in soils; organic chemicals were accumulating in the upper reaches of food chains; greenhouse gases were accumulating in the atmosphere.

Robèrt took a systems view of these problems, much like the ecological approach described in Chapter One. Recognizing that human life is embedded in complex biogeochemical cycles, he analyzed relationships among human activities and natural conditions. He focused not only on contemporary imbalances but also on *trends.* Although pollutants in the environment were worrisome, the fact that pollutants were *steadily increasing* in concentration was more worrisome. Although the loss of certain species and habitats was worrisome, the *ongoing loss* of biodiversity was more worrisome. He viewed these and similar trends as system errors, which if uncorrected would propel society toward disaster—a "republic of grass and insects."

Finding solutions requires asking the right questions. Asking the right questions starts with knowing where you're going and how to define success. Success—in this case, sustainability—is defined according to basic principles: matter and energy are conserved; matter has a tendency to disperse (the principle of entropy, the second law of thermodynamics); the value of goods for human use grows out of their concentration, structure, and purity; photosynthesis is the primary producer in the system; and humans are inherently a social species. From these principles emerged the *system conditions* that define sustainability (Holmberg, Robèrt, and Eriksson, 1996). In a sustainable society, wrote Robèrt, nature is not subject to systematically increasing

1. Concentrations of substances extracted from the earth's crust
2. Concentrations of substances produced by society
3. Degradation by physical means

And in that society

4. People are not subject to conditions that systematically undermine their capacity to meet their needs.

Health can be defined on an individual level, but from a systems perspective, and in the context of these system conditions, we also need to define health on a global level. The system conditions are requirements not only for sustainability but also for population health.

A fundamental feature of the earth's ecosystems is complexity. Accordingly, the path to sustainability is complex and necessary decisions are not self-evident. Simply reacting to today's perturbations or imbalances is likely to create new problems. Instead, Robèrt took advantage of a systematic approach called *backcasting:* envisioning a successful outcome in the future, looking back from it to the present, and identifying the strategies that would be required to reach that success. Robèrt called for backcasting from the four system conditions and letting that process guide decisions (Holmberg and Robèrt, 2000). The actions that would follow are not surprising:

1. In producing goods, use more abundant minerals instead of scarce ones, use all mined materials efficiently, and systematically reduce dependence on fossil fuels.
2. Systematically phase out certain persistent and unnatural compounds in favor of ones that are normally abundant or that break down more easily in nature, and use all substances produced by society efficiently.
3. Draw resources only from well-managed ecosystems, systematically pursuing the most productive and efficient use both of those resources and land, and exercising caution in all kinds of modification of nature, for example, overharvesting and introductions.
4. Check whether our behavior has consequences for people, now or in the future, that restrict their opportunities to lead a fulfilling life.

These actions, and the tools that emerge from them, can be viewed as a long-range, systems-based approach to prevention. In fact these four actions conform closely to the precautionary principle described earlier in this chapter. Robèrt's approach is called The Natural Step Framework (Robèrt, 2002). It has been widely discussed and accepted in his native Sweden and in other parts of the world and applied both to corporate operations (Nattrass and Altomare, 1998) and to community development (James and Lahti, 2004).

The goals of preventive and precautionary actions should be (1) reducing and eliminating exposures to potentially harmful substances, activities, and other conditions, where feasible; (2) redesigning production processes, products, and human activities so as to minimize risks in the first place; (3) establishing public health goals for restoring human and ecosystem health; (4) providing information and education to citizens to promote empowerment and accountability; and (5) establishing a research agenda to characterize risks more comprehensively, provide *early warnings* that make possible rapid interventions to prevent damage to health, and develop safer technologies. In addition, application of the tools discussed here for preventive and precautionary decision making must be combined with efforts to address institutional, financial, and technical barriers to prevention and precaution.

Secondary Prevention Interventions

Secondary prevention interventions increase the ability of public health professionals to identify early warnings of risks and understand intervention impacts. This result can be achieved through screening, health tracking, and postmarketing surveillance. These activities can be considered *monitoring programs* that are designed to function at several levels: individual, population, and system.

Screening. At the individual level, screening identifies precursors of disease (a genetic defect or biomarker) or elevated exposures to an identified hazard (such as elevated blood lead). It can identify at-risk individuals and allow them to receive early therapeutic interventions or to be removed from the source of the risk (or have the source removed from them). A concern with this type of screening is potential discrimination against people on the basis of genetic or other susceptibility, which could prevent them from securing certain types of jobs or insurance.

Health Tracking and Public Health Surveillance. The predominant view of public health surveillance programs is that they work to identify public health concerns that need further investigation and examination or intervention so that rapid control and prevention programs can be developed, implemented, and evaluated. Surveillance (which focuses on the population level) focuses on tracking rates of cancer, birth defects, asthma, infectious disease, poisonings, and other diseases in a population. Such population-level screening allows greater examination of the risk factors for disease and identification of clusters of diseased individuals and of the factors that place them at risk. Given the results of such screening, targeted prevention programs (to reduce heart disease, for example) can be established. Surveillance can also focus on emissions of pollutants into water, air, or workplaces. Yet another surveillance target is ecosystem functioning. Such *ecological surveillance* uses ecosystem data as a surrogate for potential impacts in humans.

In addition to health tracking, public health programs are increasingly interested in what has been called *biomonitoring*, or *body burden testing*. This involves periodic testing of body fluids (blood, urine, and breast milk) and adipose tissue to examine levels and trends in specific indicator contaminants. The U.S. Centers for Disease Control and Prevention, through its National Exposure Survey, has been collecting biomonitoring information for several years, and the CDC notes some important prevention benefits of this activity, including: identification of who is in danger and who is at greater risk of exposures to dangerous chemicals, improved assessment of the efficacy of previous actions taken to protect health, improved decision making to plan for future exposure prevention, and improved emergency response.

Postmarketing Surveillance. In cases where a new technology may have great benefits and where its potential impacts are uncertain but likely reversible or not widespread, it may be acceptable to allow development of the technology to continue, with responsibility placed on the proponents to institute postmarketing surveillance and to make public any risk information that is developed through the use of the technology. Such an approach is commonplace in pharmaceutical regulation. Postmarketing surveillance includes undertaking toxicological and epidemiological tests to characterize potential risks more effectively. This approach can be applied as a way to measure the impacts (positive or negative) of both technologies and public health interventions as well as to identify early warnings of risks.

Primary Preventive and Health-Promoting Measures

Centerpieces of a preventive approach to environmental health are the concepts of *pollution prevention* and *cleaner production.* These two concepts involve changes to production systems and products to reduce pollution at the source (in the production process or product development stage). This includes reducing the raw material, energy, and natural resource inputs (dematerialization) as well as reducing the quantity and harmful characteristics of toxic substances used (detoxification) in production systems and products. A central aspect of pollution prevention and cleaner production is understanding the service that a production system, product, or activity provides (for example, chlorinated solvents provide degreasing in some production processes, carpeting provides floor covering) and seeking out safer alternatives to provide that same service.

According to the 1990 Pollution Prevention Act, pollution prevention involves activity that "(i) reduces the amount of any hazardous substance, pollutant, or contaminant entering any waste stream or otherwise released into the environment . . . prior to recycling, treatment, or disposal; and (ii) reduces the hazards to public health and the environment associated with the release of such substances, pollutants, or contaminants." It includes "equipment or technology modifications, process or procedure modifications, reformulation or redesign of products, substitution of raw materials, and improvements in housekeeping, maintenance, training, or inventory control." (See Box 29.8 for an example.)

Box 29.8. A Pollution Prevention Success Story: Toxics Use Reduction in Massachusetts

The Massachusetts Toxics Use Reduction Act (TURA) of 1989 is an example of a successful preventive and precautionary approach to the risks posed by toxic chemical use. The Act requires that manufacturing firms using specific quantities of some 190 industrial chemicals undergo a biyearly process to identify alternatives to reduce waste and the use of those chemicals. Companies come to understand what they are trying to achieve with a toxic chemical and how they are using it, measure impacts and progress, and systematically search for and analyze alternatives.

The Toxics Use Reduction Act does not instruct industrial facilities to identify the "safe" levels of use, emissions, or exposure for these chemicals. Any amount of use is considered too much. The Act does instruct firms to identify ways to redesign production processes and products and identifies six methods that can be applied for toxics use reduction. Several aspects of the toxics use reduction process make it a good example of using alternatives assessment to stimulate precautionary action:

- *Goal-setting.* The Commonwealth of Massachusetts has established a goal of a 50 percent reduction in toxic by-products (waste) through toxics use reduction techniques. The Act also instructs companies to set goals and priorities for toxics use reduction.
- *Alternatives assessment required.* Companies are required to complete a well-defined alternatives assessment process, with the result that they understand why they use a specific chemical (what service it provides) and how it is used in the production process. Companies also conduct a comprehensive financial, technical, environmental, and occupational health and safety analysis of viable alternatives. The environmental and health and safety analysis must ensure that toxics use reduction does not result in risks being shifted from workers to consumers or communities or vice versa. The firm is not required to undertake any particular option, but in many cases the economic and environmental or health and safety benefits provide enough justification for action.
- *Training and support.* Toxics use reduction plans must be certified by "planners" who have undergone a forty-eight-hour training course, and who receive subsequent continuing education, which seeks to give them the skills and mentality to examine options comprehensively. Technical and research support is provided to firms to complete the alternatives assessment and identify and examine potential options.
- *Follow-up.* Once a year, companies are required to measure their progress at reducing their use of toxic chemicals. This information is made publicly available.

Between 1990 and 2000, some 550 firms continuously participated in the Toxics Use Reduction Program and have reduced their total amount of toxic and hazardous waste by 58 percent and their use of the targeted toxic chemicals by 40 percent.

At the same time, the state saw a 90 percent drop in Toxics Release Inventory releases. In 1997, the state conducted an analysis of the Act, demonstrating that it had saved Massachusetts industry some $15 million over a seven-year period. This figure does not include the public health and environmental benefits gained through the program. In reviews of the toxics use reduction planning experience, regulated companies noted the importance of planning when asking simple questions about processes and opening doors to other problems.

Source: Adapted from Toxics Use Reduction Institute, 2004.

Cleaner production takes the pollution prevention definition a step further by involving the entire *life cycle* of a product, service, or other activity; it considers opportunities to reduce impacts from the extraction of raw materials, from the use of a product or service (including its subsidiary processes such as transport and packaging), and from a product's ultimate disposal. Environmental impacts can occur throughout this life cycle, as seen in Figures 29.2 and 29.3.

Cleaner production takes a cyclical view of production, identifying opportunities to prevent exposure and environmental impacts at all stages of the life cycle. Often the greatest impacts in the life cycle of a product or activity occur at its beginning (for example, mining) and its end (for example, incineration).

Two critical aspects of the pollution prevention and cleaner production approach are *materials accounting*—understanding why potentially harmful materials are used in a production process or product and how materials flow through the

FIGURE 29.2. THE PRODUCT LIFE CYCLE.

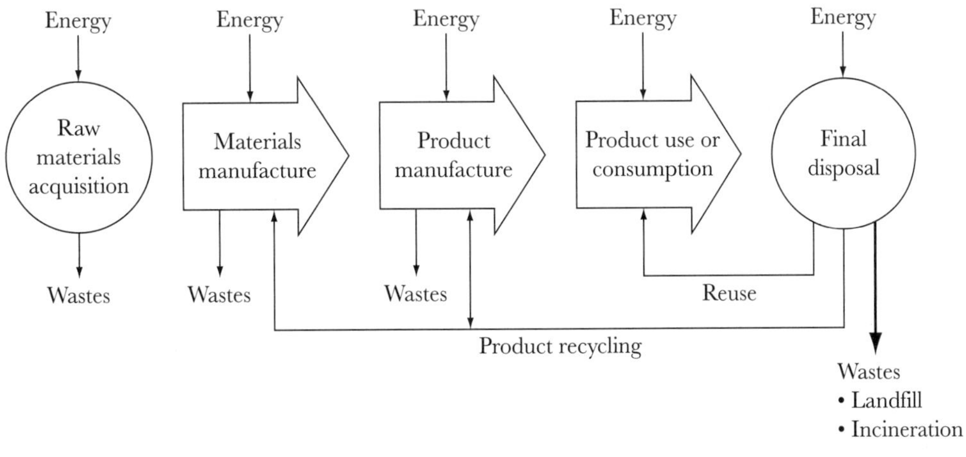

Source: Thorpe, 1999, p. 3.

FIGURE 29.3. CLEAN PRODUCTION IS BASED ON A CIRCULAR VISION OF THE ECONOMY.

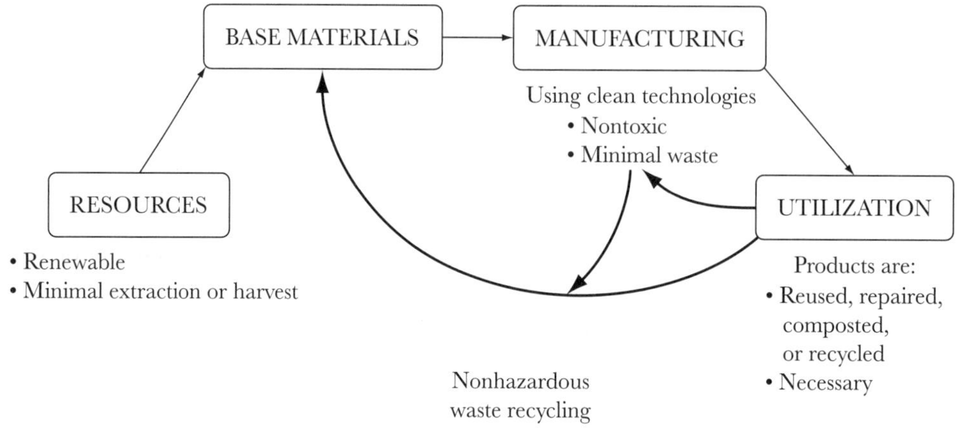

Source: Thorpe, 1999, p. 4.

product or production process life cycle—and *planning, identifying and examining a wide range of alternatives* (both existing and on the horizon) that could substantially reduce the impacts of that activity.

Because the release of pollution represents an inefficiency in a production process, application of pollution prevention and cleaner production approaches can have substantial economic and health benefits. Numerous case studies from around the world demonstrate the successes of prevention methods in practice (see Box 29.9). Application of pollution prevention can co-optimize environmental and occupational health and at the same time reduce other environmental impacts associated with production, such as water and energy use. Given these benefits many countries around the world have established cleaner production programs, and they have demonstrated success in reducing industrial and product-related pollution while reducing costs. The United Nations has established a network of *national cleaner production centers* in developing countries to provide technical support for building industrial production capacity in an environmentally friendly manner.

Box 29.9. Examples of Cleaner Production

- Clothes cleaning operations that use water instead of perchloroethylene (a chlorinated solvent)
- A program for controlling weeds on school grounds that uses manual weeding, soil aeration, and caulking

- A brewery whose organic wastes feed chickens whose wastes provide manure for a mushroom farm and energy to power the brewery
- A car-leasing program (*zip cars*) in which the individual does not own a car but has access to different types of cars, as needed
- A windup and solar-powered radio that is made out of recycled material, particularly useful in developing nations where batteries are not readily available
- A community whose living spaces, schools, retail outlets, and workplaces were designed to ensure close proximity, social connections, limited pollution, and access via foot, bicycle, or public transportation

The goals of cleaner production can be achieved through a number of subsidiary policy tools and techniques, such as the following (also see Thorpe, 1999):

- *Industrial ecology:* using wastes (material and energy) from one industrial process as inputs in another industrial process, a type of materials sharing often found in nature. In this way, for example, an industrial park can become a closed-loop system, with no waste ultimately generated and materials shared among the area's manufacturers.
- *Extended producer responsibility:* requiring product producers to assume environmental protection responsibility for their products throughout the full product life cycle, including taking products back when the useful life is finished. Extended producer responsibility provides an incentive to make products that are longer lasting and more durable; that are upgradable, reusable, and recyclable; and that minimize the use of toxic materials (because the producers will be responsible for managing these materials that become wastes at the end of the product life cycle).
- *Green chemistry:* developing chemical products that reduce or eliminate the generation of hazardous substances in their design, manufacture, and application. A subset of green chemistry is developing bio-based materials, those made from plant or other organic matter, and designing sustainable products.
- *Taxes, subsidies, and technical support:* using economic and information mechanisms to encourage voluntary compliance, discourage problematic behaviors and activities, and foster sustainable practices. These mechanisms might include *ecological taxes* on problematic products (such as cigarettes) and emissions (such as greenhouse gases), fees (such as on chemicals use), and liability for environmental degradation, so that when impacts do occur there is some accountability. Subsidies and technical support can assist firms and cities that wish to implement cleaner and safer technologies. Because governments are among the largest institutional purchasers of products and materials, *green public procurement*—whereby governments specify safer and more environmentally friendly materials in bidding processes—can have an enormous impact on the market for cleaner products and processes.

- *Integrated chemicals policy:* taking a comprehensive approach to managing the presence of chemicals in production processes, products, and the environment. For example, understanding the limitations of current efforts to manage the impacts of industrial chemicals on health, including the lack of information about most chemicals and the high levels of proof needed before action can be taken, the European Union is fundamentally reorienting its chemicals management efforts through a new policy called REACH—Registration, Evaluation, and Authorization of Chemicals. Under REACH, European manufacturers and importers of chemicals will need to provide, within eleven years, basic screening-level toxicity data, use data, and risk data on most chemicals in commerce produced in quantities of more than one ton per year or they will not be allowed to continue marketing the chemicals. Chemicals produced in large quantities and those of high concern will be evaluated by governments to determine additional research and policy intervention needs. Those chemicals that are persistent and bioaccumulative; are carcinogenic, reproductive toxicants, or mutagens; and those that present other concerns, such as respiratory sensitization or disruption of the hormone system, will be treated like drugs, meaning that any manufacturer that wants to use them or put them into products will have to demonstrate that there is no safer feasible or cost-effective alternative or that the risk can be safely controlled. The REACH program builds on several existing global programs designed to address chemicals that are *persistent organic pollutants,* or POPs. These are chemicals that persist and bioaccumulate and can travel far distances from where they are produced, for example, to Arctic areas, where native populations have in their body tissues some of the highest POPs levels recorded. In addition, in 2004 the United Nations Stockholm Convention on Persistent Organic Pollutants went into force in the signatory nations. It calls for an international phaseout of twelve industrial, pesticidal, and combustion by-product chemicals (such as DDT and PCBs), and also establishes a process for adding chemicals to the phaseout list.

The pollution prevention and cleaner production approach can be extended to a number of human activities that might affect the environment and health, including the following:

- *Pesticide use.* The use of pesticides in agriculture and general pest control is among the most important environmental risks to health, particularly that of children. The question is, How can the pest-control benefits of pesticide use be achieved through less chemically intensive techniques? The technique of integrated pest management (IPM) involves managing the root sources of pest infestations with a wide range of approaches, applying biological and physical controls and using only judicious amounts of the least toxic pesticides possible. As described in Chapter Twenty, the IPM approach can be applied not only in agriculture but also in pest control in buildings (schools, hospitals, and homes) and in lawns and flower gardens.

- *Construction.* Although shelter is a critical human need, construction uses more materials and creates more waste than most any other human activity. The built environment is becoming an important source of risk to health—ranging from exposure to dander from cockroaches to exposure to toxic chemicals and also raising waste disposal issues. *Green building* involves following basic principles for more healthy and environmentally friendly design that minimizes hazardous and nonhazardous materials, is energy efficient yet allows sufficient fresh air ventilation, minimizes buildup of allergens, and sites residential areas so as to minimize environmental impacts and improve air quality (for example, communities can be designed so as to minimize air pollution from transport and production facilities).
- *Energy production.* Energy production and use is another important global source of environmental and health impacts, as discussed in Chapter Fifteen. Substantial reductions in energy use could be achieved through simple conservation measures—making homes and buildings more energy efficient, increasing the fuel economy of cars, increasing the availability of public transport, and so forth. Renewable energy efforts focus on identifying alternative energy sources—such as wind, solar, and biomass power—that can reduce the reliance on nonrenewable fuels and also reduce global emissions of greenhouse gasses.
- *Land-use planning.* As noted in Chapter Sixteen, sprawl has been recently identified as an important cause of safety and health effects. Improved land-use planning can help communities avoid the problems of sprawl, poor transport infrastructure, and sedentary lifestyle that are important risk factors for injury and disease.
- *Restoration of contaminated sites.* Recent years have witnessed much discussion about the reuse of formerly contaminated sites. To avoid the types of problems that led to the original contamination, pollution prevention principles can be applied to ensure that new industries provide good jobs while minimizing their potential impacts on health and the environment.

Goal Setting for Environmental Health

Foresight involves outlining the type of world we wish to live in and the establishment of long-term goals for protection of health. Goal setting, coupled with development of short- and medium-term objectives, public policies (to address barriers to goal implementation and to minimize social disruptions), and metrics and indicators, focuses attention not on what futures are likely to happen but rather on how desirable futures can be achieved, a concept called *backcasting* (see Box 29.7).

Goal setting is a fairly common practice in public health. Examples are the smallpox eradication campaign, smoking cessation goals, and goals for reductions in certain types of disease, such as cancer. The U.S. Public Health Service's *Healthy People 2010* report lists two broad public health goals: increasing quality and years of healthy life and eliminating health disparities. The report contains some 450 objectives in twenty-eight focus areas, including environmental health, food safety, and occupational safety and health. The U.S. Department of Health and Human Services encourages public health practitioners to incorporate these goals into their activities and use them as a framework to promote healthy communities (U.S. Department of Health and Human Services, Public Health Service, 2000).

Several nonprofit groups have developed goals to reduce the environmental impacts of industrial activities. For example, the four system conditions of the Natural Step (see Box 29.7), provide a set of measures by which firms and governmental agencies can benchmark their progress toward more sustainable practices.

The northern European countries have been leaders in developing goal-setting processes for environmental health. These processes provide an excellent example of how prevention and precaution can serve as a compass, directing society toward practices that are ecologically sound, health promoting, and sustainable. In 1997, the Swedish Parliament passed a set of Environmental Quality Objectives for the millennium (Box 29.10). The overarching goal of these objectives it "to hand over to the next generation a society in which the main environmental problems have been solved." The goals that have been developed are issue based (water quality, forests, and so forth). They include implementation steps and measures to track progress.

Box 29.10. Sweden's Environmental Quality Goals

1. Reduced climate impact
2. Clean air
3. Natural acidification only
4. A non-toxic environment
5. A protective ozone layer
6. A safe radiation environment
7. Zero eutrophication
8. Flourishing lakes and streams
9. Good-quality groundwater

10. A balanced marine environment
11. Thriving wetlands
12. Sustainable forests
13. A varied agricultural landscape
14. A magnificent mountain landscape
15. A good built environment

Source: Swedish Environmental Protection Agency, Environmental Objectives Secretariat, 2005.

In some countries, such as The Netherlands, goal setting occurs at the firm or sector level; sectors establish five-year environmental plans (including goals and metrics) and enter into *covenants* with regulators that provide firms in each sector with the flexibility to achieve the plan's goals. If they fail to do so, however, regulations are imposed.

Environmental Health Indicators

An *environmental health indicator* is a feature of the environment that can be measured in order to characterize "magnitude of stress, habitat characteristics, degree of exposure to a stressor, or degree of ecological response to the exposure" (International Joint Commission, 1995). Indicators have several purposes. They provide decision makers with information about the health status of a community or a population, raise awareness and understanding about environmental degradation, and not least, measure progress toward established environmental health goals. By tracking progress and noting benchmarks, public health professionals, politicians, and the general public can assess the efficacy of current practices, programs, and policies and strategize ways to develop and implement more preventive approaches. For example, if a program intended to reduce the incidence of an environmentally mediated disease is found to be ineffective in meeting its objective, then public officials and the general public should implement alternative programs that have promise of succeeding.

Environmental health indicators may measure hazards, exposures, health effects, or intervention effectiveness and may assess health indirectly or directly. For example, the indicators laid out in *Healthy People 2010* will provide data on a variety of health issues. Outdoor air quality, for example, will be assessed through such means as direct measurement of hazardous air pollutants (ozone, particulate matter, and lead), and water quality will be examined through such means as the number of beach closings due to the presence of harmful bacteria.

A second type of environmental health indicator—indicators of ecosystem health (such as frog die-offs)—can be used as a surrogate for what may be occurring in human populations and can be particularly useful for diseases or illnesses that have long latency periods in humans but that occur earlier in animals with shorter life spans. Such indicators consider ecosystem vigor (the input available to an ecosystem), biodiversity, and resilience.

Environmental and Health Impact Analyses

Environmental impact analysis and health impact analysis (EIA/HIA) involve a comprehensive examination of risks and alternatives before a particular project, policy, or activity that may adversely affect health or ecosystems proceeds. The goals of EIA and HIA are to foster better decisions and the consideration of a broad range of alternative courses of action and potential impacts before an activity begins. The process of conducting these analyses starts with a broad scoping exercise in which potential direct and indirect impacts on health and on ecosystems are identified, along with historical or social resources. A full range of alternatives to the policy, project, or activity is then examined, including the option of not moving forward at all. The best option is then chosen, and procedures are put in place to minimize risks and monitor for problems. EIA and HIA are procedural, designed to internalize preventive and precautionary thinking in decisions, rather than substantive, requiring that a specific action to be taken (see Box 29.11).

Box 29.11. Noise and Health: Health Impact Analysis in Practice

Noise may be defined as unwanted sound. It has been identified as a physical, psychological, and environmental stressor. Specifically, noise has been linked to annoyance, sleep disturbance, cardiovascular disease, and impacts on children's health, with anxiety and learning disorders as secondary impacts.

The United Kingdom is in the process of reconciling its noise policies with the European Environmental Noise Directive of 2002. To that end, a health impact analysis was performed on the Mayor of London's Ambient Noise Strategy to minimize the health effects of noise on those living and working in London. In this case the HIA consisted of compiling existing relevant research into one publication. The following overview of this compilation can serve as a reference for policymakers concerned with noise and public health.

- Noise barriers around areas of heavy traffic helped in reducing annoyance, as did the creation of green spaces within the city environment and education programs focused on the source of the noise.
- Sleep disturbances are commonly caused by unfamiliar noises, often shifting sleepers from a deep sleep to a light sleep. Although those living near airports may

assume it is aircraft noise that disrupts their sleep, research shows that in fact traffic noise has a greater effect on sleeping habits, to the point that proximity to major roads is a predictor of insomnia.

- Noise probably affects the cardiovascular system by stimulating hormones, though the threat is relatively low compared to other risk factors, such as smoking. It is not yet known how the body would adjust to this stimulation when subject to loud noises on a continuous basis.
- The effect of noise on children has been well documented. Continuous loud noises in the home can lead to difficulty with learning, thinking, and understanding speech, as well as problems with memory, reading, problem solving, and attention.
- The physically and mentally ill are vulnerable to slower healing times in noisy environments.
- Those who are twenty-five to thirty-four years old, have children, and live in apartments are seven times as likely as older, childless property owners to be affected by noise, in some cases leading to responses of anger, depression, or fear.

Source: Adapted from London Health Commission, 2003.

Information Dissemination and Education

Information is a critical factor in prevention. Taken together, information and education are important public health tools that are relatively low cost yet can have substantial impacts in reducing environmental and health effects from activities. Information allows us to understand the risks of materials and activities and their alternatives; identify gaps in knowledge; identify the pollutants or activities of gravest concern; compare hazards and preventive actions across sectors, countries, and companies; and improve enforcement of environmental and health policies. Most important, information is critical to public empowerment and accountability—if people know about risks and the options for preventing them, they can take personal actions to reduce them or can hold government authorities or those who create the risks accountable for prevention. Information can also discourage behaviors that lead to risks, providing an incentive for those creating risks to consider and internalize the impacts of their activities and seek alternatives.

In occupational health, hazard communication has proved an important tool for helping workers to understand the potential impacts of chemicals used in their workplaces and to demand safer working conditions. Prior informed consent—a policy that gives a country an opportunity to deny access to a pesticide or hazardous chemical restricted in other countries—is an important tool for developing countries to use in making decisions on risks. So-called right-to-know laws in many countries have proven useful in encouraging business managers to reduce their pollution. For example, the U.S. Emergency Planning and Community Right to Know Act of 1986 requires that manufacturing firms using toxic chemicals report yearly on their wastes and emissions to the Toxics Release Inventory, a publicly accessible database. This database gives its users a better understanding of the pollution caused by a particular facility and has been an important incentive for facility pollution prevention activities. Finally, product labeling—for example, to identify products that are produced using organic methods, that contain potentially hazardous materials, or that are environmentally friendly—allows consumers to choose the products with the lowest impacts for a particular need.

A Preventive and Precautionary Environmental Health Research Agenda

Awareness and understanding are critical to prevention. That is why environmental health research needs to be a central part of any prevention strategy. A prevention-oriented research agenda will include tools for rapid identification of environmental hazards and potential exposures. It will develop tools to broaden our understanding of the unique susceptibility of some populations to environmentally related illnesses and of the linkages between genes and environment that can increase susceptibility. It will broaden our understanding of the complex determinants of environmentally related disease, including the proximate and root cause risk factors for specific impacts and the interactions between broad categories of risks (chemical, physical, climate, social); increase our knowledge of the cumulative effects of multiple risks; and allow us to project the long-term implications of today's actions for future generations (through, for example, integrated assessment methods). It will lead us to examine and develop a range of preventive options to reduce environmental risks while achieving good living standards for all people. It will also address metrics and surveillance techniques (such as health indicators) to measure progress toward reducing environmental risks and achieving more sustainable forms of development as well as identifying early warnings of impacts. An example of an aggressive, long-term, preventive and precautionary environmental health research agenda is the European Commission's 2003 Environment and Health Action Strategy, focused on understanding impacts of environmental hazards on children's health and on developing actions and evaluation to prevent impacts (European Commission, 2003).

Conclusion: Sustainable Development

The overarching goal of environmental efforts has been identified as achieving *sustainable development.* The application of prevention and precaution represent important steps toward this long-term goal. The 1987 Brundtland Commission, headed by former World Health Organization director and Norwegian prime minister Gro Harlem Brundtland, defined sustainable development as "development that meets the needs of the present without compromising the ability of future generations to meet their own needs" (World Commission on Environment and Development, 1987, p. 43). Sustainable development is traditionally viewed as having three pillars: environmental protection (conserving resources and promoting health ecosystems), economic efficiency (producing products and services that provide economic benefit), and social equity (ensuring that all people have a fair opportunity to meet their needs). In this respect, rather than being a static formula, sustainable development is a process of change in which exploitation of resources, investments, technology, and institutional policies are made consistent with present as well as future needs. Sustainable development emphasizes a long-term view and equity, improving the quality of life for everyone (ensuring the rights of the poor and of future generations). It stresses qualitative development over quantitative growth.

Sustainable development contains two subsidiary concepts: sustainable production and sustainable consumption. *Sustainable production* is defined as the production of goods and services using processes and systems that are nonpolluting; conserving of energy and natural resources; economically viable; safe and healthful for employees, communities, and consumers; and socially and creatively rewarding for all working people. *Production* can mean the creation of goods and services—through industrial processes, agricultural operations, commercial activities, and social and community activities—undertaken by both public and private actors. *Sustainable consumption,* in contrast, is defined as the consumption of safe and environmentally compatible products and services; it ensures social equity, minimizes pollution and waste, and conserves the material and energy resources of the planet. The consumers may be individuals or industries or governments, any entity that purchases and uses materials.

These two concepts are important because together they form the basic means of avoiding environmental degradation. The production of polluting products, activities, or services and the consumption of them lead to impacts on health. Achieving more sustainable forms of production (as outlined earlier in this chapter) and reducing consumption or consuming more sustainably can lead us toward more sustainable forms of development. A focus on consumption can unfairly focus on developing nations, which currently have about 75 percent of the world's population but use only about 25 percent of its resources. If these developing nations begin to consume at the rate of developed countries, the environmental and health impacts could be devastating. The fair way to respond to this dilemma is to find ways to allow developing nations to develop well, and at the same time to reduce the consumption in industrialized countries and the impacts of consumptive activities worldwide.

Like prevention, the challenge of sustainable development requires systems thinking—understanding the interactions among environment, economy, and society so as to identify root causes of degradation and to focus on sustainable solutions. Similarly, the barriers to a more preventive and sustainable approach to environmental health are generally not technical or economic. They are primarily political and cultural. Thus, understanding these challenges as well as our opportunities is critical as we move forward to a better understanding of the preventable causes of disease and a healthier, cleaner, and safer future.

Thought Questions

1. Select a contemporary environmental health problem, and outline what a preventive approach to that problem might look like. Who would need to be involved, and what types of interventions would be necessary?
2. Given the discussion of the different levels of prevention, which level do you think corresponds most closely to current U.S. and international environmental and health policies? Does this level seem to be the best choice?
3. Describe some situations in which use of the precautionary principle would promote innovation in a business or industrial context.
4. What are some barriers to prevention and precaution in environmental health, and how might you overcome these barriers?

References

Curl, C., Fenske, R., and Elgethun, K. "Organophosphorus Pesticide Exposure of Urban and Suburban Preschool Children with Organic and Conventional Diets." *Environmental Health Perspectives*, 2003, *111*, 377–382.

Environmental Defense. Homepage. [www.environmentaldefense.org]. 2005.

Epstein, P. R. "Is Global Warming Harmful to Health?" *Scientific American*, Aug. 2000, pp. 50–57.

European Commission. "Communication from the Commission to the Council, the European Parliament and the European Economic and Social Committee, Brussels, 11.6.2003." COM (2003) 338 Final. [http://europa.eu.int/comm/environment/health/index_en.htm]. 2003.

European Environment Agency. *Late Lessons from Early Warnings: The Precautionary Principle 1898–1998.* [http://www.eea.eu.int]. 2002.

Fagin, D., and Lavelle, M. *Toxic Deception: How the Chemical Industry Manipulates Science, Bends the Law, and Endangers Your Health.* Secaucus, N.J.: Birch Lane Press, 1996.

Graham, J., and Weiner, J. (eds.). *Risk Versus Risk: Tradeoffs in Protecting Health and the Environment.* Cambridge, Mass.: Harvard University Press, Belknap Press, 1995.

Heerings, H. *Asbestos: Deep in the Very Fibres of Society.* Amsterdam: Contrast Advies, for Greenpeace Netherlands, 2000.

Hill, A. B. "The Environment and Disease: Association or Causation." *Proceedings of the Royal Society of Medicine,* 1965, *58,* 295–300.

Holm, S., and Harris, J. "Precautionary Principle Stifles Discovery." *Nature,* 1999, *400,* 398.

Holmberg, J., and Robèrt, K.-H. "Backcasting from Non-Overlapping Sustainability Principles: A Framework for Strategic Planning." *International Journal of Sustainable Development and World Ecology,* 2000, *7,* 308.

Holmberg, J., Robèrt, K.-H., and Eriksson, K.-E. "Socio-Ecological Principles for Sustainability." In R. Costanza, S. Olmlan, and J. Martinez-Alier (eds.), *Getting Down to Earth: Practical Applications of Ecological Economics.* Washington, D.C.: Island Press, 1996.

Institute of Medicine. *The Future of Public Health.* Washington, D.C.: National Academies Press, 1988.

International Joint Commission: Canada & United States. *1993–95 Priorities and Progress Under the Great Lakes Water Quality Agreement.* Windsor, Ont.: International Joint Commission, Aug. 1995.

James, S., and Lahti, T. *The Natural Step for Communities: How Cities and Towns Can Change to Sustainable Practices.* Gabriola Island, B.C.: New Society, 2004.

Kriebel, D., and others. "The Precautionary Principle in Environmental Science." *Environmental Health Perspectives,* 2001, *109,* 871–876.

Landrigan, P. J., and others. "Environmental Pollutants and Disease in American Chidden: Estimates of Morbidity, Mortality, and Costs for Lead Poisoning, Asthma, Cancer and Developmental Disabilities." *Environmental Health Perspectives,* 2002, *110,* 721–728.

Leavell, H., and Clark, E. G. *Preventive Medicine for the Doctor in His Community.* New York: McGraw-Hill, 1958.

Levy, B. S., and Wegman, D. H. (eds.). *Occupational Health: Recognizing and Preventing Work-Related Disease and Injury.* (4th ed.) Philadelphia: Lippincott, 2000.

London Health Commission. *Noise and Health: Making the Link.* [http://www.londonshealth.gov.uk/pdf/noise_links.pdf]. 2003.

Lubchenco, J. "Entering the Century of the Environment: A New Social Contract for Science." *Science,* 1998, *279,* 491–497.

Markowitz, G., and Rosner, D. "Deceit and Denial: The Deadly Politics of Industrial Pollution." Berkeley: University of California Press, 2002.

Nattrass, B., and Altomare, M. *The Natural Step for Business: Wealth, Ecology and the Evolutionary Corporation (Conscientious Commerce).* Gabriola Island, B.C.: New Society, 1998.

Nestle, M. *Safe Food: Bacteria, Biotechnology, and Bioterrorism.* Los Angeles: University of California Press, 2003.

O'Riordan, T., Cameron, J., and Jordan, A. (eds.). *Reinterpreting the Precautionary Principle.* London: Cameron and May, 2001.

Perrow, C. *Normal Accidents: Living with High-Risk Technologies.* New York: Basic Books, 1984.

Raffensperger, C., and Tickner, J. (eds.). *Protecting Public Health and the Environment: Implementing the Precautionary Principle.* Washington, D.C.: Island Press, 1999.

Robèrt, K.-H. *The Natural Step Story: Seeding a Quiet Revolution.* Gabriola Island, B.C.: New Society, 2002.

Suk, W., and others. "Human Exposure Monitoring and Evaluation in the Arctic: The Importance of Understanding Exposures to the Development of Public Health Policy." *Environmental Health Perspectives,* 2004, *112,* 113–120.

Swedish Environmental Protection Agency, Environmental Objectives Secretariat. "Environmental Quality Objectives." [http://www.miljomal.nu/english/objectives.php]. 2005.
Thorpe, B. *Citizen's Guide to Cleaner Production.* Lowell, Mass.: Lowell Center for Sustainable Production, 1999.
Tickner, J. "Democratic Participation: A Critical Element of Precautionary Public Health Decision-Making." *New Solutions,* 2001, *11,* 93–111.
Tickner, J. "Precaution and Preventive Public Health Policy." *Public Health Reports,* 2002, *117,* 493–497.
Tickner, J. *Precaution, Environmental Science, and Preventive Public Policy.* Washington, D.C.: Island Press, 2003.
Tickner, J., Kriebel, D., and Wright, S. "Precaution: A Compass Towards Improved Decision-Making." *International Journal of Epidemiology,* 2003, *32,* 489–492.
Toxics Use Reduction Institute. Homepage. [www.turi.org]. 2004.
U.S. Department of Health and Human Services, Public Health Service. *Healthy People 2010: Understanding and Improving Health.* Washington, D.C.: U.S. Department of Health and Human Services, 2000.
U.S. Environmental Protection Agency. *What Do We Really Know about the Safety of High Production Volume (HPV) Chemicals.* Washington, D.C.: U.S. Environmental Protection Agency, Office of Pollution Prevention and Toxics, 1998.
Vreugdenhil, H. J., and others. "Effects of Prenatal PCB and Dioxin Background Exposure on Cognitive and Motor Abilities in Dutch Children at School Age." *Journal of Pediatrics,* 2003, *142*(5), 593–594.
Winslow, C. "The Untilled Fields of Public Health." *Modern Medicine,* 1920, *2,* 183–191.
World Commission on Environment and Development. *Our Common Future.* New York: Oxford University Press, 1987.
World Health Organization. *The World Health Report 2002: Reducing Risks, Promoting Healthy Life.* Geneva: World Health Organization, 2002.

For Further Information

Publications

Anastas, P., and Warner, J. *Green Chemistry: Theory and Practice.* London: Oxford Science, 1998.
Ashford, N., and Caldart, C. *Technology, Law, and the Working Environment.* Washington, D.C.: Island Press, 1997.
Geiser, K. *Materials Matter.* Cambridge, Mass.: MIT Press, 2001.
Jackson, T. (ed.). *Clean Production Strategies.* Boca Raton, Fla.: Lewis, 1993.
Jackson, T. *Material Concerns: Pollution, Profit, and Quality of Life.* New York: Routledge, 1996.
O'Brien, M. *Making Better Environmental Decisions: An Alternative to Risk Assessment.* Cambridge, Mass.: MIT Press, 2000.
O'Riordan, T., and Cameron, J. (eds.). *Interpreting the Precautionary Principle.* London: Earthscan, 1994.

Web Sites

The Science and Environmental Health Network is a U.S.-based nongovernmental organization dedicated to defining and applying the precautionary principle in practice:

Science and Environmental Health Network. Homepage. [http://www.sehn.org]. 2005.

The Lowell Center for Sustainable Production, at the University of Massachusetts Lowell, researches, develops, and promotes more sustainable forms of production. It has created several prevention- and precaution-oriented programs, including the Sustainable Hospitals Project and the Chemicals Policy Initiative:

Lowell Center for Sustainable Production. Homepage. [http://www.sustainableproduction.org]. 2005.
Sustainable Hospitals Project. Homepage. [http://www.sustainablehospitals.org]. 2005.
Chemicals Policy Initiative. Homepage. [http://www.chemicalspolicy.org]. 2005.

The Environmental Research Foundation publishes *Rachel's Environment and Health Weekly*, a newsletter dedicated to analyzing environmental and sustainability concerns and promoting sound solutions:

Environmental Research Foundation. Homepage. [http://www.rachel.org]. 2005.

The United Nations Cleaner Production program features a database of case studies of companies adopting more sustainable forms of production and products. The United Nations Environment Programme, Division of Technology, Industry, and Economics, Chemicals branch, has information on various global chemical reduction and notification initiatives:

United Nations Environment Programme, Division of Technology, Industry, and Economics, Production and Consumption Branch. "Cleaner Production (CP) Activities." [http://www.uneptie.org/pc]. 2005.
United Nations Environment Programme, Division of Technology, Industry, and Economics. "Chemicals." [http://www.chem.unep.ch]. 2005.

The Pesticide Action Network and the Northwest Coalition for Alternatives to Pesticides provide information and technical support for understanding pesticide risks and alternatives:

Pesticide Action Network North America. Homepage. [http://www.panna.org]. 2005.
Northwest Coalition for Alternatives to Pesticides. Homepage. [http://www.pesticide.org]. 2005.

Clean Production Action provides technical and research support and advocacy to promote cleaner production:

Clean Production Action. Homepage. [http://www.cleanproduction.org]. 2005.

The Institute for Agriculture and Trade Policy promotes more sustainable agricultural practices:

Institute for Agriculture and Trade Policy. Homepage. [http://www.iatp.org]. 2005.

The Trust for America's Health has been a leading advocate for better health surveillance and a proponent of national health tracking:

Trust for America's Health. Homepage. [http://healthyamericans.org]. 2005.

The CDC's National Center for Environmental Health has been a world leader in biomonitoring to understand human exposure to toxic substances:

Centers for Disease Control and Prevention, National Center for Environmental Health. Homepage. [http://www.cdc.gov/nceh].

CHAPTER THIRTY

THE PRACTICE OF ENVIRONMENTAL HEALTH

Sarah Kotchian

From earliest recorded times, human beings have recognized the need for guidelines, ordinances, and infrastructure to ensure the protection of the environment and human health. The practice of environmental health has grown and evolved as it has been informed over the years by the public health sciences of epidemiology and biostatistics and the emerging disciplines of toxicology and exposure and risk assessment. In addition, the public at large has demanded an increasing role in the design and delivery of community environmental health services. Environmental health activities are carried out in a variety of settings, from local and state governments to federal and tribal governments and in the private sector. This chapter begins with a historical overview of environmental public health services from ancient times through the modern recognition of the critical role of community involvement. It describes the organization and delivery of environmental health services, describes standards for service delivery, and outlines a process for community environmental health planning. The final portion of the chapter presents case studies of environmental health practice in various settings and offers students information on career opportunities in environmental health.

The History of Environmental Health Regulations and Services

The need for environmental health practices has been recognized since ancient times. In the Bible the book of Leviticus mentions food protection, housing quality, and quarantine. Engineers and public officials in ancient Rome planned for the supply of water and disposal of wastes, and government in medieval England used quarantine to limit the spread of disease. Later, social reformers advocated for improved housing conditions and clean drinking water. In England in 1842, for example, Edwin Chadwick published an influential report on sanitary conditions, and the 1871 Report of the Royal Sanitary Commission documented important environmental health protections. Counterparts in the United States published a similar report for Massachusetts and campaigned effectively for the establishment of a state board of health in Massachusetts in 1869. By the end of the nineteenth century in the United States, forty of the forty-five states could claim health departments.

The late nineteenth century and the first six decades of the twentieth century constituted the first of the modern eras of environmental health practice. C.E.A. Winslow, writing in 1923 in *The Evolution and Significance of the Public Health Campaign,* defined *public health,* which includes environmental health, this way: "Public health is not a concrete intellectual discipline, but a field of social activity. It includes applications of chemistry and bacteriology, of engineering and statistics, of physiology and pathology and epidemiology, and in some measure of sociology, and it builds upon these basic sciences a comprehensive program of community service" (p. 1). During the first fifty years of the twentieth century, states passed numerous public health laws regulating water and sewage treatment, protection of food, provision of safe housing and human and solid waste disposal, and reduction of insect and rodent-borne diseases, resulting in a corresponding decrease in human morbidity and mortality and an increase in life expectancy.

During this same period state legislatures expanded the resources available to state departments of health to assess the health status of citizens and environmental threats to health, and to develop policies and programs to improve health and environmental quality. Health departments were normally headed by physicians, with nurses overseeing the immunization programs and sanitary engineers inspecting the construction and maintenance of safe water supplies, the purveyance of milk and meat, and the sanitary operation of food preparation and service facilities. Practitioners of environmental health services, known as *sanitarians,* were trained to be generalists, with the capability to anticipate, prevent, and respond to a broad spectrum of environmental health threats and with traditional functions in vector control, proper management and disposal of sewage, and food protection. Environmental health and personal public health services coexisted until the 1960s as partners in state health departments and in the increasing number of local health departments modeled after the state system.

The rapid industrialization that had begun during the late nineteenth century continued after World War II. Additional widespread pollution of land, water, and air and the creation of new pollutants such as synthetic organic compounds helped to usher in the second modern era of environmental health protection. Scientists such as Rachel Carson and other environmental leaders brought to public attention the worsening condition of the environment and the impacts of pollutants on bird populations, natural habitats, and human health. As public outcry increased, the U.S. Congress responded over the next fifteen years by passing a great number of environmental laws, including the Safe Drinking Water Act, the Clean Air Act, the Occupational Safety and Health Act, the Consumer Product Safety Act, the Marine Mammal Protection Act, and the Toxic Substances Control Act (see also Chapter Thirty-Three). These federal acts were often complemented on the state level by similar state laws.

At the same time, the public demanded increased accountability from agencies responsible for environmental regulation. Public health professionals testified successfully before Congress for the establishment of the U.S. Environmental Protection Agency (EPA). In the states, elected officials responded by creating separate state-level environmental agencies, giving these agencies the responsibility for enforcement of new environmental laws and regulations on air, water, and hazardous waste. In some cases, traditional environmental public health activities, such as food protection and sanitary sewage disposal, were also transferred to these new agencies. These agencies were variously known as departments of environment, environmental quality, environmental regulation, or environmental protection; most dropped the word *health* from their titles. The separate agencies benefited from increased visibility and enhanced funding for environmental concerns and did not have to compete for funds with other functions in a health department.

This combination of new legislation and increased public attention created a watershed period for the practice of environmental health, with both positive and negative consequences. Although the increased visibility and funding were important in supporting necessary environmental health programs, over the next forty years the separation between health and environmental agencies resulted in the creation of separate data systems, uncoordinated planning, and the loss of a comprehensive picture of the community's health and environment. Whereas in the first half of the twentieth century, nurses and sanitarians tended to be closely connected to one another and to their small communities and familiar with the issues of the residents, population growth and the growth of agencies have interfered with this intimate local knowledge. In addition, many environmental health specialists became increasingly isolated from their public health counterparts in state and local departments of health (as their agencies grew apart as well), losing valuable affiliations that would later take years to reestablish.

Along with the new, medium-specific environmental laws (laws that pertained to air, or water, or land) came a generation of environmental health specialists who devoted their careers to one specific area of the environment, such as solid waste, hazardous waste, air quality, or drinking water. Their training often did not include training in general public health concepts or in the use of public health tools such as epidemiology and effective public health campaigns. In addition, this specialized training and focus, necessitated by complicated, single-medium federal regulations on air and water, made it more difficult for professionals in environmental health to have the time or the information to see their community's big picture. As a result, some of the programs developed by these professionals were not sensitive to community knowledge, culture, or concerns and were also not as effective as they might have been in addressing the overall health and environment because they focused on one isolated component.

The Rise of Citizen Involvement in Environmental Planning and Practice

The 1970s and 1980s saw a convergence of factors, including the ongoing negative impacts of rapid industrialization and urban growth, urban flight, and the disenfranchisement of citizens from environmental policymaking and enforcement decisions. In the wake of environmental discoveries such as the widespread contamination in Love Canal, New York; Times Beach, Missouri; and Woburn, Massachusetts, average citizens demanded a stronger role in decision making and greater transparency and accountability from the governmental agencies that were supposed to be protecting their health and environment. Watchdog groups, such as the Center for Health, Environment and Justice, headed by Lois Gibbs, and national environmental advocacy organizations, such as the Natural Resources Defense Council, gained membership and influence to ensure that agencies fulfilled their mandates and that citizen voices were heard and their input incorporated. Faith organizations, indigenous rights organizations, and other citizen groups combined their efforts and their strategies to create the environmental justice movement, insisting that social, economic, racial, and environmental concerns were interrelated and needed to be addressed with the central involvement of those who bore the greatest burden (see also Chapter Eight). This became the third era of environmental health practice, in which agencies needed to learn how to address the environmental justice and equity concerns of their multicultural communities more effectively and in which they began to develop new techniques and assign specific personnel for incorporating community involvement and communicating risk (see also Chapter Thirty-Four).

Federal laws were written or amended to require environmental impact statements, analysis of environmental justice, and public involvement in the development of policies, permits, and hazardous waste site remediation plans. In the academic community, researchers focused on effective community empowerment and strategies for effectively assessing and communicating risk in diverse communities, and they redirected some research in order to engage in community-based participatory research. Agencies struggled with retraining their existing staff to work in ways that were more culturally sensitive, and sought to hire employees drawn from the communities they served. In recent years citizen frustration over the inability of accountable agencies to document and address the link between environmental exposures and health outcomes has led to a number of initiatives to reconnect environmental and public health, a movement aided greatly by the use of applied, computer-enhanced information in epidemiology, risk assessment, toxicology, and risk communication.

The Organization and Delivery of Environmental Health Services

How is the practice of environmental health organized today? Not surprisingly, because both universal and community-specific needs exist, environmental health services in the United States are provided at federal, tribal, state, and local levels and in the private sector. The federal laws governing various aspects of the environment are enforced by numerous federal agencies, including the Environmental Protection Agency, the Department of Agriculture, the Food and Drug Administration, and others. Many federal laws contain provisions that supercede state law in order to provide equal environmental health protection to all citizens. Some federal Acts, such as the Clean Air Act, permit delegation of authority to states and, under certain circumstances of local home rule, to local jurisdictions. State governments have the authority to enact further environmental legislation as long as it does not conflict with federal law. Many of these state laws provide additional protections or address areas not covered by federal law. Within states, municipalities and counties have the authority, usually given by the state legislature, to enact local laws to protect the health and environment for their citizens.

Who decides what agencies should provide environmental health services, how agencies should be organized, and what services should be provided? Historically, environmental health agencies have come into being through a combination of public health leadership, citizen advocacy, and political will. Their creation begins with the perception of a need to protect the public from environmental hazards and the desire for a governmental unit charged with the provision of those services that will be responsive to elected officials and the public. The specific services provided are built around a core set of environmental health services, such as food protection, water sanitation, and air quality protection, with additional services added as determined by public health data and public interest. Ideally, the community-specific tailoring of local agencies can be a method of ensuring that the highest-priority services for that community are provided. Yet this necessary and desirable local political process has also resulted in a patchwork of services that are not coordinated and that leave large gaps in the core public health functions of assessment, assurance, and policy development.

Because the authority for environmental health services has developed over many decades and in multiple locations, the organization and delivery of these services is now complex and is not easily understood by environmental health professionals themselves, much less by the general public. In the early 1990s, the federal Health Resources and Services Administration (HRSA) commissioned two reports to catalogue the diversity of environmental health service organization and delivery. These reports analyzed the structure and function of state environmental health activities and found several pervasive problems. The first report (Burke, Shalauta, and Tran, 1995a) described the existing structure, authority, and funding for state environmental health services. The researchers found that federal environmental laws had driven the design and authority of state regulatory agencies but that there was no standardization in the way the agencies were organized to enforce these laws. The report further noted that many of the regulatory agencies had become oriented toward specific media and often lacked the necessary public health support, such as epidemiology, public health evaluation, and applied research, that would allow them to gain a larger perspective on the environment and health.

The second report (Burke, Shalauta, and Tran, 1995b) documented that regulatory enforcement generally took precedence over environmental health prevention, as reflected by approximately four times more funding for enforcement. The report recommended reevaluation of this imbalance, a broader view of the relationship between health and the environment, better health training for environmental professionals, and "improved cooperation between the many health and environmental agencies in the complex 'Environmental Web' to assure that they do not lose sight of their fundamental mission—the protection of the public health" (p. 24).

Standards for Environmental Health Practice

Although many environmental health programs are indeed local, this evolution across time and geographic location has resulted in a lack of consistency in the quality of programs and services provided to the public, and in an inability to measure effectiveness in order to improve these services. In the last two decades of the twentieth century and the first years of the twenty-first, a number of reports and initiatives have assessed public health services and systems, developed performance standards and indicators, and designed tools that agencies and the public can use to assess and improve public health system capacity. For example, in 1987 the Institute of Medicine (IOM) conducted a review of the U.S. public health system and then issued the *Future of Public Health,* a report that cited a number of problems and made recommendations for strengthening the system. This report outlined the three core functions of public health—assessment, policy development, and assurance:

Assessment

- The committee recommends that every public health agency regularly and systematically collect, assemble, analyze, and make available information on the health of the community, including statistics on health status, community health needs, and epidemiologic and other studies of health problems.

Policy Development

- The committee recommends that every public health agency exercise its responsibility to serve the public interest in the development of comprehensive public health policies by promoting use of the scientific knowledge base in decision making about public health and by leading in developing public health policy. Agencies must take a strategic approach, developed on the basis of a positive appreciation for the democratic political process.

Assurance

- The committee recommends that public health agencies assure their constituents that services necessary to achieve agreed upon goals are provided, either by encouraging action or by other entities (private or public sector), by requiring such action through regulation, or by providing services directly.
- The committee recommends that each public health agency involve key policymakers and the general public in determining a set of high-priority personal and communitywide health services that governments will guarantee to every member of the community. This guarantee should include subsidization or direct provision of high-priority personal health services for those unable to afford them [IOM, 1988, pp. 141–142].

TABLE 30.1. THE TEN ESSENTIAL SERVICES OF PUBLIC HEALTH.

1. Monitor health status to identify health problems.
2. Diagnose and evaluate health problems and health hazards.
3. Inform, educate, and empower people about health issues.
4. Mobilize partnerships to identify and solve health problems.
5. Develop policies and plans that support individual and statewide health efforts.
6. Enforce laws and regulations that protect health and ensure safety.
7. Link people to needed personal health services and assure the provision of health care when otherwise unavailable.
8. Assure a competent public and personal health care workforce.
9. Evaluate effectiveness, accessibility, and quality of personal and population-based health services.
10. Research for new insights and innovative solutions to health problems.

Source: The ten essential services have been widely disseminated and can be found on numerous Web sites; see, for example, CDC, 2004.

Following the publication of this report a group of federal agencies and organizations known as the Core Public Health Functions Steering Committee met in 1994 to define the workforce competencies needed to carry out these three core functions, and further defined a set of ten essential services of public health (Table 30.1), the services necessary to support the three core functions. The wording of these ten essential services was modified slightly by the National Center for Environmental Health (NCEH) at the Centers for Disease Control and Prevention (CDC), to make it more relevant to the environmental health practice community, but the essential nature of the services remains the same.

Each of these services represents an important component of the overall public health infrastructure. For instance, monitoring health, the first essential service, which requires the creation of an environmental health surveillance system, is a priority because it allows public health officials to detect environmental hazards and related illnesses, assess the need for additional services, develop necessary programs and regulations, and ensure that necessary public health protection is provided. Using data from this surveillance system, public health professionals can advocate before policymaking bodies to obtain the necessary legal support and resources for programs to address community needs. The development of spatial data technology (geographic information systems) in recent years has made it more practical for public health officials to map the occurrence of hazards and illnesses in their communities and to use these maps in dialogues with citizens and elected officials to create awareness and the political will to address specific concerns (see Chapter Thirty-One). For example, in the Albuquerque Environmental Health

Department in the 1990s, it was customary for the department director to present each newly elected city councilor with an environmental health map of his or her district, with color-coded information on the location of restaurants inspected, mosquito complaints received, dog bites, noise complaints, and other public nuisances. The map was a visual reminder of the need for services as well as documentation of the department services provided with taxpayer support.

To reinforce, support, and standardize public health systems, the CDC's Public Health Practice Program Office (PHPPO) developed a set of performance standards tools that can be used to assess the capacity of state and local agencies and local boards of health to provide the ten essential services of public health. These free tools (CDC, 2005) describe the standards of performance, ask a series of questions, and provide indicators for each of the essential services, allowing public health professionals and their communities to assess their capacity to provide the ten essential services of public health and to identify service gaps that need to be filled. For example, the questions ask whether the local public health system maintains such data as environmental exposures and workplace injuries and whether it contributes such data to population health registries. Consideration is being given to developing similar tools for tribal and international use. Although not specifically written for environmental health agencies, the standards and indicators need only slight modification in order to be useful for environmental health officials and their communities.

A number of states and local communities have assessed their capacity using the CDC performance standards tools. As a result of its assessment, the State of Florida developed a committee to make recommendations on workforce quality. The State of New York is incorporating assessment results from all New York counties into a state public health improvement plan. The State of New Mexico spent 2003 using both the state and local CDC performance standards tools in the majority of its counties and has developed follow-up recommendations to be incorporated into the state health plan.

As the challenges facing public health agencies grew and available funding became more constrained, there were efforts over the last three decades of the twentieth century to define an effective public health agency and to set goals for the health of the nation. In order to support the development of consistent public health services and to raise public awareness of national public health goals, the U.S. Department of Health and Human Services (DHHS), with broad input, created a set of model standards for public health services and established a set of national health indicators, to be revised and published once each decade. The most recent health objectives for the nation, published as *Healthy People 2010*, include environmental quality among the top ten health indicators. Several specific objectives address environmental exposures. For example, one objective (8-1a) aims to reduce the proportion of persons exposed to excess ozone in air, and another (27-10) aims to reduce the proportion of nonsmokers exposed to environmental tobacco smoke. Additional environmental objectives address outdoor air quality, water quality, toxics and waste, healthy homes and healthy communities, infrastructure and surveillance, and global environmental health. (For information on all the Healthy People 2010 indicators, including specific, measurable environmental health indicators, see Healthy People, 2005.)

Developing Tools for Community Environmental Health Planning and Practice

With the increased emphasis on community involvement came agencies' desire for standard tools that could be used strategically, systematically, and meaningfully to involve their communities in policy and planning. The National Association of County and City Health Officials (NACCHO), in conjunction with other national public health organizations such as the American Public Health Association (APHA), the Association of Schools of Public Health, and the Association of State and Territorial Health Officials, took the lead in 1991 in publishing *Assessment Protocol for Excellence in Public Health* (APEXPH), which led public health agencies through a series of steps to assess their own strengths and needs and to work in partnership with their communities to respond to community health concerns and to design more effective health programs.

Environmental health agencies, although valuing the APEXPH tool, found that it did not fully address their need to identify specific community environmental health problems and to design, in concert with the public, environmental health programs that would build on community strengths and focus on community priorities. With funding from the CDC National Center for Environmental Health, NACCHO supported a multiple-year effort by a committee of professionals in environmental health that resulted in PACE-EH (Protocol for Assessing Community Excellence in Environmental Health) (NACCHO, 2004). This protocol takes local health departments and their communities through a thirteen-step process (Table 30.2) of characterizing the community, assembling a community environmental health assessment team, generating a list of environmental issues for analysis, developing locally meaningful indicators for those issues, ranking the issues and setting priorities for action, and then evaluating progress and planning for the future. A number of other agencies, such as the U.S. Environmental Protection Agency, have also developed tools for community involvement that center around the core value of community empowerment and voice in the design of environmental health services and healthier communities.

TABLE 30.2. THE PACE-EH PROCESS.

Task 1	Determine community capacity.
Task 2	Define and characterize the community.
Task 3	Assemble a community-based environmental health assessment team.
Task 4	Define the goals, objectives, and scope of the assessment.
Task 5	Generate a list of community-specific environmental health issues.
Task 6	Analyze issues with a systems framework.
Task 7	Identify locally appropriate indicators.
Task 8	Select standards against which local status can be compared.
Task 9	Create issue profiles.
Task 10	Rank issues.
Task 11	Set priorities for action.
Task 12	Develop action plan(s).
Task 13	Evaluate progress and plan for the future.

Note: Detailed instructions for each of the thirteen tasks in the PACE-EH process task are outlined in the *PACE-EH Guidebook* (NACCHO, 2004).

Putting PACE-EH to Work: A Case Study on Community, Democracy, and the Environment

A number of communities have now implemented PACE-EH, both in the United States and internationally. The process is time intensive because it requires extensive community outreach and involvement and because, ideally, it is managed by the citizens themselves, with staff support from the local health agency. Let's look at how one local health department demonstrated its commitment to citizen-driven public health policy.

The Island County Health Department in the State of Washington provides public health services for the five islands that make up the county. In 2001, the department, with funding from the National Center for Environmental Health, Environmental Health Services Branch, initiated a process to conduct PACE-EH for its local jurisdiction. Tim McDonald, the department director, had chaired the national committee that oversaw the development of the PACE-EH document, and he was determined to have his health department model the PACE-EH principles and practices. The department hired Celine Servatius, an environmental health scientist, to lead the project. She began a series of public meetings and spent several months encouraging citizens to apply to serve on the citizen environmental health assessment team (EHAT) that would oversee the project. The EHAT membership was approved by the county board of health, and embarked on a several-year, thirteen-step process to identify and prioritize Island County's environmental health concerns.

From a long list of community issues, the EHAT selected the following four environmental health issues for initial in-depth study and reporting: vector/zoonotic disease, with an emphasis on West Nile virus; community physical activity (specifically, making Island County's communities more walkable); illegal dumping; and drinking-water quality, with a focus on arsenic in drinking water. According to Servatius, "each of the four issues has been analyzed within a systems framework to identify and understand the connections among health status, affected populations, contributing factors and behaviors, environmental agents/conditions, exposure factors, and public health protection factors. All four [EHAT] subcommittees have also selected locally appropriate indicators for their issue" (Island County Environmental Health Initiative, 2003). When the process is complete, the Island County Health Department will have a community-based health priorities action plan to guide its health programs and resource allocation. In addition, the department hopes to have fostered a stronger relationship with the citizens of Island County around environmental health issues, gained an understanding of community concerns, facilitated community interest in environmental health issues, and developed partnerships to address the issues and concerns identified through the PACE-EH process.

Notes from the Field

What do professionals in environmental health do? The next few pages offer a journey with several practitioners from urban, rural, and small city environmental health departments. They describe their career trajectories, their daily activities, and their place within the larger system of environmental public health.

Urban Environmental Health

Large urban areas pose an expanded set of challenges for the professional in environmental health. Their dense populations and large geographic areas usually require that environmental health staff work out of several different locations, with a central coordinating office. Aging housing stock and crumbling public works infrastructure lead to additional issues of lead exposures, rodent infestations, housing-related injuries, raw sewage, and potential drinking-water contamination. Heavy workloads may result in fewer inspections of each site than might occur in smaller jurisdictions, and underscore the need to focus on education and on the most effective interventions.

Urban environmental health services are often found within a larger department of health. In the Philadelphia Department of Health, for instance, the

Environmental Health Services division oversees programs in animal management and licensing, rat infestation and vector control, regulation of food establishments, and inspection of public and private institutions. Its main offices are co-located with other divisions that address injury, air quality, and noise and vibration concerns, allowing coordination of environmental issues. Health department administrators must oversee a large number of separate issues in their department, including, for example, disease control, drug and alcohol abuse, lead poisoning, tuberculosis, mental health, and ambulatory care, and are often unable to give much time and attention to environmental health when faced with other health crises. As a result, Environmental Health Services has learned to operate fairly independently and must make a special effort to coordinate with other health services; this poses an ongoing challenge in creating a comprehensive collaborative approach to meeting community needs. Some services have addressed this challenge by co-locating staff from various programs in the same field offices to encourage communication and coordination of efforts.

Randall Hirschhorn, Retired Director, City of Philadelphia Environmental Health Services

Randall Hirschhorn began his career in 1970, during the summer before his last year at Rutgers University as an undergraduate environmental health major. He was selected for an environmental internship in the City of Camden, New Jersey, and was assigned to a community group run by an Episcopal priest who asked him to do a survey of environmental issues and major sources of pollution. Hirschhorn spent the summer walking the streets of Camden, talking to citizens about their concerns and reading news articles, and compiling the issues in a final report. In the process, he became enthusiastic about a career in public service. After graduating in 1971, he began a master's degree program in environmental education and also happened upon a Philadelphia job fair at which he learned about a sanitarian position with the Philadelphia Department of Health. "I thought I knew what a sanitarian was, but I wasn't exactly sure," he recounts. He was hired for the position, expecting to stay only a few years. He met his future wife during the course of his sanitarian duties, and although later offered positions in Alaska and New Mexico with the U.S. Public Health Service, decided to make his home and career in Philadelphia.

Hirschhorn was willing to learn many aspects of environmental health and was promoted over the years, heading various sections of the program at different times. He also continued his education, acquiring master of science and master of public administration degrees in addition to his master of education degree. He was selected to be a sanitarian supervisor, and later volunteered to work in a new program in infectious waste management, one of the first such programs in the country. He became the assistant chief of vector control, working on a grant from the CDC for urban rat control and childhood lead poisoning prevention, a program that continued to flourish under his leadership despite later federal cutbacks. From there, he became chief of food protection for five years, and finally, in 1990, he was appointed to the position of director of environmental health for the City of Philadelphia, a post he held until his retirement.

After losing one-quarter of its population to yellow fever in the epidemic of 1793, Philadelphia had been one of the first cities in the United States to establish a board of health (1794) and a health department (1804). An avid student of history, Hirschhorn is quick to articulate the contributions of environmental health over the past two centuries, as sanitarians overcame urban challenges of tenement housing, adulterated food, poor water quality and sewage disposal, and insect- and rodent-borne diseases. His department now continues to provide comprehensive services in food protection, vector control, environmental engineering, and animal management to the nation's fifth largest city, with 1.5 million people within a thirty-square-mile area.

Hirschhorn has seen many changes over the years. One of the major changes has been the shift in expertise needed, from an early focus on staff able to conduct milk and food inspections to today's need for staff who can also address such matters as emergency response, hazardous materials incidents, infectious wastes, bioterrorism, safe drinking water, and watershed protection. He has also seen and contributed to the diversification of the workforce. When he first joined the department, it was made up largely of white males; it gradually diversified to males of different races and, finally, improved in gender diversity. He is proud of his role in recruiting and encouraging women in environmental health at a time when there was little support for them. The federal Comprehensive Education and Training Act (CETA) in the late 1970s provided funds to local jurisdictions to hire more college-educated sanitarians, and although the funds were later discontinued, this brief period of funding allowed a more diverse workforce to gain a foothold and to prove their abilities in this challenging field.

Other observed changes include the transition from pencils and paper to hand-held computers and the change in emphasis from inspection to education, both of the regulated industry and of the general public. In recent years, Hirschhorn says, the environmental health staff are paying greater attention to the impact of the environment on the health of children, including risks related to lead, home injuries, and indoor air. Sanitarians who might enter a home on a rat complaint see many other potential risks and are able to address those issues with family members.

He has also noted some changes for the worse over the past decade. There has been a trend to appoint people with no background in public and environmental health to positions of environmental health authority and a worrisome trend toward privatizing some environmental health activities; together these trends may result in a public health approach that lacks coordination and comprehensiveness.

One of the things of which he is most proud is his staff's ability to design programs based on what they want the future to look like. For example, in 1994, he asked his staff to envision their city in 2001 without foodborne illness. From that exercise, they determined that they needed increased computerization, mandatory education for the food industry, and additional staff. When an outbreak of foodborne illness the next year brought attention to the problem and an offer of additional staff, Hirschhorn turned down the staff but successfully pressed for the mandatory industry education.

When enforcement cases went to court, he asked the judge for enforcement cost recovery rather than for fines, keeping track of the revenues earned. Armed with this data, he later made an economic case for the self-sufficiency of his staff, given this cost recovery, and was able to market a new fee schedule that covered the department's costs of plan review and inspections and allowed him to receive authorization to hire additional staff. He considers an ability to think in economic terms and an acknowledgment of the importance of marketing environmental health to be critical for departments seeking to enhance programs in this age of budgetary cutbacks. Thirty-three years after his undergraduate internship, still actively involved in creating the environmental health future he would like to see, Hirschhorn remains excited about public service and careers in environmental health.

Gerry Barron and Allegheny County: An Environmental Health Career in a Comprehensive Local Health Department

In 1970, with his undergraduate degree in biology in hand, Gerry Barron and his wife left Boston temporarily so that Barron could pursue a master of public health degree at the University of Pittsburgh. Three and a half decades later they are still in Pittsburgh, and Barron continues to innovate in the practice of local environmental health.

During his master's program, which offered a concentration in environmental health, Gerry came to know Al Brunwasser, director of the Environmental Health Bureau in the Allegheny County Health Department. Brunwasser had an eye for students of promise, and he offered Barron a position as a sanitarian trainee. It was the 1970s, environmental issues were at the forefront, and Pittsburgh already had a long, proud history of civic involvement in collaborating to protect the environment. In the 1940s, with Pittsburgh under a cloud of pollution from the steel and other manufacturing industries, David Lawrence, the city's mayor, and

Richard King Mellon, a wealthy industrialist, called together the major industries, the health department, and other community leaders to develop solutions that would be healthy for both people and the economy; one of the results was the first smoke regulation in the country.

That community-wide awareness and support led to the growth of the comprehensive environmental health program into which Barron was hired, with traditional public health programs for food protection, housing sanitation, drinking water, wastewater, swimming pools, solid waste oversight, and air pollution. Brunwasser was a good mentor, encouraging Barron to take on challenges, and Barron had a personality that allowed him to see these challenges as opportunities to learn. Over the next twenty years, he became chief of the food protection program, worked in housing and wastewater, and became deputy director for environmental health. When the opportunity arose to become the deputy director for medical services for the Allegheny County Health Department, Barron took it, even though it represented a change in career orientation.

Over the years, with Barron's guidance and vision, the health department has reorganized to recognize the natural connections among its various public health programs. The food protection program is co-located with infectious diseases. The housing program personnel work alongside the personnel for the lead; Women, Infants, and Children (WIC); and dental programs, in recognition that these family and community health programs serve the same clientele. The department also administers federal programs for air quality and state programs for drinking water, wastewater, and solid waste, and has added programs for injury control and school sanitation. The department also regulates the licensure and training of plumbers, in order to reduce the risk of cross-connections in the public drinking-water supply. Barron insists that department staff maintain dialogue with the regulated communities. The food protection, plumbing, air quality, and drinking-water programs all have their own advisory committees, which include industry representation. The Allegheny County Health Department now has approximately 450 employees and provides services to the 130 municipalities throughout a county with a population of 1.2 million. The department is headed by Bruce Dixon, a physician and professor of medicine at the University of Pittsburgh, who is employed by Allegheny County, another indication of a strong community partnership.

After thirty-three years with the health department, Barron is now deputy director for all department operations, and he still looks forward to the challenges of environmental and public health. "Every day is different," he says. "You're not sure what's going to happen that day." He ensures that the public health programs have a strong base in science. Entry-level field personnel are required to have an undergraduate major in science, and a master's degree in public health or public administration is required for upper-level administrative positions. He continues the tradition of mentoring staff and graduate students, looking for those who are willing to see challenges as opportunities and to move around to learn new skills. He enjoys creative visioning, in his own words, "I like to spend time on what should be, and work to get there." He delegates the daily decision making in the programs and the management of personnel, purchasing, and contracting to the managers and supervisors, and spends much of his time in overseeing the implementation of strategic plans and in creating and maintaining an effective community network. Not only does this network allow him to gather support for necessary programs but also, Barron says, "you need to be able to respond quickly; you should have a system that will pick up and deal with community issues." His network serves as a radar system that allows him to listen to others and hear about issues and illnesses, gathering information about new initiatives and interventions that are needed. The appointed board of health that oversees the health department provides an additional measure of citizen direction and involvement.

He continues to learn and develop his own skills. He holds a joint appointment at the University of Pittsburgh School of Public Health and serves as director of the Pennsylvania Preparedness Leadership Institute. Several years ago he successfully spearheaded an effort to apply for a community environmental health capacity-building grant from the CDC's National Center for Environmental Health. The funds from this grant allowed the department to hire Jo Ann Glad, a registered nurse with a master of public health degree, as a full-time epidemiologist. She has begun to build the partnerships and the infrastructure to support a comprehensive community-wide health and environmental data system. When asked what continues to bring him satisfaction after so many years, Barron replies, "It's all about social justice. Everyone has the same right to clean water, clean air, and access to health care. It's really about helping others who can't speak for themselves, who don't have as much say." There is a "nobility of service" in public health, he says, that is deeply satisfying. Gerry Barron is an example of those outstanding leaders who have dedicated a lifetime of service to local environmental public health.

Island County Health Department: Painting a Picture of an Improved Environment and Public Health

Island County, Washington is another rewarding place in which to practice environmental health. The county consists of five islands northwest of Seattle; one of them, Whidbey Island, is the longest island in the contiguous forty-eight states. With the majority of its 75,000 residents living on two of the islands, Island County, despite its rural appearance, is one of the most densely populated counties in the state. A visitor from the mainland might arrive at the southern end of Whidbey Island by ferry and drive past beautiful rolling hills and farms, greeted by glimpses of ocean amid the tall evergreens and surprised by the flight of one of many bald eagles that inhabit the island, before arriving at the main office of the Island County Health Department, located in the center of the island.

Washington, like many other states, has a law requiring counties to have a local board of health and to provide public health services for county residents. Island County Health Department was created under this law, and is empowered to enforce state rules promulgated by the Washington State Board of Health and the Washington Secretary of Health, as well as enforcing any local ordinances that the county finds necessary to control and prevent dangerous or infectious diseases, control nuisances, and provide for general health and sanitation. The health department has approximately forty-five full-time-equivalent employees, and about twenty of them are engaged in environmental health work. Its programs include personal health services, community assessment and development, environmental health services, and human services, including mental health, substance abuse prevention, and developmental disabilities. The health department has made a significant effort to locate where the people live, rather than near other government offices, and has three additional offices in order to serve the citizens as close to their homes as possible.

The department is headed by Tim McDonald, who came to Whidbey Island several decades ago. After receiving a bachelor of science degree in microbiology from the University of Washington, McDonald worked for a consulting company and for the EPA as a microbiologist, eventually moving on to work as a microbiologist in the water quality section of the Seattle/King County Health Department. He joined the Island County Health Department in 1980 as an environmental health specialist, becoming the environmental health director in 1984 and the department director in 1987. While working, he earned a master of public health degree in the University of Washington's extended degree program, which meets the needs of public health professionals who are already working in the field full time. He is also a registered sanitarian.

One of the benefits of working in a county health department is the opportunity for collaborating on solutions to public health challenges. For instance, the health department has established a methamphetamine team, with environmental health professionals who address the environmental contamination, law enforcement officers who address the criminal justice system response to illegal drug labs, and substance abuse counselors who arrange services for the individuals involved. In another example of intradepartmental collaboration mental health professionals and public health nurses work together to address the physical, mental, and emotional challenges of isolated elders on the islands.

Because Island County is formed from glacially deposited soil atop volcanic bedrock and is surrounded by saltwater, it confronts the problem of saltwater intrusion into freshwater sources. The physical and geological characteristics of these islands provide interesting challenges for an environmental health practitioner. State planning law requires growth to occur in existing cities, preserving many rural areas, but this population density brings with it other environmental challenges such as the quality and quantity of available drinking water. Island County has been granted sole source aquifer designation, with 72 percent of the population depending on one of the two aquifers as the sole source of drinking water. As part of its long-term public health responsibilities, the health department must protect these sources from both contamination and overuse. A groundwater resource team, including a hydrogeologist, is charged with reviewing all proposed developments to assess the adequacy of the drinking water source and to make recommendations so that land use is compatible with water availability. Because of its location, Island County has needed to address these limitations sooner than other health departments, and it is now sharing its experience and knowledge with other health departments around the country.

The county is also the home of world-renowned Penn Cove blue mussels, a significant economic asset, so the health department works with other agencies, including the Washington State Department of Health, to protect these commercial mussel beds from chemical and biological contamination. The department's environmental health section also provides services in food protection, liquid waste, solid and chemical waste, and vector control. In 2001, the department was awarded a grant from the CDC to work with residents to conduct a citizen-led process to assess and prioritize island environmental concerns (as described earlier in this chapter in the discussion of PACE-EH).

What is a day like for a member of the environmental health staff in the Island County Health Department? After a morning staff meeting and the scheduling of appointments in the field, an environmental health professional might inspect restaurants, give a class in food protection, inspect a site proposed for an on-site liquid waste system, or meet with developers to review plans. Each staff member spends approximately 25 percent of the day in the office, answering questions from the public, returning telephone calls, catching up on related paperwork, and entering data into the health department's environmental and public health data system.

Because Island County has unusual environmental health challenges combined with a small health department staff, Director McDonald feels it is especially important to have personnel who are on the cutting edge of environmental health knowledge. Entry-level staff have a minimum of a bachelor's degree in science and often must acquire more specialized education relevant to their job assignment. McDonald advises those interested in a career in environmental health, whether in his department or elsewhere in the country, to obtain a bachelor's degree from a good institution and to begin working to gain experience in environmental health. Once employed, they can then seek support from their employer to pursue an advanced public health degree or additional professional credentials in a specific technical area.

When hiring, McDonald and his supervisors look for individuals with strong communication skills, past experience in another public health agency or related environmental health experience, and proven ability to work with the public. One outstanding example of such an individual is Keith Higman, the environmental health manager for Island County, who is pursuing his master of public health degree while working for the department. Higman earned a bachelor's degree in environmental science and worked for the Washington State Fisheries Department, for the county planning department on wetlands issues, and for the Island County Health Department as an environmental health specialist in drinking water before being hired by McDonald to head the department's environmental health division. McDonald cited outstanding communication and cognitive skills and ability to work with the public as some of Higman's strong leadership assets. More recently, Higman was appointed by the state governor to the Washington State Board of Health, where he is able both to contribute to state health policy, and to apply what he learns to issues in Island County.

Mentoring staff and building a strong public health team are priorities for McDonald. He says the members of his management team understand that they are only as good as the people who work for them, and they work hard to encourage and retain their staff. Because it is difficult to compete with the larger counties in the region in terms of salary, McDonald has instituted a policy that permits employees to devote 10 percent of their time to an area of special environmental or public health interest. The department also pays the cost of the professional license and one professional association membership, one college course per quarter, and specialized training related to job assignments if such training is needed. McDonald strongly encourages his staff to take advantage of opportunities to participate in professional activities, and models that involvement through his own contributions. For instance, he is a member of the American Public Health Association and the National Association of County and City Health Officials, chairing the latter association's environmental health advisory committee. He has served as president of the Washington State Association of Local Public Health Officials and cochaired the Washington State Public Health Finance Committee. He is a strong advocate for public health among state elected officials, working to build their commitment to funding a strong public health infrastructure as an essential component of quality of life.

A combination of job satisfaction, opportunities for professional growth, the quality of life in Island County, and perhaps in great measure McDonald's leadership example means that Island County Health Department does not experience large staff turnover. When asked why he remains committed to working in environmental and public health, McDonald says, "I don't think there's a better way to impact the world in a positive fashion than in public health. To really carry out public health, someone has to apply it locally; we are the part of the paintbrush that actually touches the canvas. You become involved in the community; you assist people. You can actually see the results of applying prevention and population-based science." And, McDonald adds, his staff make all the difference: "the people I work with are such a fantastic team; they support each other through the challenges and the tough times." It is clear that McDonald and his staff enjoy working together as a team, being part of that paintbrush that in partnership with the citizens, is painting a picture of an improved environment and public health for Island County. (For more information, see Island County Health Department, 2005.)

Iowa Department of Health: Ensuring an Improved Environment and Health Through Collaboration

States have unique challenges and opportunities when fulfilling their role of ensuring the delivery of environmental health services to statewide populations, and they organize their environmental health functions in many different ways. The Iowa Department of Public Health, for instance, shares the responsibility for various aspects of environmental health with sister departments of inspection and appeals and natural resources, and much of this responsibility is carried out through counties and local boards of health. Iowa is a home rule state, and the Iowa Code requires each county to have a county board of health with five members, including a physician, appointed by the county's board of supervisors. Two cities with populations over 25,000 have also established their own city boards of health, with members appointed by the city council. Therefore, Iowa, with 99 counties and 2 cities, has 101 local boards of health to address the needs of a state population of 2.9 million.

A person interested in working as an environmental health specialist has many options in Iowa. The Iowa Department of Inspections and Appeals regulates food safety and has contracts with approximately 75 percent of the jurisdictions to provide food protection services. The Iowa Department of Natural Resources requires local boards of health to oversee construction of private wells and on-site septic systems and has only two staff members that support the local boards in these programs. The Iowa Department of Public Health has a direct responsibility to local boards of health and oversees indoor air quality, lead poisoning prevention, swimming pools, tattoo establishments, tanning facilities, and funeral homes. In addition, the Iowa Code places requirements on local boards of health to address dog bites and vicious animals as well as dead animal disposal.

As manager of the Office of Technical Assistance in the Iowa Department of Health's Division of Health Protection and Environmental Health, Ken Sharp is responsible for providing technical support and consultation to local boards of health as they design and implement programs. Sharp's office recently conducted an environmental health workforce survey and estimates that 180 to 200 people are employed statewide in environmental health. Environmental health personnel at the county level may be located in a variety of offices; they may work in zoning, emergency management, weed control, engineering, or secondary roads, as well as in health or environmental offices. There may be one person handling all of a county's environmental health issues and that same person may work on nonenvironmental issues as well. The survey found 50 percent of the workforce to have a four-year degree, and 25 percent of the workforce to have a degree in the sciences. Statewide, this workforce experiences an annual 10 to 15 percent turnover, which is costly in both economic and health terms. Sharp's office works directly with these county personnel to provide necessary training and support. The workforce training needs are great; many of the rural counties do not require a science degree, and the salaries are often low as well. Few resources are available at the county level for training. Sharp's office helps field staff to improve their skills; develop a local response to citizen requests on issues for which there is no established program, such as mold, nuisance, or landlord complaints; and improve the quality of services provided to citizens.

The CDC awarded a grant to the Iowa Department of Health in 2001 to improve statewide capacity in environmental health services. The department was able to give minigrants to counties to improve their environmental health services and to develop trainings, fact sheets, and other resources to help the often isolated field staff. Through implementation of twenty-six minigrants totaling $270,000, thirty counties were able to purchase equipment, develop plans and tools, and establish education and marketing programs that have given them greater capacity to carry out the core functions and essential services of environmental health.

Ken Sharp's own career reflects the variety of environmental health opportunities. After receiving a bachelor's degree in environmental science, he worked for almost two years on a flood recovery team in Iowa for a CDC well survey conducted in nine Midwest states, doing water well surveys, fieldwork, inspecting construction standards, and taking samples. He spent the next five years doing environmental case management in the lead poisoning prevention program and was part of a team that established a training program for certification of lead inspectors and lead abatement contractors, before creating the Office of Technical Assistance. After ten challenging and interesting years in environmental health, Ken Sharp remains enthusiastic about his daily work. Sharp says, "there have never been two days identical in the last ten years. I like the variety of the challenges, and the satisfaction of being able to help people." The profession itself is rewarding as well; Sharp says: "This profession seems to be unique in its willingness to help each other out. Other environmental health colleagues are willing to share their experiences and to be called upon for technical assistance and guidance." It is because Iowa does not have stringent preentry requirements, Sharp believes, that most of the field personnel have experienced the frustration of having to start from the ground up in their jurisdictions and are willing to acknowledge the challenges others face and to offer support. In a recent example, a public health nurse assumed responsibility for an environmental health program in one of Iowa's counties, and Sharp's office was able to support her in sorting out programs, procedures, and policies and in setting guidelines on what qualifications to look for when hiring environmental health employees.

Sharp advises those interested in a career in environmental health to become familiar with the daily work involved and to develop an understanding of the kinds of skills that are necessary to do the job well. Sharp says, "there's a tremendous amount of public and professional interaction, and you have to be willing to talk to people." Sharp likes to hire employees who are diplomatic, honest, and open. He says:

> As we look more at the core competencies for environmental health and how they apply to the field, that set of competencies is as important as competencies in science and research. We need to be able to communicate the message. Faced with a scientist who is a poor communicator, I would rather take someone with a desire and interest and strong interpersonal and problem-solving competencies and teach him or her the science. When we have done that, these people have done a fantastic job of creating a wonderful program. You can take all the science in the world, and if you can't communicate it, it is not going to do you a whole lot of good in real-life practice.

Sharp's office has now incorporated questions related to these competencies in its interview process.

As is clear from the example of the State of Iowa, environmental health services are delivered at the state and local level through a variety of settings. Environmental health personnel in most states can expect to be called upon for both their technical and interpersonal skills, and can also expect to collaborate with citizens, other local and state agencies, private businesses, elected officials, and boards of health as they seek to improve public health and quality of life for the citizens they serve.

Stephanie Moraga-McHaley, Environmental Epidemiologist, Albuquerque, New Mexico

Stephanie Moraga-McHaley knew what she was interested in, but she didn't know what it was called. During her coursework at the University of New Mexico, she had taken courses in geology and knew that she liked the science but that she didn't want to be a geologist. She was interested in the human aspects of science but didn't want to go into medicine. When she and her husband, Curtis, moved to Colorado with a small toddler, interrupting her undergraduate career, she began searching the Web sites of Colorado universities and found the environmental health undergraduate program at Colorado State University in Fort Collins. The national and international media and popular press were full of stories of Ebola, hantavirus, and other diseases, and here was the opportunity to study what she came to understand was the field of environmental health. She went back to school at age twenty-eight to take some additional preliminary courses, was accepted into the program, and completed both her undergraduate and graduate degrees there while raising two small children.

During her studies in environmental health, Moraga-McHaley took several courses in toxicology, organic chemistry, environmental health practice, epidemiology, and biostatistics. She also took a class in science communication, which trained her in communicating about science with the general public, a skill that has proven useful in her later work. As part of her program she did an internship with the Colorado Department of Health and Environment, working on an EPA-funded childhood lead study and assembling a library of information on lead. She worked alongside community health workers and phlebotomists, conducting interviews with citizens on lead exposures and assisting with home environment assessments. She visited homes that were in such poor condition that lead seemed to be the least of the residents' problems. She went on to complete her graduate work, concentrating in environmental epidemiology and writing her thesis on farm-related illness and injuries in children.

When she moved back to Albuquerque with her family, Moraga-McHaley was hired by the Albuquerque Environmental Health Department to conduct investigations of foodborne illness outbreaks and to perform other environmental health field activities such as inspection of food facilities, pools, and spas. Her fluency in Spanish was helpful in communicating desired improvements in some of the restaurants she visited. One of her outbreak investigations focused on hepatitis A in a day-care facility; another involved an outbreak of an environmentally transmitted skin condition at the local correctional facility. Following three years at the department, she and her family moved to Spain for a year, where her husband worked as an environmental engineer. Although she did not work during this time, she was able to observe occupational health issues, such as musculoskeletal injuries related to the olive industry, and to add to her store of knowledge on the variety of ways in which environmental health is practiced. On moving back to New Mexico in 2003, she was hired to coordinate establishment of an occupational health registry for the State of New Mexico, a National Institute for Occupational Safety and Health–funded joint project between the University of New Mexico and the New Mexico Department of Health. She works in conjunction with the Council of State and Territorial Epidemiologists to develop a manual on how to create an occupational health surveillance system using occupational health indicators. To stay current in the field, she belongs to several listservs on issues such as pesticides and silicosis, attends workshops and seminars, and reads articles and information on the Internet.

Moraga-McHaley recommends the environmental health field to others interested in the intersection of science and health. "Environmental health is a good degree," she says, "because it has so many facets to it. There are so many possible career opportunities, from working with an oil company to a nonprofit or private environmental group to a public agency." Wherever they choose to work, she advises, professionals in environmental health need to be able to see both sides to every story and to remain objective. She encourages interested students to find out as much as possible about the various opportunities in order to determine the work environment best suited to their personalities and interests. She also recommends that people consider learning more about international environmental health. She says, "It's fascinating to see what's going on in other countries, how they address their environmental health issues, and what their epidemiological focus is." One day, when their children are grown, she and her husband would like to collaborate in environmental health internationally, preferably in Latin America. They are both currently trying to maintain and improve their Spanish by taking classes, and Moraga-McHaley would like to do some more coursework in public health. In the interim, she continues to find daily satisfaction in being able to study the science behind a health issue and to recommend interventions that will improve the situation. "There's nothing better," she says, "than a new set of data." As an environmental epidemiologist, Moraga-McHaley obviously enjoys the challenges and rewards of an always changing field.

Careers in Environmental Health

So you think you might enjoy a career in environmental health? You have many exciting options open to you. Environmental health services are delivered through a variety of federal, tribal, state, and local governmental agencies, within and outside traditional departments, through nongovernmental organizations, and through private businesses and academic institutions. The breadth of these services requires a diverse array of professionals in environmental health, with undergraduate and graduate training in biology, chemistry, geology, engineering, public health education, public relations, nursing, epidemiology, statistics, public health administration, and other disciplines. Technicians with associate degrees and community health workers are also valuable in delivering services and working with citizens to identify and resolve community environmental health concerns. Increasingly, as our understanding grows about the interconnections between the social, economic, and built environments and health and about the need to work collectively across disciplines to create healthy communities, the environmental health practice community includes those with backgrounds in architecture and planning, economic development, and community empowerment and capacity building.

Where do you find the training you need for a career in environmental health? You might begin by learning the location of accredited graduate and undergraduate environmental health programs near your home. Accredited programs offer their students the advantage of a curriculum, a faculty, and resources that meet nationally adopted standards. Accreditation is conducted by the National Environmental Health and Protection Accreditation Council (EHAC) (see EHAC, 2005, for the criteria for accreditation). Most of these programs require field practica or internships with agencies as part of the student's preparation. The Bureau of Health Professions of the DHHS Health Resources and Services Administration has published a document that may be useful to both students and agencies in creating meaningful internship experiences (White and Bock, 1996).

You will want to be aware of the expectations of your future employers for the competencies they believe you should be bringing to their workforce. In 2001, the National Center for Environmental Health funded a workgroup to define the core competencies for local environmental health practitioners. In addition to expectations for technical competence, this group defined fourteen core competencies under three general skill headings: assessment, management, and communication. Table 30.3 lists these fourteen competencies (more detailed information can be found at NCEH and APHA, 2001).

When you graduate with a combination of these competencies and a degree in environmental health—or in chemistry, biology, community health, health education, or another related discipline—there are a number of places you might seek to work. Local and state health departments and environmental health agencies and also tribes and industry are looking for science-trained individuals to educate, monitor, assess, and assist with environmental health compliance. You

TABLE 30.3. CORE COMPETENCIES FOR LOCAL ENVIRONMENTAL HEALTH.

A.	Assessment
	Information gathering
	Data analysis and interpretation
	Evaluation
B.	Management
	Problem solving
	Economic and social issues
	Organizational knowledge and behavior
	Project management
	Computer and information technology
	Reporting, documentation, and record keeping
	Collaboration
C.	Communication
	Educate
	Communicate
	Conflict resolution
	Marketing

Source: NCEH and APHA, 2001.

might enter the field as a food protection specialist, inspecting all the various sources of food in a community, from bakeries and meat markets to grocery stores and food-processing plants. You might become an air or water quality technician or engineer, working with community pollution sources on engineering design, pollution prevention, plan review, air or water quality monitoring, calculation of emissions, and enforcement of regulations. If you are interested in the intersection of health, environment, economic development, and community planning, you might seek a position with an agency that focuses on land-use and transportation planning or offer those skills to an existing public health agency that is interested in expanding its efforts in community-based comprehensive health planning.

If you are interested in environmental health within the larger field of public health, you might consider a master's degree in public health. Graduate programs of public health accredited by the Council on Education for Public Health have a required core course in environmental health. The Council on Linkages

Between Academia and Public Health Practice has adopted and regularly revises a list of skills and competencies expected of professionals in public health. With a graduate degree in public health, you might be employed as an epidemiologist in a mid- to large-sized agency, assessing exposures, estimating and communicating risk, investigating diseases caused by environmental factors, and working collaboratively with others across multiple agencies to develop policies and interventions to reduce exposures. Graduate public health training also prepares you for leadership of a program or agency and equips you with the skills to assess community needs, build constituencies, develop policies and plans, evaluate program effectiveness, and advocate for policy change. If you are technologically adept, you might enjoy working with data systems, geographic information, and generating statistics and maps to assist community members and elected policymakers in improved decision making for health. One of the best ways to evaluate the many exciting work possibilities is to visit a variety of agencies and talk with the professionals about their daily job satisfaction and challenges.

Once you are working in the field of environmental health, you will want to plan for ongoing training and education to improve your skills and to enhance your career development. Many training opportunities are available at low or no cost online. (For further detail on resources for career development, education, and training, see Public Health Foundation, 2005, and TRAIN, 2005.) One thing is certain: with the ever-changing environmental issues and emerging threats to community and environmental health, you will have daily opportunities and challenges to provide effective environmental health services that will keep your community healthy.

Thought Questions

1. How would you tell someone else about the history of environmental health and the link between environmental health and public health?
2. What were some of the factors that led to increased emphasis on the importance of community involvement in environmental health planning?
3. What are some of the common barriers to community environmental health planning?
4. What are some of the tools that are readily available to communities and agencies to conduct community environmental health planning?
5. Discuss the links between democracy, environment, economic development, and equity. What barriers remain to creating healthy people in healthy communities? Can you think of additional steps that need to be taken to address these barriers to achieve healthy environments for all?

References

Burke, T. A., Shalauta, N. M., and Tran, N. L. *The Environmental Web: Impact of Federal Statutes on State Environmental Health and Protection, Services, Structure and Funding.* Rockville, Md.: U.S. Department of Health and Human Services, 1995a.

Burke, T. A., Shalauta, N. M., and Tran, N. L. *Who's in Charge? 50-State Profile of Environmental Health and Protection Services: Organization, Programs, Functions/Activities and State Budgets.* Rockville, Md.: U.S. Department of Health and Human Services, 1995b.

Centers for Disease Control and Prevention, National Public Health Performance Standards Program (NPHPSP). "The Essential Public Health Services." [http://www.phppo.cdc.gov/nphpsp/10EssentialPHServices.asp]. 2004.

Centers for Disease Control and Prevention, Public Health Practice Program Office. "National Public Health Performance Standards Program." [http://www.phppo.cdc.gov/nphpsp]. 2005.

Healthy People. Homepage. [http://www.healthypeople.gov]. 2005.

Institute of Medicine. *The Future of Public Health.* Washington, D.C.: National Academies Press, 1988.

Island County Environmental Health Initiative. "Island County Environmental Health Initiative Quarterly Progress Report, July 2003." CDC Cooperative Agreement #U38/CCU020425-02. Coupeville, Wash.: Island County Health Department.

Island County Health Department. "Island County: Public Health and Human Services." [http://www.islandcounty.net/health]. 2005.

National Association of City and County Health Officials. *PACE-EH Guidebook.* [http://pace.naccho.org]. 2004.

National Center for Environmental Health and American Public Health Association. *Environmental Health Competency Project: Recommendations for Core Competencies for Local Environmental Health Practitioners.* [http://www.apha.org/ppp/Env_Comp_Booklet.pdf]. 2001.

National Environmental Health and Protection Accreditation Council. Homepage. [http://www.ehacoffice.org]. 2005.

Public Health Foundation. Homepage. [www.phf.org]. 2005.

TRAIN (a project of the Public Health Foundation). Homepage. [www.train.org]. 2005.

White, L. E., and Bock, S. *Designing Environmental Internships: A Guide for Successful Experiences.* Rockville, Md.: U.S. Department of Health and Human Services, 1996.

Winslow, C.E.A. *The Evolution and Significance of the Modern Public Health Campaign.* New Haven, Conn.: Yale University Press, 1923.

For Further Information

Publications

Lehr, J. H. (ed.). *Standard Handbook of Environmental Science, Health and Technology.* New York: McGraw-Hill, 2000.

Nadakavukaren, A. *Our Global Environment: A Health Perspective.* (5th ed.) Prospect Heights, Ill.: Waveland Press, 2000.

Salvato, J. A., Nemerow, N. L., and Agardy, F. J. (eds.). *Environmental Engineering.* (5th ed.) San Francisco: Jossey-Bass, 2003.

Larry Gordon was one of the most influential environmental health leaders of the twentieth and early twenty-first centuries. A collection of his papers (and his autobiography) can be found at www.ncleha.org. For his views on some of the priority challenges facing environmental health practitioners in the twenty-first century, see

Gordon, L. J. "Environmental Health and Protection: Century 21 Challenges." *Journal of Environmental Health,* 1995, *67*(6), 28–34.

Organizations

The CDC's National Center for Environmental Health is a national resource on many topics related to environmental health. Within NCEH, the Environmental Health Services Branch provides specific support for environmental health practice. See:

Centers for Disease Control and Prevention, National Center for Environmental Health. Homepage. [www.cdc.gov/nceh]. 2005.
Centers for Disease Control and Prevention, National Center for Environmental Health, Environmental Health Services. Homepage. [http://www.cdc.gov/nceh/ehs/default.htm]. 2005.

The National Association of County and City Health Officials provides numerous excellent resources to local environmental health agencies. Its Web site also provides detailed information on community environmental health assessment using PACE-EH:

National Association of County and City Health Officials. "Community-Based Environmental Health Assessment." [http://www.naccho.org/topics/environmental/CEHA.cfm]. 2004.

The National Environmental Health Science and Protection Accreditation Council provides information on the process of accreditation and links to accredited graduate and undergraduate environmental health academic programs.

National Environmental Health Science and Protection Accreditation Council. Homepage. [http://www.ehacoffice.org]. 2005.

The Association of Environmental Health Academic Programs provides information on accredited programs as well as scholarship and award information for students of environmental health. AEHAP's Web site also contains links to professional organizations of interest to students, such as the Society for the Advancement of Chicanos and Native Americans in Science:

Association of Environmental Health Academic Programs. Homepage. [http://www.aehap.org]. 2005.

The National Conference of Local Environmental Health Administrators is a forum and a resource for managers of local environmental health programs and for others interested in current environmental health issues. The organization's Web site contains papers and articles of importance to environmental health and an excellent links page for additional environmental health information:

National Conference of Local Environmental Health Administrators. Homepage. [http://www.ncleha.org]. 2005.

The American Public Health Association is the largest organization of public health professionals in the world. The APHA Section on Environment provides a professional home for a broad spectrum of people working in environmental health. The section convenes annually, in conjunction with the APHA annual meeting, and invites students and other professionals in environmental health to submit papers for an annual educational program.

American Public Health Association, Section on Environment. Homepage. [http://depts.washington.edu/aphaenv]. 2004.

The National Environmental Health Association is a professional society for those working in environmental health. NEHA sponsors an annual education conference and numerous credentialing programs and publications and publishes the *Journal of Environmental Health.*

National Environmental Health Association. Homepage. [www.neha.org]. 2005.

CHAPTER THIRTY-ONE

GEOGRAPHIC INFORMATION SYSTEMS

Lance A. Waller

Georeferenced data, that is, data measurements associated with particular geographic locations, often play a critical role in assessments of various aspects of environmental health. In fact the phrase "global to local" in the title of this book builds on the notion of spatial *scale,* referring to the defined space within which a phenomenon occurs, which in turn defines the geographic extent of potential outcomes and potential remediation, or other intervention efforts. Mapping spatially referenced exposure, populations at risk, and environmental factors (for example, stream flow, wind speed and direction, emissions locations, and monitoring sites) serves to manage data geographically, allows linkages among multiple indicators measured by different agencies over the same study area, and provides valuable background information for interpreting the environmental context of public health data.

We can begin to build on these ideas by considering the following key components of an environmental health response to an accidental release of a toxic agent: where is the exposure of interest, and where is the population at risk? The greatest concerns arise when areas of high exposure overlap areas of high population density. Although neither a quantitative assessment of exposure nor an in-depth epidemiological assessment, the simple act of laying a map of exposure over a map of population density provides a valuable exploratory tool, identifying areas of highest immediate concern.

The role of maps in public health extends back at least to John Snow's maps of cholera mortality in London (Snow, 1855). Most public health students have encountered the story of Snow, a physician who mapped cholera deaths during the 1854 outbreak in London, noted an aggregation near a public water pump on Broad Street, and petitioned for the removal of the handle to the pump in the interest of public health. The story provides a powerful motivator for understanding the potential of geographically linking data sets—in Snow's case, victims' homes and the locations of public pumps. (Such a brief summary of the incident minimizes some of its nuances and the role of maps, drawn by Snow and others, in the public health response; Brody and others, 2000, provide an insightful discussion of the variety of maps considered in the public health response to the 1854 epidemic.)

The dramatic story of Snow's map often serves as a call for increased use of maps and mapping in environmental health with the goal of identifying previously unknown connections between environmental exposures and public health problems. Indeed, if John Snow could accomplish his study with little more than time, ink, and paper, one wonders what explorations might be accomplished with today's computers. Indeed, such specialized computer tools are now available. A *geographic information system,* or *GIS,* is a computer software system (or more accurately, a set of linked software packages) that enables the collection, management, linkage, display, and analysis of georeferenced data. The first formal GISs arose out of the Canada Geographic Information System, devised in the 1960s to aid in the Canada Land Survey (Longley, Goodchild, Maguire, and Rhind, 2001). Since then, GISs have developed and evolved to address a wide spectrum of applications, grown to accommodate vast stores of georeferenced data, and advanced in both usability and versatility.

This chapter provides an introduction to the use of georeferenced data and geographic information systems within the field of environmental health. Important considerations include the role of maps in environmental health, the role of cartographic principles in an age of computer-generated maps, the basic features and operations of GISs, illustrations of the types of environmental health analyses enabled by GISs, and some limiting factors in such analyses.

Components of Georeferenced Data

Georeferenced data consist of location, attributes, and support. *Location* refers to the geographic location where a data measurement is taken. An *attribute* is a measurement taken at a given location. Note that several attributes may exist at a single location, for example, the particulate matter level, the nitrogen oxides level, and the ozone level. *Support* denotes the type of location associated with the attribute measurement. Geographic support is often classified in terms of *points* (single locations), *lines* (segments such as roads or rivers), and *areas* (typically, political divisions such as states, counties, or census tracts, but also watersheds or ecotones). Support provides a context for interpreting attribute values and a reference location for mapping. Data with point support are located as points on a map. Data with line support are associated with lines or curves on a map. Examples include the traffic density on a particular road segment and contaminant levels in a stream.

It is helpful to think of a data set as consisting of a table of values (as in a spreadsheet) linked to a map of data locations. Suppose each row in the data table corresponds to a set of attribute measurements associated with a single location. Each column corresponds to a particular type of attribute measurement across locations, for example, the particulate matter level at each of a number of air sampling sites. The linkage between the table and the map is such that selecting a location on the map results in selection of the associated row of attribute values in the table, and the selection of a row of the table corresponds to selection of the associated location on the map.

The multiple components of georeferenced data imply multiple components of data accuracy. In particular, quality assessments of georeferenced data must consider location accuracy and support accuracy as well as attribute accuracy. A precisely measured attribute value associated with the wrong location can be as deleterious to analysis as a mismeasured attribute value.

Basic GIS Operations

There are a variety of GIS packages available, with a range of features, interfaces, and interoperability. However, all GISs contain certain core features allowing basic operations on spatial data. Three of the most important operations are layering, buffering, and spatial queries.

As its name implies, *layering* is linking two separate databases by their underlying geography. For example, suppose we have a census database that provides summary information on population demographics for census tracts in a given county. Suppose we then obtain a second database providing the location and flow levels for a given stream network in the same county. Finally, suppose we have a third database providing both a point location for each residence where a case of a specific disease was reported in the county during a given year and a concentration value associated with a tap-water sample from each residence. We have three different data sets, but we can overlay the respective maps of locations by layering the data in a GIS. Conceptually, this corresponds to overlaying transparent maps of each set of locations so that we may view them together (see Figure 31.1). More important, we can now reference elements of one layer by their proximity to elements in another layer, for example, we can identify which streams are near homes with high tap-water concentration values.

FIGURE 31.1. HYPOTHETICAL EXAMPLE OF THE GIS LAYERING OPERATION.

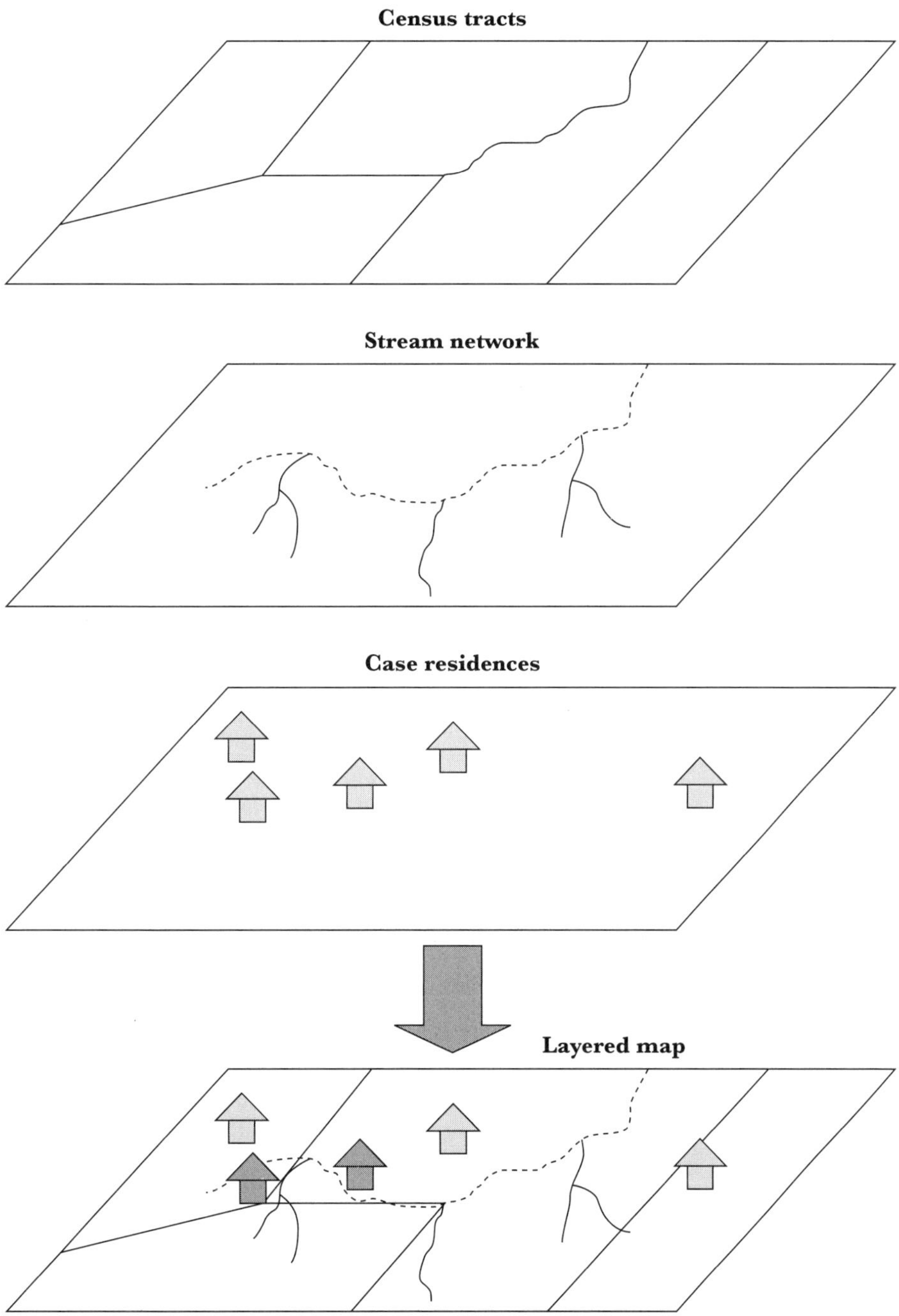

Buffering involves selection of data items by their position relative to other locations. For example, suppose we wish to identify the census tracts falling within 1 km of a selected stream segment. We select the particular stream segment on our stream map and then define a *buffer* zone around it of the prescribed distance. Most GISs implement equidistant buffers around points, lines, and areas (see Figure 31.2 for examples), but some GISs allow the user to adjust buffer zone dimensions, so that they correspond to wind direction, for example.

At its heart any GIS either implements or accesses a relational database system, allowing the sorting, combining, and selecting of data values. In addition to standard database queries, such as, "Find all records with concentrations above 5 ppm," a GIS can also conduct *spatial queries,* such as, "Display all homes within 1 km of a selected stream segment." For example, suppose we wish to identify case residences within 1 km of the dashed stream segment in Figure 31.1. Layering places the case residence data in geographic context with the stream data, and buffering identifies which case residences are within the prescribed distance (for example, the darkest houses in Figure 31.1). We may also conduct combined queries incorporating both location and attribute data, such as, "Display all records with concentrations above 5 ppm [an attribute value] and within 1 km of the selected stream segment [a relative location value]."

Combining all three operations (layering, buffering, and spatial queries) allows one to process complex queries, such as, "Display all census tracts with disease rates above 5 cases per 100,000 person-years at risk, that are within 1 km of the selected stream segment and have concentration values above 5 ppm." This query requires layering to combine the stream, health, and population databases, buffering to identify census tracts within the prescribed distance from the stream, and a combined spatial and data query to identify the desired records.

Geographic Information About Exposure: Why Map Exposure?

Having defined the basic structure of georeferenced data and basic GIS operations, we next consider the role of geography in environmental health. Building on the earlier example of considering an appropriate public health response to an accidental toxic release, we find that spatial questions abound: Where was the release? Which way was the wind blowing? What streams are nearby? Where are exposures the highest? Who lives in that area? Who works in that area? What are the possible evacuation routes? Can the spill be contained? Expanding our view to other environmental health concerns, we find similar sets of questions: for example, Where are pesticides applied? Which pesticides were applied in each

FIGURE 31.2. EXAMPLES OF BUFFERS AROUND POINT (TOP), LINE (MIDDLE), AND AREA (BOTTOM) FEATURES.

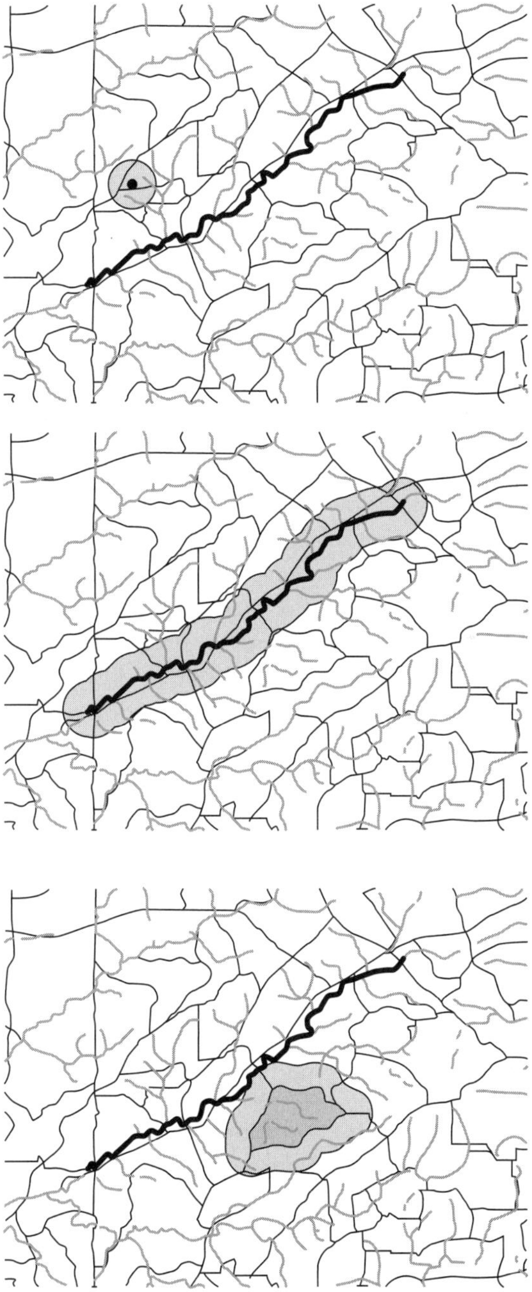

Buffer around a point feature

Buffer around a line feature

Buffer around an area feature

location? What quantity was applied? Who lives nearby? Who works nearby? Are environmental hazards sited in minority neighborhoods? How many children live near a proposed landfill? An accurate map of exposure values may answer, in whole or in part, many of these questions.

To start, consider what information can be contained in a map of exposure. First, most exposure maps are maps of *ambient* exposures, the level of a contaminant existing at a given location. Note, however, that the ambient exposure is only one component of the *personal* exposure received by a person at that location. Other factors influencing personal exposure are the individual's respiration rate, presence or absence of protective clothing, and the like, suggesting that two people at the same location may receive very different personal exposures from the same ambient exposure (see Chapter Four).

Next, consider what data are required to map ambient exposures. In the case of airborne exposures, we might use point monitoring stations that provide detailed ambient levels at each point. Construction of a map requires interpolation to all points in the study area based on the observed data. The accuracy of the monitoring data combined with the accuracy of the interpolation method will affect the accuracy of the overall exposure map. (There are many statistical techniques for spatial interpolation; Webster and Oliver, 2001, and Waller and Gotway, 2004, chap. 8, provide details and additional references.)

In the absence of measured exposure values, it is common to use geographic *proximity* as a surrogate for relative exposure, that is, we generally assume that individuals residing (or working) closer to a source of contamination sustain a higher exposure than individuals farther away. Although proximity rarely (if ever) provides an accurate surrogate for exposure values, the relative ranking may be sufficiently accurate for some exploratory classifications, for example, into *high* and *low* exposure regions. Although accurate exposure assessments strengthen the clinical relevance of any measured associations between exposure and health, assessing proximity may be useful for pilot studies, preliminary classifications, and other exploratory uses.

Geographic Information About Health: Why Map Disease?

Just as maps of exposure suggest answers to questions of interest in environmental health, maps of disease incidence and prevalence also provide insight into patterns and trends in the data. Typical questions include: Where is disease incidence or prevalence highest? Where is it lowest? How do observed local incidences or prevalences correspond to a map of exposure?

Maps of disease may be *dot maps*, with point locations of each case, or *choropleth maps*, indicating counts or estimated rates in nonoverlapping regions such as states, counties, or census tracts. Choropleth maps are more common than point maps due to confidentiality restrictions; a map that reports aggregate counts of cases from census regions reveals less individual information than a map of case residence addresses does. Although not particularly cartographically progressive, choropleth maps summarize information and are easily created and (more important) easily interpreted by public health professionals (Pickle and others, 1994).

As with exposure maps, many factors complicate the construction of maps of health outcomes. First, most people move about during the day, making it difficult to assign individuals to fixed locations on a map. Especially important in environmental health is the difference between residential location (where one sleeps), and occupational location (where one works). The location of interest corresponds to the relevant exposures, but these are often unknown and under study. In addition, residential location may be more readily available (from billing or other mailing records) than occupational location. Another complication arises because increasing geographic resolution by choosing small regions often erodes the statistical precision of the local estimates within each region due to reduced local sample size. Several statistical methods exist for stabilizing local estimates from small sample sizes (Lawson and Williams, 2001; Waller and Gotway, 2004), but few are widely available in standard statistical software.

Data Quality and Cartography: Good Maps of Good Data

The discussion in the preceding sections suggests that mapping exposure and health data may provide answers to relevant questions. However, it also raises some worries regarding the accuracy of mapped values; recall, for instance, the concerns about ambient versus personal exposures and rate estimates from small areas. One of the greatest strengths of a GIS is its ability to link disparate data sets collected over the same study area. For instance, we may wish to link exposure, health, and demographic data over a specific region. These three data sets have likely been collected separately by different agencies, perhaps over different time periods, and for different reasons. As a result, the primary strength of a GIS also raises an important weakness: the accuracy of any conclusions we draw from our map depends on the quality of the individual data components. Unlike a designed study with a single research team in charge of collecting, processing, analyzing, and interpreting the data, most GIS applications draw heavily from existing data sources for both location and attribute data such as census counts, stream locations, and so forth.

In addition to requiring quality data, a good map also requires careful thought about and selection of cartographic symbols, colors, and the like. For instance, the standard order of hues in the spectrum (red, orange, yellow, green, blue, indigo, violet) may strike the novice mapmaker as a sensible choice for displaying ordered categories on a map, but shifts from light to dark tints of the same hue (from light red to dark red, for example) are actually much easier for map readers to interpret as representing increasing values. You can test this for yourself. Try to decide quickly, and without referencing the entire spectrum, whether green is "bigger" than orange. Now, try to decide quickly whether light red is "bigger" than medium red. (Monmonier, 1996, provides an introduction to important cartographic concepts that should be required reading for anyone planning to make wide use of GIS techniques or mapping in general.)

GIS Applications: What Can We Do with a GIS?

The discussion so far has outlined data structures and operations in a GIS setting. Next we briefly consider two specific applications of GIS features and operations, addressing ongoing research programs in environmental health.

The first application is a comparison of physical activity levels between users and nonusers of parks in DeKalb County, Georgia. An important component of the study design is to sample park nonusers from neighborhoods that are demographically similar to the park users' neighborhoods and approximately the same distance from parks as the park users' neighborhoods are, in order to remove transportation time and demographics as drivers and potential confounders of the observed differences in physical activity patterns. The study design samples park users by interviewing individuals in the park, but it is not clear how the study might sample nonusers.

We can use a two-stage approach to gathering the required samples. First, the sample of park users provides the geographic distribution of park users' residences, defining a *catchment* area for the park. Second, by mapping residence locations of sampled park users onto a street map layer in our GIS and then layering census block groups (subdivisions of census tracts) over it, we assign each residence to its associated census block group. The U.S. Census provides summary demographic information for each block group, and this allows us to identify additional block groups within the park's catchment area that have similar demographics and from which we may draw potential nonusers. More specifically, by buffering around park boundaries and applying a spatial query, we can identify the subset that contains the demographically matched block groups that are within the same geographic catchment area as the park users.

Note that this example employs all three GIS operations and differs somewhat from the "standard" conceptual use of GIS to identify proximity exposure surrogates to insert into a statistical model measuring links between the (surrogate) exposure and the disease outcome. In addition, in this example standard GIS operations enhance the implementation of a fairly standard epidemiological study design (a case-control study in which the *cases* are park users) by identifying potential *controls* (park nonusers).

The second application of GIS operations to be considered is part of an assessment of an environmental justice claim. In June of 1998, Father Schmitter and Sister Chiaverini of the St. Francis Prayer Center in Flint, Michigan, citing Title VI of the U.S. Civil Rights Act of 1964, alleged environmental justice violations in the proposed siting of a new steel recycling minimill for the Select Steel Corporation of America. In August of 1998, the U.S. Environmental Protection Agency (EPA) agreed to investigate the claim. (For a full collection of EPA documents relating to the case, see EPA, Office of Civil Rights, 2005.)

The proposed minimill was to produce up to 43 tons per hour of specialty metals and, according to the EPA's review, had the potential to emit 100 tons per year of criteria pollutants, including particulate matter, lead, carbon monoxide, and oxides of nitrogen. The complaint filed with the EPA alleged that "the vast majority of the people within 3 miles of the proposed site are minority Americans and will be burdened with a disparate impact of pollution in an already deeply polluted area." Following the filing of this complaint, the *Detroit News* reported its own study of the area within a one-mile radius of the proposed site, describing the "overwhelmingly white makeup of the surrounding neighborhood's demographics." The EPA's report gives demographics for the one-, two-, three-, and four-mile radii, yielding populations that are 13.8, 37.2, 51.1, and 55.2 percent minority, respectively.

How can a GIS clarify the situation? Figure 31.3 displays a map of census block groups for the 1990 U.S. Census (the most recent census at the time of the EPA investigation), indicating the proposed minimill location and associated one-, two-, and three-mile buffers. Block groups are shaded according to the proportion of census responders who self-identified their race as "black" (the most common nonwhite racial classification for this county). The map immediately indicates the discrepancies between the reports. The proposed location is northeast of the city of Flint, and a large proportion of the county's nonwhite population resides within the city. Within one mile the population is predominantly white (as claimed in the newspaper reports), whereas the three-mile buffer begins to include the more densely populated block groups, with higher proportions of nonwhite (predominantly black) residents. Even though similar information is revealed in the EPA's report in the form of a table, a GIS quickly provided the same table accompanied by the map in Figure 31.3. Owing to results such as this, the EPA has added tools to its Web sites linking EPA, Census, and U.S. Geological Survey (USGS) data, enabling users to create similar maps online.

FIGURE 31.3. MAP OF GENESEE COUNTY, MICHIGAN, SHOWING 1990 CENSUS BLOCK GROUPS AND MINIMILL LOCATION.

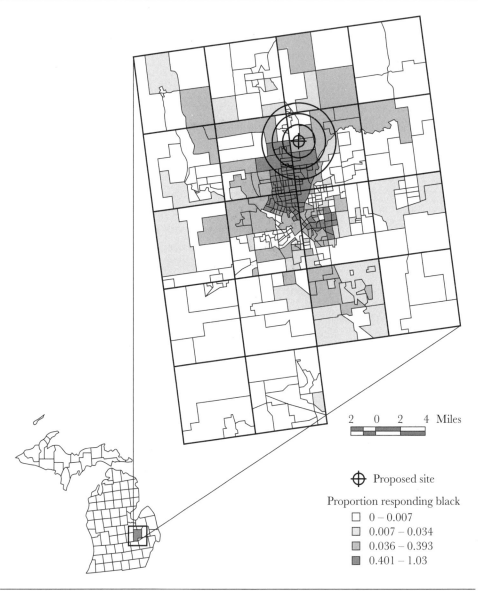

Note: Block groups are shaded according to the percentage of census respondents self-identifying their race as "black." The location of the proposed steel recycling minimill is accompanied by one-, two-, and three-mile buffers.

GIS Limitations

Many introductions to the use of GISs in public health offer long lists of advantages but often little discussion of limitations or complications. The previous sections of this chapter illustrate several compelling reasons to incorporate a GIS into the environmental health toolbox, and it is only fair to discuss the other side of the coin.

First and foremost, as mentioned earlier, the ability to combine multiple data sets collected by different agencies for different reasons is both a strength and a potential weakness of a GIS, because assessments of data quality often become murky when multiple data sets of differing quality are combined. Moreover, in this assessment we must consider the quality of *location* data as well as the quality of *attribute* data.

Second, most GIS studies are, unsurprisingly, *observational* rather than *experimental*. That is, measures of associations are based on observed data, and epidemiological concerns about types of bias, confounding, and effect modification should always define the suitable context for interpretation of GIS results.

Third, spatial data often include spatial correlations between observations (nearby observations being more similar than those taken far apart). Such correlations violate many standard statistical assumptions and require specialized statistical techniques for analysis, many of which are not currently available in either GIS or standard statistical software packages (Cromley and McLafferty, 2002; Waller and Gotway, 2004).

Fourth, the availability of data (both location and attribute) varies widely. Some studies may require development of a *base map* of locations before any study data can be assigned to locations. Data from global positioning systems (GPSs) and aerial and satellite imaging can aid the development of base maps, but these data require time and expertise to combine and prepare for use.

Finally, basic operations such as layering and buffering can be complicated when the layers use different projections of the earth's surface to the map plane or have different levels of resolution. For example, if we zoom in on the Mississippi river on a national map we may find that its course is defined by only a few line segments at the county level, much less detail than we would find on a local map. Or we may have population demographics for census block groups and hospital discharge data for hospital catchment areas whose borders do not coincide with block group boundaries. Combining data from such *misaligned* data sets often requires assumptions and calculations above and beyond standard GIS operations.

Conclusion

In summary, geographic information systems provide a valuable set of tools for managing, merging, querying, and displaying geographically referenced data in order to answer questions about environmental health. The basic operations outlined here may be combined in myriad ways, resulting in a broad set of tools for exploring, summarizing, and displaying such data. Longley, Goodchild, Maguire, and Rhind (2001) provide many examples of the use of GISs in an array of disciplines, and Cromley and McLafferty (2002) explore public health applications in more detail. Other texts addressing the use of GIS in public health include Albert, Gesler, and Levergood (2000), Kahn and Skinner (2003), and Melnick and Fleming (2002).

However, as noted previously, the use of GISs still requires appreciation of common limitations in both public health and geography. There is much to be gained by training public health professionals to "think spatially" and, similarly, much to be gained by training GIS professionals to "think epidemiologically." Innovative applications of GIS in environmental health most often arise from collaborations between individuals familiar with GIS capabilities and individuals trained in public health research. A final consideration is that it is always helpful to frame research goals in terms of questions to be answered, to frame analytical methods by the questions they answer, and then to match capabilities.

Thought Questions

1. Although the issue of *data quality* is always important in environmental health research, do the GIS structure and operations raise issues that may not arise in a controlled laboratory setting?
2. Describe how the basic operations of a GIS might help you do the following:

   - Investigate the health impact of an accidental release of a toxic agent into a stream.
   - Design a mosquito-spraying program targeting control of the spread of West Nile virus.
   - Develop a sampling plan for controls in an environmental case-control study.
   - Evaluate and prioritize potential locations for new air-monitoring stations.
   - Define commuting patterns resulting from various development plans, and project the impact of lane blockages in various parts of the street network.

   In each case discuss the data layers needed and the questions that various GIS operations may answer.

References

Albert, D. P., Gesler, W. M., and Levergood, B. (eds.). *Spatial Analysis, GIS, and Remote Sensing Applications in the Health Sciences.* Chelsea, Mich.: Ann Arbor Press, 2000.

Brody, H., and others. "Map-Making and Myth-Making in Broad Street: The London Cholera Epidemic, 1854." *Lancet,* 2000, *356,* 64–68.

Cromley, E. K., and McLafferty, S. L. *GIS and Public Health.* New York: Guilford Press, 2002.

Kahn, O., and Skinner, R. (eds.). *Geographic Information Systems and Health Applications.* Hershey, Penn.: Idea Group, 2003.

Lawson, A. B., and Williams, F. L. *An Introductory Guide to Disease Mapping.* Hoboken, N.J.: Wiley, 2001.

Longley, P. A., Goodchild, M. F., Maguire, D. J., and Rhind, D. W. *Geographic Information: Systems and Science.* Hoboken, N.J.: Wiley, 2001.

Melnick, A. L., and Fleming, D. *Introduction to Geographic Information Systems for Public Health.* Boston: Jones & Bartlett, 2002.

Monmonier, M. *How to Lie with Maps.* (2nd ed.) Chicago: University of Chicago Press, 1996.

Pickle, L. W., and others. "The Impact of Statistical Graphical Design on Interpretation of Disease Rate Maps." *Proceedings of the American Statistical Association's Section on Statistical Graphics.* Alexandria, Va.: American Statistical Association, 1994.

Snow, J. *On the Mode of Communication of Cholera.* London: John Churchill, 1855.

U.S. Environmental Protection Agency, Office of Civil Rights. Homepage. [http://www.epa.gov/civilrights/index.html]. 2005.

Waller, L. A., and Gotway, C. A. *Applied Spatial Statistics for Public Health Data.* Hoboken, N.J.: Wiley, 2004.

Webster, R., and Oliver, M. A. *Geostatistics for Environmental Scientists.* Hoboken, N.J.: Wiley, 2001.

For Further Information

National Center for Health Statistics. "GIS and Public Health." [http://www.cdc.gov/nchs/gis.htm]. 2004.

World Health Organization. "Public Health Mapping." [http://www.who.int/csr/mapping/en]. 2005.

CHAPTER THIRTY-TWO

RISK ASSESSMENT

Scott Bartell

Risk assessment is the process of identifying and evaluating adverse events that could occur in defined scenarios. Scenarios may be broadly or narrowly defined and may include many possible events. One well-known risk assessor (Kaplan, 1997) describes risk assessment as an attempt to answer three questions for a particular scenario: What can happen? How likely is it to happen? and, What are the consequences if it does happen? Risk assessment is used in many fields, including public health, engineering, economics, computer science, medicine, and law.

In the environmental health setting, risk assessors focus on health impacts that might result from being exposed to a particular agent or from working in, living in, or visiting a particular environment. For example, risk assessors might analyze the health risks of drinking water with chemical and microbial contaminants, of eating fish contaminated with mercury or polychlorinated biphenyls (PCBs), of breathing particulate matter and other airborne contaminants, or of being exposed to natural and man-made sources of ionizing radiation. Environmental health risk assessment can be viewed as a quantitative framework for evaluating and combining evidence from toxicology, epidemiology, and disciplines, with the goal of providing a basis for decision making (Box 32.1).

Box 32.1. Is Risk Assessment a Science?

Although it relies heavily on science-based information, risk assessment does not generate new empirical evidence on health effects in the way that toxicology and epidemiology do. Instead, risk assessment can be viewed as a synthesis of existing scientific information, often aimed at addressing specific regulatory or policy issues. This is why risk assessment has been referred to as a mixture of "science and judgment" (National Research Council [NRC], 1994).

Chloroform ingestion is used as an example throughout this chapter. Chloroform is a by-product of chlorinating drinking water (a *disinfection by-product,* or DBP, as explained in Chapter Eighteen), and appears at average concentrations of 1 to 90 μg/L in U.S. drinking water systems (Toxicology Excellence for Risk Assessment, 1998). Although chlorination of drinking water supplies is one of the most effective public health interventions ever conceived, due to its virtual elimination of cholera and other waterborne diseases, exposure to chloroform and other disinfection by-products may increase cancer rates in humans (Environmental Protection Agency [EPA], 2001). What are the risks of consuming typical levels of chloroform in drinking water? This chapter illustrates approaches that risk assessors might use to answer that and other questions about environmental health risks.

The Environmental Health Risk Assessment Process

Although risk assessment did not blossom until probability theory was developed in the seventeenth century, gamblers and philosophers have grappled with the concept of risk since the time of ancient Greek civilization (Bernstein, 1996). The application of risk assessment to environmental health issues is much more recent, beginning largely in the 1970s, when new environmental laws in the United States created a need for science-based decisions on the questions raised by environmental pollution. It would be very costly, and probably impossible, to achieve a society entirely free of pollution, so risk assessment is used to help us determine acceptable limits for concentrations of pollutants in air, water, soil, and biota and in emissions from vehicles and industry.

In 1983, the conceptual framework for environmental health risk assessment was formalized in a National Research Council (NRC) report, *Risk Assessment in the Federal Government,* commonly referred to as the *red book.* The red book divides risk assessment into four elements: hazard identification, dose-response

FIGURE 32.1. RISK ASSESSMENT FRAMEWORK.

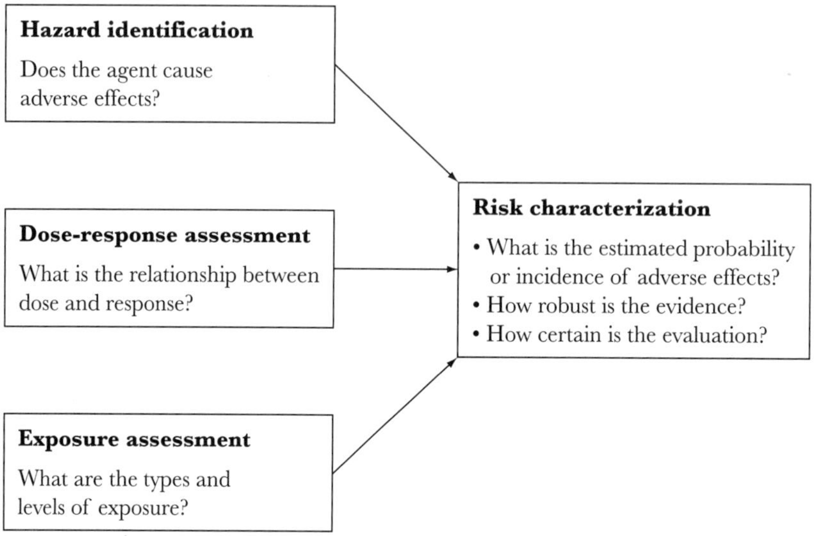
Hazard identification
Does the agent cause adverse effects?
Dose-response assessment
What is the relationship between dose and response?
Exposure assessment
What are the types and levels of exposure?
Risk characterization
• What is the estimated probability or incidence of adverse effects?
• How robust is the evidence?
• How certain is the evaluation?

Source: Adapted from Omenn, 2003.

assessment, exposure assessment, and risk characterization. Figure 32.1 shows how the four elements of risk assessment fit together.

Hazard identification is the process of identifying and selecting the environmental agent(s) and health effect(s) for assessment. This process includes causal inference for particular health outcomes, based on the strength of the toxicological and epidemiological evidence for causation. Sometimes the scope of inquiry is limited to a single agent and single health effect from the outset, leading to a fairly straightforward hazard identification process. At other times, however, the scope of inquiry may be very broad, typically leading to the selection of key agents and their most important health effects for risk assessment purposes. In the 1970s, there was widespread concern about the potential contributions of environmental pollution to rising cancer rates, so early assessments focused primarily on cancer.

For example, there is clear evidence from controlled experiments that high levels of chloroform in drinking water can cause cancer in laboratory animals (EPA, 2001). In humans, a number of observational studies have associated chlorinated drinking water consumption with a slight increase in bladder, rectal, and colon cancer; however, it is not clear how much, if any, of the cancer increase was caused by chloroform exposure, and studies that did not find an association between disinfection by-products and cancer may have been less likely to be published (EPA, 2001). Another example is chemical contaminants in fish. Although hundreds of contaminants, including pesticides, metals, dioxins, and PCBs, are typically present in low concentrations in fish and a wide variety of potential health effects are hypothesized from exposure to each of those contaminants, risk assessments for fish consumption tend to focus on the health outcomes of most concern or most clearly associated with the contaminants, such as neurodevelopmental deficits associated with methylmercury exposure (Rice, Schoeny, and Mahaffey, 2003).

Published reviews of the scientific literature can be helpful for identifying environmental health hazards and their potential health effects. The Agency for Toxic Substances and Disease Registry maintains and publicly distributes detailed *toxicological profiles* for over 250 hazardous substances commonly found at contaminated sites. Additional reviews are available from the EPA's Integrated Risk Information System and from the National Institute for Occupational Safety and Health's Registry of Toxic Effects of Chemical Substances and may also be found in scientific journals.

Dose-response assessment attempts to describe the quantitative relationship between exposure and disease. Typically, this consists of the development or selection of a mathematical model that predicts the level of toxic response for any dose. In some cases direct evidence of the level of response at the dose of interest is available, and a mathematical dose-response model is unnecessary. However, that is rare; dose-response assessments frequently rely on mathematical models in order to estimate responses for exposures that fall between experimental dose groups, or for observational data for which doses are typically continuous with few or no repetitions. Mathematical models may also be used to adjust effect estimates for differences in species, gender, race, and other factors that may confound the observed dose-response relationship, or may be used to directly incorporate specific toxicological mechanisms that affect the shape of the dose-response curve.

One well-known dose-response model for cancer is the *linearized multistage* model. This model, like many other cancer dose-response models, assumes that every molecule of exposure adds more risk of cancer. In contrast, *threshold* models assume that nobody exposed at a level below a critical threshold dose will develop cancer as the result of exposure. At low risks the linearized multistage model predicts a nearly linear relationship between the dose (d) and the probability of response (π_d):

$$\pi_d \approx \pi_0 + \beta_1 d$$

where π_0 is the estimated probability of response without any exposure, and β_1 is the effect of the dose.

Table 32.1 shows the results of a toxicological study of kidney tumors in male rats exposed to chloroform. In this study rats were randomly assigned to one of

TABLE 32.1. CARCINOGENIC EFFECTS OF CHLOROFORM ON MALE RATS.

Dose (mg/kg/day)	Number of Rats Tested	Number of Rats with Kidney Tumors	Proportion Affected
0	301	4	0.013
19	313	4	0.013
38	148	4	0.027
81	48	3	0.063
160	50	7	0.140

Source: Haas, 1994.

five groups, each of which was supplied with drinking water containing a different concentration of chloroform. The five concentrations were 0, 200, 400, 900, and 1,800 mg/L, corresponding to estimated doses of 0, 19, 38, 81, and 160 mg/kg/day (milligrams of chloroform per kilogram of body mass per day). Although other methods are sometimes used to extrapolate results from one species to another, many risk assessments assume equivalence on a mg/kg/day basis. A common statistical method called *maximum likelihood estimation* can be used to determine that $\beta_1 = 0.00011$ (mg/kg/day)$^{-1}$ provides the best fit to the rat data for the multistage model (Haas, 1994). In other words, the multistage model predicts that every mg/kg/day of chloroform exposure contributes an additional lifetime cancer risk of approximately 0.011 percent. Alternative dose-response models are described later in this chapter.

Exposure assessment includes the estimation or measurement of the magnitude, duration, and timing of human exposures to the agent of concern (NRC, 1994). This requires explicit definition of the exposed population and the routes by which it might be exposed to the agent. Exposure assessment is often quite difficult to conduct, due to inherent difficulties in measuring complex, time-varying behavior such as the frequency and amounts of water consumed by an individual or the amounts and origins of soil and dust that she unintentionally ingests or inhales or that contacts her skin.

Although ideal exposure assessment would produce a full profile of each individual's exposures over time, in practice most exposure assessments are limited to estimating summary values, such as time-averaged exposure rates. In addition, many exposure assessments rely on default assumptions about media contact rates, such as water and soil ingestion rates, rather than attempting to estimate specific exposure factors for every individual or population of interest. (Exposure assessment is described in more detail in Chapter Four.)

Consider ingestion of chloroform in drinking water at a concentration of 90 μg/L, the upper end of the range described earlier in this chapter. Although skin absorption and inhalation during bathing and other water-related activities may contribute to overall chloroform exposure, first consider exposure through drinking-water ingestion alone. The EPA (1997) recommends a default assumption that adults drink two liters of water each day. This value is probably an overestimate for most people but is not unrealistic for those who drink lots of water and is commonly used in preliminary risk assessments. A 70 kg individual consuming two liters of drinking water containing 90 μg/L chloroform every day throughout his or her entire lifetime will have an average daily chloroform dose of $2 \times 90/70 = 2.6$ μg/kg/day, or 0.0026 mg/kg/day.

Risk characterization is the final step of risk assessment. It consists of combining the information from the other three steps in order to estimate the level of response for the identified health effects(s) at the specific level of exposure to the agent(s) of interest in the defined population. Mathematically, the approach consists of substituting the specific dose amount into the dose-response equation and computing the response level. The risk that is contributed by the exposure itself is often of more interest than the overall probability of response, so analysts often summarize the result in terms of the *relative risk* (π_d / π_0), the *additional risk* ($\pi_d - \pi_0$, also known as the *attributable risk*), or the *excess risk* $[(\pi_d - \pi_0)/(1 - \pi_0)]$. Each of these risk measures adjusts the estimated probability of response in an exposed individual by the background probability of response (the response among the unexposed) in a different manner.

Combining the results of risk characterization, dose-response assessment, and exposure analysis in the chloroform example, one might conclude that chloroform in drinking water is a potential carcinogen in humans and estimate that the attributable risk of kidney cancer in a frequent consumer of drinking water containing 90 μg/L of chloroform might be about 0.0026 mg/kg/day $\times$ 0.00011 $(\text{mg/kg/day})^{-1} = 3 \times 10^{-8}$, or about 3 in 100 million.

The red book (NRC, 1983) and subsequent reports (NRC, 1994) emphasize that uncertainties associated with risk estimation should be assessed and discussed as part of the risk characterization step. Qualitative uncertainties, such as those relating to the carcinogenicity of low exposures to chloroform, were mentioned in the hazard identification section of this chapter. Substantial uncertainty also exists regarding the true shape of the dose-response model, particularly its reliability at the extremely low dose used for the drinking water example. Some toxicologists argue that chronic renal tubule injury is the likely mode of action for chloroform carcinogenicity and that a threshold model would be more appropriate for that mechanism, predicting no additional cancer risk at typical drinking-water exposure levels (EPA, 2001). The extrapolation from rats to humans on the basis of mg/kg/day of exposure introduces another major source of uncertainty (Box 32.2). The exposure assessment example was stated for a hypothetical concentration and drinking-water ingestion rate, but the actual concentration and drinking-water ingestion rate might not be perfectly known for a specific population of interest.

Box 32.2. Low-Dose Extrapolation: A Misnomer

A common feature of environmental health risk assessment is *extrapolation* from health outcomes at high exposures to predict health risks at lower exposure levels. In fact most toxicology and epidemiology studies include observations in individuals who are unexposed as well as in individuals who are exposed at higher doses. Risk estimation should actually be called low-dose *interpolation* when data for both lower and higher doses are used to fit the dose-response model.

Although qualitative uncertainty analysis is necessary and useful, the impacts and relative importance of the many sources of uncertainty are seldom obvious. In response, techniques for quantitatively characterizing the impacts of these uncertainties have proliferated during the past few decades. Quantitative uncertainty analysis techniques are summarized later in this chapter.

Risk Management

Risk managers are faced with the challenge of judging the significance of risks, comparing risks and costs for different risk management strategies, discussing these assessments with stakeholders, and finally, making appropriate decisions or recommendations. The red book (NRC, 1983) advises that risk assessment and risk management activities should be separated to ensure that the best science is used, although clearly risk assessment and risk management activities should be mutually informative.

Consider the chloroform example, which suggested an attributable kidney cancer risk of roughly 3 in 100 million. In comparison, the estimated lifetime risk of any type of cancer in the United States is about 38 percent in women and 46 percent in men (Ries, 2004). Although 3×10^{-8} is clearly a "drop in the bucket" compared to overall cancer rates, nobody would care to be among the few extra cases in that "drop." What should a risk manager do, faced with information like this? There are many different philosophies on risk management; several common approaches that rely on risk estimation are described here.

De Minimus Risk

Many risk managers and regulatory policies rely on the concept of *de minimus* risk, the idea that some risks are so small that they are acceptable or insignificant from a societal perspective. In practice the value of 1 in 1 million is often used as a threshold for excess cancer risks; activities that pose risks below this threshold are considered acceptable under this paradigm. However, activities or exposures that cause risks above the threshold are not necessarily unacceptable under this paradigm, which is sometimes used to screen out extremely small risks so that more attention can be paid to activities that pose larger risks. Using the cancer risk estimates in the chloroform example, a risk manager might conclude that the risks posed by chloroform are societally acceptable under the principle of de minimus risk.

Safety assessment relies on a similar principle. However, because procedures that do not directly assess the magnitude of risk are often employed in safety assessment (see Box 32.3), it might be more accurate to say that safety assessment relies on a philosophy of de minimus *exposure.*

Box 32.3. Risk Assessment Versus Safety Assessment

Although closely related, risk assessment and safety assessment differ in several important ways. Safety assessment is commonly used by regulatory agencies to select reasonably safe exposure limits or concentration limits in food, water, air, or other parts of the environment. Although safety assessment often relies on hazard identification and exposure assessment, its aim is to answer the question, What dose or concentration is safe? rather than to assess the likelihood of adverse health effects at a given dose or concentration. Historically, safety assessment for noncarcinogens has relied on the selection of a specifically tested dose that is not associated with statistically significant increases in adverse health effects. This no-observed-adverse-effect-level (NOAEL) is then typically divided by *uncertainty factors,* sometimes as high as 1,000, in order to determine a dose limit with a margin of safety to allow for potential differences in susceptibility across species and across individuals. In recent years many safety assessments have replaced the NOAEL with a model-based estimate of the dose at which the extra risk is 1 percent, 5 percent, or 10 percent, depending on the severity of the outcome. Identifying this *benchmark dose* relies on both dose-response modeling and risk management decisions regarding the acceptable level of risk for each health outcome.

Risk-Benefit Analysis

Some risks result from activities that are otherwise beneficial. For example, even though it may increase cancer risks, chlorination has the benefit of reducing the risk of waterborne diseases caused by a variety of microbes. Although an informal comparison between the magnitude of cholera outbreaks from untreated water systems and the magnitude of cancer risk from disinfection by-products might produce figures sufficiently uneven to suggest that chlorination is preferable to no treatment of drinking water, sophisticated quantitative techniques, such as calculating *quality-adjusted life years,* are also available for comparing more risks and benefits for disparate health outcomes (Schwartz, Richardson, and Glasziou, 1993; Ponce and others, 2000). It is important to examine risks and benefits in a balanced manner. For example, it would be more meaningful to compare risks from *all* disinfection by-products (not just the risks from chloroform) to the benefits of chlorination.

Cost-Benefit Analysis

Although the financial costs of risk abatement have always been of concern to affected businesses, they are increasingly considered by risk managers. In fact cost-benefit analysis is legally required in promulgating certain types of environmental health regulations (see Chapter Thirty-Three). This approach is generally most useful—and most controversial—when abatement costs are compared to *willingness to pay* values (Tolley, Kenkel, and Fabian, 1994) or other estimates of the dollar value of those illnesses or deaths avoided by abating the risk.

Decision Analysis or Alternatives Analysis

It has been argued that the best decisions are made after considering all the relevant potential consequences of a variety of options, rather than focusing only on particular consequences of a single option (Clemen, 1997; O'Brien, 2000). For example, the financial costs, health risks, and health benefits of a variety of disinfection methods might be assessed and compared in order to make a thoroughly informed decision about what method to choose in a particular setting. This approach differs from the first three approaches discussed here in that the focus is on the comparison of options, rather than on a single activity or exposure. Decision analysis may contain elements of the other approaches, such as cost-benefit analysis, and may be done qualitatively or quantitatively.

The Precautionary Principle

The precautionary principle is the idea that serious risks should be avoided or mitigated when possible, even when those risks are unlikely or uncertain (see Chapter Twenty-Nine). The precautionary principle may be most useful for situations in which little information is currently available to support risk estimation, situations such as global warming, bioterrorism, and the direct genetic modification of organisms. Although often advocated as an alternative to risk assessment, the precautionary principle is compatible with risk estimation and is perhaps better described as a risk management approach.

Dose-Response Modeling

Dose-response models play an important role in environmental health risk assessment, as they determine interpolations between tested doses. Although the multistage linearized model is a commonly used dose-response model for carcinogenesis, there are many competing models. Ideally, model selection should be based on biological considerations and well-characterized mechanisms of toxicity. In practice this is more difficult than it might seem, and assessors often rely on the multistage model or other familiar approaches.

The multistage model postulates that a sequence of k critical subcellular events must occur for transformation from a normal cell to a tumor. Critical events might include mutation, changes in gene expression, or cell proliferation. Those events $i = 1, 2, \ldots, k$ are modeled as independent Poisson processes with lifetime rates $(\alpha_i + \delta_i d)$, where α_i is the background rate of process i, δ_i is the rate change per unit dose for process i, and d is the dose. Under this model the probability of cancer (π_d) is equal to the probability that at least one event of each critical type occurs:

$$\pi_d = (1 - e^{-\alpha_1 - \delta_1 d})(1 - e^{-\alpha_2 - \delta_2 d}) \ldots (1 - e^{-\alpha_k - \delta_k d}).$$

Rather than identifying specific critical events and estimating their rates, analysts typically rely on a linearized approximation to the model just displayed, one that uses a smaller number of parameters:

$$\pi_d \approx 1 - \exp(-\beta_0 - \beta_1 d - \beta_2 d^2 - \cdots - \beta_k d^k).$$

These parameters, β, $\beta_1, \ldots \beta_k$, are statistically estimable using dose-response data sets with at least $k + 1$ dose groups; this approach does not require external estimates of the specific event rates or even identification of the types of critical events (Guess and Crump, 1978). For data sets with few dose groups, β_1 typically dominates the function, and probabilities of cancer are nearly linear at low doses, resulting in the approximation shown earlier in this chapter. EPA risk assessments often refer to an upper bound estimate of β_1 called the *potency*, and use it in place of the best estimate of β_1 for estimating risk. Conservative regulatory assessments often rely on upper bound parameter estimates, intentionally overestimating health risks in order to be more protective of public health (EPA, 1990).

Although the multistage model is biologically motivated, the linearized version does not use quantitative information on specific toxic events. In contrast, *mechanistic, biologically based,* or *biologically motivated* dose-response models attempt to model the dose to disease process in more detail, in the hope of providing a better understanding of the true shape of the dose-response curve and a better basis for extrapolating results from laboratory animals to humans. Examples include toxicodynamic models that predict the influence of toxicants on critical events, such as stochastic cell proliferation models for carcinogenesis (Moolgavkar and Knudson, 1981) or neurodevelopment (Leroux, Leisenring, Moolgavkar, and Faustman, 1996); toxicokinetic models that model the transport, metabolism, and disposition of toxicants that enter the body (O'Flaherty, 1993); and models that include both toxicokinetic and toxicodynamic processes (Faustman, Lewandowski, Ponce, and Bartell, 1999). Although these models hold much promise, their development and use is often limited by poorly understood mechanisms of toxicity, the lack of supporting quantitative information to characterize parameters, and the computer programming effort needed for implementation.

All monotonic dose-response models can be expressed using a simple concept known as the *tolerance distribution* (Dobson, 1990). Assume that each individual has a specific tolerance for the toxicant. If exposed at or above that tolerance dose, the individual will develop the disease of interest. If exposed below that tolerance dose, she will not develop the disease. Although each individual's tolerance is unknown, the shape of the population distribution of tolerance values implies a specific dose-response curve, and vice versa. For example, assume that a population has a normal distribution of tolerance values for kidney cancer following chloroform exposure. The probability of kidney cancer for an individual randomly selected from that population is then the area under the tolerance distribution to the left of the dose, that is, the probability that the individual's tolerance is less than or equal to her dose (Figure 32.2). This model is known as the *probit model,* and it can be written as

$$\pi_d = \Phi[(d - \mu)/\sigma]$$

where π_d is the probability of disease, μ is the mean of the tolerance distribution, σ is the standard deviation of the tolerance distribution, and Φ is the cumulative standard normal distribution function. μ is also the ED_{50}, the expected dose at which 50 percent of the population develops the disease.

More generally, simple linear tolerance models can be written as

$$F^{-1}(\pi_d) = \beta_0 + \beta_1 d$$

where F^{-1} is an inverse cumulative distribution function for the tolerance distribution, and β_0 and β_1 are the distribution parameters. For the probit model, $\beta_0 = -\mu/\sigma$ and $\beta_1 = 1/\sigma$.

FIGURE 32.2. NORMAL TOLERANCE DISTRIBUTION (PROBIT MODEL).

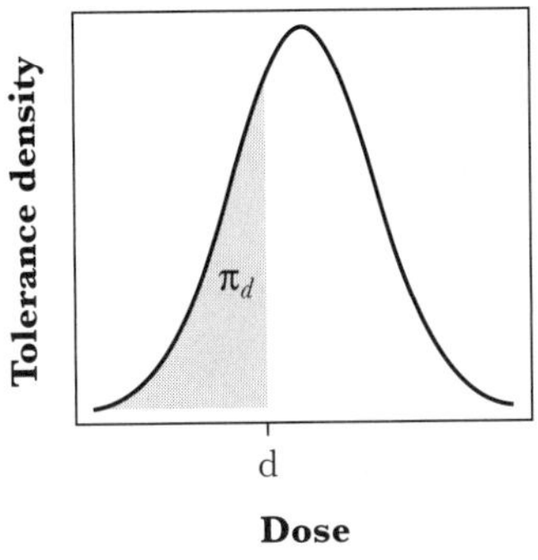

Note: The probability of response π_d is the area under the normal curve to the left of dose *d*.

These models are examples of binomial regression models. This class of models is popular among biostatisticians and epidemiologists, though they are not always aware of the tolerance distribution interpretation. The logistic tolerance distribution, with inverse cumulative distribution function $F^{-1}(\pi_d) = \log[\pi_d/(1 - \pi_d)]$, is the basis for logistic regression.

Although *goodness-of-link* tests have been developed for choosing a tolerance distribution function that best fits the data (Collett, 1999), these tests are rarely helpful when there are few dose groups, as in the chloroform example. In such situations it is not uncommon for different dose-response models to fit the data equally well, as shown in Figure 32.3. Because these models predict roughly similar probabilities of cancer, the choice of model might not be very important for some applications. However, when interpolating to extremely low probabilities and using upper bounds on risk estimates, small differences in model predictions may become magnified (NRC, 1983). Although such differences in estimated risk may be small on an absolute scale, they can have large impacts on environmental policy and cleanup costs for contaminated sites.

A wide variety of dose-response models have been developed and continue to be developed for cancer and other end points. Recent innovations include fitting different mathematical models to different parts of the dose-response curve in an attempt to model low-dose mechanisms separately, and particularly to model hormesis (Hunt and Bowman, 2004) or carcinogens that act through cytotoxicity or other nonmutagenic mechanisms (EPA, 1996). Hormesis is a phenomenon in which a toxicant reduces the probability of an adverse response at low doses compared to a zero dose but increases the probability of an adverse response at higher doses, creating a dose-response curve that is not monotonic. Hormetic

FIGURE 32.3. THREE DOSE-RESPONSE MODELS (LOGIT, PROBIT, AND THREE-PARAMETER MULTISTAGE) FIT TO THE CHLOROFORM DOSE-RESPONSE DATA IN RATS.

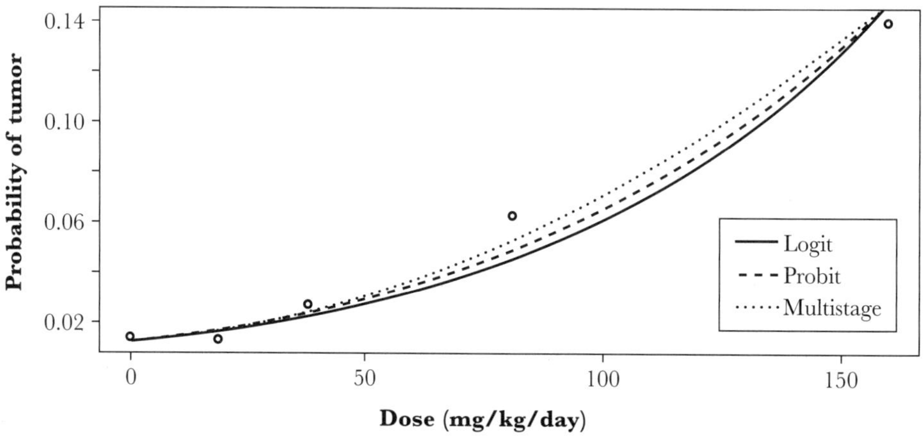

Note: Study data are plotted as circles and models are shown as lines.

effects have long been debated in relation to alcohol and heart disease and in relation to radiation and cancer; some researchers have suggested that hormetic effects may exist for most or all toxicants (Calabrese and others, 1999), but this hypothesis remains controversial.

Nonparametric regression (also called semiparametric regression) is an appealing but entirely different approach to dose-response modeling. Rather than relying on a mathematical function or functions to describe the shape of the dose-response curve, nonparametric regression relies heavily on the dose-response data set itself to determine the shape of the curve. One semiparametric regression approach uses a smoothing spline, a linked series of restricted cubic polynomial functions, to fit a dose-response curve to a data set. Figure 32.4 shows an example of a smoothing spline regression model for human lung cancer and silica exposure in a nested case-control analysis of 65,980 silica-exposed workers from ten cohorts (Steenland and others, 2001). A logistic regression model and a categorical analysis based on exposure quintiles for the same data are also plotted in the same figure. Note that the smoothing spline suggests some features that are hidden or less obvious in the other models, such as two slight dips in the dose-response curve.

The primary advantage of nonparametric regression is its ability to show such features of data sets without imposing many a priori restrictions on the shape of the model. However, revealed "features" are sometimes just artifacts of study

FIGURE 32.4. CUBIC SMOOTHING SPLINE, LOGIT MODEL, AND CATEGORICAL MODEL FIT TO NESTED CASE-CONTROL DATA ON SILICA EXPOSURE AND LUNG CANCER.

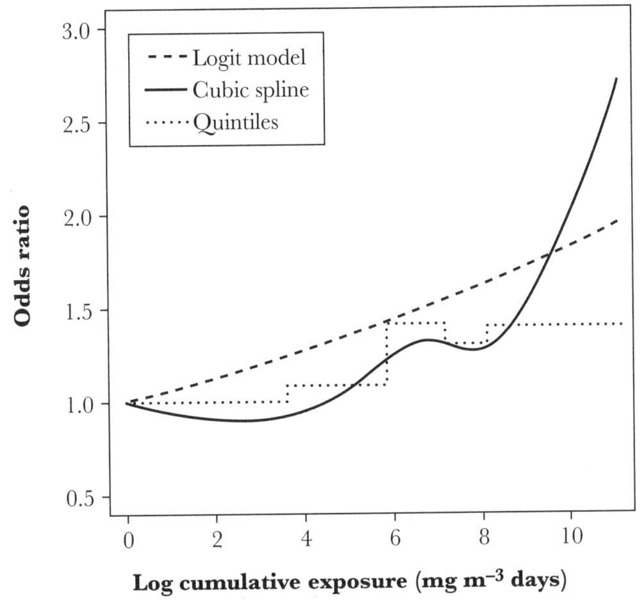

Note: The odds ratio is $\pi_d(1 - \pi_0)/[\pi_0(1 - \pi_d)]$, and is approximately equal to the relative risk when π_d and π_0 are small, as in this situation.

design or random error rather than reflections of the true dose-response curve. If confidence bounds for the dose-response curve rule out random error as a potential explanation for odd features, careful attention should be given to the data in those ranges, perhaps suggesting new hypotheses about confounding or mechanisms of toxicity.

Nonparametric regression is rarely applied to data from controlled experiments, as these studies typically rely on few dose groups, providing little information on the shape of the dose-response curve.

Uncertainty Analysis

Uncertainty analysis was highlighted as an important component of risk assessment in the red book, and has since been the subject of much interest from researchers and practitioners (Morgan, Henrion, and Small, 1990). At its simplest, uncertainty analysis consists of a qualitative description of the sources of uncertainty in a risk assessment and their potential impacts. However, uncertainty analysis is often quantitative, providing a range or distribution of reasonable risk estimates. Approaches to quantitative uncertainty analysis include probabilistic analysis and interval analysis.

Interval analysis (Alefeld and Herzberger, 1983; Ferson, 1996) is a relatively simple approach for describing uncertainty quantitatively. The idea of this approach is to estimate the risk twice, once using best-case parameter estimates and then again using worst-case parameter estimates. One advantage of this approach is its simplicity. It is relatively easy to conduct, does not require specialized software (although interval analysis software is available), is easy to explain, and provides potentially useful quantitative information about the uncertainty in the results of a given risk assessment. The primary disadvantage of this approach is that the interval provides no information about the relative plausibility of individual risk estimates within the interval. It is possible that every point in the interval is equally likely, and possible that an estimate near the center of the interval is most likely and that estimates near the ends of the interval are less likely. Moreover, single points for the best-case and worst-case parameter estimates may be difficult to define when they are not bound by physical restrictions such as proportions limited to the range of 0 to 100 percent.

Although they are seldom identified as such by risk analysts, statistical confidence intervals and prediction intervals are examples of another type of interval analysis. Such an interval, based on frequentist or Bayesian statistical methods, provides a range of estimates that is likely to include the true value. Procedures for finding these intervals are developed using mathematical statistics, resulting in intervals that seek to capture the true risk estimate with a fixed level of confidence (commonly 95 percent) (DeGroot, 1989). Frequentist methods dominated the statistical literature during the last century and serve as the basis for the most commonly used statistical software packages. However, frequentist statistical methods can be difficult to develop for complicated models, leading analysts to rely on approximations or to substitute simpler models. Moreover, traditional frequentist methods tend to divide model parameters into those that are known exactly and those that are completely unknown; there are few frequentist mechanisms for dealing with parameters that are partially understood or can only be guessed. Bayesian statistical methods, an alternative approach, readily handle parameter uncertainty, educated guesses, and complex models, and allow a formal probability-based interpretation of results (Greenland, 2001).

Probabilistic risk analysis describes risk using one or more probability distributions indicating the plausibility of an entire range of risk estimates. A number of philosophies and approaches are used to characterize these probability distributions, including formal statistical methods, but the most popular method among environmental health risk assessors is an informal approach called *Monte Carlo simulation.*

The Monte Carlo approach to probabilistic risk assessment requires additional steps after the initial quantitative risk assessment. First, probability distributions are selected to represent uncertainty, or variability, in the model parameters. Dependence among parameters may be specified using a variety of approaches, including multivariate distributions, conditional distributions, and rank correlations. Some analysts prefer to distinguish variability, which reflects known differences among individuals at risk, from uncertainty, which reflects lack of knowledge regarding the true values of model parameters. Next, plausible sets of parameter values are randomly and repeatedly selected according to the specified probability distributions and correlation structure. A risk estimate is calculated and recorded for each set of parameters. After risk estimates have been calculated for many (sometimes tens of thousands or hundreds of thousands) sets of parameters, the collection of risk estimates approximates the distribution of uncertainty regarding the risk. This Monte Carlo distribution shows the range and relative plausibility of various risk estimates after taking into account uncertainty in all the model parameters.

Although Monte Carlo simulation is a flexible method for conducting probabilistic risk assessment, it is sometimes not the most efficient approach. For some models, exact distributions can be determined explicitly. For example, the sum of a set of normal distributions is normally distributed, and the product of lognormal distributions is lognormally distributed. (Alternative methods for determining the exact or approximate distribution of functions of random variables are available in standard statistical references; see, for example, DeGroot, 1989; Evans, Hastings, and Peacock, 1993.)

Some argue that the relative plausibility of an entire range of risk estimates is impossible to determine reliably and that attempts to do so may mislead and confuse risk managers and stakeholders. Moreover, correlations between parameters are difficult to characterize and are often overlooked, introducing substantial errors in uncertainty propagation (Ferson, 1996).

Criticism of Risk Assessment

It is not difficult to criticize risk assessment; in fact criticism arises whenever risk estimates are used as a basis for regulatory policy or site cleanup decisions. One underlying source of controversy is that risk assessments are typically based on both empirical evidence and hypotheses, or science and judgment (NRC, 1994).

Although the empirical evidence for a given risk assessment, such as toxicological or epidemiological studies, is sometimes challenged on the basis of its scientific merits, much of the debate is often focused on the judgments, the untested hypotheses and default values that are relied on in the absence of clear evidence. Controversies are common over the use of conservative default assumptions in both exposure assessment and dose-response assessment, the inadequacy of data and models for assessing the effects of exposing the same individual to multiple toxicants, and the wisdom of basing policy decisions on highly uncertain risk estimates.

Conservative default assumptions are not inherent to environmental health risk assessment methodology, but they have traditionally been advocated or required by the EPA, particularly in its Superfund site assessment process (EPA, 1990). EPA default exposure parameters and scenarios are often based on the concept of the *maximally exposed individual* or of *reasonable maximal exposure,* leading to exposure estimates that intentionally overestimate the average exposure that occurs in the assessed population. The rationale for this approach is the goal of protecting the entire population, including subsets that may be especially susceptible due to higher exposures. However, these two terms have never been well defined and have been criticized as an intrusion of risk management into risk assessment, due to the fact that population risks are generally overestimated when conservative default values are used.

Another frequently criticized conservative default used by the EPA is the default potency model used for cancer dose-response assessment. Two conservative assumptions are used in this model. One is the use of the multistage linearized model as a default. When applied to typical toxicological data, this model results in linear risk estimates at low doses. Many alternative models are sublinear, predicting lower response rates than the multistage model in the low-dose range, or they include a threshold exposure that must be exceeded in order to induce a response. Moreover, the default EPA approach to risk characterization relies on the statistical upper bound estimate rather than the maximum likelihood estimate for the linear component of the dose-response model, further biasing the resulting population risk estimates toward higher values. Although the conservatism is intentional, it has been argued that these approaches conflate risk assessment with risk management, essentially presenting "half of an uncertainty analysis" without the best prediction of the true risk.

Another source of controversy is the typical reliance on dose-response models derived either from high-dose experiments in laboratory animals or from observational epidemiology in humans (see Box 32.4). Skeptics question the accuracy of human health risk estimates derived from high-dose experiments in rodents. Epidemiological dose-response models can be equally controversial, as these studies are usually observational rather than experimental, raising doubts about causal interpretations. Moreover, in practice only a subset of possible illnesses is studied for any toxicant, implying that risk estimates for known diseases may underestimate the overall burden of health effects truly caused by a given exposure.

Box 32.4. Toxicology and Epidemiology in Environmental Health Risk Assessment

Although toxicology and epidemiology are both used to study the health effects of environmental pollution, each approach has several important limitations for supporting environmental regulations. Environmental epidemiology, for practical and ethical reasons, is usually observational rather than experimental, raising questions about reliability due to the potential for uncontrolled confounding. Moreover, pollutant exposures and health effects must have already occurred in large populations in order for epidemiologists to study their associations, yet environmental regulations often seek to prevent environmental health problems before they begin. Because careful epidemiological studies are often expensive, time-consuming, and limited by ethical concerns, their widespread application to thousands of chemicals is impractical. Toxicological experiments are relatively quick and inexpensive to conduct in rodents, even for chronic health effects such as cancer. However, these experiments on rats, mice, or other laboratory animals may not always be relevant to humans. Viewed in isolation, neither observational human epidemiology nor experimental laboratory animal toxicology provides ideal information on environmental health. However, when observations in humans are confirmed by experimental evidence in laboratory animals, or vice versa, much stronger conclusions result.

Because risk assessors typically intend to address specific policy questions, they often limit their analyses to highly specific circumstances and the most significant health outcomes, resulting in more manageable but less comprehensive assessments. In practice it is sometimes difficult to strike an appropriate balance between thoroughness, which can lead to "paralysis by analysis," and focus, which can overlook important health effects or potential interactions of toxicants.

Some critics feel that environmental health risk assessment as currently practiced is fundamentally flawed and should be abandoned in favor of other approaches (O'Brien, 2000). Typical arguments directly target the moral implications of specific risk management approaches such as de minimus risk, regulatory safety assessment procedures that blur the boundaries between risk assessment and risk management, or the lack of consideration for social issues, such as unequal distribution of the costs and benefits of proposed environmental regulations. Although O'Brien and others propose alternatives analysis and the precautionary principle as alternatives to risk assessment, these approaches can be seen as alternative risk management strategies that may or may not rely on formal risk assessment, as described earlier in this chapter.

Risk assessment is inherently susceptible to criticism because it is, at heart, an attempt either to estimate an unmeasured past or present or to predict an unknown future. There are many reasonable approaches that might be taken for any particular risk assessment, and people often disagree on the best approach. When risk assessment is used as the basis for environmental health regulations or other important decisions, even small changes in risk estimates can have large economic consequences. As long as risk assessment remains a central component of environmental health regulation, debate on its methods and predictions is sure to continue.

Thought Questions

1. What role, if any, should risk assessment have in regulating pollution? Are small risks ever acceptable?
2. What are the advantages and disadvantages of the different risk management approaches described in this chapter?
3. Is it important for risk assessment and risk management to be separated, or is safety assessment a reasonable approach?

References

Alefeld, G., and Herzberger, J. *Introduction to Interval Computations.* New York: Academic Press, 1983.

Bernstein, P. L. *Against the Gods: The Remarkable Story of Risk.* Hoboken, N.J.: Wiley, 1996.

Calabrese, E. J., Baldwin, L. A., and Holland, C. D. "Hormesis: A Highly Generalizable and Reproducible Phenomenon with Important Implications for Risk Assessment." *Risk Analysis,* 1999, *19,* 261–281.

Clemen, R. T. *Making Hard Decisions: An Introduction to Decision Analysis.* (2nd ed.) Pacific Grove, Calif.: Duxbury Press, 1997.

Collett, D. *Modelling Binary Data.* Boca Raton, Fla.: Chapman & Hall/CRC, 1999.

DeGroot, M. H. *Probability and Statistics.* (2nd ed.) Reading, Mass.: Addison-Wesley, 1989.

Dobson, A. J. *An Introduction to Generalized Linear Models.* (2nd ed.) Boca Raton, Fla.: Chapman & Hall/CRC, 1990.

Evans, M., Hastings, N., and Peacock, B. *Statistical Distributions.* (2nd ed.) Hoboken, N.J.: Wiley, 1993.

Faustman, E. M., Lewandowski, T. A., Ponce, R. A., and Bartell, S. M. "Biologically Based Dose-Response Models for Developmental Toxicants: Lessons from Methylmercury." *Inhalation Toxicology,* 1999, *11,* 559–572.

Ferson, S. "What Monte Carlo Methods Cannot Do." *Human and Ecological Risk Assessment,* 1996, *2,* 990–1007.

Greenland, S. "Sensitivity Analysis, Monte Carlo Risk Analysis, and Bayesian Uncertainty Assessment." *Risk Analysis,* 2001, *21*(4), 579–583.

Guess, H. A., and Crump, K. S. "Best-Estimate Low-Dose Extrapolation of Carcinogenicity Data." *Environmental Health Perspectives,* 1978, *22,* 149–152.

Haas, C. N. "Dose-Response Analysis Using Spreadsheets." *Risk Analysis,* 1994, *14*(6), 1097–2000.

Hunt, D. L., and Bowman, D. "A Parametric Model for Detecting Hormetic Effects in Developmental Toxicity Studies." *Risk Analysis,* 2004, *24*(1), 65–72.

Kaplan, S. "The Words of Risk Analysis." *Risk Analysis,* 1997, *17*(4), 407–417.

Leroux, B. G., Leisenring, W. M., Moolgavkar, S. H., and Faustman, E. M. "A Biologically-Based Dose-Response Model for Developmental Toxicology." *Risk Analysis,* 1996, *16*(4), 449–458.

Moolgavkar, S. H., and Knudson, A. G., Jr. "Mutation and Cancer: A Model for Human Carcinogenesis." *Journal of the National Cancer Institute,* 1981, *66*(6), 1037–1052.

Morgan, M. G., Henrion, M., and Small, M. *Uncertainty: A Guide to Dealing with Uncertainty in Quantitative Risk and Policy Analysis.* New York: Cambridge University Press, 1990.

National Research Council. *Risk Assessment in the Federal Government: Managing the Process.* Washington, D.C.: National Academies Press, 1983.

National Research Council. *Science and Judgment in Risk Assessment.* Washington, D.C.: National Academies Press, 1994.

O'Brien, M. *Making Better Environmental Decisions.* Cambridge, Mass.: MIT Press, 2000.

O'Flaherty, E. J. "Physiologically Based Models for Bone-Seeking Elements, 4: Kinetics of Lead Disposition in Humans." *Toxicology and Applied Pharmacology,* 1993, *118,* 16–29.

Omenn, G. S. "The Evolution of Risk Assessment and Risk Management." *Human and Ecological Risk Assessment,* 2003, *9*(5), 1155–1167.

Ponce, R. A., and others. "Use of Quality-Adjusted Life Year Weights with Dose-Response Models for Public Health Decisions: A Case Study of the Risks and Benefits of Fish Consumption." *Risk Analysis,* 2000, *20*(4), 529–542.

Rice, D. C., Schoeny, R., and Mahaffey, K. "Methods and Rationale for Derivation of a Reference Dose for Methylmercury by the US EPA." *Risk Analysis,* 2003, *23*(1), 107–115.

Ries, L.A.G., and others (eds.). *SEER Cancer Statistics Review, 1975–2001.* National Cancer Institute. [http://seer.cancer.gov/csr/1975_2001]. 2004.

Schwartz, S., Richardson, J., and Glasziou, P. P. "Quality-Adjusted Life Years: Origins, Measurements, Applications, Objectives." *Australian Journal of Public Health,* 1993, *17*(30), 272–278.

Steenland, K., and others. "Pooled Exposure-Response Analyses and Risk Assessment for Lung Cancer in 10 Cohorts of Silica-Exposed Workers: An IARC Multicentre Study." *Cancer Causes & Control,* 2001, *12,* 773–784.

Tolley, G., Kenkel, D., and Fabian, R. (eds.). *Valuing Health for Policy.* Chicago: University of Chicago Press, 1994.

Toxicology Excellence for Risk Assessment. *Health Risk Assessment/Characterization of the Drinking Water Disinfection Byproduct Chloroform.* [http://www.tera.org/news/Chloroform.PDF]. 1998.

U.S. Environmental Protection Agency. *Risk Assessment Guidance for Superfund, Vol. 1: Human Health Evaluation Manual (Part A).* EPA/540/1-89/002. Washington, D.C.: U.S. Environmental Protection Agency, Office of Emergency and Remedial Response, 1990.

U.S. Environmental Protection Agency. "Proposed Guidelines for Carcinogen Risk Assessment." *Federal Register* 61, no. 79 (Apr. 23, 1996), 17960–18011.
U.S. Environmental Protection Agency. *Exposure Factors Handbook,* Vol. 1: *General Factors.* Washington, D.C.: U.S. Environmental Protection Agency, Aug. 1997.
U.S. Environmental Protection Agency, Integrated Risk Information System. "Chloroform: CASRN 67-663." [http://www.epa.gov/iris/subst/0025.htm]. 2001.

For Further Information

RiskWorld. Homepage. [http://www.riskworld.com]. 2005.
Society for Risk Analysis. Homepage. [http://www.sra.org]. 2005.
U.S. Environmental Protection Agency, Integrated Risk Information System. Homepage. [http://www.epa.gov/iris]. 2005.

CHAPTER THIRTY-THREE

ENVIRONMENTAL HEALTH POLICY

Barry L. Johnson

This chapter presents an overview of the ways in which policies are developed and implemented in order to prevent or reduce the adverse effects of environmental hazards. Much of the discussion focuses on the United States, but similar policies are found in many other countries. Indeed, global pollution of the environment has led to common approaches to environmental health policy development and promising international cooperation in controlling some environmental hazards. The policies discussed in this chapter include federal environmental statutes, accompanying government regulations, and nonregulatory efforts by public interest groups and individuals. This body of actions can be termed *environmental health policy.* These policies are important to understand because they have contributed to reducing the toll of environmental hazards on human health and ecological systems. Knowledge of the means by which environmental health policy is made and implemented is vital for its contribution to public health practice.

What is a policy? A standard dictionary provides two useful definitions. *Policy* (according to *Merriam-Webster's Collegiate Dictionary,* eleventh edition) is "a definite course or method of action selected from among alternatives and in light of given conditions to guide and determine present and future decisions," or a "plan embracing the general goals and acceptable procedures especially of a governmental body." In a sense, making environmental health policy is no different from making family or business policy. Many families choose as a matter of policy to budget their expenditures. Some businesses adopt a policy of servicing all customer complaints within forty-eight hours. In both of these examples, alternatives were considered and an action was selected to guide future actions.

Policy Considerations

Environmental health policy comprises actions, selected from alternatives, that are intended to reduce or eliminate the harmful effects of environmental exposures. One way to consider this kind of policy is to consider its uses, users, and nonusers, yielding the following five considerations.

Directness. Some policies directly address environmental health. Examples include U.S. Environmental Protection Agency (EPA) standards that regulate contaminant levels in an environmental medium, such as levels of air pollutants in ambient air. Other policies are primarily environmental, but even though they do not have a health focus, they indirectly affect human health or environmental quality. For example, the National Environmental Policy Act, articulates a national policy of environmental protection, which could have many indirect benefits for human health. And still other policies are not even environmental, but they incidentally have a major impact on environmental health. For example, energy policy has an impact on which fuels are used, affecting air quality and therefore respiratory health. This chapter addresses primarily those environmental health polices that directly affect human health, because they present a direct course of action toward controlling the adverse consequences of environmental hazards on human health.

Level of government. Environmental health policies span the spectrum of government. This chapter emphasizes federal government policies, such as the Clean Water Act and its approach to controlling emissions of contaminants into bodies of water. However, state and local governments also develop environmental health regulations. At a minimum, states enact statutes needed to comply with federal statutes and regulations. For instance, states will enact statutes and provide resources to meet the provisions of the Clean Air Act that require state actions. Some states go further, enacting statutes that reflect state priorities. And local governments establish environmental health polices through ordinances, such as prohibitions on smoking tobacco products in public facilities. In general, environmental health policies become more specific and targeted as they transition from federal to state to local government.

Primary strategy. Policymakers such as legislators and government officials have developed several primary strategies as environmental health policy. Some strategies aim to reduce the effects of hazards directly, some do so in a prospective manner (for example, air pollution regulations), others do so through retrospective action (for example, cleanups of uncontrolled hazardous waste sites). Other policies do not directly regulate a hazard but provide information to the public about the hazard, in effect, relying on individuals to make informed health decisions. Examples of this laissez-faire approach to controlling the effects of hazards include health warnings on tobacco products; the Toxics Release Inventory, a public database compiled by the EPA of environmental pollution data provided by industrial facilities; and workers' right to know, a provision of the Occupational Safety and Health Act that requires employers to inform employees of workplace hazards.

The prime actor in the policy. There can be several prime actors in the development of environmental health policies. Although this chapter emphasizes the role of government as the prime actor, private parties may also play a significant role. For example, the American Conference of Governmental Industrial Hygienists (ACGIH), a professional society, develops recommended exposure limits for substances found in workplaces. Private industry uses the ACGIH exposure limits as voluntary guidelines for workplace controls when OSHA standards are not in effect. Similarly, the International Organization for Standardization (ISO) develops recommended guidelines that industry and some government agencies adopt. As discussed later in this chapter, individuals can be prime actors in establishing an environmental health policy through litigation with a government agency or a business. Consider the plaintiff who sued a restaurant chain when a cup of hot coffee spilled on her leg after purchase. The coffee's temperature was sufficiently high to cause burns and scars. Litigation compensated the woman for her injuries and also contributed to a decrease in the temperature of the coffee served by the restaurant chain. Litigation by an individual therefore contributed to control of an environmental hazard.

What doesn't get regulated. This chapter focuses on policies that relate to regulations and standards as the primary means to control environmental hazards. Not described are important environmental issues for which regulatory policies do not exist. Examples of nonregulated environmental hazards include indoor air in personal residences, which is not covered under the Clean Air Act; emissions of carbon dioxide, a major greenhouse gas implicated in global warming; and tobacco products, for which labeling is required but safety is not regulated. These three examples alone illustrate that the effects from unregulated environmental hazards can rival the public health impact of regulated hazards.

Developing policy, according to our chosen definition, involves identifying alternatives that might be applied to specific situations. From the alternatives, policymakers (for example, a legislative body, tribal council, or parent) determine the best alternative (applying stated criteria), communicate their decision to interested parties, and apply the policy when future circumstances arise where a response must be based on policy. (The example in Box 33.1 reveals some potential complexities.)

Box 33.1. The EPA's Arsenic Standard

Reassessment of the U.S. standard for arsenic in water is an example of a risk assessment that got caught in the thickets of environmental politics and policies. The Public Health Service set the standard for arsenic in drinking water at fifty parts per billion (ppb) in 1947, well before the establishment of the EPA in 1970. This level was maintained for more than fifty years, even though scientific evidence was mounting that lower arsenic limits were necessary to protect the public's health. Decreasing the standard from 50 ppb to a lower level led to a brouhaha that involved the EPA, Congress, the administrations of two presidents, federal courts, environmental groups, and business associations.

In 1993, the World Health Organization (WHO), recommended that arsenic levels in drinking water not exceed 10 ppb. The EPA chose not to follow WHO's recommendation, a decision opposed by environmental and public health groups. These groups brought pressure on Congress to force the EPA to revise its arsenic standard. Opposed to any change in the arsenic standard were mining interests and some municipal water suppliers in Western states. Their opposition was based on the economic impact of a lower arsenic standard.

Congress sided with the groups advocating a lower arsenic standard. The Safe Drinking Water Act Amendments of 1996 directed the EPA to update the arsenic standard by January 1, 2001. As a matter of science, the EPA asked the National Academy of Sciences (NAS) to review the toxicology and human health literature on arsenic and recommend courses of action. In 1999, the NAS recommended that the EPA standard be lowered from 50 ppb. Two years later, in January 2001, as the Clinton administration was preparing to leave office, the EPA proposed a rule lowering the arsenic standard to 10 ppb. On January 20, 2001, George W. Bush succeeded Clinton in office and soon appointed a new EPA administrator. In March, as its first environmental policy action, the new administration withdrew the proposed arsenic rule. This provided environmental and public health groups with an easy platform from which to criticize the new administration, and indeed, considerable criticism followed. The ensuing clamor led the U.S. House of Representatives to vote to support the Clinton-era 10 ppb proposed rule. In July 2001, the NAS issued a second report on arsenic, finding it to be carcinogenic and recommending a level of less than 10 ppb as a standard. Subsequent to the NAS report, the Bush administration reversed itself and in November 2001 reinstated the arsenic rule proposed by the Clinton administration.

Meanwhile, environmental health policy on arsenic was also advanced by private action. In 2002, the EPA announced industry's voluntary action to phase out pressure-treated wood containing arsenic (CCA wood; see Chapter Twenty-Eight).

The revised EPA standard of 10 ppb for arsenic in drinking water was litigated by the State of Nebraska and the City of Alliance, Nebraska. They argued that regulating drinking water quality was a state, not federal, responsibility. In June 2003, a three-judge panel of the U.S. Court of Appeals, District of Columbia Circuit, held in favor of the EPA, concluding that plaintiffs had failed to show that the EPA's actions were in violation of the U.S. Constitution. The EPA arsenic standard was defended before the court by the U.S. Justice Department and the Natural Resources Defense Council, a national environmental advocacy organization. The court's decision removed barriers to enforcing the new, lower standard adopted by EPA, ending the political brouhaha between the Clinton and Bush administrations.

Environmental Health Policymaking

The laws and regulations that affect environmental health have their basis in the U.S. Constitution. The sections that follow discuss this constitutional foundation, the establishment and functions of the regulatory agencies primarily concerned with environmental health, and finally, the most important of the environmental health policy laws that have been enacted by the U.S. Congress.

Constitutional Basis

One way to set environmental health policy is to enact laws, which in turn contain defined policies and embedded purposes. For example, the federal National Environmental Policy Act of 1969 states that "Congress recognizes that . . . each person should enjoy a healthful environment and that each person has a responsibility to contribute to the preservation and enhancement of the environment." Similarly, laws enacted by states and ordinances set forth by counties and municipalities may contain embedded environmental health policies. States' environmental laws often emulate federal laws on specific environmental hazards, for example, hazardous waste management. An example of a local environmental health policy is a local government's decision to have county health departments apply pesticides to control mosquito infestation. Because legislated environmental policies bear the weight of law, it is important to have some understanding of the basic elements of government and the U.S. federal government in particular, because federal environmental laws form much of the environmental framework in the United States and are emulated in some other countries.

The following comments about the structure of the U.S. government are drawn from the U.S. Constitution and illustrated with regard to setting environmental health policy. Moreover, much of what follows also applies to the structure of state government and, to a lesser extent, to county and municipal governments.

Legislative Branch. Article I, Section 1, of the U.S. Constitution states, "All legislative Powers herein granted shall be vested in a Congress of the United States, which shall consist of a Senate and House of Representatives." Legislation enacted by Congress generally contains language that authorizes the executive branch to undertake specified actions. For example, the Environmental Protection Agency and the Food and Drug Administration (FDA) are authorized (indeed, mandated) in the Food Quality Protection Act (FQPA) of 1996 to implement changes in the way pesticides are registered in the United States and to change risk assessment procedures in order to give greater protection to children exposed to pesticides. *Authorizing legislation,* such as the FQPA, must also contain language that authorizes the appropriation by Congress of public funds that can then be used by a federal department or agency as it carries out its legislative mandates. *Appropriations legislation* authorizes specific amounts of public monies in the U.S. Treasury to be used by the executive branch in the conduct of authorized programs. Congressional appropriations committees are responsible for developing appropriations legislation, commencing with their consideration of the president's annual budget request to Congress. When the standard for arsenic in drinking water was changed (discussed earlier in Box 33.1), Congress played a key role by enacting the Safe Drinking Water Act and later by passing an Amendment to that Act that required the EPA to update the arsenic drinking water standard.

Executive Branch. Article II, Section 1, of the U.S. Constitution states, "The executive Power shall be vested in a President of the United States of America." The executive branch of the federal government, headed by the president of the United States, implements legislation enacted by Congress and signed into law by the president or enacted by Congress through an override of a presidential veto, including legislation affecting environmental health policy. The implementation agenda is accomplished by such components of the executive branch as the Environmental Protection Agency and the Department of Health and Human Services (DHHS). Again using the example of the Food Quality Protection Act of 1996, that statute directed the EPA, DHHS, and Department of Agriculture to revise specific polices and procedures bearing on the review and approval of pesticides and the potential impact of pesticides on children. Upon receipt of such directives, affected departments and agencies must interpret the language in the new statute or in the Amendments to an existing statute. Some legislation is deliberately written in vague terms, a product of failure by Congressional committees to negotiate more specific language. In such circumstances the executive branch must attempt its own interpretation of congressional intent. Ultimately, the judicial branch is often required to interpret legislative intent and executive branch implementation. In the case of the arsenic standard, for example, Congress directed the EPA to develop an updated arsenic water quality standard.

Judicial Branch. The U.S. Constitution, Article III, Section 1, states, "The judicial Power of the United States, shall be vested in one supreme Court, and in such inferior Courts as the Congress may from time to time ordain and establish." The courts established under the powers granted by the Constitution are known as constitutional courts. Judges of these courts are appointed for life by the president, with the advice and consent of the U.S. Senate. The constitutional courts consist of the U.S. Supreme Court, district courts, and the courts of appeals. Federal courts have had a profound effect on establishing environmental health policies. Because many environmental laws (for example, the Clean Air Act) require the federal government to regulate specific environmental toxicants, controversies can arise that become the fodder for litigation. For instance, disputes may arise over how the government (for example, the EPA) interprets its authorities in law, over specific regulatory decisions (for example, a national ambient air quality standard), or over questions of fairness in a regulation (for example, environmental justice issues). In the matter of the arsenic water quality standard, federal courts found that in promulgating such a standard the EPA had met its legal obligation.

Emergence of the U.S. Public Health Service

The role of the U.S. federal government in matters of public health dates from the late eighteenth century. For a young nation the sea was a vital source not only of security but also of food and commerce, and mariners were therefore essential to the nation's increasing prosperity. Ships transported goods and cargo between the Atlantic coast and European ports. In those postrevolutionary years, U.S. mariners traveled widely, contracting diseases at sea and in port and rarely able to find adequate health care in port cities. Because they could become health care burdens in the port cities, their well-being became a priority for the nascent federal government. In response, Congress in 1798 passed the Act for the Relief of Sick and Disabled Seamen, which established a loose network of marine hospitals, mainly in port cities, to care for sick and disabled mariners (Mullan, 1989).

A century later the Public Health Service Act of 1912 created the modern Public Health Service (PHS) and broadened the government's public health responsibilities by authorizing PHS investigations into human diseases (such as tuberculosis, malaria, and leprosy), sanitation, water supplies, and sewage disposal (National Institutes of Health, 2003). This Act provided the first policy framework for federal research and services in public health, advancing the nation's health services beyond those needed only by mariners.

In the 1950s, the PHS's environmental health programs and budgets expanded. Correspondingly, expectations grew, especially within environmental groups, that the PHS would become the federal government's leader in protecting the public against environmental hazards. However, as early as 1954, the PHS water pollution budget was decreased, eliciting criticism from some environmental organizations. Hope was replaced by disappointment. Seeds of discontent with PHS leadership of environmental health programs were being sowed. One U.S. surgeon general, in a report to Congress, presaged the eventual PHS relinquishment of a primary role in environmental health policy. He wrote, "When we are dealing with the possible harmful effects of the byproducts of industry and the wastes of nuclear technology, our goal is not *conquest* but *containment*" (Mullan, 1989, emphasis added). In retrospect this is a revealing comment from the leader of the PHS. It implies that primary disease prevention methods (that is, hazard elimination) could not, or would not, be applied to environmental problems. Would such a statement have been made about an infectious disease? Of course not. The surgeon general's comment gives us an insight into the disease-focused tradition of the PHS.

The traditional public health approach to prevention of disease and disability consists of science, consensus, and services. Science is required to identify and evaluate conditions that may cause disease or disability. Public health authorities then seek consensus on the public health significance of identified causes of disease or disability, as part of establishing a plan of preventive action. Finally, services from federal public health agencies to state and local agencies aim to prevent or mitigate identified causes of morbidity or mortality. The traditional public health approach to mitigating environmental hazards has been a nonregulatory approach, in which agencies develop consensus recommendations and pass them along to state and municipal governments for their consideration and possible adoption. Over time, a new approach, employing regulations and standards, has supplanted this traditional public health approach.

Establishment of the U.S. EPA

A key player in the emerging national commitment to environmental protection appeared in 1968 with the election of Richard M. Nixon to the presidency. As president, Nixon perceived that the Republican Party needed to expand its voting base. He correctly perceived the significance of the postwar migration from cities to suburbs, areas where the air was cleaner, green spaces were available, and housing was less expensive. Republican Party strategists thought suburbanites were more oriented to environmental quality and therefore ripe for Republican Party outreach in support of environmental protection (Landy, Roberts, and Thomas, 1994, p. 22). Moreover, in 1970, the inaugural Earth Day celebration had drawn dramatic attention to environmental issues and raised public concern for the environment, a situation ripe for political cultivation.

Nixon became a reluctant supporter of a stronger federal role in protecting the environment. He signed into law the National Environmental Protection Act of 1969, the Clean Air Act Amendments of 1970, and the Occupational Safety and Health Act of 1970. On July 9, 1970, Nixon, as head of the executive branch, submitted to Congress his reorganization plan that would establish the Environmental Protection Agency. Congress had sixty days to react to the proposal. Because neither the House nor the Senate expressed opposition to the plan within the prescribed time, Nixon's plan took effect on September 17, 1970 (Landy, Roberts, and Thomas, 1994, p. 32). It soon became apparent that establishing the EPA was the easy accomplishment. More difficult was to define the EPA's responsibilities. The White House disagreed with environmental groups and their congressional allies over the mission of the EPA and how the agency should relate to Congress. As related by Landy, Roberts, and Thomas (1994, pp. 33–34), the White House expected the EPA to pursue its mandate so as not to hinder industrial expansion and resource development. In contrast, the environmental community wanted the EPA to champion environmental values via statutes that bound the executive branch to limit environmental hazards.

The EPA was eventually cobbled together from other federal agencies' environmental activities, including programs in air pollution, solid waste, pesticides, drinking water, and radiological health taken over from the PHS (Mullan, 1989) and water pollution control programs from the Department of the Interior. Since its creation the EPA has been the prime federal agency both in protecting the environment and in protecting human health against specific environmental hazards. Indeed, the current mission of the EPA (2004) is ". . . to protect human health and the environment." The EPA's authority to protect human health comes from specific pieces of legislation, each addressing an environmental *medium* (such as air or water) or an environmental process (such as hazardous waste). Through its risk assessment policies and procedures, the agency both seeks voluntary cooperation from the private sector and promulgates *command-and-control* regulations. These endeavors are intended to reduce or prevent human contact with specified environmental hazards. Less exposure means a reduced potential for adverse human health effects and improved environmental quality. These benefits must be balanced by estimating the costs of proposed regulatory actions.

Key Federal Environmental Health Statutes

A large number of federal statutes have some relevance to protecting environmental quality and human health. In this chapter we limit our attention to the following federal statutes, which directly address air and water quality, food safety, and waste disposal:

- Clean air: Clean Air Act
- Clean water: Clean Water Act; Safe Drinking Water Act
- Food safety: Federal Meat Inspection Act; Food, Drug, and Cosmetic Act; Federal Insecticide, Fungicide, and Rodenticide Act
- Waste disposal: Resource Conservation and Recovery Act; Comprehensive Environmental Response, Compensation, and Liability Act

These statutes have substantial implications for public health practice and environmental health policymaking.

Box 33.2. Clean Air Act

The Clean Air Act, as amended, is intended to protect human health and the environment from emissions that pollute outdoor air.

Clean Air Act. The first federal air pollution statute was the Air Pollution Control Act of 1955. Currently, after several Amendments, it is known as the Clear Air Act, or CAA. The CAA, as amended, is a comprehensive, complex statute that controls air pollution emissions and regulates government, business, and community lifestyles that affect the releases of air contaminants into the environment (McCarthy, Parker, Schierow, and Copeland, 1999). As explained in Chapter Fourteen, air pollutants are emitted into the atmosphere from many sources and are broadly characterized by the EPA as deriving from mobile or from stationary sources. Examples of the former are vehicles powered by internal combustion engines; examples of the latter are industrial smokestacks, utility companies, incinerators, industrial boilers, and residential furnaces. Specific air pollutants are determined by the nature and quantity of the fuel combusted (for example, gasoline, coal, oil, municipal waste) and the physics of combustion. The 1970 Amendments established procedures by which the EPA sets national air quality standards. The states have the primary responsibility to ensure compliance with the air quality standards.

The CAA adopted the policy of developing National Ambient Air Quality Standards (NAAQS) for individual air contaminants and also established two kinds of air quality standards. *Primary standards* deal with protection of human health, including the health of sensitive populations such as children, elderly persons, and persons with infirmities (for example, asthma). *Secondary standards* set limits to protect public welfare, including protection against decreased visibility, damage to buildings, and deleterious ecological effects. The CAA requires standards for six so-called criteria air pollutants (carbon monoxide, lead, nitrogen oxides, ozone, particulate matter, and sulfur oxides), and 188 hazardous air pollutants.

Box 33.3. Clean Water Act

The Clean Water Act, as amended, provides grants for water treatment plants and authorizes regulations that apply to industrial and municipal dischargers of water contaminants.

Clean Water Act. The federal government's involvement with setting water quality standards began with the Public Health Service Act of 1912 (Weise, 2003), evolving over time toward more comprehensive, focused federal water quality statutes. The principal federal law now governing control of pollution in U.S. bodies of water is the Federal Water Pollution Control Act, enacted in 1948, which is now called the Clean Water Act (CWA) (Copeland, 1999). The CWA now consists of two major provisions. One authorizes federal financial assistance for municipal sewage plant construction. The other sets out the regulatory requirements that apply to industrial and municipal sources of water contaminants (Copeland, 1999). The CWA, as amended, also regulates pollutants discharged to surface waters from *point sources* (that is, pipes, ditches, and other discrete conveyances of pollutants), unless a permit is obtained under this provision of the Act. *Nonpoint sources* (for example, stormwater runoff from agricultural lands) are covered by the Water Quality Act of 1987, which amended the Clean Water Act.

Under the CWA the EPA establishes national standards, or effluent limitations, through regulations containing *best practicable technology* and *best available technology* effluent standards. States can be delegated the authority to issue discharge permits to industrial and municipal generators of water contaminants, and the attendant enforcement authority (Copeland, 1999). In addition, states must establish water quality standards, based on designated use. These standards serve as backups to federally set technology-based requirements.

Box 33.4. Safe Drinking Water Act

The Safe Drinking Water Act is the primary federal law for protecting public water systems from harmful contaminants.

Safe Drinking Water Act. The Safe Drinking Water Act (SDWA) of 1974 was established to protect the quality of drinking water in the U.S. This law focuses on all waters actually or potentially designated for drinking use, whether from surface or underground sources (Tiemann, 2003). The 1974 Act followed congressional findings that chlorinated organic chemicals were contaminating major surface and underground water supplies, that widespread underground injection operations were a threat to aquifers, and that the infrastructures of public water supply systems were increasingly inadequate to protect the public's health (Randle, 1991). The 1974 law gave the EPA substantial discretionary authority to regulate drinking-water contaminants and gave states the lead role in implementation and enforcement. The SDWA, as amended, requires the EPA to develop and promulgate three kinds of standards for specific contaminants in water supplies: a maximum contaminant level goal (MCLG), a maximum contaminant level (MCL), and a secondary maximum contaminant level (SMCL). MCLGs consider only public health and not the detection limits of water treatment technology, which must be a consideration in establishing MCLs. SMCLs are based not on human health concerns but on concerns such as water taste, cloudiness, and odor. MCLGs and SMCLs are recommendations, not enforceable under the CWA. MCLs, in distinction, are legally enforceable. It is a policy that a cost-benefit analysis and a risk assessment are required before a standard can be set.

Box 33.5. Federal Meat Inspection Act

A goal of the Federal Meat Inspection Act is to prevent adulterated or misbranded livestock and meat products from being sold as food.

Federal Meat Inspection Act. Public ignorance of conditions in the meatpacking industry began to change in the early years of the twentieth century, thanks in large part to Upton Sinclair's 1906 novel *The Jungle,* which graphically described unsanitary conditions in Chicago meatpacking plants. Sinclair's book, much like Rachael Carson's *Silent Spring* fifty-six years later, served to turn a spotlight on a major environmental health problem. On June 30, 1906, Congress enacted the Federal Meat Inspection Act (FMIA). That Act was substantially amended by the Wholesome Meat Act of 1967.

The primary goals of the FMIA, as amended, are to prevent adulterated or misbranded livestock and products from being sold as food and to ensure that meat and meat products are slaughtered and processed under humane and sanitary conditions. These requirements apply to animals and their products produced and sold within the states and also to imports, which must be inspected under equivalent foreign standards (U.S. Congress, 2002).

Box 33.6. Food, Drug, and Cosmetic Act

The Food, Drug, and Cosmetic Act, as amended, gives the FDA the authority to regulate food additives, drugs, and therapeutic devices.

Food, Drug, and Cosmetic Act. The Food and Drugs Act of 1906 prohibited the manufacture and interstate shipment of adulterated and mislabeled foods and drugs. The law enabled the federal government to initiate litigation against alleged illegal products, but it lacked affirmative requirements to guide compliance with the law. In June 1938, President Franklin D. Roosevelt signed into law the Food, Drug, and Cosmetic Act (FDCA). This law contained many significant changes, including the following: drug manufacturers were required to provide scientific proof that new products could be safely used before putting them into commerce; food standards were required to be established when needed; the addition of poisonous substances to foods was prohibited except where unavoidable or required in production; cosmetics and therapeutic devices were regulated for the first time ("The Story of the Laws Behind the Labels . . . ," 1981). In 1949, Congress held lengthy hearings on the FDCA, which led to three substantive Amendments: the Pesticide Amendment of 1954, the Food Additives Amendment of 1958, and the Color Additive Amendments of 1960. These Amendments effectuated an environmental health policy that no substance or therapeutic device may be introduced into the U.S. food supply or medical practice without a prior determination that it is safe. Moreover, these Amendments placed the burden of proof for product safety on manufacturers; thus the FDA became a reviewer of manufacturers' premarket data, with the authority to reject products or request more data from manufacturers.

Box 33.7. Federal Insecticide, Fungicide, and Rodenticide Act

The Federal Insecticide, Fungicide, and Rodenticide Act is intended to protect human health and the environment through required registration and labeling of pesticide products.

Federal Insecticide, Fungicide, and Rodenticide Act (FIFRA). The Federal Insecticide, Fungicide, and Rodenticide Act (FIFRA), as amended, requires the EPA to regulate the sale and use of pesticides in the United States through registration and labeling of the estimated 21,000 pesticide products currently in use (Schierow, 2003). The Act directs the EPA to restrict the use and application of pesticides as necessary to prevent unreasonable adverse effects on people and the environment, taking into account the costs and benefits of various pesticide uses. FIFRA prohibits the sale of any pesticide in the United States unless it is registered and labeled to indicate approved uses and restrictions. The EPA registers each pesticide for each approved use, for example, to control boll weevils on cotton. In addition, FIFRA requires the EPA to re-register older pesticides, evaluating them with data that meet current regulatory and scientific standards. If a pesticide is proposed for use on a food crop, the EPA must determine whether a "safe" level of pesticide residue, called a *tolerance,* can be established. If a tolerance is not granted to the manufacturer, the pesticide is restricted for use on food. The burden of proof is upon pesticide manufacturers to establish the safety of their product.

The Food Quality Protection Act of 1996 amended FIFRA in several substantive ways, notably introducing the new policy that children's health is to be protected by requiring the EPA to consider more safety factors in its risk assessments of pesticides (see Chapter Twenty-Eight).

Box 33.8. Resource Conservation and Recovery Act

The Resource Conservation and Recovery Act requires the EPA, working with states, to regulate solid and hazardous waste management.

Resource Conservation and Recovery Act. The Solid Waste Disposal Act of 1965 was the first federal environmental statute to address the public health problem of waste disposal. Later Amendments to the Act led to its being renamed the Resource Conservation and Recovery Act (RCRA). RCRA regulates solid and hazardous waste management. It defines solid and hazardous wastes, authorizes the EPA to set emission standards for facilities that generate or manage hazardous waste, and establishes a permit program for hazardous waste treatment, storage, and disposal facilities (McCarthy and Tiemann, 1999).

Most states have assumed, under EPA approval and financial support, much of the responsibility for regulating the management of solid and hazardous wastes, including the key provision of issuing permits to waste management facilities.

Individual facility operators are required to perform the monitoring, testing, analysis, and reporting necessary to abate hazards to human health or the environment. Of note, RCRA prohibits open solid waste dumps, a provision enforced by those states approved by the EPA. The policy of prohibiting open dumping brought to an end in the United States an environmental practice that dates from antiquity.

Box 33.9. Comprehensive Environmental Response, Compensation, and Liability Act

The primary purpose of the Comprehensive Environmental Response, Compensation, and Liability Act is to remediate uncontrolled hazardous waste sites and assess site effects on human health.

Comprehensive Environmental Response, Compensation, and Liability Act. The Comprehensive Environmental Response, Compensation, and Liability Act (CERCLA; also known as Superfund) was enacted in 1980 and was reauthorized by the Superfund Amendments and Reauthorization Act of 1986. The original enactment in 1980 followed the discovery of releases of hazardous substances from abandoned landfills into community residences—in particular in the community of Love Canal, New York, which was evacuated following the discovery that it overlay an abandoned chemical dump (Johnson, 1999).

The intent of the law is to provide for liability, compensation, and emergency response when hazardous substances are released into the environment and when inactive hazardous waste disposal sites require cleanup (Reisch, 1999). CERCLA's basic purposes are to provide funding and enforcement authority for remediating hazardous waste sites, responding to public health concerns, conducting emergency removal of chemical spills, and identifying *potentially responsible parties* (PRPs). Embedded in CERCLA is the policy that polluters should pay for the environmental and public health consequences of their actions, and the EPA has strong authority to recover from PRPs their share of remediating CERCLA hazardous waste sites. CERCLA also established the Hazardous Substances Superfund, a trust fund intended by Congress to be a source of funds for site remediation when other sources, such as PRPs, were unavailable.

The RCRA and CERCLA statutes differ in the kind of waste management each covers. RCRA covers the controlled storage, treatment, and disposal of solid and hazardous wastes, whereas CERCLA pertains only to the management of uncontrolled hazardous waste.

Environmental Health Policymaking in Practice

No description of a law can fully convey how the law functions in practice. Any of the major environmental statutes is subject to interpretation, political pressures, and even the effects of evolving scientific knowledge over time. Several sets of factors influence how environmental health policies are promulgated and implemented.

The Role of Science

Environmental health policies must be predicated on applicable and appropriate science bases. For example, regulations that limit levels of air pollutants must be based on empirical data about the health effects of exposure to these pollutants—data that come from toxicology, epidemiology, chemistry, physics, and other sciences. Science provides the platform on which environmental polices are built.

However, the science base is rarely complete. For any given exposure, data may not be available about specific health effects, about health effects of exposures at specific dose levels of interest, about responses among specific subgroups of the population, or about effects of concomitant exposures to other substances. For example, for many substances we have information about the effects of very high dose exposures in animals and moderately high dose exposures in the workplace, but little or no information about the effects of such low-dose exposures as typically occur in the community. Moreover, data may not be available about the feasibility or cost of implementing a regulation or even about the availability of technical alternatives. These limits bedevil policymakers.

Risk Assessment

Partly for this reason, risk assessment has assumed a central role in environmental health policymaking. As described in Chapter Thirty-Two, risk assessment can be defined as the process of estimating, usually in quantitative terms, the harm that will result from exposure to an environmental hazard (Fiorino, 1995). In 1980, a Supreme Court decision changed how U.S. regulatory agencies developed risk assessment in support of environmental and workplace standards. The Occupational Safety and Health Administration (OSHA) had proposed a stringent new benzene standard, limiting the permissible workplace exposure level to one part per million (ppm). In response, industry had sued OSHA, claiming that the standard was not justified because only a small number of benzene-induced leukemias would be averted, and at huge cost. The Supreme Court held that OSHA had failed adequately to quantify the health risk of workers potentially exposed to benzene. OSHA, the EPA, and other federal regulatory agencies interpreted the court's decision as a mandate for them to undergird their regulatory actions with the results of quantitative risk assessment. Regulatory agencies now, as a matter of policy, use quantitative risk assessment as their primary tool for determining the degree of risk posed by environmental hazards. This policy is not without its critics. Risk assessment can be a lengthy process, subject to court challenges and political influences. On the positive side, properly conducted risk assessments can serve as the basis for science-based risk management decisions on how to control specific environmental hazards.

Who Interprets the Science?

Typically, regulatory agencies form internal committees to review and act on scientific data pertaining to their tasks. This effort is normally part of a risk assessment approach. Such committees consist of specialists in toxicology, epidemiology, statistics, chemistry, physics, and other academic fields. Published scientific articles and reports are reviewed and debated as to their relevance and quality. When gaps in data are discovered, committees must decide whether the gaps are sufficient to prevent establishing a standard.

In some cases federal agencies play a major part in producing or collecting the scientific data used in regulatory policymaking. In other cases regulated parties play a major role. Some statutes require the EPA to develop the data upon which its standards are based. For example, the CAA, CWA, SDWA, and CERCLA all require the EPA to develop the science base for its standards, placing the burden of proof on the agency. In contrast the FDCA, FIFRA, FMIA, and RCRA place this burden on the entities whose products or activities are regulated. The FDCA requires manufacturers of drugs, cosmetics, food additives, and therapeutic devices to provide the FDA with product safety data for review and approval. Similarly, FIFRA requires pesticide producers to provide the EPA with data for pesticide safety review. RCRA requires waste management operators to provide the EPA with data on their operations in support of their compliance with hazardous waste regulations.

From Science to Policy

Regulatory agencies use science-based risk assessments as the basis of risk management policies and practices. But risk management is based on far more than science; risk management is the mortar in which economic, social, political, and scientific considerations are ground into policy by a bureaucratic pestle. Science, as the basis of a proposed regulation or standard, can only point to a risk management strategy. Questions of the social and economic costs of a proposed regulation or standard must also be answered, along with issues of political reaction. Consider a proposed standard for a drinking-water contaminant. Risk managers must ask: Is it feasible to clean the water to this level? How much will it cost public water systems to implement the standard? Will there be opposition to the standard? From whom?

As regulatory agencies' decisions become public, political influences come into the picture. It is common to have scientists who represent special interest groups such as industrial trade associations present scientific data or interpretations that they assert will contradict the government's science base and its interpretation. Some debates about regulatory science eventually find their way into litigation, where courts must attempt to sort out whose science should prevail. It is common for courts to obtain the services of scientists whom they consider objective and unbiased in their fields of scientific expertise.

The public can also play a significant role through advocacy, monitoring, and enforcement of proposed or enacted environmental policies. As discussed later in this chapter, public groups and individual citizens can engage in litigation with government agencies for failure to perform specified environmental health responsibilities under specific statutes. However, there are other opportunities for the public to influence environmental health policymaking. These mechanisms include citizen participation in public surveys, voter initiatives, negotiated rule making, citizen review panels, advisory commissions, written comment processes, and site-specific dispute resolution (Fiorino, 1995, pp. 96–97).

Consider the involvement of the public in the Superfund statute. Upon the discovery of hazardous waste underneath Love Canal, New York, and other residential areas of the United States, citizen groups formed to advocate the relocation of residents to noncontaminated residential areas. These same groups caught the attention of national news media, leading to legislative action by Congress and administrative action by the White House. Upon enactment of CERCLA, community groups were formed by people who lived near Superfund sites. These groups participated in public hearings convened by the EPA and state agencies, serving as monitors of site cleanup progress and public health interventions. Individual citizens served on various advisory committees. Public involvement has arguably led to better informed Superfund policies and remediation of hazardous waste sites.

An important interest in the policymaking process is environmental justice, which evolved in the United States from concerns in communities of color that environmental hazards were being imposed on them due to discriminatory actions by government and business interests. In particular, historical environmental justice concerns were associated with the location of hazardous waste sites in minority communities (Johnson, 1999; also see Chapter Eight in this volume). Environmental justice advocates have successfully seen to it that government environmental policies enforce nondiscriminatory imposition of environmental hazards.

The Question of Cost

The U.S. public looks skeptically at personal health decisions that are based on financial cost; for example, an unpopular aspect of health maintenance organizations is that costs are seen as driving health care decisions. Nevertheless, cost-benefit analyses have become a standard part of environmental health policymaking. Cost-benefit analysis appears in environmental statutes as a result of legislative directives and federal court decisions and in business operations when decision quality relies on having a sense of costs associated with the business's products, working conditions, and consumer affairs. On the surface, consideration of costs and benefits to the public is important and reasonable. But current cost-benefit analysis necessarily forces decisions about the worth of human life, estimates technology costs using projection models, and can force decisions when adequate information is lacking on the costs and benefits to different races, cultures, and age groups. Cost-benefit analysis will remain a public policy cloth—but with frayed edges until better health benefits data become available.

Global Regulatory Developments

Increasingly, the United States has entered into regional and global treaties on trade that can influence—and indeed overturn—U.S. environmental regulations. For example, the North American Free Trade Agreement (NAFTA), a treaty among Canada, Mexico, and the U.S., contains provisions for arbitrating disputes among the treaty's partners. This dispute resolution mechanism can lead to setting aside U.S. environmental regulations. Similarly, the World Trade Organization can overturn U.S. environmental regulations. For example, U.S. restrictions on the importation of shrimp from countries where nets that can kill endangered sea turtles are used were set aside by the WTO (Friends of the Earth, 2003). The U.S. policy was deemed to be in violation of free trade. Whether U.S. environmental regulations should be sacrificed on the altar of free trade is a policy question awaiting resolution (Rao, 2000; Esty, 1994; Gallagher, 2004).

Regulation and Its Alternatives

In the United States, over the course of many years but particularly since the 1960s, policies have evolved that target specific environmental health hazards, for example, chemical contaminants in drinking-water supplies. The most frequently used policy approach has been to pass laws and subsequent regulations that control the risk of exposure to select environmental hazards. In general this body of environmental law gave federal agencies such as the EPA the authority to *command* actions and *control* workplace and community sources of environmental hazards—hence the term *command and control* for this policy paradigm. Generators of pollution, such as manufacturers and utilities, that are required to comply with specific regulations are called the *regulated community*. The processes used by regulatory agencies to establish regulations and standards must comply with the Administrative Procedures Act of 1946. This Act requires federal agencies to provide advance notice and opportunity for comment on proposed regulations (often this includes holding public hearings), and agencies must document the basis for their decisions in a public record (Andrews, 1999, p. 66).

Command-and-control regulations employ three broad strategies: quality standards, emissions standards, and product prohibition. *Quality standards* stipulate the maximum levels of pollution permitted in air, water, soil, workplace, or other locations. Typically, states are responsible for maintaining their airsheds and waterways within permissible levels, and employers bear this responsibility for their workplaces. The CAA and the SDWA contain air and water quality provisions, respectively. *Emission standards* prescribe the acceptable pollution discharges from sources of air or water contamination (Rosenbaum, 1998, pp. 181–182). For example, the CWA limits the materials facilities may emit into waterways. *Product prohibition* provides regulatory agencies such as the EPA and FDA with the authority to ban products such as pesticides and drugs that fail to meet product safety requirements.

Command and control is a controversial policy. The regulated community often objects to the alleged economic impact of quality and emission standards, usually arguing that the costs to them far outweigh the benefits to the public. One response in recent years, as noted earlier, has been the requirement by Congress that regulatory agencies conduct cost-benefit analyses of proposed regulations. Even after cost-benefit analyses are conducted and regulatory actions became final, litigation often occurs when the regulated community disagrees with the final regulatory action. Because command-and-control regulations mandate legally enforceable actions that polluters must take, it is certain that litigation and confrontation will continue.

Beginning in the 1980s and '90s, several factors combined to challenge the command-and-control approach to environmental health policy. First, the political climate shifted toward an antiregulatory posture, part of a broader shift away from "big government" that began with the Reagan administration. Second, some of the limitations of command-and-control policies became clear; they can be inefficient, time consuming, and ineffective. Both industry and, to a lesser extent, environmental and health groups have endorsed more flexible federal policies toward environmental health hazards. Industry has historically opposed any regulations viewed as bad for business. Environmental groups have noted that command-and-control regulation takes too long and can be subject to industry influences, and have favored alternatives in some situations. Several policy alternatives to command-and-control regulation have therefore emerged, including voluntary action by business, litigation, market mechanisms, consumer pressure, and public education.

Voluntary Action by Business

Corporations and other businesses can adopt voluntary actions to eliminate workplace, community, and home environmental hazards. Voluntary actions are those not mandated by government agencies. A policy of voluntary action may reap benefits for businesses, such as increased income, better community relations, and less litigation, depending of course on the nature of the voluntary action.

For example, a manufacturing plant might voluntarily decrease the amounts of pollution released into the community environment beyond the levels required by environmental emission standards such as clean water discharge standards. Sometimes, voluntary actions to reduce emissions are a response to public awareness of the data supplied by a plant or facility to the Toxics Release Inventory (TRI). Some companies have taken extra efforts to decrease their TRI emissions in order to improve their community image (Graham, 2000). Although reporting certain levels of emissions to the EPA under the TRI regulations is mandatory, reducing the amounts of emissions beyond air and water quality standards is voluntary. If emissions released into the environment are thought of as waste, making them an indicator of inefficient production, finding ways to decrease those emissions may benefit a company economically.

Litigation

Substantial and numerous issues in environmental health policy have been established or modified through litigation. Courts have served as arbiters—and sometimes, by default, policy decision makers—on many wide-ranging environmental issues. Plaintiffs have included government agencies, private industry, environmental groups, and individual citizens. In the case of standards for arsenic in drinking water, the state of Nebraska litigated a claim against the EPA, alleging that the revised arsenic water quality standard was unconstitutional. Similarly, the EPA has litigated municipalities' failure to meet Clean Water Act standards. In these examples of "proactive" litigation, courts have become final authorities on how appropriately government agencies have met their legal environmental responsibilities.

Private industry has also turned to courts for relief from allegedly burdensome regulations. In the case of benzene exposure noted earlier, affected industries sued OSHA over its proposed regulation to control benzene levels in the workplace. The legal challenge made its way to the Supreme Court, which agreed with the industry plaintiffs. The court sent OSHA home with an assignment to engage in quantitative risk assessment when it attempted to regulate carcinogens (Rodricks, 2003). The court's decision completely changed the way federal regulatory agencies assess the risk from environmental hazards. Quantitative risk assessment became part of regulatory policy at the EPA, OSHA, and other federal regulatory agencies.

Environmental groups have been particularly effective in litigation, taking advantage of environmental statutes that contain citizen suit provisions, including the CAA, CWA, RCRA, and CERCLA (Andrews, 1999, p. 418). This strategy dates back to the 1970s, when national environmental organizations developed the capacity to engage in litigation with the EPA and other regulatory agencies under citizen suit provisions of several environmental statutes. For example, in 1971 the Environmental Defense Fund (now called Environmental Defense) successfully sued the EPA to force the agency to hold public hearings on whether or not to ban DDT. Similarly, the Natural Resources Defense Council sued the EPA in 1973 and 1974 for failing to develop standards to control toxic water pollutants; in the resulting court settlement the EPA agreed to develop standards for sixty-five water contaminants (Andrews, 1999, p. 241). Individuals can sue federal agencies when specifically permitted to do so under the relevant law. Such citizen lawsuits have continued to the present, leading to a significant body of law that has resulted from citizen litigation provisions in air, water, and waste removal statutes.

Market Mechanisms

Incentives are a powerful motivator of human behavior. In the sports world some players' contracts stipulate that exceeding performance goals will result in extra salary. For example, a baseball pitcher who wins twenty games, has an earned run average less than 3.0, and is voted to the All-Star team might be paid more for achieving these goals, if it is so stipulated in his contract. Similarly, salespersons who exceed sales goals are often paid extra. Incentives can be part of a carrot-and-stick approach to performance.

Pollution trading credits (PTCs), also called *cap and trade credits,* use market mechanisms based on a similar approach. The idea is relatively simple. A regulatory body (for example, the EPA) grants individual polluting facilities (for example, an electric power plant) an annual allocation of PTCs that equals the maximum amount of pollution that they can release into the environment. Facilities must hold credits equal to their actual emissions. However, if a given facility releases less pollution than its emissions allocation, the difference in trading credits can become a commodity to be sold to other facilities. This provides an economic incentive for a facility to overachieve in order to market its PTCs. This is the free enterprise system being used to drive gains in environmental quality.

Consumer Pressure

In a society based on a consumer economy, consumers can markedly influence environmental policies. If individuals and groups express a preference for purchasing environmentally sensitive products (sometimes called *green* products), they can help determine what products remain in commerce. For example, consumer preferences for household detergents with low or zero phosphorus content will help reduce water pollution and algal growth in waterways. Similarly, companies, small businesses, and government agencies can voluntarily adopt polices that favor purchasing green products. Also, consumers can preferentially purchase *no sweat* products, those not made in sweatshops, where exploited workers experience low wages, no health or other benefits, and unsafe working conditions.

Antismoking campaigns are an example of consumer power becoming environmental health policy in action. Antismoking activists have been quite successful in lobbying local governments and businesses to ban or restrict tobacco smoking in public and some private premises. A contemporary example is the restriction on tobacco smoking in restaurants. Many local governments have required restaurants and other food service establishments either to ban tobacco smoking altogether or, in some localities, to provide areas where smoking is prohibited. Where consumers have a choice between restaurants with no smoking at all and those with restricted smoking areas, they can exert pressure by selecting no-smoking establishments, thereby promoting an increase in the number of such restaurants. Similarly, it was pressure from airline customers that eventually led to no-smoking polices on domestic and international flights, illustrating how consumer power can have a global impact. The essential point to be made is that market pressure can influence policy for both environmental protection and societal good.

Public Education

An informed public can make a significant difference in reducing the effects of exposure to environmental hazards. For example, informed individuals can choose to purchase green products and services, patronize companies and business enterprises that have evidenced environmental contributions, and advocate for the importance of nurturing environmental health policies. Acting on the basis of environmental information is activism in practice. But how does an individual acquire such information? And from whom?

U.S. environmental organizations such as the Sierra Club, Natural Resources Defense Council, Environmental Defense, and Physicians for Social Responsibility have emphasized public education policies. These and similar organizations provide scientific documents, news alerts, and policy recommendations of relevance to environmental health policies and practices. Because environmental organizations have achieved considerable credibility with the public, their public education actions and products have great political and personal impact. These organizations' educational materials are now typically accessible on the Internet. For example, the Environmental Health program of Physicians for Social Responsibility (2005) offers an online brochure on reproductive disorders and birth defects. Using the information in the brochure, people can make lifestyle choices that will reduce exposure to environmental hazards (for example, solvent-based paint) to fetal development.

Policy Cornucopia

Regulation will probably remain the anchor policy in controlling environmental hazards. Without the weight of law to control environmental hazards, pollution sources are unlikely to be abated voluntarily in amounts sufficient to make a real difference in environmental quality. Further, regulatory frameworks level the playing field by treating all sources of pollution the same. That is to say, water and air quality standards apply equally to contaminants released by big corporations and by small businesses. Without regulations and standards, based on statutes, developed countries would become no different from developing countries, where pollution controls are largely nonexistent.

However, as history has shown, workplace and community environmental regulations are only one approach to environmental health protection. Regulations are often opposed by the regulated community, which has the economic and political wherewithal to block or alter them. Moreover, regulations are not always the optimal approach to protecting environmental health. A range of approaches, from regulation to voluntary action to consumer pressure, will continue to characterize the environmental health policy landscape.

Conclusion

This chapter has described environmental health policymaking and implementation in ways that might imply an orderly, effective process. In fact, developing regulations and standards is far from orderly. During the preliminary phase of policy development, special interest groups of all stripes exert great pressure on policymakers such as members of Congress to support a particular point of view. After a statute has been signed into law, regulations and standards must be developed, even when statutory language is vague. Again, special interest groups attempt to sway regulatory agencies by presenting data and interpretations during public hearings held in compliance with administrative law procedures. The example of setting a standard for arsenic in drinking water illustrates how politics, litigation, lobbying by special interest groups, and science all come into play when contentious regulations are developed and promoted.

Thought Questions

1. Select one of these laws: the Clean Air Act, Clean Water Act, Safe Drinking Water Act, or Federal Meat Inspection Act. Describe the law's purpose and the policies that have been promulgated as a result. Describe the law's impact, both in terms of environmental health and in terms of economics, on you personally. Then assume the law you selected does not exist. Discuss the ramifications of having no law, and discuss any actions you would take to protect your personal health.
2. Rachel Carson's book *Silent Spring,* published in 1962, is given much credit for shaping the U.S. public's concerns about environmental hazards. Discuss, in your opinion, (a) why the book had such a significant effect and (b) whether such a book would achieve the same sociopolitical prominence today.
3. What should government regulatory agencies do when the scientific data are insufficient for developing an environmental standard?

References

Andrews, R.N.L. *Managing the Environment, Managing Ourselves: A History of American Environmental Policy.* New Haven, Conn.: Yale University Press, 1999.

Copeland, C. "Summaries of Environmental Laws Administered by the EPA: Clean Water Act." [http://www.ncseonline.org/NLE/CRSreports/BriefingBooks/Laws/e.cfm]. 1999.

"Court Upholds Tougher Rule on Arsenic Limits in Water." *New York Times,* June 21, 2003.

Esty, D. C. *Greening the GATT: Trade, Environment and the Future.* Washington, D.C.: Institute for International Economics, 1994.

Fiorino, D. J. *Making Environmental Policy.* Berkeley: University of California Press, 1995.

Friends of the Earth. "WTO Scorecard." [http://www.foe.org]. 2003.

Gallagher, K. P. *Free Trade and the Environment: Mexico, NAFTA, and Beyond.* Palo Alto, Calif.: Stanford University Press, 2004.

Graham, M. "Regulation by Shaming." *Atlantic Monthly,* Apr. 2000, pp. 36–40.

Johnson, B. L. *Impact of Hazardous Waste on Human Health: Hazard, Health Effects, Equity, and Communications Issues.* Boca Raton, Fla.: Lewis, 1999.

Landy, M. K., Roberts, M. J., and Thomas, S. R. *The Environmental Protection Agency: Asking the Wrong Questions: From Nixon to Clinton.* New York: Oxford University Press, 1994.

McCarthy, J. E., Parker, L. B., Schierow, L., and Copeland, C. "Summaries of Environmental Laws Administered by EPA: Clean Air Act." [http://www.cnie.org/nle/leg-8/d.html]. 1999.

McCarthy, J. E., and Tiemann, M. "Summaries of Environmental Laws Administered by EPA: Solid Waste Disposal Act/Resource Conservation and Recovery Act." [http://www.cnie.org/nle/leg-8/h.html]. 1999.

Mullan, F. *Plagues and Politics: The Story of the United States Public Health Service.* New York: Basic Books, 1989.

National Institutes of Health. *Images from the History of the Public Health Service.* Rockville, Md.: National Library of Medicine, 2003.

Physicians for Social Responsibility. "Children's Environmental Health: Birth Defects." [http://www.envirohealthaction.org/children/birth_defects/]. 2005.

Randle, R. V. "Safe Drinking Water Act." In J. G. Arbuckle and others (eds.), *Environmental Law Handbook.* Rockville, Md.: Government Institutes, 1991.

Rao, P. K. *The World Trade Organization and the Environment.* New York: St. Martin's Press, 2000.

Reisch, M. "Summaries of Environmental Laws Administered by the EPA: Superfund." [http://www.ncseonline.org/NLE/crsreports/BriefingBooks/Laws/j.cfm]. 1999.

Rodricks, J. V. "What Happened to the Red Book's Second Most Important Recommendation?" *Human and Ecological Risk Assessment,* 2003, *9*(5), 1169–1180.

Rosenbaum, W. A. *Environmental Politics and Policy.* (4th ed.) Washington: Congressional Quarterly, 1998.

Schierow, L. "Summaries of Environmental Laws Administered by the EPA: Federal Insecticide, Fungicide, and Rodenticide Act." [http://www.ncseonline.org/NLE/CRSreports/BriefingBooks/Laws/l.cfm]. 2003.

"The Story of the Laws Behind the Labels, Part II: 1938—The Federal Food, Drug, and Cosmetic Act." *FDA Consumer,* June 1981.

Tiemann, M. "Summaries of Environmental Laws Administered by the EPA: Safe Drinking Water Act." [http://www.ncseonline.org/NLE/CRSreports/BriefingBooks/Laws/g.cfm]. 2003.

U.S. Congress. House. Agriculture Committee. *Federal Meat Inspection Act of 1906.* [http://agriculture.House.gov/glossary/federal_meat_inspection_act_of 1906.htm]. 2002.

U.S. Environmental Protection Agency. Homepage. [http://www.epa.gov]. 2004.

Weise, J. *Historic Drinking Water Facts.* Anchorage, Alaska: ADEC Division of Environmental Health, Drinking Water and Wastewater Program, 2003.

For Further Information

A number of the books listed in the references are of general interest. R.N.L. Andrews's *Managing the Environment, Managing Ourselves,* a scholarly work of lasting value, offers an outstanding description of past and current policies on U.S. environmental management. D. J. Fiorino's *Making Environmental Policy* (chaps. 1, 2, and 3) presents a good explanation of policymaking challenges and the federal institutions engaged in environmental policymaking. There is currently no available book on the history of the U.S. Environmental Protection Agency, but M. K. Landy, M. J. Roberts, and S. R. Thomas's *The Environmental Protection Agency: Asking the Wrong Questions from Nixon to Clinton,* comes close. It is required reading for persons wanting to know how the EPA has evolved. B. L. Johnson's *Impact of Hazardous Waste on Human Health* is the only book that describes the policy challenges presented by management of uncontrolled hazardous waste sites.

In addition, many persons consider the Clean Air Act to be the major federal environmental statute in regard to policymaking. For an excellent review of the policy challenges in the management of air contaminants, see

National Research Council. *Air Quality Management in the United States.* Washington, D.C.: National Academies Press, 2004.

Risk assessment drives many environmental policies. The following crisp little book describes the history and practice of risk assessment better than any other:

Rodricks, J. V. *Calculated Risks: The Toxicity and Human Health Risks of Chemicals in Our Environment.* New York: Cambridge University Press, 1992.

Finally, for an excellent review of environmental policy during a period of political changes and challenges to U.S. federal environmental policymaking, see

Vig, N. J., and Kraft, M. W. *Environmental Policy in the 1990s* (2nd ed.) Washington, D.C.: Congressional Quarterly, 1994.

CHAPTER THIRTY-FOUR

RISK COMMUNICATION

Vincent T. Covello

Members of a community learn that a nearby factory has contaminated the local groundwater with solvents through three decades of improper handling. Workers learn that mercury levels in their workplace periodically exceed applicable standards. Consumers learn that detectable levels of pesticides are found in many of the fruits and vegetables they buy. In each case people understand that an environmental exposure may place their health at risk, and they are concerned. Even if the risk turns out to be low, the concern may still be high. To understand risk and to act on it appropriately, people need information. Risk communication is the practice of providing this information.

Risk communication has been variously defined. For example, according to the National Research Council (1989), *risk communication* is "an interactive process of exchange of information and opinion among individuals, groups, and institutions." Risk communication is successful to the extent that "it raises the level of understanding of relevant issues or actions for those involved and satisfies them that they are adequately informed within the limits of available knowledge" (p. 4).

In this chapter, *risk communication* is defined as a science-based approach that is typically used to guide communication with diverse audiences in high-stress, high-concern, or controversial situations. It refers to any public or private communication that informs individuals about the existence, nature, form, severity, or acceptability of risks. Many parties may employ risk communication—a local public health agency managing a toxic chemical spill, a manufacturing company that has just disclosed air emissions in the annual Toxics Release Inventory, a school system confronting an outbreak of symptoms among children and teachers, a food company just found to be selling contaminated food, or a nongovernmental agency active in disaster relief. In each case concerned stakeholders—members of the public, employees, customers, newspaper reporters—need more information, and ideally the opportunity to participate in active dialogue, so they can satisfy their need to assess and respond to the risk.

Goals of Risk Communication

The purpose of risk communication changes according to the nature of the issue. In some cases its purpose is to inform and to disseminate information about risk. In other cases its purpose is to involve people in a two-way communication process designed to build consensus. Whatever the issue, the overarching goals of risk communication are

- Knowledge and understanding
- Trust and credibility
- Cooperation and constructive dialogue

Effective risk communication provides the public with timely, accurate, clear, objective, consistent, and complete information about risks. It creates an informed population that

> Is involved, interested, reasonable, thoughtful, solution oriented, cooperative, and collaborative
>
> Is appropriately concerned about the risk involved
>
> Takes appropriate actions and engages in appropriate behavior

Risk Communication and Risk Management

Effective risk communication is key to effective risk management. It establishes public confidence in an organization's ability to deal with risk. Effective risk communication is a key responsibility of managers. Policymakers, the media, and the public all expect timely and quality information. Although events are by nature difficult to predict, risk communication strategies can be planned.

Risk communication is essential when decisions are being made about an issue of concern. It enables people to participate in determining how risks should be managed. Communication is also a vital part of implementing decisions—whether explaining policies and decisions to people, informing and advising people about risks that they can control themselves, or dissuading people from risky behavior.

Risk Communication and Crisis Management

Until something dramatic goes wrong, the elaborate infrastructures and mechanisms that protect health, safety, and the environment on a daily basis often go unnoticed. In the heat of a crisis, quality risk communication will directly influence events. Poor risk communication in a crisis can fan emotions and undermine confidence. Good risk communication in a crisis can rally support, calm a nervous public, provide needed information, and encourage appropriate behaviors. Communicate badly in a crisis and one may be perceived as incompetent, uncaring, or dishonest. Communicate well in a crisis and one can reach many people with clear and credible messages.

Risk Communication and Risk Perception

Basic to risk communication is the concept of risk itself. In the scientific literature the term *risk* refers typically to the uncertainty of an outcome. It is a combination of likelihood and impact. For the public, however, the term *risk* has a broader meaning. As noted by Peter Sandman, for the public,

$$\text{Risk} = \text{Hazard} + \text{Outrage}.$$

This equation sums up the observation that an individual's perception or assessment of risk reflects his or her understanding of the danger at hand (for example, the statistical probability of injury, illness, or death) and his or her sense of outrage about it. Outrage may take on strong emotional overtones. It predisposes an individual to react emotionally to risk information (for example, with fear, anger, or hostility), which can in turn significantly amplify levels of worry.

According to risk perception and risk outrage theory, the concerns that people have and their perceptions of risk are often determined more by outrage and emotional factors than by the potential for actual, typically physical, harm or hazard. For example, ten times more Americans died in traffic crashes in 2001 than died in the World Trade Center attacks, but the attacks elicited far more outrage. Psychologists and others have identified a number of factors that affect levels of outrage, as shown in Box 34.1.

Box 34.1. Outrage Factors

Voluntariness. Risks from activities considered to be involuntary or imposed (for example, exposure to chemicals or radiation from a terrorist attack using chemical weapons or "dirty bombs") are judged to be greater, and are therefore less readily accepted, than risks from activities that are seen to be voluntary (for example, smoking, sunbathing, or mountain climbing).

Controllability. Risks from activities viewed as under the control of others (for example, releases of nerve gas in a coordinated series of terrorist attacks) are judged to be greater, and are less readily accepted, than risks from activities that appear to be under the control of the individual (for example, driving an automobile or riding a bicycle).

Familiarity. Risks from activities viewed as unfamiliar (such as infection with an exotic-sounding disease) are judged to be greater than risks from activities viewed as familiar (such as household work).

Fairness. Risks from activities believed to be unfair or to involve unfair processes (for example, inequitable siting of certain facilities) are judged to be greater than risks from fair activities (for example, vaccinations).

Benefits. Risks from activities that seem to have unclear, questionable, or diffused personal or economic benefits (for example, waste disposal facilities) are judged to be greater than risks from activities that have clear benefits (for example, jobs, efforts with monetary benefits, or automobile driving).

Catastrophic potential. Risks from activities viewed as having the potential to cause a significant number of deaths and injuries closely grouped in time and space (for example, a major terrorist attack using biological, chemical, or nuclear weapons) are judged to be greater than risks from activities that cause deaths and injuries scattered or random in time and space (for example, automobile accidents).

Understanding. Poorly understood risks (such as the health effects of long-term exposure to low doses of toxic chemicals or radiation) are judged to be greater than risks that are well understood or self-explanatory (such as pedestrian accidents or slipping on ice).

Uncertainty. Risks from activities that are relatively unknown or that pose highly uncertain outcomes (for example, genetic engineering) are judged to be greater than risks from activities that have outcomes relatively well known to science (for example, automobile accidents, for which actuarial statistics are available).

Delayed effects. Risks from activities that may have long latency periods between exposure and adverse health effects (for example, cancer due to exposure to low doses of radiation) are judged to be greater than risks from activities viewed as having immediate effects (for example, poisonings).

Effects on children. Risks from activities that appear to put children specifically at risk (for example, drinking milk contaminated with radiation or toxic chemicals or exposure of pregnant women to radiation or toxic chemicals) are judged to be greater than risks from activities that do not involve children (for example, workplace accidents).

Effects on future generations. Risks from activities that seem to pose a threat to future generations (for example, exposures to toxic chemicals or radiation that may have genetic effects) are judged to be greater than risks from activities that do not endanger future generations (for example, skiing accidents).

Victim identity. Risks from activities that produce identifiable victims (for example, a worker exposed to high levels of toxic chemicals or radiation; a child who falls down a well; a miner trapped in a mine) are judged to be greater than risks from activities that produce statistical victims (for example, statistical profiles of automobile accident victims).

Dread. Risks from activities that evoke fear, terror, or anxiety (for example, exposure to cancer-causing agents, to AIDS, or to smallpox) are judged to be greater than risks from activities that do not arouse such feelings or emotions (for example, common colds and household accidents).

Trust. Risks from activities associated with individuals, institutions, or organizations lacking in trust and credibility (for example, activities of governments with poor antiterrorist track records) are judged to be greater than risks from activities associated with those that are trustworthy and credible (for example, activities of regulatory agencies that achieve high levels of compliance among regulated groups).

Media attention. Risks from activities that receive considerable media coverage (for example, anthrax attacks via the postal system; accidents at nuclear power plants) are judged to be greater than risks from activities that receive little coverage (for example, on-the-job accidents).

Accident history. Risks from activities with a history of major accidents or incidents or frequent minor accidents or incidents (for example, leaks at a waste disposal facility) are judged to be greater than risks from activities with little or no such history (for example, recombinant DNA experiments).

Reversibility. Risks from activities considered to have potentially irreversible adverse effects (for example, exposures to a toxic substance or radiation known to cause birth defects) are judged to be greater than risks from activities considered to have reversible adverse effects (for example, sports injuries).

Personal stake. Risks from activities viewed by people as placing them (or their families) personally and directly at risk (for example, living near a waste disposal site) are judged to be greater than risks from activities that appear to pose no direct or personal threat (for example, disposal of waste in remote areas).

Ethical or moral nature. Risks from activities believed to be ethically objectionable or morally wrong (for example, providing diluted or outdated vaccines for use in an economically distressed community) are judged to be greater than risks from ethically neutral activities (for example, taking medication with possible side effects).

Human versus natural origin. Risks generated by human action, failure, or incompetence (for example, disasters caused by negligence, inadequate safeguards, or operator error) are judged to be greater than risks believed to be caused by nature or "acts of God" (for example, exposure to geological radon or cosmic rays).

Risk Communication and High Stress

When people are stressed, they often have difficulty hearing, understanding, and remembering information. Stress can greatly reduce a person's ability to process information. The challenge for risk communicators therefore is to

- Overcome the barriers that stress creates.
- Produce accurate messages for diverse audiences in high-stress situations.
- Achieve maximum communication effectiveness within the constraints posed by stress.

Risk communication solutions to the problems created by high stress include

Conciseness—developing a limited number of key messages: ideally, no more than three key messages (or one key message with three parts) that address the underlying concern or specific question

Brevity—keeping individual key messages brief: ideally, using fewer than three seconds or fewer than nine words for each key message and fewer than nine seconds or twenty-seven words for the entire set of three key messages

Clarity—developing messages that can be easily understood by the target audience: typically, for communications to the general public, written at a sixth- to eighth-grade reading level

Additional solutions include

- Placing messages within the message set so that the most important messages occupy the first and last positions in the communication (what is most important will depend on the specific audience and specific context)
- Citing third parties or sources perceived as credible by the receiving audience
- Developing key messages and supporting information that address such important risk perception and outrage factors as trust, benefits, control, voluntariness, dread, fairness, reversibility, catastrophic potential, effects on children, memorability, morality, origin, and familiarity
- Using graphics, visual aids, analogies, and narratives (for example, personal stories) designed to increase substantially an individual's ability to hear, understand, and recall a message
- Balancing a negative key message with positive, constructive, or solution-oriented key messages, employing a ratio of least three positive messages to each negative message

- Avoiding unnecessary, indefensible, or nonproductive uses of absolutes and of the words *no, not, never, nothing,* and *none*

Risk Communication and Trust

Risk messages are typically judged not only by their content but by the trustworthiness of the source of information: *who is telling me this, and can I trust them?* When the answer to the trust and credibility question is no, communications are likely to fail, no matter how well intentioned and well delivered.

Trust can only be built up over a number of years; its foundation is a consistent track record of listening, caring, competence, honesty, and accountability. Experts no longer command the levels of trust observed in the past. Reliance on scientific credentials alone to establish trust is unlikely to prove effective. Trust is easily lost; once lost it is difficult to regain. Trust is more likely to be strong when

- Organizations are clear about their goals, objectives, and values.
- There is openness and transparency around decisions.
- Decisions are clearly grounded in evidence.
- Public values and concerns are taken into account in making decisions.
- Sufficient information is provided to allow individuals to make balanced judgments.
- Mistakes are quickly acknowledged and acted upon.
- Actions speak louder than words (judgments about trust often depend more on what is done than on what is said).
- Outrage and the legitimacy of fear and emotion are acknowledged.

The most important factors involved in trust are perceived listening, caring, and compassion; honesty, openness, candidness, and transparency; expertise, competence, and wisdom; perseverance, dedication, and commitment; objectivity, fairness, goodwill, and consistency.

Principles of Effective Risk Communication

Public health officials and others who engage in risk communication may benefit from applying guidelines such as the ones that follow. Each guideline is accompanied by key examples of methods for achieving it.

Accept and Involve Stakeholders as Legitimate Partners

- Demonstrate respect for people affected by risk management decisions by involving them early, before important decisions are made.

- Address in the decision-making process the broad range of factors involved in determining public perceptions of risk, concern, and outrage.
- Involve all parties that have an interest or a stake in the risk in question.
- Use a variety of communication channels to engage and involve people.
- Adhere to the highest ethical standards; recognize that people hold you professionally and ethically accountable.
- Strive for win-win outcomes.

Listen to People

- Do not make assumptions about what people know, think, or want done about risks.
- Take the time before taking action to find out what people are thinking: use techniques such as interviews, facilitated discussion groups, information exchanges, availability sessions, advisory groups, toll-free numbers, and surveys.
- Let all parties that have an interest or a stake in the issue be heard.
- Let people know that what they said has been understood and what actions will follow.
- Identify with your audience, and try to put yourself in their place, to be empathetic.
- Acknowledge the validity of people's emotions.
- Emphasize communication channels that encourage listening, feedback, participation, and dialogue.
- Recognize that competing agendas, symbolic meanings, and broader social, cultural, economic, or political considerations often exist and complicate the task of risk communication.

Be Truthful, Honest, Frank, and Open

- If an answer is unknown or uncertain, express willingness to get back to the questioner with a response by an agreed-upon deadline.
- Disclose risk information as soon as possible (emphasizing appropriate reservations about reliability); fill information vacuums.
- Do not minimize or exaggerate the level of risk; do not overreassure.
- Make corrections quickly if errors are made.
- When in doubt, lean toward sharing more information, not less, or people may think something significant is being hidden or withheld.
- Discuss data and information uncertainties, strengths, and weaknesses, including ones identified by other credible sources.
- Identify worst-case estimates as such, and cite ranges of risk estimates when appropriate.
- Do not speculate, especially about worst cases.

Coordinate, Collaborate, and Partner with Other Credible Sources

- Take the time to coordinate all interorganizational and intraorganizational communications.
- Devote effort and resources to the slow, hard work of building bridges, partnerships, and alliances with other organizations.
- Use credible and authoritative intermediaries between you and your target audience.
- Consult with others to determine who is best able to take the lead in responding to questions or concerns about risks; establish and document agreements.
- Do not attack those with higher perceived credibility.
- Cite credible sources that believe what you believe; issue communications together with, or through, other trustworthy sources.

Meet the Needs of the Media

- Be accessible to reporters; respect their deadlines.
- Prepare a limited number of key messages in advance of media interactions; take control of the interview and repeat or bridge to your key messages several times.
- Provide information tailored to the needs of each type of media, such as sound bites and visuals for television.
- Provide background materials on complex risk issues.
- Say only those things that you are willing to have repeated by the media: everything you say is on the record.
- Keep interviews short; agree with the reporter in advance about the specific topic, and stick to this topic during the interview.
- Tell the truth.
- If you do not know the answer to a question, focus on what you do know, and tell the reporter what actions you will take to get an answer.
- Stay on message; bridge to important messages.
- Be aware of and respond effectively to media pitfalls and trap questions.
- Avoid saying, "no comment."
- Follow up on media reports with praise or criticism, as warranted.
- Work to establish long-term relationships of trust with specific editors and reporters.

Speak Clearly and with Compassion

- Use clear, nontechnical language appropriate to the target audience.
- Use graphics and other pictorial material to clarify messages.

- Avoid embarrassing people.
- Respect the unique communication needs of special and diverse audiences.
- Understand that trust is earned; do not ask or expect to be immediately trusted by the public.
- Express genuine empathy; acknowledge, and say, that any illness, injury or death is a tragedy and to be avoided.
- Personalize risk data; use stories, narratives, examples, and anecdotes that make technical data come alive.
- Avoid distant, abstract, unfeeling language about harm, deaths, injuries, and illnesses.
- Acknowledge and respond (in words, gestures, and actions) to emotions that people express, such as anxiety, fear, anger, outrage, and helplessness.
- Acknowledge and respond to the distinctions that the public views as important in evaluating risks.
- Use risk comparisons to put risks in perspective; avoid comparisons that ignore distinctions people consider important.
- Identify specific actions that people can take to protect themselves and to maintain control of the situation.
- Be sensitive to local norms, such as speech and dress.
- Strive for brevity, but respect people's desire for information, and offer to provide needed information within a specified period of time.
- Always try to include a discussion of actions that are under way or can be taken.
- Promise only that which can be delivered, then follow through.

Plan Thoroughly and Carefully

- Begin with clear, explicit objectives, such as providing information, establishing trust, encouraging appropriate actions, stimulating emergency response, or involving stakeholders in dialogue, partnerships, and joint problem solving.
- Identify important stakeholders and subgroups within the audience; respect diversity and design communications for specific stakeholders.
- Recruit spokespersons with effective presentation and personal interaction skills.
- Train staff, including technical staff, in basic, intermediate, and advanced risk and crisis communication skills; recognize and reward outstanding performance.
- Anticipate questions and issues.
- Prepare and pretest messages.
- Carefully evaluate risk communication efforts, and learn from mistakes.
- Share what you have learned with others.

Risk Communication and Message Mapping

One of the most important tools used by risk communicators is the *message map*. As illustrated in template form in Table 34.1, a message map is a matrix for displaying detailed, hierarchically organized responses to anticipated questions or concerns. It is a visual aid that provides at a glance the organization's messages for high-concern or controversial issues.

Developing and using message maps achieves several important risk communication goals:

- Identifying stakeholders early in the communication process
- Anticipating stakeholder questions and concerns before they are raised
- Organizing one's thinking, and developing prepared messages in response to anticipated stakeholder questions and concerns
- Developing key messages and supporting information within a clear, concise, transparent, and accessible framework

TABLE 34.1. TEMPLATE FOR RISK COMMUNICATION MESSAGE MAP.

Stakeholder: ____________________

Question or concern: ____________________

Key Message 1	**Key Message 2**	**Key Message 3**
Supporting Fact 1-1	**Supporting Fact 2-1**	**Supporting Fact 3-1**
Supporting Fact 1-2	**Supporting Fact 2-2**	**Supporting Fact 3-2**
Supporting Fact 1-3	**Supporting Fact 2-3**	**Supporting Fact 3-3**

Promoting open dialogue about messages both inside and outside the organization

Providing user-friendly guidance and direction to spokespersons

Ensuring that the organization has a central repository of *accurate, timely, consistent, and relevant* messages

Encouraging the organization to *speak with one voice*

The process used to generate message maps may be as important as the end product. Message-mapping exercises—involving teams of subject matter experts (for example, scientists), communication specialists, and individuals with policy, legal, and management expertise—often reveal a diversity of viewpoints within an organization for each major question, issue, or concern. Gaps in message maps often should be seen as early warnings of message incompleteness. As such, they represent opportunities for focused efforts by issue management teams. Message-mapping exercises may also suggest needed changes in strategies, policies, or performance.

Seven steps are involved in constructing a message map.

Identify Stakeholders

The first step is to identify stakeholders—interested, affected, or influential parties—for the selected issue of high concern. Stakeholders can be distinguished further by prioritizing them according to their potential to affect outcomes and their credibility with other stakeholders. For example, stakeholders in an environmental health crisis might include (in no particular order)

Victims

Victims' families

Other directly affected individuals

Emergency response personnel

Public health personnel (local, county, state, national)

Law enforcement personnel

Hospital personnel

Families of emergency response, law enforcement, and hospital personnel

Government agencies (all levels)

Politicians and legislators

Unions

The media (all types)

Legal professionals

Contractors

Consultants

Suppliers and vendors

Ethic and minority groups

Groups with special needs (for example, elderly, disabled, or homebound populations)

Health agency employees

Advisory panels

Nongovernmental organizations

Educators

Scientific community

Religious community

Business community (for example, tourism, food, and recreation services)

Professional societies

General public

Identify Stakeholder Concerns

The second step in message mapping is to identify a complete list of the specific concerns of each important stakeholder group. Stakeholder questions and concerns typically fall into three groupings:

Overarching questions: for example, What is the most important thing that the public should know about this issue?

Informational questions: for example, What is the budget allocated for your response?

Challenging questions or statements: for example, Why should we trust what you are telling us? How many more people have to die or suffer before you take appropriate action?

Lists of specific stakeholder concerns and questions are typically generated through empirical research, including

Analyzing media content (print, radio, television)

Analyzing Web-site material

Reviewing documents, including public meeting records, public hearing records, and legislative transcripts

Reviewing complaint logs, hotline logs, toll-free-number logs, and media logs

Conducting focused interviews with subject matter experts

Holding facilitated discussion sessions with individuals intimately familiar with the issue

Conducting focus groups

Conducting surveys

Nearly all concerns and questions that will be raised by any stakeholder in any controversy, conflict, crisis, or high-concern situation can be predicted by using these techniques.

Among the most important stakeholders are the media. Box 34.2 presents a list of seventy-seven questions commonly asked by journalists in a disaster. This list was produced by analyzing the questions posed by reporters at over 2,500 press conferences.

Box 34.2. Seventy-Seven Questions Commonly Asked by Journalists During a Crisis

In a crisis journalists are likely to ask six general types of questions (who, what, where, when, why, how) that relate to three broad topics: (1) what happened; (2) what caused it to happen; (3) what does it mean.

Specific questions likely to be asked at press conferences include the following:

1. What is your name and title?
2. What are your job responsibilities?
3. What are your qualifications?
4. Can you tell us what happened?
5. When did it happen?
6. Where did it happen?
7. Who was harmed?
8. How many people were harmed [or injured or killed]?
9. Are those that were harmed getting help?
10. How are those who were harmed getting help?
11. What can others do to help?
12. Is the situation under control?
13. Is there anything good that you can tell us?
14. Is there any immediate danger?

15. What is being done in response to what happened?
16. Who is in charge?
17. What can we expect next?
18. What are you advising people to do?
19. How long will it be before the situation returns to normal?
20. What help has been requested or offered from others?
21. What responses have you received?
22. Can you be specific about the types of harm that occurred?
23. What are the names of those that were harmed?
24. Can we talk to them?
25. How much damage occurred?
26. What other damage may have occurred?
27. How certain are you about damage?
28. How much damage do you expect?
29. What are you doing now?
30. Who else is involved in the response?
31. Why did this happen?
32. What was the cause?
33. Did you have any forewarning that this might happen?
34. Why wasn't this prevented from happening?
35. What else can go wrong?
36. If you are not sure of the cause, what is your best guess?
37. Who caused this to happen?
38. Who is to blame?
39. Could this have been avoided?
40. Do you think those involved handled the situation well enough?
41. When did your response to this begin?
42. When were you notified that something had happened?
43. Who is conducting the investigation?
44. What are you going to do after the investigation?
45. What have you found out so far?
46. Why was more not done to prevent this from happening?
47. What is your personal opinion?
48. What are you telling your own family?
49. Are all those involved in agreement?
50. Are people overreacting?
51. Which laws are applicable?
52. Has anyone broken the law?
53. What challenges are you facing?
54. Has anyone made mistakes?
55. What mistakes have been made?
56. Have you told us everything you know?
57. What are you not telling us?

58. What effects will this have on the people involved?
59. What precautionary measures were taken?
60. Do you accept responsibility for what happened?
61. Has this ever happened before?
62. Can this happen elsewhere?
63. What is the worst-case scenario?
64. What lessons were learned?
65. Were those lessons implemented?
66. What can be done to prevent this from happening again?
67. What would you like to say to those that have been harmed and to their families?
68. Is there any continuing danger?
69. Are people out of danger? Are people safe?
70. Will there be any inconvenience to employees or to the public?
71. How much will all this cost?
72. Are you able and willing to pay the costs?
73. Who else will pay the costs?
74. When will we find out more?
75. What steps need to be taken to avoid a similar event?
76. Have these steps already been taken? If not, why not?
77. What does this all mean? Is there anything else you want to tell us?

Analyze Stakeholder Concerns

The third step in message map construction is to analyze the lists of specific concerns to identify common sets of underlying general concerns. Case studies indicate that most high-concern issues are associated with no more than fifteen to twenty-five primary underlying general concerns. (Box 34.3 provides a sample list of general concerns.) As part of this step, it is often useful to create a matrix, or table, that matches stakeholders with their concerns or questions. The vertical axis of this table lists stakeholders (in priority order). The horizontal axis lists concerns or questions for each stakeholder. Those concerns or questions that appear in the largest number of cells should receive priority attention for message mapping.

Box 34.3. A Sampling of General Concerns

Health concerns

Safety concerns

Ecological or environmental concerns

Economic or financial concerns

Property value concerns
Quality-of-life concerns
Wildlife concerns
Pet or livestock concerns
Equity or fairness concerns
Cultural or symbolic concerns
Legal or regulatory concerns
Honesty, openness, transparency, or access to information concerns
Accountability concerns
Future generation concerns
Ethical concerns
Competency or expertise concerns
Listening, caring, or empathy concerns
Trust concerns

Develop Key Messages

The fourth step in message map construction is to develop key messages in response to each stakeholder question, concern, or perception (see Table 34.2). Message map development and construction by the message-mapping team should be guided by the theories and principles of risk communication discussed earlier in this chapter.

Key messages are typically developed through brainstorming sessions with a message-mapping team. As noted earlier, the message-mapping team typically consists of a subject matter expert, a communications specialist, members with expertise in policy, legal, and management perspectives, and a facilitator. The brainstorming session produces message narratives, usually in the form of complete sentences, that become key messages on the message map. Alternatively, the brainstorming session may produce key words for each message, and those key words are then entered on the message map. Key words serve as an aid to memory for those delivering the messages. Each key message should have one to three key words, but no more than three.

Key messages should address the information that the target audience

Most needs to know
Most wants to know

TABLE 34.2. SAMPLE RISK COMMUNICATION MESSAGE MAP.

Stakeholder: General public
Question: How contagious is smallpox?

Key Message 1	Key Message 2	Key Message 3
Smallpox spreads slowly compared to measles and flu.	This allows time to trace those who have come into contact.	Vaccination shortly after contact will generally prevent disease.
Supporting Fact 1-1	**Supporting Fact 2-1**	**Supporting Fact 3-1**
People are infectious only when the rash appears.	The incubation period for the disease is 10–14 days.	People who have never been vaccinated are the most important to vaccinate.
Supporting Fact 1-2	**Supporting Fact 2-2**	**Supporting Fact 3-2**
Smallpox infection requires hours of face-to-face contact.	Resources are available for tracing contacts.	Adults who were vaccinated as children may still have some immunity.
Supporting Fact 1-3	**Supporting Fact 2-3**	**Supporting Fact 3-3**
There are no carriers without symptoms.	Finding people who have been exposed and vaccinating them has proved successful.	Adequate vaccine is on hand.

The most important message map is the *core message map*, the map that contains and displays the organization's overarching messages on an issue. The core message map addresses

What the organization believes people should know about the issue or topic

What the organization wants people to know, regardless of the questions that are asked

What the content of the opening statement will be for a presentation or press conference on the issue or topic

It is critical that the core message be delivered to the intended audience. One technique for ensuring message delivery is *bridging*. An example of a bridging statement is, "I want to remind you again . . ." The core message map can also serve as a port in a storm, when questioning becomes aggressive, for example.

Develop Supporting Information for the Messages

The fifth step in message map construction is to develop supporting facts, information, or proofs for each key message. The same principles that guide key message construction should guide the development of supporting information. Proofs, especially when they are highly complex, do not necessarily need to be included in the body of the message map. Instead, they are often attached to the map as an appendix. In addition, proofs are often held in reserve to support a particular message if it is challenged.

Test the Messages

The sixth step in message map construction is to conduct systematic message testing, using standardized message-testing procedures. This step aims to ensure message consistency and coordination. Message testing should begin by asking subject matter experts not directly involved in the original message-mapping process to validate the accuracy of technical information contained in the message map. Message testing should then be done with

- Surrogates for internal and external target audiences
- Partner organizations

Plan Message Delivery

The seventh, and final, step is to plan for the delivery of the prepared message maps through

- A trained spokesperson
- Appropriate communication channels
- Trusted individuals or organizations

Once developed, message maps can be used to structure press conferences, media interviews, information forums and exchanges, public meetings, Web sites, telephone hotline scripts, and fact sheets or brochures focused on frequently asked questions.

Guidelines for Using Message Maps

- Translate all scripted messages into key words that can easily be accessed and recalled by spokespeople. (Most people have difficulty memorizing or delivering scripts; however, they can deliver agreed-upon key words, using their own words to form whole sentences.)
- Use one or all of the three key messages on the message map as a media sound bite.
- Repeat messages and bridge to the core message map, the map that contains the most important information to be conveyed, frequently during interviews.
- Present sound bite messages in fewer than nine seconds for television and fewer than twenty-seven words for the print media.
- When responding to specific questions from a reporter or a stakeholder about a key message, present the supporting information from the message map in fewer than nine seconds or twenty-seven words.
- If time allows, present the key messages and the supporting information contained in a message map to people by using the *triple T model:* (1) summarize what you are going to tell them (that is, the three key messages); (2) tell them more (that is, the supporting information); (3) summarize again what you told them (that is, repeat the three key messages).
- Stay on the prepared messages in the message map; avoid "winging it."
- Take advantage of opportunities to reemphasize or bridge again to key messages.
- Keep messages short and focused.
- Be honest; tell the truth.

In short, message maps are a viable tool for risk communicators. They ensure that risk information has an optimum chance of being heard, understood, and remembered. Just as important, they encourage agencies and organizations to develop a consistent set of messages and to speak with one voice.

Conclusion

The World Trade Center tragedy of September 11, 2001, the SARS outbreak in 2003, and other recent events have given public health professionals and organizations throughout the world a heightened recognition of the need to enhance their risk communication skills. These threats and the concomitant risks posed to human populations and the environment are a call for organizations to reassess their knowledge of the risk communication literature and to elevate their level of risk communication skill and risk preparedness.

Thought Questions

1. What are decision makers to do when public risk perceptions are at odds with expert opinion?
2. Given the need to be extremely concise and clear when communicating in high-risk situations, how can one avoid oversimplification?
3. Given the importance of expressing empathy and caring when communicating in high-risk situations, what are decision makers to do if they feel no empathy?
4. Are there conditions that justify lying or withholding risk information? What is the relationship between risk communication and ethics?
5. Is there an inherent conflict between the goals of risk communication and the goals of journalists? If so, can these conflicts be resolved?

References

National Research Council, Committee on Risk Perception and Communication. *Improving Risk Communication.* Washington, D.C.: National Academies Press, 1989.

For Further Information

Adams, J. *Risk.* London: University College London Press, 1995.

Bennett, P. G., and Calman, K. C. (eds.). *Risk Communication and Public Health: Policy, Science and Participation.* New York: Oxford University Press, 1999.

Chess, C., Hance, B. J., and Sandman, P. M. *Planning Dialogue with Communities: A Risk Communication Workbook.* New Brunswick, N.J.: Rutgers University, Cook College, Environmental Media Communication Research Program, 1989.

Covello, V. T. "Best Practice in Public Health Risk and Crisis Communication." *Journal of Health Communication,* 2003, *8,* 5–8.

Covello, V. T., McCallum, D. B., and Pavlova, M. T. *Effective Risk Communication: The Role and Responsibility of Governments and Nongovernmental Organizations.* New York: Plenum, 1989.

Covello, V. T., and Sandman, P. M. "Risk Communication: Evolution and Revolution." In A. Wolbarst (ed.), *Solutions to an Environment in Peril.* Baltimore, Md.: Johns Hopkins University Press, 2001.

Fischhoff, B. "Helping the Public Make Health Risk Decisions." In V. T. Covello, D. B. McCallum, and M. T. Pavlova (eds.), *Effective Risk Communication: The Role and Responsibility of Government and Nongovernmental Organizations.* New York: Plenum, 1989.

Fischhoff, B. "Risk Perception and Risk Communication Unplugged: Twenty Years of Process." *Risk Analysis,* 1995, *15*(2), 137–145.

Fischhoff, B., and others. "How Safe Is Safe Enough? A Psychometric Study of Attitudes Towards Technological Risks and Benefits." *Policy Sciences,* 1978, *9,* 127–152.

Hance, B. J., Chess, C., and Sandman, P. M. *Industry Risk Communication Manual.* Boca Raton, Fla.: CRC Press/Lewis, 1990.

Kahnemann, D., and Tversky, A. "Prospect Theory: An Analysis of Decision Under Risk." *Econometrica,* 1979, *47*(2), 263–291.

Krimsky, S., and Plough, A. "Environmental Hazards: Communicating Risks as a Social Process." Dover, Mass.: Auburn House, 1988.

Morgan, G., and Fischhoff, B. *Risk Communication: A Mental Models Approach.* New York: Cambridge University Press, 2001.

Morgan, G., and others. "Communicating Risk to the Public." *Environmental Science and Technology,* 1992, *26*(11), 2048–2056.

National Research Council. *Understanding Risk: Informing Decisions in a Democratic Society.* Washington, D.C.: National Academies Press, 1996.

Peters, R. G., Covello, V. T., and McCallum, D. B. "The Determinants of Trust and Credibility in Environmental Risk Communication: An Empirical Study." *Risk Analysis,* 1997, *17*(1), 43–54.

Powell, D., and Leiss, W. *Mad Cows and Mother's Milk: The Perils of Poor Risk Media Communication.* Montreal: McGill-Queen's University Press, 1997.

Renn, O., and others. "The Social Amplification of Risk: Theoretical Foundations and Empirical Applications." *Journal of Social Science Issues,* 1992, *48,* 137–160.

Royal Society. *Risk: Analysis, Perception, Management.* London: Royal Society, 1992.

Sandman, P. M. "Hazard Versus Outrage in the Public Perception of Risk." In V. T. Covello, D. B. McCallum, and M. T. Pavlova (eds.), *Effective Risk Communication: The Role and Responsibility of Government and Nongovernmental Organizations.* New York: Plenum, 1989.

Slovic, P., Krauss, N., and Covello, V. "What Should We Know About Making Risk Comparisons?" *Risk Analysis,* 1990, *10,* 389–392.

United Kingdom Interdepartmental Liaison Group on Risk Assessment (UK-ILGRA). *Risk Communication: A Guide to Regulatory Practice.* London: United Kingdom Interdepartmental Liaison Group on Risk Assessment, Health and Safety Executive, 1998.

Wildavsky, A., and Dake, K. "Theories of Risk Perception: Who Fears What and Why." *Daedalus,* 1990, *112,* 41–60.

Wildavsky, A., and Douglas, M. *Risk and Culture: An Essay on the Selection of Technological and Environmental Dangers.* Berkeley: University of California Press, 1983.

CHAPTER THIRTY-FIVE

HEALTH CARE SERVICES

Robert Laumbach
Howard M. Kipen

Although much of public health focuses on prevention, clinical care is an essential part of the story. In primary care, clinicians diagnose illnesses, administer treatments, and help their patients with recovery and restoration of function. They also offer routine preventive services such as immunizations, screening, and education. In environmental and occupational health, the clinical role is similar.

Diagnosing illnesses that relate to environmental exposures is an important clinical function, one that sometimes involves thorny questions: To what was the patient exposed? Did the exposure cause this case of illness? Treating environmentally related illnesses is often identical to treating the same illnesses when they result from other causes, although some environmental ailments, such as lead poisoning, have specialized treatments. Finally, the clinician's public health role is broad and varied in environmental and occupational health, involving collaboration with many other professionals to achieve primary, secondary, and tertiary prevention.

What is the *environment* for a clinician? Historically, the care of patients with potentially hazardous exposures arose in the workplace environment. Occupational medicine traces its roots to an Italian physician of the late Renaissance, Bernardino Ramazzini (1633–1714), who systematically observed the diseases of metalworkers, miners, painters, glassmakers, and others with work-related disorders. As the industrial revolution was beginning in England, Thomas Morson

Legge (1633–1714), the first "medical inspector of factories," investigated poisoning by such substances as lead and arsenic among various occupational groups. Alice Hamilton (1869–1970), the first occupational medicine clinician in the United States and a crusader for safer workplaces, studied lead poisoning among bathtub enamelers, mercury poisoning among hatters, "vibration dead finger" in jackhammer operators, and anemia in workers exposed to benzene. Occupational nursing arose at about the same time. In 1888, a nurse named Betty Moulder cared for Pennsylvania coal miners and their families—and launched a profession. Occupational health nursing expanded as industry grew in the late nineteenth and early twentieth centuries, and *factory nurses* tended to workers injured and made ill on the job. It is easy to understand why these pioneering clinicians, beginning with Ramazzini, focused on the workplace. It was an environment with especially concentrated and long-term exposures. Workers, like the proverbial canaries in the coal mine, demonstrated some of the most severe environmental health problems.

More recently, clinical attention has broadened from the workplace to the general environment. Clinicians play roles in diagnosing and treating lead poisoning in substandard housing, asthma in polluted cities, and pesticide poisoning in farm children. In the environmental arena, clinicians also play an invaluable role in preventive efforts, ranging from advocacy for protective health standards to patient education.

What illnesses (and injuries) do clinicians in environmental and occupational health diagnose and treat? The answer is broad and varied. Whereas some clinical specialties focus on a specific *organ system* (think of gastroenterology or dermatology) and others focus on a specific group of *patients* (think of pediatrics or geriatrics), this clinical specialty is defined by a set of *causes.* In this, environmental and occupational medicine and nursing are like the specialty of infectious diseases. Many different exposures are involved, and many different diseases can result, affecting all organ systems. Toxic exposures can affect the skin, causing dermatitis; they can be inhaled, affecting the airways or the lungs; they can circulate through the body, affecting the nervous system, the kidneys, or the liver. Physical exposures such as noise can impair hearing, and excessive radiation exposure can increase the risk of cancer. Repetitive motion can injure joints, and stressful environments can contribute to mental illness. The clinical concerns in environmental health are nearly unlimited.

One way to think about these diseases is shown in Table 35.1. Some environmental and occupational diseases are in effect trademarks; they are unique, easy to identify, and clearly related to exposures. For example, silicosis in a foundry worker who is exposed to silica dust is a classic occupational disease. Other diseases

TABLE 35.1. CATEGORIES OF ENVIRONMENTAL AND OCCUPATIONAL DISEASES.

Category	Features	Examples
Unique conditions clearly related to exposures	• A specific, characteristic clinical syndrome • Often a clear history of exposure to the offending agent • Often a biomarker of exposure	• Asbestosis or mesothelioma from asbestos • Silicosis from silica • Lead poisoning from lead • Pesticide poisoning from organophosphate pesticides
Well-recognized conditions that may be caused by many factors, both environmental and nonenvironmental	• An environmental case looks clinically like a nonenvironmental case • Causation difficult to prove in individual cases; diagnosis often probabilistic	• Lung cancer in an asbestos worker • Encephalopathy in a long-term solvent worker • Asthma in a resident of a moldy house
Poorly understood conditions that may involve environmental factors	• Often no objective signs or lab results • Often considerable media attention	• Multiple chemical sensitivity • Nonspecific building-related illness (sick building syndrome) • Gulf War syndrome

that may have an environmental or occupational cause are not unique; they can and do occur without environmental exposures. For example, a person living in a moldy house may develop asthma, but her friend or neighbor, living in a house with no excess mold, may also develop asthma. In these cases one of the clinician's principal challenges is to decide whether the environmental exposure contributed to the disease. Finally, still other diseases are less well understood, and a role for environmental exposures may be only suspected. For example, *multiple chemical sensitivity* is a poorly understood condition that cannot be confirmed by any findings on physical examination or laboratory tests. There is debate about what this condition is and about the role of chemical exposures in triggering it.

This chapter describes the importance of clinical practice in environmental health. It begins with diagnosis, moves next to treatment, and then discusses the many public health functions clinicians perform. It then turns to some of the fascinating ethical issues that arise in clinical practice in environmental health, introduces the professions that make up the field, and ends with mention of some emerging issues.

The Clinical Role in Environmental and Occupational Health

The environmental medicine clinician diagnoses, treats, and prevents medical conditions that arise from or are affected by the environment.

Diagnosis

To accomplish these tasks, the clinician must determine whether some environmental factor is causing or contributing to the health problems of an individual or population. This *causal connection* then allows specific treatment or prevention interventions, such as removal from or reduction in exposure. The diagnostic process may be divided into roughly three parts: assessing the patient's exposure, characterizing the patient's disease, and evaluating the causal link between exposure and disease.

Assessing Environmental Exposure. Assessing exposure to disease-causing agents is a cornerstone of environmental medicine. Environmental exposures are measured in many ways, as described in Chapter Four. The clinician needs not only to establish that an exposure has occurred but also to assess its magnitude. Not every encounter with a chemical, even a hazardous one, is sufficient to threaten a patient's health.

The starting point for this assessment is the *exposure history*—the patient's account of his or her exposures (Goldman and Peters, 1981; Becker, 1982; American Lung Association, 1983; Agency for Toxic Substances and Disease Registry, 1992). Clinicians who focus on environmental and occupational exposures are skilled in taking a detailed history and in assessing what exposures it reveals. For example, suppose a patient complains of headaches and confusion following exposure to organic solvents at work. The clinician would elicit a detailed description of the workplace, the patient's duties, the solvents used, the air-handling system, the use of personal protective equipment, the presence of symptoms in other patients, and changes in workplace procedures, among other factors (Box 35.1).

Box 35.1. Six Questions to Ask About Exposure

1. What is the agent?
2. When did the exposure occur?
3. How long did the exposure persist?
4. What is the relationship between the exposure over time and any observed or anticipated disease manifestations (for example, latency)?
5. What is the concentration or intensity of the exposure?
6. Is there any clinical evidence (symptoms or signs) to substantiate the exposure?

A second important source of exposure information is measurement of contaminants in the environment. To continue the previous example, the patient with solvent exposure might report that his or her employer has measured workplace air levels of certain solvents. Reviewing these records might confirm excessive exposures. However, the absence of high measured air levels does not rule out excessive exposure. Measurements might have been taken at times when exposures were low or at inappropriate locations in the workplace, or the patient's main exposure might be percutaneous rather than airborne. For these reasons, exposure data must be carefully interpreted in view of the patient's history.

Historical environmental test results can be used to estimate past, current, or future exposure. Estimation of past exposure is critical for assessing causation of existing disease or determining the risk of disease at a later time. When historical data are unavailable, contemporary testing may be used to estimate past exposure or the potential for exposure in the future. The environmental medicine clinician plays a valuable role in decisions about what to test for and when, where, and how to conduct the testing. First, the clinician can help to identify potential causative agents suggested by the clinical diagnosis, reducing the virtually limitless number of agents that might be tested for. Using the patient's work or environmental history, the clinician can also help to determine when and where representative exposures are likely to occur. Decisions about how to test include selecting an appropriate test method and determining how many tests to conduct. In making such decisions the clinician frequently collaborates with other professionals, such as industrial hygienists. When available, highly accurate methods, such as those validated by the U.S. Environmental Protection Agency (EPA) or the National Institute for Occupational Safety and Health (NIOSH), are used. The usefulness of environmental testing is often limited, however, because typically a relatively small number of samples is obtained. Environmental testing is costly, and rarely are sufficient samples available to provide statistically valid estimates of the mean and variability of exposure.

Exposure pathways are a useful conceptual framework for understanding the complexities of the movement of an agent from a source, through a medium, to a point of contact with an individual (see Chapter Four). *Exposure* may be defined as contact between a chemical, physical, or biological agent and the outer boundary of the human body. Contact with the human body may occur through any one of, or any combination of, three principal *routes of exposure:* inhalation, skin absorption, and ingestion. (In some circumstances other routes of exposure, such as eye contact or parenteral exposure, may be relevant.) In occupational and environmental medicine it is important not to overlook any of these routes of exposure in estimating actual or potential exposure. Ideally, exposure is quantified by measuring the concentration of the agent in the medium in contact with the body, usually averaged or integrated over time of contact. Thus, for example, the closer we can get to quantifying the concentration of a cancer-causing air contaminant in the air inside the lung at the site of interaction with lung tissue and during a particular time period, the better our estimate of exposure. In reality we might be lucky if the average concentration of the agent at an air-monitoring station miles away is what is known. Because it is rarely, if ever, feasible to measure personal exposure concentrations over extended periods of time, it is important to realize that what available measurements typically do is help us to estimate actual exposure. The concentration of an agent in a medium and the location of an individual may both vary greatly over space and time, making precise exposure assessment difficult at best. When possible, environmental health clinicians evaluating an exposure-disease relationship may visit the site of exposure to inform their interpretation of sampling or other data.

A third approach to exposure assessment—one that overcomes some of the limits of environmental testing—is to conduct clinical tests of exposure. By measuring the level of a contaminant at the place where it most matters, in the patient's tissues, these tests integrate all routes of entry and provide clinically meaningful information. Many biomarkers of exposure exist, including direct measurement of chemicals in body fluids (for example, heavy metals or organic chemicals such as dioxins and PCBs) and also indirect measures (for example, carboxyhemoglobin levels can indicate carbon monoxide exposure and blood cholinesterase can indicate organophosphate or carbamate exposure). Although these biomarkers of exposure are useful, they too have limitations. For example, some toxins are cleared rapidly—carboxyhemoglobin within hours of a carbon monoxide exposure, mercury within weeks or months of ingestion. Clinical testing must therefore be timed in accordance with the toxicology of the chemical and the history the patient provides.

The Dose-Response Relationship. The toxicological law of dose-response, that "the dose makes the poison," was introduced in Chapter Two. This law refers to the general fact that greater doses of a toxic agent cause greater responses (toxic effects). Although this is generally true, for agents that act through an immunological mechanism to cause an allergic response, the dose-response relationship may be less straightforward. Many people who are not prone to developing or able to develop an allergic reaction, for genetic or other reasons, will not respond adversely to the substance at any dose. However, those who are susceptible are more likely to become specifically reactive (sensitized) to the specific agent with increasing dose. After sensitization has occurred, severe reactions may occur with exposures that are much lower than the previous level required for sensitization.

Diagnosing Disease. A *disease* is a clear alteration of organ function; usually detectable by pathology or laboratory evaluation (except for psychiatric disorders). As noted earlier, a disease related to environmental exposures may not be notably distinct from a run-of-the-mill case of the same disease. The clinician identifies and differentiates specific diseases based on symptoms, signs, and laboratory data that have varying degrees of specificity. A specific diagnosis is usually necessary before the question of a possible environmental cause can be addressed. For example, *lung disease* is not specific enough, because the more specific diagnoses of asthma, emphysema, or lung cancer have different sets of causes. Tests that are commonly used in environmental medicine for making diagnoses are discussed later in this chapter.

Often patients present not with an apparent disease but with symptoms. Symptoms, defined as the patient's subjective experience of illness, are often due to disease but can also occur in the absence of objectively definable disease. For reliably establishing a diagnosis, symptoms are generally considered less satisfactory than signs (physical examination or laboratory findings). In general, the poorly understood conditions that may be environmental (the category forming the bottom row of Table 35.1) are defined by symptoms, with few if any characteristic signs or tests. However, even in this era of sophisticated medical testing protocols, it is estimated that 70 percent of significant patient problems can be identified, although not necessarily confirmed, through a thorough patient history.

Laboratory Tests Diagnosing Environmental Diseases. Common laboratory tests include routine blood chemistries, blood cell counts, microbiological and serological tests for infection, and imaging studies such as X-rays, CT scans, MRIs, or angiograms. These tests are used in one of three ways in the diagnostic process in environmental and occupational health. First, and most commonly, they are routinely used to characterize a disease process. For example, chest X-rays and pulmonary function tests are used to diagnose lung diseases and neurobehavioral tests are used to diagnose nervous system dysfunction. A second and also important use of laboratory tests is to estimate exposure to potentially toxic substances, as described earlier. Tests used for this purpose include measures of an agent in the body (for example, blood lead levels). It is critical to understand that such tests determine only exposure and not disease or health effect. A third, and less common, type of laboratory test is used to substantiate a specific exposure-effect relationship. *Challenge* tests are used to measure skin or respiratory sensitization, or to document physiological change in different environments (such as lung function tests conducted at a workplace suspected of aggravating asthma). This type of test is especially important when considering environmental causes of asthma and dermatitis. Other indicators of early biochemical or physiological effects include elevated serum proteins, which may signal subclinical lung injury; beta-2 microglobulin and other markers of renal tubular injury; and depressed leukocyte counts, which can follow benzene exposure.

Establishing Causation. For the clinician, causal reasoning is the means of establishing that environmental factors (work, chemical exposures, lifestyle, medications, and so forth) cause or contribute to disease. Clinicians can consult texts and other resources to see which, if any, exposures are known to cause a particular disease, a test sometimes referred to as general causation. Establishing *general causation* means determining that sufficient scientific evidence exists to support a conclusion that the disease can be caused by the exposure under consideration. The next step, establishing *specific causation,* refers to the determination that the exposure in question did cause the disease in a particular person. Specific causation is established by considering specific circumstances: results of an etiologic lab test, individual susceptibility information, dose, latency, temporal sequence, improvement with reduced exposure (or aggravation with challenge), and alternative or competing causes. When the circumstances are compelling or there is an outbreak but no documentation of a causal role for a specific agent, scientists may undertake clinical or epidemiological research to attempt to verify causation. Less formal research techniques may also be applied. For example, observation of changing patterns of exposure and disease over time in a single individual may be useful for establishing causation for conditions whose manifestations wax and wane, such as environmental asthma. Figure 35.1 shows some of these patterns.

Establishing General Causation: Reviewing the Literature. The amounts of toxicological and epidemiological data available for specific agents vary greatly. For many of the 60,000 specific chemical agents in commerce in the United States, no data on associations between exposure and disease are available. However, extensive literature is available for the relatively few substances for which serious hazards or potential hazards have been recognized. The amounts of data on physical and biological agents also vary widely. A number of peer-reviewed scientific journals publish studies that may provide useful data for establishing general causation. Scientific reviews and editorial opinions may provide overviews of the more important or controversial exposure-disease relationships. Other sources of information include governmental and nongovernmental agencies. Fortunately, modern information technology facilitates access to available information for environmental clinicians, specialists and nonspecialists alike.

In addition to scientific studies, clinicians also have access to case reports or case series in the medical literature. Case reports lack controls and thus are not as

FIGURE 35.1. DETERMINING CAUSATION.

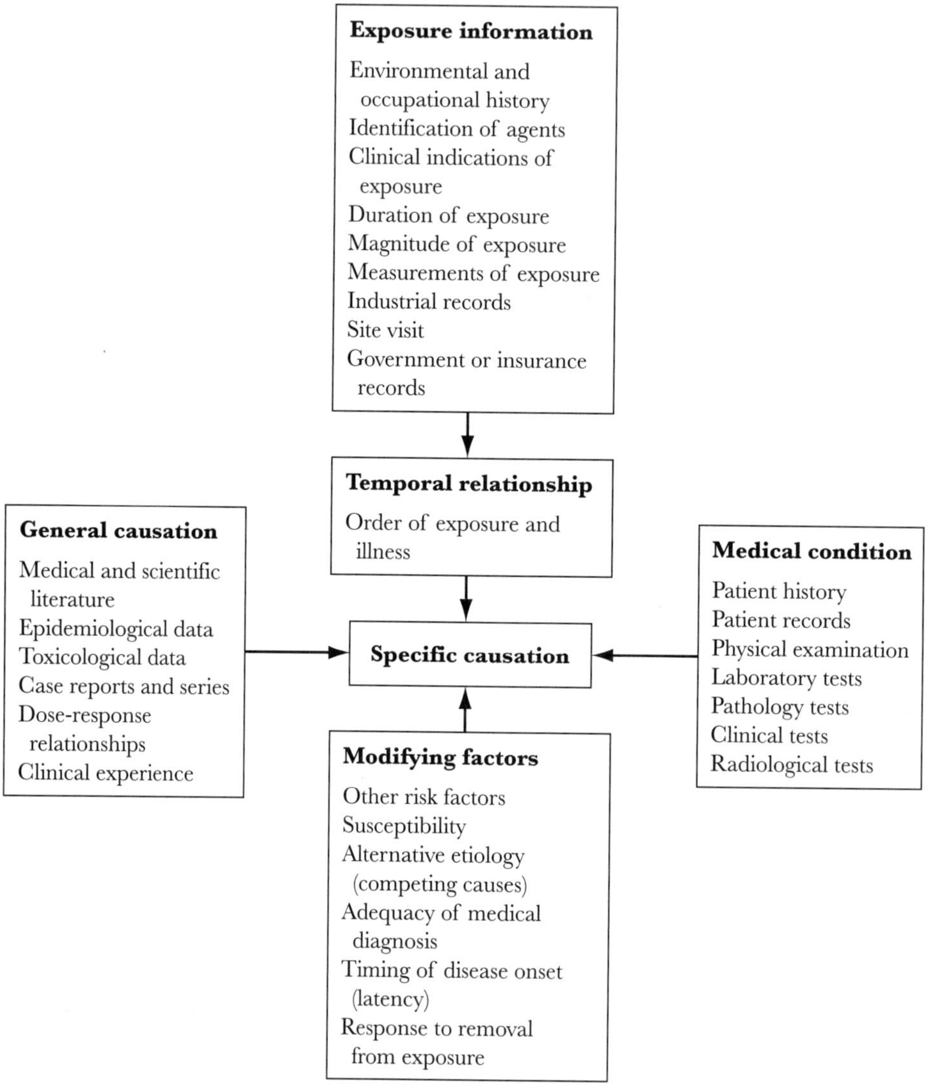

informative as controlled epidemiological studies. However, case reports are often all that is available on a particular subject, because they usually do not require substantial, if any, funding to accomplish, and the human exposure in question may be rare and difficult to study systematically. These reports can suggest relationships between exposure and disease that have not yet been established by epidemiological studies. For example, an apparent association between asbestos and lung cancer was first reported in a 1939 case report, although the first controlled epidemiological study on the association was not published until the 1950s. There are other instances in which epidemiological studies have confirmed associations first reported in case studies (for example, benzene-induced leukemia and vinyl chloride–induced liver angiosarcoma have been demonstrated), but there are also instances in which controlled studies have failed to confirm initial case reports (for example, Bendectin-induced miscarriage and a relationship between breast implants and autoimmune disease have not been demonstrated). Although causal attribution based on case studies must be regarded with caution, such studies may be carefully considered in light of other available information, including toxicological data.

Nine criteria advanced by A. B. Hill (1965) are now widely used to examine the strength of the epidemiological and toxicological literature linking an agent to a disease:

Hill's Considerations for Assessing Causality

1. Strength of association
2. Consistency of association
3. Specificity of association
4. Temporality of association
5. Biological gradient (dose response)
6. Plausibility of the association
7. Coherence of the association
8. Corroborating experimental evidence
9. Analogy to established associations

These are not truly criteria, as there is no specification of how many need to be satisfied or how well they need to be satisfied in order to consider an association to be causal. Nonetheless, they do provide a useful frame for considering general causation. Examining the literature with these criteria in mind helps the clinician establish or reject general causation.

Clinician Decision Making: The Probabilistic Basis of Diagnosis. Medical diagnosis is not an exact science. Clinicians make probabilistic judgments on a day-to-day basis, even when they have supplemented a patient's history and physical examination with the results of extensive laboratory tests. Laboratory, clinical, and physiological tests are important for defining any given disease but rarely provide perfect information.

Each diagnostic test has performance characteristics known as sensitivity and specificity. *Sensitivity* is the probability that when disease is present the test will correctly detect the disease. *Specificity* is the probability that when disease is absent the test will correctly give a negative result. These test characteristics assist diagnostic reasoning in a population of patients, but they cannot confirm or exclude disease in individual patients. For this, clinicians must consider the predictive value of a test—the probability that a test gets it right. *Positive predictive value* is the probability that a positive test result signals true disease, and *negative predictive value* is the probability that a negative test result signals true absence of disease. To calculate these values, information about the patient (and an imagined population of patients with similar risk factors) must be incorporated. For example, the positive predictive value of a symptom of chest pain for a heart attack is very low in a twenty-five-year-old because severe atherosclerosis is rare in this age group and other causes of chest pain (for example, musculoskeletal causes) are more common. Similarly, interstitial fibrosis on a chest X-ray, whatever its sensitivity and specificity as a true underlying finding of pathological fibrosis, has a much higher predictive value for a diagnosis of asbestosis in a member of the insulators union than in someone with no history of asbestos exposure. In the latter case the fibrosis is more likely to have an immunological, infectious, or other cause.

When sensitivity and specificity are known in general for a particular test, sign, or symptom and when the overall prevalence of the condition is known for the population group from which the patient comes, then one can estimate the predictive value of the test, sign, or symptom for that person for that condition. This is done according to a rule known as Bayes' theorem, which has been translated into nomograms (tables) for general use.

In practice, diagnostic reasoning is usually a complex process that is based on multiple symptoms, signs, and test results. Not all of these findings are statistically independent of one another, thus preventing straightforward addition of the probabilities, as in a Bayesian model. However, clinicians routinely make qualitative estimates, taking into account the predictive values of various diagnostic tests. Bayesian reasoning is one of the major tools used by clinicians to reach a diagnosis.

Other Diagnostic Considerations. The possibility of *multiple causes* for a clinical condition is a critical consideration. It is a commonly held misconception that the existence of causes other than exposure to the toxic agent in question excludes a role for that exposure. Although this is sometimes the case, in reality the converse can also be true. For example, epidemiological studies dealing with occupational asbestos exposure and cigarette smoking indicate that together they have a synergistic effect on lung cancer risk. In other words, these two toxic agents have been found to interact in a multiplicative manner, so that their combined effects are much greater than the sum of the effects each one has on its own.

Differences in individual susceptibility or vulnerability may explain why one person gets sick from an environmental exposure that has no effect on another person. True individual *susceptibility* is based on genetic differences in such areas as immunological reactivity, enzyme metabolism, and gender. A number of other acquired factors, such as age, body mass, interacting simultaneous exposures, and preexisting disease, may contribute to an individual's *vulnerability* to a harmful environmental agent. The fact that individual genetic factors affect disease is generally recognized (and discussed in Chapter Six). However, established links between specific genes and disease are relatively few at this time. Links between genes and susceptibility to diseases caused by environmental exposures are fewer still. Information on gene-environment-disease relationships is not yet used on a routine clinical basis in environmental medicine, although it is an active area of research.

The Legal Context for Determining Causation. Determining causation is important not only in public health preventive efforts but also in the legal setting. In U.S. civil courts, a person who claims to have been harmed by an environmental exposures must generally prove the claim to a reasonable degree of (medical) certainty, often translated as at least a 51 percent probability (or "more likely than not"). (A much higher standard, beyond a reasonable doubt (95 percent probability), is applied in criminal cases.) Epidemiological evidence is probabilistic rather than deterministic, and this is often difficult to translate into situations that demand yes or no answers and preventive actions. The clinician is often faced with the challenge of testifying about causation, a process discussed further in Chapter Thirty-Six.

In almost all instances, integration of all the factors we have been discussing into an opinion on causality cannot be reduced to mathematical formulae. There are inevitable gaps in information, including lack of knowledge about individual characteristics such as susceptibility and vulnerability. Thus clinical judgment is critical to opinions on diagnosis and specific causation for the individual patient, regardless of the strength or weakness of the scientific population basis for general causation.

Treatment

The cornerstone of treatment, as well as prevention, in environmental medicine is removal of the patient from exposure to an agent or situation that is causing or aggravating disease. When it comes to treating environmental or occupational ailments, ranging from asthma from isocyanates to cognitive dysfunction from solvents to carpal tunnel syndrome from improper tool use, most treatments are identical to those used for similar conditions without environmental causes. However, the environmental medicine clinician does have special expertise for a few treatments. These include chelation therapy for lead or other heavy metal intoxication and methods of reducing exposure through the use of engineering controls, administrative controls, and personal protective equipment. Environmental and occupational medicine (EOM) clinicians are frequently expert in primary prevention techniques such as the use of skin barrier creams, gloves, and respirators. EOM clinicians also often have specialized skills in the administrative aspects of treatment and recovery. Examples include assessing impairment and disability, defining restrictions for safely returning people to work or other exposure after an illness or injury, and prescribing rehabilitation appropriate to the demands of a given job. The Americans with Disabilities Act requires employers to make reasonable workplace accommodations for certain types of disabilities, often requiring expert guidance from EOM clinicians.

The Clinician's Public Health Function

In addition to traditional clinical roles of diagnosis and treatment, EOM clinicians play several important public health roles. First, they must always be alert for new conditions and particularly alert for new causes of recognized conditions. This requires a high index of suspicion, familiarity with the medical literature, and an orientation toward contributing new knowledge. Second, many clinicians conduct formal surveillance of different population groups, looking for indicators of exposure or disease. Surveillance is often targeted to populations known to have some potential for exposure to a toxic agent, and the surveillance aims to verify that the exposure is not causing a detectable increase in disease. States or other entities may conduct surveillance for time-space clusters of disease (most often cancer); finding a cluster prompts evaluation looking for an environmental or other cause. A related public health function is reporting. Many diseases with an environmental (occupational) etiology, for example, metal poisonings and occupational lung diseases, are reportable to state or other authorities.

An important public health function is health education, and this responsibility is shared by EOM clinicians. Because the nuances of environmental disease causation are often not common knowledge, many environmental clinicians educate both their colleagues and their patients. Many serve in advisory roles for voluntary organizations such as local affiliates of the American Lung Association or on government boards and commissions that address environmental health issues. In these roles, clinicians make their expertise available to authorities responsible for public health decision making. Collaboration and coordination with state, local, and federal health officials are key functions of EOM clinicians in their roles as sentinels for and investigators of apparent disease outbreaks. Finally, clinicians collaborate with other professionals, such as industrial hygienists, to effect primary prevention—a core public health function.

The case study in Box 35.2 sums up key parts of the discussion so far.

Box 35.2. Case Study: A Twelve-Year-Old Boy with Cough and Wheezing

A twelve-year-old boy visits his primary care clinician for intermittent wheezing, breathlessness, and nighttime cough, symptoms present for several months. The child also has a runny nose that is being treated with an over-the-counter allergy medication. The mother has asthma and the father smokes cigarettes. Heavy diesel truck traffic from a nearby cement factory passes in front of their home in an inner-city neighborhood. The mother is concerned because several children in the neighborhood take medication for breathing problems.

The physical exam reveals wheezing throughout the lung fields. Peak expiratory flow rate is 300 liters per minute, compared to predicted normal of 400 ($\pm$20 percent), indicating mild airway obstruction.

Differential Diagnosis

The environmental clinician's first objective is to establish the diagnosis. A useful pathophysiological classification for wheezing in children is allergic versus nonallergic. Allergic wheezing, which usually occurs in children who have other allergies, such as allergic rhinitis or allergic skin rashes, suggests asthma. Nonallergic wheezing can accompany a respiratory infection and is more likely to occur in children with cystic fibrosis, bronchopulmonary dysplasia, and some congenital conditions. The differential diagnosis for wheezing in a child also includes gastroesophageal reflux disease, foreign body obstruction, vocal cord dysfunction, structural abnormalities of the trachea, and tumor.

Further Testing

Asthma, the leading diagnosis in this case, is a chronic inflammatory disorder characterized by variable obstruction of the airways, with symptoms that include wheezing, breathlessness, chest tightness, and coughing. Asthma can be confirmed by additional testing that demonstrates its specific pathophysiology. In this case, pulmonary function tests performed a few days after the initial office visit verify reversible airway obstruction.

Skin-prick testing, performed by an allergist, demonstrates skin flare reactions to dust mites, tree pollens, grass pollens, and cat dander. These results indicate an allergic basis for the child's asthma but should be correlated with the clinical history to determine whether he is currently exposed to these allergens.

Exposure History

Asthma can be triggered by exposure to specific allergens or to nonimmunological agents such as smoke, dust, diesel fumes, other chemical irritants, cold air, or exercise. The causal relationship between these environmental triggers and asthma exacerbation can often be established by the patient's history of exposure followed by rapid onset of symptoms. Establishing a causal connection between exposure and onset of asthma as a chronic disease state, in contrast to exacerbation of preexisting asthma, is far more challenging, due to the potential latency between exposure and disease. The number of environmental agents that cause asthma exacerbation in children is far larger than the number of agents identified as causes of new onset asthma. When one or both parents have asthma or atopy, these conditions are much more likely to occur in the child, indicating a strong genetic basis for asthma, although specific genes are yet to be identified.

Environmental tobacco smoke and specific allergens, such as dust mite and cockroach antigens, are among the few well-established environmental risk factors for developing asthma. This child's history reveals no pets or insects in the house, but the child's father smokes tobacco in the home, and there is wall-to-wall carpeting, which may contribute to increased dust mite allergens.

Increased outdoor air pollutants, such as ozone, sulfur and nitrogen oxides, and particulate matter, have been associated with increased asthma morbidity. Studies have shown that children living near high-traffic roadways have higher rates of wheezing and asthma. Experimental evidence suggests that diesel exhaust particles may augment allergic responses, but the role of diesel exhaust in asthma causation or exacerbation is yet to be clearly defined.

Treatment and Prevention

Medical treatment and management of asthma is beyond the scope of this case study, which focuses on the unique role of the environmental clinician in preventing or reducing exposure to environmental factors that may cause or exacerbate asthma. Steps that this child and his family can take to reduce exposure to allergens and pollutants include

- Not allowing smoking in the house or family cars
- Reducing house dust mites by modifying the home environment
- Limiting outdoor activities during smog alerts to times when ozone levels are lowest (mornings)
- Limiting outdoor activities when tree and grass pollen counts are highest

Reducing cigarette smoking and allergen exposure in the home may not only act as secondary prevention, preventing exacerbation of the child's asthma, but may also promote primary prevention of asthma in his siblings.

Actions to prevent exposures to relevant agents need not be limited to modifying the home environment or staying indoors when outdoor pollutant or allergen levels are high. In this case the mother, with the clinician's assistance, became actively involved with a community group concerned about poor air quality and increased asthma in the neighborhood. As a result of their work with local public health officials, politicians, community leaders, and the management of the cement factory, the diesel trucks were routed away from residential neighborhoods.

Ethical Issues in Environmental and Occupational Medicine and Nursing

Because employers and those potentially responsible for exposures pay for much of the research, clinical evaluation, and patient care related to environmental medicine, real or perceived ethical conflicts are not uncommon in this field. The party responsible for an exposure is potentially being asked to pay for care or damages, or both, and this produces a set of issues different from the issues elsewhere in medicine. The costs of preventing and treating environmental disease in exposed populations can be very large. Great injustices have occurred since the industrial revolution and continue to occur because entities with influence over clinicians and over their causal determinations also have a significant financial or political stake in the outcome of those determinations, sometimes leading to biased decision making. This recently occurred in the town of Libby, Montana, in a case of environmental asbestos exposure to workers, where scandalous disregard for open and honest sharing of information and respect for the public's health was displayed. At the same time, some claims of environmentally induced illness, such as claims of nervous system effects from allegedly toxic mold or of systemic effects from leaking breast implants, are not yet substantiated by convincing causal associations in the medical literature or in the eyes of the courts, even though such effects have long been widely alleged and (perhaps prematurely) accepted by society.

Straightforward codes of ethical conduct for EOM clinicians have been promulgated by a number of organizations, including the American College of Occupational and Environmental Medicine (ACOEM), American Association of Occupational Health Nurses (AAOHN), Association of Occupational and Environmental Clinics (AOEC), and the International Commission on Occupational Health (ICOH). These codes address such themes as confidentiality of medical information (especially diagnoses, as opposed to work capacity) except when required by law or in legal proceedings, the right of the individual to complete knowledge about his or her medical findings, and the right of the individual to know about contractual relationships of practitioners so that he or she can assess potential biases and conflicts. These codes are discussed further in Chapter Seven.

Environmental Medicine Clinicians and Practice Venues

In some sense all clinicians are environmental clinicians because patients frequently relate information or ask questions about the relationship of their environment to their clinical state. However, only a minority of clinicians are actually trained in the disciplines of environmental medicine. Relatively few clinicians have a working knowledge of the disciplines that take a population approach to environmental health, such as toxicology, epidemiology, and environmental hygiene.

Nurses with special training in environmental and occupational health (EOH) nursing may become members of the AAOHN and gain certification for their added competencies. Many work in the occupational setting, although federal, state, and local health authorities also employ many EOH nurses, along with nurses specializing in infectious disease and in general prevention.

Mental health professionals, especially neuropsychologists, sometimes specialize in problems related to toxic exposures. This specialization assists them in accurately determining whether observed effects are consistent with toxicity. Specialists in rehabilitation are often asked to participate in treatment of those recovering from toxic exposures, and they may need to deal not only with physical limitations but also with concerns related to potential future exposures to lower levels of a given agent.

In the United States and many other countries, following medical school and at least one year of general clinical training, a physician can continue training in a two-year residency in preventive medicine with a concentration in occupational medicine. Although this leads to an American Board of Preventive Medicine (ABPM) exam in occupational medicine, a majority of the residency programs in the United States have added the words and the focus of "Environmental Medicine" to this accredited residency training.

Many who choose occupational medicine residency training have prior training in a primary care specialty or experience in the military, which has a long record of emphasis on environmental and occupational exposures. Unfortunately, as stated earlier, most community practitioners, even those who are very sophisticated, are not well versed in EOM. For various social and historical reasons, occupational medicine is better integrated with other medical specialties in many European and Asian countries than it is in the United States, although outside of workplace clinicians, a relative dearth of clinical expertise in environmental conditions still prevails around the world. (The American Board of Environmental Medicine, created in the 1990s, follows the alternative practices of the physician group formerly known as Clinical Ecologists. This board is not one of the member boards of the American Board of Medical Specialties—as the ABPM is, for example—and has no accredited training programs listed in the Graduate Medical Education Directory published by the American Medical Association.)

Specialists in environmental and occupational medicine work in a variety of settings. A decreasing number are employees of large corporations, responsible for the health and safety of workers at either a clinical or an administrative level. Some are employed in clinics run by national, state or provincial, municipal, or labor organizations. Others work for private entities that contract their medical services to private businesses. Those employed in all these settings tend to practice in the occupational medicine sphere and may not even be available to address questions arising from the general environment.

Individuals who practice with a focus on environmental health tend to work either for government entities or in academic settings. Often they were originally trained in occupational health. In the United States, the Centers for Disease Control and Prevention (now including the Agency for Toxic Substances and Disease Registry) has a relatively large number of clinicians who are trained in the scientific principles of public and environmental health, and most of the fifty states also have some capacity here. International organizations, such as the World Health Organization, are also developing environmental health capabilities. Academic faculties are often engaged in research but also address issues of environmental disease in individuals or outbreaks. In the United States the Environmental Protection Agency is often the agency that takes the lead in characterizing an environmental problem, but it consults with clinicians for the Public Health Service or nongovernmental entities in addressing clinical questions.

Employers or workers' compensation carriers cover diagnosis and treatment of environmental diseases that arise out of work, but there is no standard source of funding outside the workplace setting. Most health insurance systems in the United States do not pay for preventive care in this area. Unless the patient already has a disease, insurance generally does not provide financial compensation for a clinical provider addressing the possibility of environmental disease. For example, medical insurance will not pay for a clinician site visit or for the lab costs of environmental testing of a home or a water supply, or for any indicated remediation work. Medical insurance may pay for biological monitoring, such as a blood lead level, if there is accompanying illness.

As suggested throughout this chapter, beyond the individuals and families who are concerned or directly affected by a diagnosis of an environmental etiology for a condition, there are likely to be other individuals and entities with their own concerns. When lead paint or mold in a rented house is causing health effects, then someone other than the sick person or his or her health insurer may be asked to remedy the situation or even to pay damages. In the United States this frequently leads to an adversarial legal proceeding. Clinicians should be aware of this and be reassured that they are rarely the targets of these court proceedings (as distinguished from malpractice proceedings) but should also understand that the legal system sometimes demands more specification of the documentation behind a clinical opinion than one provides in a typical office or even consultation note. Open discussions with the representatives of the legal system before agreeing to provide an opinion can often help clinicians avoid subsequent confusion.

Challenges to Our Understanding

There are many influences on symptoms (emotional state, perceptions, level of available information, group processes) that do not necessarily correspond completely with disease state or exposure (Kipen and Fiedler, 2002). An illness is how a person experiences a disease, both medically (with symptoms such as pain or fatigue) and behaviorally (with behaviors such as withdrawal, sadness, or loss of interest in life). It is clear that illness outbreaks that are generally not recognized to be specific diseases, such as illness in Gulf War veterans, nevertheless produce a symptomatic illness burden on those afflicted, even though the pathology is not documented. Again, psychological factors can play a huge role in the presentation of illness related to environmental causes, whether or not there is an underlying identifiable disease. It is less clear that psychological stress can induce disease, although in the case of heart disease, there is substantial evidence in support of this association.

As this discussion of symptoms and illness versus disease implies, there are many determinants of the health perceptions and symptoms of both individuals and populations (Kipen and Fiedler, 2002). Although presence or absence of disease is the major clinical focus, stressful circumstances are well known to influence the perceptions of illness. An expanding literature also suggests that stress, or psychological factors, can worsen the objective markers of diseases such as asthma (Lehrer and others, 2002) or heart disease. In the extreme case of post-traumatic stress disorder (PTSD), life-threatening stress is felt to cause an anxiety syndrome manifested by both symptoms and neuroendocrine physiological variation. Anxiety and the related concept of hyperventilation have also been suggested to play a role in the symptoms of some individuals with perceived hypersensitivities to chemicals (Tarlo and others, 2002).

Recognition of novel conditions and causes is still ongoing. Historically, some established occupational toxic agents were only slowly recognized to represent hazards in the larger environment. This was true of asbestos, for example, where time after time the impact of relatively low doses (descending from factories to construction sites to bystander workers and to take-home exposures) was not predicted, or was even actively denied, until cases could be counted. Some of the particular toxicity of asbestos at nonoccupational concentrations relates to its environmental persistence, but this is also true of lead paint dust and radon. We must not be overly constrained by existing knowledge and must be aware that we do not know everything there will be to know about toxicology dose-response relationships.

In a similar vein, despite our knowledge about the impact of single toxic agents, we are substantially ignorant about the impact of mixtures of these agents on human health. Our present toxicology paradigms are especially inadequate for assessing risks of mixtures. Thus, without casting aside what we do know or speculating wildly, it makes sense to leave open the possibility of new or greater effects from mixtures of agents.

Sometimes environmental outbreaks are recognized as clusters (in space or time, or both) of a new or a common illness. However, in the case of the routinely monitored diseases (cancer and birth defects), examples of an etiologic association being found outside a workplace are uncommon. Sometimes outbreaks are recognized through a massive or obvious exposure, as happened with diarrheal disease from cryptosporidium in the water supply in Milwaukee in 1993, although even then it was a run on antidiarrheal agents from pharmacies that indirectly alerted public health authorities. Environmental outbreaks of disease are often somewhat singular. Although close examination reveals shared features among, for example, an outbreak of unexplained symptoms at a high school (Jones and others, 2000; Wessely, 2000), grain dust inducing asthma in Barcelona (Anto and others, 1993), and respiratory problems in responders to the 2001 World Trade Center attacks, all also have unique aspects in the exposure or in the clinical state. Thus the astute environmental medicine clinician will strive to balance a respect for what is well known with an appreciation for new possibilities not precisely described in available texts. When a patient's history, physical findings, and test results do not conform to recognized patterns of disease presentation, it is often instructive to consult one's colleagues, not only in medicine and nursing, but also in the public health sciences.

Thought Questions:

1. Discuss the various relationships that a given disease can have to an exposure, and how they integrate with concepts of causation.
2. Discuss the determinants and manifestations of exposure to a chemical agent in the water supply in regard to disease causation.

3. Discuss the differences and overlaps between symptoms, illness, and disease.
4. Discuss general versus specific causation, and describe how these types of causation might apply to a diagnosis of lung cancer in a pesticide applicator.
5. Describe how treatment in an environmental medicine setting is often related to public health resources and personnel.

References

Agency for Toxic Substances and Disease Registry. *Case Studies in Environmental Medicine: Taking an Environmental History.* Washington, D.C.: Agency for Toxic Substances and Disease Registry, 1992.

American Lung Association, Occupational and Environmental Health Committee. "Taking the Occupational History." *Annals of Internal Medicine,* 1983, *99,* 641–651.

Anto, J. M., and others. "Preventing Asthma Epidemics Due to Soybeans by Dust-Control Measures." *New England Journal of Medicine,* 1993, *329,* 1760–1763.

Becker, C. E. "Key Elements of the Occupational History for the General Physician." *Western Journal of Medicine,* 1982, *137,* 581–582.

Goldman, R., and Peters, J. M. "The Occupational and Environmental Health History." *Journal of the American Medical Association,* 1981, *246,* 2831–2836.

Hill, A. B. "The Environment and Disease: Association or Causation?" *Proceedings of the Royal Society of Medicine,* 1965, *58,* 295–300.

Jones, T., and others. "Mass Psychogenic Illness Attributed to Toxic Exposure at a High School." *New England Journal of Medicine,* 2000, *342,* 96–100.

Kipen, H. M., and Fiedler, N. "Environmental Factors in Medically Unexplained Symptoms and Related Syndromes: The Evidence and Challenge." *Environmental Health Perspectives,* 2002, *110*(suppl. 4), 597–600.

Lehrer, P., and others. "Psychological Aspects of Asthma." *Journal of Consulting and Clinical Psychology,* 2002, *70*(3), 691–711.

Tarlo, S., and others. "Responses to Panic Induction Procedures in Patients with Multiple Chemical Sensitivity/Idiopathic Environmental Intolerance: Understanding the Relationship with Panic Disorder." *Environmental Health Perspectives,* 2002, *100*(suppl. 4), 669–673.

Wessely, S. "Responding to Mass Psychogenic Illness." *New England Journal of Medicine,* 2000, *342,* 129–130.

For Further Information

Established in 1987, the Association of Occupational and Environmental Clinics, a nonprofit organization, is committed to improving the practice of occupational and environmental health through information sharing and collaborative research. The AOEC's Web site contains a directory of clinics in North America as well as excellent downloadable educational materials, including PowerPoint lectures:

Association of Occupational and Environmental Clinics. Homepage. [http://www.aoec.org]. 2005.

The Agency for Toxic Substances and Disease Registry (ATSDR) is a branch of the CDC, within the Center for Environmental Health. It has created a series of thirty-eight educational case studies on chemical-specific topics (such as benzene), on disease topics (such as environmental triggers of asthma), and on more general topics (such as disease clusters and taking an environmental history). ATSDR also provides online access to its toxicological profiles, offering detailed information on the toxicity of specific agents; see

Agency for Toxic Substances and Disease Registry. "Case Studies in Environmental Medicine." [http://www.atsdr.cdc.gov/HEC/CSEM]. 2004.
Agency for Toxic Substances and Disease Registry. "Toxicological Profile Information Sheet." [http://www.atsdr.cdc.gov/toxpro2.html#-A]. 2005.

The American College of Occupational and Environmental Medicine (ACOEM) is the largest membership organization for occupational and environmental physicians in North America. Among its useful clinical resources are a code of ethics as well as the Web site for the *Journal of Occupational and Environmental Medicine;* see

American College of Occupational and Environmental Medicine. "About ACOEM." [http://www.acoem.org/general]. 2005.

CHAPTER THIRTY-SIX

LEGAL REMEDIES

Douglas A. Henderson

In 1998, while filling your car with gasoline, you notice a warning on the pump that gasoline vapors have been "shown to cause cancer in laboratory animals." Three years later you are diagnosed with fatal lung cancer. Can you sue the gas station for your medical expenses, pain, suffering, and likely death? Or is it medically—and legally—unreasonable to think that you developed cancer by simply filling your car with gasoline? And what if you don't have cancer? Can you still sue just for inhaling vapors? Can you sue for *cancerphobia,* the fear of getting cancer? Now, suppose the truck delivering gasoline to the station crashes near your home, spilling 5,000 gallons of gasoline on your front lawn. Can you force the trucking company to clean up the spill? Or is that the responsibility of the U.S. Environmental Protection Agency? And to what extent can you recover the decrease in the value of your property caused by the spill?

All of these questions address the legal remedies available to exposed individuals and property owners. *Remedies* are the requirements and procedures to repair injury, collect and distribute compensation, and deter wrongs. As a subject of inquiry, remedies appear disordered and confusing. They reflect a patchwork of laws: cases decided during the industrial revolution, confusing statutes enacted by Congress and state legislatures, both slanted and sincere judicial interpretations, and bewildering regulations promulgated by multiple regulatory agencies. From another perspective, remedies are what happens when prevention—the main focus of environmental and public health—fails and an exposure occurs that results in some damage to human health and the environment.

Unfortunately, for even the simplest of environmental exposures, it is difficult to know which laws apply, how they apply, when they apply, and where they apply. A sixty-five-year-old retired coal miner suffering from pneumoconiosis (black lung disease) is presumptively entitled to compensation and his family to death benefits, if warranted, under the Black Lung Benefits Act. But a sixty-five-year-old retired ship worker suffering from mesothelioma has no such remedy available under any law, even though his mesothelioma undisputedly resulted from his employment. Unlike the coal miner the ship worker must hire a lawyer, file a lawsuit, and spend years fighting for information about his asbestos exposure—only then just to have the chance to present his case to a jury, assuming of course the defendant has not filed for bankruptcy.

The same confusion arises in property exposure cases. A leak of perchloroethylene (PERC) from an underground storage tank is regulated under the Resource Conservation and Recovery Act (RCRA), the federal hazardous waste law, but a spill of polychlorinated biphenyls (PCBs) from an aboveground electrical transformer is regulated by the Toxic Substances Control Act (TSCA). To recover cleanup costs for the PERC spill, a property owner might file a *cost recovery* lawsuit, not under RCRA but under another law, the Comprehensive Environmental Response, Compensation, and Liability Act (CERCLA). As enacted by Congress, RCRA cannot be used to recover cleanup *costs;* it permits an individual only to seek an *injunction* in a federal court to force compliance with the applicable regulatory requirements. And adding to the legal confusion, CERCLA does not provide the actual cleanup standard for the PCB spill, because that is set by the TSCA, which controls the cleanup of certain substances, namely, PCBs and asbestos.

The legal system in the United States, as in many nations, offers two general approaches to remedies. First, a citizen can demand that another citizen or firm compensate him for his losses. This is known as the *tort system,* and claimants generally have to go to great lengths to prove their tort claims have merit. Second, if a group of victims is considered deserving, society can set up mechanisms to compensate them more or less automatically, relieving them of some of the burdens of proving their case and delivering more rapid relief.

Both of these general approaches to remedies are covered in this chapter. The focus here is not prevention but exposure—what remedies, if any, does the legal system offer to those exposed or about to be exposed? These remedies, it turns out, differ considerably for personal injury and property damage, both of which are addressed in separate sections. Following this, the chapter turns to the reasons why the tort system, with the concept of fault as its foundation and with transactional costs eating up much of the compensation, continues to survive over various *no-fault* alternatives that distribute compensation largely without blame and for far lower costs. Not covered in this chapter are two related issues—the legal rights and remedies available to federal, state, and local governments to remedy harms, and the laws and regulations designed to *prevent* environmental exposures. Rather, the goal here is to consider why Congress and the states provide guaranteed compensation to certain individuals with certain environmental diseases but leave other individuals with diseases that are just as deadly to battle their way through an expensive and arbitrary legal process.

Remedies for Environmental and Toxic Exposures

Environmental exposures prompt thousands of lawsuits every year in the United States. At issue in these lawsuits is a range of both toxic and nontoxic chemicals, substances, and conditions. They involve natural substances such as asbestos, lead, arsenic, chromium, manganese, and silica; they involve synthetic substances such as paint thinners, pesticides, dry-cleaning solvents, and nail polish remover. The lawsuits also involve exposures to drugs such as Rezulin, Propulsid, Prozac, and Baycol and to "defective" medical devices such as breast implants, hair transplants, and tooth fillings. The exposures in these lawsuits derive from everyday occurrences, from talking on a cell phone, inhaling urban air, and smelling carpet emissions to eradicating cockroaches, drinking water, eating hamburgers, and wearing latex gloves.

But exposure lawsuits are not just about chemicals. In Eastern Pennsylvania, one hepatitis-infected carton of lettuce at one Chi-Chi's restaurant killed several individuals, sickened thousands, generated concern in restaurants throughout the world—and prompted more than 800 lawsuits. Mold, ubiquitous throughout the world, is today the subject of thousands of lawsuits in the United States. A more recent development is lawsuits against fast-food restaurants owing to their alleged contribution to obesity.

Challenges Associated with Exposure Lawsuits

Exposure lawsuits differ from traditional personal injury and property damage lawsuits in several ways. Instead of, for example, acute, immediate physical injuries resulting from an automobile accident, the harm in the typical exposure lawsuit is a disease, sickness, condition, or in some instances, the fear resulting from the exposure. Still other differences raise fundamental legal issues (Cranor, 1993). For example, environmental exposures are often invisible to the naked eye, and concentrations as low as one part per million (a measurement equivalent to one inch in sixteen miles) may cause some physical irritation or injury.

Another distinguishing factor in exposure lawsuits is timing. Injuries resulting from environmental exposures typically take years or decades to manifest. For instance, it may take ten to twenty years for exposure to asbestos to result in asbestosis and thirty to fifty years for it to result in mesothelioma. Complicating matters further, some individuals exposed to asbestos may never experience a related injury or disease. In addition, the diseases caused by environmental exposures are frequently indistinguishable from naturally occurring illnesses, a unique challenge for a legal system based on the plaintiff's proving his or her case. Compounding all this is a serious lack of basic knowledge about the thousands of chemicals and compounds to which people may be exposed. Although hundreds of thousands of substances are used in commerce, very little is known about the majority of these substances, contrary to what many people would assume. For many substances, even fundamental questions about carcinogenicity remain unanswered. All these unique circumstances challenge a legal system founded on examining direct, immediate, and easily detectable impacts.

Understanding Remedies

For every potential lawsuit, a range of factors determine whether it can be filed, when it can be filed, how it can be filed, and where it can be filed. For environmental exposures, several additional issues are important, including

- Whether the exposure or injury involves *personal injury* or *property damage*—this is the key screening variable in remedy law
- For personal injury or property damage, the type of specific substances or media involved (for example, dioxin, soil, and so forth)
- For personal injury or property damage, the type of relief being sought (for example, monetary damages, an injunction to stop certain behavior, and so forth)
- For personal injury or property damage, the means through which injury or exposure occurred (for example, a vaccine, air release, and so forth)
- For personal injury, the type of damage that occurred (for example, black lung disease, birth-related brain injury, AIDs, and so forth)
- For personal injury, whether the exposure or injury occurred while the person was at work and, if so, the position of that person (for example, employee, coal miner, and so forth)

Largely as a result of these differences, learning which remedies are available for a particular type of case is complicated (Kole and Nye, 1999).

Personal Injury Remedies for Environmental Exposures

Several types of remedies may be available to an exposed or injured individual attempting to recover expenses, seek compensation, and punish wrongdoers. No single remedy works for all exposures; a wide variety of factors influence which remedies are legally permitted. By far the most frequently used remedies for personal injury recovery are tort remedies—and negligence in particular. Any exposed or injured individual, however, needs to consider whether one or more of the no-fault compensation programs covers his or her damage.

Common Law Theories of Recovery

A *tort* is simply a civil wrong, distinguished from wrongs resulting from criminal behavior and wrongs resulting from a breach of contract. A tort is legal shorthand for a number of theories of common law recovery. Negligence is the best known of these; among the others are nuisance, trespass, fraud, battery, slander, false imprisonment, and defamation. The tort system is based largely on the concept of *fault.* The driving principal in tort law is that the person or entity causing the injury should pay to remedy the harm.

Traditional Tort Theories to Remedy Personal Harms. The most common theory of recovery in environmental exposure cases is *negligence.* To establish a claim for negligence, a plaintiff must prove several key elements by a preponderance of the evidence. Namely, a plaintiff must prove the defendant had a duty to conform to a *standard of care* to protect others, the defendant breached that duty, the plaintiff sustained actual damages, and the breach of the duty by the defendant actually caused the plaintiff's injuries. Stated differently, *negligent* behavior is behavior that falls below what a reasonably prudent person would do confronting the same facts and circumstances.

Perhaps the most common negligence lawsuit is one for medical malpractice. While intending to remove a bunion from a left toe, a surgeon cuts off the right toe—and the patient is a professional athlete. In this case all the elements of negligence are met. The surgeon owed a duty of care to remove the correct bunion, and the loss of a toe damages a professional athlete. As for other elements of liability, it is clear that the surgeon's breach of the duty to remove the correct bunion *caused* the damage. With these findings a jury would likely find the surgeon liable for negligence.

Injured parties also rely on other tort theories. In virtually all states, when a manufacturer puts a product into the *stream of commerce* (that is, sells a product), the legal system typically holds the manufacturer strictly liable if the product is defective or *unreasonably dangerous.* When a product injures somebody owing to a design or manufacturing defect, the injured party may have a claim against the manufacturer under the law of *product liability,* as this area of the law is known. When a hot water heater explodes, spraying scalding water across a porch, the injured owner may be able to sue the manufacturer for defective design or manufacturing. And subject to several limited defenses, the manufacturer may be strictly liable for the defect; in other words, the manufacturer may have no defenses to liability. Contrary to what many might think, a manufacturer may be liable for a product's defective design even if the manufacturer is *not* negligent. The goal of product liability law is to force manufacturers to internalize the costs of any damage caused by their products. The focus is not on the reasonableness of the manufacturer but on the adequacy of the product.

Under product liability law an injured party may claim the manufacturer failed to warn or inadequately warned about the dangers of its products, even if those products were designed and manufactured properly. A *failure-to-warn* claim is a common cause of action for injuries sustained from prescription drugs, over-the-counter drugs, and chemical exposures. Failure-to-warn cases are, however, legally complex, with often unpredictable results. For example, even though it unquestionably complied with Food and Drug Administration labeling requirements for a particular drug, a drug manufacturer may still be liable for failure to warn if a jury concludes the labeling was insufficient. If a defendant can establish that its actions were in compliance with law, that demonstration will not usually constitute a complete defense to liability but rather represents only strong evidence that the defendant's actions were reasonable.

In many exposure cases, however, the law of product liability provides no remedy because the exposure may result from a substance, chemical, or other exposure not considered a *product.* In mold exposure cases, for example, the mold is not a product placed into commerce, although product liability claims may be brought against the manufacturer of the equipment, flooring, or furniture where mold is growing. Wet plasterboard, a defective heating and ventilation system, or a leaking window may have visible mold, but mold in itself is likely not a product. In addition, in a successful product liability case, an injured party must identify the type of product causing the harm and know the manufacturer of the product. For lead or asbestos exposure, it is often impossible to know which company produced the lead or asbestos, even assuming the lead and asbestos would be considered a product subject to product liability law.

Old and New Damages. Under any theory of liability—product liability, negligence, or fraud—if there are no damages, a plaintiff has no case. In a personal injury action the damages sought by plaintiffs are often relatively straightforward.

Plaintiffs may seek to recover medical costs and lost wages (both past and future); they may seek recompense for pain and suffering, wrongful death (if applicable), and attorney fees; and they may seek punitive damages. Assuming liability has been established, the calculation of damages for personal injury—although sometimes challenging for certain individuals—usually is not the most difficult issue in an exposure case involving personal injury. In addition to monetary relief, an exposed or injured person may seek *equitable relief,* which usually means an order from the court that the defendant must take some action or refrain from taking some action. The sought-after relief may be a temporary restraining order, a temporary injunction, or a permanent injunction. Finally, in the context of environmental health, several innovative kinds of damages have been the subject of lawsuits, especially when the medical outcome of an exposure has not (yet) appeared. In the aftermath of a hazardous environmental exposure, lawsuits have sought damages for such things as a fear of future diseases, such as cancer (known as *cancerphobia*); an increased risk of future disease; and costs of ongoing or future medical monitoring.

Cancerphobia. Along with traditional damages, some plaintiffs seek recovery for cancerphobia in environmental health cases. Here the damages sought by a plaintiff are not for getting cancer and not for being at an increased risk for cancer from an exposure. Rather, a cancerphobia claim is about the *fear of* contracting cancer, and the money damages are intended to compensate for that fear. For these plaintiffs, in other words, the emotional distress resulting from an environmental exposure is as real as the actual disease, assuming it were to materialize.

For centuries the common law has permitted plaintiffs to recover for the emotional distress resulting from a physical injury. For instance, the emotional distress of seeing a toe severed by a defective lawn mower is traditionally permitted to be recovered in a tort suit. In other instances, known as *bystander* cases, individuals may recover for emotional distress if they were not personally injured but were near family members or close friends when they were injured. It is under this line of cases that a parent may be able to recover for emotional distress after seeing a child killed or significantly injured.

Courts are reluctant about, but not adamantly opposed to, awarding damages for fear-of claims, whether the fear in question is fear of cancer, fear of AIDS, or fear of becoming a lawyer. A few courts have held that "mere" exposure is sufficient to establish a claim for cancerphobia. But most courts reject this approach, noting that in today's modern civilization, exposure to potentially hazardous substances is a fact of life and that permitting plaintiffs to win damages for mere exposure would cripple the economy and debilitate an already troubled judicial system. For this reason many courts require plaintiffs to show at least a physical impact to recover for cancerphobia or other *emotional distress* lawsuits, and among these courts, most require a plaintiff to prove a resulting physical injury of some sort, such as a rash, headache, or related injury. The physical impact requirement is simply a device to make sure only meritorious claims for emotional distress are compensated. Individuals believing they have been exposed to a hazardous substance and filing a lawsuit to recover for fear of exposure but lacking any evidence of exposure are not likely to prevail in most jurisdictions in the United States. Still other courts, perhaps a majority, require a plaintiff to show more than impact to claim damage in fear-of cases. In these jurisdictions a plaintiff not only must prove a physical injury, such as a rash or headache, resulting from the emotional distress but also must prove that his or her reaction was reasonable under the circumstances. For instance, a court is unlikely to conclude that simply by pumping gas a plaintiff could suffer the requisite physical injury and the requisite reasonable emotional distress to establish the elements of a claim for cancerphobia.

For most courts considering a fear-of claim, simple exposure to a hazardous or toxic substance, product, or condition does not constitute damage under the law. Has an individual been *damaged* when there are absolutely no signs or symptoms after exposure to a toxic substance? For most courts, the answer is no. In most AIDS needlestick cases, unless the plaintiff can show evidence of HIV infection, it is unlikely the plaintiff can recover for a fear of AIDS cause of action. In the asbestos context, if a plaintiff can show only pleural thickening and not asbestosis, a claim for fear of disease likely, though not always, will fail legally.

Increased Risk of Disease. Along with cancerphobia claims, exposed individuals sometimes file *increased risk of disease* claims. Here the damage is the probability that through one or more exposures caused by the defendant, the plaintiff faces an increased risk of contracting a disease. In these cases plaintiffs present no symptoms or physical indications of the disease, only the knowledge of being at an increased probability of getting the disease. Legally, this is a claim for risk of future injury, not present exposure. As a general rule courts are reluctant to accept increased risk of disease cases. Most courts believe that if increased risk claims were permitted, those who do not develop the illness would be overcompensated and those who do would be undercompensated, at least over the long run (Kanner, 2000).

The few courts that accept these claims invoke a number of legal tests to screen out unmeritorious claims. A few require plaintiffs to prove to a *reasonable medical certainty* that they will develop the disease, although offering no definition of these terms. Other courts, perhaps a majority, require plaintiffs to prove they will *more probably than not* acquire the disease, a threshold established through expert testimony that the disease is more than 50 percent likely to occur. In most cases, largely because of the enormous technical challenges involved, experts are unwilling or unable to opine that an individual's risk of contracting a disease has increased by a set percentage.

Medical Monitoring. Rather than fighting over fear of cancer or increased risk, many exposed but unaffected plaintiffs seek to recover the costs of medical surveillance, also known as *medical monitoring* costs. The award of medical monitoring costs to *asymptomatic* plaintiffs is a difficult issue philosophically, medically, and legally. The results in court cases range across the board, from a simple no to elaborate multipart tests for calculating medical monitoring costs. At this point in the development of the case law, the majority rule appears to be that medical monitoring claims for the asymptomatic claimant are likely not legally recognized, even if those individuals are undeniably exposed to highly toxic or hazardous substances. For most courts, it makes more sense legally and economically for a plaintiff to wait until symptoms of the disease manifest before any recovery is permitted through the legal system. If a plaintiff has undertaken medical monitoring prior to actually exhibiting symptoms, that individual should be able to recover the costs for that surveillance at the time the symptoms appear.

In interpreting an asbestos case, for example, the U.S. Supreme Court rejected a claim for medical monitoring. After reviewing the available case law and considering the policy implications of awarding damages to asymptomatic plaintiffs, the Court declined to award medical monitoring costs. The Court held that without symptoms, a plaintiff has no claim for medical monitoring. According to the Court, the fundamental reason for not permitting medical monitoring costs was that health care monies would then be used to monitor currently healthy individuals when those funds would be better reserved for assisting the truly injured. For other courts the benefits of medical monitoring for individuals exposed to environmental exposures have warranted recovery, even if the individuals have no symptoms of the disease or injury. However, before a recovery for medical surveillance is permitted, a number of requirements must be met, and these requirements vary from court to court. Generally, however, these courts have required a plaintiff to establish the following to recover on a medical monitoring claim:

- Exposure was to greater than normal background levels of an established hazardous substance.
- Exposure was caused by defendant's negligence.
- Exposure has resulted in a "significantly increased risk of contracting the disease."
- Monitoring procedures exist that make early detection possible.

- Monitoring is different from what would ordinarily be carried out during routine medical care.
- Early detection has an established clinical value.

With each of these conditions established, courts will sometimes award lump sum payments for medical surveillance. Usually, though, courts award only periodic payments or funds to cover limited medical monitoring.

Fundamental Challenges Associated with the Common Law Tort System

As suggested by the range of innovative damages sought by plaintiffs today, exposure cases raise significant problems for the traditional tort system.

Causation. Without question, the most difficult issue in exposure law is *causation*—that is, Did the exposure (or repeated exposures or a combination of exposures) actually cause the injury? Exposure cases are won and lost on the issue of causation, because a defendant will be held liable only for those harms actually and legally caused by the defendant. Causality is generally not an issue when an individual breaks a leg during an automobile accident. But for the accident, the leg would not have been broken. Environmental exposure cases are, however, different. Causation is difficult to prove for numerous reasons (Kanner, 2002):

- The toxic properties of many hazardous substances are not known.
- Information on the plaintiff's frequency, duration, and amount of past exposures to most substances is not available.
- Not all individuals react the same way to similar exposures to disease-producing agents or chemicals.
- Multiple exposures in a variety of settings have contributed to or caused the injury.

For these and other reasons, juries in exposure cases are often at a loss when trying to assess the weight and importance of scientific evidence.

In environmental exposure cases, courts typically break causation into two components: (1) general causation, and (2) specific causation. *General* causation is the requirement that the specific substance, exposure, or process is capable of producing the general type of injury. Does benzene exposure cause cancer generally? If so, the court will proceed to the second element, specific causation. *Specific* causation is the requirement that under the specific facts of the case in dispute, the actual exposure more likely than not caused the disease. Did low-level exposure to benzene while filling up a car with unleaded gasoline cause cancer in that individual—who also smoked a pack of cigarettes a day and who worked in a dry-cleaning store where perchloroethylene, a suspected carcinogen, was used regularly?

The 200 or so reported legal decisions addressing causality in environmental exposure cases defy easy description. Just as scientists disagree over the fundamental meaning of causation, courts struggle with the type and sufficiency of evidence necessary to *prove* or capable of *proving* causation, and often the battleground—as in science—is epidemiological research studies. A few courts are reluctant to delve into the meaning of epidemiology, toxicology, and the scientific method. These courts, believing these issues to be a fundamental fact question, permit parties to explain the issues to a jury and let the science fall where it may. For many courts, epidemiological studies that do not address the substance at issue in the case or the disease or injury at issue in the case will be considered uninformative. Epidemiological studies that are not statistically significant may likewise be rejected. If the reported cases are any measure, the judicial system's reliance on epidemiology has not made causation decisions any easier.

Yet a majority of courts, especially federal courts, operating under stricter rules of civil procedure regarding the testimony of experts (Box 36.1), take their role as gatekeepers more seriously. For these courts, *relative risk*—a standard measure in epidemiology—constitutes fair game for the legal system. Among the reported decisions interpreting relative risk in environmental exposure cases, the bottom line is not clear. Some courts require plaintiffs to show a relative risk of greater than 2.0 (that is, a doubling of the risk), whereas still other courts require a showing of a relative risk greater than 4.0. Still other courts, perhaps the most sophisticated of the pack, look to relative risk only as a measure of causality that should be considered in the context of other factors, especially those developed by A. B. Hill (see Chapters Three and Thirty-Five).

Box 36.1. Who Is an Expert in Exposure Cases?

Under the evidentiary laws of almost every state, if a matter is *beyond the ken* of the ordinary citizen, then an expert is required to clarify the issues and offer opinions regarding those issues. Before or after trial the distinction between an expert and a fact witness is critical in exposure cases, as in all other cases. A *fact witness* testifies to personal knowledge, and a fact witness is not usually permitted to present opinions, which essentially amount to speculation. In contrast, an *expert* offers opinions, which may or may not be based on facts admitted into evidence. An expert is someone who through experience, expertise, or education has gained a unique perspective on an area of technical subject matter.

In exposure lawsuits, experts are necessary to offer opinions on whether the exposure caused the damage and, if so, to what extent. Establishing causation in toxic exposure cases is the number one area where expert testimony is critical. Expert testimony is also critical in establishing damage—whether the contamination interferes with the use of the property or whether filling up a car with gasoline could lead to cancer.

For many years courts took a relaxed view of the definition of *expert.* Then, in 1993, the Supreme Court, in *Daubert* v. *Merrill Dow,* held that a plaintiff must prove that the opinion of its expert witness is (1) relevant and (2) reliable. And perhaps more important, the Court held that the trial court was required to act as a *gatekeeper* to screen out expert testimony that did not meet this standard. The Court also provided a nonexclusive list of factors a trial court should consider in this gatekeeping function:

- Whether the theory or technique used by the expert can be, and has been, tested
- Whether the theory or technique has been subjected to peer review and publication
- What the known or potential error rate of the theory or technique used is
- The degree to which the theory or technique or conclusion is accepted in the relevant scientific community

Daubert has become the standard in federal courts, but not all states have accepted *Daubert.* Several have specifically rejected *Daubert,* finding that judges are not required to scrutinize experts closely, leaving those matters for the jury. These courts have continued to rely on a *general acceptance* standard, meaning that if a plaintiff can show its theory meets a general acceptance standard it can be admitted.

The Court's decision in *Daubert,* subsequently explained in two additional cases, *Joiner* and *Kumho Tire,* now forms the most important standard for expert testimony in federal courts. Lawsuits in federal court regularly include numerous motions trying to strike experts or limit their testimony. To be reliable, all testimony must be by an expert with appropriate qualifications, experience, and knowledge, and the particular method used by the expert must be acceptable scientifically. If a plaintiff cannot convince a court that its expert testimony is both relevant and reliable, then it will not be admitted for use in the proceeding. If the defense is successful in striking the testimony of the plaintiff's expert witness, the case may be over, because the plaintiff may not be able to offer another expert to testify on this issue.

In lawsuits over environmental exposures, proving causation is challenging for yet another reason—the existence of multiple defendants. In the typical exposure case numerous defendants may have produced the substance or equipment at issue. At trial the plaintiff is required to prove that one or more of the defendants caused the injury. But this is often a difficult burden, especially given the historical conditions at work. For example, fifty different companies may have produced the lead-based paint used in apartment buildings, making it impossible to tell which company produced the paint at issue in a particular lawsuit. To prove its case, however, a plaintiff must make out a case for liability against a manufacturer of lead-based paint.

A final reason causation is so difficult to establish in exposure cases is just as basic. In proving an exposure caused a disease, injury, or condition, a plaintiff is required to offer expert testimony that none of the plaintiff's own prior exposures, eating habits, drug habits, exercise habits, family history, or risk-taking behaviors caused the very disease attributed to the defendant's actions or omissions. Canceling out competing explanations for the injury, an element of the plaintiff's case, is often technically and legally challenging. It will be tough for a plaintiff to prove that his or her cancer resulted from the benzene vapors escaping from the service station pump when the plaintiff also works at a dry cleaner that uses PERC and when he or she smokes a pack of cigarettes a day.

Latency. The second major legal challenge presented by environmental exposures is *latency.* In an automobile accident, the exposure (the crash) and the damage (the broken leg or dented fender) occur nearly simultaneously. But in an exposure case it may take years or decades for the exposure to result in a symptom, disease, or disorder. It may take thirty years for exposure to asbestos to result in pleural thickening, which may—or may not—be a result of asbestos exposure and may—or may not—result in asbestosis that likely resulted from asbestos exposure.

The delay between initial exposure and discernable injury creates a fundamental problem for the legal system. The legal system is premised on the notion that if a party has a legally recognizable claim, that party should bring the claim when he or she discovers or should have discovered the injury or learns about the claim—or the party should forever waive that right after a set period of time. As a matter of public policy a defendant should not have to worry about any past exposures it may have caused after a reasonable period of time has run.

Statutes of limitations are the legal barriers created to bar stale claims. A statute of limitations is nothing more than a time frame within which a legal claim must be brought, and these statutes vary widely from state to state. In some states the statute of limitations for personal injury claims allows only a year from the date the individual "discovered" or "should reasonably have discovered" the injury, but other states allow as long as three years for the very same exposure. The period allowed by a statute of limitations for a property damage case may be as short as four years from the time the injury occurred to the property, irrespective of when the damage was discovered. Every year in every state, plaintiffs lose their cases because they failed to file their claims before the statute of limitations period expired. Once that period is over a plaintiff is forever barred from bringing the claim. Given the implications, lengthy legal battles frequently occur over the time when an injury was discovered or reasonably should have been discovered.

The potential delay between toxic exposures and injuries or damage creates two perverse results. First, exposed individuals may be prevented from recovering medical expenses related to an environmental exposure because they waited too long to file a claim, even though they may have been symptom free and may never have been told by a physician that they had a disease. Second, knowing the harsh effects of statutes of limitations, exposed individuals often race to file lawsuits so they do not miss the limitation period, even when it is clear to all involved they do not have any real symptoms or injury. The end result is that precautionary filers clog the courts while the truly injured wait for their day in court. Nowhere is there a better example of this than in asbestos lawsuits (Box 36.2).

Box 36.2. The Elephantine Mass of Asbestos Litigation

Asbestos exposure has been called the "worst occupational health disaster in U.S. history," and asbestos litigation represents a legal crisis of unprecedented proportions in the United States. As of 2002, 600,000 individuals had filed personal injury lawsuits involving asbestos (Carroll and others, 2002; Biggs, 2003). Between 1999 and 2001, the number of claims for asbestos exposure tripled, and between 2000 and 2002, roughly 50,000 to 70,000 new claims were filed (Biggs, 2003; Congressional Budget Office, 2003).

The costs of this situation are staggering. One estimate puts the total spent by defendants and insurers at $70 billion. And of that $70 billion, $21 billion went to defendants' lawyers and an additional $20 billion went to plaintiffs' lawyers (White, 2004). As a point of reference, the total amount paid to lawyers in the recent tobacco settlement was only $13 billion, paid out over twenty-five years.

Why Is Asbestos Litigation So Different?

The asbestos cases are different from other mass tort cases involving environmental exposures for a number of reasons (White, 2004). First, the sheer number of plaintiffs distinguishes asbestos litigation. According to one estimate, 1 to 3 million people will eventually file asbestos lawsuits. In comparison, the breast implant litigation involved only 440,000 plaintiffs (White, 2004).

Second, the number of defendants is unparalleled. Upward of 9,000 companies in the United States are now defendants in asbestos exposure lawsuits. No other mass tort has had more than twenty or so major defendants. Along with the number of cases, the list of defendants continues to grow. Although 300 companies were targeted by plaintiffs in the 1980s, more than 8,400 companies have been named as defendants in asbestos cases today. At least one company in nearly every U.S. industrial sector is now involved in asbestos litigation (Biggs, 2003).

Third, the ease of forum shopping, seeking a favorable venue, is making the crisis worse. For example, although Mississippi has only 1 percent of the U.S. population, approximately 20 percent of the pending cases have been filed in Mississippi, because Mississippi courts are believed to be more pro-plaintiff (Biggs, 2003). Apparently, this forum shopping does pay off. Asbestos verdicts in Mississippi, West Virginia, and Texas were on average $3 million higher than awards in other jurisdictions (White, 2004). Elected judges, lax procedural rules, sympathetic juries, and an active plaintiffs' bar largely explain these regional differences.

Fourth, unimpaired plaintiffs have had significant success in asbestos lawsuits to date. In fact most asbestos plaintiffs today are unimpaired, showing no signs of serious asbestos impact, a perverse result of the impact of statutes of limitations on filings (White, 2004). Indeed, the number of mesothelioma cases, which virtually everyone recognizes as caused by asbestos, represent only a tiny fraction of all asbestos cases (Carroll and others, 2002). To date, about 65 percent of the compensation in asbestos lawsuits has gone to nonmalignant claimants (Carroll and others, 2002).

Fifth, unlike what has happened in other mass torts, the procedural options for resolving difficult exposure cases have failed to work. For example, the bankruptcy of asbestos manufacturers has not slowed the filing of asbestos lawsuits. When a key defendant files for bankruptcy, plaintiffs' lawyers simply target peripheral industries with some alleged role in asbestos. After asbestos manufacturers were bankrupt, any company handling asbestos became a target of plaintiffs. Likewise, class action settlements, another procedural device that has been successful in certain other settings, have not worked to resolve the asbestos crisis. Even though the Supreme Court has called for a national solution to the problem, on at least two occasions when the Court has reviewed massive settlement class actions for asbestos claims, it has rejected the settlements on legal grounds, noting that future asbestos claimants would be compromised by the settlement.

Proposed Solutions

For more than thirty years there have been repeated calls to resolve the asbestos litigation crisis, but none of the proposals have been successful to date. According to Michael Green (1999), professor of law at Wake Forest University, "Everyone knows that the system is broken, judges know it, commentators know it, asbestos victims know it, their families know it, the experts who testify over and over and over again know it, and the lawyers who are litigating these cases know it."

The 1980s saw several proposals by asbestos defendants, insurers, and Congress to resolve the crisis (Biggs, 2003). The best known have been the proposal to form the Center for Claims Resolution (CCR), an entity created by twenty-one asbestos producers in 1988 to resolve asbestos claims, and the Georgine settlement of 1993, a class action settlement intended to resolve the vast majority of claims. The Georgine settlement, and the similar Fibreboard settlement, were overturned by the U.S. Supreme Court, and the CCR stopped settling new asbestos claims in 2001. The most recent legislative proposal, the Fairness in Asbestos Injury Resolution Act (FAIR Act), is currently before Congress.

As of 2005, the use of asbestos is still legal in the United States, a fact that boggles the minds of many observers of the asbestos litigation crisis.

Procedural Innovations

A few courts have developed procedural solutions to address these issues. With respect to the harsh implications resulting from short limitation periods for personal injury, some courts in some asbestos cases have held that exposure is not damage for purposes of the statute of limitations. For these courts a plaintiff can file a claim only when he or she shows concrete symptoms of a disease. To ensure that asbestos-exposed but symptom-free plaintiffs are not barred from filing their claims by a statute of limitation, other courts have created *plural registries,* which permit plaintiffs to sign up as potential plaintiffs, after which the case is administratively frozen. These registries permit symptom-free plaintiffs to preserve their cases without currently clogging the judicial system with their claims.

Another procedural technique used by judges in tort cases is bifurcation—separating some issues from others, especially contentious ones, and considering them sequentially. In tort cases the general rule has been for courts to bifurcate issues of causality from issues of damages. Procedurally, this means a plaintiff first has to prove that an exposure caused an injury, before offering evidence and making arguments about damages. If a plaintiff proves exposure, then another trial is held to determine damages. In asbestos cases some judges have employed *reverse* bifurcation, which requires a plaintiff to prove damages first, followed by a trial on liability. The goal in reverse bifurcation is to ensure that damage has occurred before considering the issue of responsibility.

Another procedure, used for many types of cases, not only exposure cases, is to file a *class action* in order to pursue a large number of claims at once. The key legal issue in class action law is whether common issues of law and fact predominate. In environmental exposure cases, putative members of a class may differ considerably from each other. For example, among people exposed to groundwater contamination, there are salient differences between smokers and nonsmokers and between those who use pesticides in their backyards and those who do not.

Statutory Remedies for Personal Injury

For certain exposures and health outcomes, Congress and state legislatures have enacted specific statutes to compensate people who have been harmed. These statutory remedies fall into three general types: no-fault programs, such as workers' compensation; partial-fault programs, such as the Federal Employees Liability Act; and compensation funds. These three approaches vary in their eligibility requirements, claims processing, and exclusivity (that is, whether claimants can also file tort suits).

No-Fault Programs: Workers' Compensation

Largely because of the limitations of the traditional tort system, Congress and state legislatures have enacted several *no-fault* programs. These programs, which differ widely in scope and structure, address only a few personal injuries, diseases, and exposures.

The best known of the administrative no-fault systems for personal injury is the workers' compensation system. Workers' compensation guarantees medical and income benefits to those who are injured on the job *regardless of who is at fault.* All states have workers' compensation systems, although they differ in many respects from state to state.

Workers' compensation is an *exclusive* remedy. In exchange for the no-fault provision of this remedy—for being relieved of the burden of proving fault in cases of workplace injury or illness—workers are barred from suing their employers in tort. Following a workplace injury or illness, an employee cannot sue the employer for negligence, cannot receive compensation for pain and suffering, and cannot receive punitive damages. However, at least in theory, workers receive their compensation, including medical costs and lost wage replacement, promptly and without the need for extensive legal maneuvers. This was the trade-off crafted by state legislatures in the early twentieth century when workers' compensation systems originated.

To be covered under most workers' compensation statutes, an injury must "arise out of and be in the course of employment." Both the injury and the "in course of employment" elements are at issue in these cases. As a general rule an injury may be the result of a single traumatic event, the result of an aggravation of an existing condition, or the result of a cumulative traumatic activity. Injuries arising from inherently personal risk factors—attributes such as epilepsy, drug addictions, or physical deformities—are not covered under the definition of injuries. Death occurring during the course of employment is covered under the workers' compensation program. For injuries covered by the workers' compensation system, the employer must pay all work-related costs, including doctor bills, therapy costs, and travel expenses, and death benefits may be available in certain instances. If an employer does not provide the workers' compensation coverage sought by an employee, the employee may seek a hearing before an administrative law judge.

Workers' compensation programs may also cover *occupational diseases.* Under most state workers' compensation programs, an employee can recover for an occupational disease provided certain basic conditions are met:

- The work or employment condition directly caused the disease.
- The disease "naturally resulted" from the work experience.
- The disease is one that does not ordinarily result from an employee's exposure to conditions outside the work setting.
- The disease is not a normal disease of life endured by the general public.

If a worker contracts a disease meeting these conditions, the medical expenses and resulting disability resulting from that disease are covered under the workers' compensation program.

Still other issues arise in determining coverage under workers' compensation programs. By definition, only employees are covered by these programs. An independent contractor, for example, someone hired for a specific job, is not an employee and is not covered. In many states additional categories of workers, such as domestic servants and farm laborers, are not covered by workers' compensation programs.

Workers' compensation systems, like all legal frameworks, contain certain exceptions. Although the workers' compensation system bars employees from suing their employers, employees are free to sue third parties. Accordingly, if an employee severs his hand while using an electric saw at work, he can sue the saw manufacturer (say, in a product liability claim). And under certain circumstances—injury arising from an intentional act by the employer or while in the hire of an employer who has not been participating in the workers' compensation insurance program—the employee is permitted to sue the employer in the tort system.

Some workers' compensation systems cover only a few types of employees. For example, civilian federal employees are covered by the Federal Employees' Compensation Act (FECA), and longshore and harbor workers are covered by the Longshore and Harbor Workers' Act (LHWA). Another workers' compensation law that covers a certain type of worker is the Federal Mine Safety and Health Act, and a specific part of this Act, the Black Lung Program, addresses a certain type of injury. Coal miners, railroad workers hauling coal, and others involved with coal mining who demonstrate that they have pneumoconiosis (black lung disease) are compensated by this program, which provides monthly payments to them and their surviving dependents. To establish eligibility, a coal miner must show—by chest X-ray or a "physician's reasoned medical opinion"—that he or she has black lung and is totally disabled. The Black Lung Program is administered by the U.S. Department of Labor.

Partial-Fault Programs: FELA and the Jones Act

The remedy for certain other injured workers is not a no-fault workers' compensation program but other similar programs. For example, injured interstate railroad workers are required to seek recovery under the Federal Employers Liability Act (FELA). Like a workers' compensation program, FELA was enacted to reduce the inefficiencies of the tort system. But unlike a workers' compensation program, FELA is not a true no-fault program. FELA is best thought of as a partial-fault workers' compensation program or a relaxation of certain tort requirements. Although an injured employee must prove the railroad was negligent, FELA contains several mechanisms to make proof of negligence easier than it is under a classic tort system. If an injured employee can show the railroad violated certain federal laws, for instance, FELA becomes a strict-fault system. The Jones Act, a section of the Merchant Marine Act of 1920, is a FELA-like program for merchant marines.

Compensation Funds

Other statutes attempt to take certain exposures, certain substances, and certain injuries out of the tort system completely, or at least significantly to limit the tort liability associated with these exposures. These statutory remedies may be in addition to those provided by the tort system, but often they take the place of tort remedies. Of these *administrative compensation programs,* the most important for environmental health are the

- Smallpox Emergency Personnel Protection Act of 2003
- September 11th Victim Compensation Fund of 2001
- Radiation Exposure Compensation Act of 1990 (as amended, 2000)
- Florida Birth-Related Neurological Injury Compensation Act of 1988
- Virginia Birth-Related Neurological Injury Compensation Act of 1987
- California AIDs Vaccine Victims Compensation Fund of 1986
- National Childhood Vaccine Injury Act of 1986
- Agent Orange Veterans' Payment Program of 1984

- National Swine Flu Act of 1976
- Price-Anderson Act of 1957, an amendment to the Atomic Energy Act of 1954

These compensation frameworks vary in their breadth and structure, and few generalizations are possible (Mullenix and Stewart, 2002–2003). In all these programs, when claimants meet the program requirements, they receive compensation for their injury or exposure, without needing to prove that a defendant caused the injury.

Some of these programs have exclusivity provisions like those of workers' compensation plans. For example, under the Swine Flu Act, people contracting swine flu from a vaccine are limited to recovery from the fund. But in other programs, a claimant may be able to file a tort suit despite being covered by an administrative fund. The National Childhood Vaccine Injury Act bars civil suits that allege inadequate product warnings from the manufacturer of the vaccine. Under this Act a claimant who wants to bring other tort claims must adjudicate these claims under the National Childhood Vaccine Injury Act and then waive an award before filing a civil action to recover damages under the tort system. Under the Smallpox Emergency Personnel Protection Act a claimant may sue in tort only after exhausting that Act's program.

Other programs implement their own brand of exclusivity. Under the Agent Orange program, for example, disputes over recovery must be submitted to binding arbitration. The California AIDs fund permits plaintiffs to file tort suits along with seeking compensation from the fund, but provides that the fund is subrogated to any recovery, meaning the fund may recover if the claimant is successful in the tort suit. Under the Price-Anderson Act, claimants are required to waive all defenses in the event of a substantial nuclear accident.

Although purportedly no-fault, each of these programs differs widely in its approach to causality. For example, under the National Childhood Vaccine Injury Act, a claimant does not have to prove causation. If the claimant received one of the vaccines covered by the Act and has one of diseases identified on the vaccine table, the court will award damages. Instead of causality, the legal issue becomes whether an injury is included on the vaccine table. If it is off-table, the Act may still cover the injury but to a lesser extent and then only if the claimant presents expert testimony that the injury resulted from the vaccine exposure. Under the LHWA a worker can receive compensation without proving negligence because there is a presumption of causation if a worker can show exposure to an injurious substance and a disease and that the exposure could have caused the disease. Under the Radiation Exposure Compensation Act (RECA) Amendments of 2000, the standards of eligibility differ by an individual's status. Uranium miners, millers, and ore transporters may receive $100,000 if they can establish certain basic criteria. Under RECA, any individuals who "participated" in any atmospheric testing of nuclear weapons can receive $75,000 payment for certain diseases. In addition, RECA provides that *downwinders,* those individuals physically present in one of the areas downwind from the Nevada Test Site during atmospheric testing, can receive $50,000. There are no periodic payments under RECA. If eligible, the person receives a one-time payment.

These programs exhibit still other differences, including the ways in which funds are distributed. For some the U.S. District Courts administer funds; for the Agent Orange program the administrator is Aetna Technical Services, Inc., a private company. For the September 11th Victim Compensation Fund a *special master* determines eligibility and awards compensation. Under the National Childhood Vaccine Injury Act a special master for the U.S. Court for Federal Claims issues awards, which are appealable to that court.

Other Statutes Providing Limited Private Remedies

Individuals exposed to certain substances or hazardous situations may be able to seek certain other relief short of compensation. The two best-known examples of legislation that enables such relief are the federal Occupational Safety and Health Act and a California law known as Proposition 65.

Occupational Safety and Health Act. Even though the Occupational Safety and Health Act (OSH Act) was intended to provide the Occupational Safety and Health Administration (OSHA) with significant statutory authority to protect workers, the OSH Act also provides employees with certain, although limited, direct remedies to address occupational exposure. When construction workers are exposed to certain lead concentrations, for example, the employer may be required to provide certain medical monitoring tests. And under the lead standard, if employees notify their employer that they have developed symptoms associated with a lead-related disease or that they desire medical advice concerning the effects of past or current lead exposure on pregnancy, those employees can seek medical monitoring that must be provided by the employer. Beyond requiring the employer to provide certain monitoring, OSHA does not guarantee workers any relief for damages. However, following a request for medical monitoring, an employee also may file a workers' compensation claim related to the lead exposure.

Proposition 65. California's Safe Drinking Water and Toxic Enforcement Act of 1986, also known as Proposition 65, prohibits the discharge of listed chemicals to potential drinking water sources and prohibits exposing persons to listed chemicals without prior warning of the risks created by those substances. The Office of the California Attorney General and certain city attorney offices enforce the Act. In addition, Proposition 65 permits private citizens to file enforcement actions, provided appropriate notice is given to the offending party. Proposition 65's citizen suit provision is similar to the citizen suit provisions of other environmental statutes discussed later in this chapter. If a citizen believes that consumers—including the citizen who wishes to file the complaint—are being exposed to certain substances without proper warning of the risks of those substances, that citizen is permitted to file a complaint intended to cause the proper warnings to be displayed.

Sovereign Immunity

The *exclusive remedy* provisions of workers' compensation programs are not the only barrier to lawsuits against certain defendants, especially government defendants. Exposure claims against federal or state governments may also be barred by the concept of *sovereign immunity.* Under the Constitution of the United States and the constitutions of most states, the government can be sued only when that action is specifically permitted and in no situations can punitive damages be recovered from a government entity. Under the Federal Tort Claims Act, the federal government has waived its sovereign immunity for negligent acts of agents of the United States, and states have enacted comparable state Tort Claims Acts. Before a claimant files suit in court, these Acts typically require that claimant to present an administrative claim to the appropriate agency identifying the negligent act and damages sought. If the agency does not admit or deny the claim within six months, the claimant can then file a negligence claim.

These Tort Claims Acts permit negligence suits only in a few narrow situations. If a government employee's alleged negligent activities resulted from the "exercise or performance or the failure to exercise or perform a discretionary function or duty," those claims are not permitted by the Tort Claims Act. For example, a claim relating to the negligent design of a federal wastewater treatment system that permitted the cross-contamination of stormwater and sewage would probably be barred by the Federal Tort Claims Act. Suits based on misrepresentation are also specifically not permitted by most Tort Claims Acts. Claims against government employees who maintain that lead ingestion does not harm adults would also probably be barred. So when considering who can be sued, it is always critical to know whether the defendant has sovereign immunity.

Property Damage Remedies

The remedies for property damage resulting from environmental exposures differ fundamentally from the remedies for personal injury, as one might expect. But still there are parallels, particularly the concern over whether the tort system can handle the difficult issues created by environmental exposures. For example, just as several no-fault programs were enacted to correct the tort system's failure to remedy certain personal injuries, numerous environmental laws were enacted in the 1970s and 1980s to correct the tort system's failure to protect the environment.

Common Law Theories to Remedy Property Harms

In considering the available remedies for property damage, the first question is to determine what relief is being sought. If the goal is to recover the costs of cleaning up contamination, one set of laws applies. If the goal is to recover the diminution in property value caused by contamination, another set of laws applies. And if the goal is to force compliance with already existing laws and regulations, still another set of laws applies.

Traditional Tort Claims. Traditional tort law provides several theories of recovery to remedy property damage. An owner of property next to a leaking underground storage tank may file a claim for nuisance, trespass, negligence, strict liability, fraudulent or negligent concealment, or similar tort claims. The standard elements of negligence in a personal injury setting—for example, duty, breach, cause, and damages—also apply when the negligence involves property damage, and all the limitations of the tort system—including those concerning proof of causation, expert testimony, and statutes of limitations—likewise apply. Under a negligence theory, a gasoline station owes a duty of care to adjacent property owners to prevent leaks from underground storage tanks, and some courts would regard that duty as having been breached when the tanks leak.

The adjacent property owner also may be able to bring a *nuisance* claim, one of the most common claims brought to remedy property contamination. Nuisance comes in two types, public nuisance and private nuisance. A cause of action for *private nuisance* is a claim that the leaking underground storage tank on the adjacent property "substantially and unreasonably" interferes with the adjacent property owner's use of his property. The issue is whether the activity actually constitutes a substantial and unreasonable interference. In the case of a leaking underground storage tank, does the presence of contaminated groundwater actually constitute a substantial and unreasonable interference with the land if the property is served by a public drinking-water system and there are no streams or other water receptors on the property? A claim for public nuisance differs in the rights that are harmed. A *public nuisance* is an injury to some public good, not to private property, and the party bringing a public nuisance claim must do so on behalf of the public. Traditionally, governments brought public nuisance claims to stop the open dumping of waste materials on public lands or to prohibit some land uses. In recent years, however, public nuisance has become a favorite choice for states and municipalities trying to influence public health and environmental health policy. In the war against tobacco, for example, the attorneys general of several states filed public nuisance claims against the tobacco companies, arguing that these companies were creating a public nuisance. Several states and cities have filed public nuisance claims to stop the sale of handguns, to force the cleanup of lead-based paint, and most recently, to force electric utilities to stop burning coal and thus to reduce global climate change. Often simply the filing of these public nuisance claims prompts discussions, which may in turn lead to settlement. Instead of trying to enact statutes or promulgate regulations, these states and municipalities prefer to fight these significant public health issues out in the courts. The strategy of filing a lawsuit to address thorny public health issues—where no statute or regulation seems to work—has been called *regulation by litigation.* It is a subject with its own set of issues and concerns.

A number of other common law torts may be available to address property damage claims. A trespass claim may be available to the adjacent property owner, assuming the gasoline from the underground tank has in fact migrated onto his or her property. A *trespass* is an intentional, reckless, or negligent entry onto land owned by another. A trespass can occur when a party permits a "thing or third person" to enter the land of another. If during the construction of a shopping center the developer fails to install soil and erosion control and thus permits silt to run onto the adjacent property, the developer may be liable for trespass. The unpermitted entry of chemicals onto property is also a trespass. For a successful nuisance claim, however, contamination need not physically affect the property. Simply being next door to a contaminated site may be enough for a successful nuisance claim.

Under a *strict liability* claim a defendant may be liable for activities that are considered *abnormally dangerous* or *ultrahazardous*—a situation where no amount of care would prevent the harm. In these cases the focus is on the activity, not the injury. The prototypical abnormally dangerous activity is blasting. If a prudent person takes every known precaution prior to blasting dynamite, it is still possible that windows in the area will be cracked and dishes destroyed. Legally, because no amount of precaution can prevent the harm, the blasting becomes an abnormally dangerous activity, and the defendant has no defenses to liability.

Just what other activities are abnormally dangerous remains unclear. In a few cases a spill of hazardous substances has been held to be an abnormally dangerous activity, but in the majority of cases it has not. Just because a landfill leaks toxic waste, it does not necessarily follow that the landfill is an abnormally dangerous activity imposing strict liability. The defining activity for a landfill is not such leaking, which clearly is a significant environmental harm, but the depositing of waste. For most courts the determining factor is whether a regulatory agency would issue a permit or license to conduct the activity. Accordingly, a leaking underground storage tank is generally not an abnormally dangerous activity for most courts, because an underground storage tank is permitted by federal and state regulations. And for many courts, if a state agency will issue a permit for the activity, it cannot be abnormally dangerous, by definition.

Valuing Property Damage. A key issue in contaminated property cases is valuation. Under the common law the measure of damage for contaminated property depends on whether the injury is defined as permanent or abatable. If the property damage is considered *permanent,* the measure of damage will be the diminution in value of the property, calculated from the fair market value before and after the injury. But if the contamination is considered *abatable,* the measure of damages is the cost of repair. This legal difference can be significant. If a leaking underground storage tank is considered an abatable nuisance, then an affected property owner may be able to recover only the costs of repair. And if someone is already correcting the problems with the underground storage tank, there may be no damages for the cost of repair, even if the contamination remains in place. In this instance the arcane nature of tort law, which is keyed to the *permanent* versus *abatable* distinction, would also prevent the property owner from recovering the decrease in value to his or her property caused by the abatable contamination from the underground storage tank.

The difference between a permanent and an abatable nuisance raises still other issues in the context of contaminated property. A state statute of limitations for claiming *permanent* property damage may offer periods as short as two years or as long as six years. As a general rule these periods run from the time the property is first damaged, not from the time the property owner discovers the damage, which is the standard rule in personal injury cases. Under this rule, when a leak or other exposure first occurs it triggers the running of the period in which a claim of permanent property damage may be filed, assuming the leak is considered permanent.

But in the case of most contamination, the time of the first leak, release, or spill can be difficult or impossible to establish. When an underground storage tank is leaking, the first injury may be many years past, preventing an adjacent property owner from filing suit to seek damages. For many courts, however, this result is unacceptably harsh, and they have developed a fiction that the damage from the contamination is still continuing, assuming some of the contamination remains, even though the leak may have occurred several years in the past. Courts therefore often characterize contamination as a *continuing* nuisance so that the statute of limitations for permanent property damage will not bar meritorious claims.

Stigma Damages. Another issue raised in property damage cases is whether a plaintiff can recover *stigma* damages. Stigma damages come in several varieties. A property owner may claim that simply by being located near some undesirable activity, such as a landfill or industrial facility, his or her property has been *stigmatized*. Or the owner of a property contaminated by a leaking underground gasoline storage tank may claim that his or her property is stigmatized even though the leaking tanks and contamination have been removed and the regulatory agency has issued a letter stating "no further action" is required. The more difficult case is where property has been cleaned up, but some residual contamination below the regulatory standard remains. Does this constitute stigma? For many courts it is an open legal question whether the presence of contamination below the regulatory standard constitutes property damage.

In the context of environmental exposures the case law on stigma damages is anything but clear on whether contamination—even after it has been cleaned up—creates long-term valuation issues. A majority of courts seem to hold that if even one molecule of a substance affects a property, the owner can seek stigma damages and that the jury should determine whether and how much that stigma affects the value of the property. A few courts have permitted stigma claims where there is no physical impact, focusing on whether it is *reasonable* to believe the property is affected, but this is likely a minority position. For most courts, however, the simple act of being located next to a hazardous waste landfill or a leaking underground storage tank cannot constitute a stigma claim when nothing from the landfill or the tank has affected the property. Otherwise, simply living next to a morgue or a strip club might imply stigma damages, a result with negative public policy implications. This may, however, be a nuisance if the elements of a nuisance are met.

Statutory Remedies for Property Damages from Environmental Exposures

The perceived failure of the tort system—including the failure of claims of nuisance and trespass—to protect human health and the environment was the main reason Congress enacted a wide range of environmental laws in the 1960s, 1970s, and 1980s. These laws empowered certain regulatory agencies—in particular, the U.S. Environmental Protection Agency—to take action to protect human health and the environment. Under these environmental laws, federal and state environmental agencies were given the responsibility and resources to protect the environment. (These laws and agency functions are discussed in Chapter Thirty-Three.)

Citizen Suits. In certain situations environmental statutes permit private citizens to become, in effect, private attorneys general and to enforce the environmental requirements as if they were the regulatory authorities. Under these *citizen suit* provisions, private parties can enforce environmental regulations, traditionally the province of regulatory agencies. Although they differ from statute to statute, the citizen suit provisions limit a private party's action to those situations where the agency in charge has taken no action or has taken inadequate action. In the case of the leaking underground storage tank contaminating groundwater, for example, it may be possible to file a citizen suit under the Resource Conservation and Recovery Act (RCRA) to seek an injunction to force the remediation of contaminated groundwater when the groundwater concentrations are above the *maximum contaminant level.* Under RCRA's citizen suit provision, an adjacent property owner may be able to force the operator of the underground storage tank to install new monitoring devices or take other remedial action. Under these citizen suit provisions, attorney fees and expert witness expenses may be awarded to the prevailing party, an attractive feature to many plaintiffs.

Cost Recovery Actions. Other environmental statutes permit private parties to seek compensation for cleanup costs. Take the case of a shopping center contaminated by a tenant's improper waste disposal from a dry-cleaning facility. If required to clean up dry-cleaning solvent contamination in soil or groundwater, the landlord may be able to file a *cost recovery* claim against the tenant under CERCLA or a state Superfund regulation to recover the costs necessary to investigate or clean up the groundwater. Under CERCLA a private party can recover the costs incurred in investigating and remediating contaminated sites.

In fact the most common environmental lawsuit throughout the 1980s and 1990s was the cost recovery action, brought by the government and by private parties. As thousands of contaminated sites were identified in the 1980s and 1990s, the U.S. Environmental Protection Agency (EPA) took action to force *potentially responsible parties* (PRPs) to clean up these sites. If these PRPs would not assist in the cleanup, the EPA would clean up the site itself and then file a cost recovery action. PRPs that settled with the EPA would then file a cost recovery action against the nonsettling parties to recover their share of the cleanup. To win a cost recovery claim, the claimant must meet a number of procedural and substantive requirements, including the requirement of public notice prior to cleanup.

Complexity of Environmental Laws. Whether the subject is contaminated sites, wetlands, or air quality, the applicable environmental statutes are complex. Few environmental laws are intuitive. Almost all the standard environmental laws contain intricate liability frameworks, complex technical definitions, and numerous exclusions, all often implemented by an agency through formal and informal guidance. To illustrate, a spill of PCBs on a concrete floor would be governed by the

Toxic Substances Control Act, but a spill of PERC on unpaved soil might be governed by CERCLA, depending on the quantity of PERC released. A release of either PERC or PCBs from an underground storage tank would be regulated by the Resource Conservation and Recovery Act, but a release of PERC from an aboveground storage tank would not be regulated by that Act. At the same time, an airborne release of PERC or PCBs would be regulated by CERCLA or the Clean Air Act, or both, depending on the quantity of PERC and PCBs and on the molecular weight of the PCBs released. Unfortunately, the only way to know these differences is to know the fine technical distinctions in the law.

For private parties seeking to clean up a contaminated site, the hypertechnical hurdles contained in most environmental laws create very real legal challenges. Because *petroleum products* are excluded from CERCLA's definition of *hazardous substances,* CERCLA cannot be used to recover cleanup costs when the cleanup involves only petroleum contamination. Legally, this means the owner of property contaminated by a leaking underground gasoline storage tank on an adjacent property cannot use CERCLA to recover associated cleanup costs. However, if lead, which is included in CERCLA's *hazardous substance* definition, were also contained in the groundwater plume from the underground storage tank, it might be possible to use CERCLA to recover costs associated with the contamination. But CERCLA has additional limitations. It cannot be used to recover for diminution in property value resulting from contamination or to recover medical monitoring expenses. To recover the petroleum contamination cleanup costs, a property owner would be required to file a tort claim, such as negligence, nuisance, or trespass. To effect a complete recovery for many property damages, accordingly, an injured party must file both common law and statutory claims.

Implications and Discussion

The chief complaint about the tort system is its ineffectiveness. According to the Congressional Budget Office (2003), available data show that in the tort system, people who file claims receive an average of 46 cents from each direct dollar spent (with the other 54 cents going to attorney's fees and insurance expenses). Others estimate that 54 percent of total tort costs are expenses rather than transfers: 19 percent to claimant's attorney fees, 14 percent to defense costs, and 21 percent to defense administrative costs. Of the 46 percent of the funds that is actually compensation for injured parties, 22 percent is for awards for economic loss and 24 percent is for awards for pain and suffering (Tillinghast-Towers Perrin, 2004).

Second, along with this perceived inequity, the tort system also appears to overcompensate less-injured claimants and undercompensate more-injured claimants. In the context of automobile accidents, it has been estimated that for losses less than $500, people receive almost four and a half times their loss in the tort system, but people with over $25,000 in expenses receive only about a third of their costs (Hager, 1998). That litigation costs in the tort system add up quickly is not surprising. A board-certified toxicologist typically charges $250 to $500 per hour, and it is not unusual for a toxicologist to spend several weeks reviewing medical records, researching the scientific and medical literature, and otherwise preparing for a deposition or a trial. If the toxicologist spends two weeks on a case, the cost of this one expert may exceed $18,000. With the typical exposure case having ten to fifteen experts on each side, the costs skyrocket.

A third criticism leveled against the tort system is its arbitrariness. An individual claiming asbestos exposure in a Mississippi court is, other things being equal, far more likely to recover damages than is an individual claiming asbestos exposure in a New Jersey court. A fourth criticism concerns the tort system's lack of speed. It is not unusual for lawsuits to take years to reach final resolution. It may be seven to fifteen years from the time the case is filed before an asbestos exposure claimant has his day in court. Yet another criticism is the nature of the participants. Under the tort system, judges and juries decide the key issues, legal and technical, although they may have absolutely no expertise or experience with the subject matter at hand. Particularly in the context of punitive damage, awards by juries often do not reflect the true state of the scientific literature.

Largely as a result of these perceived shortcomings, a number of changes to the current tort system have been proposed. Several state legislatures have taken measures to reduce the filing of claims by shortening statutes of limitations, capping legal fees, and setting limits for punitive damage and noneconomic loss awards (Furrow and others, 2000). Strategies taken by other legislatures to control the tort system include increasing the plaintiff's burden of proof, forcing more pretrial review of cases, and requiring mandatory alternative dispute resolution.

No-Fault Proposals

Theoretically a strong medicine for the tort system, no-fault programs have turned out to be no panacea, and the actual strengths and weaknesses of these programs remain largely undocumented. Ironically, in one empirical evaluation of no-fault automobile accident programs, the number of collisions actually increased following the enactment of a no-fault liability program (Cummins, Phillips, and Weiss, 2001). Apparently, without the threat of tort liability, drivers actually acted more carelessly. This may explain why no-fault programs exist in only twenty-six states plus the District of Columbia and Puerto Rico, and it may also explain why several other states have recently repealed no-fault automobile insurance programs (Hager, 1998).

The lack of strong evidence one way or the other on the efficiency and effectiveness of no-fault programs reflects the small universe of substances, injuries, and damages covered by these programs. The best available data show that the *transaction costs* for no-fault systems are proportionately much smaller than in the tort system. According to the National Academy of Social Insurance, only 23 cents out of every dollar of workers' compensation claims goes to administrative costs. Under the National Childhood Vaccine Injury Act, administrative costs are estimated to be 15 percent of the total compensation award (Congressional Budget Office, 2003). In an assessment of the Virginia Birth-Related Neurological Injury Compensation Act of 1987, only 10.3 percent of total spending went to dispute resolution (Bovbjerg, Sloan, and Rankin, 1997).

Despite the main selling point of more dollars going to compensation, the existence of a no-fault program may not equate to less litigation. The best example of this may be the National Childhood Vaccine Injury Act, the most frequently cited example of a model no-fault program. As of 1999, there were more than 1,000 published decisions, including 1 decision by the U.S. Supreme Court and 38 opinions from U.S. Courts of Appeals (Ridgway, 1999). At issue in these disputes are challenges to an applicant's compliance with the filing requirements, disagreement over the cause of the injury, doubts over the credibility of witnesses, and disputes over the amount of compensation (Mariner, 1992). Similarly, a leading assessment of the Florida Birth-Related Neurological Injury Compensation Act concludes its success as a no-fault program is only "modest" (Studdert, Fritz, and Brennan, 2000). Implementation of this no-fault program failed to steer cases away from the tort system; litigation over negligence in birth-related neurological injuries occurred almost as frequently in the years after the plan as before it.

Why Does the Tort System Survive?

Why are some injuries or exposures covered by a no-fault administrative compensation fund while others are not? Clearly, no single event motivates Congress or state legislatures to move certain injuries out of the tort system (Culhane, 2003). One cynical explanation is that plaintiffs' lawyers exert undue influence on policy. No doubt special interests influence how Congress and state legislatures enact public policy, but in the case of no-fault programs, it is doubtful that one group holds the legislative reins tightly enough to perpetuate the tort system.

A more likely basic explanation for the continued survival of the tort system is legislative inertia. The tort system is the default system in the United States, for better or worse, and unless or until a legal crisis comes along that forces elected officials on both sides of the aisle to believe that change is required, that system will not change. In the case of asbestos litigation—a situation that everyone agrees is a crisis—the lack of any legislative change to the tort system and the lack of a no-fault system are probably explained by several realities, including the absence of congressional agreement on the elements of a no-fault system for asbestos claims and the continued success of plantiffs' lawyers in filing lawsuits under the current system. For many environmental exposures, advocates of no-fault systems or administrative compensation funds have been unable to organize enough votes to revise the system.

However, congressional reluctance to alter the tort system may also simply reflect the superior theory underlying the tort system—deterrence and corrective justice. In the tort system a plaintiff files suit to compensate a loss, and if the plaintiff wins, the culpable party pays for the injury, not the plaintiff and not the federal government. And if society knows the culpable party paid for the injury, that result will deter others from committing the same type of injury, at least theoretically.

In contrast, the theory driving no-fault systems is equality in distribution of compensation. The costs of remedying a wrong are paid out of a common fund funded by taxes or other mechanisms. The main attribute is efficient compensation allocation, not blame, not deterrence, and not corrective justice. A second attribute is a framework in which professionals, whether special masters, bureaucrats, or claims processors, make the key decisions. A no-fault or administrative compensation system focuses on addressing the victim's injuries. It does not address whether all the losses—economic and noneconomic—are being recovered.

In deciding to keep the tort system, Congress and the state legislatures may simply be embracing the tort system's fundamental focus on deterrence and corrective justice. Even with its gross ineffectiveness in getting compensation to the truly injured, the tort system may be preferred over a no-fault framework on the purely philosophical grounds that no administrative system should replace the tort system when culpable parties are available to pay for the wrongdoing causing the harm. Because no-fault offers little deterrence, it is unlikely to replace the tort system.

Similarly, it may be that the tort system survives because it guarantees that an individual will have his or her day in court. Few legal protections in the United States are as sacred as a citizen's day in court, and it may be that any displacement of the tort system by no-fault programs impermissibly dilutes a citizen's day in court. Other things being equal, Congress probably views juries as more fundamental to democracy than regulatory decision makers. Again, it may be that Congress continues to keep the tort system because it keeps the jury system at the forefront of legal decision making. It may be that Congress and the state legislatures realize that but for plaintiffs' lawyers operating in the tort system, tobacco reform would have been unlikely. Given a choice between the tort system with judges and juries making decisions and a bureaucracy charged with operating an administrative compensation framework, Congress apparently gives the nod to juries.

What Prompts the Creation of No-Fault Frameworks or Administrative Compensation Funds?

The main reason some injuries are taken out of the tort system apparently is a legislative concern about the survival of a class of defendants if a no-fault or compensation system is *not* implemented. In the case of the National Childhood Vaccine Injury Act, for example, Congress was concerned that a safe and effective supply of vaccines could not be established if vaccine producers were defending lawsuits. In some cases, Congress enacts a social insurance program, such as the Price-Anderson Act, or an administrative compensation fund, but the motivation is the same.

Concern for the financial health of a certain category of defendants prompted the creation of the September 11th Victim Compensation Fund. A few days after the September 11, 2001, tragedy, Congress enacted the Air Transportation Safety and Stabilization Act, which provided substantial financial incentives to the airline industry and limited the personal injury liability associated with the terrorist hijackings and crashes. In return for limiting the airline industry's liability, Democrats in Congress pushed for a no-fault compensation fund, which became the September 11th Victim Compensation Fund. According to one observer, the fund was part of the bailout of the airline industry following the disaster (Diller, 2003). The fund provides that victims of the September 11 attack can receive an allocated compensation provided they agree not to file claims against the airline industry.

By enacting any administrative compensation program, legislatures are also sending a message. By protecting those with personal losses from September 11, for example, Congress was also reassuring Americans that if they were to fall victim to a terrorist attack, their families would be well cared for (Diller, 2003). The same can be said about the smallpox vaccine program for emergency workers. Congress wanted to ensure that if any of these workers died from the vaccine, their families would at least not be destroyed financially.

Historically, Congress has also enacted no-fault or administrative compensation programs to encourage certain behaviors. In the case of the smallpox vaccinations, Congress wanted to make sure that anyone receiving the smallpox vaccination would not be required to pursue claims through the normal tort system. In the case of black lung and certain other diseases, Congress enacted administrative compensation funds because of concern for workers so clearly affected by one exposure. But it is still difficult to understand why dock workers exposed to asbestos have no administrative compensation system while miners exposed to coal dust do.

No matter how many perspectives are considered, there are still no logical explanations for addressing some matters outside the tort system and leaving others matter within the tort system. For example, emergency workers exposed to asbestos more than seventy-two hours after the September 11, 2001, World Trade Center collapse were not provided compensation as a matter of law, but those exposed to asbestos-containing dust a few hours after the collapse were. Victims of the Oklahoma City bombings received no compensation from the U.S. government; their families were required to file suit to try to collect damages. Yet the average award from the September 11th Victim Compensation Fund is $1.6 million per estate.

Conclusion

Environmental public health aims to prevent hazardous exposures and to control the risks of those exposures that do occur. When exposures nonetheless occur, appropriate remedies serve important purposes. As a matter of social justice, remedies help to compensate people who have been harmed. And as a matter of public health, remedies can represent incentives that prevent additional exposures.

Remedies may result from private actions in the tort law system or from social mechanisms such as compensation funds. Neither approach is perfect. Tort law has been criticized for being inefficient, costly, and arbitrary, although tort actions have provided compensation to many harmed by environmental exposures and may be credited with helping to reduce exposures to such hazards as asbestos and second-hand cigarette smoke. Administrative compensation schemes may also appear inconsistent and arbitrary. Individuals with nearly identical diseases and exposed to nearly identical substances often have vastly different legal remedies available. An individual with a work-related disease is eligible for workers' compensation, and an individual with the identical disease resulting from environmental exposures may end up with no recovery options. Nevertheless, systems such as the Black Lung Program have provided compensation to thousands of disease victims in a manner that is generally equitable, transparent, and economically efficient. Each of these approaches to remedies needs to be improved.

Despite the best preventive efforts, hazardous exposures are likely to continue to occur, and fair and efficient remedies are likely to remain necessary.

Thought Questions

1. Should judges or juries decide issues of causation in exposure cases, or is that decision best left to professionals?
2. Who has improved environmental health more: plaintiffs' lawyers, regulators, or elected representatives?
3. Why does the tort system survive, given that a no-fault liability framework has demonstrably lower costs?
4. Is there really a litigation crisis in mass tort exposure cases—involving, say, breast implants, asbestos, or tobacco—or is the problem simply that too many hazardous exposures are permitted to occur?

References

Biggs, J. L. "Proposed Resolution Regarding the Need for Effective Asbestos Reform." Statement of Jennifer L. Biggs, FCAS, MAAA Chairperson, Mass Torts Subcommittee, American Academy of Actuaries, July 10, 2003.

Bovbjerg, R. R., Sloan, F. A., and Rankin, P. J. "Administrative Performance of 'No-Fault' Compensation for Medical Injury." *Law & Contemporary Problems,* 1997, *60,* 71–115.

Carroll, S. J., and others. *Asbestos Litigation Costs and Compensation: An Interim Report.* Santa Monica, Calif.: Rand, 2002.

Congressional Budget Office. *The Economics of U.S. Tort Liability: A Primer.* Washington, D.C.: Congressional Budget Office, 2003.

Cranor, C. F. *Regulating Toxic Substances: A Philosophy of Science and the Law.* New York: Oxford University Press, 1993.

Culhane, J. G. "Tort, Compensation, and Two Kinds of Justice." *Rutgers Law Review,* 2003, *55,* 1027–1107.

Cummins, J. D., Phillips, R. D., and Weiss, M. A. "The Incentive Effects of No-Fault Automobile Insurance." *Journal of Law & Economics,* 2001, *44,* 427–461.

Diller, M. "Tort and Social Welfare Principles in the Victim Compensation Fund." *DePaul Law Review,* 2003, *53,* 719–768.

Furrow, B. R., and others. *Health Law.* (2nd ed.) Hornbook Series. St. Paul, Minn.: West, 2000.

Green, M. Prepared Statement of Professor Michael Green Concerning S. 758, The Fairness in Asbestos Compensation Act of 1999. Hearing of the Subcommittee on Administrative Oversight and the Courts of the Senate Committees on the Judiciary, October 5, 1999. [http://judiciary.senate.gov/oldsite/10599mg.htm]. 1999.

Hager, M. M. "No-Fault Drives Again: A Contemporary Primer." *University of Miami Law Review,* 1998, *52,* 793–830.

Kanner, A. "Theories of Recovery in Toxic Tort Litigation." *Trial Lawyer,* 2000, *23,* 130–158.

Kanner, A. *Environmental and Toxic Tort Trials.* Dayton, Ohio: LexisNexis, 2002.

Kole, J. S., and Nye, S. *Environmental Litigation.* (2nd ed.) Chicago, Ill.: American Bar Association, 1999.

Mariner, W. K. "The National Vaccine Injury Compensation Program." *Health Affairs,* 1992, *11*(1), 255–265.

Mullenix, L. S., and Stewart, K. B. "The September 11th Victim Compensation Fund: Fund Approaches to Resolving Mass Tort Litigation." *Connecticut Insurance Law Journal,* 2002–2003, *9,* 121–152.

Ridgway, D. "No-Fault Vaccine Insurance: Lessons from the National Vaccine Injury Compensation Program." *Journal of Health Politics, Policy and Law,* 1999, *24,* 59–90.

Studdert, D. M., Fritz, L. A., and Brennan, T. A. "The Jury Is Still In: Florida's Birth-Related Neurological Injury Compensation Plan After a Decade." *Journal of Health Politics, Policy and Law,* 2000, *25,* 499–526.

Tillinghast-Towers Perrin. *U.S. Tort Costs: 2003 Update: Trends and Findings on the Costs of the U.S. Tort System.* New York: Tillinghast-Towers Perrin, 2004.

White, M. J. "Asbestos and the Future of Mass Torts." NBER Working Paper 10308. [http://papers.nber.org/papers/w10308.pdf]. Feb. 2004.

Name Index

A

Aaron-Thomas, A., 323
Abdel-Rahman, A. A., 550*b*
Abel, D., 114
Aber, J. D., 4, 19
Abraham, J. L., 333, 334
Abraham, M. H., 639
Abram, D., 783
Abylkassimova, Z., 275
Ackermann-Liebrich, U., 345
Adler, N. E., 393
Agarwal, A., 227
Agricola, G., 649
Aha, Rabbi, 212
Akesson, A., 313
Akhmedova, S., 134
Akiva, R., 210
Al-Mufti, A. W., 598
Alavanja, M.C.R., 566, 567
Albalak, R., 309, 310, 375
Albers, J. W., 278
Albert, D. P., 938
Albert, M. J., 488
Alefeld, G., 954
Alexander, C., 108, 110
Allen, D., 436
Allen, D. E., 757
Allen, D. T., 787
Alm, J., 315
Altman, I., 99, 104, 108
Altomare, M., 875
Altshuler, D., 136
Anane, R., 704
Andersen, L. B., 425
Anderson, A., 617
Anderson, D. H., 793
Anderson, W. P., 786
Andrews, R.N.L., 980, 982
Andrulis, D. P., 397
Anisimov, S., 134
Annas, G. J., 677
Annest, J. L., 350
Anto, J. M., 1029
Anton, M. T., 793
Antonovsky, A., 99
Appleyard, D., 109
Aquinas, T., 199
Arghababian, R. V., 753
Armstrong, B. K., 700, 701
Arquette, M., 179
Arvanitidou, M., 489
Astakhova, L. N., 692
Astrop, A., 323
Atherholt, T. B., 253, 254
Atkinson, J. O., 807
Ausubel, J. H., 6
Autier, P., 749
Aw, J., 251, 252
Azizi, F., 809

B

Babisch, W., 438
Baccarelli, A., 31
Back, K., 109
Bailey, R., 725
Bais, A., 701
Baker, D., 661
Baker, D. B., 254
Baker, S. P., 726
Bakir, F., 598
Balakrishnan, K., 309, 310
Balbus, J., 414
Balk, S. J., 822
Bammer, G., 382
Band, L., 486
Banken, R., 382
Barker, R. G., 97, 101, 112
Barker, S. B., 786
Barlow, S. E., 434

Barnes, D. F., 367
Barron, G., 909–911
Barry, M., 564
Bartell, S., 940
Bartram, J., 466, 502, 503
Baum, A., 108
Baxter, P. J., 759
Beaglehole, R., 99
Beasley, R., 315
Beauchamp, T. L., 148
Becalski, A., 42
Bechtel, R. B., 97, 99
Beck, A. M., 785, 786, 787
Becker, A. B., 191
Becker, C. E., 1013
Behrens, W. W., 408
Belkic['], K., 437
Bell, M. L., 331, 332, 333, 334, 347
Bellet, S., 436
Bellinger, D., 832
Bellow, S., 389
Bende, M., 632
Bennet, G. W., 548, 551, 552, 553, 555, 556, 558
Bennett, L. W., 793
Benson, M., 768
Bentham, G., 260
Berent, S., 278
Berglund, M., 313
Berkman, L. F., 109, 398
Berkowitz, G. S., 808, 832, 835
Berman, D. S., 793
Bernard, B. P., 655
Bernard, S. M., 250, 251
Bernstein, P. L., 941
Berry, C. L., 333, 334
Betazzi, P.A., 31
Bhuiyan, S. I., 318
Bickers, D. R., 701
Bienbaum, A., 793
Biggs, J. L., 1045*b*, 1046*b*
Bikir, F., 808
Bisesi, M., 73, 99
Bjorn, L. O., 701
Black, R. E., 306
Blackburn, R., 225
Blair, S. N., 433, 434
Blancet, T., 726
Blanchard, A., 104, 116, 119
Blanchard, F. T., 564
Block, G., 432
Blomberg, R. D., 724
Blot, W. J., 808
Blue, I., 409
Blumenthal, G. M., 832
Board, P. G., 134
Bock, S., 920
Bodin, M., 794*b*
Bohonos, J. J., 757
Bolen, E., 617
Boorman, G. A., 497
Borda, A. I., 598
Bornehag, C. G., 631, 642
Bouma, M., 257
Bouman, B.A.M., 318
Boutin, B. K., 497
Bovbjerg, R. R., 1061
Bowman, D., 951
Boy, E., 375
Brauer, M., 429
Breiman, R. F., 488
Brener, N. D., 618*b*
Brennan, T. A., 1061
Brenner, S. A., 757
Briassoulis, G., 820
Briggs, D., 806
Brill, M., 105, 108
Brimblecombe, P., 331, 625
Brison, R. J., 424
Brissette, I., 398
Brock, J. W., 818
Brody, H., 927
Broeckaert, F., 343
Broman, S., 835
Bronzaft, A. L., 107
Brook, R. D., 343
Brooks-Gunn, J., 408
Broom, L. A., 756
Brown, B., 110, 438
Brown, L., 225, 227, 232
Brown, P., 685
Browne, A., 787
Brownson, R. C., 564
Bruce, N., 309, 310, 375
Brundtland, G. H., 889
Brunekreef, B., 429
Bryant, D., 228
Buck, G. M., 312
Buechley, R. W., 246
Buescher, M. D., 550*b*
Bullard, R. D., 120, 174
Bullinger, M., 108, 439
Bunn, F., 724
Burch, J., 756
Burdick, P. A., 829
Burdon, J. G., 315
Burke, G., 723
Burke, T. A., 900
Burton, S., 409
Burton, W. N., 632
Burwell, D., 173
Buse, K., 298
Bush, G. W., 283, 776, 964*b*
Bush, M. B., 3
Butler, J. C., 488
Butter, M. E., 290, 310
Butterfield, B., 787
Butts, W. L., 548, 551, 552, 553, 555, 556, 558
Byers, E. S., 794

C

Caballero, B., 306
Cabello, F., 487
Cai, M., 246
Cairnes, H., 783
Calabrese, E. J., 952
Calderón-Garcidueñas, L., 340
Caldwell, G., 56
Caldwell, M. M., 702
Camann, D. E., 564
Cameron, J., 864
Cameron, P. A., 768
Campbell, A., 101
Campbell, C., 811b
Campbell, C. G., 832
Cannuscio, C. C., 435
Canon, L. K., 109
Cantor, N., 557
Cardone, S., 793
Carlin, J. B., 315
Carlson, J. E., 829
Carrillo, J. A., 808
Carroll, M. D., 434
Carroll, S. J., 1046*b*
Carson, R., 545, 567, 570, 897, 972
Carter, A. O., 757
Cassel, C. K., 148
Cassel, J., 99
Cassis, G., 781
Castaneda, A. R., 318
Castells, M., 119
Casterline, J. B., 398
Caulfield, F., 251
Cave, B., 382

Chadwick, E., 896
Champion, H. R., 768
Chan T'sai, 200
Chapin, F. S., III, 4
Chavis, B. F., Jr., 172
Checkley, W., 233, 254, 255
Cheek, A. O., 31
Chen, D., 393
Cheng, M. F., 497
Cherniak, M., 172
Chiaverini, Sister, 935
Childress, J. F., 148
Chilima, D. M., 306
Chiou, H. Y., 827
Chiu, H. F., 497
Chivian, E., 232
Choi, S. M., 31
Chorus, I., 466
Chotani, H., 726
Christoffel, T., 724
Churchman, A., 99
Ciccone, G., 429
Cifuentes, L., 357
Cimprich, B., 784, 791
Cincotta, R. P., 230
Cirillo, J. D., 480
Clark, E. G., 852
Clark, R. M., 497
Clarke, R., 457, 461
Claudiio, L., 133
Clauw, D. J., 278
Clemen, R. T., 948
Clement, G., 148
Clinton, B., 184, 812
Clitheroe, C., 96, 98, 100, 102
Clutton-Brock, J., 785
Cobey, J. C., 279
Codd, G. A., 466
Coffin, M., 849
Cohen, A. J., 308
Cohen, B., 420
Cohen, C., 100, 103, 107
Cohen, D. A., 395, 404, 406
Cohen, J., 223, 226, 232
Cohen, M. A., 728
Cohen, S., 108, 109, 118
Cohill, A., 119
Colan, N. B., 794
Colditz, G. A., 435
Cole, R., 482
Coleman, M. P., 246
Colford, J. M., Jr., 62, 65, 66
Collett, D., 951
Collins, F. S., 129, 132
Columbus, C., 172
Colville, F., 705, 707
Colwell, R. R., 254, 479, 480, 483, 488
Conolly, R. B., 832
Constantinides, T. C., 489
Constanza, R., 20, 21
Converse, K., 482
Cook, P. J., 728
Cookson, S. T., 643
Cooper, K. H., 434
Copeland, C., 970, 971
Corrigan, J., 118
Corvalan, C., 291
Coto, J. A., 719
Coussens, C., 129
Coutsoundis, A., 311
Covello, V. T., 988
Cowan, M. L., 770
Cox, S. E., 465
Cox, T., 228
Coyle, M., 174
Cranor, C. F., 1034
Crenson, M., 226
Cresteil, T., 832
Crick, F.H.C., 131
Cridland, N. A., 699, 700, 701
Criss, R. E., 19
Cromley, E. K., 937, 938
Cropper, M., 322
Crump, K. S., 949
Culerrier, R. M., 701
Culhane, J. G., 1061
Cumberland, W. G., 103
Cumes, D., 793
Cummins, J. D., 1060
Curl, C. L., 818, 869
Curriero, F., 244, 253, 254
Curtis, C. F., 574*b*
Curtis, S., 382
Cutler, D., 406
Czarny, D., 315

D

Dahlback, A., 701
Daigle, C. C., 340
Daily, G. C., 20, 781
Dalager, N. A., 274, 275
Dalaker, J., 564
Dalgado, H., 310
Dannenberg, A. L., 724
Darby, S. C., 691
Darwin, J., 731
Dato, V., 592
Davies, H. G., 128, 134
Davis, D. L., 332, 333, 334
Davis, J. R., 564
Davis-Berman, J., 793
Davisson, M. L., 19
Davy, J., 36
Dawson, K. S., 786
Day, J. F., 549*b*, 550*b*
Dayananda, Swami, 207
de Bruycker, M., 761, 762
de Kok, T., 99
de Ville de Goyer, C., 749, 776
Dearborn, D., 642
Dearry, A., 190, 829
Deddens, J., 67
Deffeyes, K. S., 369
DeGroot, M. H., 954, 955
den Broeder, L., 382
Dennison, B. A., 829
Detels, R., 99
Devlin, R. B., 340
Dewailly, E., 816*b*
Dhara, R., 665
Dhara, V. R., 665
Diabate, S., 376
Diana, Princess, 722*b*–723*b*
Dickens, C., 332*b*, 403
Dietrich, K. N., 49
Diette, G. B., 793
Dietz, W. H., Jr., 434, 435, 829
Diez Roux, A. V., 103, 104, 617, 828
Diffey, B., 701
Dijkstra, L., 417, 425
DiLiberti, J. H., 807
Diller, M., 1063
Dixon, B., 910
Dobson, A. J., 950
Docherty, D., 482
Dockery, D. W., 339, 343, 429
Doebbeling, B. N., 437, 438
Dohrenwend, B. P., 403
Dohrenwend, B. S., 403
Doll, R., 128, 691, 696
Donaldson, M. S., 118
Dong, L., 432
Dooley, D., 102

Doos, B., 227
Dora, C., 382
Douglas, M. J., 382
Dowd, J., 367
Dowie, M., 177
Doyle, S., 395
Draper, R. J., 787
Driscoll, C.M.H., 699, 700, 701
Driver, B. L., 793
Duarte, J. M., 376
Duhme, H., 429
Duperrex, O., 724
Durkheim, É, 403
Dwight, R. H., 254
Dye, J. A., 343

E

Earls, F., 400, 405
Easterling, D. R., 461
Eastey, A. T., 793
Eberly, S., 49
Ecobichon, D. J., 301
Edwards, J., 429
Egeland, G. M., 352
Egorov, A. I., 489
Ehrenberg, R., 56
Ehrhart, J. C., 701
Ehrlich, P., 223
Eisenberg, J.N.S., 62, 65, 66
Eldredge, N., 230
Elgethun, K., 818, 869
Ellegard, A., 313, 314
Ellenbog, U., 649
Elliott, H., 150
Elliott, M., 396
Ellis, W. S., 460
Elvik, R., 736
Elwood, J. M., 704
Engel, L. S., 818
Engelke, P. O., 115, 425
Engelman, R., 230, 459
Engels, F., 144
Engleman, R., 233
English, D. R., 700, 701
Epstein, P. R., 232, 258, 851
Epstein, Y. M., 108
Erbring, L., 118
Eriksson, J. G., 811*b*
Eriksson, K.-E., 874*b*
Esty, D. C., 979
Etheridge, D. M., 238
Ettinger, A., 564
Etzel, R.A., 822
Evans, G. W., 10, 100, 103, 107, 108, 120, 438, 439, 784, 791
Evans, L., 732
Evans, M., 955
Evans, N. J., 691
Ewing, R., 3993
Ezzati, M., 309, 310, 375, 400

F

Faber, D. R., 170
Fabian, A. K., 105
Fabian, R., 948
Faghihi, M., 310
Fagin, D., 862
Falchero, S., 791
Falk, H., 311, 519
Fancey, R. J., 238
Fanger, P. O., 631
Fanning, A., 643
Faruque, A. S., 254, 255
Faruque, S. M., 488
Faustman, E. M., 950
Fauveau, U., 726
Fayed, D., 722b
Fehr, R., 382
Fenske, R., 869
Fenske, R. A., 818
Ferencz, C., 818
Ferguson, S. A., 726
Ferson, S., 954, 955
Festinger, L., 109, 398
Fewtrell, L., 503
Fielder, N., 1028
Fielding, J. E., 102, 103, 114
Finch, C. F., 768
Fine, J., 279
Fineberg, H. V., 181
Fiorino, D. J., 978
Firket, J., 332
Fischer, G., 260
Fisher, B., 110
FitzGerald, J. M., 643
Flegal, K. M., 434
Fleming, C., 700, 701
Fletcher, T., 333, 334
Floor, W. M., 367
Fly, F., 179
Foegeding, P. M., 582
Folkman, A., 617*b*
Folkman, K. L., 617*b*
Ford, T., 381, 454, 465, 477, 479, 483, 488, 496, 498, 504, 506
Forgas, J. P., 100
Forjuoh, S. N., 725
Forman, J., 805
Forman, V. L., 406
Fortune, C. R., 564
Fox, J. E., 31
Fox, S., 783
Fradin, M. S., 549*b*, 550*b*
Frank, A. L., 702
Frank, L. D., 115, 393, 425, 828
Frankenhaeuser, M., 436
Frazier, A. L., 435
Frederickson, L. M., 793
Freedman, S., 486
Freeman, N.C.G., 564
Freese, B., 369
Friedman, B., 436
Friedman, E., 786
Friedman, G. D., 720
Friedman-Jiménez, G., 671
Fritz, L. A., 1061
Frohberg, K., 260
Frumkin, H., 99, 324, 393, 671, 705*b*, 781, 788, 795, 828
Fry, S. A., 692
Fuchs, G., 254, 255
Furlong, C., 134
Furrow, B. R., 1060
Futterman, L. G., 835

G

Gabbe, B. J., 768
Gahan, J. B., 573*b*
Galanti, M. R., 275
Gale, J. L., 808
Gale, P., 502, 503
Galea, S., 191, 387
Gallagher, K. P., 979
Gallichhio, L., 312
Galvez, M., 805
Gansier, T., 705*b*
Garces, R. F., 119
Garcia, R., 564
Gardner, G., 225, 232
Gardner, M. J., 691
Garfield, R. M., 270
Garland, C. A., 110
Garner, C. H., 768

Garner, P., 323, 405, 736
Gauderman, W. J., 347
Gauna, J., 174
Gay, J. M., 481
Geldreich, E. E., 481
Geller, E. S., 787
Gerber, G. J., 787
Gerlach-Spriggs, N., 788
Gerr, F., 655
Gershenfeld, H. K., 278
Gesler, W. M., 938
Gibbons, L. W., 434
Gibbs, L., 898
Gibson, J. L., 808
Gifford, R., 97
Gill, A. C., 725
Ginsberg, G., 832
Ginsburg, M. J., 726
Githeko, A., 257
Glacken, C. J., 145
Glad, J. A., 911
Gladen, B. C., 820
Glass, D. C., 108
Glass, G. E., 258, 259
Glass, T., 398
Glasziou, P. P., 948
Gleick, P. H., 457, 461
Golden, R. J., 31
Goldman, R., 1013
Goldstein, S., 390
Golley, F. B., 4, 10
Golshan, M., 310
Gomes, M. E., 796
Goodchild, M. F., 927, 938
Goodland, R., 223, 224
Goodstein, D., 369
Goodyear, N. N., 434
Gordis, L., 339
Gordon, S., 436
Gore, A., 812, 859*b*
Gortmaker, S. L., 829
Gotway, C. A., 932, 933, 937
Gould, P., 310
Gourney, J. G., 807
Graham, J., 867
Graham, M., 981
Graitcer, P. L., 724
Grandolfo, M., 705
Grant, E., 404
Grant, L. D., 702
Gray, W., 247
Greco, D., 762
Green, B. L., 247
Green, M., 1046*b*
Green, T. L., 791
Greenland, S., 46, 954
Greenway, R., 794
Griffin, M., 793*b*, 794*b*
Griffiths, R. K., 429
Grifo, F., 230
Grimes, D. J., 479, 504, 506
Grosselet, F. P., 701
Grossman, M., 112
Gschwend, P. M., 470
Gubler, D. J., 256, 257
Guenther, A., 251
Guess, H. A., 949
Guha-Sapir, D., 750
Guidotti, T., 99
Guillette, L. J., 567
Gulluck, T., 238
Gurunathan, S., 564

H

Haas, C. N., 944
Haddon, W., 720, 721, 722
Hager, M. M., 1060, 1061
Haggerty, R., 806
Hahn, R. A., 434
Haile, R. W., 63, 65
Haines, M., 438, 439
Haley, R., 278
Hall, E. J., 691
Hallegraeff, G. M., 254
Halweil, B., 225, 232
Hamilton, A., 650, 651*fig*, 1011
Hamilton, E., 783
Hamilton, G. C., 544, 553
Handy, S., 436
Hanfling, M. J., 724
Hanina ben Dosa, R., 212
Hanna, K., 129
Hanusa, B. H., 108
Harada, H., 807, 808
Hardell, L., 705*b*
Hardin, G., 151
Hardoy, J. E., 407
Hardy, R. J., 436
Harley, N. H., 699
Harper, L. C., 701
Harpham, T., 409
Harris, J., 867
Harris, P. Q., 793, 794
Harrison, K., 768
Hartig, T., 791, 794*b*
Hastings, N., 955
Hatzis, T., 820
Hau, W., 406
Haughton, G., 407
Hayes, T. B., 567
Haythornthwaite, C. A., 104, 105, 118
Head, J., 439
Heal, G. M., 20
Heckt, K., 617*b*
Hedberg, G., 437
Heerwagen, J. H., 783, 791, 792
Hein, H. O., 425
Helmrich, S. P., 434
Henderson, D. A., 1032
Henderson, J. A., 178
Hennessy, D. A., 437
Henriksen, T., 701
Henrion, M., 953
Herbst, A. L., 809
Hering, J. G., 470
Herzberger, J., 954
Hess, J. J., 715
Higman, K., 914
Hill, A. B., 46, 47, 66, 1019, 1042
Hill, B., 871, 872
Hill, J. O., 434
Hinrichsen, D., 221, 223, 224, 225, 228, 231
Hipp, J., 181
Hippocrates, 331, 649
Hirschhorn, R., 907–909
Hobbs, T. R., 793
Hodgson, M. J., 625, 631, 638, 642
Hoet, P.H.M., 332
Hogan, D. E., 757
Hogrefe, C., 251, 252
Holder, Y., 716
Holdren, J., 223
Holm, S., 867
Holman, E. A., 110
Holmberg, J., 874*b*, 875
Honeyman, M. K., 791
Hooper, C., 705
Hooper, K., 816*b*
Hoppin, J. A., 566, 567
Horan, T., 104, 116, 119
Hore, P., 564
Horowitz, M., 244, 245
Hosier, R. H., 367

Houghton, J., 16, 242
Howard, C. R., 49
Hricko, A., 814
Hrudey, E. J., 476
Hrudey, S. E., 476
Hshieh, P., 574*b*
Hsu, C. C., 820
Hu, F. B., 434
Hu, H., 648
Huang, S., 315
Hubby, M. M., 809
Huer, H. H., 702
Hull, R. B., 791
Hummon, N., 705
Huna, R., 201
Hunt, A., 333, 334
Hunt, D. L., 951
Hunter, C., 407
Hunter, N. L., 788
Hunter, P. R., 317, 489
Hüttenmoser, M., 785
Hwang, H. L., 820
Hyer, L., 793
Hygge, S., 108, 439

I

Iacono, S., 116
Ichihashi, M., 701
Ilyasd, M., 701
Imboden, D. M., 470
Ising, H., 438
Ismail, K., 278
Ismail, S. J., 306
Israel, B. A., 191
Ittelson, W. H., 97, 111

J

Jaakkola, J. J., 630
Jackson, C. R., 807
Jackson, R., 393
Jackson, R. J., 827, 828
Jacobs, G., 323
Jacobs, J., 112
Jacobson, A., 705*b*
Jacobson, J. L., 820, 832
Jacobson, S. W., 832
Jacobsson, K. A., 437
James, S., 875*b*
Jameton, A., 143
Jansen, J., 626, 628
Jarczyk, J., 793
Jargowsky, P., 393
Jarvik, G. P., 128, 134
Jarvis, W. R., 643
Jencks, C., 398
Jenkins, P. L., 829
Jennings, G. R., 786
Jensen, T. K., 818
Jerstad, L., 793, 794
Jeyaratnam, J., 301
Jinabhai, C. C., 311
Jines, J. D., 574*b*
Job, R. F., 439
Jodelet, D., 111
Johnson, B. L., 961, 975
Johnson, C. L., 434
Johnson, D., 108
Johnson, M., 288, 315
Johnson, N. F., 548, 550, 552, 553, 554
Johnson, S. P., 407
Joint, M., 437
Jones, T., 1029
Jordan, A., 864
Jordan, C. M., 49
Jorm, A. F., 786
Judah, R., 207
Judson, B., 333, 334

K

Kahane, C. J., 725
Kahle, S. C., 465
Kahn, O., 938
Kahn, P. H., Jr., 785
Kalnay, E., 246
Kalstein, L. S., 246
Kamada, N., 273
Kamel, F., 566, 567
Kaminoff, R., 105
Kammen, D. M., 309, 310, 367, 375
Kanellou, K., 489
Kang, H. K., 274, 275
Kanner, A. D., 796
Kant, I., 148
Kaplan, R., 115, 118, 782, 783, 784, 791, 792
Kaplan, S., 115, 118, 783, 791, 792
Kapp, C., 573, 574*b*
Karasek, R., 660
Karim, E., 301
Karpati, A., 404
Karter, M. J., 730
Kasperson, J., 225
Kasperson, R., 181, 182
Katcher, A. H., 785, 786, 787
Katsouyannopoulos, V., 489
Katspiyanni, K., 761
Kattenberg, A., 246
Kaufman, P. R., 420
Kaufman, R. E., 788
Kavanaugh, A., 119
Kavats, R. S., 263
Kawachi, I., 398
Keary, B. S., 310
Keifer, M. C., 545
Kelada, S. N., 134
Keller, B., 273
Kellerman, A. L., 719, 724
Kellermann, A. L., 715
Kellert, S. R., 785
Kelly-Schwartz, A. C., 395
Kelsey, J. L., 436
Kelsey, K. T., 272
Kemm, J., 382
Kendall, H., 227, 229
Kenkel, D., 948
Kennedy, B. P., 398, 793
Kent, J., 249, 250
Kessler, R. C., 403
Keug, E., 727, 728
Khabib, O., 277
Kickbusch, I., 298
Kiesler, S., 116
Kilbourne, E. M., 244
Kilner, T., 768
Kimmel, C. A., 831
King, C. H., 480
King, G., 398
King, M. L., Jr., 173
Kinicki, A., 396
Kinney, P. L., 428
Kipen, H. M., 1010, 1028
Kiszewski, A. E., 550
Kjaergaard, S. K., 632
Kjellström, T., 99, 291, 382
Klare, M. T., 372, 461
Klebanoff, M. A., 818
Kleeman, M. J., 251, 252
Kling, R., 116
Knudson, A. G., 689
Knudson, A. G., Jr., 950
Knutson, T. R., 247

Koenig, K. L., 768
Kofler, W. W., 439
Kogevinas, M., 761
Koh, D., 301
Kohn, L. T., 118
Kole, J. S., 1035
Kondo, I., 134
Konig, K. A., 172
Kopits, E., 322
Koren, H., 73, 99
Korpea, K., 791
Kossenko, M. M., 695
Kostis, J., 436
Kotchian, S., 895
Koty, R. L., 632
Kovats, R. S., 250, 262
Kovats, S., 245, 246
Krajinovic, M., 135
Kramer, J. E., 820
Kranner, A., 1039, 1041
Krantz, D. S., 103, 108
Kreiger, J., 191
Krewski, D., 343
Kricker, A., 700, 701
Kriebel, D., 867, 873*b*
Krieger, N., 441
Kripke, M. L., 701
Krohne, R. M., 3
Krug, E., 717
Kruglyak, A. K., 136
Kruppa, B., 438
Krzyzanowski, M., 308
Kuester, S., 618*b*
Kuller, L. H., 245, 246
Kundi, M., 705*b*
Kuo, F. E., 784, 789
Kurihara, Y., 247

L

Labruna, M. B., 376
Lacombe, M., 382
Laflammer, L., 726
Lahit, T., 875*b*
Lakish, R., 206
Lamb, R. J., 791
Lander, E., 136
Landrigan, P. J., 805, 807, 810, 813, 829, 861*b*
Landsbergis, P. A., 661
Landy, M. K., 969
Lange, J. L., 272
Langendoen, S., 437
Langenfields, R. L., 238
Langer, E. J., 108
Langford, I. H., 260
Langholz, B., 430
Lanphear, B. P., 49
Laortanakul, P., 438
Larsen, S., 701
Larson, L., 787
Lasker, R. D., 187, 188
Latham, S. M., 259
Lathan, S. M., 260
Latkin, C. A., 406
Lau, B. P., 42
Laumbach, R., 1010
Lavalle, M., 174
LaVeist, T. A., 617*b*
Lavelle, M., 862
Lawrence, C. E., 820
Lawrence, D., 909
Lawson, A. B., 933
Layng, E. M., 787
Le Couteur, D. G., 134
Leach, G., 367
Leatherman, S., 247, 249
Leavell, H., 852
Lechat, M. F., 750, 762
LeChevallier, M. W., 253, 254
LeCount, E. R., 436
Lee, A., 768
Lee, B. M., 31
Lee, C., 170, 171, 173, 174, 188
Lee, C. Y., 745
Lee, I. M., 435
Lee, S. H., 62
Legge, T. M., 1010–1011
Legler, J. M., 807
Legters, L. J., 574*b*
Leigh, J. P., 664
Leikin, J. B., 820
Leisenring, W. M., 950
Lele, S., 244, 253, 254
Lemberg, L., 835
Lengeler, C., 573*b*
Leong, S. T., 438
Lepore, S. J., 108
Lercher, P., 438
Lerer, L., 382
Leroux, B. G., 950
Lestina, D. C., 731
Leung, R. C., 315
Leung, R. W., 434
Leventhal, T., 408
Levergood, B., 938
Levi, L., 102
Levin, H., 638
Levin, R., 487
Levine, D., 793
Levy, B. S., 269, 854
Levy, P., 189
Levy, S. B., 481
Lewis, C. A., 110, 788
Lewis, D., 42
Lewis, R. G., 564
Li, G., 726
Li, W. F., 128, 134
Lillibridge, D. R., 757, 758
Lim, H. W., 701
Lin, S., 429
Linden, C., 313
Lindheim, R., 99
Linquist, A. W., 573*b*
Linthicum, K. J., 259
Lipman, R. M., 703
Lippmann, M., 347
Lipscomb, J. W., 820
Lipton, R. B., 632
Litman, T., 440
Liu, J., 311
Liu, Z., 134
Lochner, K., 398
Loffredo, C. A., 818
Loh, P., 428
London, L., 301
Longley, P. A., 927, 938
Longmire, A. W., 756
Longnecker, M. P., 574*b*
Loomis, D., 55
Lopez, A. D., 291, 404, 718
Lopman, B. A., 486
Lord, C. C., 556
Loretti, E. M., 246, 247
Loughlin, L. L., 574*b*
Lubchenco, J., 21, 232, 858
Luby, S. P., 717, 726
Lucier, G., 574*b*
Ludwig, J., 728
Lund, A. D., 724
Lund, E., 275
Lundberg, U., 436
Lushbaugh, C. C., 692
Lutz, S. M., 420
Lyman, P., 118
Lynch, K., 111

M

Maantay, J., 178
Mabaso, M. L., 573*b*
Mac Kenzie, W. R., 476, 502
McBride, W. G., 808
McCally, M., 148
McCarthy, D., 170, 247
McCarthy, J., 244, 249
McCarthy, J. E., 970, 974
McCarty, C. A., 701
McCaru, A. T., 727
McCauley, L., 278
McConnell, R., 545
McDonald, J. E., 734
MacDonald, J. M., 420
McDonald, T., 905, 912, 914, 915
McDonald, T. A., 816*b*
MacDorman, M. F., 807
Mace, G., 230
McEwen, B. S., 120, 393
McEweN, J., 99
McFeters, G. A., 480
McGee, K., 717
McGeehin, M. A., 311
McGuire, V., 49
Macher, J., 638
Macintyre, S., 617*b*, 829
McKenzie, R. L, 701
MacKenzie, W. R., 253, 254
McKeown, R. E., 159
McKibben, B., 21
MacLachian, C., 174
McLafferty, S. L., 937, 938
McLuhan, T. C., 783
Maclver, S., 829
McMahan, S., 102
McMichael, A. J., 246, 252, 253
McMichael, M., 408
McMichael, T., 232, 233, 382
McNeil, E. B., 794
McNeill, J. R., 399
McNeill, W., 544
McSwane, D., 581
Maddrey, A. M., 278
Madigann, M. T., 468
Maes, S., 660
Magnusson, D., 100, 101
Maguire, D. J., 927, 938
Mahaffey, K. R., 350, 943
Mahan, C. M., 274
Maimondes, 200
Mair, J. S., 726
Makii, M. M., 809
Malilay, J., 756
Mandel, S., 432
Mang, M., 791
Manguin, S., 574*b*
Mangus, L. G., 725
Mankiller, W., 171
Mannino, D. M., 807
Maranadi, M., 310
Marans, R., 179
Mariner, W. K., 1061
Markowitz, G., 861*b*
Markowitz, M. E., 49
Marks, J. S., 434
Marmot, M., 393
Marsh, D. M., 717, 726
Marshall, M. M., 489
Martinez, E., 481
Marx, J. D., 793
Marx, K., 144
Mascie-Taylor, C.G.N., 301
Masera, O. R., 367
Masuda, Y., 320
Mathee, A., 289, 299
Matheson, M. P., 438
Mathews, K.E.J., 109
Matson, P. A., 4
Matthews, E., 374
Mattson, R. H., 788
Mattsson, M. O., 705*b*
Mayer, S. E., 39
Mead, P. S., 486, 582
Meadows, D. H., 408
Meadows, D. L., 408
Meehan, T., 724
Mehta, S., 309
Meis, M., 438
Meister, E. A., 288, 289
Mekalanos, J. J., 488
Mekel, O., 382
Melanson, E. L., 434
Meliker, J., 288
Melillo, J. M., 4, 21, 232
Mellick, G. D., 134
Mellon, R. K., 910
Menaghan, E., 396
Mendell, M. J., 630, 632
Mendola, P., 312, 831
Menne, B., 245
Menzies, D., 631, 643
Mercier, J.-R., 382
Merzel, C., 397
Meselson, M., 279
Messerli, F. H., 835
Metcalf, J. S., 466
Mettler, F. A., 684, 686, 691, 693, 695, 696
Meyer, O., 43
Meyer, P. A., 311
Meyer, P. S., 6
Meyers, N. M., 785, 786, 787
Meyrowitz, J., 104
Michaelson, S. M., 703
Michelson, W. H., 101
Middaugh, J. P., 352
Mild, K., 705*b*
Milgram, S., 108, 111, 117
Mill, J. S., 148
Miller, C., 618*b*
Miller, G., 406
Miller, G. W., 24
Miller, R. W., 808
Miller, T. R., 728, 731
Millqvist, E., 632
Millson, M. E., 757
Minami, M., 793
Miranda, M., 808
Mishra, V., 306
Mitchell, H., 187
Mitchell, J., 227
Mitchell, R., 468
Mitlin, D., 407
Mittler, B. S., 835
Mizell, L., 437
Moah, J., 702
Moe, C., 46
Moeller, R. B., Jr., 272
Mohammed, 212
Molhave, L., 632
Moller, H., 818
Monet, C., 332*b*
Monmonier, M., 934
Montgomery, M. R., 398
Moolgavkar, S. H., 950
Mooney, C., 617*b*
Mooney, H. A., 4, 21, 232
Moore, B. C., 481
Moore, E., 792
Moore, M., 310
Moos, R. H., 109
Moraga-McHaley, S., 918–919
Morel, F.M.M., 470
Morgan, J. J., 470

Morgan, M. G., 953
Morland, K., 420, 617*b*, 828
Morris, R. D., 487, 497
Morton, F. A., 573*b*
Mouchet, J., 574*b*
Moulder, B., 1011
Moulder, J. E., 704
Moyer, J. A., 793
Mueller, B. A., 424
Muellman, R. L., 719
Muir, J., 783
Muirhead, C. B., 275
Mullan, F., 968, 969
Mullan, J., 396
Muller, p., 545
Munn, T., 232
Murphy, R. S., 350
Murray, C. J., 718
Murray, C.J.L., 291, 404
Murray, S., 374
Myatt, T. A., 643
Myers, N., 230, 249, 250

N

Nabhan, G. P., 785
Nadakavukaren, A., 544
Nadziejko, C., 340
Naidoo, R., 311
Naifeh, M., 564
Nantulya, V. M., 400
Narain, S., 227
Nardell, E. A., 643
Narlioglou,, 820
Nasar, J. L., 110
Nash, R., 783
Nattrass, B, 875*b*
Naumovitz, D., 489
Ndegwa, W., 257
Needleman, H. L., 809
Neel, J. V., 691
Neese, R., 788
Negroponte, N. P., 104
Nelson, A. C., 436
Nelson, J. H., 550*b*
Nelson, M., 187
Nemery, B., 332
Nemmar, A., 332
Nestle, M., 856*b*
Neufeld, L., 375
Neugut, A. I., 270
Newman, O., 110
Ng'ang'a, L. W., 316
N'Goran, E. K., 376
Nicholls, N., 242, 247, 249
Nicholson, D. W., 690
Nie, N. H., 118
Nielsen, D., 228
Nightingale, F., 147, 864
Niland, J., 73
Nixon, R. M., 968, 969
Noji, E. K., 246, 247, 745, 748, 757, 761, 762, 768
Normile, D., 692
Northridge, M. E., 428, 817
Norton, E. H., 173
Norton, W. D., 253, 254
Nriagu, J., 288, 311, 318
Nyberg, F., 430
Nye, S., 1035
Nystrom, L., 437

O

O'Brien, M., 948, 957
O'Connor, D. R., 476
Oddy, W. H., 815
Odero, W., 323, 405, 736
O'Donnell, M. P., 100
Odum, E. P., 2, 5, 15, 18
O'Fallon, L. R., 190, 829
O'Flaherty, E. J., 832
Ogden, C. L., 434
Ohbu, S., 561
Olden, K., 134, 807
Oldenburg, R., 113
Oliver, M. A., 932
Olson, B. H., 254
O'Meara, E. S., 818
Omenn, G. S., 942
Onalaja, A., 133
O'Neill, B., 726
O'Neill, M. S., 180
Ordonez, J. V., 808
Orians, G., 791
Orians, G. H., 783
O'Riordan, T., 864
Orloff, K., 519
Ortega, Y., 489

P

Pacyna, J. M., 318
Paffenbarger, R. S., Jr., 434
Pai, N., 62, 65, 66
Palmer, S., 382
Pan, W., 315
Pandis, S. N., 344, 346
Parcelsus, 25–26
Parker, E. A., 191
Parker, J., 468
Parker, L. B., 970
Parry, J., 382
Parry, M. L., 260
Parsons, R., 784
Pascual, M., 254, 255, 259
Passineau, J. B., 793
Pastor, M., Jr., 181
Patel, I. C., 787
Patz, J. A., 238, 244, 250, 251, 252, 253, 254, 259, 260, 262, 263
Paul, H., 722
Paulson, A. S., 820
Paykel, E. S., 403
Payment, P., 479
Payne, R., 374
Peacock, B., 955
Peacock, J., 794*b*
Pearlin, L., 396
Pearson, J., 793
Pearson, R. L., 430
Peden, M., 717, 726
Pedersen, O. F., 632
Pedigo, L. P., 570, 571
Pedley, S., 480
Peers, J., 436
Pelletier, D. L., 306
Pendall, R., 393
Penris, M., 382
Pereira, M. C., 376
Perera, F. P., 180
Perez-Padilla, R., 309, 310, 375
Perkins, D., 110
Perlman, M., 787
Peron, E. M., 791
Perry, M., 648
Pervin, L. A., 100
Pesatori, A. C., 31
Peters, J. M., 1013
Petruccelli, B. P., 272
Pettenkofer, M. von, 628, 632
Pettitt, L., 103
Philen, R. M., 598
Phillips, R. D., 1060
Piacitelli, L., 67
Pianka, E. R., 8

Pickle, L. W., 933
Pierce, M., 808
Pimental, D., 227, 229
Plakun, E., 793
Plapp, F. W., Jr., 278
Pliny the Elder, 649
Plkum, E., 794*b*
Plog, B. A., 73
Polen, M. R., 720
Poli de Figueredo, L. F., 725
Pollack, R. J., 550
Pommer, L., 631
Ponce, R. A., 948
Poole, C., 828
Pope, C. A., III, 343, 429
Popper, K., 46
Porter, D., 145
Porter, K. G., 480
Posada de la Paz, M., 598
Postel, S., 457, 460
Poston, W.S.C., 617*b*
Pott, P., 649
Potter, J. D., 129
Potter, V. R., 147
Potts, P., 128
Powell, C. V., 315
Power, J., 232
Pretty, C., 793*b*
Pretty, J., 793*b*, 794*b*
Preusser, D. F., 724
Proshansky, H. M., 97, 105
Prothrow-Stith, D., 398
Pruss, A., 62, 65
Pucher, J., 417, 425, 436
Purcell, A. T., 791
Put, G. V., 382
Putnam, R. D., 109, 111, 190, 191

Q

Quinlan, P. J., 73

R

Racioppi, F., 382
Racz, A., 553
Raffensperger, C., 865
Ragland, D. R., 434
Raglin, J. S., 435
Rakitsky, V., 573*b*
Ramazzini, B., 649, 1010, 1011
Ramlow, J. M., 245, 246
Ranchi, E., 317
Randall, A., 787
Randers, J., 408
Randle, R. V., 972
Rankin, P. J., 1061
Rao, P. K., 979
Rapp, R., 345
Rashad, I., 112
Raudenbush, S. W., 400, 405
Razzak, J. A., 715, 717, 726
Reasoner, D. J., 479
Reddy, A.K.N., 367
Rees, G., 502
Rees, W., 21, 22
Rees-Jones, T., 722
Reich, M. R., 400
Reich, W. T., 147
Reid, C., 786
Reigart, J. R., 550
Reilly, W., 184
Relf, D., 787
Renner, M., 281
Repetti, R. L., 120
Ressel, G. W., 434, 435
Retting, R. A., 726
Revell, G.R.B., 791
Revenga, C., 228
Rex, M., 701
Rheingans, R., 362
Rheingold, H., 104, 116
Rhind, D. W., 927
Rhoads, G., 564
Rice, D. C., 943
Rice, D. H., 481
Rich, R., 110
Richardson, J., 948
Richardson, J. R., 24
Ricks, R. C., 692
Ridenour, D. A., 480
Ridgway, D., 1061
Ries, L.A.G., 946
Rivlin, L. G., 97, 104
Robert, J.-H., 875*b*
Robert, K.-H., 873*b*, 874
Roberts, D. R., 550, 574*b*
Roberts, I., 724
Roberts, J., 350
Roberts, N. J., Jr., 703, 969
Roberts, T., 582
Robey, B., 224
Robinson, T. N., 829
Robson, M. G., 544
Rocchini, A. P., 434
Rodenbeck, S., 519
Rodenburg, E., 228
Rodes, C., 429
Rodin, J., 108
Rodo, X., 254, 255, 259
Rodricks, J. V., 982
Rogan, W. J., 574*b*, 820
Rogers, H., 519
Rohweder, M., 374
Roman, I., 436
Roodman, D., 226
Rooney, C., 246
Roosevelt, F. D., 973
Rosa, R. R., 643
Rose, J., 244, 253, 254
Rose, J. B., 479, 504, 506
Rosen, G., 145
Rosen, J. F., 49
Rosen, J. S., 253, 254
Rosenberg, D. M., 376
Rosenthal, J., 230
Rosenthal, N. E., 702
Rosenzweig, C., 260
Rosner, D., 861*b*
Roszak, T., 796
Rothenberg, R. B., 434
Rothman, K., 46, 56
Rothmann, J., 807
Rousseau, J.-J., 402–403
Roy, E., 310
Rucker, T. D., 397
Rucklehaus, W., 185
Rukstinat, C. J., 436
Russo, T. J., 829
Rutledge, L. C., 550*b*
Rutter, D., 705
Rutter, M., 835
Ryan, P. B., 72

S

Saatkamp, B. D., 367
Sacks, O., 788
Sadd, J., 181
Safe, S. H., 31
Salem, R., 225
Sallis, J. F., 828, 829
Salzberg, S., 207, 211
Samet, J. M., 308, 331, 343, 429
Sampson, R. J., 400, 405
Samrakandi, M. M., 480

Samueloff, S., 244, 245
Sandstrom, T., 340
Sapsin, J. W., 726
Sarasin, A., 701
Sartory, D. P., 479
Satterthwaite, D., 401, 407
Savage, E. P., 564
Scchoeny, R., 943
Schachter, S., 109
Scheck, C., 396
Scherer, R., 312
Schieber, R. A., 393
Schierow, L., 970, 974
Schipper, K., 210
Schlesinger, R. B., 344
Schlossberg, M., 395
Schmid, T. L., 115
Schmitter, Father, 935
Schnall, P. L., 661
Schnohr, P., 425
Schoggen, P., 101, 112
Schrader, G., 40*b*
Schrenk, H. H., 332
Schroeder, H. W., 791
Schroll, M., 425
Schulte, P., 56
Schultz, C. H., 768
Schultz, R., 108
Schulz, A. J., 191
Schwartz, B. S., 632
Schwartz, E., 134
Schwartz, J., 343
Schwartz, S., 948
Schwartz, S. M., 818
Schwarzenbach, R. P., 470
Schwela, D., 308
Scorpio, R., 768
Scudder, T., 382
Seager, J. R., 289, 299
Seaman, J., 750
Seaman, S. W., 42
Seeman, T. E., 120, 398
Seidler, F. J., 832
Seinfeld, J. H., 344, 346
Selevan, S. G., 831
Selikoff, I., 652
Sellens, M., 793*b*, 794*b*
Sellin, B., 376
Selye, H., 106
Semenza, J. C., 254, 567
Sen, A., 192
Serpell, J., 786
Sexton, K., 179
Sexton, M., 312
Shabecoff, P., 177
Shalauta, N. M., 900
Shallow, S., 582
Shapiro, J., 699
Shapiro, S. E., 278
Sharma, A., 227
Sharp, B., 573*b*
Sharp, K., 916–917
Shea, K. M., 481, 831, 832
Shelley, P. B., 403
Shelton, G. C., 793
Sheng, Z. Y., 761
Shinar, D., 437
Shniderman, C. M., 794
Shoemaker, C. A., 787
Shore, R. E., 699
Shotts, E. B., 480
Shriver, K., 436
Shumaker, S., 101
Shy, C., 55
Sidel, V. W., 269
Sieber, W. K., 631, 637
Siegel, J., 786
Sigsgaard, T., 631, 642
Silbergeld, E. K., 818
Silva, M., 705
Silva, P. A., 835
Silver, R. C., 102
Simonsen, N., 55
Sims, J., 289, 310
Singal, M., 56
Singer, J. E., 108, 436
Singh, A., 480
Sinnett, M., 49
Skinner, R., 938
Slemr, F., 238
Slesin, L., 702
Sliney, D. H., 701, 702, 705, 707
Sloan, F. A., 1061
Slotkin, T. A., 832
Small, M., 953
Smallwood, S. M., 420
Smith, A. G., 574*b*
Smith, A. H., 630
Smith, G. S., 724
Smith, K. R., 21, 309, 310, 367
Smith, M., 134, 135
Smith, R. L., 6, 9, 10, 11
Smith, T. M., 6, 9, 10, 11
Snow, J., 863–864, 926–927
Soares, S. R., 340
Socrates, 783
Sommer, R., 108
Sonawane, B. R., 816*b*
Sonnenschein, C., 31
Sooman, A., 617*b*, 829
Soto, A. M., 31
Spanjaard, H., 277
Spielberg, S. P., 811b
Spielman, A., 550
Spreng, M., 438
Springer, A. D., 487
Srinivasan, S., 829
Standfield, S., 717
Stannard, J. N., 695
Stansfeld, S., 438, 439
Stauffer, B., 238
Steele, L. P., 238
Steenland, K., 46, 55, 67, 952
Stellar, E., 120
Stelzen, J., 794
Stelzer, J., 793
Sterling, C. R., 489
Stern, P. C., 181
Stevens, W., 275
Stewart, J., 393
Stewart, W. F., 632
Stockard, J., 395
Stokols, D., 96, 97, 98, 99, 100, 101, 102, 103, 104, 107, 110, 117
Stolberg, S. G., 574*b*
Stone, R. S., 685
Stone-Scott, N., 684
Storey, E., 629
Stover, E., 279
Streenland, K., 664
Streifel, A. J., 643
Studdert, D. M., 1061
Stumm, W., 470
Sturm, R., 395
Sudakin, D. L., 550*b*
Suk, W. A., 136, 318, 857
Sullivan, R., 544
Sullivan, W. C., 789, 790
Sundell, J., 631, 642
Sundstrom, E., 108
Sundstrom, M. G., 108
Susskind, L., 189
Swarz, D. J., 197
Swift, C.C., 178

Syme, S. L., 99, 109
Szabo, M. P., 376

T

Takala, J., 665
Talbot, J. F., 792
Talbott, E. O., 438
Tan, G., 246
Tanaka, H., 99
Tansley, A., 4
Targ, N., 186
Taussig, H., 808
Taylor, A. F., 784, 789
Taylor, H. R., 701
Taylor, L. H., 259, 260
Taylor, M. C., 134
Taylor, P., 497
Taylor, P. R., 820
Taylor, R. A., 110, 179
Taylor, R. B., 108
Taylor, S. E., 120
Teeuw, K., 632
Tegegn, Y., 246, 247
Ten Brinke, J., 631
Ten Eyck, R. P., 756, 770
Tenforde, T. S., 705, 706, 707
Tennessen, C. M., 784, 791
Teret, S. P., 726
Ternesten-Hasseus, E., 632
Tester, P. A., 254
Teuscher, J., 755
Teutsch, J. M., 434
Thackrah, C. T., 540
Thomas, E. P., 289, 299
Thomas, S. A., 786
Thomas, S. R., 969
Thomas-Larmer, J., 189
Thoreau, H. D., 783
Thornberry, N. A., 690
Thorpe, B., 879, 880, 881
Thun, M. J., 705*b*
Tickner, J. A., 849, 864, 865, 866, 867, 868
Tiemann, M., 972, 974
Tilson, H. A., 820
Timmerman, R., 232
Tinsworth, D. K., 734
Tolley, G., 948
Tomatis, L., 573*b*
Toole, M. J., 748, 753
Tran, N. L., 900
Travis, B. V., 573*b*
Tren, R., 574*b*
Trevathan, W. R., 550*b*
Trevejo, R. T., 258
Trichopoulos, D., 761
Trimble, S., 785
Triola, D. Y., 414
Tripathi, B. J., 703
Tripathi, R. C., 703
Triplehorn, C. A., 548, 550, 552, 553, 554
Troiano, R. P., 434
Tronko, M. D., 692
Trout, D. B., 638
Truman, L. C., 548, 551, 552, 553, 555, 556, 558
Truppi, L. E., 246
Tsai, S. S., 497
Tucker, G. J., 793, 794
Tuleya, R. E., 247
Turner, B. L., 225
Turusov, V., 573*b*

U

Ulmer, R. C., 724
Ulrich, R. S., 784, 791, 792
Unger, D. G., 105
Upadhyay, U. D., 224
Upton, A. C., 683, 684, 686, 691, 693, 695, 696, 699
Ussher, J. H., 752
Utzinger, J., 376

V

Vahter, M., 313
Valins, S., 108
Van Bruggen, J., 246
van der Doef, M., 660
van der Kaay, H., 257
Van Dolah, F. M., 254
Van Donsel, D. J., 481
van Kempen, E. E., 438
van Kerkhoff, L., 382
Van Vliet, P., 429
Vandegrift, D., 395
Vandenbroucke-Grauls, C. M., 632
Varian, H. R., 118
Vayer, J. S., 770
Vecchia, P., 705
Veneman, A. M., 619
Venkateswarlu, D., 666
Venn, A. J., 429
Verhoef, J., 632
Vernick, J. S., 726
Vilenchik, M. M., 689
Villaveces, A., 725
Vitousek, P. M., 21, 232
Vlahov, D., 387
Vogele, J. P., 403
Vreugdenhil, H. J., 859

W

Wackernagel, M., 21, 22, 149
Wade, T. J., 62, 65, 66
Wadman, M. C., 719
Waite, M., 317
Wakeford, R., 691, 696
Walker, E. D., 671
Wallace, J. M., Jr., 617*b*
Wallace, R. B., 437, 438
Waller, L. A., 926, 932, 933, 937
Walters, S., 42
Wandersman, A., 104, 105, 110
Wang, G., 434, 435
Wang, J., 134
Warady, B. A., 793
Ward, M. H., 818
Ware, G. W., 545
Wargocki, P., 631
Warner, S. B., 788
Warshaw, L. J., 632
Watanabe, K. K., 275
Watson, J. D., 131
Watson, R. T., 241, 243
Wayne, P., 251
Webster, R., 932
Wechsler, H., 617*b*, 618*b*
Weed, D. L., 159
Wegman, D. H., 673, 854
Wegner, J., 3
Weich, S., 806
Weidemann, S., 105, 108
Weidner, I. S., 818
Weiner, J., 867
Weise, J., 971
Weiss, B., 813
Weiss, E. S., 187, 188
Weiss, M. A., 1060
Weitzman, E. R., 617*b*
Wellenius, G. A., 340
Wellman, B., 104, 105, 118

Wells, M., 102
Wells, N. M., 784
Welsch, F., 832
Wesseling, C., 545
Wessley, S., 1029
Wesson, D. E., 768
West, C., 375
West, K. P., 306
West, P. C., 179
Whitacre, D. M., 545
White, L. E., 920
White, L., Jr., 199, 200, 201
White, M. J., 1045*b*, 1046*b*
Whitman, W., 403
Whitmore, R. W., 564
Whitney, K. D., 832
Whittemore, A., 49
Whyte, A., 232
Wicklund, K., 424
Wiesenthal, D. L., 437
Wiles, R., 811*b*
Williams, A. F., 724
Williams, D. R., 397
Williams, F. L., 933
Williams, J., 279
Wilson, E. O., 781, 782, 785, 789
Wilson, S. H., 128, 134, 136, 807
Wilson, W. J., 393
Windrem, R., 273
Wing, S., 486, 617*b*, 828
Winslow, C.E.A., 850, 896
Wirtz, R. A., 550*b*
Withaneachi, D., 724
Witman, J. P., 793, 794
Wojcik, A., 690
Wolbarsht, M., 702
Wolcott, M., 482
Wolf, T., 245
Wolf, U., 382
Wolkoff, P., 636, 638
Wondolleck, J., 189
Woodcock, A., 316
Woods, J. E., 636, 637
Wooley, R. E., 480
Woolhouse, M. E., 259, 260
Worrest, R. C., 702
Wright, S., 867
Wu, M. T., 312

Y

Yaffee, S., 189
Yakimovsky, A., 134
Yamamoto, M., 134
Yan, L., 480
Yanez, L., 318
Yang, C. Y., 497
Yannai, R., 209
Yashar, S. S., 700, 701
Yassi, A., 99
Yi, S.-L., 788
Yoked, T., 395
Yokoro, K., 273
Yoo, S. D., 31
Yu, M. L., 820
Yuan, L., 643
Yung, J. W., 6

Z

Zahm, S. H., 818
Zegeer, C. V., 393
Zeni, O., 704
Zhang, J., 818
Zhou, H., 818
Zinsser, H., 544
Ziska, L. H., 251, 252
Zmuidzinas, M., 98, 100
Zoeller, T. R., 31
Zwi, A., 323, 405, 736
Zwingle, E., 457

Subject Index

A

AAIN (American Association of Industrial Nurses), 145
AAOHN (American Association of Occupational Health Nurses), 145, 1025, 1026
AAOHN's Code of Ethics, 147
AAP (American Academy of Pediatrics), 813
ABM (Anti-Ballistic Missile) Treaty, 283
Abnormally dangerous (or ultrahazardous), 1055–1056
ABPM (American Board of Preventive Medicine), 1026, 1027
Absorption of toxic compound, 33–34
Accommodation approach to climate change, 261
ACGIH (American Conference of Governmental Industrial Hygienists), 963
Acid Rain Program (EPA), 354–355
ACOEM (American College of Occupational and Environmental Medicine), 145, 1025
ACOEM's Code of Ethics, 147
Active air delivery-absorber system, 80
Acute exposures, 88
Acute radiation syndrome, 693–695, 694*t*
Additional risk, 945
Administrative compensation programs, 1050–1052
Administrative strategies (hazard control), 83
Advocacy approach, 282–284
Aerodynamic diameter, 341
Aetna Technical Services, Inc., 1052
African Americans: environmental racism against, 172, 177–184; multiple/cumulative effects of exposure on, 180–181; pedestrian fatality rates among, 423. *See also* Racial differences
African countries: continuing high fertility rate in, 223; DALYs in developed countries compared to, 306; globalizing health difficulties in, 299; health risks of dried fish/meats sold in, 310–311; vulnerability to climate change by, 243–244. *See also* Developing countries
Age structure (population), 9–10*fig*
Agency for Toxic Substances and Disease Registry (2000), 311, 943
Agenda 21 (Earth Summit, 1992), 231
AGI (acute gastrointestinal infection), 485–486
Agriculture: climate change, malnutrition, and productivity of, 260; GAPs (good agricultural practices) [FDA], 612; no-till, 567; occupational hazards of, 668, 670; waste produced by, 525
Agriculture development programs: environmental health risk factors associated with, 302*t*–303*t*; pesticide hazards of, 300*b*–301*b*; Third World health impact of, 299–304; vector-borne disease increase due to, 301; water scarcity and, 460

AIDS/HIV, 483, 523*b*, 1039
Air pollutants (exposure assessment): asbestos, 639–640; biomass, fossil fuels, and indoor chemistry, 640; carbon dioxide, 640–641; ETS (environmental tobacco smoke), 639; microbial agents, 638; radon, 640; VOCs (volatile organic compounds), 638–639
Air pollutants (sources/health effects): air toxics, 351; carbon monoxide, 347–348; inhalation route, 88, 816–817; lead (Pb), 348–351; mercury, 351–352; nitrogen oxides, 238, 240*t*, 344–345; PM (particulate matter), 308, 341–343, 342*fig*; sulfur dioxide, 343–344; tropospheric ozone, 346–347. *See also* Carbon dioxide; VOCs (volatile organic compounds)
Air pollution: ambient, 334–335, 336*t*–338*t*, 399; Donora disaster (1948), 332, 333*b*; environmental health ethics controversy regarding, 161*b*; history of, 331–332; indoor, 309–311, 374–375, 379*t*; London fog disaster (1952), 332*fig*–333*b*, 332*fig*–333*fig*, 334*fig*; prevention and control of, 352–357; related to transportation, 425–432; sampling apparatus for evaluating, 81*fig*; SES (socioeconomic status) and susceptibility to exposure of, 179*b*–180*b*; sources and health effects of major outdoor, 340–352; studies on health and, 339–340; Third World and effects of, 308–312; types of ambient, 334–339; weather, health, and, 250–252. *See also* Pollution
Air Pollution Control Act (1955), 970
Air pollution prevention/control: additional approaches to, 356–357; recommended pathways for, 352–353; regulatory approaches to, 353–355; related to other environmental problems, 357; technological controls, 355–356
Air Transportation Safety and Stabilization Act (2001), 1063
Air-conditioning systems, 633–637
Albert Lasker Public Service Award, 650, 652
Albuquerque Environmental Health Department, 902–903, 918–919
ALDF (American Lyme Disease Foundation), 556
Allele, 129
Ambient air pollution: classifying, 335, 339; described, 334–335; sources, health effects, and regulations on, 336*t*–338*t*
Ambient Noise Strategy (London), 886*b*
Ambient standards, 353–354
American Cancer Society's Cancer Prevention Study (CPS) II, 339, 343
American Heart Association, 434
American Public Health Association (APHA), 904, 920, 921
ANA (American Nurses Association) Code for Nurses, 147
Analytical (or etiologic) studies, 48–49
Anecdotal (or convenience) sampling, 79
Animal testing, 42–44, 43*fig*
Animal-facilitated therapy, 787
Animals: decomposers, 12–13; food chain role of, 12; herbivores (plant feeders), 12, 14*fig*; heterotrophs (other feeders), 12; nature contact through, 785–787; omnivores (plants and animal feeders), 12; as reservoir for pathogens, 481–482; testing toxicity using, 42–44, 43*fig*
Anthropogenic chemical contaminants, 464*t*, 466–467. *See also* Pesticides
Anti-personnel landmine convention, 279*b*
Anticipation of hazards, 73, 74–75
Antimalarial campaign, 573*b*–574*b*
Antipersonnel landmines, 279, 280*fig*
AOEC (Association of Occupational and Environmental Clinics), 1025
APEXPH (*Assessment Protocol for Excellence in Public Health*), 904
APHA (American Public Health Association), 904, 920, 921
Aquatic system engineering, 462*t*–463
Arable land deterioration, 227
Arctic Climate Impact Assessment, 242
Arboviruses (climate change effects), 257–258
Arsenic contamination, 463, 826–827
Arsenic poisoning, 319*t*–320
Arsenic standard (EPA), 964*b*–965*b*
Asbestos exposure, xxxvii, 525, 639–640, 860*b*
Asbestos litigation, 1045*b*–1047*b*
ASHRAE (American Society of Heating, Refrigerating and Air-Conditioning Engineers), 633, 637, 640
ASHRAE Standard 62, 640–641
Asthma: fossil fuel combustion in home and, 642; home moisture and, 641; occupational, 643, 654–655; transportation-related air pollution and, 429
Atmosphere changes, 238–239*fig*, 241–242
ATSDR (Agency for Toxic Substances and Disease Registry), *xxxib*, 824, 827
Attentional fatigue, 784
Attributable risk, 945
Automobiles. *See* Motor vehicles
Autotrophic ecosystem, 13
Autotrophic systems, 13
Autotrophs, 11–12
Avian flu outbreak (2004), 766
Awareness of environmental problems, 282

B

Backcasting, 854
BACT (best available control technology), 354, 971

Bacterial foodborne illness, 586–591
Bacterial waterborne diseases, 487–489*fig*
Bad Bug Bood (FDA), 586
Bangladesh: arsenic poisoning in, 320*b*; diseases following cyclone (1991) in, 756; sea-level rise in, 249*fig*
Barcelona asthma clusters (1980s), 57
Basel Convention (1989), 541
BCME (bis-chloromethyl ether), xxxvii
Bean v. Southwestern Waste Management, 172
Bedbugs, 548–549
Behavior settings, 112–113*fig*
Benchmark dose, 947*b*
Bethel New Life, Inc., 187, 189
Bhopal disaster (1984), 665*b*, 762
Bhutan urbanization, 395*b*
Bias: defining, 51; information, 52; recall, 50, 52; selection, 51–52
Bicycling, 419*fig*, 424
Bills of Mortality (U.K.), xxxiv–xxxv
Bioavailable substances, 470
Biodiversity, 229–230
Bioethics, 147, 148*b*
Biofilm (or slime), 481, 504
Biogeochemical (or nutrient) cycles, 16
Biological agents, 278–279
Biological monitoring, 82
Biological system, 24
Biomagnification, 598
Biomarkers, 90, 91*b*–92*b*
Biomass fuels, 373–375
Biomonitoring, 876–877
Biophilia, xxxviii, 782–783
Bioterrorism: disaster preparedness in case of, 764–766; food safety and threat of, 619–620; preparedness/emergency response to, 771–774. *See also* Terrorism
Biotransformation process, 34–39
Birds: as pests, 558–559; as reservoir for pathogens, 481–482
Bis-chloromethyl ether, xxxvii
Black Death, xxxiii
Blacksburg Electronic Community, 119
BLS (Bureau of Labor Statistics), 666
BMI (body mass index), 434
Body burden testing, 876–877
Breast feeding, 815*b*–816*b*
BRIs (building-related illnesses), 628–629*t*
Brundtland Commission, 150, 192, 888–889
BSE (bovine spongiform encephalopathy) [UK outbreak], 490, 618–619
Buffering operations (GIS), 930, 931*fig*
Built environments: applying pollution prevention/cleaner production approach to, 883; diagnostic strategies/prevention for, 644–645; disorders associated with, 628–632; environmental design and control, 632–633; heating, ventilating, and air-conditioning systems of, 633–637, 634*fig*, 644; investigating complaints about, 626*b*–628; specific types of, 641–643. *See also* Housing; Indoor environments
Business sector voluntary actions, 981
BWC (Biologic and Toxin Weapons Convention), 283–284

C

C. perfringens, 587–588
CAA Amendments (1990), 335, 970
CAA (Clean Air Act) [1970], 348*b*, 899, 970–971, 980
California AIDS fund, 1051
California Air Resources Board, 429
California Interfaith Partnership for Children's health and the environment, 197, 215*b*–216*b*, 805-46
California landslides (1998), 248*fig*
California's Proposition 65, 1052–1053
Cancer: basal cell carcinoma of skin, 700*fig*; cell phones and, 705*b*; estimated risks from exposure to ionizing radiation, 697*t*; occupational, 655–656; transportation-related air pollution and lung, 430. *See also* Carcinogens
Cancerphobia, 1032, 1038–1039
Candidate gene approach, 134
Cap and Trade credits, 982–983
CAPE (Canadian Association of Physicians for the Environment), 149
Caracas business district, 401*fig*
Carbon cycle, 16–18, 17*fig*
Carbon dioxide: as ambient air pollution source, 335; ASHRAE Standard 62 for, 640–641; biomarkers used to measure exposure of, 91*b*–92*b*; examining changes in levels of, 5; fertilization effect of, 260; greenhouse effect and level of, 17–18, 230–231, 238–239*fig*, 240*t*; Kyoto Protocol (1997) regarding, 230–231; ventilation and levels of indoor, 628, 632. *See also* Air pollutants (sources/health effects)
Carbon monoxide, 347–348
Carboxyhemoglobin (COHb), 347–348
Carcinogens: described, 30; testing for toxicity, 42–44, 43*fig*; toxicokinetic process of chemical, 35*b*. *See also* Toxicity
Cardiovascular disease, 658–659
Carnivores (flesh feeders), 12
Carpal tunnel syndrome, 655
Carrying capacity, xxxix, 9, 226*b*
Cars. *See* Motor vehicles
Case-control studies, 50
CAST (Council for Agricultural Science and Technology), 582
Catalytic converter, 356
Categorical dose-response model, 953*fig*
Catholic Hospital Association, 197, 215
Catskill/Delaware watershed, 20
Causality: as legal issue, 1041–1044; of phthalate plasticizers in toys, 872*b*–873*b*; prevention and, 871–872. *See also* Prevention

CBO (Congressional Budget Office), 1059
CBPR (community-based participatory research), 189, 190*b*
CCA (chromated copper arsenic), 826–827
CCL (Contaminant Candidate List) [EPA], 500
CCP (critical control point), 608, 609
CCR (Center for Claims Resolution), 1046*b*–1047*b*
CDC (Centers for Disease Control and Prevention): cancer clusters investigated by, 56; clinicians working for, 1027; ED (endocrine disrupter) surveys conducted by, 831; elevated blood lead levels definition by, 350*b*; food safety regulated by, 582, 602, 613–614, 619; on growing physical inactivity, 433; on increased car use, 722; on public health approach to injury prevention, 716; public health preparedness role by, 776; toxicologists working at, 25
CDC's Emerging Infections Program, 582
CDC's National Pharmaceutical Stockpile (NPS) program, 773
CDC's Public Health Practice Program Office (PHPPO), 903
Cell phones, 704*fig*, 705*b*
Census sample, 78
Center for Health, Environment, and Justice, 898
CERCLA (Comprehensive Environmental Response, Compensation, and Liability Act) [Superfund], 975*b*, 978, 1058–1059
CETA (Comprehensive Education and Training Act), 908
CF (constant flow) systems, 635
CFC-12 level, 240*t*
CFOI (Census of Fatal Occupational Injury), 664
Chemical food contamination: ciguatoxin, 599; food allergens, 598–599; mercury, 599–600*b*; overview of, 597–598; scombrotoxin, 599. *See also* PCBs (polychlorinated biphenyls); Pesticides
Chemical hazards anticipation, 74
Chemical water contamination: anthropogenic, 464*t*, 466–467; classes of chemical contaminants, 464*t*; deposition, storage, and bioconcentration of, 468–471; health effects of, 471*t*–472; naturally occurring, 465–466; transformations due to, 467–468
Chemical weapons, 276–278*b*
Chemical Weapons Convention (CWC) [1997], 277
Chernobyl accident (1986), 275*b*, 362, 377, 692, 762
Child labor, 667*fig*, 668, 670, 672*b*
Childhood obesity, 827–829
Children: changing patterns of disease in, 806–807; environmentally related disease burden on, 291, 291*t*–292*t*, 294*fig*; exposure to diseases in homes/schools, 641–642; increasing physical inactivity of, 433; lead poisoning of Third World, 312; nature contact role in development of, 785; parent's religious values used in development of, 207–214; pedestrian injuries/fatalities among, 423–424; pesticide exposure of, 564, 569–570; policy consequences of property rights for health of, 213–214; protected from harm, 209–210; religious traditions facilitating environmental health of, 214; Safe Routes to School program for, 442*b*; 7discount rate required by OMB on value of, 213; studies on genetic effects of radiation on, 690–691; transportation air pollution threatening health of, 429; unique susceptibility of, 810*b*–811*b*; valuing future generations through, 210–213. *See also* Pediatric environmental disease; Playgrounds; Women
Children's Health Fund, 421
Chimney-Sweepers Act (1788) [England], 649
China: changing definitions of urban in, 390, 391*b*; employment patterns in, 653; growing energy demand in, 370*b*; ship breaking practice of, 542
Chlorine gas exposure, 29*b*–30*b*
Chloroform: carcinogenic effects on male rats, 943–944*t*; described, 941; exposure assessment of, 944–945; hazard identification of, 942–943; risk management of, 946–949; three dose-response models fit to dose-response data on, 952*fig*
Cholera mortality maps (London, 1854–55), xxxv–xxxvi, 926–927
Choropleth maps, 932–933
Chronic exposures, 88
CI (confidence interval), 53
Ciguatoxin, 599
Cities: environmental health issues in, xxxiii, 387–413; building healthy, 407–409; Caracas business district, 401*fig*; characteristics of, 389–390; environmental health significance of, 395–402*fig*; environmental impact on health by, 402–407; Manila substandard housing, 402*fig*; megacities, 387–388; nature contact in the inner, 789*b*, 790*fig*; physical environments of, 398–402*fig*, 399*b*, 401*fig*; population factors of, 396–397; services and resources of, 397; social environments of, 397–398; urban sprawl of, 392*b*–395*b*. *See also* Communities; Urbanization
Civil Rights Act (1964), 935
Civil rights movement, 170
Class action lawsuits, 1047
Clean Air Act (1970): command-and-control regulations of the, 980; NAAQS requirement of, 348*b*; overview of the, 970–971; state authority under, 899
Clean Air Act Amendments (1990), 335, 970

Clean Water Act (CWA), 971
Cleaner production: based on circular vision of the economy, 880*fig*; described, 879; examples of, 880*b*–881*b*; extending application of, 882–883; goals of, 881–882
Clear Air Act (CAA), 970–971
Climate change: changes in atmosphere affecting, 238–239*fig*, 241–242; current state of, 230–231; effects on vector-borne diseases by, 255*b*–256*b*; environmental health ethics controversy regarding, 161*b*; ethical and political considerations of, 262–263; factors affecting, 238; food productivity, malnutrition, and, 260; projected changes in global temperature, 243*fig*; projected sea-level rise and, 242–243; public health approach to, 261; regions particularly vulnerable to, 243–244; sea-level and, 242–243, 246–249; variations of surface temperature across two time frames, 241*fig*; vector-borne diseases and, 255–260; water scarcity due to, 461–462; waterborne diseases and, 253–254. *See also* Global warming; Weather
Clinical Ecologists, xxxix, 1027
Clinical trials (randomized clinical trials), 48–49
Clinical practice: environmental medicine and practice venues for, 1026–1028; environmental and occupational aspects of, xxxix, 1013–1025*b*
Cluster investigation, 56–57
CMAQ (Congestion Mitigation and Air Quality), 441
Coal, 369, 371
Coal mining: pollution of, 369; worker's compensation for occupational diseases of, 1049–1050
Coalition on the Environment and Jewish Life, 215
Cockroaches, 550–551
Cohort studies, 49–50
Collaborative problem-solving, 186–192
Columbia Center for Children's Environmental Health, 180
Command-and-control regulations, 980–981
Committee on Atherosclerosis, Hypertension, and Obesity in the Young, 434
Common law tort system: causation issue of, 1041–1044; expert testimony in, 1042*b*–1043*b*; no-fault proposed alternative to, 1048–1050, 1060–1061, 1063–1064; procedural innovations of, 1047; resistance to changing, 1061–1063; theories of recovery, 1036–1041. *See also* Lawsuits
Communication: of information between hospital/disaster site, 770–771; prevention strategies of dissemination, education, and, 887–888. *See also* Dissemination; Message mapping; Risk communication
Communities: Albuquerque Environmental Health Department's work with, 902–903, 918–919; Allegheny County's work with, 909–911; consumer pressure from within, 983; environmental justice, 185; Iowa Department of Health's work with, 915–918; Island County Health Department's work with, 905–906, 911–915; PACE-EH process involving, 904–906, 905*t*; solid waste and right-to-know by, 526*b*; valuing future generations, 210–213. *See also* Cities; Religious communities
Community health: environmental justice as part of, 177–192; WHO's definition as positive, 187
Compensation funds, 1050–1052
Competitive inhibition, 37
Concentration: continuum of dose, exposure, and, 84*b*–86*b*, 88; described, 85
Confidentiality issues, 162*b*
Confounder variables: defining, 49; SES (socioeconomic status) as, 51
Confounding, 52
Confucian tradition, 211
Conjugation, 36
Connectivity, 417
Construction debris, 524
Construction occupational injuries, 670
Consumer advisories (food safety), 615–616
Consumer Confidence Reports, 501
Consumer pressure, 983
Contaminated sites: restoration of, 883; Superfund assessment of, 956
Contextual analysis: levels of, 100, 101*t*; principle 1: interdependencies influencing environment-health relationship, 101–102; principle 2: synergistic effect on health by different environments, 102; principle 3: health is result of interaction among environmental features, 102–103
Convenience (or anecdotal) sampling, 79
Convention on Biological Diversity (Rio Convention), 230
Convention to Combat Desertification, 227
Conventional weapons, 271–272*b*
Core Public Health Functions Steering Committee (1994), 902
Core Writing Team, 241, 243
Corn borer, 547*fig*
Correlational (or ecological) studies, 48
Cost-benefit analysis, 948
Council on Education for Public Health, 921
Council on Linkages Between Academia and Public Health Practice, 921–922
CPS (Cancer Prevention Study) II [ACS], 339, 343
Creative class, 113–114
Crisis management. *See* Disaster management
Cross-contamination, 606–607*b*

Cross-sectional (or prevalence) studies, 50–51
Crowding, 108
Cryptosporidiosis, 253
CSPC (Consumer Product Safety Commission), 873*b*
CTBT (Comprehensive Nuclear-Test-Ban Treaty), 282
Cubit smoothing spline, 953*fig*
Cultural conflict issues, 161*b*
Cumulative impacts: EPA's framework for, 180–181; EPA's framework for risk assessment of, 180–181, 189; vulnerability in context of, 181–182, 183*fig*, 184
CVDs (cardiovascular diseases), 307–308
CWA (Clean Water Act), 971
CWC (Chemical Weapons Convention) [1997], 277, 283

D

DALYs (disability-adjusted life years): comparing Third World and Second World, 291, 304, 306; indoor pollution resulting in, 310; injuries leading to, 322*t*, 404; lead poisoning and, 312; waterborne diseases resulting in, 482
Data analysis: cost-benefit of risk management, 948; determining permissible levels of exposure, 66–68; EIA/HIA system of, 886–887*b*; environmental psychology, 100, 101*t*–103; HACCP system of, 607–609*b*, 610–613, 856*b*; interval risk, 954; issues of epidemiology, 52–54; options analysis, 721*t*–722; pooled analysis, 66–67; probabilistic risk analysis, 954–955; risk benefit analysis, 947–948; risk management decision analysis, 948; uncertainty analysis, 953–955
Daubert v. Merrill Dow, 1043*b*
Day-care exposure, 823–825
DBPs (disinfection by-products), 468, 497
DDE, 59
DDT, 59, 545, 561, 572, 573*b*–574*b*, 982
De minimus risk, 947
Decision making: energy, 367*fig*, 378–383; environmental health indicators used in, 885–886; precautionary principle flow of, 870*b*–871*b*; risk management, 948
"Declaration of the Environmental Leaders of the Eight on Children's Environmental Health" (1997), 149
Decomposers, 12–13
Deep well injection, 534–536
Deer Island System (Boston), 472, 475*fig*, 476
DEET, 549–550, 819–820
Defensible space, 110
Deforestation report (Earth Summit, 1992), 229
DeKalb County (Georgia) park mapping, 934
Deontology, 148*b*
Denver urban sprawl, 394*fig*
Dermal contact: exposure assessment of, 92–93; as exposure route, 88
Dermatologic conditions, 662
Descriptive studies, 47
Desertification report (Earth Summit, 1992), 227–228
Detroit News, 935
Developed countries: DALYS in Africa compared to, 306; dropping rate in fertility levels among women in, 222; endocrine disruptors in drinking water of, 321; expected to sign Kyoto Protocol, 262; indoor environments regulated in, 626; injuries in, 717–739; mitigating role in energy consumption by technology, 226; per capita energy use in, 363–365*b*, 364*t*; road traffic deaths in, 725–726; YLDs (2002) in, 204*fig*. *See also* United Kingdom; United States
Developing countries: access to safe drinking water in, 316*t*–320; agriculture development health impact in, 299–304; air pollution health impact on, 308–312; Bangladesh, 249*fig*, 320*b*, 756; changing disease burden in, 290–294; described, 288; disease burden in, 290–294; environment and nutrition in the, 304–308; globalization impact on health in, 295–299; hazards of, 289–290; health impact of urbanization of, 313–316; increasing energy consumption/more pollution by, 226; India, 542, 665*b*–667*fig*, 762; injuries in, 717–739; injuries related to environmental risk factors in, 321–323, 322*t*; Manila substandard housing, 402*fig*; nuclear power as energy source in, 376–377; pesticide hazards in, 300*b*–301*b*; risk overlap in, 290; road traffic deaths in, 725–726; vehicular mortality in, 322–323; YLDs (2002) in, 204*fig*. *See also* African countries
DHHS (U.S. Department of Health and Human Services), 433, 772–773, 774, 776, 777, 903, 920
DHS (Department of Homeland Security), 774
Dichotomous variables, 53
Digital divide, 119
Direct exposure assessment methods, 90–92
Direct reading instruments, 79
Disaster health care needs: disposition of dead bodies, 775–776; earthquakes, 760–762; epidemics, 775; floods, 752–753; industrial disasters, 762–764, 763*fig*; terrorism, 764–766; tornadoes, 757–758; tropical cyclones (hurricanes and typhoons), 753–757; volcanic eruptions, 758–759
Disaster management: austerity issue of, 767; health care needs as part of, 751–766; information systems for, 750–751; on-site medical care, 770; past problems in natural, 748–750; risk

communication role in, 770–771, 990; terrorism preparedness/ emergency response, 771–774; triage and rationing, 767–770
Disaster preparedness: environmental conditions/health challenges of, 745–747; future of public health, 776–777; practical issues in disaster response, 766–774; public health approach to, 747–751. *See also* Public health
Disasters: health care needs in specific, 751–766; public concerns associated with, 775–776; selected natural (1970–2004), 746*t*; short-term effects of major natural, 749*t*; three components of defining, 748
Diseases: BRIs (building-related illnesses) or SBS (sick building syndrome), 628–629, 630*t*–632; categories of environmental and occupational, 1012*t*; changing pattern in children, 806–807; confounding relationship between exposure and, 52; CVDs (cardiovascular diseases), 307–308; dose-response assessment of exposure and, 943; drinking water pathogens and, 473*t*; epidemiological study of exposures relating to, 46–70; geographic information/ mapping, 932–933; HIV/AIDS, 483, 523*b*, 738–739*t*, 1039; home moisture connection to, 641–642; legal claims of increased risk of, 1039–1040; occupational risk of infectious, 662–663; rodent-borne, 255*b*–256*b*; spread through transportation, 416*b*; Third World and changing burden of disease, 290–294; urban environment and transmission of infectious, 406–407; vector-borne, 255–260, 301, 416*b*, 483–484*t*, 766. *See also* Environmental health; Pediatric environmental disease; Waterborne diseases
Disproportionate impacts: described, 177; proximity to pollution sources, 177–178; susceptible and sensitive populations, 179; unique exposure pathways, 178–179
Dissemination: of information between hospital/disaster site, 770–771; as prevention strategy, 887–888; risk communication and, 833*b*–834*b*. *See also* Communication; Risk communication
Distribution (toxic compounds), 34
DMATs (disaster medical assistance teams), 774
DNA: identifying sequence variations in, 132; ionizing radiation damage to, 689–691; MW/RFR damage to, 704; UVR absorption in, 701
Documenting environmental problems, 281
DoD (Department of Defense), 773, 774
Donora air pollution disaster (1948), 332, 333*b*
Dose: continuum of concentration to exposure to, 84*b*, 86*b*, 88; defining, 85*b*; measuring, 85*b*–86*b*
Dose-response: assessment of, 943; modeling used to determine, 949–953*fig*, 956–957
Dot maps, 932
DOT (U.S. Department of Transportation), 421, 422, 438
Doubling time, 7
DPSEEA (driving forces, pressures, state, exposures, effect, actions) model, xlviii–xlix
Dracunculiasis Eradication Program (WHO), 485*b*
Dracunculiasis (guinea worm disease), 483, 484*t*, 485*b*
Drinking water: contamination of, 463–482; endocrine disruptors in, 321; EPA's arsenic standard for, 964*b*–965*b*; estimated population exposure to arsenic in, 319*t*; improper disposal of waste materials and, 539–541; MCL (maximum contaminant limit) for, 319*t*, 320, 499, 500, 972; provision of in early cities, xxxiv; regulatory framework for monitoring quality of, 498–502; safe, 316*t*–320, 490–498, 505–506*fig*, 972. *See also* Freshwater; Water
Drowning prevention/countermeasures, 733*t*
DU (depleted uranium), 276
DUMBELS, 565
Duplicate diet study, 92
Dust spot efficiency, 633–634

E

E. coli: food poisoning due to, 582, 583, 588–589*b*, 612; water sources and outbreaks of, 476–477*b*, 587
The Earth Charter, 149*b*
Earth Summit (1992), 226–227
Earthquakes, 760–762
EBS (environmental and behavior studies), 97. *See also* Environmental psychology
Ecological footprint concept, 21–22
Ecological medicine: clinical practice of, 1013–1025*b*, 1026–1028; ethical considerations of, 152*b*
Ecological (or correlational) studies: epidemiological, 48; as hypothesis-generating studies, 48
Ecologists, 3–4
Ecology: common theme of definitions of, 3; core study focus of, 3; ecosystem, 10–19*fig*; examining concept of, 4–6; links with environmental health, xxxviii–xxxix; population, 6–10*fig*; services/ functions performed by, 20*t*–21
Economics: burden of pediatric environmental disease, 807–808; as energy decision making issue, 381; "home finance" meaning of, 3
Ecopsychology, 796
Ecosystem coupling, 13
Ecosystem ecology: basic components of, 11*fig*; coupling heterotrophic and autotrophic, 13; defining concept of, 4–6;

described, 10–11; energy flow through, 11–13; energy flow through populations and individuals, 14*fig*–15
Ecosystem services: described, 20; values of various, 20*t*–21
Ectotherms, 14
EDs (endocrine disruptors), 31*b*, 321, 831
Educational approaches, 887–888, 983–984
EEA (European Environment Agency), 859*b*
Effect modification, 52
The Effects of the Principal Arts, Trades and Professions (Thackrah), 650
EGP (Environmental Genome Project), 133–136
EHAC (National Environmental Health Science and Protection Accreditation Council), 920
EHAT (environmental health assessment team), 905–906
EIA/HIA (environmental impact assessment and health impact assessment), 886–887*b*
EIS (environmental impact statement), 441
El Niño: impact on sea levels by, 233, 254; vector-borne disease outbreaks and, 257, 258*b*–259*b*
El Niño Southern Oscillation (ENSO), 254, 258*b*–259*b*
Electricity generation: coal as source of, 369, 371; U.S. emissions and costs of, 380*t*–381. *See also* Energy sources
ELF (extremely low frequency) EMFs (electromagnetic fields), 705–707
ELSIs (ethical, legal, and social implications), 131*b*
Emergent properties (plant community), 5
Emerging Infections Program (CDC), 582
Emigration, in population ecology), 10
Emissions standards, 354, 431*t*
Emotional distress lawsuits, 1039
Employees. *See* Occupational health; Workplace
The End of Nature (McKibben), 21
Endocrine disruptors (EDs), xxxvii, 31*b*, 321, 831
Endotherms, 14
Energy: developing countries demand of, 363–365*b*, 364*t*; health risks associated with sources of, 365–378; human activities requiring, 362; patterns of human use of, 363–364, 366*t*; per capita use by sector/region (1999), 364*t*
Energy decision making: economic issues of, 381; energy ladder issues of, 367*fig*, 379–381; externalities issues of, 378–379; health impact assessment factor of, 381–383
Energy flow: humans, fossil fuels, and, 15; *P*/*R* ratio calculating, 13; properties in ecosystems, 15; *R*/*A* (respiration to assimilation) ratio calculating, 14–15; through ecosystems, 11–13; through populations and individuals, 14*fig*–15
Energy ladder, 367*fig*, 379–381
Energy policies: applying pollution prevention/cleaner production approach to, 882–883; as public health policy, 382*b*
Energy sources: biomass, 373–375; coal, 369–371; decision making issues regarding, 378–383; health risks associated with, 365–378; hydroelectric, 375–376; natural oil, 372–373; new renewable, 377–378; nuclear fission, 161*b*–162*b*, 376–377; petroleum, 371–372; by region, 366*t*. *See also* Electricity generation; Fossil fuels
ENSO (El Niño Southern Oscillation), 254, 258*b*–259*b*
Envelope integrity, 635–636
Environment: animate and inanimate factors of, 3; defining, 129; health care service context of, 1010–1011; impact of population growth on, 221–224*b*, 225–226*b*; impacts of war on the, 271–281; indoor and built, 625–645; links between health and, 782–785; religious traditions regarding, 199–203; Third World nutrition and the, 304–308; urban physical, 398–402*fig*, 399*b*, 402*fig*
Environment-host-vector triangle, 720
Environmental Defense Fund (now Environmental Defense), 430, 858*b*, 859*b*, 982, 984
Environmental distress syndrome, 232–233
Environmental epidemiology: described, 54–55, 99; investigation of clusters in, 56–57; recreational water quality studies example of, 62*b*–66*b*
Environmental ethics: climate change and, 262–263; controversies in, 161*b*–163; ecological medicine, 152*b*; general principles of, 150–160; global health concept of, 148; promoting awareness of, 149; sustainability concept of, 148, 150*b*–151. *See also* Ethics
Environmental ethics principles: interconnections affecting health, 153–154; realistic understanding, 159–160; respect for all life principle of, 154–156; respectful participation, 157–158
Environmental exposure. *See* Exposure
Environmental hazards: anticipation of, 74–75; vulnerability, health disparities and, 183*fig*
Environmental health: challenges to perceptions of, 1028–1029; chimney sweeps case (1775) of, 128; clinical role in occupational and, 1013–1025*b*; core competencies for working toward, 921*t*; defined, xxx–xxxi, *xxxib–xxxiib*; EIA/HIA (environmental impact analysis and health impact analysis) of, 886–887*b*; ELSIs (ethical, legal, and social implications) and, 131*b*; emerging issues in,

xl–xliv; ethics in, 143–163, 1025–1026; goal setting for, 883–885; history of, xxxii–xl; indicators of, 885–886; linking genes and environmental exposures, 136–138, 137*fig*; new generation of research on, 133–136; -omics technologies, 138–140; religious approaches to, 197–216; steps toward the greening of, 795–797; Sweden's goals for, 884*b*–885*b*. *See also* Diseases; Gene-environment interactions; Health

Environmental health policy: alternatives to regulation, 979–984; considerations of, xl, 962–964; constitutional basis of, 965–967; described, 961; emergence of U.S. Public Health Service (PHS), 967–968; key federal environmental health statutes, 970–975; moving from science to, 977–979. *See also* Public policies; Regulatory approaches

Environmental health policymaking: cost issues considerations of, 979; determining scientific interpretation, 977; global regulatory developments and, 979; moving from science to policy, 977–979; risk assessment role in, 976–977; role of science in, 976

Environmental health practice: careers in, 919–922; core competencies for, 921*t*; field work examples of, 906–919; history of regulations and services, 896–898; increasing citizen involvement in, 898–899; organization and delivery of services and, 899–900; PACE-EH process of, 904*t*–906; standards for, 901–906; ten essential services of, 902*t*. *See also* Public health; Public policies; Regulatory approaches

Environmental health practice cases: Gerry Barron's work, 909–911; Iowa Department of Health, 915–918; Island County Health Department (Washington), 905–906, 911–915; Philadelphia Department of Health, 906–907; Randall Hirschborn's work, 907–909; Stephanie Moraga-McHaley's work, 918–919

Environmental impact statements, 899

Environmental justice: case study on practice of, 911; CBPR (community-based participatory research) on, 189, 190*b*; collaborative and integrated problem solving used in, 186–192; community-based participatory research on, 190*b*–192; disproportionate impacts concept and, 177–184; EPA Office of Environmental Justice role in, 184*b*–185*b*; using GIS operations to investigate, 935; legal, public policy, and research implications of, 184–186; nondiscriminatory policies supported by, 978–979; ReGenesis Revitalization Project case of, 187*b*–189*b*; religious principles regarding, 206–207

Environmental justice communities, 185

Environmental justice issues: examples of community-based, 175*t*–176*t*; meaning and implications of, 185

Environmental justice movement: community-driven process of, 174–177; core concepts of, 171; origins of, xli, 170, 171–172

Environmental psychology: assumptions of, 96; importance of "context" and "settings" in, 97; on neighborhood changes and influence on health, 103–105; on neighborhood features, 105–119; overview of, 97–98. *See also* EBS (environmental and behavior studies)

Environmental psychology analysis: levels of, 100, 101*t*; three principles of contextual, 101–103

Environmental psychology cases: The Trio of Tripping Pedestrian Revisited, 98*b*; A Trio of Tripping Pedestrians, 96*b*–97*b*

Environmental racism: described, 172; disproportionate impacts concept and, 177–184

Environmental response machinery, 130

Environmentally responsive genes, 135–136, 137*fig*

EOH (environmental and occupational health), 1026

EPA (Environmental Protection Agency): on air pollutants from transportation-related sources, 426, 427*fig*; arsenic standard of, 964*b*–965; CCL (Contaminant Candidate List) of, 500; on chemical toxicity testing issues, 858*b*–859*b*; community involvement tools developed by, 904; conservative default assumptions used by, 956; cumulative risk assessment framework by, 180–181, 189; CWA requirements of, 971; environmental health functions of, 899; environmental health policies of, 962; environmental justice report by, 178; environmental justice role by, 184*b*–185; epidemiological studies published by, 47; establishment and development of, 897, 968–969; FIFRA requirements of, 974; food safety regulated by, 614; industrial disaster recommendations by, 764; injection wells regulated by, 535; level of exposure permitted by, 67; litigation by, 981–982; NAAQS created by, 335; noise standards by, 439; Office of Environmental Justice established by, 173; pesticide regulation under, 567–570; pesticide use/poisonings estimated by, 559, 565; pests as defined and categorized by, 545–546; RCRA requirements of, 525, 541, 974–975; SDWA requirements of, 972; 7discount rate

required by OMB on value of children, 213; surface water/groundwater as defined by, 456–457; SWTR (Surface Water Treatment Rule) promulgated by, 493; Total Coliform Rule of, 500–501; toxicologists working at, 25; water standards established by, 319*t*, 320, 499–502; water-ingestion for adults recommended by, 945; WPS (Worker Protection Standard) of, 570
EPA's Acid Rain Program, 354–355
EPA's Integrated Risk Information System, 943
EPA's Toxic Release Inventory (TRI), 355, 859*b*, 963, 981, 989
EPCRA (Emergency Planning and Community Right-to-Know Act) [1986], 526*b*
Epidemics (disaster), 775
Epidemiological studies: correlational (or ecological), 48; descriptive, 47; etiologic (or analytic), 48–49; observational, 49–51
Epidemiological triangle, 720
Epidemiology: analysis issue in, 52–54; bias issue in, 51–52; described, 46; determining permissible exposure levels/risk assessment, 66–68; environmental health risk assessment use of, 957*b*; environmental and occupational, 54–66; future directions in, 68–69; Hill's hypothesis criteria used in, 46–47, 66; Popperian causality framework used in, 46
Equitable relief, 1038
Ethics: consensus statements on, 149*b*; controversies in environmental health, 161–163; defining, 143–145; ecological medicine, 152*b*–160*b*; environmental health, 145–146; environmental/occupational medicine and nursing, 1025–1026; general principles of, 150; global equity principles of, 156–157; selected theories on, 148*b*–149*b*; sustainability and, 150*b*–151*b*; thinking objectively about, 144–145; typical elements of professional codes of, 146*b*–148*b*. *See also* Environmental ethics; Moral/morality
Ethnic churning, 181
Etiologic (or analytical) studies, 48–49
ETS (environmental tobacco smoke), 631, 634, 639
European Centre for Health Policy, 382
European Charter on Environment and Health, *xxxib–xxxiib*
European Commission, 379
European Commission's 2003 Environment and Health Action Strategy, 888
Evaluation of hazards: air pollution sampling apparatus for, 81*fig*; described, 73, 78; instruments used for, 79–81, 82; population sampling for, 78–79
Evangelical Environmental Network, 215
The Evolution and Significance of the Public Health Campaign (Winslow), 896
Excretion, 37–38
Executive Order 128–98, 173, 184, 185
Executive Order on Children's Environmental Health and Safety (1997), 812–813
Expert testimony, 1042*b*–1043*b*
Exploring the Dangerous Trades (Hamilton), 650
Exponential growth model, 6–8, 7*fig*
Exposure: acute, chronic, subchronic, 88; asbestos, 525, 639–640, 860*b*, 1045*b*–1047*b*; concentration to exposure to dose continuum, 84*b*–86*b*, 88; confounding relationship between disease and, 52; defining, 85; dose-response assessment of disease and, 943; environmental and occupational epidemiology study of, 54–69; environmental pediatrics and routes/settings of, 814–829; epidemiological study of disease related to, 46–70; future directions of research studies on, 68–69; during gene-environment interactions, 129–130*fig*; geographical information about, 930, 932; lead, 60, 312*b*–313*b*, 675*b*–677*b*; legal remedies for environmental/toxic, 1034–1035; linking genes and environmental, 136–138, 137*fig*; misclassification (or mismeasurement) of, 63; pesticide use patterns and human, 562–564; reasonable maximal, 956; research on air pollution, 339–340; settings of pediatric, 821–829; transportation-related air pollution, 425–432
Exposure assessment: described, 84–86, 944–945; determining exposure profile, 86, 88; determining permissible levels of exposure, 66–68; differences between industrial hygiene and, 72–73, 84; EPA's framework for cumulative, 180–181; evaluation of hazards, 73, 78–81*fig*, 82; improving pediatric environmental, 830–831; indoor environment pollutants, 637–641; for ingestion and skin absorption, 92–93; methods used for, 88–93; quantifying hazardous exposure task of, 72. *See also* Industrial hygiene; Occupational hazards; Risk assessment
Exposure assessment methods: carbon monoxide exposure assessment, 91*b*–92*b*; direct, 90–92; indirect, 58, 59*fig*, 88–89; inputing or modeling exposure, 88–90; JEM (job-exposure matrix), 58, 59*fig*, 89; measuring biomarkers, 90–91; measuring environmental exposures, 90; measuring personal exposures, 90
Exposure lawsuits: challenges associated with, 1034–1035; understanding remedies available for, 1035

Exposure measurements: concentration, 84*b*–86*b*; example of, 87*fig*; overview of, 57–60, 90
Exposure pathways: described, 88; disproportionate impact of unique, 178–179
Exposure profile, 86, 88
Exposure routes: ingestion, 88, 92–93, 817–819; inhalation, 88, 816–817
Exposure scenarios, 89
Exposure-response analyses, 67
Exposure-response curve, 67

F

Factory Act (1833), 650
Failure-to-warn claims, 1037
Falls: injuries from, 656*b*–658*b*; prevention/countermeasures for, 732*t*
False positives, 867, 869–870
FAO (Food and Agriculture Organization) [UN], 228
Fast-food consumption: settings of, 112–113*fig*; Third World health and increasing, 315–316
FBI (Federal Bureau of Investigation), 772
FCCC (United Nations Framework Convention on Climate Change), 262
FDA Food Code, 586–587, 613*fig*
FDA (Food and Drug Administration): environmental health functions of, 899; food safety regulations by, 611–613, 616; foodborne illness estimates by, 582; labeling requirements of, 1037; mercury advisory by, 352; recommendations for avoiding mercury in fish, 600*b*; toxicologists working at, 25
FDCA (Food, Drug, and Cosmetic Act) [1938], 973
FDCA (Food, Drug, and Cosmetic Act) Amendments, 973
Federal Aviation Administration, 439
Federal Highway Administration, 437, 439, 442
Federal Insecticide, Fungicide, and Rodenticide Act (FIFRA), 567, 568–569, 614, 973*b*–974
Federal Meat Inspection Act [1906], 972*b*–973
Federal Tort Claims Act, 1053
Federal Water Pollution Control Act (1948), 971
FELA (Federal Employers Liability Act), 1050
FEMA (Federal Emergency Management Agency), 772, 774
Feminist ethics, 148*b*
Fertility: legal issues of lead exposure and, 675, 677; occupational exposure and, 675*b*–677*b*
Fertility rates: African continuing high, 223; dropping rate in developed countries, 222; replacement-level, 221
FFDCA (Federal Food, Drug, and Cosmetic Act), 567–570
FIFRA (Federal Insecticide, Fungicide, and Rodenticide Act), 567, 568–569, 614, 973*b*–974
The Fight Bac! Campaign, 614–615*fig*
First National People of Color Environmental Leadership Summit (1991), 173
First World, 288–289
Fisheries, 228–229
Fixing energy, 11
Fleas, 552
Flood health care needs, 752–753
Florida Birth-Related Neurological Injury Compensation Act, 1061
FMIA (Federal Meat Inspection Act) [1906], 972*b*–973
Food: climate change, malnutrition, and productivity of, 260; organic/natural and, 601*b*–602*b*, 869–870; safe food as healthy, 617*b*–618*b*; transportation systems for distribution of, 420
Food allergens, 598–599
Food chain, 12
Food contamination sources: bacteria, 586–591; bioterrorism as, 619–620, 764–766; chemical, 597–601; cross-contamination and, 606–607*b*; dead bodies from disasters, 776; NRC report on pesticides as, 810; overview of, 584*fig*–586; parasites, 594; pesticides, 601, 817–819; viral, 592–594*b*
Food diary, 92–93
Food and Drugs Act (1906), 973
Food environment, 828
Food irradiation, 616–617
Food Quality Protection Act (1996), 974
Food safety: careers in, 620–621; case study on proximate/root cause prevention, 856*b*; described, 581; emerging threats to, 618–620; HACCP (Hazard Analysis Critical Control Point) system for, 607–609*b*, 610–613, 856*b*; healthy food environment and, 617*b*–618*b*; pros and cons of natural/organic foods, 601*b*–602*b*; recent initiatives in, 614–618*b*; regulatory agencies on, 610–614. *See also* Foodborne illness
Food web, 12
Foodborne illness: investigating outbreaks of, 594*b*–597*b*; magnitude of, 581–583; preventing outbreaks of, 602–607*b*. *See also* Food safety
FoodNet (Foodborne Disease Active Surveillance Network), 582
Forest destruction, 229
Fossil fuels: assessment of indoor exposure, 640; environmental health ethics controversy regarding, 161*b*; growing demand in China of, 370*b*; home combustion of, 642; human reliance on energy from, 15; military consumption of, 281; reducing environmental impacts of, 373; types and uses of, 368*t*–369, 371–373. *See also* Energy sources
Fossil water, 459
FQPA (Food Quality Protection Act) [1996], 568, 602, 614, 812
Framingham Heart Study, 835
Freshwater: contamination of, 463–482; contamination of Third World, 318–320, 319*t*;

decreasing availability of, 228; estimates of U.S., 459–460; improper disposal of waste materials and, 539–541; terminology related to, 454–457; waterborne diseases and ecosystem of, 253–254. *See also* Drinking water; Oceans; Water
Friendship-environmental relationship, 109
Frogs (*Rana* genus), 6
Fungal waterborne diseases, 489–490
Future of Public Health (IOM), 901

G

GAPs (good agricultural practices) [FDA], 612
Gauley Bridge disaster (Hawk's Nest incident), 650, 652
Gender differences: in health impacts of physical inactivity, 433–435; mortality by development level, risk factor, and, 292*t*–293*t*; Third World indoor air pollution exposure, 310. *See also* Women
Gene chip technology, 504–505
Gene-environment interactions: described, 128–129; genetic variation and, 132–133; linking genes and environmental exposures, 136–138; research being conducted on, 133–136; susceptibility, risk, and exposure during, 129–130*fig*. *See also* Environmental health
Genes: environmentally responsive, 135–136, 137*fig*; linking environmental exposures and, 136–138, 137*fig*
Genesee County (Michigan) mapping, 935–936*fig*
Genetic susceptibility: described, 129–130*fig*; environmentally responsive genes and, 135–136, 137*fig*; to lead toxicity, 132*b*–133*b*
Genetic variation, 132–133
Genetically modified organisms, 161*b*
Genetics: ELSIs (ethical, legal, and social implications), 131*b*; genomics included in definition of, 129
Genomics: described, 129; EGP (Environmental Genome Project) research on, 133–136; environmental health ethics controversy regarding, 162*b*; HGP (Human Genome Project) research on, 131–132
Georeferenced data, 927–928
Ghirardelli Square (San Francisco), 114*fig*
GIS (geographic information systems): applications of, 934–936*fig*; basic operations of, 928–929*fig*, 930, 931*fig*; data quality/cartography included in, 933–934; described, xlii, 178, 927; georeferenced data used in, 927–928; limitations of, 937; mapping diseases, 932–933; public health facilitated by, 902–903
Global warming: accepted as real trend, 69; climate change compared to, 239; current state of, 230–231; described, 18; environmental health ethics controversy regarding, 161*b*; projected ozone increase associated with, 252*fig*. *See also* Climate change
Globalization: xliii; impact on health in developing countries, 295–299; risk transition to overnutrition and, 307–308
GMPs (good manufacturing practices) [FDA], 612
Goodness-of-link tests, 951
Government policies. *See* Public policies; Regulatory approaches
Green buildings, 261
Green chemistry, 881
Green exercise, 793*b*–794*b*
Green revolution, 300
Greenhouse effect: carbon dioxide levels and, 17–18, 230–231, 238–239*fig*, 240*t*; climate change and, 230–231; main gases involved in, 240*t*; positive radiative forcing resulting in, 238–239*fig*
Groundwater: definition of, 456–457; Ogallala Aquifer source of, 457–458*fig*, 459
Gulf War I, 271, 272*b*, 276, 278
Gulf War II, 276
Gulf War syndrome (GWS), 278*b*
GWUDI (groundwater under the direct influence of surface water), 457

H

H2E (Hospitals for a Healthy Environment), 149
Haber-Bosch process, 18
HACCP (Hazard Analysis Critical Control Point), 607–609*b*, 610–613, 856*b*
Haddon matrix, 422, 721*t*
HAN (Health Alert Network), 776
Hand washing, 604–605*fig*
Handbook of Pediatric Environmental Health (AAP), 813
Haplotypes, 133
HapMap Project, 133
Harm prevention value, 209–210
Harvard Medical School, 650
Harvard School of Public Health, 428, 628, 650
Harvard University's Center for Health and the Global Environment, 232
Hazard identification, 942–943
Hazardous wastes: CERCLA's definition of, 1059; definition of, 525; early recognition of, xxxviii; EPCRA giving community right-to-know about, 526*b*; evaluation of, 73, 78–81*fig*, 82; generated in the U.S., 526; international trafficking in, 541*b*–542*b*; landfilling disposal of, 527; mechanistic approach to assessing, 832; military operations producing, 280–281; prevention case studies on specific environmental, 859*b*–863
Hazards Communication Act, 678–679
HCFC-22 level, 240*t*
HCWH (Health Care Without Harm), 149

Health care facilities, 643
Health care services: clinical role in environmental/occupational health, 1013–1025*b*; environment in context of, 1010–1011; ethical issues in environmental/occupational, 1025–1026; practice venues of, 1026–1928. *See also* Public health
Health Care Without Harm, 215
Health Cities program (WHO), 408–409
Health disparities, environmental hazards, vulnerability relationship, 183*fig*
The Health Disparities Research Program (NIEHS), 186
Health hazards anticipation, 74
Healthy People 2010, 903–904
Healthy worker effect, 51
Hearing loss, 660–662
Heat stress, 244–246*fig*
"Heat stroke" deaths, 245*t*–246
Hebrew Bible, 207, 211
Hepatitis A virus, 592
Hepatotoxins, 30
Herbivores (plant feeders), 12, 14*fig*
Heterotrophic ecosystem, 13
Heterotrophs (other feeders), 12
HGP (Human Genome Project), 131–132
HIA (health impact assessment), 381–383
HICs (high-income countries): injuries in, 717, 718; road traffic deaths in, 725–726. *See also* Developed countries
Highway-railroad crossings, 737*b*–738*b*
Hiroshima (1945), 273
HIV/AIDS: lawsuits over exposure to, 1039; public's anxiety over medical waste due to, 523*b*; waterborne diseases contributing to deaths by, 483
Home injury prevention, 738–739*t*
Homelessness, 400
Homicide rates, 404
Hormetic effects, 951–952
Horticultural therapy, 788
Host-vector-environment triangle, 720
Hot tub lung, 480*b*
Housing: fossil fuel combustion in, 642; moisture and disease link in, 641–642; pediatric exposure in, 821–823; programs to improve, 408; shortages of, 400. *See also* Built environments
HOV (high occupancy vehicle) lanes, 443
HPS (hantavius pulmonary syndrome), 558
HPV (high production volume) chemicals, 805
HRSA (Health Resources and Services Administration), 776, 900
Hubbard Brook experiment (New Hampshire), 19
Hubbert peak, 369
The Human Genome Project, 131–132
Humus, 12
Hurricane Isabel (2003), 755*fig*
Hurricane Ivan (2004), 754*fig*
Hurricane Mitch (1999), 247
Hurricanes (typhoons), 753–757
HVAC (heating, ventilating, and air-conditioning) systems, 633–637, 634*fig*, 644
Hydrodynamics, 462
Hydroelectric power, 375–376
Hydrologic cycle: described, 454–455*fig*; pesticide movement in the, 469*fig*
Hydrolysis, 36
Hypotheses: ecological studies as generating, 48; Hill's criteria for plausibility of, 46–47, 66; Popperian philosophy on, 46

I

IAEA (International Atomic Energy Agency), 283
IAFP (International Association for Food Protection), 595*b*–597*b*
IARC (International Agency for Research on Cancer), 47
ICOH (International Commission on Occupational Health), 1025
ICPD (International Conference on Population and Development) [UN], 231
IEA (International Energy Agency), 363–364, 370*b*
Ignorance, 863
ILO (International Labour Organization), 652, 653, 665
Imageability (environment memorability), 111
Immigration, in population ecology, 10
Incineration, 533–534, 535*fig*
Incivilities (physical and social), 110
Increased risk of disease claims, 1039–1040
Indels (DNA insertions and deletions), 132
Indeterminacy, 862
India: Bhopal disaster (1984) in, 665*b*, 762; child worker in, 667*fig*; occupational health in, 665*b*–666*b*; ship breaking practice of, 542
Indicator approach, 477–478*t*, 479
Indira Gandhi Children's Hospital, 280*fig*
Indirect exposure assessment methods: described, 88–89; JEM (job-exposure matrix) used for, 58, 59*fig*, 89
Indoor air pollution, 309–311, 374–375, 379*t*
Indoor chemistry, 640
Indoor environments: applying pollution prevention/cleaner production approach to, 883; determinants of people's symptoms and air quality of, 631*t*; diagnostic strategies/prevention for, 644–645; exposure assessment of specific pollutants of, 637–641; historical changes in use/purpose of, 625–626; investigating building complaints about, 626*b*–628; regulated in developed countries, 626. *See also* Built environments
Indoor neighborhood settings, 106–108
Industrial disasters, 762–764, 763*fig*
Industrial hygiene: anticipation of occupational hazards, 73, 74–77; control of occupational hazards, 82–83; described, 73;

differences between exposure assessment and, 72–73, 84; evaluation of occupational hazards, 73, 78–82; quantifying hazardous exposure task of, 72; recognition of occupational hazards, 73, 77. *See also* Exposure assessment
Industrial hygiene evaluations: electronic manufacturing facility, 75*b*–76*b*; leaking underground storage tanks at old gas station, 76*b*–77
Industrial Poisons in the United States (Hamilton), 650
Infectious diseases: HIV/AIDS, 483, 523*b*, 1039; occupational risk of, 662–663; spread through transportation, 416*b*; urban environment and transmission of, 406–407. *See also* Diseases; Vector-borne diseases
Information bias, 52
Informed consent controversy, 162*b*
Infrared radiation, 702–703
Ingestion: case study on pesticides in food/water, 817–819; exposure assessment for, 92–93; as exposure route, 88
Inhalation exposure, 88, 816–817. *See also* Air pollution
Injuries: defining, 715, 716; global DALYs (2002) due to, 322*t*, 404, 717–718*t*; ionizing radiation, 689; pedestrian, 422–424; radiation, 685*t*, 689–696, 694*t*; related to environmental risk factors, 321–323; related to transportation, 421–425*t*; types of, 717; urban environments and, 404–406. *See also* Motor vehicle crashes; Occupational injuries/illnesses
Injury control: described, 715; options analysis in, 721*t*–722; public health approach to, 716–727; in special settings, 733–739*t*; three E's of, 723–726
Injury prevention: of burns, 728, 730*t*; of drowning, 733*t*; of falls, 732*t*; of home injuries, 738–739*t*; of intentional injuries (violence), 727–728, 729*fig*, 730*t*; of playground injuries, 734–735*fig*; of poisoning, 731*t*
Injury pyramid, 718–719*fig*
Insect pests, 548
Insect repellants: organophosphate, 40*b*–42*b*, 58–60; overview of, 549*b*–550*b*. *See also* Pesticides
Institute of Transportation Engineers, 442
Integrated Risk Information System (EPA), 943
Intergovernmental Panel on Climate Change, xliv, 242, 243
Intergovernmental Panel on Forests, 229
International Campaign to Ban Landmines, 279
International Federation of Red Cross and Red Crescent Societies, 246
International HapMap Project, 133
Internet: stimulation overload from, 117–118; virtual communities of, 106*t*, 115–119
Interval risk analysis, 954
Invasive species, 8–9
IOM (Institute of Medicine), 47, 275, 285, 641, 864, 901
Ionizing radiation: acute radiation syndrome, 693–695, 694*t*; average amounts received annually by U.S. residents, 688*t*; carcinogenic effects of, 695–696; described, 686–688; estimated risks of fatal cancers from exposure to, 697*t*, 700*fig*; genetic effects of, 689; quantities and dose units of, 687*t*; risk assessment of, 696–698; somatic effects of, 691–695; types and mechanisms of injury, 689
Iowa Department of Health, 915–918
IPCC (UN Intergovernmental Panel on Climate Change), xliv, 242, 243
IPM (integrated pest management), 548, 570–576
Iroquois Nation traditions, 211
Island County Health Department (Washington), 905–906, 911–915
Isolation of hazard, 82
ISTEA (Intermodal Surface Transportation Efficiency Act), 440

J

James Bay poisonings (Quebec), 462*t*, 468
JARC (Job Access Reverse Commute), 421
JEM (job-exposure matrix), 58, 59*fig*, 89
Johannesburg Summit (2002), xliii–xliv
Johnson Controls, UAW v., 675, 677
Joint Commission on Accreditation of Healthcare Organizations, 643
Jones Act (Merchant Marine Act of 1920), 1050

K

K-species, 8
Karasek job strain model, 660, 661*fig*
Killer bees, 416*b*
Kin-Buc landfill (New Jersey), 537–538*fig*
Koran, 207
Kosovo war refugee camp (1999), 748*fig*
Kuwait Oil Fires, 271–272*b*
Kyoto Protocol (1997), 230–231, 262

L

Land-use planning, 883
Landfills: health concerns related to, 536–541; solid waste disposal in, 527, 530–532*fig*, 533
Landmarks: described, 111; Space Needle (Seattle), 111, 112*fig*
Landscapes, 789, 791–793
Lasker Public Service Award, 650, 652
Late Lessons from Early Warnings (EEA), 859–860
Latency legal issue, 1044–1046*b*
Latino pedestrian fatality rates, 423
Lawsuits: asbestos, 1045*b*–1047*b*;

challenges associated with exposure, 1034–1035; class action, 1047; emotional distress, 1039; no-fault proposed alternative to, 1060–1061, 1063–1064; personal injury, 1036–1047; as prevention approach, 981–982; property damage, 1053–1059. *See also* Common law tort system; Legal remedies
Layering operations (GIS), 928–929*fig*
LD_{50} (or lethal dose for 50 percent), 26, 42–44, 43*fig*
Lead (Pb), xxxvii, 348-51; and job discrimination, *677b*; epidemiologic study of, 60; genetic susceptibility to toxicity, *132b-133b*; health effects of, *312b-313b, 675-677b*; in gasoline, *348b-350b*; in lead arsenate pesticide (1900s), *546fig*; routes of exposure, *675b*; SES and, 60; Third World and, 311-312; toxicity in children, 821-23; workplace exposure, *675b-677b*
League of Nations Health Committee, 650
A Leg to Stand On (Sacks), 788
Legal remedies: for environmental and toxic exposures, 1034–1035; implications and discussion of, 1059–1964; personal injury statutory, 1048–1053; statutory property damage, 1057–1059; understanding, 1035. *See also* Lawsuits
Legibility of image, 111
Legionella outbreaks, 488, 503–504
Legionnaires' disease, 55, 56
Lesotho Highlands Water Project (South Africa), 382–383
LET (linear energy transfer), 689
Leviticus, xxxii–xxxiii, 896
Liberty Mutual 2002 Workplace Safety Index, 666
Lice, 552–553
LICs (low-income countries): drownings in, 733; injuries in, 717, 719, 732, 739; road traffic deaths in, 725–726. *See also* Developing countries
Life domains, 101
Life expectancy gap, 289
Lifeguard lung, 480*b*
Lifestyles, 3
Linearized multistage model, 943
Listeria Monocytogenes, 590–591*b*
Litigation. *See* Legal remedies
Liverpool Sanitary Act (1846), xxxv
Logistic model, 7–8
Logit dose-response model, 952*fig*–953
London fog disaster (1952), 332b–333*b*, 332*fig*, 334*fig*
Love Canal (New York), 978
Low-dose extrapolation, 946*b*
Lung cancer, 430
Lyme disease, 556

M

Maastricht Treaty (1994), 864
MACT (maximum achievable control technology), 354
Mad cow disease (BSE), 490, 618–619
Madrid neuropathy outbreak (1981), 55
Malaria, 257, 483, 484*t*, 573*b*–574*b*
Malibu wildfire (1996), 763*fig*
Malignancies/radioactive fallout relationship, 274*b*–275*b*
Malnutrition, 260
Manhattan Project (1942), 276
Manila substandard housing, 402*fig*
Mapping. *See* GIS (geographic information systems)
Market mechanisms, 982–983
Material accounting, 879–880
Maximally exposed individual, 956
Maximum likelihood estimation, 944
MCL (maximum contaminant limit), 319*t*, 320, 499, 500, 972
MCLGs (Maximum Contaminant Level Goals), 499, 972
MCS (multiple chemical sensitivity), 663
Media. *See* Message mapping
Medical monitoring claims, 1049–1050
Medical waste container, 524*fig*
Medical wastes, 523–524*fig*
Megacities, 387–388
Mental health: animal-facilitated therapy and, 787; noise pollution associated with, 438–439; occupational stress impact on, 660; SAD (seasonal affective disorder), 702; Third World urbanization and rising problems with, 315; transportation relationship to, 436–437. *See also* Nature contact; Stress
Merchant Marine Act (1920), 1050
Mercury, 351–352, 468, 599–600*b*
Merrill Dow, Daubert v., 1043*b*
Message mapping: analyzing stakeholder concerns, 1003–1004*b*; communication goals of, 998–999; guidelines for using, 1007; identifying stakeholders, 999–1000; key message development, 1004–1006; planning message delivery, 1006; questions commonly asked by journalists during crisis, 1001*b*–1003; sample risk communication message map, 1005*t*; supporting information for, 1006; systematic message testing, 1006; template for risk communication, 998*t*. *See also* Communication
Messaging online, 118
Meta-analyses, 66, 67
Metabolomics, 140
Metapopulation (population of populations), 10
Methane level, 238, 240*t*
METS (metabolic equivalents), 432*t*
Metta Sutta, 211
Mi-shebeyrach l'cholim (Jewish prayer for the sick), 201–202
Mice, 558
Microbiological water contaminants: deposition, storage, and bioconcentration, 481–482; environmental pathogens as, 479–480*b*; idealized wastewater treatment system, 475*fig*; indicator approach to, 477–478*t*, 479; pathogens, infectious doses, and diseases due to, 473*t*; sanitation options, 474*fig*; sources of, 472,

476; transformations due to, 480–481
Microwave radiation, 703–705, 704*fig*
MICs (middle-income countries): drownings in, 733; injuries in, 717, 719, 732, 739. *See also* Developed countries
Militarism, 270–271
Millennium Ecosystem Assessment, 259
Milwaukee *E. coli* outbreak (1993), 476, 502
Minamata Bay contamination (Japan, 1950s)
Mine Ban Treaty, 279*b*, 284
Mines Act (1842), 650
Mining industry: occupational hazards of, 668, 669*fig*; waste generated from, 525, 539*fig*–540; worker's compensation for occupational diseases of, 1049–1050
Minority groups: environmental hazards, vulnerability and health disparities of, 183*fig*; environmental racism against, 172, 177–184; Executive Order 12898 directive to identify, 173, 184, 185. *See also* Racial differences
Misclassification (or nondifferential error), 52
Mode shares: of commuting to work in the U.S., 418*fig*; defining, 417; percentage of trips by bicycling/walking, 419*fig*; of trips in urban areas by country, 418*t*
Model uncertainty, as obstacle to prevention, 862
Mold exposure, xxxii–xxxiii, 825–826
"Mold in Schools" (EPA), 826
Monte Carlo simulation, 955
Moral/morality, 143. *See also* Ethics
Morbidity. *See* DALYs (disability-adjusted life years)
De Morbis Artificum Diatriba (Ramazzini), 649
Mortality: declining U.S. HIV-related, 406; gun-related deaths in the U.S., 271; London fog disaster (1952), 332*fig*–333*b*, 334*fig*; pedestrian injuries and, 422–424; transportation-related air pollution and, 429–430; vehicular, 322–323, 422; war morbidity and, 270; WHO estimates on air pollution, 334
Mosquito-borne diseases, 256–258, 416*b*
Mosquitoes, 553–554
Motor vehicle crashes: Haddon matrix applied to, 721*t*; pedestrian injuries and mortalities due to, 422–424; prevention of, 735–738*b*; Princess Diana's death in, 722*b*–723*b*; Third World mortality from, 322–323; three E's of injury control applied to, 723–726; U.S. injuries and mortality due to, 422. *See also* Injuries
Motor vehicles: carbon monoxide produced from, 347–348; HOV (high occupancy vehicle) lanes for, 443; leaded gasoline used in, 348*b*–351; nitrogen oxide produced from, 344–345; road rage and, 437; TDM (transportation demand management) for, 443*t*–444*t*; VMT (vehicle miles traveled), 417, 422, 431, 722. *See also* Transportation
MRI (magnetic resonance imaging) systems, 705, 706
MSDSs (material safety data sheets), 679
MTO (Moving to Opportunity for Fair Housing), 408, 409
Multiple chemical sensitivity, 1012
Multistage dose-response model, 949–952*fig*
Municipal solid waste, 520–522*fig*, 521*fig*, 528*fig*
Musculoskeletal disorders (MSDs), 655
Mutagens (or toxicants, carcinogens), 30
MW/RFR (microwave and radiofrequency radiation), 703–705, 704*fig*

N

NAAG (National Agriculture Assessment Group), 260
NAAQS (National Ambient Air Quality Standards), 335, 343, 348*b*–349*b*, 353, 970–971
NACCHO (National Association of County and City Health Officials), 904
Nagasaki (1945), 273, 274*fig*
National Academy of Sciences (NAS), 424, 601, 858, 964*b*
National Academy of Social Insurance, 1061
National Association of Evangelicals, 197
National Center for Environmental Health (NCEH), *xxxiib*, 902, 920
National Childhood Vaccine Injury Act, 1051, 1061
National Children's Study, 835–836
National Conference of Catholic Bishops (1981), 201, 202, 214
National Council of Catholic Women, 197
National Council of Churches of Christ, 215
National Electronic Injury Surveillance System, 664
National Health Interview Survey, 664
National Health and Nutrition Examination Survey III, 434
National Institute on Deafness and Other Communication Disorders, 438
National Institute for Occupational Safety and Health's Registry of Toxic Effects of Chemical Substances, 943
National Law Journal, 174
National Lead Company, 860*b*
National Religious Partnership for the Environment, 215
National Research Council (NRC), 343, 689, 690, 691, 699, 809, 941, 988
National Toxicology Program (NTP), 574*b*
NATO (North Atlantic Treaty Organization), 277, 279

Natural gas, 372–373
Natural history, 3
Natural Resources Defense Council, 429, 898, 984
The Natural Step Framework, 873*b*–875*b*
Natural/organic foods, 601*b*–602*b*, 869–870
Nature contact: domains of, 785–795; health benefits of, 782–785; historical interest in, xxxvi; steps toward increasing, 795–797. *See also* Mental health; Populations
Nature contact domains: animals, 785–787; landscapes, 789, 791–793; plants, 787–789*b*; wilderness experiences, 793–795
Nature (journal), 131
Nature (neighborhood), 114–115, 116*t*, 117*fig*
NAWQA (National Water Assessment Program), 467
NCEH (National Center for Environmental Health), 902, 920
NCRLC (National Catholic Rural Life Conference), 819
NCRP (National Council on Radiation Protection and Measurements), 686, 692, 696, 699, 707
NDMS (National Disaster Medical System), 773–774
Negligence, 1036
NEHA (National Environmental Health Association) Code of Ethics, 146–147
Neighborhood features: described, 105–106; indoor settings, 106–108; neighborhoods as wholes, 111–115; outdoor settings, 108–110; presence of nature, 114–115, 116*t*, 117*fig*; virtual, 106*t*, 115–119
Neighborhoods: childhood obesity and design of, 827–829; concepts of, 103–104; features of, 105–119; health and changing, 103–105; incivilities and stigmatization of, 110; new definition of, 105; traditional definitions of, 104. *See also* Society
Nephrotoxins, 30
NESHAP (National Emissions Standards for Hazardous Air Pollutants), 354
Neuropathy outbreak (Madrid, 1981), 55
Neurotoxic disorders, 659–660
New Kanawha Power Company, 172
New pediatric morbidity, 807
New York Academy of Medicine, 188
New York City: homicides in, 404; overdose risk in, 405; urban sprawl of, 392*fig*; water source protection by, 490–493; water supply system of, 492*fig*
NHANES II (National Health and Nutrition Examination Survey) [1976–1980], 349*b*
NHANES III (National Health and Nutrition Examination Survey) [1982–1984], 350*b*
NHANES IV (National Health and Nutrition Examination Survey) [1988-–1994], 350*b*
NHTSA (National Highway Traffic Safety Administration), 422
NIEHS (National Institute of Environmental Health Sciences), 186
NIH (National Institutes of Health), EGP project launched by, 134–136
NIMBY (not in my backyard), 200
NIOSH (National Institute for Occupational Safety and Health), 656, 658, 660, 668, 670
Nitrogen cycle, 18–20*fig*
Nitrogen oxides: children's sensitivity to, 817; greenhouse effect and level of, 238, 240*t*; sources and health effects of, 344–345
NMRT-WMD (National Medical Response Team—Weapons of Mass Destruction), 774
No-fault programs: conditions prompting creation of, 1063–1064; overview of, 1048–1050; proposals for, 1060–1061
NOAEL (no-observable-adverse-effect-level), 947*b*
No-till agriculture, 567
Noise pollution: EIA/HIA (environmental impact analysis and health impact analysis) of, 886*b*–887*b*; health effects of, 438–439; hearing loss from, 660–662; stress due to high level of, 107; transportation related to, 437–439
Nondifferential error (or misclassification), 52
Nonparametric regression, 952–953
Noroviruses, 592–594*b*
North Carolina Agricultural Extension Service, 556
NPDWR (National Primary Drinking Water Regulations), 499
NPS (National Pharmaceutical Stockpile) program [CDC], 773
NPT (Non-Proliferation Treaty), 282–283
NRC (National Research Council), 343, 689, 690, 691, 699, 809, 941, 988
NRC Committee on Pesticides in the Diets of Infants and Children (1993), 8323
NRC's *Risk Assessment in the Federal Government*, 941–942
NTP (National Toxicology Program), 47
Nuclear power: Chernobyl accident (1986), 275*b*, 362, 377, 762; developing countries interest in, 376–377; environmental health ethics controversy regarding, 161*b*–162*b*
Nuclear weapons: environmental contamination from dismantling/disposal of, 275–276; malignancies associated with radioactive fallout, 274*b*–276; Nagasaki (1945) after detonation of, 274*fig*; proliferation of, 272–273. *See also* War
Nutrient cycles: concept of, 15–16; generalized, 16*fig*
Nutrition: environmental impact on Third World, 304–308; fast-food consumption, 112–113*fig*, 315–316; risk transition to overnutrition, 307–308. *See also* Undernutrition

O

Obesity: childhood, 827–829; environmental health ethics controversy regarding, 162*b*; physical inactivity and, 434–435
Observational studies, 48, 49–51
Observational study design: case-control, 50; cohort, 49–50; cross-sectional or prevalence, 50–51; three principle types of, 49–50
Occupational cancer, 655–656
Occupational Disease Commission (Illinois), 650
Occupational epidemiology: described, 55–56; investigation of clusters in, 56–57; silica-exposed worker study example, 59*fig*, 60–62*t*; of workplace injuries/illnesses, 656*b*–658*b*, 657*fig*, 663–670, 733–734
Occupational hazards: anticipation of, 73, 74–77; control of, 82–83; evaluation of, 73, 78–82; exposure magnitude, frequency, and duration of exposure to, 86–92; exposure to pesticides, 564; injuries and illnesses as, 656*b*–670; recognition of, 73, 77; regulatory approach to, 677–679. *See also* Exposure assessment
Occupational health: challenges to perceptions of, 1028–1029; clinical role in environmental and, 1013–1025*b*; epidemiology of, 55–57, 59*fig*, 60–62*t*; ethical issues in, 1025–1026; history of, xxxiv, 649–652; issues of, 648–649; Karasek job strain model, 660, 661*fig*; regulatory approach to, 677–679. *See also* Workplace
Occupational injuries/illnesses: categories of environmental and, 1012*t*; epidemiology of, 656*b*–658*b*, 657*fig*, 663–670, 733–734; lead exposure and reproductive health, 675*b*–677*b*; prevention of, 673–679; types of, 656*b*–658*b*, 657*fig*; workers' compensation coverage of, 1048–1050. *See also* Injuries
Occupational lung diseases, 654–655
Oceans: climate change and rising sea-level, 242–243, 247–250; deterioration of, 228–229; El Niño impact on, 233, 254; hydrologic cycle and, 454–455*fig*, 469*fig*; red tides, 254; waterborne diseases and changes in marine ecosystems, 254. *See also* Freshwater; Water
Odwalla apple juice contamination, 598*b*
Office materials, 636
Ogallala Aquifer, 457–458*fig*, 459
Oikos (house or home), 3
Oklahoma City bombings, 1064
Older workers, 673
OMB (Office of Management and Budget), 213
-Omics technologies, xlii, 138–140
Omnivores (plants and animal feeders), 12
"On Air, Water, and Places" (Hippocrates), 331
OPCW (Organization for the Prohibition of Chemical Weapons), 277
OPIDN (organophosphate-induced delayed neuropathy), 565
Options analysis, 721*t*–722
Organ system toxicity classification, 31–32
Organic/natural foods, 601*b*–602*b*, 869–870
Organophosphate insecticides, 40*b*–42*b*, 58–60
OSHA (Occupational Safety and Health Administration), 67, 438, 645, 658, 677, 678–679, 963, 982, 1052
Ottawa Convention, 279*b*
Ouagadougou Water Supply Project, 382
Our Common Future (1987), xliii
Outdoor neighborhood settings, 108–110
Overall life situation, 101
Overnutrition, 307–308
Ownership limits, 213–214
Oxidation, 36
Ozone: climate change affecting levels of, 250–251; projected increase in, 252*fig*; tropospheric, 346–347
Ozone alert day, 357
Ozone season, 251–252
Ozone shield, 232

P

P450 genes, 36
PACE-EH (Protocol for Assessing Community Excellence in Environmental Health), 904*t*–906
Pan American Health Organization, 488
Parameter uncertainty, 862
Parasites (foodborne illness), 594–597*b*
Parent compound, 90
Participant selection bias, 51–52
Passive air delivery-absorber system, 80–81*fig*, 82
PCBs (polychlorinated biphenyls), 60, 351, 470–471, 537, 538, 540, 600–601, 660, 820–821, 859, 1058–1059. *See also* Chemical food contamination
PDD (Presidential Decision Directive) 39, 62, 772–73
PDP (Pesticide Data Program), 602*b*
Pedestrian injuries/mortalities, 422–424
Pediatric environmental disease: assessment/communication about, 829–834*b*; case studies in, 813–829; economic burden of, 807–808; historical perspective of, 808–813; National Children's Study (2000) on, 835–836; new pediatric morbidity and, 807; unique susceptibility of children to, 810*b*–811*b*. *See also* Children; Diseases
Pediatric environmental disease exposure: dilemma of breast feeding and, 815*b*–816*b*; routes of, 814–821; settings of, 821–829
Pediatric environmental health specialty units, 813

PERC (tetrachlorethylene), 823, 824, 825, 1059
Perfluoromethane level, 240*t*
Personal exposure measurements, 90
Personal hygiene, 604–605*fig*
Personal injury lawsuits: asbestos, 1045*b*–1047*b*; causation issue and, 1041–1044; common law theories of recovery, 1036–1041; latency issue of, 1044–1045; statutory remedies for, 1048–1053
Personal protective equipment (PPE): described, 82–83*fig*; Ghanaian workers without adequate, 565*fig*; during industrial disasters, 763–764
Pest control: early history of, 544–545; IPM (integrated pest management) approach to, 548, 570–576; regulation approach to, 567–570; sanitation and solid waste management as, 572
Pesticide Data Program (PDP), 602*b*
Pesticides: applying pollution prevention/cleaner production approach to, 882–883; classifications by chemical structure, 561–562; classifications by target, 559*b*–560*b*; developing countries and chemical hazards of, 300*b*–301*b*; early history of, 544–545, 546*fig*; environmental health ethics controversy regarding, 162*b*; food/water contaminated by, 601, 817–819; general use and restricted use of, 562*b*–564*b*, 569; hydrologic cycle and movement of, 469*fig*; modern equipment for applying, 547*fig*; NCR report on infants/children's diet contaminated by, 810; patterns of human exposure and use of, 562–564; regulation of, 567–570; tolerance levels of, 974; toxicity of, 564–567; water supplies infiltrated by, 318. *See also* Anthropogenic chemical contaminants; Insect repellants
Pesticides in the Diets of Infants and Children (NRC), 601, 809
Pests: bedbugs, 548–549; cockroaches, 550–551; corn borer, 547*fig*; defining, 545; EPA's seven categories of, 545–546; fleas, 552; insect, 548; lice, 552–553; mosquitoes, 553–554; termites, 554–555; ticks, 555–556; vertebrate, 556–559
Petroleum, 371–372
PFASs (personal fall arrest systems), 658
Pharmacogenetics, 138
Phase I reactions, 36
Phase II reaction, 36
Phenotypes, 132
Philadelphia Department of Health, 906–907
Philadelphia pneumonia outbreak (1976), 55, 56
Photochemical smog, 346
PHPPO (Public Health Practice Program Office), 903
PHS. *See* U.S. Public Health Service (PHS)
Phthalate plasticizers, 872*b*–873*b*
Physical inactivity: gender differences in health impact of, 433–435; transportation relationship to, 432*t*–436
Physical incivilities, 110
Phytosociology, 4–5
Plant community: defined, 4; phytosociological study of, 4–5
Plants: autotrophs, 11–12; decomposers feeding on decomposed, 12–14; food chain role of, 12; heterotrophs (other feeders) feeding on, 12; nature contact through, 787–789*b*; phytosociological study of, 4–5
Playgrounds: case study on arsenic exposure from, 826–827; injuries on, 734–735*fig*; as source of toxic emissions, 814*fig*. *See also* Children
Pleural registries, 1047
Plutonium, 276
PM (particulate matter): diseases associated with, 308; distribution of, 342*fig*; sources and health effects of, 341–343
Point source, 463
Poisoning: arsenic, 319*t*–320; food, 581–583, 594*b*–597*b*, 602–607*b*; prevention of, 731*t*. *See also* Toxicity
Politically induced uncertainty, 862
Pollution: coal mining, 369; developing countries contribution to, 226; disproportionate impact of proximity to sources of, 177–178; indoor and built environment, 625–645; noise, 107, 437–439, 660–662, 886*b*–887*b*; prevention activities related to, 877–879*b*, 882–883. *See also* Air pollution; Water contamination; Water pollution
Pollution Prevention Act (1990), 854, 877
Polygenic disease, 129
Polymorphism, 132
Pooled analysis, 66–67
Poor Laws (Great Britain), xxxv
POPs (persistent organic pollutants), 470, 882
Population Action International, 459
Population age structure, 9–10*fig*
Population ecology: carrying capacity application to, 9; energy flow through populations/individuals, 14*fig*–15; exponential growth model of, 6–7*fig*; on k-species and r-species impact, 8–9; logistic model of, 7–8; on population pressure on resources and environment, 221–234
Population growth: exponential growth model on, 6–7*fig*; impact on resource use and the environment, 221–234; logistic model on, 7–8; in megacities, 387–388; metapopulation concept of, 10; population age structure and predicting, 9–10*fig*; poverty and, 231–232; replacement rate (R_o) measuring, 9; replacement-level fertility and, 221; in wealthy vs. less wealthy countries, 388*fig*
Population momentum, 9

Population sampling, 78–79
Population-environment scorecard: on arable land, 227; on biodiversity, 229–230; on climate change, 230–231; on forests, 229; on freshwater, 228; on oceans, 228–229; organizations contributing data for, 226–227; on population and poverty, 231–232
Populations: carrying capacity and, 9, 226*b*; city, 396–397; ecological system services provided to, 20–21; energy sources used by, 15; exposure pathway from source to, 88; less wealthy countries' urban vs. rural, 389*fig*; measuring impact of, 223*b*–224*b*; prevention and susceptible, 861; special working, 670–673; susceptible and sensitive, 179; urbanization and, 224–225; water scarcity and, 459–460. *See also* Nature contact
Positive radiative forcing, 238–239*fig*
Postmarketing surveillance, 877
Potency, 949
Poverty: energy ladder related to, 367*fig*, 379–381; Population-environment scorecard on, 231–232; rapid population growth and increased, 227. *See also* SES (socioeconomic status)
PPE. *See* Personal protective equipment (PPE)
P/R ratio, 13
Pre-preliminary exposure assessment, 74
Precautionary principle: critiques of the, 867–870; decision-making process flow, 870*b*–871*b*; definitions of the, 865; described, 833, 863–864; goals of actions based on, 875–876; implementing the, 865–866; risk management use of, 948–949; roots of the, 864–865
Preemptive war, 270
Prevalence (or cross-sectional) studies, 50–51
Prevention: decision-making process flow of precautions and, 870*b*–871*b*; environmental and health impact analyses (EIA/HIA) and, 886–887; environmental health indicators used in decision-making, 885–886; environmental health intervention model of, 851*fig*; information dissemination and education as part of, 887–888; of complex environmental health risk, 857–863; precautionary environmental health research agenda as part of, 888; precautionary principle applied to, 833, 850–873; primary health-promoting measures and, 877–883; secondary interventions, 876–877; sustainable development attained through, 888–890; tools for applying preventive/precautionary approach to, 873–888. *See also* Causality; Public health interventions
Prevention case studies: food safety, 856*b*; lack of knowledge of chemical toxicity, 858*b*–859*b*; natural step/systems thinking for environmental health/sustainability, 873*b*–875*b*; on phthalate plasticizers in toys, 872*b*–873*b*; on specific environmental hazards, 859*b*–863; TURA (Massachusetts Toxics Use Reduction Act) [9189], 878*b*–879*b*; uncertainty as obstacle of, 861–868
Prevention goals: establishing precautionary actions and, 875–876; natural step/systems thinking for sustainability, 873*b*–875*b*; setting environmental health, xlv-xlix, 883–885*b*; sustainable development, 888–890
Prevention of harm, 209–210
Prevention levels: applied to environmental risk, 852–855, 853*b*; primary, 82, 261, 527–528, 852, 853*b*; primordial, 853–854; root cause (or distal primary), 855–856*b*; secondary, 852, 853*b*; tertiary, 852, 853*b*
Preventive war, 270
PRIA (Pesticide Registration Improvement Act) [2003], 569
Price-Anderson Act, 1051
Primary prevention: climate change, 261; described, 852, 853*b*; occupational hazard, 82; pollution prevention/cleaner production concepts of, 877–883; root cause (or distal primary), 855–856*b*; of waste, 527–528
Primordial prevention, 853–854
Prions, 490
Private nuisance claims, 1054
Probabilistic risk analysis, 954–955
Probit model, 950–951*fig*, 952*fig*
Procedures to Investigate Foodborne Illness (IAFP), 597*b*
Product life cycle: cleaner production of, 879–883; illustration, 879*fig*
Product/process: cleaner production of, 879–883; personal injury remedies for liability of, 1036–1047; substitution of, 82, 674, 853, 854
Property damage: statutory remedies for, 1057–1059; tort actions regarding, 1053–1056; valuing, 1056–1057
Property rights, 213–214
Proposition 65 (California), 1052–1053
Protected group identification, 173, 184, 185
Protective devices: controlling safety hazards using, 82–83*fig*; personal protective equipment (PPE), 82–83*fig*, 565*fig*, 763–764
Protozoal waterborne diseases, 489
Proximate primary prevention, 855–856*b*
Proximity, 417
PRPs (potentially responsible parties), 975
PSR (Physicians for Social Responsibility), 149
Psychological disorders. *See* Mental health
PTBT (Partial Test Ban Treaty), 282

PTCs (pollution trading credits), 982–983
PTSD (post-traumatic stress disorder), 247, 1028
Public education approaches, 887–888, 983–984
Public health: challenges of growing energy demand in China and, 370*b*; DDT in antimalarial campaign trade-off for, 573*b*–574*b*; defining, 850; dissemination and education as tools of, 887–888; energy generation/use as threat to, 362; health impact assessments on transportation for, 441; IOM *Future of Public Health* report on, 901. *See also* Disaster preparedness; Environmental health practice; Health care services; U.S. Public Health Service (PHS)
Public Health Act (1848), xxxv
Public Health Foundation, 922
Public health interventions: applied to microbial contamination of food, 856; climate change and, 261; controlling air pollutants through, 356–357; disaster preparedness through, 747–751, 776–777; injury control through, 716–727; nature contact facilitated by, 796–797; prevention model using, 850–856; secondary prevention strategies for, 876–877. *See also* Prevention; Regulatory approaches
Public nuisance claims, 1054–1055
Public policies: alternatives to regulation, 979–984; cleaner production supported by, 881–882; climate change and considerations of, 262–263; consequences for children's health of property, 213–214; drivers of energy policy, 382*b*; environmental justice implications for, 184–186; Executive Order 12898, 173, 184, 185; key federal environmental health statutes, 970–975; preemptive and preventive war, 270–271. *See also* Environmental health policy; Environmental health practice; Regulatory approaches
PulseNet, 614

Q

QSARs (quantitative structure activity relationships), 44
Quarantine, 416*b*

R

R-species, 8–9
R/A (respiration to assimilation) ratio, 14–15
Racial differences: disproportionate impacts concept and, 177–184; environmental justice and, 172–173; health and social segregation related to, 398; pedestrian fatality rates and, 423. *See also* African Americans; Minority groups
Radiation: cancer and cell phone, 705*b*; Chernobyl accident (1986), 275*b*, 362, 377, 692; effects on developing embryo, 696; ELF (extremely low frequency) EMFs (electromagnetic), 705–707; historical background, 683–686; infrared, 702–703; injuries from, *685t*; ionizing, 686–699; microwave, 703–704; two forms of, 683, 684*fig*; ultrasound, 707–708; UVRs (ultraviolet radiation), 699–702; visible light, 702
Radioactive fallout, 274*b*–276
Radiological weapons, 276
Radon, 640
Ramazzini Institute, 652
Rana pipiens (leopard frog), 6
Rana silvatica (wood frogs), 6
Random error, 53–54
Randomized clinical trials, 48–49
Rats, xxiii, 556–557
RCRA (Resource Conservation and Recovery Act) [EPA], 525, 541, 974*b*–975, 1058
De Re Metallica (Agricola), 649
REACH program, 882
Reasonable amaximal exposure, 956
RECA (Radiation Exposure Compensation Act) Amendments (2000), 1051–1052
Recall bias, 50, 52
RECLAIM (Regional Clean Air Incentives Market), 354, 355
Recognition of hazards, 73, 77
Recreational water standards, 501–502
Recycling solid waste, 528*fig*, 529*b*–530*b*
Red Book (NRC), 941–942, 945, 946
Red tides, 254
Reduction (biotransformation), 36
Refugees: created by war, 270; Kosovo war refugee camp (1999), 748*fig*
ReGenesis Revitalization Project (South Carolina), 187*b*
Registry of Toxic Effects of Chemical Substances, 943
Regulatory approaches: to air pollution prevention/control, 353–355; alternatives to, 979–984; command-and-control, 980–981; to energy decision making, 379; environmental impact statements requirements, 899; history of environmental laws passed in the U.S., 897; to occupational safety, 677–679; to pesticides, 567–570; to transportation issues, 440–441; to ventilation systems, 632–633; to water quality monitoring, 498–502. *See also* Environmental health policy; Environmental health practice; Public health interventions; Public policies
Relative risk, 945
Religious communities: environmental health perspective of, 199–201; guiding principles of environmental health followed by, 203–207; increase of environmental health activities by, 197–198*fig*; parents' societal obligations to child development facilitated by, 207–214; successful

partnerships between environmental health and, 214–216*b*. *See also* Communities
Religious environmental principles: on demands of justice, 206–207; on God loving all people, 203–205; on sacred nature of human development, 205–206
Remedies, 1032. *See also* Legal remedies
Repetitive strain injuries, 655
Replacement rate (R[U]o[u]), 9
Report of the Royal Sanitary Commission (1871) [England], 896
Report of the Walkerton Commission of Inquiry (O'Connor), 476
Reproduction disorders, 659
Reproductive health. *See* Fertility
Research: on air pollution and health, 339–340; CBPR (community-based participatory research), 189, 190*b*; environmental health ethics controversy regarding, 162*b*; environmental justice implications for, 184–186; nature contact, 795–796; preventive and precautionary environmental health agenda used in, 888; vulnerability impact on agenda for, 186. *See also* Science
Resource Conservation and Recovery Act (RCRA), 525, 541, 974*b*–975, 1058
Resource wars, 461*t*
Resources: ecological footprint concept and, 21–22; impact of population growth on, 221–224*b*; population-environment scorecard on, 226–232; urban services and, 397. *See also* Water
Right-to-know standard, 678–679, 887–888
Rio Convention, xliii, 230
Rio Declaration, xliii, 149*b*, 865
Rio Plus Five Conference (1997), 227
Risk: calculating relative, additional, and attributable, 945; *de minimus*, 947; defining, 990; during gene-environment interactions, 129–130*fig*; outrage and perception of, 990–992*b*; precautionary principle as creating new, 869; prevention and complexity of environmental health, 857–863; uncertainty in environmental, 861–868. *See also* Vulnerability
Risk assessment: criticism of, 955–958; defining, 940; dose-response, 943; dose-response modeling, 949–953*fig*; environmental health policymaking role in, 976–977; EPA's framework for cumulative, 180–181, 189; evaluation of hazards and, 73, 78–81*fig*, 82; extrapolation from, 946*b*; pediatric environment disease and, 829–833; precautionary principle applied to, 833; safety assessment vs., 947*b*; science element of, 941*b*; terminology and framework used in, 941–946, 942*fig*; toxicology and epidemiology in environmental health, 957*b*; uncertainty analysis of, 953–955; World Trade Center terrorism pediatric exposure, 833*b*–834*b*. *See also* Exposure assessment
Risk Assessment in the Federal Government (NCR), 941–942
Risk Assessment and Risk Management (1997), 181
Risk benefit analysis, 947–948
Risk characterization, 945
Risk communication: crisis management and, 990; defining, 988–989; goals of, 989; high stress and, 993–994; importance of, 833; message mapping tool for, 998*t*–1007, 1005*t*; perception of risk and, 990–992*b*; principles of effective, 994–997; risk management and role of, 770–771, 989–990; trust and, 994; World Trade Center exposures and, 833*b*–834*b*. *See also* Communication
Risk management: cost-benefit analysis, 948; *de minimus* risk concept of, 947; decision analysis or alternatives analysis, 948; precautionary principle used in, 948–949; red book recommendations on, 946; risk benefit analysis as part of, 947–948; risk communication role in, 989–990
Risk outrage factors, 991*b*–992*b*
Risk outrage theory, 990–992*b*
Risk overlap, 290
Risk transition, 289–290, 857
Road rage, 437
Road traffic injury, 735. *See also* Motor vehicle crashes
Roadway design improvements, 441–442
Rodent-borne diseases, 255*b*–256*b*
Routes of exposure, 88

S

SAD (seasonal affective disorder), 702
SADM (special atomic demolition munitions), 273
Safe drinking water: distribution of, 489; EPA's arsenic standard for, 964*b*–965*b*; idealized scheme for, 506*fig*; MCL (maximum contaminant limit) for, 319*t*, 320, 499, 500, 972; point-of-use treatment or bottled water, 498; regulatory framework for monitoring quality of, 498–502; source protection of, 490–493; Third World access to, 316*t*–320; water treatment for, 472, 475*fig*, 476, 494–497, 505–506*fig*
Safe Drinking Water Act (1974), 499–500, 501, 971*b*–972, 980
Safe Drinking Water Act Amendments (1996), 964*b*
Safe Routes to School program, 442*b*
Safety assessment, 947*b*. *See also* Risk assessment
Safety belt law, 724–725
Safety engineering anticipation, 74
Safety hazards anticipation, 74
Salmonella, 591, 612, 619
Sample collection instruments, 79

Sampling: active and passive, 80–82; exposure evaluation and population, 78–79
Sanitary Conditions of the Labouring Populations (1842), xxxv
Sanitary landfills, 530–532*fig*, 533
SARS outbreak (2003), 766, 1007
SBS (sick building syndrome), 628–629, 630*t*–632, 663
Scales, spatial, in environmental health, xliv–xlv
Schools: case study on mold in, 825–826; toxicity in buildings, 642–643
Science: environmental health policymaking role of, 976; interpretation of, 977; moving to policy from, 977–979; precautionary approach as being against norms of, 867–868; prevention and limitations of, 858; research use of appropriate, 868; risk assessment use of, 941*b*. *See also* Research
Science (journal), 131, 792
Scombrotoxin, 599
Screening, 876
SDWA (Safe Drinking Water Act) [1974], 499–500, 501, 971*b*–972, 980
Sea-levels: climate change and rising, 242–243, 246–249, 247–250; effects on vector- and rodent-borne diseases, 256*b*
Second World: described, 288; globalization impact on health in, 295–299; risk overlap in, 290. *See also* Developing countries
Secondary prevention: described, 852, 853*b*; health tracking/public health surveillance as, 876–877; postmarketing surveillance and, 877; screening as, 876
SEHN (Science and Environmental Health Network), 149
Selection bias, 51–52
Sense of place: impact on mental/physical well-being, 99; neighborhoods as wholes and, 111–115
September 11, 2001, 102, 399, 619, 765, 833*b*–834*b*, 1007, 1064. *See also* Terrorism
September 11th Victim Compensation Fund, 1052, 1063, 1064
SES (socioeconomic status): as confounder variable, 51; energy ladder and, 367*fig*, 379–381; Executive Order 12898 directive to identify low-income, 173, 184, 185; lead exposure and, 60; susceptibility to air pollution exposure and, 179*b*–180*b*; workers with low, 671–672. *See also* Poverty
Settings: behavior, 112–113*fig*; defining, 100–101; environmental psychology study of context and, 97; indoor neighborhood, 106–108; outdoor neighborhood, 108–110; third places, 113–114*fig*, 115*fig*
Ship breaking practice, 542
Sick building syndrome (SBS), 628–629, 630*t*–632, 663
Sierra Club, 984
Silent Spring (Carson), xxxvi–xxxvii, 545, 567
Silica-exposed worker study, 59*fig*, 60–62*t*
SIP (state implementation plan), 353
Six Cities study, 343
Skin absorption exposure assessment, 92–93
SLEV (Saint Louis encephalitis virus), 257
SLUDGE (mnemonic for organophosphate toxicity), 565
Smallpox Emergency Personnel Protection Act, 1051
Smokescreen uncertainty, 862
SNPs (single nucleotide polymorphisms), 132, 133, 135
Social capital: in context of cities, 398; environmental justice collaborative problem solving and, 190–191; positive social climate as form of, 109
Social contacts: nature contact as facilitating, 785; outdoor neighborhood settings impact on, 108–110
Social environments (cities), 397–398
Social incivilities, 110
Society: mobility as defining modern, 414–415; obligation of parent's to child development in, 207–214. *See also* Neighborhoods
Solid waste: community right-to-know regarding, 526*b*; described, 520; municipal, 520–522*fig*, 521*fig*; pest control by management of, 572; recycling, 528*fig*, 529*b*–530*b*; special waste, 522–526*b*
Solid Waste Disposal Act (1965), 974
Somalia'a water supply, 460
Source water, 457
South Coast Air Quality Management District, 430
Southwestern Waste Management, Bean v., 172
Sovereign immunity, 1053
Space design, 636
Space Needle (Seattle), 111, 112*fig*
Spatial queries (GIS), 930
Spatial scales, xliv–xlv
Special waste: agricultural, 525; asbestos, 525; construction debris, 524; hazardous waste, 525–526; medical, 523–524*fig*; mining waste, 525, 539*fig*–540
Special working populations: children, 667*fig*, 668, 670, 672*b*; older workers, 673; socially/economically disadvantaged workers, 671–672; women workers, 670–671
Species toxicological specificity differences, 33
Spore-forming bacteria, 587–588
Sprawl Index, 393*b*, 395*b*
Stakeholders: concerns of, 1000–1002, 1003–1004*b*; identification of, 999–1000
Standard of care, 1036
Staphylococcus aureus, 591
Starvation (ethical controversy), 162*b*
"Statement on the Precautionary Principle" (1998), 833

Statistical significance, 54
Stewardship vs. dominion tradition, 199
Stimulation overload, 117–118
Stimuli: described, 100, 101–102; environmental stressors as, 106–107
Stockholm Convention on Persistent Organic Pollutants (2001), 573*b*
Stockholm International Peace Research Institute, 269
STPP (Surface Transportation Policy Project), 423
Stress: Karasek job strain model on, 660, 661*fig*; nature contact reducing, 784, 786–787; occupational psychological disorders and, 660; psychological, 107; PTSD (post-traumatic stress disorder), 247, 1028; risk communication and high, 993–994; September 11, 2001 studies on chronic, 102. *See also* Mental health
Stressors: airplane coming in for landing over LA school, 107*fig*; environmental, 106–108
Strict liability claim, 1055
Sub-Saharan Africa. *See* African countries
Subchronic exposures, 88
Subclinical toxicity, 809
Substitution: of occupational hazard, 82; as prevention strategy, 674, 853, 854
Sulfur dioxide, 343–344
Sulfur hexafluoride levels, 240*t*
Summa Theologica (Thomas Aquinas), 199
Superfund Act (1980), 975*b*, 978, 1058–1059
Superfund Amendments and Reauthorization Act (1986), 975
Superfund site assessment (EPA), 956
Surface water, 456–457
Surpraorganisms, 5
Surveillance: of environmental problems, 281; health tracking and public health, 876–877; as part of disaster response, 750–751; postmarketing, 877
Surveillance cycle, 750
Survey of Occupational Injuries and Illnesses (Bureau of Labor Statistics), 663
Susceptibility: xli; children and their unique, 810*b*–811*b*; genetic, 129–130*fig*, 135–136, 137*fig*; prevention and subpopulation, 861; SES and air pollution exposure, 179*b*–180*b*. *See also* Vulnerability
Sustainability: xliii–xliv; environmental ethics regarding, 148, 150*b*–151; natural step/systems thinking for, 873*b*–875*b*; as prevention goal, 888–890
Sustainable consumption, 889
Sustainable production, 889
Sweden's environmental quality goals, 884*b*–885*b*
Swine Flu Act, 1051
SWS (Safe Water System), 318
SWTR (Surface Water Treatment Rule) [EPA], 493
Symptom-defined disorders, 663
System (or epistemic) uncertainly, 862
Systems biology, described, 137
Systems thinking, 873*b*–875*b*

T

Talmud, 202, 207, 210, 213
Tanzania, urbanization in, 395*b*
TDM (transportation demand management), 443*t*–444*t*
TEA-21, 441
Technology: air pollution controls using, 355–356; BACT (best available control technology), 354, 971; evolution of waste-management, 536; gene chip, 504–505; MACT (maximum achievable control technology), 354; mitigating role in energy consumption by, 226
TEL (tetraethyl lead), 348
Temperature: effects on vector- and rodent-borne diseases, 255*b*; extremes of weather, 244–246*fig*; foodborne illness and improper, 587–588, 603*fig*–604, 606; mortalities from European heat wave (2003), 245*t*; ozone season and, 251–252; projected changes in global, 243*fig*; urban heat island profile, 246*fig*; variations across two time frames of surface, 241*fig*
Termites, 554–555
Terrorism: disaster preparedness in case of, 764–766; food safety and threat of, 619–620; Oklahoma City bombings, 1064; preparedness/emergency response to, 771–774. *See also* Bioterrorism; September 11, 2001
Tertiary prevention, 852, 853*b*
Thermal stress, 244–246*fig*
Third places, 113–114*fig*, 115*fig*
Third World. *See* Developing countries
Three Mile Island, 362
Ticks, 555–556
Tier 2 standards, 431
Tiered toxicity testing, 43*fig*
Title VI (Civil Rights Act of 1964), 935
Tokyo radiation accident (1999), 692
Tokyo subway Sarin attack (1995), 767
Tolerance: defining, 974; distribution models on, 950–953*fig*
Torah, 201, 207
Tornadoes, 757–758
Tort Claims Acts, 1053
Total Coliform Rule (EPA), 500–501
Toxic compounds: biotransformation pathways of chlorphyrifos, 41*fig*; classifications of, 28*t*–32; determining relative toxicity of, 26; exposure to, 33–39; interactions leading to toxicity of, 39–42; LD_{50} (or lethal dose for 50 percent) of, 26; testing for toxicity, 42–44, 43*fig*; toxicokinetics (from environment to body) of, 39; toxicological specificity of, 33
Toxic Wastes and Race in the United States (UCC, 1987), 172, 184

Toxicants (or mutagens), 30. *See also* Carcinogens
Toxicity: asbestos, 525, 639–640; breast feeding dilemma over, 815*b*–816*b*; food contamination, 586–607*b*; HPV (high production volume) chemicals, 805; lead, 132*b*–133*b*, 311–312, 348*b*–351, 675*b*–677*b*; pesticide, 564–567; prevention and lack of knowledge issue, 858*b*–859*b*; subclinical, 809; unique susceptibility of children to, 810*b*–811*b*. *See also* Carcinogens (or toxicants, mutagens); Poisoning
Toxicity classification examples: chemical carcinogenesis, 35*b*; endocrine disruptors, 31*b*; organophosphate insecticides, 40*b*–42*b*; rail crash releasing chlorine gas, 29*b*–30
Toxicity classifications: chemical class, 29; listed examples of, 28*t*; source of exposure class, 29–30*b*; target organ class, 30–32*b*
Toxicity testing: enhancing pediatric environmental, 831–832; EPA's Toxic Release Inventory (TRI), 355, 859*b*; lack of knowledge and chemical, 858*b*–859*b*; tiered, 43*fig*
Toxicogenomics, 138–139
Toxicokinetic process: absorption, 33–34; of chemical carcinogenesis, 35*b*; distribution, 34; excretion, 37–38; improving pediatric models for, 832; metabolism conversion, 34–35; toxicokinetics (from environment to body), 39
Toxicological profiles, 943
Toxicological specificity, 33
Toxicologist, types of, 24–25
Toxicology: described, 24; environmental health risk assessment use of, 957*b*; environmental public health context of, 27–28; interdisciplinary nature of, 25*fig*
Traffic accidents. *See* Motor vehicle crashes
TRAIN (Public Health Foundation), 922
Transportation: air quality and, 425–432; benefits of, 419–421; disease spread through, 416*b*; evolution of, 414–416*b*; improving roadway design, 441–442; injuries related to, 421–425*t*; integrated solutions to health problems related to, 439–444*t*; mental well-being and, 436–437; noise pollution related to, 437–439; physical inactivity and, 432*t*–436; TDM (transportation demand management) of, 443*t*–444*t*; terminology and trends of, 417–419*fig*; urban sprawl and changes in, 392*fig*–395*b*. *See also* Motor vehicles
Trauma Score, 768
Treaty on the Non-Proliferation of Nuclear Weapons, 282–283
Trespass, 1055
TRI (Toxic Release Inventory) [EPA], 355, 859*b*, 963, 981, 989
Triage process: adjuncts to, 769–770; disaster management using, 767–769; mechanics of, 769
Trio of Tripping Pedestrians case, 96*b*–97*b*, *98b*
Tropical cyclones (hurricanes and typhoons), 753–757
Tropospheric ozone, 346–347
Trust-risk communication relationship, 994
TSDFs (treatment, storage, and disposal facilities), 172
TSP (total suspended particles), 341, 343
TURA (Massachusetts Toxics Use Reduction Act) [9189], 878*b*–879*b*
12-hour push packages, 773
Typhoons (hurricanes), 753–757

U

UAW v. Johnson Controls, 675, 677
UCC (United Church of Christ) Commission for Racial Justice study (1987), 172
U.K. Clean Air Act (1956), 333*b*
Ultrahazardous (or abnormally dangerous), 1055–1056
Ultrasound, 707–708
UN Agreement on Straddling Fish Stocks and Highly Migratory Fish Stocks, 228
UN Committee on Economic, Cultural and Social Rights, 316
UN Department of Economic and Social Affairs, Population Division, 222, 224, 225, 313
UN Division for Sustainable Development, 229
UN Framework Convention on Climate Change (1997), 230–231
UN Population Fund, 224
UN Scientific Committee on the Effects of Atomic Radiation, 377
UNAIDS studies, on AIDS pandemic, 222, 223
UNCED (United Nations Conference on Environment and Development) [1992], 226–227
Uncertainty analysis of risk, 953–955
Uncertainty, as obstacle to prevention, 861–863
Undernutrition: environmental health ethics controversy regarding, 162*b*; mortality and DALYs, 292*t*–293*t*. *See also* Nutrition
Understanding Risk (National Academy of Sciences), 181
UNDP (United Nations Development Programme), 226
UNEP (United Nations Environment Programme), 242, 295, 299
UNESCO (United Nations Educational, Cultural and Scientific Organization), 459
UNFAO (United Nations Food and Agriculture Organization), 228
UNFCCC (United Nations Framework Convention on Climate Change), 262
UNICEF (United Nations Children's Fund), 320, 465
UNICPD (United Nations International Conference on Population and Development), 231

Union Carbide, 172
Union Carbide disaster (India, 1984), 665*b*, 762
UNIPCC (United Nations Intergovernmental Panel on Climate Change), 242
United Kingdom: Ambient Noise Strategy (London) in, 886*b*; BSE (bovine spongiform encephalopathy) outbreak in, 490, 618–619; cholera mortality maps (1855) in, 926–927; EAI/HIA of noise pollution by, 886*b*–887*b*; fatality rates by travel mode (1992), 425*t*; first use of mechanical ventilation indoors in, 632; London fog disaster (1952), 332*fig*–333*b*, 332*fig*–333*fig*, 334*fig*; Report of the Royal Sanitary Commission (1871) of, 896. *See also* Developed countries
United Nations Conference on Environment and Development (Rio Declaration), 149*b*, 865
United Nations Stockholm Convention on Persistent Organic Pollutants (2004), 882
United States: air lead concentrations (1977–1996) in the, 349*fig*; deep well injection regulated/classified in, 535; estimates of freshwater in, 459–460; gun-related deaths in the, 271; history of environmental laws passed in the, 897–898; key federal environmental health statutes of the, 970–975; Kyoto Protocol objections by, 262; leaded gasoline and blood lead levels in the, 348*b*–351; mode share of commuting to work in the, 418*fig*; municipal solid waste produced in the, 521*fig*, 522*fig*, 528*fig*; NMRT-WMD (National Medical Response Team—Weapons of Mass Destruction) dispersed in, 774; nuclear weapons produced by, 273; number of municipal sanitary landfills in, 531; ventilation regulation in, 632–633. *See also* Developed countries
UNSCEAR (United Nations Scientific Committee on the Effects of Atomic Radiation), 686, 690, 691, 692, 693, 696, 699
Upstream thinking in environmental health, xlv–xlix
Urban: Census Bureau definition of, 390*b*–391*b*; changing definitions in China, 390, 391*b*; environmental health issues in cities, xxxiii, 387–413; multiple meanings of, 390
Urban heat island profile, 246*fig*
Urban sprawl: characteristics of, 828; Denver area, 394*fig*; New York Metropolitan Area, 392*fig*; overview of, 392*b*–393*b*, 395*b*
Urbanization: dramatic growth of, 387–389; health impact of Third World, 313–316; infectious diseases transmission and, 406–407; measuring, 395*b*; multiple meanings of, 390; population impact on, 224–225. *See also* Cities
U.S. Catholic Bishops Conference, 215
U.S. Census Bureau, 390*b*–391*b*, 934
U.S. Civil Rights Act (1964), 935
U.S. Clean Air Act (1963), 333*b*
U.S. Department of Defense (DOD), 773
U.S. Department of Health and Human Services (DHHS), 433, 772–773, 774, 776–777, 903, 920
U.S. Department of Homeland Security (DHS), 774
U.S. Department of Transportation (DOT), 421, 422, 438
U.S. Emergency Planning and Community Right to Know Act (1986), 887–888
U.S. General Accounting Office, 439
U.S. Occupational Safety and Health Administration (OSHA), 67, 438, 645, 658, 677, 678–679
U.S. Public Health Service (PHS), 967–968. *See also* Public health
USDA (U.S. Department of Agriculture), 420, 602*b*, 610–611, 616, 619
USGS (U.S. Geological Survey), 459, 466, 467, 482, 935
Utero exposure, 820–821
Utilitarianism, 148*b*
UVRs (ultraviolet radiations), 699–702

V

V. cholerae, 488, 489*fig*, 504
Variables: confounder, 49, 51; dichotomous, 53
VAV (variable air volume) systems, 635
VDTs (video display terminals), 705, 706
Vector-borne diseases: agricultural development programs and increase of, 301; climate change impact on, 255–259; importance of prompt diagnosis of, 766; land-use change, microclimate, and, 259; mosquito-borne diseases, 256–258, 416*b*; related to water, 483–484*t*; some effects of weather/climate on, 255*b*–256*b*. *See also* Infectious diseases
Vector-host-environment triangle, 720
Vegetarianism, 161*b*
Ventilation: as control strategy, 82; regulations governing, 632–633
Ventilation for Acceptable Indoor Air Quality, 633
Vertebrate pests, 556–559
Vietnam War, 271, 276–277
"View Through a Window May Influence Recovery from Surgery" (*Science*), 792
Vinyl chloride, xxxvii
Violence: countermeasures for, 730*t*; intentional injuries from, 727–728; typology of, 729*fig*. *See also* War
Viral waterborne diseases, 486–487
Viroids, 490
Virtual neighborhoods, 106*t*, 115–119

Visible light, 702
Vital statistics, xxxiv–xxxv
VMI (vendor managed inventory), 773
VMT (vehicle miles traveled), 417, 422, 431, 722
VOCs (volatile organic compounds), 250–251, 335, 345, 426, 537, 631, 636, 638–639. *See also* Air pollutants (sources/health effects)
Volcanic eruptions, 758–759
Vorsorgeprinzip, 864
VTPI (Victoria Transport Policy Institute), 425, 442
Vulnerability: climate change and regions with, 243–244; definition of, 181–182; direct bearing on research agenda, 186; environmental hazards, health disparities and, 183*fig*; global risk shaped by environmental, 192; social, 181–182, 184. *See also* Risk; Susceptibility

W

Walk-through facility, 77
Walkerton *E. coli* outbreak (2000), 476, 477*b*
Walking School Buses project, 442*b*
War: definition of, 269; direct/indirect impacts on human health by, 269–270; environmental health ethics controversy regarding, 162*b*; impacts on the environment, 271–281; impacts on health by preparation for, 270–271; possible solutions to environmental problems of, 281–284. *See also* Nuclear weapons; Violence
Waste: health concerns related to, 536–541; international trafficking in hazardous, 541*b*; management strategies for solid, 527; primary prevention of, 527–530; solid, 520–562*b*; treatment and disposal of, 530–536. *See also* Water treatment
Waste tires, 529*fig*–530*b*
Water: fossil, 459; groundwater and surface, 456–457; hydrologic cycle of, 454–455*fig*, 469*fig*; interconnections between health and, 456*fig*; regulatory framework for monitoring quality of, 498–502; scarcity of, 457–463. *See also* Drinking water; Freshwater; Oceans; Resources
Water contamination: bioterrorism as source of, 619–620, 764–766; chemical, 463–472; improper disposal of waste materials and, 539–541; microbiological, 472–482; pesticide, 601, 817–819; risk characterization for, 502–503; Third World, 318–320, 319*t*
Water pollution: environmental health ethics controversy regarding, 161*b*; Third World drinking supply contaminated by, 318–320, 319*t*
Water Quality Act (1987), 971
Water quality monitoring: Consumer Confidence Reports, 501; EPA recreational water standards, 501–502; gene chip technology used in, 504–505; SDWA (Safe Drinking Water Act), 499–500, 501; Total Coliform Rule (EPA), 500–501
Water scarcity: agriculture and, 460; climate change and, 461–462; human impacts on aquatic systems resulting in, 462*t*–463; Ogallala Aquifer, 457–458*fig*, 459; political implications of, 460–461*t*; population and, 459–460; as serious health threat, 457
Water stress, 459
Water treatment: Boston's Deer Island system of, 472, 475*fig*, 476; disinfection approaches to, 496*t*; disinfection by-product toxicity (DBPs), 468, 497; disinfection resistance to, 494, 496; multibarrier approach to, 495*fig*; steps taken in, 494; wastewater reuse approach to, 505–506*fig*. *See also* Waste
Waterborne diseases: AGI (acute gastrointestinal infection), 485–486; bacterial, 487–489*fig*; climate change associated with, 253–254; freshwater ecosystems and, 253–254; fungal, 489–490; *Legionella* outbreaks, 488, 503–504; marine ecosystems and, 254; protozoal, 489; *V. cholerae*, 488, 489*fig*, 504; vector-borne, 483–484*t*; viral, 486–487; viroids and prions, 490; WHO on global burden of, 482–483. *See also* Diseases
Weather: air pollution, health, and, 250–252; effects on rodent-borne diseases, 255*b*–256*b*; effects on vector-borne diseases by, 255*b*–256*b*; health and extremes of, 244–250. *See also* Climate change
Western Inscription (Chang T'sai), 200
Wet desert, 4
"What Would Jesus Drive?" campaign, 197, 198*fig*, 215
Whittier College GIS environmental justice project, 178
WHO (World Health Organization): air pollution mortality estimates by, 334; arsenic levels recommendations of, 964*b*; on climate change and malaria, 257; on community health as positive concept, 187; definition of health, xxxi; on disease burden in Third World, 290, 291; ecosystem and meningitis epidemic reported on by, 233; emerging infectious diseases report by, 259; on food irradiation, 616; health as defined by, 202; injury as defined by, 716; on life expectancy gap, 289; malaria mortality/morbidity figures by, 483; MCL (maximum contaminant limit) set by, 319*t*, 320; mercury guidelines of, 468; on obesity health risk, 827; on Third World vehicular mortality, 322–323; water standards published by, 503
Wholesome Meat Act (1967), 972

WHO's Dracunculiasis Eradication Program, 485*b*
WHO's Global Burden of Disease Initiative, 334
WHO's Healthy Cities program, 408–409
WHO's *World Health Report 2002,* 482, 857
Wilderness experiences, 793–795
Wilderness rapture, 793
Wildfire disaster (Malibu, 1996), 763*fig*
Wildfowl pathogen reservoir, 481–482
WMO (World Meteorological Organization), 242
WNV (West Nile virus), 257–258, 554, 766
Women: breast feeding dilemma and, 815*b*–816*b*; lead-exposure and reproductive health of, 675*b*–677*b*; radiation exposure of pregnant, 696; as workforce members, 670–671. *See also* Children; Gender differences
Women of Reform Judaism, 197
Woods Hole Oceanographic Institution, 466
Workers' compensation, 1048–1050
Workplace: epidemiology of injuries/illnesses in the, 656*b*–658*b*, 657*fig*, 663–670, 733–734*t*; health and safety problems in, 653–663; Karasek job strain model on, 660, 661*fig*; prevention of injuries and illnesses in, 673–679; special working populations of, 670–673; varieties of environments of, 652–653. *See also* Occupational health
World Bank, 226
World Commission on Environment and Development (Brundtland Commission), xliii, 150, 192, 888–889
The World Health Report for 1996, 483
World Health Report (WHO), 482
Worst case sampling, 79
WPS (Worker Protection Standard) [EPA], 570
WRI (World Resources Institute), 227, 228
WTC (World Trade Center) tragedy (2001), 102, 399, 619, 765, 833*b*–834*b*, 1007, 1064

X

X-rays, 683–684, 685*t*, 687
Xenobiotic, 33

Y

YLD (years lived with disability), 291, 294*fig*
Yusho disease, 820

Z

ZIPERS (Zuckerman Inventory of Personal Reactions), 791